THE ROUTLEDGE INTERNATIONAL HANDBOOK OF PERINATAL MENTAL HEALTH DISORDERS

The Routledge International Handbook of Perinatal Mental Health Disorders comprehensively presents the leading, global research in understanding and clinically treating perinatal mental health disorders.

In this wide-ranging book, Wenzel invites a global community of scholars and practitioners working in perinatal mental health to discuss contemporary empirical research in the field and how this can be applied in practice. Presented in five parts, the book begins by laying out the historical context of the field before exploring prenatal and postpartum mental health disorders, such as depression, anxiety, alcohol and drug misuse, eating disorders, and insomnia. Chapters describe different interventions, such as mindfulness-based interventions, integrative interpersonal psychotherapy, and cognitive behavioral therapy, before addressing specific special issues, such as fathers' experiences, 2SLGBTQ+ individuals, and perinatal mental health disorders in migrant women. Designed to have international relevance, each chapter includes case studies and sections on cultural considerations, and clinical dialogue is used throughout to illustrate specific applications of contemporary empirical research to clinical practice.

This handbook is essential reading for clinicians who have an interest in issues associated with perinatal mental health disorders, as well as students of clinical social work, clinical psychiatry, clinical psychology, obstetrics and gynecology, nursing, and midwifery.

Amy Wenzel, PhD, ABPP, is the author or editor of over 25 books and treatment manuals and over 100 peer-reviewed articles and book chapters, many on the topic of perinatal psychology. Dr. Wenzel currently divides her time between clinical work, training and consultation, and scholarship.

ROUTLEDGE INTERNATIONAL HANDBOOKS

For more information about this series, please visit: www.routledge.com/Routledge-International-Handbooks/book-series/RIHAND

THE ROUTLEDGE INTERNATIONAL HANDBOOK OF PERINATAL MENTAL HEALTH DISORDERS

Edited by Amy Wenzel

R Routledge
Taylor & Francis Group

NEW YORK AND LONDON

Designed cover image: PeopleImages © Getty Images

First published 2025
by Routledge
605 Third Avenue, New York, NY 10158

and by Routledge
4 Park Square, Milton Park, Abingdon, Oxon, OX14 4RN

*Routledge is an imprint of the Taylor & Francis Group, an informa
business*

Library of Congress Cataloging-in-Publication Data
Names: Wenzel, Amy, editor.
Title: The Routledge international handbook of perinatal
mental health disorders / edited by Amy Wenzel.
Description: New York, NY : Routledge, 2025. | Series: Routledge
international handbooks | Includes bibliographical references and index.
Identifiers: LCCN 2023059303 (print) | LCCN 2023059304 (ebook) |
ISBN 9781032074320 (hbk) | ISBN 9781032074351 (pbk) |
ISBN 9781003206903 (ebk)
Subjects: LCSH: Postpartum depression. | Mental illness. | Mental health.
Classification: LCC RG852 .R68 2025 (print) |
LCC RG852 (ebook) | DDC 618.7/6—dc23/eng/20240411
LC record available at https://lccn.loc.gov/2023059303
LC ebook record available at https://lccn.loc.gov/2023059304

ISBN: 978-1-032-07432-0 (hbk)
ISBN: 978-1-032-07435-1 (pbk)
ISBN: 978-1-003-20690-3 (ebk)

DOI: 10.4324/9781003206903

Typeset in Sabon
by Apex CoVantage, LLC

This handbook is dedicated to the multitude of perinatal women whom I have treated throughout my career, who faced their perinatal mental health disorders with grace and dignity, ultimately transcending their struggle and attaining great clarity and wisdom.

CONTENTS

Contents

EDITOR BIOGRAPHY

Amy Wenzel, PhD, ABPP, is the author or editor of over 25 books and treatment manuals and over 100 peer-reviewed articles and book chapters, many on the topics of perinatal psychology and cognitive behavioral therapy. She is Founder and Director of the Main Line Center for Evidence-Based Psychotherapy, a trainer-consultant with the Academy of Cognitive Therapy, and an affiliated faculty member of the Beck Institute for Cognitive Behavior Therapy. Dr. Wenzel has been awarded numerous grants to conduct empirical research from agencies such as the National Institutes of Health, the American Foundation for Suicide Prevention, and the National Alliance for Research on Schizophrenia and Depression (now the Brain & Behavior Research Foundation). Moreover, she has trained and supervised hundreds of clinicians to become certified cognitive behavioral therapists (many of whom specialize in perinatal mental health), she lectures internationally on perinatal mental health, she has been featured in several video demonstrations published by the American Psychological Association, and she is on the editorial boards of *Cognitive and Behavioral Practice*, *Cognitive Behaviour Therapy*, and the *Journal of Rational Emotive and Cognitive Behavior Therapy*. Dr. Wenzel currently divides her time between clinical work, training and consultation, and scholarship.

CONTRIBUTORS

Fiona Alderdice, PhD, is the Senior Social Scientist at the National Perinatal Epidemiology Unit, University of Oxford, and Honorary Professor at Queen's University Belfast. She has an undergraduate degree and PhD in Psychology from Queen's University Belfast. She is a Fellow of the Higher Education Academy and a long-standing Cochrane reviewer. Her research focuses on assessing maternal and infant needs and experience by developing population surveys to benchmark perinatal health and well-being nationally and internationally and developing standardized measures and evaluating interventions to promote psychological well-being in the perinatal period.

Kelly C. Allison, PhD, is Professor of Psychology in Psychiatry at the Perelman School of Medicine at the University of Pennsylvania and Director of the Center for Weight and Eating Disorders. She received her BA from the University of Notre Dame and her MA and PhD from Miami University. Dr. Allison has authored over 170 research articles and chapters, as well as two books in the areas of chrononutrition, night eating syndrome, binge-eating disorder, the role of weight and eating behaviors on women's health, bariatric surgery outcomes, and clinical trials for weight and disordered eating.

Zafiro Andrade-Romo, MD, MSc (she/her), is a Mexican feminist lesbian, a medical doctor in the tradition of Latin American Social Medicine, and with strong training in Latin American Feminism. She is a PhD candidate in the University of Toronto's Dalla Lana School of Public Health in the Department of Social and Behavioural Health. She has 13 years of experience in LGBTQ+ health and has participated in research projects in Mexico, Brazil, Nigeria, Peru, and Canada. Her research program focuses on the mental health and well-being of lesbian, bisexual, trans, and queer women. Her research interests include women's migration, mixed methods, and STIs.

Cara Angelotta, MD, is Vice Chair for Education in the Department of Psychiatry Behavioral Sciences, the Lisa A. Rone, MD Professorship in Psychiatric Education and Research at Northwestern University Feinberg School of Medicine, and the Program Director for the psychiatry residency program. She is a graduate of the Feinberg School of Medicine. She completed her residency at Cornell University and fellowship training at Columbia University.

Ellen Bartolini, PsyD, PMH-C, is a licensed clinical psychologist with the Developing Brain Institute Children's National Hospital, Washington, DC. Dr. Bartolini provides clinical services across the prenatal and postpartum period and specializes in treating parents and families coping with complex prenatal medical diagnoses. Dr. Bartolini has extensive experience in treating grief, loss, and medical trauma. She is Assistant Professor of Psychiatry and Pediatrics at The George Washington University (GWU) School of Medicine & Health Sciences. Dr. Bartolini earned her PsyD from Widener University's Institute for Graduate Clinical Psychology and completed her postdoctoral fellowship through The Johns Hopkins University School of Medicine.

Cynthia L. Battle, PhD, is Professor of Psychiatry & Human Behavior at the Warren Alpert Medical School of Brown University and Associate Director of the Psychosocial Research Program at Butler Hospital. Her research focuses on women's mental health, in particular developing and testing novel nonpharmacologic interventions for mental health conditions during pregnancy and the postpartum period. She received her PhD in clinical psychology from the University of Massachusetts Amherst and completed NIH-funded postdoctoral training in treatment intervention research at Alpert Medical School of Brown University.

Emma Bränn, PhD, has a background in cell biology and molecular biology and holds a PhD in reproductive medicine from Uppsala University, conducted at the Department of Women's and Children's health. Her main research field is perinatal depression, and currently she is employed as a postdoc at Karolinska Institutet, the Institute of Environmental Medicine.

Sabrina J. Chan, BS, is a clinical research coordinator in the Dekel Lab at Harvard Medical School and Massachusetts General Hospital. She earned her bachelor's degree in Behavioral Neuroscience at Northeastern University, completing her undergraduate honors thesis examining the efficacy of intranasal oxytocin in promoting maternal-infant bonding behaviors in a sample of mothers at risk for postpartum depression. Her research interests are broadly in the field of psychiatry and currently center on maternal mental health with a focus on childbirth-related post-traumatic childbirth (CB-PTSD).

U'nek Clarke, LICSW, LCSW-C, PMH-C, is a Lead Perinatal Behavior Health Specialist for the DC Mother-Baby Wellness Program with the Developing Brain Institute at Children's National Hospital and an affiliated pediatric clinic, TheARC. She is instrumental in program operations, providing therapy, assessment, community engagement, and advocacy for expanding mental health treatment, especially for Black women and BIPOC populations. She is certified in perinatal, infant, and early childhood mental health and child-parent psychotherapy. She speaks and trains on perinatal mood and anxiety disorders internationally. She was recently honored by ZERO TO THREE with the Infant and Early Childhood Mental Health Emerging Leadership Practice Award.

Elizabeth Cox, MD, is a reproductive psychiatrist in private practice based out of North Carolina. She is a member of the adjunct faculty at the University of North Carolina at Chapel Hill, where she formerly served as Medical Director of UNC Women's Mood Disorders at

Wake Med North and Residency Education Director of Women's Mood Disorders. She is an active member of Postpartum Support International and helps lead continuing medical education curriculum training other clinicians in reproductive psychiatry.

Grace E. DeCost, MS, received her master's degree from Drexel University. After completing her master's degree, she first worked as a research assistant at Brown University's Center for Alcohol and Addiction Studies and then soon after took a position as a Research Project Coordinator in the Department of Medicine at Women and Infants Hospital. Presently, she is Research Project Manager in the Department of Pediatric Hematologic Malignancies at the Dana Farber Cancer Institute. She has expertise in data collection and maintenance, clinical research, compliance with FDA regulations, and project development.

Sharon Dekel, PhD, is Assistant Professor of Psychology at Harvard Medical School and Director of the Postpartum Traumatic Stress Laboratory at Massachusetts General Hospital. She is known internationally for her research on childbirth-related posttraumatic stress. She serves as the PI of the largest NIH-funded investigation that assesses traumatic childbirth and PTSD to inform novel preventive therapies, and she also has a private practice. She earned a PhD in Clinical Psychology from Columbia University, completed her clinical internship training at Columbia Medical Center, and continued to a research postdoctoral fellowship in a leading trauma lab in Israel.

Nathalie Dieujuste, BA, is a graduate student in the clinical psychology PhD program at the University of Denver. In 2016, she received her BA in psychology with a minor in human development and family studies from Auburn University. She has worked as a project manager and research coordinator with the Rocky Mountain Regional VA Medical Center and the University of Colorado Anschutz Medical Campus. She is a National Science Foundation Graduate Research Fellow.

Sona Dimidjian, PhD, is Director of the Renée Crown Wellness Institute and Professor in the Department of Psychology and Neuroscience at the University of Colorado Boulder. Her current research projects focus on preventing depression and supporting wellness among new and expectant mothers, promoting healthy body image and leadership among young women, and enhancing mindfulness and compassion among youths, families, and educators. She also has a long-standing interest in expanding access, scaling, and sustaining effective programs, using both digital technology and community-based partnerships. She received her BA in psychology from the University of Chicago and her PhD in clinical psychology from the University of Washington.

Kelly Elliott, PhD, is Assistant Research Professor and leads the Baby S.T.E.P.S. (Supporting Teachers, Educators, Parents, and Service Providers) lab at the Graduate School of Professional Psychology at the University of Denver. Her applied clinical research focuses on the evaluation of prevention and early intervention services for families across perinatal and early childhood periods, and she is also committed to the implementation and evaluation of specialized training programs to support workforce development. She is a certified Integration of Working Models of Attachment Parent-Child Interaction Therapy trainer and received a Scholarship of Teaching and Learning Fellowship.

Elizabeth H. Eustis, PhD, received her doctorate in clinical psychology from the University of Massachusetts Boston. She completed her predoctoral internship at The Warren Alpert Medical School of Brown University and her postdoctoral fellowship at the Center for Anxiety and Related Disorders at Boston University. She was previously a research assistant professor at Boston University. Currently, she is an adjunct research assistant professor at Boston University and works full-time at Big Health, a digital therapeutics company. She has expertise in cognitive behavioral therapies for anxiety, perinatal mental health, and digital mental health interventions.

Natalie Feldman, MD, is a Women's Mental Health Fellow and Dupont Warren research fellow at Brigham and Women's Hospital/Harvard Medical School. Dr. Feldman completed her medical school at the University of Chicago Pritzker School of Medicine, and her psychiatry residency at Brigham and Women's Hospital. Her research interests include perinatal mental health, with a focus on anxiety and trauma.

Gracia Fellmeth, DPhil, qualified in Medicine and Public Health before completing doctoral studies and establishing herself as a clinical researcher in perinatal mental health at the National Perinatal Epidemiology Unit, University of Oxford. Her research focuses on improving the identification of perinatal mental health conditions and understanding the key determinants of mental health conditions, with a particular focus on women living in low- and middle-income countries.

Anne Fritzson, MA, is a doctoral student in Clinical Psychology at the University of Colorado, Boulder. The majority of her research focuses on interventions to support the mental health of youth and their families, with a special interest in LGBTQ and perinatal populations. She is currently examining the impact of social connection and sense of belonging on body image and mental health in historically minoritized communities.

Millicent Fugate, MD, graduated from the University of Kentucky College of Medicine, where she stayed to complete her psychiatric residency training. She then moved to Providence, Rhode Island, to pursue further training in reproductive psychiatry with Brown University Women's Mental Health Fellowship. She is currently working at The Motherhood Center of New York, where she provides psychiatric services in both the Day Program and outpatient clinic. She is passionate about the treatment of perinatal mood and anxiety disorders including the complex interplays between biological, psychological, and societal factors contributing to the elevated risk of psychiatric conditions in the perinatal period.

Megan Galbally, PhD, is a clinical academic and the current Professor/Director for the Centre for Women's and Children's Mental Health at Monash Health and Monash University as well as the Program Director for Monash Mental Health Program, the largest Mental Health Program in Victoria providing mental health services across the lifespan. She is the current National Chair of the Section of Perinatal and Infant Psychiatry, RANZCP, Chair of the Gender Equity Working Group, RANZCP, and a member of the Clinical Academic Psychiatry Steering Group, RANZCP. She currently holds honorary positions at the University of Melbourne, the University of Western Australia, Murdoch University, and the University of Notre Dame. She currently leads an ongoing longitudinal pregnancy cohort study, Mercy Pregnancy and Emotional Wellbeing Study, with women and children, followed up from early pregnancy to now at eight years of age.

Jennifer M. Goldberg (they/she) is completing their PhD in Social and Behavioural Health Sciences at the Dalla Lana School of Public Health, University of Toronto, where they received their MPH in Family and Community Medicine. Their research program takes a critical, interdisciplinary approach to investigating 2SLGBTQAI sexual and reproductive health equity, drawing from public health, critical midwifery, and gender studies, using theoretically informed critical qualitative methodologies to examine social and political forces of health. They are a Registered Midwife in Ontario, Canada, and will be starting a Postdoctoral Fellowship at the McMaster Midwifery Research Centre in 2024.

Ashlee B. Grierson, PhD, is a postdoctoral registered psychologist working with the NSW Department of Education. In her role, she works to provide psychological expertise in education and learning support and delivers evidence-based interventions to children, adolescents, parents, and carers. She has a research background in Internet cognitive behavioral therapy and digital interventions for sleep–wake and circadian rhythm disorders, as well as in the development and evaluation of two self-guided Internet based interventions for perinatal depression and anxiety (This Way Up).

Sophie Grigoriadis, PhD, MD, FRCPC, has been working in Women's Mood Disorders with a focus on times of hormonal transitions for over 20 years. She is a psychiatrist and Professor in the Department of Psychiatry, the University of Toronto, Canada. She completed a psychiatry residency, MA and PhD in Psychology, Clinical Programme, and an internship in Clinical Psychology. She takes a holistic approach, considering biological, psychological, and social factors in the causes and treatments of mental health conditions. She has an active clinical practice and clinical research program. Dr. Grigoriadis has not only authored peer-reviewed papers, books, chapters, and co-authored treatment guidelines, but also written standards of care used by front-line clinicians.

Lauren Gross, PsyD, is a Postdoctoral Fellow at the University of New Mexico's Center for Development and Disability. She earned her doctorate at the Graduate School of Professional Psychology (GSPP) at the University of Denver. At GSPP, Lauren was involved in various research projects in the area of Perinatal to 5 Mental Health, including being a part of designing and conducting the WePlay(TM) Denver program, a parent-child playgroup at the Children's Museum of Denver. Currently, Lauren provides assessment and therapy services for families with young children around the state of New Mexico.

Tomasz Gruchala, BS, is a Polish-American medical student at the Northwestern University Feinberg School of Medicine in Chicago, Illinois. He received his BS from the University of Alabama in 2020 and began the MD program at Northwestern in 2021. He is active in both clinical and basic science research, examining topics within psychiatry and pathology, and anticipates pursuing a career in forensics after completing a medical residency and fellowship.

Juliana L. Restivo Haney, MPH, is a clinical psychology PhD student at West Virginia University (WVU). Juliana's research and clinical interests include perinatal anxiety, trauma, and OCD. She is passionate about reproductive health psychology, family and cultural influences on mental health, and increasing access to evidence-based psychological treatments for populations with historically limited access to care. Previously, Juliana worked in the Department of Global Health at Boston University School of Public Health (BUSPH) as well as at Harvard Medical School as the Program Manager of two global mental health research programs.

Siân Harrison, PsyD, is a clinical psychologist and social scientist at the National Perinatal Epidemiology Unit at the University of Oxford. Her primary research interests are in the field of perinatal mental health, in particular the determinants of depression, anxiety, and posttraumatic stress during pregnancy and the postpartum period and the assessment of these common mental disorders in perinatal populations. She has extensive experience in designing, implementing, and evaluating national maternity surveys, instrument development, and systematic reviewing.

Gali Hashmonay, MD, studied at the Sackler School of Medicine in Tel Aviv, Israel, and completed a residency in General Psychiatry at SUNY Downstate Medical Center. She completed her fellowship in Women's Mental Health at Brigham and Women's Hospital. She joined the Department of Psychiatry as an Instructor at Harvard Medical School with areas of interest including the psychological impact of the reproductive experience, as well as the female experience of psychosis.

Gretchen Heinrichs, MD, FACOG, DTMH (she/her/hers), completed medical school and OBGYN residency at the University of Colorado. For 16 years, she was Associate Professor of OBGYN at Denver Health, teaching residents and medical students and working with refugees, immigrants, and the underserved. She has a degree in Clinical Tropical Medicine and worked extensively in global health with communities in Mexico, India, Rwanda, the Philippines, and Guatemala and with Doctors Without Borders in Nigeria. She received a Federal DOJ grant to provide clinical and psychological care for survivors of Female Genital Cutting in Colorado. She currently works as an OBGYN in Santa Fe, NM.

Laurel M. Hicks, PhD, is a researcher at the University of Colorado Boulder in the Renée Crown Wellness Institute. She is passionate about wellness and ensuring *all* people are provided equal opportunity to thrive in their lives and threads together research, clinical, and policy pathways to ensure that there are both micro- and macro-level changes. She specifically focuses her research on improving wellness in the perinatal year through mindfulness, yoga, and peer-based programs and especially works to ensure that interventions are inclusive and relevant to all communities, especially those who are exposed to violence (community, interpersonal, racial) and/or trauma.

Brooke Dorsey Holliman, PhD, is Assistant Professor in the Department of Family Medicine in the School of Medicine. She specializes in the use of qualitative and mixed methods in health services research and is skilled at health policy and program evaluation. Dr. Dorsey Holliman's research focuses on health disparities and inequalities due to socioeconomic status, race/ethnicity, and social and structural factors. Prior to joining the University of Colorado, she was the founding Director of the Qualitative Core for the Mental Illness Research Education and Clinical Center at the Rocky Mountain Regional VA Medical Center.

John R. Holmberg, PsyD, gained a doctoral degree in clinical psychology from Baylor University prior to completing a clinical fellowship at the Yale University Child Study Center. He was a research faculty on several evidence-based preventive intervention programs (e.g., Nurse-Family Partnership, Fostering Healthy Futures) at the University of Colorado prior to becoming a research associate professor at the University of Denver's Graduate School of Professional Psychology. He is the director of the Caring for yoU and Baby (CUB) Clinic and focuses on clinical instruction, mentorship, and the development of research and clinical programs to address mental health issues in parents and children.

Nathaniel Holmes, BA, is a clinical research coordinator at the University of Pennsylvania Center for Weight and Eating Disorders. He graduated with Latin honors from Washington University in St. Louis, where he majored in psychology and drama. While there, he completed his thesis where he investigated the university's prevalence of muscle dysmorphia. Under the supervision of Dr. Kelly C. Allison, he is currently working on a multisite, National Institutes of Health-funded study investigating the underlying physiological and behavioral mechanisms associated with weight regain following a period of weight loss.

Catherine Hunt is an undergraduate student in psychology at the Université of Moncton, New Brunswick, Canada. Her research focuses on gender attitudes, co-parenting, and relationship satisfaction among new parents. She has experience working with autistic children and their families.

Jacqueline Jacobs, MA, is a doctoral student at the University of Denver's Graduate School of Professional Psychology. She is currently completing her pre-doctoral internship at the University of Denver consortium on the Right Start for Infant Mental Health team. There, she provides services for children aged birth to 5 years, their parents, and pregnant individuals. Her research interests include intergenerational transmission of trauma, parent-child relationships, early-childhood adversity, and perinatal substance use.

Kathleen M. Jagodnik, PhD, is Research Fellow in Psychiatry at Harvard Medical School and Massachusetts General Hospital, and in Information Science at Bar-Ilan University in Israel. She earned her BS degree in Computer Science, Chemistry, Philosophy, and Classical Languages (Latin and Ancient Greek) from John Carroll University in University Heights, Ohio, USA, and her MS and PhD degrees in Biomedical Engineering from Case Western Reserve University in Cleveland, Ohio. Her research interests include maternal mental health with a focus on childbirth-related posttraumatic stress disorder (CB-PTSD), information science, and scientific and societal communication, as well as computational biology and bioinformatics.

Linda Jüris, PhD, is a Swedish psychologist specialized in exposure therapy. She has worked mainly with OCD and complex anxiety disorders for almost 25 years. As well as running a highly specialized private practice in Uppsala, Sweden, she teaches at several universities, supervises other OCD specialists and clinics, and takes part in research projects as a clinical expert on OCD. Dr Jüris is a former president of the Swedish Association of Behaviour Therapy (SABT). Also, she is one of the experts for the Swedish OCD association.

Kathleen Kendall-Tackett, PhD, IBCLC, FAPA, is a health psychologist, International Board-Certified Lactation Consultant, and the CEO of Praeclarus Press, a small press specializing in women's health. Dr. Kendall-Tackett is Editor-in-Chief of the journal *Psychological* Trauma and was the Founding Editor-in-Chief of *Clinical Lactation*. She is a Fellow of the American Psychological Association in Health and Trauma Psychology and Past President of the APA Division of Trauma Psychology. She has authored over 500 articles or chapters and is the author or editor of 42 books.

Brieanne Kidd Kohrt, PhD, PMHC, is a licensed clinical psychologist specializing in perinatal mental health, complex trauma and crisis behaviors, and psychological evaluations for immigration court. She is a certified bilingual perinatal psychologist within the Developing Brain Institute at Children's National in Washington, DC, and holds an Associate Clinical Professor appointment in the Department of Psychiatry & Behavioral Sciences at George Washington University. Dr. Kohrt's research focuses on mental health capacity building for low-resource settings in Latin America, with a focus on the use of task-sharing models to expand access to psychosocial care. She has active projects in Guatemala and Perú.

Laurel E. Kordyban, BS, is Maternal Data Specialist at the Colorado Department of Health and Environment. She specializes in maternal health data system improvements. Laurel is passionate about ensuring equitable access to health information for people to make informed healthcare decisions. Her background is in perinatal clinical psychology and developmental neuroscience research. She holds a Bachelor of Science in Neurobiology with Women's Health and Global Health certificates from the University of Wisconsin—Madison and a graduate certificate in Social Justice from Harvard Extension School. Laurel is a Master of Public Health student at The Johns Hopkins Bloomberg School of Public Health.

Mylène Lachance-Grzela, PhD, is Associate Professor of Psychology in the School of Psychology at the University of Moncton, New Brunswick, Canada. Her research is focused on understanding the psychological well-being of couples and families as they navigate various life transitions. She is also a clinical psychologist who works with adults.

Siobhan A. Loughnan, PhD, is a postdoctoral early career researcher at the Centre of Research Excellence in Stillbirth (Stillbirth CRE, Brisbane, Australia) and co-leads the Care Around Stillbirth and Neonatal Death program which focuses on optimizing care for parents and families around the time of perinatal loss and in subsequent pregnancies. She has a background in digital mental health and perinatal psychology. Her contribution to this area includes the development and evaluation of three self-guided Internet-based interventions for prenatal and postpartum anxiety and depression (This Way Up Clinic) and perinatal bereavement following perinatal loss (Living with Loss, Stillbirth CRE).

Kelli K. MacMillan, DPsych (Clinical), is Senior Lecturer and Clinical Psychologist. Kelli teaches in the postgraduate psychology program at Murdoch University and practices in the public sector at the tertiary maternity and gynecological hospital for women and infants in Western Australia, King Edward Memorial Hospital for Women, Perth. Kelli holds a DPsych (Clinical) from Murdoch University, as well as a BSc (Hons) and BA (LLB), from the University of Western Australia. Kelli was a Post-Doctoral Research Fellow in perinatal mental health and is currently on the Mental Health Education Advisory Group for perinatal mental health and education across Western Australia. Kelli's research focus is on understanding factors that may influence maternal and infant outcomes, as well as child development and the family system longer term.

Kelsey Maki, PsyD, is an infant and early childhood psychologist dedicated to supporting young children's development and family mental health. Kelsey holds a BS in Education and Social Policy from Northwestern University and a PsyD in Clinical Psychology from the University of San Francisco. She completed her clinical internship with an emphasis on early childhood psychology at the University of New Mexico Health Science Center in the Center for Development and Disability. She received postdoctoral training at Children's Hospital Los Angeles with a specialty in early childhood mental health and is trained in Child-Parent Psychotherapy.

Caitlin McKimmy, MTS, MA, is a doctoral student in Clinical Psychology at the University of Colorado, Boulder. She received a master's degree in Buddhist Studies from Harvard Divinity School, where she studied religion and science, and she also worked for several years as a teacher and a learner of comparative religion and meditation traditions in India and Nepal. Since returning to the United States, she has worked to advance research investigating how mindfulness and compassion practices can transform suffering. She brings an interdisciplinary lens to her research into the clinical applications of mindfulness, well-being, and resilience in college-aged youth, and cross-cultural interventions.

Dhara T. Meghani, PhD, is Associate Professor and licensed psychologist at the University of San Francisco PsyD Program. Her research and clinical work focus on promoting perinatal, infant, and early childhood mental health using brief and solution-focused interventions. She founded Parentline, a telemental health service for parents of children birth to 5. She holds a BA in Psychology from UC Berkeley and a PhD in Clinical Psychology from the University of Massachusetts Amherst. She completed her clinical internship and postdoctoral fellowship at the UC San Francisco Clinical Psychology Training Program and is trained in Child-Parent Psychotherapy.

Samantha Meltzer-Brody, MD, MPH, is the Assad Meymandi Distinguished Professor and Chair of the Department of Psychiatry at the University of North Carolina at Chapel Hill. She also directs the UNC Center for Women's Mood Disorders. Dr. Meltzer-Brody is an internationally recognized physician-scientist in perinatal depression. Her research investigates the epidemiologic and biological predictors of perinatal depression and innovative treatment approaches. She also served as the academic PI for the novel psychopharmacologic clinical trials developing the first Food and Drug Administration-approved medication for postpartum depression (brexanolone) and also served as Co-I for the newly approved oral drug (zuranolone) for postpartum depression.

Leah A. Millard is a PhD Psychology student in the Division of Psychology and Mental Health at The University of Manchester, specializing in perinatal mental health. She is part of the university's Specialist Perinatal Mental Health and Parenting Research Unit (PRIME-RU), where she has also worked as an Honorary Research Assistant. Leah received a master's degree in Early Intervention in Psychosis from the Institute of Psychiatry, Psychology and Neuroscience at King's College London and a bachelor's degree in Psychology from Brunel University London.

Laura J. Miller, MD, is the Medical Director of Reproductive Mental Health for the Veterans Health Administration. She heads the VA Reproductive Mental Health Consultation Program and contributes to women's mental health training initiatives. She is a Professor of Psychiatry at Loyola Stritch School of Medicine. She has developed nationally award-winning women's mental health services and educational programs and has participated in numerous women's mental health policy initiatives. She has authored or co-authored more than 90 articles and book chapters related to women's mental health. She is devoted to improving women's mental health through clinical care, education, and research.

Alyssa M. Minnick, PhD, earned her PhD in health psychology, within the clinical concentration, at the University of North Carolina at Charlotte. She completed postdoctoral fellowships at the University of Pennsylvania in weight and eating disorders, as well as in sleep medicine. Her research focuses on the intersection of weight and sleep, including the impact of sleep extension on weight loss, eating behaviors, and cardiometabolic outcomes. She has also examined correlates of binge eating and body image among under-researched populations, namely college men from diverse racial/ethnic backgrounds. Her goal is to use clinical research to optimize treatment outcomes.

Gwen Vogel Mitchell, PsyD, serves as Associate Professor and Co-Director of the International Disaster Psychology: Trauma & Global Mental Health program at the University of Denver. She has worked for organizations such as Doctors Without Borders, The Center for Victims of Torture, the United Nations, and Open Society. Her areas of expertise cover direct service work in various regions including Southeast Asia, the Middle East, the Caribbean, and Africa. Dr. Mitchell's research interests include trauma recovery, post-traumatic growth, global mental health, women's health, group psychotherapy in Myanmar, moral injury, and psychological responses to disasters.

Leena Mittal, MD, FACLP, MS, FACLP, is Associate Vice Chair for Diversity Equity and Inclusion and Chief of the Women's Mental Health Division in the Department of Psychiatry at Brigham and Women's Hospital. An Instructor at Harvard Medical School, she serves as the Program Director for the Women's Mental Health Fellowship. Dr. Mittal serves as the Medical Director of Equity and Innovation for the Massachusetts Child Psychiatry Access Program for Moms (MCPAP for Moms), an innovative statewide consultation service for providers seeing pregnant and postpartum women with mental health and substance use conditions.

Molly Moore, BS, graduated from Hobart and William Smith Colleges with a BS in Psychological Sciences. She currently works as Clinical Research Coordinator at the Center for Weight and Eating Disorders at the University Of Pennsylvania Perelman School Of Medicine under the guidance of Dr. Kelly C. Allison and Dr. Namni Goel on a National Institute of Diabetes and Digestive and Kidney Diseases-funded study investigating time-restricted eating and obesity. Recently, she has worked on a study with Dr. Ariana Chao examining food insecurity, behavioral weight loss treatment, and obesity.

Tracy Moran Vozar, PhD, IMH-E (IV-R), PMH-C, is Clinical Director of Perinatal Behavioral Health for the Developing Brain Institute at Children's National Hospital and Associate Professor of Pediatrics and Psychiatry at George Washington University. She studies intersections between perinatal and early childhood mental health. She founded WePlay!, an infant development and social support group. Tracy earned her PhD in Clinical Psychology at the University of Iowa and completed her postgraduate training in infant mental health at Tulane University. Tracy previously served as Director of the Perinatal Through Five program and the Caring for You and Baby Clinic at the University of Denver.

Maya Nauphal, MA, is a PhD candidate in Clinical Psychology at Boston University and is currently completing her pre-doctoral internship at Montefiore Medical Center in New York. Maya has experience with evidence-based treatments including cognitive behavioral therapy (CBT), dialectical behavior therapy (DBT), and acceptance and commitment therapy (ACT). Her research interests include developing brief transdiagnostic interventions to increase access to mental healthcare and understanding and targeting factors that influence individuals' attitudes towards their mental health and treatment. Maya is also passionate about advocating for LGBTQ+ mental health and dismantling mental health stigma.

Michael W. O'Hara, PhD, is Professor Emeritus in the Department of Psychological and Brain Sciences at the University of Iowa, where he served for 40 years. He founded the Iowa Depression and Clinical Research Center and is the former Director of Clinical Training for the department's clinical psychology program. Dr. O'Hara received his PhD in clinical psychology at the University of Pittsburgh in 1980. He and his colleagues developed Interpersonal Psychotherapy for postpartum depression. He has over 220 peer-reviewed articles, chapters, and books. Dr. O'Hara has served as the President of the Marcé Society for Perinatal Mental Health (1996–1998) and was awarded the Marcé Medal in 2002.

M. Laura Pappa, PhD, is Director of Behavioral Health Education for the McGaw Northwestern Family Medicine Residency Erie Humboldt Park. She earned her doctoral degree at the University of Akron, Ohio, completed her internship at Illinois Masonic Medical Center in Chicago, and a fellowship in Perinatal and Women's Mental Health at Northwestern Medicine. Her clinical interests include trauma-informed care (as she is certified in Cognitive Processing Therapy), domestic violence, women's health, and reproductive psychiatry.

Patrece Hairston Peetz, PsyD, is a clinical psychologist and maternal wellness consultant with over ten years of combined clinical and academic experience, public policy experience, and qualitative and quantitative research retraining. She obtained her doctorate in clinical psychology from Wright State University, completed her predoctoral internship at Children's Hospital Colorado, and completed her postdoctoral fellowship at the University of Colorado—Anschutz campus. Through the Authentic Mamas project, she provides good services to mothers during the transition to parenthood. She has obtained certificate training from Postpartum Support International (PSI) in the treatment of perinatal mood disorders and has held leadership positions in the non-profit and public policy sectors.

Stephanie Pinch, PsyD, M.Ed, is a psychologist in a group private practice in Denver, Colorado, where she is completing her postdoctoral fellowship in early childhood. Dr. Pinch completed her clinical predoctoral internship at the University of New Mexico Health Sciences Center in the early childhood track. She is trained in Iowa Parent-Child Interaction Therapy and specializes in providing therapeutic services to parent–child relationships and infant mental health through an attachment lens to help caregivers and children connect.

Jessica Pineda, MD, received her medical degree from the Medical College of Wisconsin in Milwaukee, Wisconsin, and graduated from the Family Medicine/Psychiatry residency at The University of Cincinnati, Ohio. Specific interests include women's health and how the different stages of life, including psychosocial stressors, role transitions, and hormonal changes, impact both physical and mental health. She is currently working at Women & Infants Hospital in Providence, Rhode Island. She provides primary care services as well as outpatient psychiatric services to women planning pregnancy and pregnant and postpartum breastfeeding mothers. She is the program director for Brown University's Women's Mental Health Fellowship.

Gabriella T. Ponzini, PhD, is a postdoctoral fellow at the Durham Center of Innovation to ADAPT. Her clinical experience is focused on providing adults and adolescents with evidence-based mental health treatment for anxiety, obsessive-compulsive, and trauma-related disorders. She also has specialized experience working with complex clinical presentations in Veterans. Her research interests include increasing access to evidence-based treatments, reducing stigma towards mental illness, and engaging patients and providers in treatment adaptation and implementation.

Kaley N. Potter, BA, is a clinical psychology PhD student at West Virginia University. Her main areas of interest include cognitive biases and personality disorders. Kaley is passionate about prison reform and increasing access to mental healthcare services in correctional settings. She is also interested in developing evidence-based treatments for antisocial personality disorder. She earned her bachelor's degree in psychology and previously served as a lab manager for Dr. Nicholas Allan's Factors of Emotional/Affective Risk (FEAR) Lab at Ohio University.

Josephine Power, MBBS, MPM, FRANZCP, is a consultant psychiatrist with experience in leading and delivering perinatal and women's mental healthcare. She is the Deputy Program Director of Mental Health at Monash Health in Melbourne, Australia, and she has previously provided clinical services in neuropsychiatry within the Austin Neurology Department at the Austin Hospital also in Melbourne. As well as working clinically and leading mental health services, she is undertaking a PhD in understanding the early influences on the development of executive functioning in children at Monash University. She received her training at the University of Melbourne and completed a psychiatry fellowship at Austin Health in Melbourne.

Sharon Ben Rafael, PsyD, is a licensed clinical psychologist and founder and director of the Israeli Program for Interpersonal Psychotherapy. Certified by the International Society of Interpersonal Psychotherapy (ISIPT) as a therapist, trainer, and supervisor, she has been providing IPT training since 2010. She is the founder and chair of the Perinatal Special Interest Group at ISIPT, is certified as a cognitive behavioral therapist and supervisor, teaches at the Israeli Program for Cognitive Behavioral Therapy, serves on the faculty at "Bria" program for women's mental health, and services on the Faculty of Medicine, Tel Aviv University.

Gail Erlick Robinson, MD, is Professor of Psychiatry and Obstetrics/Gynaecology at the University of Toronto where she co-founded the Women's Mental Health Program. She won the YWCA Women of Distinction Award for her work in women's mental health. She received the Alexandra Symonds Award from the American Psychiatric Association for outstanding and sustained contributions to women's mental health and the advancement of women. In 2013, she was appointed to the Order of Ontario, and, in 2017, she received the Order of Canada for her work concerning the mental and physical health of women and the regulation of the health professions.

Lori E. Ross, PhD, (she/her) is Associate Professor in the Division of Social & Behavioural Health Sciences, Dalla Lana School of Public Health, University of Toronto. She is an interdisciplinary mixed methods researcher with a particular interest in research methodologies for social justice. Lori leads a team of scholars focused on using research to address health and social inequities for Two-Spirit, lesbian, gay, bisexual, trans, and queer (2SLGBTQ+) people. More about Lori's research can be found at www.lgbtqhealth.ca.

Mylène Ross-Plourde, PhD, is Associate Professor in the School of psychology at the University of Moncton, New Brunswick, Canada. Her research focuses on social psychology, with a particular interest in the transition to parenthood, parental roles, and paternal involvement. She also holds a license to practice as an adult clinical psychologist.

Katherine Sevar, MBChB, MPM, DCH, FRANZCP, is a psychiatrist, with a sub-specialty in Perinatal Psychiatry and Consultation and Liaison Psychiatry. Her qualifications include a Bachelor of Medicine, a Bachelor of Surgery from the University of Edinburgh in 2005, and a Master of Psychological Medicine at Monash University in 2012. She is a Fellow of The Royal Australian and New Zealand College of Psychiatrists and has experience across perinatal psychiatry, consultation and liaison psychiatry, community psychiatry, and criminal and civil forensic psychiatry. She is Adjunct Lecturer at Monash University and previously worked with the State-wide Perinatal and Infant Mental Health Unit, Washington. She is undertaking a PhD investigating perinatal depression in culturally and linguistically diverse populations through Monash University, Melbourne.

Alkistis Skalkidou, MD, was born in Athens, Greece, in 1977. She completed her medical studies at Athens University and received her PhD in Epidemiology in 2005. She then relocated to Sweden; she became a certified specialist in Obstetrics and Gynecology in 2010 in Uppsala, Sweden. She now holds a joint position as Professor of Obstetrics and Gynecology in the Department of Women's and Children's Health and a senior consultant in Uppsala University Hospital. She has served as chairman of the Gynecological Endocrinology Working Group of the Swedish Association for Obstetricians and Gynecologists and is currently President of the Nordic Marcé Society for Perinatal Mental Health. Her main research field is peripartum depression.

Mira D. H. Snider, PhD, is a postdoctoral fellow with the Center for Childhood Resilience at Ann & Robert H. Lurie Children's Hospital of Chicago. She has clinical experience with children, adolescents, and families in hospital, school, and community settings. Her work is focused on providing evidence-based mental healthcare to youth experiencing trauma- and anxiety-related disorders, and she is passionate about educating professionals who interface with youth in community settings to wield evidence-based interventions effectively. Dr. Snider's research interests include understanding how implementation strategies act upon providers and service systems to promote equitable uptake of best practices and address health disparities.

Dakota Staren, MPH, is a health policy professional with expertise in perinatal and reproductive U.S. policies. Ms. Staren received her MPH from George Washington University and has since worked at multiple organizations leading efforts to improve the healthcare system.

Kylie M. Steinhilber, PhD, is a clinical fellow in pain psychology in the Department of Anesthesiology, Perioperative and Pain Medicine at Brigham and Women's Hospital. She provides trauma-informed psychological services for those with pain conditions, particularly pain conditions that disproportionately affect women. Dr. Steinhilber is interested in understanding and ameliorating gender and racial/ethnic disparities in pain care and her program development projects aim to evaluate and improve the implementation of psychological services for women experiencing chronic pain and co-morbid mental health conditions.

Shari A. Steinman, PhD, is Associate Professor and Director of Clinical Training at West Virginia University. Her research involves understanding the cognitive mechanisms of anxiety and using this knowledge to develop new interventions and prevention programs for anxiety, OCD, and related disorders. She is particularly interested in perinatal mental health and preventing postpartum psychiatric symptoms via novel methods. Shari received her master's and doctoral degrees from the University of Virginia and her bachelor's degree from Washington University in St. Louis.

Morgan Sterling is currently pursuing her master's degree in adult clinical psychology at the University of Windsor, Canada. Her research interests revolve around women's health disorders, with a specific focus on reproductive and sexual psychology. Previously working at the Sunnybrook Research Institute, Morgan is now diving into the impact of endometriosis on sexual satisfaction for her thesis, generously funded by the Ontario Graduate Scholarship. Passionate about contributing to the field, she has previously shared her insights in the *Journal of Psychiatric Research* and *Archives of Sexual Behavior*.

Deana Stevens, PsyD, is a clinical psychologist in independent practice with over 25 years of experience providing care across the lifespan in diverse treatment settings. She is a Visiting Clinical Supervisor at Rutgers University Graduate School of Applied and Professional Psychology. Certified in Perinatal Mood and Anxiety Disorders treatment, EMDR therapy, and as a Gottman Bringing Baby Home educator, she uses an integrative approach to help growing families around issues of fertility, trauma and loss, pregnancy, and parenting. Since 2017 she has facilitated Postpartum Support International's CHAT with an Expert and served as an executive board member of Postpartum Support International New Jersey from 2017 to 2023.

Michelle W. Y. Tam, MA, (she/her) is a critical 2SLGBTQIA+ health scholar and PhD candidate in the Division of Social and Behavioural Health Science at the Dalla Lana School of Public Health, University of Toronto. She holds a Master of Arts in Gender Studies from Queen's University. Her research program integrates social science theories with critical qualitative health methodological approaches to investigate 2SLGBTQIA+ and Black, Indigenous, and People of Colour (BIPOC) healthcare access and health outcomes. As an interdisciplinary researcher, her interests include 2SLGBTQIA+ health, sexual and reproductive health, reproductive justice, critical race theory, queer theory, mixed-methods, and qualitative research.

Polina Teslyar, MD, is an instructor at Harvard Medical School, a Consultation-Liaison and Perinatal Psychiatrist at Brigham and Women's Hospital as well as the Associate Director for the Women's Mental Health Fellowship at Brigham and Women's Hospital. Dr. Teslyar is a graduate of the Tufts University School of Medicine, University of Maryland/Sheppard-Pratt Psychiatry residency program and has completed a fellowship in Consultation-Liaison Psychiatry at Brigham and Women's Hospital primarily focused on Women's Mental Health.

Amy Van Arsdale, PhD, is a psychologist in private practice in Denver, Colorado, and a clinical supervisor for the University of Denver's Graduate School of Professional Psychology PsyD program. Dr. Van Arsdale has had a clinical specialty in perinatal mental health since 2017 and completed her post-doctoral training at the Postpartum Stress Center in Rosemont, PA. She is also certified in Iowa Parent-Child Interaction Therapy (PCIT).

Dr. Van Arsdale has trained psychiatrists, birth doulas, nurses, and community groups in perinatal mental health. Additionally, she serves on the Board of Directors for Division 42 (Independent Practice) of the American Psychological Association.

Amy Wenzel, PhD, is the founder and director of the Main Line Center for Evidence-Based Psychotherapy and editor of this volume. She is the author or editor of over 25 books and treatment manuals, including *The Oxford Handbook of Perinatal Psychology* (2016), *Cognitive Behavioral Therapy for Perinatal Distress* (Routledge, 2015), and *Dropping the Baby and Other Scary Thoughts: Breaking the Cycle of Unwanted Thoughts in Motherhood* (2nd edition) (Routledge, 2021; with Kleiman, Waller, and Adler). She divides her time between scholarship, clinical practice, and training and supervision in cognitive behavioral therapy (CBT) and in the treatment of perinatal mental health disorders.

Grace L. Wheeler, MS, is a clinical psychology PhD student at West Virginia University (WVU). Grace's research and clinical interests include the treatment of anxiety disorders with cognitive-based treatments, such as cognitive bias modification interventions, with particular interest in interventions targeting emotion recognition in anxiety. Previously, Grace worked at the Center for Addiction Medicine at Massachusetts General Hospital. She received her BA in Psychology from Bowdoin College.

Pamela S. Wiegartz, PhD, is a licensed clinical psychologist and Director of Ambulatory Psychology and the Cognitive Behavioral Therapy Training Clinic at Brigham and Women's Hospital/Harvard Medical School. She specializes in anxiety and OCD, working within the Women's Mental Health division to develop and deliver evidence-based treatments for perinatal populations. Dr. Wiegartz is a member of the Association for Behavioral and Cognitive Therapies, the National Register of Health Service Psychologists, and a Fellow of the Academy of Cognitive and Behavioral Therapies. She is co-author of the popular books on anxiety: *Ten Simple Solutions to Worry* and *The Pregnancy and Postpartum Anxiety Workbook*.

Anja Wittkowski, Clin PsyD, is Senior Lecturer/Associate Professor at the University of Manchester. She is also a practicing Clinical Psychologist for Manchester's Mother and Baby Unit, the Director of the Perinatal Mental Health and Parenting (PRIME) Research Unit at Greater Manchester Mental Health NHS Foundation Trust, and the British Psychology Society representative for the Perinatal Mental Health Clinical Reference group for NHS England. Her research and clinical work span perinatal mental health and parenting. She is particularly interested in the assessment of perinatal mental health problems including bonding difficulties as well as the development and evaluation of psychological/parenting interventions.

INTRODUCTION

Perinatal Mental Health in the 2020s

Amy Wenzel

Over the past 30 years, there has been a dramatic increase in the quantity and quality of research on the psychological, emotional, and adjustment experiences of childbearing. It is now widely recognized that whereas the transition to parenthood can be a time of joy and satisfaction for many new parents, there is a substantial number of new parents who struggle with the emotional and psychological adjustment that ranges from transient to serious disturbance. Although postpartum depression has, historically, been given the greatest amount of attention, both in the empirical literature and in the media, research has documented a wide range of emotional experiences and psychological adjustments that can be problematic during the transition to parenthood. Correspondingly, many scholars and clinicians have developed assessments, treatments, and prevention programs for people at risk for the wide array of emotional distress and psychological maladjustment associated with childbearing. Scholars are now moving beyond the mere documentation of these emotional experiences and are conducting empirical research that is designed to understand the mechanisms by which they emerge. Moreover, with increasing frequency, clinicians screen for indicators of psychological maladjustment and make referrals for treatment. Thus, the emotional and psychological experience of childbearing has become a mainstream topic in the field of psychology.

I have had the privilege of watching the field grow ever since the late 1990s, as a clinical psychology graduate student serving as a research assistant for a large-scale randomized controlled trial evaluating the efficacy of interpersonal psychotherapy (IPT) for postpartum depression (O'Hara et al., 2000; see O'Hara, this volume). After implementing a program of research examining the nature and prevalence of postpartum anxiety in the 2000s, I had the distinct pleasure of serving as the editor for *The Oxford Handbook of Perinatal Psychology*, ultimately published in 2016 but assembled over the course of much of the first half of the 2010s (Wenzel, 2016). The landscape of the understanding and treatment of perinatal mental health disorders looks much different now than it did when I compiled that volume, let alone the late 1990s as my career was burgeoning. In this volume, I have aimed to capture a rich portrayal of contemporary thinking in the broad field of perinatal mental health.

I find three trends particularly striking. First is the proliferation of research and discourse on perinatal mental health disorders beyond prenatal and postpartum depression. For example, the examination of perinatal anxiety and anxiety-related conditions has now

DOI: 10.4324/9781003206903-1

received very detailed attention to many of its manifestations—pregnancy-related anxiety, generalized anxiety, panic attacks, obsessive-compulsive symptoms, and traumatic stress symptoms. As the reader will see in Chapter 15, there is advocacy for childbirth-related posttraumatic stress disorder (C-PTSD) to be considered a diagnostic category in its own right. Moreover, there is an ever-increasing body of systematic research on other categories of perinatal mental health disorders, such as eating disorders, substance use disorders, and serious mental illness, which was not the case even a decade ago. No longer must researchers extrapolate from the literature at large on these conditions; at present, studies are being conducted continually with samples of perinatal women who are at risk for, have a history of, or meet criteria for mental health disorders other than depression. It is through this research that scholars and clinicians will be able to hone screening, prevention, and treatment programs to meet the unique needs of perinatal women who, in the past, might have been overlooked.

A second trend that I observe is that women who struggle with perinatal mental health disorders have an increasing number of options for treatments. Cognitive behaviorally based intervention packages have expanded significantly, particularly those that can be culturally adapted and easily operationalized so that they can be transported to communities across the globe (e.g., WHO, 2015). In addition, Internet-based treatment options have proliferated to bring evidence-based treatment to people in rural and remote areas where there are few specialists available to deliver treatments (see Loughnan & Grierson, this volume). The advent of Internet-based programs and, more general, telemedicine, was particularly timely during the COVID-19 pandemic, when the restrictions precluded people from participating in regular in-person mental health services. From a biological perspective, there is much more research on the use of transcranial magnetic stimulation for perinatal women (e.g., Cox et al., 2020) who do not wish to introduce medications that could affect the fetus or infant and who also are uncomfortable with electroconvulsive therapy as an option in the treatment of more severe perinatal mental health disorders. Moreover, an exciting treatment that is referenced in several chapters in this handbook is brexanolone, a progesterone metabolite derivative that has been uniquely adapted to the biology of postpartum women with moderate to severe depression (Edinoff et al., 2021). Thus, researchers are working diligently to refine and adapt efficacious treatments for perinatal mental health disorders and to extend their reach to women outside of the Global North.

The third trend that is striking has already been referenced in the previous paragraph—the focus on the cultural expression of perinatal mental health disorders, and the cultural adaptation of existing treatments and dissemination to far-away communities—even those communities in which there are few specialists. Perinatal mental health specialists have worked diligently to manualize treatments, train nonspecialists and paraprofessionals to deliver the treatments, and provide ongoing supervision to ensure their fidelity. The commitment to bringing quality, evidence-based interventions to perinatal women who are struggling is, in my view, one of the most impressive accomplishments in all of the broad fields of mental health disorders. In addition, this focus on broad applicability pertains to other diverse populations, including people who are not heteronormative and people who are transexual. In fact, the reader will notice that a few of the chapters in this volume use the term *chestfeeding* rather than *breastfeeding* to demonstrate the inclusion of masculine-identified trans individuals who feed their babies from their chests regardless of whether they have had top surgery.

Overview of This Volume

The overarching aim of this handbook is to provide a comprehensive resource on clinical aspects of the understanding and treatment of perinatal mental health disorders. The handbook has a solid basis in science and contemporary empirical research, and at the same time, it emphasizes clinical application. Nearly all of the chapters include an extensive case study, some highlighting sample dialogue between clinicians and clients/patients. In addition, the handbook has been designed to have international relevance. The proposed authors of the handbook represent experts in perinatal mental health across the globe. All contributors were encouraged to include sections on cultural considerations in their chapters, and several chapters focus on perinatal mental health in diverse populations. Thus, it is expected that this volume will serve as the most comprehensive resource to date for scholars and students who have an interest in issues associated with perinatal mental health disorders, particularly from the perspective of diversity, inclusion, and cultural adaptation.

This handbook is divided into five parts. Part I includes six chapters that provide a contextual foundation for the chapters on perinatal mental health disorders, intervention for perinatal mental health, and special issues that affect perinatal mental health. In Chapter 1, Michael W. O'Hara provides a poignant overview of the history and evolution of the field, using his personal experiences and career trajectory to illustrate ways in which this field proliferated during the past two decades of the 1990s and the first two decades of the 2000s. Chapter 2, authored by Dhara T. Meghani, Tracy Moran Vozar, Kelsey Maki, U'nek Clarke, and Ellen Bartolini, describes psychological factors that have particular relevance in understanding the onset and phenomenology of perinatal mental health disorders. Chapter 3, authored by Alkistis Skalkidou and Emma Bränn, parallels Chapter 2 with a focus on the biological factors that have particular relevance in understanding the onset and maintenance of perinatal mental health disorders. Mylène Lachance-Grzela, Mylène Ross-Plourde, and Catherine Hunt turn to relationship and sexual functioning in couples undergoing the transition to parenthood in Chapter 4, highlighting the important notion that perinatal mental health affects the couple just as much as it affects the individual who gives birth. Chapter 5, authored by Kathleen Kendall-Tackett, describes the bidirectional relation between breastfeeding and perinatal mental health. Finally, in Chapter 6, Kelli K. MacMillan, Josephine Power, Katherine Sevar, and Megan Galbally provide an intricate view of the effects of perinatal mental health and child development. It is hoped that after digesting these chapters, readers will have a sophisticated understanding of the many factors at work in shaping perinatal mental health, and conversely, the many factors that are shaped by various manifestations of perinatal mental health disorders.

Part II focuses on specific prenatal mental health disorders, including both pre-existing mental health disorders in women who become pregnant and new episodes of mental health disorders that present during pregnancy. Authors of these chapters were encouraged to describe the salient features of the pathology; its prevalence; correlates and risk factors of the pathology; its effects on the partner relationship, children, and other family members; assessment of symptoms associated with pathology; evidence-based treatments; cultural considerations; and specific directions for future research. Chapter 7, authored by Elizabeth H. Eustis, Maya Nauphal, Grace E. DeCost, and Cynthia L. Battle, highlights prenatal depression, and Chapter 8, authored by Pamela S. Wiegartz, Polina Teslyar, Kylie M. Steinhilber, Natalie Feldman, Gali Hashmonay, and Leena Mittal, highlights prenatal anxiety. The authors of Chapter 9, Alyssa M. Minnick, Molly Moore, Nathaniel Holmes, and Kelly

C. Allison, turn our attention to prenatal eating disorders and body image disturbance. Prenatal alcohol and drug misuse is the subject of Chapter 10, authored by Jacqueline Jacobs, Kelly Elliott, Tracy Moran Vozar, Lauren Gross, and Dakota Staren. Part II on prenatal mental health disorders concludes with the innovative Chapter 11 by Leah A. Millard and Anja Wittkowski, with its focus on preexisting serious mental illness (notably bipolar disorder and psychosis) in women during pregnancy.

Together, the chapters on prenatal mental health disorders demonstrate that many women struggle with emotional adjustment during pregnancy, particularly if they have a history of mental health problems. Fortunately, the medical field is increasingly attuned to mental health problems in pregnancy; not only are many efficacious interventions available for women who are suffering, but there exist prevention programs for women who are deemed during pregnancy to be at risk for mental health and adjustment problems after they give birth.

Part III focuses on postpartum mental health disorders, and the chapters included in this part follow a similar format as the chapters in Part II on prenatal mental health disorders. Chapter 12 by Elizabeth Cox and Samantha Meltzer-Brody focuses on postpartum depression, and Chapter 13 by Juliana L. Restivo Haney, Gabriella T. Ponzini, Mira D. H. Snider, Kaley N. Potter, Grace L. Wheeler, and Shari A. Steinman describes the many manifestations of postpartum anxiety. In Chapter 14, Linda Jüris considers the unique clinical presentation of postpartum obsessive-compulsive disorders, including the inadvertent but important role that family members can play in exacerbating the disorder (but also in reinforcing principles of treatment). Sharon Dekel, Sabrina J. Chan, and Kathleen M. Jagodnik turn our attention to childbirth-related posttraumatic stress disorder in Chapter 15, reminding us of just how common it is that a childbearing individual experiences complications and profound fear in the events surrounding delivery. Postpartum eating disorders and body image disturbance are examined by Alyssa M. Minnick, Nathanial Holmes, Molly Moore, and Kelly C. Allison in Chapter 16, and postpartum alcohol and drug misuse is considered by Tracy Moran Vozar, Stephanie Pinch, Amy Van Arsdale, Kelly Elliot, and Dakota Staren in Chapter 17. Part III on postpartum mental health disorders concludes with a chapter on postpartum psychosis (Chapter 18), in which Anja Wittkowski considers the contemporary conceptualization of psychosis that includes manifestations of bipolar disorder and major depressive disorder with psychotic features.

These chapters capture both the continuation of psychiatric symptoms and diagnoses from pregnancy and new onset cases following childbirth. They illustrate ways in which the early postpartum period can be especially challenging for women with postpartum mental health disorders, as well as ways in which their worlds can contract over time as they struggle to establish a new cadence for daily living. Partner relationship adjustment and satisfaction often plummet during this time. Fortunately, these chapters provide hope as they describe the many interventions that have been tailored to the needs of women with postpartum mental health disorders.

Part IV turns toward intervention for many of the mental health disorders described in Parts II and III. This part is introduced by Gracia Fellmeth, Siân Harrison, and Fiona Alderdice, who present, in Chapter 19, a detailed description of screening and assessment measures and procedures for perinatal mental health disorders. Women who are identified through these screening and assessment procedures are often referred for one or more of the interventions described by the authors of the chapters in this section. Chapter 20, authored by Jessica Pineda and Millicent Fugate, describes approaches and points of concern for prenatal pharmacotherapy, and Chapter 21, authored by Sophie Grigoriadis, Morgan Sterling, and Gail Erlick Robinson, describes approaches and points of concern for postpartum pharmacotherapy. The best-researched evidence-based psychotherapies for perinatal mental health disorders are covered in the subsequent two chapters, with my summary of cognitive behavioral therapy (CBT) for perinatal mental health disorders in Chapter 22, and Sharon Ben Rafael's summary of IPT in Chapter 23. Ben Rafael's chapter moves toward the integration of IPT with other evidence-based approaches for clinical conditions like obsessive-compulsive disorder, which require interventions beyond the interpersonal framework. Similarly, Chapter 24, authored by Deana Stevens, describes a similar integrative approach, this time with psychodynamic therapy and eye movement desensitization and reprocessing for perinatal trauma. The final two chapters of this part capture treatment approaches that have received attention, particularly over the past decade, including Chapter 25's focus on mindfulness-based interventions, authored by Anne Fritzson, Laurel E. Kordyban, Caitlin McKimmy, Laurel M. Hicks, and Sona Dimidjian, and Chapter 26's focus on Internet-based interventions, authored by Siobhan A. Loughnan and Ashlee B. Grierson.

Collectively, chapters in this part demonstrate that there are many evidence-based options to treat women with perinatal mental health disorders. It is heartening that there are alternative options to pharmacotherapy for women who are uncomfortable with exposing their unborn child or infant to psychotropic medications, although it is equally as heartening that a number of these medications have been found to be safe for pregnant and breastfeeding women who do, indeed, take them. Moreover, it is encouraging that the two most researched evidence-based psychotherapies (i.e., CBT and IPT) are continually being adapted to treat perinatal mental health disorders beyond depression and that they incorporate additional elements based on theoretical principles of change and the needs of the women. Moreover, the use of Internet-based interventions has proliferated, bringing quality treatments to women even during times of pandemic, who face challenges in attending in-person treatment sessions even in non-pandemic times, and even to women who live in areas where specialists are scarce.

Finally, Part V contains chapters that speak to a number of special issues, populations, and circumstances that have relevance for perinatal mental health disorders and that can guide clinicians who work with such clients. This part leads with Chapter 27, in which John R. Holmberg and M. Laura Pappa write on the once-neglected issue of fathers' perinatal mental health. Chapter 28, authored by Michelle W. Y. Tam, Jennifer M. Goldberg, Zafiro Andrade-Romo, and Lori E. Ross, describes challenges and perinatal mental health disorders in people who identify as 2SLGBTQ+ (Two-Spirit–lesbian–gay–bisexual–transgender–queer). In Chapter 29, Laura J. Miller considers the mental health challenges faced by people who have experienced infertility and pregnancy loss. Tomasz Gruchala and Cara Angelotta turn our attention in Chapter 30 to the unique issue of neonaticide and its association with pregnancy denial. The final two chapters of the volume focus on the mental health challenges experienced by ethnically diverse women, with Patrece Hairston Peetz, Brooke Dorsey Holliman, and Nathalie Dieujuste focusing on people of color in Chapter 31, and Brieanne Kidd Kohrt, Gwen Vogel Mitchell, and Gretchen Heinrichs focusing on migrant women in Chapter 32.

It is hoped that *The Routledge International Handbook of Perinatal Mental Health Disorders* provides the reader with an up-to-date, "cutting-edge" view of the current state of research into the phenomenology and treatment of perinatal mental health disorders and highlights the significant expansion and broadening of this literature beyond a focus solely on depression.

Moreover, it is hoped that this volume pays homage to the many perinatal mental health experts—researchers and clinicians alike—whose work helps us to understand individual differences in the nature of and risk for perinatal mental health disorders as a function of many expressions of diversity. I believe that the field of perinatal mental health can serve as a shining example of the knowledge and wisdom that can be attained when experts give due attention and respect to people throughout the world, of all ethnicities, income levels, and identities, who are in need of intervention during a monumental transition in their lives.

References

Cox, E. Q., Killenberg, S., Frische, R., McClure, R., Hill, M., Jenson, J., . . . Meltzer-Brody, S. E. (2020). Repetitive transcranial magnetic stimulation for the treatment of postpartum depression. *Journal of Affective Disorders, 264*, 193–200.

Edinoff, A. N., Odisho, A. S., Lewis, K., Kaskas, A., Hunt, G., Cornett, E. M., . . . Urits, I. (2021). Brexanolone, a GABA(A) modulator, in the treatment of postpartum depression in adults: A comprehensive review. *Frontiers in Psychiatry, 12*, 699740.

O'Hara, M. W., Stuart, S., Gorman, L. L., & Wenzel, A. (2000). Efficacy of interpersonal psychotherapy for postpartum depression. *Archives of General Psychiatry, 57*, 1039–1045.

Wenzel, A. (Ed.). (2016). *The Oxford handbook of perinatal psychology*. Oxford University Press.

World Health Organization. (2015). *Thinking healthy: A manual for psychosocial management of perinatal depression: WHO generic field-trial version 1.0. series on low-intensity psychological interventions*. World Health Organization. https://iris.who.int/bitstream/handle/10665/152936/WHO_MSD_MER_15.1_eng.pdf?sequence=1

PART I

Context

1

PERINATAL MENTAL HEALTH

Historical Context and Evolution of the Field

Michael W. O'Hara

The field of perinatal mental health has evolved rapidly over the past several decades. However, mental health problems in the time surrounding childbirth have been recognized for millennia, most famously by Hippocrates about 2,400 years ago (Jones, 1923). He described a woman who had given birth to twin daughters. By the first day postpartum she was not sleeping and was "silent, sulky and refractory." He noted by the sixth day postpartum she was wandering at night, not sleeping. By the eleventh day, "she went out of her mind and then was rational again." She died on the seventeenth day postpartum (pp. 282–283). This case and one other have been brought up repeatedly as evidence that Hippocrates was describing postpartum psychosis (Hamilton, 1962); however, in my view, it is just as likely that these patients were experiencing delirium.

Documenting the evolution of the field from its ancient origins to the present is well beyond the scope of this chapter. But at what point in history to begin? The year 1980 might be a good starting point. It was the year of the founding of the International Marcé Society and the Society for Reproductive and Infant Psychology in the United Kingdom. It was also the year that I finished my dissertation and took a position as an assistant professor at the University of Iowa, the beginning of a 44-year career focused on perinatal mental health. Also, by that time, the International Society of Psychosomatic Obstetrics and Gynaecology had been founded (1962) as well as its North American counterpart (1970). The organizing principle of this chapter is to highlight key issues that have dominated the field over the years, particularly from 1980 to the present. Even with a time frame of only 44 years, the amount of work to be discussed is still overwhelming. As a consequence, I will concentrate on work with which I am most familiar, particularly research and clinical care in the United States. This is a very personal chapter.

Personal Context

Let me begin with a bit of personal history to contextualize much of the work by psychologists in the United States during the 1980s. My interest in depression developed very early in life because both of my parents suffered from depression. In the case of my father, it was bipolar depression. He was hospitalized several times because the treatment of bipolar

DOI: 10.4324/9781003206903-3

depression was not very advanced in the early 1960s. My mother suffered from depression and committed suicide by overdose when I was 13 years old and the oldest of six. She and my father would take turns going to the hospital for their illnesses. It is likely that my mother suffered from postpartum depression (undiagnosed) following the birth of several of her six children (over a nine-year period). Because of my mother's death and my father's hospitalization, we were sent to live with various aunts and uncles until my father recovered sufficiently to gather us together again. My specific interest in studying depression was dormant until college upon taking a course in abnormal psychology and subsequently reading Aaron Beck's 1967 book, *Depression: Causes and Treatment*. This book had a very large impact on my decision to study depression in graduate school because in part it helped me understand my parents' suffering and provided an approach to treating depression without medication.

I was lucky to be admitted to the University of Pittsburgh in 1975 to work with Lynn Rehm, who was intensely interested in the psychology of depression, particularly among women. We carried out several treatment trials evaluating self-control therapy for depression in women and some basic research on the self-control model of depression (Rehm, 1977). In contrast to the complexity of treatment trials today, we were able to advertise for depressed women right after the New Year each year and complete our trials in less than a year. In graduate school, I participated in three treatment trials over three years. One anecdote stands out. The *Wall Street Journal* ran a very small story about our recruitment for one of our depression trials. Back then, potential participants would be required to call us and either speak to one of the research assistants directly or leave a message on the answering machine. Because of the *Wall Street Journal* article, we received hundreds of calls from all over the United States. It was my job to call these individuals back and let them know that they had to live within commuting distance of the clinical psychology center at the University of Pittsburgh to be in our trial. Our success in recruiting women for our trials and the overwhelming response from the *Wall Street Journal* article made it clear to me that there was a great need for psychological treatments for depression, particularly for ones that had research validation.

My own work in graduate school focused on testing causal models of depression, particularly the self-control model (Rehm, 1977; O'Hara & Rehm, 1979). One of the problems with the then-extant psychological models of depression was that many of the core features of the models were similar to depressive symptoms (e.g., negative view of self and future in the cognitive model; helplessness; hopelessness in the learned helplessness model; negative self-monitoring in the self-control model). Measures of these psychological constructs were highly correlated with measures of depression, which at the time was taken as evidence of the validity of these models. However, it was also argued that measures of depression and measures of the psychological models were often measuring the same thing but in slightly different ways. One of the keyways to disentangle measures of depression model constructs and depression symptoms was to conduct a prospective study. These types of studies were often very difficult to do because research subjects often had to be followed for long periods of time. Moreover, it was often not clear as to a suitable time in the future to remeasure depression. One possible solution was to identify an upcoming life event and obtain measures of depression and relevant psychological constructs both before and after the event. The problem was that stressful life events are rarely predictable. My solution to this problem set the stage for the rest of my career. It occurred to me that childbirth was a very significant life event for women that was highly predictable. Because most women received prenatal care, it was relatively easy to identify and recruit subjects during pregnancy and then follow them through pregnancy and into the postpartum period. My assumption was that childbirth would activate psychological vulnerabilities that might be present and thus increase the risk of depression in the period following childbirth. This approach has become very common over the years, but with a few exceptions it was not frequently used at that time (1970s) to test psychological models of depression. At this early stage in my career, my interest was not so much in postpartum depression per se but in using the perinatal context to study psychological models of depression.

Early Studies

The early psychological studies (the 1980s) of pregnant and postpartum women tested psychological models of depression, particularly the learned helplessness model focusing on attributional style (Cutrona, 1983; Manly et al., 1982; O'Hara et al., 1984, 1982). To one degree or another, these studies found that learned helplessness measured during pregnancy accounted for variance in postpartum depressive symptoms over and above depressive symptoms measured during pregnancy. Other studies focused on stressors associated with parenting, marital adjustment, maternal expectations, infant perceptions, parenting self-efficacy, social support, and prepartum life stress (Atkinson & Rickel, 1984; Cutrona & Troutman, 1986; O'Hara et al., 1984; O'Hara, 1986; Whiffen, 1988). These studies evaluating the role of traditional depression risk factors (e.g., poor marital adjustment, life stressors, social support) and risk factors unique to postpartum depression (e.g., infant temperament, maternal expectations) found that a variety of hypothesized risk factors accounted for depression level and depression diagnosis in the postpartum period over and above that associated with depression level during pregnancy. Despite positive findings from these early studies, the predominant risk factor for postpartum depression was prepartum depression. That is to say, the level of depression during pregnancy was significantly and often highly correlated with the level of depression measured in the postpartum period. Almost all studies of postpartum depression going forward included measurement of depression during pregnancy as a way of controlling for baseline risk for depression in the postpartum period.

One of the tasks of a new assistant professor is to decide on a program of research that builds on a dissertation or to take off in a different direction. My plan was to continue to focus on postpartum depression by improving my study design and attempting to answer new questions. Along with graduate students, Danny Neunaber and Ellen Zekoski, I began recruiting women from the prenatal clinic in the Department of Obstetrics and Gynecology at Iowa. My task was to sit in an exam room (feeling somewhat uncomfortable) until one of the nurses brought a patient to see me. All patients were eligible for the study if they were in the second trimester of pregnancy. If the patient was willing to come in the room with me, I would pitch the study to her. We recruited about 100 women this way, all face to face. The innovations in this study included following up with women until six months postpartum, completing diagnostic interviews with all women during pregnancy and at nine weeks postpartum, evaluating the relative contributions of cognitive-affective and somatic depressive symptoms, and obtaining maternal ratings of the child at age 4½ years (O'Hara et al., 1984; Philipps & O'Hara, 1991). In these studies, we found that a psychological model of depression accounted for significant variance in postpartum depression symptoms and diagnosis, that depression severity was generally higher in pregnancy than in the

11

postpartum period, that somatic symptom severity was much higher during pregnancy and during the postpartum period, and that the effect of postpartum depression on child outcomes was largely mediated through later depressive episodes. Near the conclusion of the project (around 1983), I was introduced by Dr. George Winokur, a very prominent psychiatrist and Head of Psychiatry at the University of Iowa, to an organization called the Marcé Society. I learned that he was a founding member and that he had published several papers on postpartum psychosis. He encouraged me to reach out to a San Francisco psychiatrist, Dr. James Hamilton, who was organizing the next biennial meeting.

The International Marcé Society for Perinatal Mental Health (aka Marcé Society)

The Marcé Society convened in Oakland, California, for its third biennial meeting in 1984. This meeting introduced me to the Marcé Society and many prominent British researchers, such as Channi Kumar, Margaret Oates, Ian Brockington, and John Cox of EPDS (*Edinburgh Postnatal Depression Scale*) fame. Another important attendee was Jane Honikman, who went on to found Postpartum Support International (PSI). It was striking that there were few Americans at this meeting despite the best efforts of Dr. Hamilton to entice them to attend. Nevertheless, I had the opportunity to present my research to the leading British and European perinatal mental health researchers of the day. For me, there were two major consequences of meeting these colleagues. I was invited to come to London the following year to present new research and also to write a review chapter on postpartum depression (O'Hara & Zekoski, 1988) for the second edition of *Motherhood and Mental Illness* (Kumar & Brockington, 1988). Following meetings in Nottingham, Keele, York, Cambridge, Amsterdam, and London again, I became the first American and the first psychologist to be president of the Marcé Society. At the time, presidents were selected by Marcé leadership, not elected. So, it was Eugene Paykel, president of the Marcé Society (and Head of Psychiatry at Cambridge), who asked me to become President-elect at the Cambridge meeting in 1994. The biennial meeting, which I oversaw, was held at the University of Iowa in Iowa City in June 1998 (Stuart et al., 1998). Subsequent meetings in Manchester (2000), Sydney (2002), Oxford (2004), Keele (2006), Sydney (2008), Pittsburgh (2010), Swansea (2012), Paris (2014), Melbourne (2016), Bengaluru, India (2018), Iowa City (2020), and most recently London (2022) reflect the increasing internationalization of the Marcé Society. Upcoming biennial meetings will be held in Barcelona (2024) and South Africa (2026). Dr. Lavinia Lumu, a Black psychiatrist from Johannesburg, South Africa, is the current president-elect. What started as a mainly White British and English language enterprise in 1980 has blossomed into a truly international and diverse society, with regional groups reflecting different countries and languages. Another feature of the Marcé Society is that members come from a diversity of professions beyond psychiatry and clinical psychology, including obstetrician-gynecologists, pediatricians, nurse practitioners, health visitors, clinical social workers, support group leaders, and perinatal activists.

Regional groups became a feature of the Marcé Society in the early 2000s, with the establishment of the Australasian and Francophone societies. Since that time, regional groups have emerged in Germany, Spain, Italy, Japan, the Nordic countries, Portugal, the United Kingdom, and Ireland. Regional groups are now forming in North Africa and the Middle East, Poland, South Africa, and Chile/South America. Surprisingly, Marcé of North America (MONA) did not become an official regional group until 2018. For many years

Marcé leadership and members bemoaned the fact that there was not a strong Marcé presence in North America, despite having many leading perinatal mental health researchers and clinicians. It was not until Katherine Wisner organized a perinatal mental health meeting in Chicago in 2013 that a push began to establish a North American group. Our name at that time was the Perinatal Mental Health Society. Following very successful and well-attended meetings in Chicago in 2015 and 2017, the founding members (me included) led by Dr. Wisner voted to seek recognition as MONA to represent the United States, Canada, and Mexico. The first official meeting of MONA was held in Chapel Hill in 2019, hosted by Samantha Melzer-Brody (as president); a virtual meeting was held in 2021, hosted by Crystal Clark of Northwestern University. Jennifer Payne of the University of Virginia will host the next meeting in Alexandria, Virginia, in October 2023. As an aside, members of regional groups are automatically members of the International Marcé Society.

How Do We Understand Perinatal Mental Health Disorders?

In the United States, the *Diagnostic and Statistical Manual of Mental Disorders* published by the American Psychiatric Association has sometimes been called *Psychiatry's Bible* (Horwitz, 2021). This *Bible*, first published in 1952 (DSM-I; American Psychiatric Association, 1952), has guided clinician diagnosis of mental disorders up to the present. In today's world and for many decades into the past, clinicians, researchers, public health officials, insurance providers, and especially patients and families have depended upon the presence of relevant diagnoses in the DSM for the classification of mental illness, legitimacy of research investigations, development of public health policy, deciding of reimbursement to clinicians, and a way of understanding personal suffering. However, perinatal mental health disorders have had an uneven history in the various versions of the DSM. For example, in DSM-III (American Psychiatric Association, 1980), postpartum psychosis is listed in the Index but only under the category of atypical psychosis and only if the episode does not meet the criteria for any other disorder (p. 203). There is no mention of postpartum or prenatal depression. The DSM-III-R (American Psychiatric Association, 1987) similarly labeled postpartum psychosis as an atypical psychosis (p. 211). Manic and depressive episodes occurring in the postpartum had the following description in the DSM-III-R,

> Some investigators consider a postpartum Manic Episode to have an "organic" etiology. However, because of the difficulty of distinguishing the psychological and physiologic stresses *associated* with pregnancy and delivery, in this classification such episodes are not considered Organic Mood Syndromes, and should be diagnosed as Manic Episodes
>
> *(p. 216)*.

The exact same wording was applied to postpartum depressive episodes (p. 221). In sum, there was no support in the DSM-III-R for labeling postpartum depression, mania, or psychosis as such.

The guidance regarding postpartum disorders changed rather dramatically with the DSM-IV (American Psychiatric Association, 1994), such that a postpartum onset specifier could be added to major depressive, manic, mixed episode, bipolar I and II, and brief psychotic disorder episodes if the episode began within four weeks of childbirth (p. 386). These specifiers were not diagnoses but did allow the recording of postpartum onset, even if limited to the first four weeks after delivery. In addition, there was a text that provided some elaboration about the nature of postpartum disorders (pp. 386–387). Nevertheless, patients, clinicians, and researchers remained unhappy with such a limited definition of postpartum onset, particularly considering that many investigators use the first 12 months postpartum as the risk period for postpartum depression. Little changed in DSM-IV-TR (American Psychiatric Association, 2000) aside from a more elaborate discussion of the postpartum onset specifier (pp. 422–423). For survivors of postpartum depression and those in advocacy and support groups (e.g., PSI, www.postpartum.net/), recognition of postpartum depression, now more broadly perinatal depression, is critical to legitimize their suffering and reduce stigma. It is important to remember that postpartum (perinatal) mental health disorders have often not been taken seriously by mental health professionals.

In preparation for the DSM-5 (led by Dr. David Kupfer), the APA established what were called Study Groups that addressed general issues, such as life span developmental approaches, and, importantly, gender and cross-cultural issues. The Gender and Cross-Cultural DSM-5 Study Group included Kimberly Yonkers (a prominent perinatal psychiatrist) as Chair and Ellen Frank (a prominent perinatal psychologist and wife of David Kupfer) as a member (American Psychiatric Association, 2013). As a small aside, Ellen was my classmate in the clinical psychology program at the University of Pittsburgh. There was great hope that the Study Group would recommend extending the timeframe for the postpartum onset specifier or even recommend a specific diagnosis for postpartum depression. Dr. Frank gave a presentation on the work of the Study Group at the 2010 biennial meeting of the Marcé Society, which was held in Pittsburgh under the leadership of Dr. Katherine Wisner. Dr. Frank's presentation, ambiguously titled "Will postpartum onset disorders disappear from DSM-5?" was marked with great anticipation, particularly among members of PSI, which was holding its annual meeting in conjunction with the Marcé Society meeting. During the course of Dr. Frank's presentation, when it became clear that many of the hopes of the Marcé and PSI members would not be realized, there was palpable anger, including boos coming from those in attendance. Fortunately for Dr. Frank, she had to leave the meeting immediately after her presentation. The DSM-5 (American Psychiatric Association, 2013), however, did extend the period for "peripartum" (to include pregnancy and postpartum) onset to include all of pregnancy and, again, up to four weeks after delivery. In justifying its decision, the DSM-5 authors pointed out that as many as half of postpartum depressions begin during pregnancy (pp. 186–187). The latest version of the DSM (DSM-5-TR) was published in 2022 (American Psychiatric Association, 2022). It contains additional information on sex and gender, along with enhanced discussions of the range of mood disorders and peripartum onset. Nevertheless, DSM-5-TR still asserts that the high-risk period for mood disorders, including psychosis, is pregnancy and the first four weeks after delivery. However, there is still no diagnosis of postpartum depression in the DSM. Finally, it should be noted that the ICD-11 (Radoš et al., 2024) uses depression onset within six weeks of childbirth as its criterion to label postpartum depression (Coded as 6E20, Mental or behavioral disorders associated with pregnancy, childbirth, and the puerperium, without psychotic symptoms). In the section "Sex- and Gender-Related Diagnostic Issues" in DSM-5-TR (pp. 268–269), it is briefly noted that OCD may have an onset or exacerbation during the peripartum period, but little else is said. Similar language is found in DSM-5 (p. 240).

Perinatal depression is not the only mental health condition experienced by women that has had a difficult time being fully recognized in the DSM. There was no mention of premenstrual dysphoric disorder in DSM-III (American Psychiatric Association, 1980). In the

DSM-III-R (American Psychiatric Association, 1987), it was called late luteal phase dysphoric disorder (p. 369) and included in "Appendix A: Proposed Diagnostic Categories Needing Further Study." In DSM-IV (American Psychiatric Association, 1994), it was relabeled premenstrual dysphoric disorder (p. 715) but only included in "Appendix B: Criteria Sets and Axes Provided for Further Study." In the DSM-IV-TR (American Psychiatric Association, 2000), premenstrual dysphoric disorder continued in the same appendix (p. 771). Premenstrual dysphoric disorder (p. 171) finally entered the DSM as a fully recognized disorder with DSM-5 (American Psychiatric Association, 2013). Thirty-three years elapsed between the publication of DSM-III and the full recognition of premenstrual dysphoric disorder as a serious mental illness suffered by millions of women. Some of this was due to the slow progress of the science, but much of it was probably due to the fact that premenstrual mood problems were often deemed as normal by the psychiatric establishment.

Prevalence of Perinatal Depression

What is the prevalence of depression during pregnancy and in the months following childbirth, and is the prevalence different from that of similarly situated women who have not experienced childbirth in the preceding months? In my first major review of the literature (O'Hara & Zekoski, 1988) covering studies up through 1986, Zekoski and I reported that using standard diagnostic criteria, the prevalence rate for postpartum depression ranged from 8.2% (Cutrona, 1983) to 14.9% (Kumar & Robson, 1984). Findings for depression prevalence during pregnancy were similar (O'Hara & Zekoski, 1988). It should be noted that then as now, investigators used varying time frames for prevalence estimates during pregnancy and after delivery, making comparisons across studies difficult. Also, it was not until later (O'Hara & Swain, 1996) that systematic reviews along with quantitative (rather than qualitative) analyses became a common way to aggregate the results of studies of prevalence. Another issue addressed in the O'Hara and Zekoski review was whether women were at increased risk for depression after delivery. Several studies addressed this issue, and there was little evidence that depression was more common in postpartum women than women who had not recently given birth (O'Hara et al., 1984; Watson et al., 1984). At that time, we commented in the review, "The revelation that depression is no more common after delivery than at other times provides little solace to the puerperally depressed woman. Several studies have documented the long duration of many postpartum depressions" (p. 35). We went on to comment on the suffering of women and their families and the negative long-term effects on the infant that were documented elsewhere in the volume (Murray, 1988). For me, the major takeaway was that depression during pregnancy and following childbirth is a major public health problem that deserves public resources for clinical care and research.

Over the ensuing decades, hundreds of studies were published in the United States and around the world that documented the prevalence of depression in pregnancy and after delivery. In 1996, Annette Swain and I (O'Hara & Swain, 1996) published a quantitative summary of postpartum depression prevalence studies based on a total of 59 studies (12,810 subjects). We reported an overall prevalence of 13%. Interestingly, there was not much difference in rates between self-report (14%) and interview-based measures (12%). In 2005, Gavin et al. published a very influential systematic review of the prevalence and incidence of perinatal depression. Out of 109 articles, only 28 met their inclusion criteria, which included the criterion that a diagnosis of depression must have been made. Studies based on self-report were excluded. They reported that as many as 19.2% of women experience a major or minor episode of depression ("minor" defined as having only three or four symptoms of major depression) in the first three months after delivery (7.1% major depression). They made several important points in their article. The first was that there was a wide confidence interval around their estimates, and the second was that larger and more representative studies should be undertaken to delineate periods of peak prevalence and incidence of perinatal depression (Gavin et al., 2005). Another influential systematic review was published by Fisher et al. (2012) on the prevalence of perinatal disorders in low- and lower-middle-income countries. The authors reported an overall prevalence of "common perinatal mental disorders" (mostly depression) during pregnancy of 15.6% and 19.8% in the postpartum period. The rate of postpartum depression was not very different from that reported by Gavin et al. More recent systematic reviews yielded similar results. Shorey et al. (2018) analyzed results from 58 studies from around the world, including numerous studies from Asia, Africa, and the Middle East, covering 37,294 women and found a global prevalence for postpartum depression of 17%. Finally, Liu et al. (2022) reported on a systematic review of 27 studies covering 133,313 women and found a global prevalence of postpartum depression of 14%. What have we learned over the past 40 years about the prevalence of postpartum depression? It is probably somewhere in the range of 13% to 19% but may be more or less in some cultural settings. We have also learned that postpartum depression is common across all countries and cultures that have been studied. It is a global phenomenon. As a point of comparison, various versions of the recent DSMs have reported rates of major depression not much different from those for postpartum depression. For example, DSM-IV-R (American Psychiatric Association, 2000) indicated a point prevalence of major depression for women to range from 5% to 9% (compared to Gavin et al. 7.1% in the first three months after delivery). At the time of the Gavin et al. review, there were three studies that compared perinatal and non-perinatal women (Cox et al., 1993; O'Hara et al., 1990; Cooper et al., 1988). There was almost no evidence from these three studies that there was a higher prevalence of depression in recently delivered women compared to a sample of women who had not recently delivered (Gavin et al., 2005, Table 2). More recent studies (Vesga-Lopez et al., 2008; Davé et al., 2010) based on very large samples do offer some evidence that there may be a small increased risk of depression associated with childbearing, but the evidence is still rather weak (O'Hara & McCabe, 2013).

Screening and the Advent of the
Edinburgh Postnatal Depression Scale

The EPDS (Cox et al., 1987) has become something of the de facto tool to screen for postpartum depression. It has garnered over 14,000 citations in the literature. It has been translated into dozens of languages and is used around the world. Indeed, picture versions of the EPDS have been developed for use with illiterate women. There is no doubting the profound impact of this simple instrument. In their 1987 paper, Cox, Holden, and Sagovsky noted that existing depression scales were not very useful in identifying women with clinically relevant postpartum depression because they had poor specificity; that is, they yielded too many false positives. In that article, Cox et al. cited two of my early studies (O'Hara et al., 1983, 1984) in which we used the *Beck Depression Inventory* (BDI; Beck et al., 1961) to measure depression severity in pregnancy and the postpartum period. Cox et al. were correct in noting that many women in our studies with elevated scores were not clinically depressed based on Research Diagnostic Criteria (Spitzer et al., 1978). However, in my earlier work, I was not screening per se but rather using the BDI as a measure of the severity of pregnancy and postpartum depression symptoms. It worked well in that regard. Most of the other studies cited by Cox et al. had similar purposes. Nevertheless, Cox et al. were correct in believing that a specific tool was needed to screen postpartum women, a tool that would be easy to administer and score. The EPDS fulfilled those objectives – ten simple (and colloquially worded) items that were scored zero to three (0 – 30 total range). They found that using a threshold of 12/13 was reasonably sensitive and specific for iden-tifying clinically relevant depression.

It is worth reading this paper because Cox et al. made several important points in their discussion that have current resonance. First, they said that an above-threshold score on the EPDS should be further assessed by a primary care worker to confirm the presence of a clinical depression. They also said that a score just below the threshold should not be taken to mean the absence of depression. Finally, they stated that a 9/10 threshold might be considered for use by primary care workers. Perhaps the first research use of the EPDS was an important study led by Jeni Holden (Holden et al., 1989), in which she used the EPDS to identify postnatally depressed women for a clinical trial. The depression intervention was delivered by British health visitors who would be similar to advanced practice nurses in the United States. They were trained to deliver a brief counseling intervention based on Rogerian or nondirective counseling methods in the homes of women during their regularly scheduled home visits. The trial was successful and demonstrated that the EPDS could be successfully used in clinical practice and that nonmental health professionals could be trained to effectively deliver brief interventions to women in the community. This approach to depression treatment was widely adopted in the United Kingdom (Hanley, 2015) and by one of my colleagues, Dr. Lisa Segre, at the University of Iowa (Segre et al., 2015).

The EPDS and the practice of universal perinatal depression screening was not without its critics in the United Kingdom. For example, in 1991 a conference organized by John Cox was held at the University of Keele entitled, "Prevention of Depression After Childbirth: Use and Misuse of the *Edinburgh Postnatal Depression Inventory*." It was largely a British affair with only me and Peter Boyce (Australia) representing the rest of the world. It resulted in a book published a few years later (Cox & Holden, 1994). Sandra Elliott, a British psychologist, argued that the EPDS was often used without careful thought as to what to do next. Even in the United Kingdom, which has a reasonably good health and mental health system (at least in the past), there was not always a place to refer women who scored above the threshold on the EPDS, nor was there a clear understanding of the best times to screen women with the EPDS or other instruments for that matter (Elliott, 1994). These concerns would echo what U.S. professional organizations would argue over the next decade and one-half.

It would be quite a while before systematic perinatal depression screening would become common in the United States. Our first efforts at systematic screening for postpartum depres-sion began in 1996 and were done in support of our first postpartum treatment trial (O'Hara et al., 2000). We systematically reached out and screened women from four counties in Iowa that included the cities of Des Moines, Iowa City, Cedar Rapids, and Davenport. Using the state of Iowa birth register, we identified 20,620 women who had recently delivered. The self-report screen that we used was the *Inventory to Diagnose Depression* (IDD; Zimmerman & Coryell, 1987). It was a lengthy questionnaire that allowed us to make a provisional diagnosis of major depression. We used the IDD as a research screening tool in another trial as well, but it was not suitable for clinical use because of its length and complexity.

Beginning in 2001, the U.S. Health Resources and Services Administration (HRSA) required all Healthy Start Programs (104 sites) to begin perinatal depression screening for pregnant and postpartum women served by the programs (Segre et al., 2012). In support of this mandate, HRSA offered Healthy Start Programs the opportunity to apply for grants to implement comprehensive perinatal depression screening and referral. Our group was contacted by the Des Moines Healthy Start Program to seek our assistance in applying for one of the available grants in the fall of 2000. Because so little work had been done nationally to support screening, I was surprised that HRSA and the National Healthy Start Program were in a position to mandate screening on a large-scale basis. I called Maribeth Badura, the director of the National Healthy Start Program, and asked her if she and her colleagues knew anything about perinatal depression screening. She admitted to me that there was not a great deal of knowledge in the Healthy Start Program about perinatal depression screening and then asked if I could help in reviewing the applications for funding. At the same time, my colleague, Dr. Lisa Segre, and I were brought on as consultants for the Des Moines Healthy Start Program (one of the grant recipients) to support their effort to implement perinatal depression screening. This began a collaborative effort that went on for over a decade. We developed a training program about perinatal mental health, screening, and treatment that was delivered monthly to the Healthy Start home visitors who were expected to screen women in their homes using the EPDS. Two developments emerged from our early efforts. First, HRSA officials requested that I provide workshops to 11 Healthy Start Programs (in 2004–2005) that had requested technical assistance from HRSA regarding perinatal depression screening (programs mostly located in eastern and southern states). Dr. Segre and I developed a two-day training program similar to what we had provided to the Des Moines Healthy Start Program. We undertook an evaluation of the training program at the end of training with program staff (N = 442) and at six months and five years with program directors (N = 11). Program staff rated their level of knowledge of core curriculum topics (e.g., perinatal depression, screening and referral, management of depression) before and after training. They also rated the usefulness of the knowledge of core curriculum topics to their work in Healthy Start (Segre et al., 2013). By the end of the training, there were significant improvements in curriculum topic knowledge and high ratings of the usefulness of the material presented. Program directors overall rated the training as very useful and that they largely met the training goals originally set by them during the pre-consultation process. Outcomes with the program directors five years later yielded similar results.

In 2009, Dr. Gerald Joseph became president of the American College of Obstetricians and Gynecologists (ACOG). His special focus for his presidential year was postpartum depression. Early on in this presidential year, he charged one of the practice committees to examine whether ACOG should recommend perinatal depression screening. At the annual meeting of the North American Society for Psychosocial Obstetrics and Gynecology in February 2010, he reported that the practice committee had declined to recommend routine perinatal depression screening, much to the disappointment of all of us in attendance. The committee stated the following, "At this time there is insufficient evidence to support a firm recommendation for universal antepartum or postpartum screening. There are also insufficient data to recommend how often screening should be done" (American College of Obstetricians and Gynecologists, 2010, p. 394). Nevertheless, the tide was already beginning to turn regarding screening. The American Academy of Pediatrics recommended postpartum depression screening later in 2010, followed by the Association of Women's Health, Obstetrics and Neonatal Nurses and ACOG in 2015. Finally, in 2016 the U.S. Preventive Services

Task Force (Siu et al., 2016) stated the following, "The USPSTF recommends screening for depression in the general adult population, including pregnant and postpartum women. Screening should be implemented with adequate systems in place to ensure accurate diagnosis, effective treatment, and appropriate follow-up" (p. 380). This was the most important recommendation because of the very large influence of USPSTF recommendations on all of medical practice. Also, at around the same time, several states began to require (e.g., New Jersey, Illinois) or encourage (e.g., California, Massachusetts) screening. State Medicaid agencies were also allowed to cover maternal depression screening during well child visits (e.g., Colorado, Illinois). Despite all of the progress to date, there are still major gaps in screening across the United States (Griffen et al., 2021).

Interventions for Perinatal Mental Health Disorders

By the early 1990s, I had published numerous papers on the epidemiology and causal factors associated with postpartum depression. The most recent ones at that time reported on a large controlled prospective study of pregnant and postpartum women and matched controls, which included follow-up assessments of children up to three years of age (O'Hara et al., 1990; O'Hara, Schlechte, Lewis, & Varner, 1991; O'Hara, Schlechte, Lewis, & Wright, 1991). The findings from these studies were complex and extensive, but there were several of specific importance. First, the prevalence of major depression was not significantly different between pregnant and postpartum women and their matched controls, but mood symptoms (from BDI and a *Visual Analog Scale*) clearly differentiated the two groups during pregnancy and after delivery (O'Hara et al., 1990). Second, among childbearing subjects, a vulnerability-life stress model of depression was supported in a hierarchical multiple regression. Hormonal variables were largely unrelated to the diagnosis of postpartum depression with the exception of estradiol (lower at week 26 gestation and day 2 postpartum) (O'Hara, Schlechte, Lewis, & Varner, 1991). Third, a constellation of depression risk factors measured during pregnancy was associated with the development of the postpartum blues soon after delivery (O'Hara, Schlechte, Lewis, & Wright, 1991). Also, there were higher levels of total and free estriol late in pregnancy and early in the postpartum period among women experiencing the postpartum blues than women who did not experience the postpartum blues after delivery (O'Hara, Schlechte, Lewis, & Wright, 1991). For me, these papers represented a culmination of a research program that I had launched in 1979. I believed at that time there was little in the way of further research that would illuminate our understanding of postpartum depression. I was wrong, of course, but my beliefs set me off in a new direction – interventions for suffering women.

In April 1979, my academic advisor, Dr. Lynn Rehm, organized a conference with support from the National Institute of Mental Health (NIMH) to examine current behavioral treatments for depression (Rehm, 1981). At the time there were many psychological treatments for depression, reflecting different behavioral approaches and strategies, as well as cognitive approaches. This conference took place in Pittsburgh at the same time that NIMH was actively planning what became known as the NIMH Treatment of Depression Collaborative Research Program (Elkin et al., 1985). It was at this conference that I learned about interpersonal psychotherapy (IPT). I had been trained in cognitive therapy (CT), behavior therapy (BT), and self-control therapy in graduate school. IPT was new to me, and I was surprised to learn in the course of the meeting that it along with CT and antidepressant medication (imipramine) would be the three treatments to be included in the NIMH collaborative study. By that time there had been a good amount of evidence for CT and also BT (Blaney, 1981). The work on IPT was not as extensive. In fact, Steven Hollon, one of the speakers, expressed skepticism regarding the specific efficacy of IPT in direct contrast to CT (Hollon, 1981). I speculated at that time that Dr. Gerald Klerman, one of the developers of IPT and a very influential psychiatrist, might have played a role in ensuring that IPT along with CT was included in this trial, the main purpose of which was to validate psychotherapy as a treatment for major depression. It struck me as strange that two psychotherapeutic approaches developed by psychiatrists would be used in a trial comparing psychotherapy to antidepressant medication. Nevertheless, the trial proceeded at three locations, Oklahoma City, Pittsburgh, and Washington, D.C. The first major report was not published until about ten years later (Elkin et al., 1989). The findings were complex, but, overall, the antidepressant condition had the best outcomes, and IPT fared better than CT with the more severely depressed patients.

It was only a few years later that I decided to seek NIMH funding for a postpartum depression treatment trial. My first major task in designing the trial was to decide on the intervention. Given that NIMH had essentially endorsed IPT and CT in the treatment of depression collaborative study (Elkin et al., 1989), I felt obligated to choose one or the other of these two psychotherapies. My dilemma was that I felt confident in my ability to deliver CT and train others but that there were two important reasons that I might want to choose IPT. First, and most important, the data from the collaborative trial suggested that IPT might be superior to CT, particularly for more severely depressed patients. Second, the focus of IPT on interpersonal disturbances, such as interpersonal role disputes, role transitions, and grief and loss, seemed particularly applicable to the postpartum context. Because of these considerations, I chose IPT and thus began a long journey to obtain NIMH funding. In the early 1990s, there were no restrictions on how many times an investigator could submit a revised application. I submitted a total of five revisions of my initial application over several years before it was funded in 1995. After the first couple of failures in funding, I had the good fortune to be introduced to Dr. Scott Stuart, a newly arrived psychiatrist and faculty member at the University of Iowa. Dr. Stuart had done his residency at Pittsburgh and was trained in IPT by Dr. Cleon Cornes, who had been one of the IPT therapists in the NIMH collaborative study. We have had a fruitful collaboration for over 30 years. Dr. Stuart brought IPT credibility to my research team, and he and I undertook a small pilot study to test IPT with postpartum depressed women (Stuart & O'Hara, 1995). The pilot trial was successful, and funding came soon thereafter. Although we were funded to undertake our trial, there was still a good bit of skepticism on the part of the reviewers and NIMH staff. For example, there was a strong belief that postpartum depression was not a serious problem and that women in our trial would get better soon without treatment. There was also skepticism that we could recruit sufficient numbers of women to have adequate power to test our hypotheses. As a consequence, we were funded for only two years and had to reply for funding for years at a time for a total of six years of funding.

Several key findings emerged from this trial (O'Hara et al., 2000). First over a 12-week period, depressed women in the IPT condition showed statistically significant improvement in depression symptom level on self-report and clinician-rated measures relative to women in the waiting list group. These findings were mirrored in measures of social adjustment as well. What was striking was that there was little improvement in the women who waited for treatment. We provided it for them after the waiting period, and they improved to the same degree as the women who were initially treated with IPT. A second purpose of the trial was to evaluate the impact of treatment on the children of the women in the trial (Forman et al., 2007). We went into the homes of the women and did careful assessments of the infants and mother–infant interactions both before and after treatment or waiting. We also recruited a sample of non-postpartum depressed mothers as a comparison. Following treatment mothers in the IPT condition reported significantly less parenting stress than mothers who waited for treatment. However, there were no differences in mother–infant interactions. Depressed mothers (from both treatment conditions) showed less responsiveness to their infants, experienced more parenting stress, and viewed their infants more negatively than the non-postpartum depressed mothers. These findings were largely replicated 18 months later. In sum, there was little evidence that effective treatment for postpartum depression had a significant positive impact on infants of these mothers. An important implication of these findings was that the mother–infant relationship must be addressed in addition to maternal depression.

Our team went on to undertake numerous new studies of the treatment and prevention of postpartum depression. For example, we undertook a trial with colleagues from Brown University in which postpartum depressed women were assigned to one of three conditions, IPT, sertraline with clinical management, and placebo with clinical management (O'Hara et al., 2019). A significant innovation in this trial was the inclusion of breastfeeding women. This was one of the first randomized double-blind placebo-controlled trials of an antidepressant medication that included postpartum depressed breastfeeding women. The findings of the study were complex, but there were some significant takeaways. First, although each of the interventions performed well, there was some evidence that the sertraline condition produced the best results based on the general depression scale of the *Inventory of Depression and Anxiety Symptoms* (Watson et al., 2007). Another notable finding was that breastfeeding women were significantly more likely to complete the trial than non-breastfeeding women. It may have been that breastfeeding women were especially motivated to complete the trial to benefit their newborn infant.

We completed a trial testing yoga as a treatment for postpartum depression (Buttner et al., 2015), a trial evaluating listening visits for low-income perinatal depressed women in their homes (Segre et al., 2015), a trial evaluating a coach-supported cognitive behavioral therapy online intervention for postpartum depressed women veterans (Solness et al., 2021), and an online preventive intervention delivered during pregnancy for women at high risk for postpartum depression (Duffecy et al., 2022). Finally, we have a paper under review describing a trial in which we evaluated a "flexible" form of IPT for postpartum depression (Stuart et al., 2023). All these studies had one common aim: to reduce the suffering of depressed pregnant and postpartum women.

What I Have Left Out

This chapter has not addressed perinatal anxiety disorders. In our own work, we often had measures of anxiety occasionally (Stuart et al., 1998). Around that same time, Dr. Amy Wenzel, the editor of this volume and a scholar of perinatal anxiety disorders (Wenzel & Stuart, 2011), joined my laboratory as a graduate research assistant. She brought with her an intense interest in anxiety and anxiety disorders, and it would seem that collaborating with me and my colleagues on a postpartum depression treatment trial led to a marrying of interests. Later, my colleagues and I developed a brief scale to detect postpartum anxiety, consisting of three scaled items, feeling panicky, feeling restless, and having problems sleeping. These three items had very good psychometric characteristics (O'Hara et al., 2012). Perinatal anxiety disorders and their treatment are addressed fully in other chapters of this volume. However, in reviewing recent systematic reviews and meta-analyses, I was struck by how few trials of cognitive behavioral therapy actually had subjects who carried a diagnosis of a specific anxiety disorder (Li et al., 2022; Maguire et al., 2018). The vast majority of studies simply used elevated anxiety scores or relied on elevated levels of depressive symptoms.

Although my lab published data on the hormonal basis of postpartum depression in the 1990s (O'Hara, Schlechte, Lewis, & Varner, 1991; O'Hara, Schlechte, Lewis, & Wright, 1991), as well as one treatment trial with a medication arm, our lab had largely a psychological/psychosocial orientation to perinatal mental health. I look to my psychiatrist colleagues, such as Dr. Katherine Wisner at George Washington University and Dr. Samantha Meltzer-Brody at the University of North Carolina at Chapel Hill, for guidance on biology and medical treatments.

Conclusion

As I look back on my career, I cannot help but reflect on the success of my former graduate students. During the first 20 years of my career at the University of Iowa, I had only one graduate student who had an interest in perinatal mental (Dr. Laura Gorman). Dr. Gorman went on to serve as a research scientist in our laboratory and was instrumental in managing many of our trials and traveling to Europe on my behalf for our work on the Transcultural Study. Later came a flood of great graduate students with specific interests in perinatal mental health, Dr. Tracy Moran Vozar, associate professor of psychiatry and behavioral sciences and pediatrics, School of Medicine and Health Sciences, George Washington University; Dr. Kimberly Hart, clinical professor, Department of Psychiatry, University of Iowa; Dr. Crystal Schiller, assistant professor, Department of Psychiatry, UNC-Chapel Hill; Dr. Sheehan Fisher, associate professor, Department of Psychiatry, Northwestern University; Dr. Jennifer McCabe, associate professor, Psychology Department, University of Western Washington; Dr. Rebecca Grekin, Private Practice, Ann Arbor, Michigan; Dr. Emily Kroska, clinical associate professor, Department of Psychological and Brain Sciences, University of Iowa; Dr. Michelle Miller, assistant professor, Department of Psychiatry, Indiana University, and Dr. Kristen Merkitch, private practice, Indianapolis, Indiana. Finally, I cannot exclude Dr. Amy Wenzel, though not technically one of my graduate students, I still claim. Whatever I have accomplished in my career in perinatal mental health will live on in the lives and the work of my wonderful students and colleagues. And none of this would have been possible without the support of my wife, Dr. Jane Engeldinger. Jane was a constant companion in all my adventures and a leader in her own right in psychosocial obstetrics and gynecology. She kept me sane and focused. What more can I say!

References

American College of Obstetricians and Gynecologists. (2010). Screening for depression during and after pregnancy: Committee opinion no. 453. *Obstetrics & Gynecology, 115*, 394–395.

American Psychiatric Association. (1952). *Diagnostic and statistical manual of mental disorders* (1st ed.).

American Psychiatric Association. (1968). *Diagnostic and statistical manual of mental disorders* (2nd ed.).

American Psychiatric Association. (1980). *Diagnostic and statistical manual of mental disorders* (3rd ed.).

American Psychiatric Association. (1987). *Diagnostic and statistical manual of mental disorders* (3rd ed., rev.).

American Psychiatric Association. (1994). *Diagnostic and statistical manual of mental disorders* (4th ed.).

American Psychiatric Association. (2000). *Diagnostic and statistical manual of mental disorders* (4th ed., text rev.).

American Psychiatric Association. (2013). *Diagnostic and statistical manual of mental disorders* (5th ed.). https://doi.org/10.1176/appi.books.9780890425596

American Psychiatric Association. (2022). *Diagnostic and statistical manual of mental disorders* (5th ed., text rev.). https://doi.org/10.1176/appi.books.9780890425787

Atkinson, A. K., & Rickel, A. U. (1984). Postpartum depression in primiparous parents. *Journal of Abnormal Psychology, 93*(1), 115–119.

Beck, A. T., Ward, C. H., Mendelson, M., Mock, J., & Erbaugh, J. (1961). An inventory for measuring depression. *Archives of General Psychiatry, 4*(6), 561–571.

Blaney, P. H. (1981). The effectiveness of cognitive and behavior therapies. In L. P. Rehm (Ed.), *Behavior therapy for depression: Present status and future directions* (pp. 1–32). Academic Press.

Buttner, M. M., Brock, R. L., O'Hara, M. W., & Stuart, S. (2015). Efficacy of yoga for depressed postpartum women: A randomized controlled trial. *Complementary Therapies in Clinical Practice, 21*, 94–100.

Cooper, P. J., Campbell, E. A., Day, A., Kennerley, H., & Bond, A. (1988). Non-psychotic psychiatric disorder after childbirth: A prospective study of prevalence, incidence, course and nature. *British Journal of Psychiatry, 152*(6), 799–806.

Cox, J., & Holden, J. (Eds.). (1994). *Perinatal psychiatry: Use and misuse of the Edinburgh postnatal depression scale*. Gaskell.

Cox, J., Holden, J., & Sagovsky, R. (1987). Detection of postnatal depression: Development of the 10-item *Edinburgh Postnatal Depression Scale. British Journal of Psychiatry, 150*, 782–786. https://doi.org/10.1192/bjp.150.6.782

Cox, J. L., Murray, D., & Chapman, G. (1993). A controlled study of the onset, duration and prevalence of postnatal depression. *British Journal of Psychiatry, 163*(1), 27–31.

Cutrona, C. E. (1983). Causal attributions and perinatal depression. *Journal of Abnormal Psychology, 92*, 161–172. https://doi.org/10.1037/0021-843X.92.2.161

Cutrona, C. E., & Troutman, B. R. (1986). Social support, infant temperament, and parenting self-efficacy: A mediational model of postpartum depression. *Child Development, 57*, 1507–1518.

Davé, S., Petersen, I., Sherr, L., & Nazareth, I. (2010). Incidence of maternal and paternal depression in primary care: A cohort study using a primary care database. *Archives of Pediatrics & Adolescent Medicine, 164*(11), 1038–1044.

Duffecy, J., Grekin, R., Long, J. D., Mills, J. A., & O'Hara, M. W. (2022). Randomized controlled trial of Sunnyside: Individual versus group-based online interventions to prevent postpartum depression. *Journal of Affective Disorders, 311*, 538–547.

Elkin, I., Parloff, M., Hadley, S., & Autry, I. (1985). The NIMH treatment of depression collaborative research program: Background and research plan. *Archives of General Psychiatry, 42*, 305–316.

Elkin, I., Shea, M. T., Watkins, J. T., Imber, S. D., Sotsky, S. M., Collins, F. L., . . . Parloff, M. B. (1989). NIMH treatment of depression collaborative research program: I. General effectiveness of treatments. *Archives of General Psychiatry, 46*, 971–982.

Elliott, S. A. (1994). Uses and misuses of the *Edinburgh postnatal depression scale* in primary care: A comparison of models developed in health visiting. In J. Cox & J. Holden (Eds.), *Perinatal psychiatry: Use and misuse of the Edinburgh postnatal depression scale* (pp. 221–232). Gaskell.

Fisher, J., de Mello, M. C., Patel, V., Rahman, A., Tran, T., Holtona, S., & Holmes, W. (2012). Prevalence and determinants of common perinatal mental disorders in women in low- and lower-middle-income countries: A systematic review. *Bulletin of the World Health Organization, 90*, 139–149.

Forman, D., O'Hara, M. W., Stuart, S., Gorman, L., Larsen, K., & Coy, K. C. (2007). Effective treatment for postpartum depression is not sufficient to improve the developing mother-child relationship. *Development and Psychopathology, 19*, 585–602.

Gavin, N. I., Gaynes, B. N., Lohr, K. N., Meltzer-Brody, S., Gartlehner, G., & Swinson, T. (2005). Perinatal depression: A systematic review of prevalence and incidence. *Obstetrics & Gynecology, 106*(5 Part 1), 1071–1083. https://doi.org/10.1097/01.AOG.0000183597.31630.db

Griffen, A., McIntyre, L., Belsito, J. Z., Burkhard, J., Davis, W., Kimmel, M., . . . Meltzer-Brody, S. (2021). Perinatal mental health care in the United States: An overview of policies and programs. *Health Affairs, 40*(10), 1543–1550. https://doi.org/10.1377/hlthaff.2021.00796

Hamilton, J. A. (1962). *Postpartum psychiatric problems*. C. V. Mosby.

Hanley, J. (2015). *Listening visits in perinatal mental health: A guide for health professionals and support workers* (1st ed.). Routledge. https://doi.org/10.4324/9781315774220

Holden, J. M., Sagovsky, R., & Cox, J. L. (1989). Counselling in a general practice setting: Controlled study of health visitor intervention in treatment of postnatal depression. *British Medical Journal, 298*(6668), 223–226.

Hollon, S. D. (1981). Comparisons and combinations with alternative approaches. In L. P. Rehm (Ed.), *Behavior therapy for depression: Present status and future directions* (pp. 33–71). Academic Press.

Horwitz, A. V. (2021). *DSM: A history of psychiatry's Bible*. Johns Hopkins University.

Jones, W. H. S. (1923). *Hippocrates with an English translation by W. H. S. Jones*. Harvard University Press.

Kumar, R., & Brockington, I. F. (Eds.). (1988). *Motherhood and mental illness: 2 Causes and consequences*. Butterworths.

Kumar, R., & Robson, K. M. (1984). A prospective study of emotional disorders in childbearing women. *British Journal of Psychiatry, 144*, 35–47.

Li, X., Laplante, D. P., Paquin, V., Lafortune, S., Elgbeili, G., & King, S. (2022). Effectiveness of cognitive behavioral therapy for perinatal maternal depression, anxiety and stress: A systematic review and meta-analysis of randomized controlled trials. *Clinical Psychology Review, 92*, 102–129.

Liu, X., Wang, S., & Wang, G. (2022). Prevalence and risk factors of postpartum depression in women: A systematic review and meta-analysis. *Journal of Clinical Nursing, 31*(19–20), 2665–2677.

Maguire, P. N., Clark, G. I., & Wootton, B. M. (2018). The efficacy of cognitive behavior therapy for the treatment of perinatal anxiety symptoms: A preliminary meta-analysis. *Journal of Anxiety Disorders, 60*, 26–34.

Manly, P. C., McMahon, R. J., Bradley, C. F., & Davidson, P. O. (1982). Depressive attributional style and depression following childbirth. *Journal of Abnormal Psychology, 91*(4), 245–254. https://doi.org/10.1037/0021-843X.91.4.245

Murray, L. (1988). Effects of postnatal depression on infant development: Direct studies of early mother-infant interaction. In R. Kumar & I. F. Brockington (Eds.), *Motherhood and mental illness: 2 Causes and consequences* (pp. 159–190). Butterworths.

O'Hara, M. W. (1986). Social support, life events, and depression during pregnancy and the puerperium. *Archives of General Psychiatry, 43*(6), 569–573. https://doi.org/10.1001/archpsyc.1986.01800060063008

O'Hara, M. W., & McCabe, J. E. (2013). Postpartum depression: Current status and future directions. *Annual Review of Clinical Psychology, 9*, 379–407.

O'Hara, M. W., Neunaber, D. J., & Zekoski, E. M. (1984). A prospective study of postpartum depression: Prevalence, course, and predictive factors. *Journal of Abnormal Psychology, 93*, 158–171.

O'Hara, M. W., Pearlstein, T., Stuart, S., Long, J. D., Mills, J. A., & Zlotnick, C. (2019). A placebo controlled treatment trial of sertraline and interpersonal psychotherapy for postpartum depression. *Journal of Affective Disorders, 245*, 524–532.

O'Hara, M. W., & Rehm, L. P. (1979). Self-monitoring, activity levels and mood in the development and maintenance of depression. *Journal of Abnormal Psychology, 88*, 450–453.

O'Hara, M. W., Rehm, L. P., & Campbell, S. B. (1982). Predicting depressive symptomatology: Cognitive-behavioral models and postpartum depression. *Journal of Abnormal Psychology, 91*, 457–461.

O'Hara, M. W., Rehm, L. P., & Campbell, S. B. (1983). Postpartum depression: A role for social network and life stress variables. *Journal of Nervous and Mental Disease, 171*, 336–341.

O'Hara, M. W., Schlechte, J. A., Lewis, D. A., & Varner, M. W. (1991). A controlled prospective study of postpartum mood disorders: Psychological, environmental, and hormonal variables. *Journal of Abnormal Psychology, 100*, 63–73.

O'Hara, M. W., Schlechte, J. A., Lewis, D. A., & Wright, E. J. (1991). Prospective study of postpartum blues: Biologic and psychosocial factors. *Archives of General Psychiatry, 48*, 801–806.

O'Hara, M. W., Stuart, S., Gorman, L. L., & Wenzel, A. (2000). Efficacy of interpersonal psychotherapy for postpartum depression. *Archives of General Psychiatry, 57*, 1039–1045.

O'Hara, M. W., Stuart, S., Watson, D., Dietz, P. M., Farr, S. L., & D'angelo, D. (2012). Brief scales to detect postpartum depression and anxiety symptoms. *Journal of Women's Health, 21*(12), 1237–1243.

O'Hara, M. W., & Swain, A. M. (1996). Rates and risk of postpartum depression: A meta-analysis. *International Review of Psychiatry, 8*, 37–54.

O'Hara, M. W., & Zekoski, E. M. (1988). Postpartum depression. In R. Kumar & I. F. Brockington (Eds.), *Motherhood and mental illness: 2 Causes and consequences* (pp. 17–63). Butterworths.

O'Hara, M. W., Zekoski, E. M., Philipps, L. H., & Wright, E. J. (1990). A controlled prospective study of postpartum mood disorders: Comparison of childbearing and nonchildbearing women. *Journal of Abnormal Psychology, 99*, 3–15.

Philipps, L. H., & O'Hara, M. W. (1991). Prospective study of postpartum depression: 4½ year follow-up of women and children. *Journal of Abnormal Psychology, 100*, 151–155.

Radoš, S. N., Akik, B. K., Žutić, M., Rodriguez-Muñoz, M. F., Uriko, K., Motrico, E., . . . Lambregtse-van den Berg, M. (2024). Diagnosis of peripartum depression disorder: A state-of-the-art approach from the COST action riseup-PPD. *Comprehensive Psychiatry, 152456.*

Rehm, L. P. (1977). A self-control model of depression. *Behavior Therapy, 8*, 787–804.

Rehm, L. P. (Ed.). (1981). *Behavior therapy for depression: Present status and future directions.* Academic Press.

Segre, L. S., Brock, R. L., & O'Hara, M. W. (2015). Depression treatment for impoverished mothers by point-of-care providers: A randomized controlled trial. *Journal of Consulting and Clinical Psychology, 83*, 314–324. https://doi.org/10.1037/a0038495

Segre, L. S., O'Hara, M. W., Brock, R. A., & Taylor, D. L. (2012). Depression screening of perinatal women by the Des Moines Healthy Start Project: Program description and evaluation. *Psychiatric Services, 63*, 250–255. https://doi.org/10.1176/appi.ps.201100247

Segre, L. S., O'Hara, M. W., & Fisher, S. D. (2013). Perinatal depression screening in Healthy Start: An evaluation of the acceptability of technical assistance consultation. *Community Mental Health Journal, 49*, 407–411. https://doi.org/10.1007/s10597-012-9508-z

Shorey, S., Chee, C. Y. I., Ng, E. D., Chan, Y. H., San Tam, W. W., & Chong, Y. S. (2018). Prevalence and incidence of postpartum depression among healthy mothers: A systematic review and meta-analysis. *Journal of Psychiatric Research, 104*, 235–248.

Siu, A. L., US Preventive Services Task Force (USPSTF), Bibbins-Domingo, K., Grossman, D. C., Baumann, L. C., Davidson, K. W., . . . Pignone, M. P. (2016). Screening for depression in adults: US Preventive Services Task Force recommendation statement. *JAMA, 315*, 380–387.

Solness, C. L., Kroska, E. B., Holdefer, P. J., & O'Hara, M. W. (2021). Treating postpartum depression in rural veterans using Internet delivered CBT: Program evaluation of *MomMoodBooster. Journal of Behavioral Medicine, 44*, 454–466. https://doi.org/10.1007/s10865-020-00188-5

Spitzer, R. L., Endicott, J., & Robins, E. (1978). Research diagnostic criteria: Rationale and reliability. *Archives of General Psychiatry, 36*, 773–782.

Stuart, S., Brock, R. L., Ramsdell, E., Arndt, S., & O'Hara, M. W. (2023). Collaborative decision making improves interpersonal psychotherapy efficiency: A randomized clinical trial with postpartum women. *Journal of Affective Disorders Reports, 14*, 100636.

Stuart, S., Couser, G., Schilder, K., O'Hara, M. W., & Gorman, L. L. (1998). Postpartum anxiety and depression: Onset and comorbidity in a community sample. *Journal of Nervous and Mental Disease, 186*, 420–424.

Stuart, S., & O'Hara, M. W. (1995). Interpersonal psychotherapy for postpartum depression: A treatment program. *The Journal of Psychotherapy Practice and Research, 4*, 18–29.

Vesga-Lopez, O., Blanco, C., Keyes, K., Olfson, M., Grant, B. F., & Hasin, D. S. (2008). Psychiatric disorders in pregnant and postpartum women in the United States. *Archives of General Psychiatry, 65*(7), 805–815.

Watson, D., O'Hara, M. W., Simms, L. J., Kotov, R., Chmielewski, M., McDade-Montez, E. A., . . . Stuart, S. (2007). Development and validation of the *inventory of depression and anxiety symptoms* (IDAS). *Psychological Assessment, 19*(3), 253–268.

Watson, J. P., Elliot, S. A., Rugg, A. J., & Brough, D. I. (1984). Psychiatric disorder in pregnancy and the first postnatal year. *British Journal of Psychiatry, 144*, 453–462.

Wenzel, A., & Stuart, S. (2011). *Anxiety in childbearing women: Diagnosis and treatment.* American Psychological Association. https://doi.org/10.1037/12302-000

Whiffen, V. E. (1988). Vulnerability to postpartum depression: A prospective multivariate study. *Journal of Abnormal Psychology, 97*(4), 467–474.

Zimmerman, M., & Coryell, W. (1987). The *Inventory to Diagnose Depression* (IDD): A self-report scale to diagnose major depressive disorders. *Journal of Consulting and Clinical Psychology, 55*, 55–59.

2

PSYCHOLOGICAL ASPECTS OF PERINATAL MENTAL HEALTH

Dhara T. Meghani, Tracy Moran Vozar,
Kelsey Maki, U'nek Clarke, and Ellen Bartolini

The transition to parenthood is a vulnerable and dynamic time. For a childbearing parent, pregnancy presents a host of physical, physiological, psychological, emotional, and social changes. Navigating the first few months after birth can be stressful along these dimensions of functioning, and for new and multiparous parents it requires a great deal of adjustment across all facets of work and family life (Johns & Belsky, 2007; Riggs et al., 2018; Ruppanner et al., 2019). Infants are simultaneously adjusting to life outside the womb, depending heavily on their caregivers for support with sleep, feeding, and soothing and concurrently undergoing developmental changes that enhance alertness, attention, and independence. This transition initially centers on caregiving responsibilities such as feeding and changing the baby, problem solving around sleep, and providing developmentally appropriate opportunities for stimulation, learning, and play.

The shift in priorities and daily activities presents a formidable challenge, particularly for caregivers influenced by and living in societies subscribing to the discourse of *intensive mothering*,[1] a paradigm dominant in individualistic and Western child-rearing belief systems. Intensive mothering core beliefs center on the notion that mothers must spend exhaustive amounts of time and resources to raise successful and well-adjusted children (Ennis, 2014). Little time is devoted to a parent's own well-being, as the focus is largely on caring for and growing the relationship with their baby (Negron et al., 2013). The quality of the partner relationship declines during the first year of a child's life (see Twenge et al., 2003, for a review), and, absent social support and multiple caregivers, role strain and time pressure are major players that impact psychological well-being throughout the trajectory of parenthood (Ruppanner et al., 2019). Hormonal fluctuations, sleep deprivation, role integration, parental self-efficacy, financial stress, the loss of independence, and difficult infant temperament are known to contribute to feelings of stress, frustration, and even apathy in new parents (Jia et al., 2016; Radesky et al., 2013; Rallis et al., 2014; Wenzel, 2013). Left untreated, these sequelae can manifest as a number of clinical syndromes and contribute to detrimental outcomes for parents, children, and their relationships (Bauer et al., 2016; Goodman et al., 2016).

DOI: 10.4324/9781003206903-4

Overview of Perinatal Mental Health: Disorders and Challenges

Mental health challenges during the perinatal period (typically defined as pregnancy through the first year postpartum) present with varying symptomatology, duration, and severity, and gaps in knowledge remain regarding their predictability and associated risk factors, which will be discussed later in this chapter. For example, "baby blues" is an oft-used nonclinical term in many countries to normalize hormonal changes impacting mood and motivation following the transformative experience of childbirth (Rezaie-Keikhaie et al., 2020). The emotional volatility and identity displacement experienced by new mothers in this time, even if relatively brief, are not inconsequential, and overly down-played as argued by Moore (2018), who vividly describes feelings of rage, helplessness, and dread in the early moments of her postpartum life. Still, in most societies, the period of baby blues is thought to be akin to a "bee sting" that is shocking and temporarily painful but which is typically soothed by a home-based remedy, quickly forgotten as the skin heals organically.

What about parents who have an allergic reaction to this bee sting and require an outpatient visit? Many first-time parents especially tend to underestimate the vulnerability of their personal mental health or assume that symptoms of stress and low mood are requisite elements of new parenting. In some cases, these symptoms represent a minor or major mood episode with greater severity and longevity than the baby blues. These parents may be naive to mental health treatment and hesitant to make an entry due to stigma, lack of awareness, or mistrust of psychological and/or pharmacological interventions (see Dennis & Chung-Lee, 2006, for a review). Even among women who are aware and knowledgeable of signs and symptoms of perinatal mood and anxiety disorders (PMAD), barriers such as a lack of cultural understanding and warmth from healthcare providers and inflexibility of treatment services were cited as reasons for not seeking mental health support (Byrnes, 2019). Although this decision may prolong the course of and potentially worsen the severity of their symptoms, most parents are likely to seek nonclinical support if available, rise to parenting demands, and experience acceptable resolution of these transitional challenges eventually. Postpartum psychosis, in contrast, might be compared to a venomous snake bite, necessitating immediate treatment and hospitalization for the protection of mother and baby. Metaphorically speaking, one cannot be sure whether to prepare for a bee sting, a snake bite, or even a tiger in the room as might be the experience for mothers with significant trauma history, although researchers have begun to elucidate predictive markers of perinatal mental health disorders (PMHDs).

In this chapter, we begin with a brief introduction to commonly occurring PMHDs, prevalence, presentation, and impact, followed by cultural and societal pressures that exacerbate psychological risk during this time. The heart of this chapter centers on psychological factors, which are intrapsychic and interpersonal aspects that influence an individual's mental health, level of functioning, overall well-being, and emotional health. It is critical to examine and understand psychological factors that may be implicated in the development of PMHDs to design and implement focused interventions. There are many such contributions to mental health, and the factors that we emphasize in this chapter are early life experiences, history of interpersonal trauma and intimate partner violence, difficult pregnancy experiences, maladaptive cognitions, parenting self-efficacy, perfectionism, social support, and pre-existing psychological conditions. These factors may be particularly significant contributors to maternal mental health because they impact daily functioning, parenting style, and caregiving capacity and thus have impacts on the well-being of the baby. We conclude with a case study that illustrates the interconnected nature of psychological and other pregnancy-related risk factors in the development of posttraumatic stress disorder during the perinatal period.

Perinatal Mood and Anxiety Disorders

PMADs are among the most common mental health disorders diagnosed or exacerbated during the perinatal period (Fairbrother et al., 2015). Among childbearing women, the highest rates of depression and anxiety are likely to appear during the first year postpartum with symptoms that can persist well after the first year of life. New parents are vulnerable to experiencing high rates of depression and anxiety in the perinatal period with potential short- and long-term consequences to parent–child bonding and attachment, cognitive and socioemotional development, and parental well-being. Despite growing clinical and research attention to depression and anxiety during the perinatal period, the two major diagnostic classification systems – the *Diagnostic and Statistical Manual of Mental Disorders*, 5th edition Text Revision (DSM-5-TR) and *International Classification of Diseases*, 11th edition (ICD-11) – do not list diagnoses specific to pregnancy or postpartum. In the DSM-5-TR, patients who meet the criteria for a major depressive episode during pregnancy or within four weeks after giving birth can be diagnosed with a "with peripartum onset" specifier (American Psychiatric Association [APA], 2022, p. 213). The ICD-11 provides for a slightly longer window for the onset of symptoms (six weeks) in the diagnosis of a mental and behavioral diagnosis attributable to the postpartum (i.e., puerperium) period. The presentation of perinatal depression is variable and can include symptoms that resemble a major depressive disorder (e.g., sadness, fatigue, feelings of guilt and worthlessness, and suicidality). Postpartum depression (PPD) is not unique to women and is experienced by fathers as well (Cameron et al., 2016; Gavin et al., 2005). In a robust global review, Wang et al. (2021) found no significant differences in prevalence rates across women experiencing PPD during various segments of the first year after birth (1–3 months, 3–6 months, 6–12 months) and beyond, highlighting the necessity for continued screening and assessment, diagnosis, and treatment well after four to six weeks postpartum.

A systematic review of studies conducted across the world estimates the prevalence of perinatal depression at 11.9%, with higher rates among women in low- and middle-income countries (Woody et al., 2017). Pregnancy-related stress, anxiety, and depression are weighty risk factors for PPD, and the likelihood of psychiatric admission is 22 times higher postnatally compared to during pregnancy (Kendell et al., 1987). PPD is estimated to impact 10–20% of mothers and is prevalent in 17.22% of the world's population with relatively lower (but not insignificant) prevalence rates in more developed, high-income countries (Wang et al., 2021). Although prevalence rates are impacted by multiple factors such as screening and diagnostic measures utilized, study size, reporting practices, and mental health stigma, women in low- and middle-income countries, as well as racial and ethnic minorities and younger women within high-income countries, routinely experience higher rates of PPD and are less likely to receive timely care and treatment (Howard & Khalifeh, 2020). Developmental consequences of PPD can include maternal rejection, disengagement, insensitivity, and low warmth in the early postpartum period (Lovejoy et al., 2000), disorganized attachment at 12 months (Hayes et al., 2013), and externalizing problems and lower IQ at age 8 (Barker et al., 2011).

Anxiety is a frequent experience among pre- and postpartum women and tends to be more prevalent than perinatal depression (Fairbrother et al., 2015; Leach et al., 2016). Even though anxiety in the perinatal period does not have distinctive diagnostic criteria, it is characterized by symptoms such as excessive worry and intrusive thoughts and behaviors that are specific to pregnancy and parenting, including concerns about prenatal health, parenting ability and evaluation, and the health and development of the baby (Goldfinger et al., 2020; Pawluski et al., 2017). Prevalence estimates of prenatal anxiety (2.6–36.9%) and postpartum anxiety (3.7–20%) span a large range due to the lack of uniform screening and diagnostic tools and extensive variation in the timing of measurement (Leach et al., 2016). Maternal anxiety is associated with a number of obstetric and postpartum complications (Grigoriadis et al., 2018) as well as reduced maternal sensitivity, infant passivity, insecure attachment, and low parenting confidence (Marchesi et al., 2016; Parfitt et al., 2013; Prenoveau et al., 2013).

The co-occurrence of perinatal anxiety and depression is well established (Biaggi et al., 2016; Falah-Hassani et al., 2017; González-Mesa et al., 2020). Women who experience comorbid anxiety and depression in the perinatal period experience more severe symptoms, are less responsive to treatment, and are prone to worse prognoses and developmental outcomes. Biaggi et al. (2016) emphasized greater clinical attention and screening efforts during pregnancy due to the strong predictive value of prenatal anxiety on PPD. There is emerging evidence that brief, simultaneous screening of both disorders during pregnancy is feasible, effective, and necessary to provide early opportunities for prevention and treatment (Barrera et al., 2021; Cena et al., 2020).

In addition to perinatal depression and anxiety disorders, mothers are vulnerable to experiencing other new or worsening psychological disturbances during the transition. Within and surrounding PMADs, there is a spectrum of diagnoses that when they occur during the perinatal period have particular prevalence, risk factors, and sequelae, even when not specified by diagnostic manuals. Thus, this chapter includes risk factors that are associated with PMADs and a brief overview of perinatal posttraumatic stress disorder (P-PTSD), psychosis, bipolar disorder, obsessive-compulsive disorder (P-OCD), and substance use disorders (P-SUD), as they are each associated with particular psychological risk factors, and, in some cases, diagnosis of one of these disorders can serve as a psychological risk factor for the diagnosis of another. A more thorough discussion of each of these diagnoses, their symptom presentation, and their impact on individuals and the family system is included later in the volume.

Biological and Sociocultural Risks Associated With Perinatal Mental Health

Although the primary focus of this chapter concerns *psychological* factors underlying the development and persistence of PMHDs, a brief summary of evidence regarding biological and sociocultural factors that may also impose risks to one's psychological functioning is warranted. Pregnancy, recovering from delivery, and caring for a newborn are physically taxing. Those who give birth may experience fluctuating hormones (Trifu, 2019; Zappas et al., 2021) and dysregulation in their body's stress response system through the hypothalamus–pituitary–adrenal (HPA) axis (Hutchens & Kearney, 2020) that can heighten vulnerability to perinatal mental health challenges. Chronic sleep disruption, a common experience throughout pregnancy due to discomfort and during the postpartum period due to nighttime infant care (Liu et al., 2020), can additionally lead to structural and functional changes in the brain through decreased connectivity and an increase in amygdala response, an area of the brain that processes fearful and threatening stimuli (Cárdenas et al., 2020). In addition to the fatigue inherently associated with newborn care, factors related to the baby's health and temperament can impact perinatal mental health. For example, parents of preterm infants (van der Zee-van den Berg et al., 2021) or infants with health problems (Field, 2017) are at higher risk for the development of depression and anxiety in the post-partum period.

It is impossible to ignore the sociocultural context that shapes the psychological experience of pregnancy and the postpartum period. Consideration of ecological factors, including the family's cultural background, community, and broader sociopolitical context, is essential to more fully understand the factors that contribute to PMHDs. Chronic stress related to experiences of lack of access to resources, including food insecurity (Abrahams et al., 2018), housing instability (Suglia et al., 2011), financial stress (Lin & Hung, 2015; Yang et al., 2022), poor working conditions (Biaggi et al., 2016), community violence (Crear-Perry et al., 2021), and inadequate medical care (Foster et al., 2021), increases risk and susceptibility to psychological disorders in the perinatal period. Stability and equity are shaped by the sociocultural and political context; historical and current systemic discrimination based on race, ethnicity, gender, sexual orientation, religion, national origin, and other cultural identities have led to prejudiced and unfair policies that limit access to resources and care. Experiences of continued discrimination through racism, cisnormativity, and heteronormativity additionally contribute to increased levels of chronic stress and PMHDs (Crear-Perry et al., 2021; Kirubarajan et al., 2022; Prady et al., 2013) and can lead to an understandable lack of trust in systems, including medical and mental health professionals. Additionally, stigma related to mental health conditions that persists in many communities can negatively impact access to support and worsen perinatal mental health challenges (Byatt et al., 2015).

Policies that contribute to accessible care and support during pregnancy and the postpartum period can also affect stress and perinatal mental health. For example, insurance coverage gaps during the postpartum period can have dire consequences for both medical and mental healthcare (Solomon, 2021). Additional supportive policies, including paid family leave and affordable, accessible child care, can ease burdens for families, but lack of access to these supports can negatively impact mental health in the perinatal period (Crear-Perry et al., 2021). Health policy is not the only factor that can impact the level of support for families during pregnancy and postpartum; for example, the recent COVID-19 pandemic has led to elevated stress and isolation across the globe. Pregnant families and caregivers in the postpartum period across 64 countries reported increased worries regarding their health, their child's health, receiving necessary prenatal and postpartum care, adequate childcare, and financial security during the pandemic (Basu et al., 2021; Lebel et al., 2020). Families additionally reported elevated loneliness, decreased ability to tolerate uncertainty, and increased depression and anxiety due to the pandemic (Sbrilli et al., 2021). These challenges exacerbated pre-existing health disparities, increasing concerns for perinatal mental health in marginalized communities (Hill et al., 2022).

The juxtaposition of an idealized view of intensive mothering with the reality of sociocultural and political constraints surrounding family life sets the stage for a practical conundrum that is linked to negative mental health outcomes (Henderson et al., 2016; Rizzo et al., 2013). Intensive parenting is a belief system that values and perpetuates the ideas that mothers are superior to other caregivers in the child's life, that for mothers, parenting will bring joy unrivaled to other life experiences, that mothers must engage in concerted socialization and educational efforts to stimulate their child, and that children's needs must always come first (Hays, 1996). In the context of limited social support, parental leave policies that are misaligned with development and family needs, the economic demands of raising a family, and modern technological advances, a competing cultural discourse introduces the notion that mothers are unknowing and must seek the advice of experts (Aston, 2002) to successfully raise their children. To meet the expectations of an internalized intensive mothering ideology and to assuage fears of being judged by other parents, family members, and even healthcare providers, parents are increasingly accessing "on demand" support and information via parenting and baby-focused mobile phone applications, websites, and social media networks (Archer & Kao, 2018), despite many websites having questionable accuracy or providing irrelevant or incomplete information (Buultjens et al., 2012). Contrary to the opinion that having information at one's fingertips can be anxiety relieving, mothers have reported an "information overload" from the plethora of online resources, indicating that the time spent "Googling" information added additional stress (Price et al., 2018). Social network forums (e.g., Facebook groups) both lack anonymity and confidentiality and require parents to elucidate which piece of advice is most pertinent or trustworthy. These experiences are exhausting and can increase feelings of loneliness, obsessive behaviors, decision paralysis, and lowered confidence and joy, further contributing to the intrapsychic conflict of new parenting.

Psychological Factors Associated With Perinatal Mental Health

Multiple factors which transcend or interact with biological, genetic, physical, and sociocultural risks are implicated in the development of PMADs and associated symptomatology. Whereas screening and support for psychosocial stressors, mood, and anxiety are typically integrated within the prenatal appointment schedule, there is no parallel assessment or counseling process in place for new parents beyond the six-week postpartum visit. Absent professional attention, issues that initially present as minimally disruptive may contribute increasing risk to perinatal mental health, posing additional consequences for child development (Honey et al., 2003; Jones & Prinz, 2005).

Early Family Experiences

Pregnancy and the postpartum period can evoke powerful memories and dynamics of a mother's experience with her own caregivers and give rise to emotionally charged representations and expectations of her relationship to her new baby (Stern, 1995). These "ghosts" of the past can trigger unanticipated anxiety, negative feelings, or even jealousy toward the new baby, thereby significantly compromising maternal well-being in addition to the formation of the new relationship (Fraiberg et al., 1975). Parents with an ambivalent attachment style due to a history of inadequate or unpredictable support in childhood are at an especially high risk for depression during the transition to parenthood, particularly when feeling unsupported by their partners (Simpson et al., 2003). Individuals whose caregivers' parenting style was characterized by low warmth, low reciprocity, and high control are also at a substantially high risk for perinatal mental health difficulties: they are up to six times as likely to be diagnosed with anxiety during pregnancy and seven times more likely to be diagnosed with PPD (Grant et al., 2012). Though these "ghosts" can predispose parents to negative mental health outcomes, "angels" stemming from positive experiences with one's own caregivers can bolster mental health outcomes in the perinatal period (Lieberman et al., 2005). For example, mothers who reported more emotional support from their own parents during childhood were less likely to experience prenatal depression (Jeong et al., 2013) than those who reported less emotional support.

Trauma

A history of trauma, particularly experiences of intimate partner violence, physical and/or sexual abuse, or the unexpected death or illness of a friend or family member, increases risk for PMHDs (Biaggi et al., 2016; Katon et al., 2020; Mutua et al., 2020; Yang et al., 2022), including P-PTSD.

Perinatal Posttraumatic Stress Disorder

Sometimes included within PMADs under the anxiety umbrella, P-PTSD has distinct properties. There is no DSM-5-TR specifier for PTSD surrounding childbirth; however, P-PTSD is operationalized as a disorder occurring subsequent to a traumatic experience that lasts at least one month and occurs during pregnancy or the postpartum period (Cirino & Knapp, 2019). The prevalence of P-PTSD varies widely (i.e., 3–39%) according to diagnostic criteria used, precipitating traumatic event considered (e.g., miscarriage, infant loss, difficult labor/delivery), and population examined (Ayers et al., 2018; Christiansen, 2017; Farren et al., 2016; Grekin & O'Hara, 2014; Yildiz et al., 2017). Certain symptoms including detachment, loss of interest, anger, irritability, difficulty sleeping, and nightmares may appear more commonly in P-PTSD versus PTSD at other time periods (Seng et al., 2010). Risk factors for P-PTSD include pregnancy complications and vulnerabilities including prior and current abuse, prior PTSD diagnosis, and a difficult pregnancy and/or labor and delivery experience (Forray et al., 2009; Madigan et al., 2015; Muzik et al., 2013; Polachek et al., 2016). Providers often do not know when a traumatic event predisposing their clients to potential P-PTSD has occurred. Furthermore, an event that is traumatic and PTSD-inducing for one individual is not for another. Therefore, even if labor and delivery, pregnancy complications, medical procedures, or other potentially traumatizing experiences surrounding childbirth do not objectively sound traumatic to a professional, the subjective experience of an event as traumatic to the patient is what is predictive of P-PTSD.

Use of the ICD-11 (World Health Organization, 2019) criteria for complex trauma may more comprehensively describe PTSD surrounding childbirth than DSM-5-TR criteria for PTSD as complex trauma includes clinical presentations seen in response to more chronic traumatic events such as history of child abuse and ongoing domestic/intimate partner violence. Complex PTSD includes the core symptoms of PTSD (i.e., re-experiencing, avoidance, and sense of threat) and adds symptom clusters of emotional dysregulation, relationship difficulties, and negative self-concept (Cloitre, 2020). In their treatment and discussions with women diagnosed with complex PTSD, Dr. Cerith Waters and his group based in the United Kingdom reported that difficulties with emotional regulation and self-compassion were specific psychological risk factors for the perinatal population (Waters, 2022). Regarding screening for P-PTSD, Waters suggested asking during the PMADs screening process, "Has anything happened to you that you think contributed to what you've been experiencing and feeling?" thereby opening up the possibility of disclosing a traumatic event related to described symptoms. His team has recommended taking a stepped-care approach to treatment. Dr. Waters and his group, in collaboration with their perinatal PTSD patients, created a trauma-focused guided self-help workbook as a step-one intervention. For those who require more intensive treatment, they recommend stepping up to a perinatal trauma-focused cognitive behavioral therapy (CBT) model (Waters, 2022).

Traumatic experiences can interfere with brain circuits, disrupting emotion regulation and overactivating the body's alarm system (van der Kolk, 2014). This can exacerbate the aforementioned biological risk factors and HPA axis dysregulation that can occur in the perinatal period (Hutchens & Kearney, 2020) and therefore deepen one's vulnerability to mental health challenges. Given this context, the perinatal period brings heightened risk for the existing negative impact of trauma on mental health; research shows that a history of childhood abuse increased the risk for perinatal mental health difficulties over and above the increased lifetime psychiatric risk associated with trauma (Plant et al., 2013). Exposure to trauma also has a dose–response effect. Parents who reported three or more traumatic experiences had a fourfold risk of prenatal depression in comparison to parents with no trauma history (Robertson-Blackmore et al., 2013).

Experience of Pregnancy and Delivery

Factors related to pregnancy, history of pregnancy loss, and the experience of the pregnancy and labor all impact perinatal mental health. There are mixed research findings on pregnancy factors such as parity and the age of the mother. Some research reports that multiparity increases the risk for perinatal mental health difficulties (Yang et al., 2022) due to potential increased stress related to caregiving for multiple children (Shelke & Chakole, 2022), whereas others reported that first-time parents are at higher risk (Biaggi et al., 2016). Becoming a parent is a major developmental and psychological transition that may precipitate changes to one's identity, relationships, and priorities, increasing the vulnerability to isolation and low confidence in the face of the unknowns of parenting (Abdollahi et al., 2016). However, other research has not identified any significant relationship between parity and mental health (Abujilban et al., 2014), suggesting that parity itself may not be driving differences in peripartum mental health challenges but rather may be impacting mental health through other psychological factors, such as stress, social support, and parenting confidence. In terms of age, young adolescent mothers and mothers with advanced maternal age (i.e., age 40+) may have a slightly increased risk for PMHDs (Räisänen et al., 2014). In both cases, having a child outside of the culturally defined "typical" age range of motherhood may decrease support, increase loneliness, and therefore increase stress. Older mothers are additionally at risk for increased complications for their own health and their baby's health (Muraca & Joseph, 2014) and may also be othered due to ageist and ableist beliefs in society and medicine (Scala & Orsini, 2022).

Having an unplanned or unwanted pregnancy also increases the risk for anxiety and depression, though the impact lessens after the first trimester (Lee et al., 2007; Marchesi et al., 2009). The shock and uncertainty that may arise upon learning about an unplanned pregnancy, particularly as one considers how this will impact finances, health, and family and social relationships, can be stressful and therefore increase the risk for perinatal mental health challenges. However, as acceptance and a relationship with the fetus grow throughout the pregnancy, stress and depressive symptoms tend to decrease (Biaggi et al., 2016).

A history of miscarriage or stillbirth in previous pregnancies leads to increased vulnerability to perinatal mental health difficulties. This is particularly true if conceiving within six months (Gong et al., 2013) to one year after the loss (Blackmore et al., 2011), when grief associated with the loss of one's baby may feel especially intense. Perinatal loss can be traumatic and result in symptoms of P-PTSD in addition to experiences of anxiety and depression (Berry, 2022). Subsequent pregnancies can bring back memories of the loss. Parents may experience heightened worries regarding the new baby's health and guard themselves against feeling too much excitement or hope for their new baby lest they experience another loss (Hill et al., 2008). This can leave parents feeling detached with "one foot in the pregnancy and one foot out," reliving the past while attempting to remain in the present and prepare for a new baby (Côté-Arsenault & Marshall, 2000).

The evidence for the impact of pregnancy complications on perinatal mental health is mixed (Biaggi et al., 2016; Yang et al., 2022). The perception and emotional experience of complications and delivery seem to be more impactful than the objective level of complications; a negative experience of pregnancy (Agostini et al., 2015) and childbirth (Field, 2017) is associated with increased anxiety in the postpartum period. Fears related to childbirth and negative thoughts about delivery also increase the risk for anxiety throughout pregnancy and depression in the postpartum period (Räisänen et al., 2014; Rubertsson et al., 2014). During labor, feeling out of control, angry, fearful, and having low confidence in one's self and/or medical staff are all associated with postpartum mental health challenges (Polachek et al., 2014).

Self-Perceptions and Cognitions

We recognize that there is conceptual and statistical overlap among many of the concepts listed within this section, but they are parsed apart for ease of discussion.

Body Image

Normative bodily changes that occur during pregnancy can lead to body image dissatisfaction depending on the expectations of both the birthing person and the broader societal context. A meta-analysis consisting of studies from Canada and the United States noted a strong association between body image dissatisfaction and PPD (Hutchens & Kearney, 2020). A study conducted in Brazil by Meireles et al. (2022) noted lower body appreciation in the second trimester compared to the third trimester of pregnancy and even lower body appreciation in the postpartum period. Early in pregnancy, there may be increased weight gain without visibly appearing pregnant, which can lead to a sense of incongruence. After birth, having unrealistic beliefs regarding how quickly one may return to pre-pregnancy weight can negatively impact self-esteem (Meireles et al., 2022). Body image impacts self-esteem across cultures in positive and negative directions; a study in Iran also noted a strong relationship between body satisfaction and positive self-esteem in the postpartum period (Garoosi et al., 2013).

Self-Esteem and Self-Efficacy

Low self-esteem, or holding negative beliefs regarding one's self and one's value, is a well-established risk factor for additional mental health difficulties across cultures during pregnancy and the postpartum period (Onyemaechi et al., 2017). There is a reciprocal association between self-esteem and depression; self-esteem leads to increased depressive symptoms, and depression can facilitate lower self-esteem (Han & Kim, 2020). Interventions to bolster self-esteem have demonstrated effectiveness in lessening depressive symptoms (Sharifzadeh et al., 2018), making this an important target for the treatment of perinatal mental health challenges. Perceived stress level is also associated with lower self-esteem (Dolatian et al., 2013), highlighting the importance of addressing sources of stress for parents rather than self-esteem alone to bolster mental health.

Parental self-efficacy, or one's beliefs about their ability to be successful as a parent, is similarly connected to perinatal mental health. Low self-efficacy is associated with an increased risk for perinatal depression and anxiety (van der Zee-van den Berg et al., 2021). A caregiver's self-esteem and self-efficacy regarding their parenting ability are informed by societal expectations. For example, internalized beliefs associated with intensive mothering, which can contribute to increased self-blame and guilt for not doing things the "right" way as well as a global sense of failure if not successful in the all-encompassing role of motherhood, can lead to decreased self-efficacy and increased anxiety even if mothers do not report subscribing to intensive mothering ideologies on a conscious level (Henderson et al., 2016).

Cognitions

Depression, anxiety, and stress can all lead to cognitive distortions and maladaptive alterations to the way information is processed (Han & Kim, 2020). For example, parents with a history of anxiety reported less adaptive cognitive coping responses in the face of stress, such as self-blame or denial of reality (Field, 2017). However, specific cognitive styles or distortions can also lead to increased depression and anxiety symptoms. Perfectionism, which leads to unrealistically high and rigid self-standards, is often correlated with perinatal mental health difficulties (Evans et al., 2022). Both self-oriented perfectionism and societal-prescribed parenting perfectionism increase and impact anxiety in the postpartum period (Donegan et al., 2022). Donegan et al. (2022) describe self-oriented parenting perfectionism as the degree to which individuals set excessively high parenting standards for themselves (e.g., "I must always be a successful parent"), and societal-prescribed parenting perfectionism as the belief that others expect one to be a perfect parent (e.g., "Most people in society expect me to always be a perfect parent"). Perception of others' high standards is a significant predictor of PPD even when accounting for life stress, social support, and trait anxiety (Maia et al., 2012). Intolerance of uncertainty is also associated with perinatal mental health difficulties (Sbrilli et al., 2021); the inability to cope with unknowns that often accompany pregnancy, birth, and caring for an infant can lead to increased difficulty managing negative thoughts and emotions about present or potential sources of stress. Increasing tolerance for uncertainty has been shown to decrease anxiety during both pregnancy and postpartum (Donegan et al., 2022).

Expectations and Experiences Related to Parenthood

Beliefs and attitudes specifically related to parenthood have also been shown to impact perinatal mental health and can shape the way parents view themselves and their parenting skills. Attitudes toward parenthood are significant predictors of PPD and anxiety even when accounting for cognitive biases (e.g., need for approval from others, omnipotence, and perfectionism), partner relationship dysfunction, and inadequate social support (Sockol et al., 2014). Beliefs related to parenthood that can negatively impact perinatal mental health include beliefs about others' judgments (e.g., "If I make a mistake, people will think of me as a bad parent"), beliefs related to parental responsibility (e.g., "I should feel more devoted to my baby," "I am the only one who can keep my baby safe"), and beliefs related to parental role idealization (e.g., "It is wrong to have mixed feelings about my baby"; "If I fail at parenthood, I am a failure as a person").

Partner and Social Support

Familial and community support is crucial in supporting mental health in the perinatal period. Stress, conflict, and lack of support within the partner relationship contribute to PPD and anxiety (Hutchens & Kearney, 2020). Though not having partner support can also contribute to depression and anxiety symptoms (Biaggi et al., 2016), conflictual and unsupportive partners more negatively impact perinatal mental health (Marchesi et al., 2009).

Perceived lack of community social support is also predictive of PPD, anxiety, and stress (Dennis et al., 2017; Field, 2017; Lin & Hung, 2015). On the other hand, perceived social support and relational satisfaction are protective factors for perinatal mental health (Zeng et al., 2015). Positive, meaningful support from partners can also mediate the negative impact of stress and insecure attachment histories on postpartum anxiety and depression (Bilszta et al., 2008; Jeong et al., 2013; Liu et al., 2020; Simpson et al., 2003).

Preexisting Psychological Conditions as Predictors and Outcomes in the Perinatal Period

A history of mental health challenges is one of the strongest predictors of PMHDs (Jeong et al., 2013), though it is not uncommon for the initial onset of mental health difficulties to occur during pregnancy (Räisänen et al., 2014). When depression or anxiety is experienced during pregnancy, it increases the likelihood of continued mental health difficulties during the postpartum period. As mentioned earlier in this chapter, depression and anxiety are also highly comorbid, and high anxiety during pregnancy, in particular, is a strong risk factor for PPD (Biaggi et al., 2016), increasing the risk up to threefold (Mohamad Yusuff et al., 2016). In addition to histories of anxiety, depression, and trauma, histories of eating disorders and/or eating disorder symptoms during pregnancy and the postpartum period increase the risk of perinatal anxiety and depression (Micali et al., 2011). In the sections that follow, we discuss the contributions of specific mood and anxiety disorders and substance use to perinatal mental health with the intention that a history of mental health difficulties would be considered psychological factors worthy of consideration in treatment planning and outcome research. Covering all possible preexisting and comorbid conditions is outside of the scope of this chapter, so we selected those that we commonly see in practice and that are commonly co-occurring in the perinatal mental health literature. Each concern is discussed separately, in the following sections, though they can interact and co-occur.

Bipolar Disorder

Bipolar mood disorders are defined as chronic episodes of depression, hypomania, and mania. The spectrum of the disorder category includes bipolar I, bipolar II, cyclothymia, and unspecified; these will be discussed in more detail in later chapters. Although rates of bipolar disorder are similar across genders, women with bipolar disorder are more likely than men to experience depression and rapid cycling. In perinatal women with no history of prior mental illness, the prevalence of bipolar I disorder was 2.6%, and the prevalence of all bipolar spectrum disorders was 20.1% (Masters et al., 2022). As aforementioned, the DSM-5 includes a specifier of peripartum onset for mood episodes occurring during pregnancy and within four weeks of delivery (APA, 2022); on average the time frame from illness onset to diagnosis ranges from five to ten years (Bauer & Pfennig, 2005), sometimes leading to misdiagnosis and contraindicated treatment in the interim.

By nature of the disorder, misdiagnosis is common as patients often seek treatment during a depressive phase and likely do not seek treatment or attend ongoing treatment during a manic phase when patients may be more prone to seeking pleasure or risky behaviors. During the depressive cycle, symptoms mirror a major depressive episode with perinatal onset. Depressive episodes are usually more common and longer lasting than elevated mood (Battle et al., 2014). A mother presenting with these symptoms during a medical appointment is potentially misdiagnosed with PPD, especially if her additional manic symptoms do not rise to the level of hospitalization, which most do not. Providers should regularly screen for mania symptoms to distinguish them from perinatal unipolar depression, though this screening is not commonly occurring at medical appointments. A hallmark indicator of perinatal bipolar disorder is a lack of sleep that is not attributed to a baby's sleep cycle. Other symptoms of mania that may become a focus of treatment include risky behaviors, excessive energy, grandiosity, and flight of thoughts.

For several reasons, the perinatal period is a particularly vulnerable time for relapse (Clark & Wisner, 2018). Mothers face role transitions, lack of sleep, and hormone fluctuations. Research suggests there is a 23% relapse rate during pregnancy and a 52% relapse rate in the postpartum period. Relapse rates are exceptionally higher (85%) when medication is discontinued abruptly during pregnancy than when continued (37%; Viguera et al., 2007). Identified postpartum episodes of bipolar disorder were almost exclusively depressive cycles. Increased depressive symptoms during pregnancy were significantly associated with postpartum mood episodes in patients with bipolar disorder (Viguera et al., 2007).

There are numerous psychological risk factors for perinatal bipolar disorder diagnosis. As with other mental health concerns, genetics, comorbid substance use (Mei-Dan et al., 2015), and stress impact prevalence. Individuals with first-degree relatives diagnosed with bipolar disorder are more likely to be diagnosed as well. History of childhood maltreatment and abuse occurred at rates four times higher with individuals diagnosed with bipolar disorder. There is also a likelihood of more significant mood shifts, increased risk of suicide, and substance misuse (Rowland & Marwaha, 2018). Anecdotally, our team has found diagnosis of bipolar disorders using screening tools such as the *Mood Disorder Questionnaire* (MDQ; Hirschfeld et al., 2000) to be challenging, as many of our patients deny experiencing impairment, a criterion required for a positive screen on the MDQ. Removing the impairment criterion of item three and following the existence of diagnostic symptoms (i.e., scoring of items 1 and 2) likely result in more women being accurately diagnosed, though the concern becomes false positives with this method (Clark et al., 2015).

Health disparities, including poor health habits, lack of exercise, obesity, smoking, and low socioeconomic status, are also associated with serious mood disorders, thus negatively impacting pregnancy outcomes (Mei-Dan et al., 2015). Impairment in functioning during episodes can negatively affect social support, employment, access to healthcare, and overall health (Clark & Wisner, 2018). Lack of treatment during pregnancy is associated with pre-term birth, intrauterine growth restriction, low birth weight, and contrary developmental outcomes (Clark & Wisner, 2018).

Postpartum Psychosis

Postpartum psychosis is the most severe and potentially life-threatening form of PMHD. A psychotic episode surrounding childbirth is complex and should be considered a psychiatric emergency that requires immediate medical intervention and hospitalization. Postpartum psychosis is characterized by hallucinations, delusions, disorganized thoughts and speech, extreme confusion, and paranoia (Stevens, 2017). One study found that 34% of cases were characterized by agitation and mania, 40% were characterized by depression and anxiety, and the rest experienced mixed states (Kamperman et al., 2017). Due to this presentation of symptoms, the first line of treatment includes medication management with mood stabilizers or antipsychotics (Işik, 2018). Once stable, subsequent therapy including individual, group, and family approaches has been shown to be successful. Although not specifically included in the DSM-5-TR, postpartum psychosis is vaguely captured under the classification of brief psychotic disorder with the peripartum onset specifier to include symptoms presenting during pregnancy or within four weeks postpartum (American Psychiatric Association, 2022).

Psychotic symptoms present differently in women than in men, as they are impacted by the endocrine and reproductive systems. Symptoms worsen during premenstrual periods and during menopause due to fluctuations in estrogen production. Naturally, symptoms also increase during the postpartum period when estrogen levels decrease (American Psychiatric Association, 2022). The prevalence of postpartum psychosis is estimated at 0.01–0.02% in postpartum individuals. Birthing people are 23 times more likely to experience psychosis in the month following childbirth than at any other time in their lives (Işik, 2018). In one study of individuals with postpartum psychosis, 28–35% reported delusional thoughts about their baby, with 9% indicating persecutory thoughts about their child. Relatedly, the risk of suicide is 70 times higher in the first year postpartum (Işik, 2018).

Risk factors for postpartum psychosis span biological, psychological, and social indicators. Those at increased risk include individuals with a personal or family history of bipolar disorder or psychotic episodes, a history of schizoaffective disorders, primiparity, lack of social support, pregnancy and obstetric complications, lack of social support, stressful social situations, sleep deprivation, and discontinuation of medication (Grover & Avasthi, 2015). Many of the risk factors occur at a high base rate (e.g., lack of social support, stressful social situations, sleep difficulties) and are not indicative of heightened risk for only perinatal psychosis but more so for perinatal mental health difficulties, broadly speaking. Therefore, predicting the occurrence of perinatal psychosis is difficult and depends on the knowledge of the more sensitive and specific risk factors for perinatal psychosis, specifically. For example, women who have experienced a prior perinatal psychotic episode are at extremely high risk (70%) for another episode in a subsequent pregnancy and require close monitoring throughout pregnancy and into the postpartum period (Wesseloo et al., 2016). Women who have experienced a psychosis not surrounding childbirth are also at increased risk (32%; Rommel et al., 2021). Women diagnosed with bipolar disorder have a 25–50% increased risk for psychosis (Clark & Wisner, 2018). Therefore, the diagnosis of bipolar disorder in a perinatal woman is associated with negative sequelae in isolation and with additional psychological risk due to the association with more severe perinatal psychosis.

Furthermore, women who experienced complications in the first six weeks postpartum are twice as likely to develop postpartum psychosis than those who did not (Upadhyaya et al., 2014). These factors speak to the importance of accurate identification and management within various healthcare systems to reduce the risk of a crisis.

Obsessive-Compulsive Disorder

Pregnancy and the postpartum period represent a period of vulnerability for the development and/or exacerbation of OCD (Russell et al., 2013). Diagnostically, there are no specific criteria in the DSM-5-TR or ICD-11 that distinguish perinatal OCD from a general OCD diagnosis. However, available literature suggests that perinatal OCD has a distinct profile of symptoms, which emerge most commonly within the first weeks postpartum (Sharma & Sommerdyk, 2015). Obsessions tend to be more common than compulsions in perinatal OCD and generally center on concerns regarding the safety of the new baby (Abramowitz et al., 2003). Many women report intense and intrusive fears that they will accidentally or intentionally harm their baby or that their baby may become ill or die. Compulsions associated with these fears are varied and can include checking rituals (e.g., counting baby's breaths), reassurance seeking, repetitive cleaning (e.g., washing hands and bottles), and other ritualized behaviors.

Although estimates of the prevalence of perinatal OCD generally range from 3% to 5% (Viswasam et al., 2019), OCD may be undercounted in the perinatal period, as it is not routinely assessed during perinatal mental health screening. Furthermore, some postpartum women may conceal or minimize their OCD-related symptoms due to feelings of shame and/or fears of being reported to child protective services (Hudak & Wisner, 2012). This effect is likely most pronounced in women who experience obsessive and intrusive thoughts that they may harm their own baby. It should be noted that women with perinatal OCD experience such thoughts as ego-dystonic and highly distressing; unwanted thoughts of harming one's baby are not associated with actual acts of infant aggression or child abuse (Fairbrother et al., 2022). Furthermore, fears related to infant safety and related behaviors such as checking and reassurance seeking are remarkably common in the postpartum period (Brok et al., 2017). It is the intensity and persistence of those symptoms, combined with their interference in one's life and well-being, that distinguish this normal presentation from perinatal OCD.

A range of biological, environmental, and psychological factors can contribute to the development of perinatal OCD. A personal history of psychiatric disorders is an especially strong risk factor for the development of OCD symptoms in the postpartum period (Zambaldi et al., 2009); a history or current diagnosis of depression is common in women with perinatal OCD (Wisner et al., 1999). Some studies highlight the role of postpartum hormonal changes in the development of obsessive-compulsive symptoms (Karpinski et al., 2017), though reports of OCD in postpartum fathers and non-birthing parents (Abramowitz et al., 2001) would suggest that nonhormonal factors such as sleep deprivation (Sharma, 2019) play a critical role. Psychological factors such as experiential avoidance, perfectionism, and excessive responsibility taking are also related to the development and maintenance of perinatal OCD (Ojalehto et al., 2021; Oddo-Sommerfeld et al., 2016). In particular, some experts suggest that women diagnosed with perinatal OCD may have a tendency to misattribute a high degree of significance to their intrusive but normal fears of infant harm (Abramowitz, 2006). For instance, a mother who experiences an intrusive and unwanted thought of stabbing her infant with a kitchen knife may be more likely to develop symptoms of postpartum OCD if she responds to the thought by viewing herself as horrible and immoral and/or by avoiding going into the kitchen with her baby versus responding to the thought with compassion or with the understanding that she is likely tired and the thought is fleeting. Untreated, perinatal OCD can lead to persistent symptoms and functional impairment (Forray et al., 2010) with potential downstream implications for maternal well-being, family functioning, mother–infant bonding, and long-term child development. Treatment generally includes a combination of psychotherapy (e.g., CBT, acceptance and commitment therapy) and/or medication (e.g., selective serotonin reuptake inhibitors) (Brandes et al., 2004).

Perinatal Substance Use Disorders

Perinatal substance use, defined here as substance use during pregnancy and the first year postpartum, is a serious public health concern in the United States (Deutsch et al., 2021) with associated risks for mothers (e.g., viral infections, overdose) and infants (e.g., stillbirth, preterm birth, low birth weight, sudden infant death syndrome, neonatal abstinence syndrome, fetal alcohol spectrum disorders; Kramlich et al., 2018; Maralit, 2022; Renbarger et al., 2020), and overdose risk is highest in the first year after giving birth (Schiff et al., 2018). Unfortunately, perinatal substance use prevalence rates are difficult to gauge due to maternal concerns including stigma, policy, mandated reporting, and the possibility of child welfare involvement. Although it is likely that current prevalence rates underestimate the true scope of the issue due to reluctance to endorse perinatal substance use, it is evident that the frequency of perinatal substance use is on the rise (Ko et al., 2020; Schiff et al., 2017; Smid et al., 2019).

Substance use disorders have, historically, been conceptualized by many as a distinct concern from other behavioral health issues (Bell & McCutcheon, 2020). For women with perinatal substance use, a holistic understanding of behavioral health and comorbid substance use is needed for effective treatment and support (Guyon-Harris et al., 2023). From a relational and perinatal standpoint, motivations for perinatal substance use are especially related to the human need for connection, safety, and regulation (Khantzian, 2014; Tippett, 2020), as suggested by the intersection of the neurobiology of addiction and attachment (Guyon-Harris et al., 2023; Parolin & Simonelli, 2016). From a relational lens, perinatal substance use can be seen as an attempt to compensate for insecure attachment histories and regulatory issues (Lyden & Suchman, 2013; Goodman, 2008). For example, women with perinatal substance use report feeling distant or withdrawn from their infant, along with accompanied feelings of guilt or shame over not feeling as enamored with their infants as they perceive other mothers report (Guyon-Harris et al., 2023). Their experience of disconnection likely stems from neurobiological lasting impacts of substance use instead of a lack of desire for connection. Reframing the emotional experience of mothers with comorbid substance use concerns may reduce feelings of guilt and shame, thereby potentially reducing urges for substance use and supporting the healthy development of the mother–infant relationship (Guyon-Harris et al., 2023).

Case Illustration

No single case can encompass the vastness of issues pertaining to perinatal mental health. The experience of a woman who approached one of the authors to tell her story highlights many of the issues to keep in mind when working with birthing families.

Lydia and her partner, Allen, hoped to start a family right away. For months, they experienced difficulties becoming pregnant and eventually sought treatment with in vitro fertilization (IVF). They scraped finances together to be able to afford treatment. The IVF process was strenuous and painful, psychologically, physically, and financially, but it remained hopeful. Lydia became pregnant with twins, and the couple initially rejoiced. Lydia quietly experienced anxiety regarding the health of her twins and became especially fearful she would catch an illness that would harm her developing infants. She wanted to be sure she did "everything right" as a pregnant woman and read books and online materials about what she should and should not do. She spent many of her days concerned about a miscarriage and isolated herself to avoid exposure. She began washing her hands so frequently that her skin was cracking and sore, but she felt compelled to continue, fearful of germs and viruses on surfaces. She was thrilled to be pregnant but had not expected the anxiety and fear that seemed to pervade her pregnancy.

Lydia's health was generally good in early pregnancy, but she began experiencing some health difficulties in her second trimester including gestational diabetes. She was monitored more closely, seeing her physician weekly. She worried about entering the hospital setting post-pandemic for fear of exposure and tried to schedule telehealth appointments whenever possible. Her small frame struggled with the weight of carrying twins, and she had difficulty remaining active, especially while trying to remain at home. During one prenatal care appointment, her blood pressure was so high that she met the criteria for preeclampsia and her physician scheduled a cesarean section that night. She and her partner arrived at the hospital nervous but hopeful, and the cesarean section went smoothly, with their twins healthy and in need of monitoring only due to prematurity.

Overnight, Lydia's physical condition plummeted. The medical team could not control the bleeding, and she went into shock. Three procedures and numerous rounds of blood donation later, she stabilized. The providers told Lydia and Allen that Lydia nearly died. Despite her weakened state, Lydia desired to breastfeed and was connected to a pump while still receiving critical care for her own health. The ordeal was harrowing, but, as Lydia described, "Little did we know the worst was yet to come."

Once home, Lydia experienced ongoing physical health constraints including lift and physical exercise restrictions for weeks. She noticed her fears and worries regarding cleanliness now extended to her infants as well as herself and she spent a good deal of time cleaning them, herself, and her home. She worried about family members and friends visiting and denied their offerings of help out of concern about exposure to illnesses. Emotionally, she began experiencing flashbacks of her time in the hospital, as well as nightmares and social withdrawal. She recalls feeling scared all the time, as though there was a "tiger in the room" with her and her twins. Allen recalls her feeling irritable and lashing out at him and others. Their relationship suffered as she withdrew further and further from him physically and emotionally. He began experiencing depressive symptoms but did not know what to call his difficulties at the time and thought he needed to "remain strong for her," so he did not seek help. Lydia tried to describe how she felt to friends and family but was told she was "being crazy" and just needed to "get over it." After all, she had her babies and was "healthy."

She recalls being screened for depression at a follow-up appointment. She answered honestly and did not meet the cutoff score, and she knew she was not depressed. She knew something else was wrong. When no one asked her whether she was experiencing other symptoms (e.g., nightmares, flashbacks, fear, worry, withdrawal, avoidance) or difficulties, she did not know how to start the conversation. Eventually, a friend referred her to a psychiatrist. This provider was a generalist, not trained in perinatal mental health. He prescribed alprazolam daily. He worked with her on exposure to her symptoms of OCD. She found her need to "get things right," and her worries regarding cleanliness slowly dissipated. She recalls taking the medication and feeling her symptoms alleviate slightly, thinking, "Maybe this is as good as things can get." She still experienced nightmares, flashbacks, and a need to remain at home with her infants. She thought maybe this was what being a mother was going to be like.

Months later, Lydia mentioned taking alprazolam to her family physician. Her doctor asked her about her ongoing symptoms and questioned whether Lydia could be experiencing PTSD. Lydia recalls feeling disbelief, "That's what Veterans get!," but when she looked up the symptoms, she realized that was what she had been struggling with since childbirth. She researched PTSD surrounding childbirth online but only found treatments for veterans and victims of sexual trauma.

She was considering joining a support group for victims when she was introduced to one of the authors by a mutual acquaintance. Lydia learned about P-PTSD and treatment options in her area. A referral was made to a local clinician experienced in perinatal mental health and eye movement desensitization reprocessing treatment. Within a few weeks, Lydia felt initial relief followed by a significant improvement within months of starting treatment. Allen felt Lydia was doing well enough for him to seek treatment for his depression. They now advocate for public awareness of P-PTSD, realizing how long she suffered, how her partner and family was affected, and how lucky she was to be accurately diagnosed and connected with effective and accessible treatment.

In Closing

Pregnancy, childbirth, and motherhood are unparalleled developmental transitions characterized by changes in one's body, mental state, identity, family structure, emotional life, and relationships. The psychological adjustments and challenges encountered during this time may be classified as a "natural progression" with relatively benign consequences or a "substantial upheaval" that is triggered or propagated by early life experiences, traumatic events, and other psychological predispositions and risks (Redshaw & Martin, 2011, p. 305). This chapter has provided a survey of psychological aspects that impact perinatal mental health on an individual level, recognizing that these factors occur within the context of complex cultural and sociopolitical forces, biology, and neurophysiology that additionally explain variation in prevalence and trajectories of severity and responsiveness to intervention. Additional research and dissemination and sharing of findings from studies and clinical practice are key to advancing knowledge about psychological factors implicated in perinatal mental health.

Much of the early work in perinatal mental health focused on PPD at the individual level, so it makes sense that PPD remains centered on the conversation among perinatal mental health clinicians and researchers. The scope and charge of perinatal mental health practice and scholarship are actually much broader, encompassing all diagnoses, comorbidities, and complexities that are found in the general population. Hence, to work in perinatal mental health, professionals need depth and breadth in screening, assessment, diagnosis, and treatment knowledge and skills, as well as a specific understanding of how psychological factors and conditions intersect with the perinatal period. This is a tall order and requires an expansion of our training in the perinatal mental health field. In addition, much of the work that occurs needs to keep the infant in mind and present in the conversations. Rather than two distinct fields, perinatal, infant, and early childhood mental health can be seen as a developmental progression of work. To use a healthcare metaphor, this progression is more akin to a family practice model of mental health versus the current model of forced separation similar to obstetrics and pediatrics with siloed healthcare focused on the mother and that focused on the infant. A more dyadic and developmental approach is needed to further the field.

The impact of parenting on mental health is profound and multidimensional. Burgeoning neuroimaging research provides confirmatory evidence of structural and neural alterations in brain anatomy and function that are thought to be promulgated not only by prenatal hormonal and physiological changes but also as a response to caregiving experiences postnatally (Cárdenas et al., 2020). Future research may consider attempting to explain how the role of evolving cultural scripts, advances in science and technology, rapidity of information exchange, and internalized ideologies that conjure images of quintessential mothering (Tummala-Narra, 2009) affect the etiology and expression, for example, of a perinatal anxiety disorder. A prospective, longitudinal examination of the transition to parenthood that integrates neuroimaging of parents and children with clinical observation, measurement, and practice can further elucidate how changes at the neural level manifest behaviorally and functionally and can thus inform psychotherapeutic and pharmacological interventions.

In sum, broadening the scope and embracing an interprofessional, interdisciplinary approach to perinatal mental health to include the full spectrum of mental health concerns, psychological factors, and comorbidities as well as the central importance of the developing infant and developing infant–parent relationship will lead to novel research questions and training opportunities. Furthermore, asking what are the common factors needed to promote parent and infant mental health, with consideration of mothers, parenting partners, infants, and the family system, will create a richer and more integrated foundation for perinatal mental healthcare beyond what currently exists. Flipping the script to focus more on prevention and early intervention including ensuring social support, social determinants of health (e.g., safe stable housing, nutrition, medical care), and exercise are central to every perinatal woman's care plan and will greatly promote health, mental health, and well-being for mom, baby, and the family.

Note

1 The authors wish to acknowledge that the terminology (i.e., mothers, women) used within this chapter and widely in the literature on perinatal mental health is outdated and centers cisgender and heteronormative individuals. Although the literature reviewed within this chapter was conducted without an emphasis on inclusion of LGBTQIA+ families, future research needs to be more inclusive of sexual and gender minorities. The use of the term, "birthing persons", throughout would be a notable step towards inclusivity and an affirming stance.

References

Abdollahi, F., Agajani-Delavar, M., Zarghami, M., & Lye, M. S. (2016). Postpartum mental health in first-time mothers: A cohort study. *Iranian Journal of Psychiatry and Behavioral Sciences, 10*(1), e426. https://doi.org/10.17795/ijpbs-426

Abrahams, Z., Lund, C., Field, S., & Honikman, S. (2018). Factors associated with household food insecurity and depression in pregnant South African women from a low socio-economic setting: A cross-sectional study. *Social Psychiatry and Psychiatric Epidemiology, 53*, 363–372. https://doi.org/10.1007/s00127-018-1497-y

Abramowitz, J. S. (2006). The psychological treatment of obsessive – compulsive disorder. *The Canadian Journal of Psychiatry, 51*(7), 407–416. https://doi.org/10.1177/070674370605100702

Abramowitz, J. S., Franklin, M. E., Schwartz, S. A., & Furr, J. M. (2003). Symptom presentation and outcome of cognitive-behavioral therapy for obsessive-compulsive disorder. *Journal of Consulting and Clinical Psychology, 71*(6), 1049. https://doi.org/10.1037/0022-006X.71.6.1049

Abramowitz, J. S., Moore, K., Carmin, C., Wiegartz, P. S., & Purdon, C. (2001). Acute onset of obsessive-compulsive disorder in males following childbirth. *Psychosomatics, 42*(5), 429–431. https://doi.org/10.1176/appi.psy.42.5.429

Abujilban, S. K., Abuidhail, J., Al-Modallal, H., Hamaideh, S., & Mosemli, O. (2014). Predictors of antenatal depression among Jordanian pregnant women in their third trimester. *Health Care for Women International, 35*(2), 200–215. https://doi.org/10.1080/07399332.2013.817411

Agostini, F., Neri, E., Salvatori, P., Dellabartola, S., Bozicevic, L., & Monti, F. (2015). Antenatal depressive symptoms associated with specific life events and sources of social support among Italian women. *Maternal and Child Health Journal, 19*, 1131–1141. https://doi.org/10.1007/s10995-014-1613-x

American Psychiatric Association. (2022). *Diagnostic and statistical manual of mental disorders* (5th ed., text rev.). https://doi.org/10.1176/appi.books.9780890425787

Archer, C., & Kao, K.-T. (2018). Mother, baby and Facebook makes three: Does social media provide social support for new mothers? *Media International Australia, 168*(1), 122–139. https://doi-org.libproxy1.usc.edu/10.1177/1329878X18783016

Aston, M. L. (2002). Learning to be a normal mother: Empowerment and pedagogy in postpartum classes. *Public Health Nursing, 19*(4), 284–293. https://doi.org/10.1046/j.1525-1446.2002.19408.x

Ayers, S., Wright, D. B., & Thornton, A. (2018). Development of a measure of postpartum PTSD: The city birth trauma scale. *Frontiers in Psychiatry, 9*, Article 409. https://doi.org/10.3389/fpsyt.2018.00409

Barker, E. D., Jaffee, S. R., Uher, R., & Maughan, B. (2011). The contribution of prenatal and postnatal maternal anxiety and depression to child maladjustment. *Depression and Anxiety, 28*(8), 696–702. https://doi.org/10.1002/da.20856

Barrera, A. Z., Moh, Y. S., Nichols, A., & Le, H.-N. (2021). The factor reliability and convergent validity of the Patient Health Questionnaire-4 among an international sample of pregnant women. *Journal of Women's Health, 30*(4), 525–532. https://doi.org/10.1089/jwh.2020.8320

Basu, A., Kim, H. H., Basaldua, R., Choi, K. W., Charron, L., Kelsall, N., . . . Koenen, K. C. (2021). A cross-national study of factors associated with women's perinatal mental health and wellbeing during the COVID-19 pandemic. *PLoS One, 16*(4), e0249780. https://doi.org/10.1371/journal.pone.0249780

Battle, C. L., Weinstock, L. M., & Howard, M. (2014). Clinical correlates of perinatal bipolar disorder in an interdisciplinary obstetrical hospital setting. *Journal of Affective Disorders, 158*, 97–100. https://doi.org/10.1016/j.jad.2014.02.002

Bauer, A., Knapp, M., & Parsonage, M. (2016). Lifetime costs of perinatal anxiety and depression. *Journal of Affective Disorders, 192*, 83–90. https://doi.org/10.1016/j.jad.2015.12.005

Bauer, M., & Pfennig, A. (2005). Epidemiology of bipolar disorders. *Epilepsia, 46*, 8–13.

Bell, D. J., & McCutcheon, S. R. (2020). Moving the needle to promote education and training in substance use disorders and addictions: Special issue introduction. *Training and Education in Professional Psychology, 14*(1), 1–3. https://doi.org/10.1037/tep0000305

Berry, S. N. (2022). The trauma of perinatal loss: A scoping review. *Trauma Care, 2*(3), 392–407. https://doi.org/10.3390/traumacare2030032

Biaggi, A., Conroy, S., Pawlby, S., & Pariante, C. M. (2016). Identifying the women at risk of antenatal anxiety and depression: A systematic review. *Journal of Affective Disorders, 191*, 62–77. https://doi.org/10.1016/j.jad.2015.11.014

Bilszta, J. L., Tang, M., Meyer, D., Milgrom, J., Ericksen, J., & Buist, A. E. (2008). Single motherhood versus poor partner relationship: Outcomes for antenatal mental health. *Australian & New Zealand Journal of Psychiatry, 42*, 56–65. https://doi.org/10.1080/00048670701732731

Blackmore, E. R., Côté-Arsenault, D., Tang, W., Glover, V., Evans, J., Golding, J., & O'Connor, T. G. (2011). Previous prenatal loss as a predictor of perinatal depression and anxiety. *British Journal of Psychiatry, 198*(5), 373–378. https://doi.org/10.1192/bjp.bp.110.083105

Brandes, M., Soares, C. N., & Cohen, L. S. (2004). Postpartum onset obsessive-compulsive disorder: Diagnosis and management. *Archives of Women's Mental Health, 7*, 99–110. https://doi.org/10.1007/s00737-003-0035-3

Brok, E. C., Lok, P., Oosterbaan, D. B., Schene, A. H., Tendolkar, I., & van Eijndhoven, P. F. (2017). Infant-related intrusive thoughts of harm in the postpartum period: A critical review. *Journal of Clinical Psychiatry, 78*(8), e913–e923. https://doi.org/10.4088/JCP.16r11083

Buultjens, M., Robinson, P., & Milgrom, J. (2012). Online resources for new mothers: Opportunities and challenges for perinatal health professionals. *Journal of Perinatal Education, 21*(2), 99–111. https://doi.org/10.1891/1058-1243.21.2.99

Byatt, N., Levin, L., Ziedonis, D., Moore Simas, T. A., & Allison, J. (2015). Enhancing participation in depression care in outpatient perinatal care settings: A systematic review. *Obstetrics & Gynecology, 126*(5), 1048–1058. https://doi.org/10.1097/AOG.0000000000001067

Byrnes, L. (2019). Perinatal mood and anxiety disorders: Findings from focus groups of at risk women. *Archives of Psychiatric Nursing, 33*(6), 149–153. https://doi.org/10.1016/j.apnu.2019.08.014

Cameron, E. E., Sedov, I. D., & Tomfohr-Madsen, L. M. (2016). Prevalence of paternal depression in pregnancy and the postpartum: An updated meta-analysis. *Journal of Affective Disorders, 206*, 189–203. https://doi.org/10.1016/j.jad.2016.07.044

Cárdenas, E. F., Kujawa, A., & Humphreys, K. L. (2020). Neurobiological changes during the peripartum period: Implications for health and behavior. *Social Cognitive and Affective Neuroscience, 15*(10), 1097–1110. https://doi.org/10.1093/scan/nsz091

Cena, L., Palumbo, G., Mirabella, F., Gigantesco, A., Stefana, A., Trainini, A., . . . Imbasciati, A. (2020). Perspectives on early screening and prompt intervention to identify and treat maternal perinatal mental health: Protocol for a prospective multicenter study in Italy. *Frontiers in Psychology, 11*, Article 365. https://doi.org/10.3389/fpsyg.2020.00365

Christiansen, D. M. (2017). Posttraumatic stress disorder in parents following infant death: A systematic review. *Clinical Psychology Review, 51*, 60–74. https://doi.org/10.1016/j.cpr.2016.10.007

Cirino, N. H., & Knapp, J. M. (2019). Perinatal posttraumatic stress disorder: A review of risk factors, diagnosis, and treatment. *Obstetrical & Gynecological Survey, 74*(6), 369–376. https://doi.org/10.1097/OGX.0000000000000680

Clark, C. T., Sit, D. K., Driscoll, K., Eng, H. F., Confer, A. L., Luther, J. F., . . . Wisner, K. L. (2015). Does screening with the Mdq and Epds improve identification of bipolar disorder in an obstetrical sample? *Depression and Anxiety, 32*(7), 518–526. https://doi.org/10.1002/da.22373

Clark, C. T., & Wisner, K. L. (2018). Treatment of peripartum bipolar disorder. *Obstetrics and Gynecology Clinics of North America, 45*(3), 403–417. https://doi.org/10.1016/j.ogc.2018.05.002

Cloitre, M. (2020). ICD-11 complex post-traumatic stress disorder: Simplifying diagnosis in trauma populations. *The British Journal of Psychiatry: The Journal of Mental Science, 216*(3), 129–131. https://doi.org/10.1192/bjp.2020.43

Côté-Arsenault, D., & Marshall, R. (2000). One foot in-one foot out: Weathering the storm of pregnancy after perinatal loss. *Research in Nursing & Health, 23*(6), 473–485. https://doi.org/10.1002/1098-240X(200012)23:6<473::AID-NUR6>3.0.CO;2-I

Crear-Perry, J., Correa-de-Araujo, R., Johnson, T. L., McLemore, M. R., Neilson, E., & Wallave, M. (2021). Social and structural determinants of health inequities in maternal health. *Journal of Women's Health, 30*(2), 230–235. https://doi.org/10.1089/wjh.2020.8882

Dennis, C. L., Brown, H. K., Falah-Hassani, K., Marini, F. C., & Vigod, S. N. (2017). Identifying women at risk for sustained postpartum anxiety. *Journal of Affective Disorders, 213*, 131–137. https://doi.org/10.1016/j.jad.2017.02.013

Dennis, C. L., & Chung-Lee, L. (2006). Postpartum depression help-seeking barriers and maternal treatment preferences: A qualitative systematic review. *Birth (Berkeley, Calif.), 33*(4), 323–331. https://doi.org/10.1111/j.1523-536X.2006.00130.x

Deutsch, S. A., Donahue, J., Parker, T., Paul, D., & De Jong, A. R. (2021). Supporting mother-infant dyads impacted by prenatal substance exposure. *Children and Youth Services Review, 129*, 106191. https://doi.org/10.1016/j.childyouth.2021.106191

Dolatian, M., Mirrabzadeh, A., Setareh Forouzan, A., Sajjadi, H., Alawimajd, H., Maafi, F., & Mahmoudi, Z. (2013). Correlation of self-esteem with perceived self-esteem in pregnancy and strategies to cope with. *Research Journal of Shahid Beheshti University of Medical Sciences, 18*(3), 148–155.

Donegan, E., Frey, B. N., McCabe, R. E., Streiner, D. L., & Green, S. M. (2022). Intolerance of uncertainty and perfectionistic beliefs about parenting as cognitive mechanisms of symptom change during cognitive behavior therapy for perinatal anxiety. *Behavior Therapy, 53*(4), 738–750. https://doi.org/10.1016/j.beth.2022.02.005

Ennis, L. R. (2014). *Intensive mothering: The cultural contradictions of modern motherhood.* Demeter Press.

Evans, C., Kreppner, J., & Lawrence, P. J. (2022). The association between maternal perinatal mental health and perfectionism: A systematic review and meta-analysis. *British Journal of Clinical Psychology, 61*(4), 1052–1074. https://doi.org/10.1111/bjc.12378

Fairbrother, N., Collardeau, F., Woody, S. R., Wolfe, D. A., & Fawcett, J. M. (2022). Postpartum thoughts of infant-related harm and obsessive-compulsive disorder: Relation to maternal physical aggression toward the infant. *Journal of Clinical Psychiatry, 83*(2), 39944. https://doi.org/10.4088/JCP.21m14006

Fairbrother, N., Young, A. H., Janssen, P., Antony, M. M., & Tucker, E. (2015). Depression and anxiety during the perinatal period. *BMC Psychiatry, 15*(206), 1–9. https://doi.org/10.1186/s12888-015-0526-6

Falah-Hassani, K., Shiri, R., & Dennis, C.-L. (2017). The prevalence of antenatal and postnatal comorbid anxiety and depression: A meta-analysis. *Psychological Medicine, 47*(12), 2041–2053. https://doi.org/10.1017/S0033291717000617

Farren, J., Jalmbrant, M., Ameye, L., Joash, K., Mitchell-Jones, N., Tapp, S., . . . Bourne, T. (2016). Post-traumatic stress, anxiety and depression following miscarriage or ectopic pregnancy: A prospective cohort study. *BMJ Open, 6*(11), e011864. https://doi.org/10.1136/bmjopen-2016-011864

Field, T. (2017). Postpartum anxiety prevalence, predictors and effects on child development: A review. *Journal of Psychiatry and Psychiatric Disorders, 1*(2), 86–102. https://doi.org/10.26502/jppd.2572-519X0010

Forray, A., Focseneanu, M., Pittman, B., McDougle, C. J., & Epperson, C. N. (2010). Onset and exacerbation of obsessive-compulsive disorder in pregnancy and the postpartum period. *The Journal of Clinical Psychiatry, 71*(8), 13337. https://doi.org/10.4088/JCP.09m05381blu

Forray, A., Mayes, L. C., Magriples, U., & Epperson, C. N. (2009). Prevalence of post-traumatic stress disorder in pregnant women with prior pregnancy complications. *The Journal of Maternal-Fetal & Neonatal Medicine, 22*(6), 522–527. https://doi.org/10.1080/14767050902801686

Foster, V., Harrison, J. M., Williams, C. R., Asiodu, I. V., Ayala, S., Getrouw-Moore, J., . . . Jackson, F. M. (2021). Reimagining perinatal mental health: An expansive vision for structural change. *Health Affairs, 40*(10), 1592–1596. https://doi.org/10.1377/hlthaff.2021.00805

Fraiberg, S., Adelson, E., & Shapiro, V. (1975). Ghosts in the nursery: A psychoanalytic approach to the problems of impaired infant-mother relationships. *Journal of the American Academy of Child Psychiatry, 14*(3), 387–421. https://doi.org/10.1016/s0002-7138(09)61442-4

Garoosi, B., Razavi, V., & Etminan Rafsanjani, A. (2013). Investigating the relationship between depression and self-esteem in pregnant women in terms of their conception of their body. *Journal of Health and Development, 2,* 117–127.

Gavin, N. I., Gaynes, B. N., Lohr, K. N., Meltzer-Brody, S., Gartlehner, G., & Swinson, T. (2005). Perinatal depression: A systematic review of prevalence and incidence. *Obstetrics & Gynecology, 106*(5 Pt 1), 1071–1083. https://doi.org/10.1097/01.AOG.0000183597.31630.db

Goldfinger, C., Green, S. M., Furtado, M., & McCabe, R. E. (2020). Characterizing the nature of worry in a sample of perinatal women with generalized anxiety disorder. *Clinical Psychology & Psychotherapy, 27*(2), 136–145. https://doi.org/10.1002/cpp.2413

Gong, X., Hao, J., Tao, F., Zhang, J., Wang, H., & Xu, R. (2013). Pregnancy loss and anxiety and depression during subsequent pregnancies: Data from the C-ABC study. *European Journal of Obstetrics and Gynecology and Reproductive Biology, 166*(30), 30–36. https://doi.org/10.1016/j.ejogrb.2012.09.024

González-Mesa, E., Kabukcuoglu, K., Blasco, M., Körükcü, O., Ibrahim, N., González-Cazorla, A., & Cazorla, O. (2020). Comorbid anxiety and depression (CAD) at early stages of the pregnancy A multicultural cross-sectional study. *Journal of Affective Disorders, 270,* 85–89. https://doi.org/10.1016/j.jad.2020.03.086

Goodman, A. (2008). Neurobiology of addiction: An integrative review. *Biochemical Pharmacology, 75*(1), 266. https://doi.org/10.1016/j.bcp.2007.07.030

Goodman, J. H., Watson, G. R., & Stubbs, B. (2016). Anxiety disorders in postpartum women: A systematic review and meta-analysis. *Journal of Affective Disorders, 203,* 292–331. https://doi.org/10.1016/j.jad.2016.05.033

Grant, K. A., Bautovich, A., McMahon, C., Reilly, N., Leader, L., & Austin, M. P. (2012). Parental care and control during childhood: Associations with maternal perinatal mood disturbance and parenting stress. *Archives of Women's Mental Health, 15*(4), 297–305. https://doi.org/10.1007/s00737-012-0292-0

Grekin, R., & O'Hara, M. W. (2014). Prevalence and risk factors of postpartum posttraumatic stress disorder: A meta-analysis. *Clinical Psychology Review, 34*(5), 389–401. https://doi.org/10.1016/j.cpr.2014.05.003

Grigoriadis, S., Graves, L., Peer, M., Mamisashvili, L., Tomlinson, G., Vigod, S. N., . . . Richter, M. (2018). Maternal anxiety during pregnancy and the association with adverse perinatal outcomes: Systematic review and meta-analysis. *Journal of Clinical Psychiatry, 79*(5), 813. https://doi.org/10.4088/JCP.17r12011

Grover, S., & Avasthi, A. (2015). Mood stabilizers in pregnancy and lactation. *Indian Journal of Psychiatry, 57*(Suppl 2), S308. https://doi.org/10.4103/0019-5545.161498

Guyon-Harris, K. L., Jacobs, J., Lavin, K., & Moran Vozar, T. E. (2023). Perinatal substance use and the neurobiology of addiction and attachment: Implications for parenting interventions. *Practice Innovations*. Advance online publication. https://doi.org/10.1037/pri0000199

Han, J. W., & Kim, D. J. (2020). Longitudinal relationship study of depression and self-esteem in postnatal Korean women using autoregressive cross-lagged modeling. *International Journal of Environmental Research and Public Health, 17*(10), 3743. https://doi.org/10.3390/ijerph17103743

Hayes, L. J., Goodman, S. H., & Carlson, E. (2013). Maternal antenatal depression and infant disorganized attachment at 12 months. *Attachment & Human Development, 15*(2), 133–153. https://doi.org/10.1080/14616734.2013.743256

Hays, S. (1996). *The cultural contradictions of motherhood*. Yale University Press.

Henderson, A., Harmon, S., & Newman, H. (2016). The price mothers pay, even when they are not buying it: Mental health consequences of idealized motherhood. *Sex Roles, 74*, 512–526. https://doi.org/10.1007/s11199-015-0534-5

Hill, L., Artiga, S., & Ranji, U. (2022, November 1). Racial disparities in maternal and infant health: Current status and efforts to address them. *KFF*. https://www.kff.org/racial-equity-and-health-policy/issue-brief/racial-disparities-in-maternal-and-infant-health-current-status-and-efforts-to-address-them/

Hill, P. D., DeBackere, K. J., & Kavanaugh, K. L. (2008). The parental experience of pregnancy after perinatal loss. *Journal of Obstetric, Gynecologic & Neonatal Nursing, 37*(5), 525–537. https://doi.org/10.1111/j.1552-6909.2008.00275.x

Hirschfeld, R. M., Williams, J. B., Spitzer, R. L., Calabrese, J. R., Flynn, L., Keck, P. E., Jr., . . . Zajecka, J. (2000). Development and validation of a screening instrument for bipolar spectrum disorder: The mood disorder questionnaire. *The American Journal of Psychiatry, 157*(11), 1873–1875. https://doi.org/10.1176/appi.ajp.157.11.1873

Honey, K. L., Bennett, P., & Morgan, M. (2003). Predicting postnatal depression. *Journal of Affective Disorders, 76*(1–3), 201–210. https://doi.org/10.1016/s0165-0327(02)00085-x

Howard, L. M., & Khalifeh, H. (2020). Perinatal mental health: A review of progress and challenges. *World Psychiatry, 19*(3), 313–327. https://doi.org/10.1002/wps.20769

Hudak, R., & Wisner, K. L. (2012). Diagnosis and treatment of postpartum obsessions and compulsions that involve infant harm. *American Journal of Psychiatry, 169*(4), 360–363. https://doi.org/10.1176/appi.ajp.2011.11050667

Hutchens, B. F., & Kearney, J. (2020). Risk factors for postpartum depression: An umbrella review. *Journal of Midwifery & Women's Health, 65*(1), 96–108. https://doi.org/10.1111/jmwh.13067

Işik, M. (2018). Postpartum psychosis. *Eastern Journal of Medicine, 23*(1), 60–63. https://doi.org/10.5505/ejm.2018.62207

Jeong, H. G., Lim, J. S., Lee, M. S., Kim, S. H., Jung, I. K., & Joe, S. H. (2013). The association of psychosocial factors and obstetric history with depression in pregnant women: Focus on the role of emotional support. *General Hospital Psychiatry, 35*(4), 354–358. https://doi.org/10.1016/j.genhosppsych.2013.02.009

Jia, R., Kotila, L. E., Schoppe-Sullivan, S. J., & Kamp Dush, C. M. (2016). New parents' psychological adjustment and trajectories of early parental involvement. *Journal of Marriage and Family, 78*(1), 197–211. https://doi.org/10.1111/jomf.12263

Johns, S. E., & Belsky, J. (2007). Life transitions: Becoming a parent. In C. A. Salmon & T. K. Shackelford (Eds.), *Family relationships: An evolutionary perspective* (pp. 71–90). Oxford University Press. https://doi.org/10.1093/acprof:oso/9780195320510.003.0004

Jones, T. L., & Prinz, R. J. (2005). Potential roles of parental self-efficacy in parent and child adjustment: A review. *Clinical Psychology Review, 25*(3), 341–363. https://doi.org/10.1016/j.cpr.2004.12.004

Kamperman, A. M., Veldman-Hoek, M. J., Wesseloo, R., Robertson-Blackmore, E., & Bergink, V. (2017). Phenotypical characteristics of postpartum psychosis: A clinical cohort study. *Bipolar Disorders, 19*(6), 450–457. https://doi.org/10.1111/bdi.12523

Karpinski, M., Mattina, G. F., & Steiner, M. (2017). Effect of gonadal hormones on neurotransmitters implicated in the pathophysiology of obsessive-compulsive disorder: A critical review. *Neuroendocrinology, 105*(1), 1–16. https://doi.org/10.1159/000453664

Katon, J. G., Gerber, M. R., Nillni, Y. I., & Patton, E. W. (2020). Consequences of military sexual trauma for perinatal mental health: How do we improve care for pregnant veterans with a history of sexual trauma? *Journal of Women's Health, 29*(1), 5–6. https://doi.org/10.1089/jwh.2019.8154

Kendell, R. E., Chalmers, J. C., & Platz, C. (1987). Epidemiology of puerperal psychoses. *The British Journal of Psychiatry, 150*(5), 662–673. https://doi.org/10.1192/bjp.150.5.662

Khantzian, E. J. (2014). The self-medication hypothesis and attachment theory: Pathways for understanding and ameliorating addictive suffering. In R. Gill (Ed.), *Addictions from an attachment perspective: Do broken bonds and early trauma lead to addictive behaviours?* (pp. 33–56). Routledge.

Kirubarajan, A., Barker, L. C., Leung, S., Ross, L. E., Zaheer, J., Park, B., . . . Lam, J. S. H. (2022). LGBTQ2S+ childbearing individuals and perinatal mental health: A systematic review. *BJOG: An International Journal of Obstetrics & Gynaecology, 129*, 1630–1643. https://doi.org/10.1111/1471-0528.17103

Ko, J. Y., Coy, K. C., Haight, S. C., Haegerich, T. M., Williams, L., Cox, S., Njai, R., & Grant, A. M. (2020). Characteristics of marijuana use during pregnancy – Eight states, pregnancy risk assessment monitoring system, 2017. *MMWR: Morbidity and Mortality Weekly Report, 69*(32), 1058–1063. https://doi.org/10.15585/mmwr.mm6932a2

Kramlich, D., Kronk, R., Marcellus, L., Colbert, A., & Jakub, K. (2018). Rural postpartum women with substance use disorders. *Qualitative Health Research, 28*(9), 1449–1461. https://doi.org/10.1177/1049732318765720

Leach, L. S., Poyser, C., Cooklin, A. R., & Giallo, R. (2016). Prevalence and course of anxiety disorders (and symptom levels) in men across the perinatal period: A systematic review. *Journal of Affective Disorders, 190*, 675–686. https://doi.org/10.1016/j.jad.2015.09.063

Lebel, C., MacKinnon, A., Bagshawe, M., Tomfohr-Madsen, L., & Giesbrecht, G. (2020). Elevated depression and anxiety symptoms among pregnant individuals during the COVID-19 pandemic. *Journal of Affective Disorders, 277*, 5–13. https://doi.org/10.1016/j.jad.2020.07.126

Lee, A. M., Lam, S. K., Sze Mun Lau, S. M., Chong, C. S., Chui, H. W., & Fong, D. Y. (2007). Prevalence, course, and risk factors for antenatal anxiety and depression. *Obstetric Gynecology, 110*, 1102–1112. https://doi.org/10.1097/01.AOG.0000287065.59491.70

Lieberman, A. F., Padrón, E., Van Horn, P., & Harris, W. W. (2005). Angels in the nursery: The intergenerational transmission of benevolent parental influences. *Infant Mental Health Journal, 26*(6), 504–520. https://doi.org/10.1002/imhj.20071

Lin, P. C., & Hung, C. H. (2015). Mental health trajectories and related factors among perinatal women. *Journal of Clinical Nursing, 24*(11–12), 1585–1593. https://doi.org/10.1111/jocn.12759

Liu, Y., Guo, N., Li, T., Zhuang, W., & Jiang, H. (2020). Prevalence and associated factors of postpartum anxiety and depression symptoms among women in Shanghai, China. *Journal of Affective Disorders, 274*, 848–856. https://doi.org/10.1016/j.jad.2020.05.028

Lovejoy, M. C., Graczyk, P. A., O'Hare, E., & Neuman, G. (2000). Maternal depression and parenting behavior: A meta-analytic review. *Clinical Psychology Review, 20*(5), 561–592. https://doi.org/10.1016/s0272-7358(98)00100-7

Lyden, H. M., & Suchman, N. E. (2013). Transmission of parenting models at the level of representation: Implications for mother-child dyads affected by maternal substance abuse. In N. E. Suchman, M. Pajulo, & L. C. Mayes (Eds.), *Parenting and substance abuse: Developmental approaches to intervention* (pp. 100–125). Oxford University Press. https://doi-org.du.idm.oclc.org/10.1093/med:psych/9780199743100.003.0006

Madigan, S., Vaillancourt, K., McKibbon, A., & Benoit, D. (2015). Trauma and traumatic loss in pregnant adolescents: The impact of trauma-focused cognitive behavior therapy onmaternal unresolved states of mind and posttraumatic stress disorder. *Attachment and Human Development*, *17*(2), 175–98. Pmid:25703488

Maia, B. R., Pereira, A. T., Marques, M., Bos, S., Soares, M. J., Valente, J., . . . Macedo, A. (2012). The role of perfectionism in postpartum depression and symptomatology. *Archives of Women's Mental Health*, *15*(6), 459–468. https://doi.org/10.1007/s00737-012-0310-2

Maralit, A. M. (2022). Beyond the bump: Ethical and legal considerations for psychologistsproviding services to pregnant individuals who use substances. *Ethics & Behavior*, 1–12. https://doi.org/10.1080/10508422.2022.2093202

Marchesi, C., Bertoni, S., & Maggini, C. (2009). Major and minor depression in pregnancy. *Obstetrics & Gynecology*, *113*, 1292–1298. https://doi.org/10.1097/AOG.0b013e318a45e90

Marchesi, C., Ossola, P., Amerio, A., Daniel, B. D., Tonna, M., & De Panfilis, C. (2016). Clinical management of perinatal anxiety disorders: A systematic review. *Journal of Affective Disorders*, *190*, 543–550. https://doi.org/10.1016/j.jad.2015.11.004

Masters, G. A., Hugunin, J., Xu, L., Ulbricht, C. M., Moore Simas, T. A., Ko, J. Y., & Byatt, N. (2022). Prevalence of bipolar disorder in perinatal women: A systematic review and meta-analysis. *Journal of Clinical Psychiatry*, *83*(5), 21r14045. https://doi.org/10.4088/JCP.21r14045

Mei-Dan, E., Ray, J. G., & Vigod, S. N. (2015). Perinatal outcomes among women with bipolar disorder: A population-based cohort study. *American Journal of Obstetrics and Gynecology*, *212*(3), 367.e1–367.e3678. https://doi.org/10.1016/j.ajog.2014.10.020

Meireles, J. F. F., Neves, C. M., Amaral, A. C. S., Morgado, F. F. da R., & Ferreira, M. E. C. (2022). Body appreciation, depressive symptoms, and self-esteem in pregnant and postpartum Brazilian women. *Frontiers in Global Women's Health*, *3*, 834040. https://doi.org/10.3389/fgwh.2022.834040

Micali, N., Simonoff, E., & Treasure, J. (2011). Pregnancy and post-partum depression and anxiety in a longitudinal general population cohort: The effect of eating disorders and past depression. *Journal of Affective Disorders*, *131*(1–3), 150–157. https://doi.org/10.1016/j.jad.2010.09.034

Mohamad Yusuff, A. S., Tang, L., Binns, C. W., & Lee, A. H. (2016). Prevalence of antenatal depressive symptoms among women in Sabah, Malaysia. *The Journal of Maternal-Fetal & Neonatal Medicine*, *29*(7), 1170–1174. https://doi.org/10.3109/14767058.2015.1039506

Moore, W. N. (2018). The violent birth of the mother and the baby blues. *Psychodynamic Practice: Individuals, Groups and Organisations*, *24*(1), 60–63. https://doi.org/10.1080/14753634.2017.1400737

Muraca, G. M., & Joseph, K. S. (2014). The association between maternal age and depression. *Journal of Obstetrics and Gynaecology Canada*, *36*(9), 803–810. https://doi.org/10.1016/S1701-2163(15)30482-5

Mutua, J., Kigamwa, P., Ng'ang'a, P., Tele, A., & Kumar, M. (2020). A comparative study of postpartum anxiety and depression in mothers with preterm births in Kenya. *Journal of Affective Disorders Reports*, *2*, 100043. https://doi.org/10.1016/j.jadr.2020.100043

Muzik, M., Bocknek, E. L., Broderick, A., Richardson, P., Rosenblum, K. L., Thelen, K., & Seng, J. S. (2013). Mother-infant bonding impairment across the first 6 months postpartum: The primacy of psychopathology in women with childhood abuse and neglect histories. *Archives of Women's Mental Health*, *16*(1), 29–38. https://doi.org/10.1007/s00737-012-0312-0

Negron, R., Martin, A., Almog, M., Balbierz, A., & Howell, E. A. (2013). Social support during the postpartum period: Mothers' views on needs, expectations, and mobilization of support. *Maternal and Child Health Journal*, *17*(4), 616–623. https://doi.org/10.1007/s10995-012-1037-4

Oddo-Sommerfeld, S., Hain, S., Louwen, F., & Schermelleh-Engel, K. (2016). Longitudinal effects of dysfunctional perfectionism and avoidant personality style on postpartum mental disorders: Pathways through antepartum depression and anxiety. *Journal of Affective Disorders*, *191*, 280–288. https://doi.org/10.1016/j.jad.2015.11.040

Ojalehto, H. J., Abramowitz, J. S., Hellberg, S. N., Butcher, M. W., & Buchholz, J. L. (2021). Predicting COVID-19-related anxiety: The role of obsessive-compulsive symptom dimensions, anxiety sensitivity, and body vigilance. *Journal of Anxiety Disorders*, *83*, 102460. https://doi.org/10.1016/j.janxdis.2021.102460

Onyemaechi, C. I., Aroyewun, B. A., & Ifeagwazi, C. M. (2017). Postpartum depression: The role of self-esteem, social support and age. *IFE PsychologIA*, *25*(2). eISSN: 1117–1421

Parfitt, Y., Pike, A., & Ayers, S. (2013). The impact of parents' mental health on parent – baby interaction: A prospective study. *Infant Behavior and Development*, *36*(4), 599–608. https://doi.org/10.1016/j.infbeh.2013.06.003.

Parolin, M., & Simonelli, A. (2016). Attachment theory and maternal drug addiction: The contribution to parenting interventions [review]. *Frontiers in Psychiatry*, *7*. https://doi.org/10.3389/fpsyt.2016.00152

Pawluski, J. L., Lonstein, J. S., & Fleming, A. S. (2017). The neurobiology of postpartum anxiety and depression. *Trends in Neurosciences, 40*(2), 106–120. https://doi.org/10.1016/j.tins.2016.11.009

Plant, D. T., Barker, E. D., Waters, C. S., Pawlby, S., & Pariante, C. M. (2013). Intergenerational transmission of maltreatment and psychopathology: The role of antenatal depression. *Psychological Medicine, 43*, 519–528. https://doi.org/10.1017/S0033291712001298.

Polachek, I. S., Dulitzky, M., Margolis-Dorfman, L., & Simchen, M. J. (2016). A simple model for prediction postpartum PTSD in high-risk pregnancies. *Archives of Women's Mental Health, 19*(3), 483–490. https://doi.org/10.1007/s00737-015-0582-4

Polachek, I. S., M.D., Harari, L. H., M.D., Baum, M., M.D., & Strous, R. D., M.D. (2014). Postpartum anxiety in a cohort of women from the general population: Risk factors and association with depression during last week of pregnancy, postpartum depression and postpartum PTSD. *The Israel Journal of Psychiatry and Related Sciences, 51*(2), 128–134.

Prady, S. L., Pickett, K. E., Croudace, T., Fairley, L., Bloor, K., Gilbody, S., Kiernan, K. E., & Wright, J. (2013). Psychological distress during pregnancy in a multi-ethnic community: Findings from the born in Bradford cohort study. *PLoS One, 8*, e60693. https://doi.org/10.1371/journal.pone.0060693

Prenoveau, J., Craske, M., Counsell, N., West, V., Davies, B., Cooper, P., . . . Stein, A. (2013). Postpartum GAD is a risk factor for postpartum MDD: The course and longitudinal relationships of postpartum GAD and MDD. *Depression and Anxiety, 30*, 506–514. https://doi.org/10.1002/da.22040

Price, S. L., Aston, M., Monaghan, J., Sim, M., Tomblin Murphy, G., Etowa, J., . . . Little, V. (2018). Maternal knowing and social networks: Understanding first-time mothers' searchfor information and support through online and offline social networks. *Qualitative Health Research, 28*(10), 1552–1563.

Radesky, J. S., Zuckerman, B., Silverstein, M., Rivara, F. P., Barr, M., Taylor, J. A., . . . Barr, R. G. (2013). Inconsolable infant crying and maternal postpartum depressive symptoms. *Pediatrics, 131*(6), e1857–e1864. https://doi.org/10.1542/peds.2012-3316

Räisänen, S., Lehto, S. M., Nielsen, H. S., Gissler, M., Kramer, M. R., & Heinonen, S. (2014). Risk factors for and perinatal outcomes of major depression during pregnancy: A population-based analysis during 2002–2010 in Finland. *BMJ Open, 4*(11), e004883. https://doi.org/10.1136/bmjopen-2014-004883

Rallis, S., Skouteris, H., McCabe, M., & Milgrom, J. (2014). The transition to motherhood: Towards a broader understanding of perinatal distress. *Women and Birth, 27*(1), 68–71. https://doi.org/10.1016/j.wombi.2013.12.004

Redshaw, M., & Martin, C. (2011). Motherhood: A natural progression and a major transition. *Journal of Reproductive and Infant Psychology, 29*(4), 305–307. https://doi.org/10.1080/02646838.2011.639510

Renbarger, K. M., Shieh, C., Moorman, M., Latham-Mintus, K., & Draucker, C. (2020). Health care encounters of pregnant and postpartum women with substance use disorders. *Western Journal of Nursing Research, 42*(8), 612–628. https://doi.org/10.1177/0193945919893372

Rezaie-Keikhaie, K., Arbabshastan, M. E., Rafiemanesh, H., Amirshahi, M., Ostadkelayeh, S. M., & Arbabisarjou, A. (2020). Systematic review and meta-analysis of the prevalence of the maternity blues in the postpartum period. *Journal of Obstetric, Gynecologic, & Neonatal Nursing, 49*(2), 127–136. https://doi.org/10.1016/j.jogn.2020.01.001

Riggs, D. W., Worth, A., & Bartholomaeus, C. (2018). The transition to parenthood for Australian heterosexual couples: Expectations, experiences and the partner relationship. *BMC Pregnancy and Childbirth, 18*, 1–9. https://doi.org/10.1186/s12884-018-1985-9

Rizzo, K. M., Schiffrin, H. H., & Liss, M. (2013). Insight into the parenthood paradox: Mental health outcomes of intensive mothering. *Journal of Child and Family Studies, 22*, 614–620. https://doi.org/10.1007/s10826-012-9615-z.

Robertson-Blackmore, E., Putnam, F. W., Rubinow, D. R., Matthieu, M., Hunn, J. E., Putnam, K. T., . . . O'Connor, T. G. (2013). Antecedent trauma exposure and riskof depression in the perinatal period. *Journal of Clinical Psychiatry, 74*(10), e942–e948. https://doi.org/10.4088/JCP.13m08364

Rommel, A. S., Molenaar, N. M., Gilden, J., Kushner, S. A., Westerbeek, N. J., Kamperman, A. M., & Bergink, V. (2021). Long-term outcome of postpartum psychosis: A prospective clinical cohort study in 106 women. *International Journal of Bipolar Disorders, 9*(1), 31. https://doi.org/10.1186/s40345-021-00236-2

Rowland, T. A., & Marwaha, S. (2018). Epidemiology and risk factors for bipolar disorder. *Therapeutic Advances in Psychopharmacology, 8*(9), 251–269. https://doi.org/10.1177/2045125318769235

Rubertsson, C., Hellstrom, J., Cross, M., & Sydsjo, G. (2014). Anxiety in early pregnancy: Prevalence and contributing factors. *Archives of Women's Mental Health, 17*(3), 221–228. https://doi.org/10.1007/s00737-013-0409-0

Ruppanner, L., Perales, F., & Baxter, J. (2019). Harried and unhealthy? Parenthood, time pressure, and mental health. *Journal of Marriage and Family, 81*, 308–326. https://doi.org/10.1111/jomf.12531

Russell, E. J., Fawcett, J. M., & Mazmanian, D. (2013). Risk of obsessive-compulsive disorder in pregnant and postpartum women: A meta-analysis. *Journal of Clinical Psychiatry, 74*(4), 18438. https://doi.org/10.4088/JCP.12r07917

Sbrilli, M. D., Haigler, K., & Laurent, H. K. (2021). The indirect effect of parental intolerance of uncertainty on perinatal mental health via mindfulness during COVID-19. *Mindfulness, 12*(8), 1999–2008. https://doi.org/10.1007/s12671-021-01657-x

Scala, F., & Orsini, M. (2022). Problematising older motherhood in Canada: Ageism, ableism, and the risky maternal subject. *Health, Risk & Society, 24*(3–4), 149–166. https://doi.org/10.1080/13698575.2022.2057453

Schiff, D. M., Nielsen, T., Terplan, M., Hood, M., Bernson, D., Diop, H., . . . Land, T. (2018). Fatal and nonfatal overdose among pregnant and postpartum women in Massachusetts. *Obstetrics & Gynecology, 132*(2), 466–474. https://doi.org/10.1097/AOG.0000000000002734

Schiff, D. M., Zuckerman, B., Wachman, E. M., & Bair-Merritt, M. (2017). Trainees' knowledge, attitudes, and practices towards caring for the substance-exposed mother infant dyad. *Substance Abuse, 38*(4), 414–421. https://doi.org/10.1080/08897077.2017.1356423

Seng, J. S., Rauch, S. A., Resnick, H., Reed, C. D., King, A., Low, L. K., . . . Liberzon, I. (2010). Exploring posttraumatic stress disorder symptom profile among pregnant women. *Journal of Psychosomatic Obstetrics and Gynaecology, 31*(3), 176–187. https://doi.org/10.3109/0167482X.2010.486453

Sharifzadeh, M., Navininezhad, M., & Keramat, A. (2018). Investigating the relationship between self-esteem and postpartum blues among delivered women. *Journal of Research in Medical and Dental Science, 6*(3), 357–362.

Sharma, V. (2019). Role of sleep deprivation in the causation of postpartum obsessive-compulsive disorder. *Medical Hypotheses, 122*, 58–61. https://doi.org/10.1016/j.mehy.2018.10.016

Sharma, V., & Sommerdyk, C. (2015). Obsessive – compulsive disorder in the postpartum period: Diagnosis, differential diagnosis and management. *Women's Health, 11*(4), 543–552. https://doi.org/10.2217/whe.15.20

Shelke, A., & Chakole, S. (2022). A review on risk factors of postpartum depression in India and its management. *Cureus, 14*(9), e29150. https://doi.org/10.7759/cureus.29150

Simpson, J. A., Rholes, W. S., Campbell, L., Tran, S., & Wilson, C. L. (2003). Adult attachment, the transition to parenthood, and depressive symptoms. *Journal of Personality and Social Psychology, 84*(6), 1172–1187. https://doi.org/10.1037/0022-3514.84.6.1172

Smid, M. C., Metz, T. D., & Gordon, A. J. (2019). Stimulant use in pregnancy: An under-recognized epidemic among pregnant women. *Clinical Obstetrics and Gynecology, 62*(1), 168–184. https://doi.org/10.1097/grf.0000000000000418

Sockol, L. E., Epperson, C. N., & Barber, J. P. (2014). The relationship between maternal attitudes and symptoms of depression and anxiety among pregnant and postpartum first-time mothers. *Archives of Women's Mental Health, 17*(3), 199–212. https://doi.org/10.1007/s00737-014-0424-9

Solomon, J. (2021). Closing the coverage gap would improve Black maternal health. *Center on Budget and Policy Priorities*, 1–11.

Stern, D. N. (1995). *The motherhood constellation: A unified view of parent – infant psychotherapy.* Basic Books.

Stevens, G. P. (2017). A mother's love? Postpartum disorders, the DSM-5 and criminal responsibility – A South African medicolegal perspective. *Psychiatry, Psychology, and Law: An Interdisciplinary Journal of the Australian and New Zealand Association of Psychiatry, Psychology and Law, 25*(2), 186–196. https://doi.org/10.1080/13218719.2017.1395820

Suglia, S. F., Duarte, C. S., & Sandel, M. T. (2011). Housing quality, housing instability, and maternal mental health. *Journal of Urban Health: Bulletin of the New York Academy of Medicine, 88*(6), 1105–1116. https://doi.org/10.1007/s11524-011-9587-0

Tippett, J. (2020, September 15). *Regulatory systems: Neurobiology of addiction treatment.* (Virtual Presentation) University of Denver.

Trifu, S. (2019). Neuroendocrine aspects of pregnancy and postpartum depression. *Acta Endocrinologica (Bucharest), 15*(3), 410–415. https://doi.org/10.4183/aeb.2019.410

Tummala-Narra, P. (2009). Contemporary impingements on mothering. *The American Journal of Psychoanalysis*, 69(1), 4–21. https://doi.org/10.1057/ajp.2008.37

Twenge, J. M., Campbell, W. K., & Foster, C. A. (2003). Parenthood and marital satisfaction: A meta-analytic review. *Journal of Marriage and Family*, 65(3), 574–583. https://doi.org/10.1111/j.1741-3737.2003.00574.x

Upadhyaya, S. K., Sharma, A., & Raval, C. M. (2014). Postpartum psychosis: Risk factors identification. *North American Journal of Medical Sciences*, 6(6), 274–277. https://doi.org/10.4103/1947-2714.134373

van der Kolk, B. A. (2014). *The body keeps the score: Brain, mind, and body in the healing of trauma.* Viking.

van der Zee-van den Berg, A. I., Boere-Boonekamp, M. M., Groothuis-Oudshoorn, C. G. M., & Reijneveld, S. A. (2021). Postpartum depression and anxiety: A community-based study on risk factors before, during and after pregnancy. *Journal of Affective Disorders*, 286, 158–165. https://doi.org/10.1016/j.jad.2021.02.062

Viguera, A. C., Whitfield, T., Baldessarini, R. J., Newport, D. J., Stowe, Z., Reminick, A., & Cohen, L. S. (2007). Risk of recurrence in women with bipolar disorder during pregnancy: Prospective study of mood stabilizer discontinuation. *American Journal of Psychiatry*, 164(12), 1817–1824. https://doi.org/10.1176/appi.ajp.2007.06101639

Viswasam, K., Eslick, G. D., & Starcevic, V. (2019). Prevalence, onset and course of anxietydisorders during pregnancy: A systematic review and meta analysis. *Journal of Affective Disorders*, 255, 27–40. https://doi.org/10.1016/j.jad.2019.05.016

Wang, Z., Liu, J., Shuai, H., Cai, Z., Fu, X., Liu, Y., . . . Xiang Yang, B. (2021). Mapping global prevalence of depression among postpartum women. *Translational Psychiatry*, 11, 543. https://doi.org/10.1038/s41398-021-01663-6

Waters, C. (2022, September). Perinatal complex PTSD: A handbook for understanding and managing overwhelming emotions. In A. Gregoire (Chair), *Advancing and applying intergenerational mental health knowledge: Complex PTSD – a workshop for academic-clinical mutual inspiration.* Symposium conducted at the Meeting of the Marce Society.

Wenzel, A. (2013). *Strategic decision making in cognitive behavioral therapy.* American Psychological Association. https://doi.org/10.1037/14188-005

Wesseloo, R., Kamperman, A. M., Munk-Olsen, T., Pop, V. J., Kushner, S. A., & Bergink, V. (2016). Risk of postpartum relapse in bipolar disorder and postpartum psychosis: A systematic review and meta-analysis. *Bipolar Spectrum Disorder during Pregnancy and the Postpartum Period*, 173(2), 117–127. https://doi.org/10.1176/appi.ajp.2015.15010124

Wisner, K. L., Peindl, K. S., Gigliotti, T., & Hanusa, B. H. (1999). Obsessions and compulsions in women with postpartum depression. *Journal of Clinical Psychiatry*, 60(3), 176–180. https://doi.org/10.4088/jcp.v60n0305

Woody, C. A., Ferrari, A. J., Siskind, D. J., Whiteford, H. A., & Harris, M. G. (2017). A systematic review and meta-regression of the prevalence and incidence of perinatal depression. *Journal of Affective Disorders*, 219, 86–92. https://doi.org/10.1016/j.jad.2017.05.003

World Health Organization. (2019). *International statistical classification of diseases and related health problems* (11th ed.). https://icd.who.int/

Yang, K., Wu, J., & Chen, X. (2022). Risk factors of perinatal depression in women: A systematic review and meta-analysis. *BMC Psychiatry*, 22(1), Article 63. https://doi.org/10.1186/s12888-021-03684-3

Yildiz, P. D., Ayers, S., & Phillips, L. (2017). The prevalence of posttraumatic stress disorder in pregnancy and after birth: A systematic review and meta-analysis. *Journal of Affective Disorders*, 208, 634–645. https://doi.org/10.1016/j.jad.2016.10.009

Zambaldi, C. F., Cantilino, A., Montenegro, A. C., Paes, J. A., de Albuquerque, T. L. C., & Sougey, E. B. (2009). Postpartum obsessive-compulsive disorder: Prevalence and clinical characteristics. *Comprehensive Psychiatry*, 50(6), 503–509. https://doi.org/10.1016/j.comppsych.2008.11.014

Zappas, M. P., Becker, K., & Walton-Moss, B. (2021). Postpartum anxiety. *The Journal for Nurse Practitioners*, 17(1), 60–64. https://doi.org/10.1016/j.nurpra.2020.08.017

Zeng, Y., Cui, Y., & Li, J. (2015). Prevalence and predictors of antenatal depressive symptoms among Chinese women in their third trimester: A cross-sectional survey. *BMC Psychiatry*, 15, Article 66. https://doi.org/10.1186/s12888-015-0452-7

3

BIOLOGICAL ASPECTS OF PERINATAL MENTAL HEALTH

Alkistis Skalkidou and Emma Bränn

Perinatal depression, or peripartum depression, refers to an episode of major depression with onset during pregnancy or within four weeks after childbirth (*DSM-5-TRTM Classification*, n.d.). This period is in many settings extended to comprise the first 6 to 12 months postpartum. What is becoming more evident is that this diagnosis encompasses many different subgroups, or trajectories, making it difficult to characterize. These trajectories are defined by both the time of disease onset and the different characteristics (Paul & Corwin, 2019; Putnam et al., 2017; Wikman et al., 2020). Commonly, perinatal depression is subdivided into prenatal depression, referring to depression that occurs during pregnancy (also referred to as antenatal depression), and postpartum depression, referring to depression that occurs after childbirth. Perinatal depression is considered a disorder with multifactorial etiology, with biological and psychosocial components. In the next paragraphs, different biological systems studied in relation to perinatal depression and, when relevant, other mental health disorders in the perinatal period will be described, together with hypothesized pathophysiological mechanisms.

Genetics and Epigenetics

Genes represent the basic coding information in our cells. Genome-wide association studies have identified genes associated with psychiatric disorders, where over 100 loci have been found for major depression (Howard et al., 2019), although varying between populations (Giannakopoulou et al., 2021). Genome-wide association studies as of day come with no consistent findings. Twin studies have revealed that about half of the variability in perinatal depression can be explained by genetic factors (Viktorin et al., 2016). Although perinatal depression has higher heritability than other mood disorders, its genetic basis may partially overlap with some of them. Some studies have found depressive symptoms during the perinatal period to be associated with polymorphisms in the genes coding for the serotonin transporter, catechol-O-methyl-transferase, monoaminoxidase-A, brain-derived neurotrophic factor (BDNF), hemicentin-1, methyltransferase 13, estrogen receptor 1, oxytocin, and oxytocin receptor (Doornbos et al., 2009; Sanjuan et al., 2008; Y. Yu et al., 2021). Furthermore, studies have found differences

DOI: 10.4324/9781003206903-5

in mRNA content related to the glucocorticoid receptor complex, as well as the estrogen signaling (Katz et al., 2012; Y. Yu et al., 2021). Lastly, epigenetic alterations have been found in loci associated with estrogen signaling pathways (HP1BP3 and TTC9B) in women with perinatal depression (Guintivano et al., 2014; Osborne et al., 2016). Most likely, there is a genetic component to perinatal depression, and additional genome-wide association studies are warranted. However, epigenetic modifications and variance in transcription and translation of the genetic code complicate the understanding of the importance of genetic markers. Hence, multiomics analyses, carefully taking into account the timing of the symptom onset, could be beneficial.

Neurotransmitters

Neurotransmitters are the molecules that transfer information from one neuron to the next. Some of the most well-known neurotransmitters are epinephrine, norepinephrine, serotonin, dopamine, and gamma-aminobutyric acid (GABA). For each trimester during pregnancy, serotonin, epinephrine, and dopamine measured in the plasma have been shown to decrease, whereas norepinephrine in the plasma increases (Shetty & Pathak, 2002). Decreased levels of epinephrine, serotonin, and dopamine could predispose a person to depression, as depression is generally characterized by low levels of neurotransmitters in the synaptic clefts. Hence, to increase neurotransmitter levels, most antidepressants target either the reuptake or the breakdown of neurotransmitters, focusing mainly on the serotonin transporter, catechol-O-methyl-transferase, and monoaminoxidase-A.

Serotonin is one of the major neurotransmitters involved in mood regulation. It derives from the essential amino acid L-tryptophan, and throughout pregnancy, as the placenta catabolizes tryptophan, the synthesis of cerebral serotonin is reduced (Munn et al., 1999; Schrocksnadel et al., 2003). Tryptophan metabolism and activation of the kynurenine pathway may be important contributors to perinatal depression (Duan et al., 2018). Epinephrine, also known as adrenaline, is involved in our fight-or-flight response, and low levels have been associated with anxiety and depression (Montoya et al., 2016; Moret & Briley, 2011). Norepinephrine, also known as noradrenaline, acts both as a neurotransmitter and as a stress hormone and is involved in the fight-or-flight response. Whereas lower levels of norepinephrine have been associated with depression, higher levels of norepinephrine have been associated with anxiety (Boulenger & Uhde, 1982; Heninger & Charney, 1988). Hence, norepinephrine balance seems important in bipolar disorder (Kurita, 2016), and women with bipolar disorder are at high risk of postpartum psychosis (Wesseloo et al., 2016). Dopamine is involved in the reward system. Low levels of dopamine have been associated with suicide (Hoertel et al., 2021). Neurotransmitters are hard to measure in living subjects, especially in pregnant women, but positron emission tomography studies have shown that the lower the levels of allopregnanolone (a neurosteroid metabolite of progesterone and a positive allosteric modulator of the GABA receptor), the higher the levels of serotonin receptor binding. Allopregnanolone is also thought to have strong sedative, antianxiolytic properties (Sundström Poromaa et al., 2018). However, alterations in neurotransmitter levels in depressed patients could be considered a consequence of other underlying causes (e.g., genetic polymorphisms in the genes coding for the transporters and enzymes that catabolize the neurotransmitters), rather than explanatory in the pathophysiology.

The Endocrine System

The endocrine system is our messenger system, composed of hormones released into the circulatory system by internal glands such as the hypothalamus, the pituitary gland, the adrenal glands, the ovaries and testes, the thyroid and parathyroid gland, the pineal gland, and the pancreas. This messenger system regulates other biological systems through feedback loops between these glands and their hormone products.

Sex-Steroid Hormones

In women, the primary sex hormones (estrogens, such as estradiol and estriol, and progesterone) are produced mainly in the ovaries and regulated via feedback mechanisms between the hypothalamus, the pituitary, and the ovaries. Furthermore, testosterone is also produced at low levels. Throughout pregnancy, large alterations in hormonal levels occur, such as an increase in estrogen, progesterone, and cortisol (Chrousos et al., 1998). The increase in estrogens is believed to enhance mood by increased degradation of monoaminoxidase, an enzyme that degrades serotonin and, through its impact on neurotropins, such as brain-derived neurotrophic factor. Furthermore, testosterone has been shown to have an antidepressive effect (Zarrouf et al., 2009). Progesterone, on the other hand, might work in the opposite direction, leading to mood deterioration (reviewed in Douma et al., 2005). Fluctuations in these sex-steroid hormones, as well as individual sensitivity to these fluctuations, have been investigated in relation to perinatal depression (Ahokas et al., 2001; Harris et al., 1989; Klier et al., 2007; Mehta et al., 2014) as well as in other periods of hormonal fluctuations with high mental impact, such as in puberty, throughout the menstrual cycle, and in menopause. The success of estrogen therapy, which has been assessed as a treatment for postpartum depression in small studies, strengthens this hypothesis (Kettunen et al., 2021; H. J. Li et al., 2020; Moses-Kolko et al., 2009; Myoraku et al., 2018; Wisner et al., 2015). The progesterone metabolite, allopregnanolone, increases sharply during pregnancy and decreases postpartum. Studies have found lower levels of allopregnanolone in depressed pregnant women during late gestation (Hellgren et al., 2014), although there is a paucity of research on levels postpartum and on genetic susceptibility. In general, more studies are needed to fully understand the role of sex-steroid hormones and individual sensitivity to them in the pathophysiology of perinatal depression.

The Hypothalamic–Pituitary–Adrenal Axis

The main regulator of the stress response is the hypothalamic–pituitary–adrenal (HPA) axis. When under stress, the hypothalamus releases corticotrophin-releasing hormone, leading to the stimulation of the pituitary gland to release adrenocorticotrophic hormone, which further leads to the release of glucocorticoids such as cortisol from the adrenal cortex. The glucocorticoids provide a negative feedback loop suppressing hypothalamic activity.

When the placenta starts to develop, it begins to produce corticotrophin-releasing hormone (Thomson, 2013), which is not subject to negative feedback by cortisol and thereby leads to a hypercortisolemic state that has its peak after childbirth (Chrousos et al., 1998). Perinatal depression has been linked to both hypo- and hypersensitivity of the HPA axis (Kammerer et al., 2006). Corticotrophin-releasing hormone in mid-pregnancy has been shown to be lower among severely depressed women during pregnancy and higher among healthy pregnant women who will develop postpartum depression

(Hannerfors et al., 2015; Iliadis et al., 2015b), but contradictive studies find no associations between high mid-pregnancy corticotrophin-releasing hormone and postpartum depression (Meltzer-Brody et al., 2011). Although some studies find high levels of adrenocorticotrophic hormone to be associated with postpartum depression (Jolley et al., 2007) and others an increased adrenocorticotrophic hormone response in postpartum depressed women (Lara-Cinisomo et al., 2017), other studies have not found this association (Ferguson et al., 2017). Furthermore, the majority of studies report no association between cortisol levels and depression during pregnancy (Orta et al., 2018), but depressed women postpartum have been shown to, in general, have higher evening cortisol levels (Iliadis et al., 2015a). Thus, dysregulation of the HPA axis is important in the etiology of perinatal depression, but the results of the separate hormone and glucocorticoid levels are inconclusive (Y. Yu et al., 2021).

The Thyroid Axis

The thyroid gland, located in the neck, stimulated by thyroid-stimulating hormone secretes the hormones triiodothyronine and thyroxine, which influence the metabolic rate, the cardiovascular system, and protein synthesis, and in children even growth and development. During pregnancy, there is an increased need for thyroid hormones to stimulate optimal growth and development in the fetus (Eng & Lam, 2020). Both excess and insufficient levels of thyroid hormones can affect cognition and mood. However, there seems to be a bidirectional link, as depression might affect thyroid function (Hage & Azar, 2012). Some studies have analyzed thyroid-stimulating hormone levels during pregnancy in relation to subsequent postpartum diagnosis, and others have examined thyroid-stimulating hormone levels postpartum in relation to postpartum depression diagnosis, but most of them do not support an association (Szpunar & Parry, 2018). However, some studies find association between levels of thyroid-stimulating hormone during pregnancy and at delivery and depressive symptoms postpartum (Parry et al., 2003; Sylvén et al., 2013). Another study found a positive association between low-normal thyroid function and both depression and anxiety scores during pregnancy and postpartum (Konstantakou et al., 2021). Hence, the thyroid axis alterations might be more related to milder symptoms of depression postpartum than those meeting clinical diagnostic criteria.

Oxytocin and Prolactin

Oxytocin and prolactin are both peptide hormones that are secreted by the pituitary gland. During pregnancy, prolactin levels increase in preparation for breastmilk production. Prolactin stays elevated if breastfeeding continues. Studies have found associations between breastfeeding and postpartum depression, suggesting a protective role of breastfeeding (Borra et al., 2015; Cato et al., 2017, 2019; Haga et al., 2012; Watkins et al., 2011; Ystrom, 2012). At the onset of labor, increasing levels of oxytocin lead to uterus contractions. After the baby is born, oxytocin has calming effects on the mother and is thought to help reduce memories of pain; it also facilitates mother–baby attachment/bonding and trust processes. Oxytocin is related to reward processes and is involved in many aspects of social behavior. It is thought to interact with the serotonergic system and to be involved in stress responsivity by the inhibition of the HPA axis activity, leading to reduced stress response (Slattery & Neumann, 2010).

Studies have investigated the effect of intranasal oxytocin on anxiety and depression but with inconclusive results (De Cagna et al., 2019). Other studies have investigated the therapeutic potential of exogenous oxytocin for postpartum posttraumatic stress disorder, suggesting a link between posttraumatic stress disorder following childbirth and the oxytocinergic system with a protective role of oxytocin, but no clinical trials have yet been conducted (reviewed in Witteveen et al., 2020). Thus, oxytocin and prolactin represent crucial factors involved in perinatal depression pathophysiology regarding breastfeeding, dampening of the stress reaction at delivery, and mother–infant attachment/bonding. However, there are most likely large individual and circumstantial differences in how these hormones impact the mental health of perinatal women.

Leptin and Adiponectin

Leptin and adiponectin are both hormones produced by fatty tissue. Besides being involved in appetite regulation, leptin acts as a regulator of metabolic homeostasis during pregnancy and is important for placentation and maternal–fetal exchange processes. To increase nutrients provided for the fetus, leptin resistance occurs during late pregnancy (Tessier et al., 2013). Adiponectin primarily functions as a holder of energy homeostasis and is related to insulin sensitivity but does not seem to increase during normal pregnancy despite increased insulin resistance. Studies outside the perinatal period have found no or low support for the role of neither leptin nor adiponectin in major depression (Carvalho et al., 2014). However, levels of leptin at the time of delivery have been negatively associated with depressive symptoms at six months postpartum (Skalkidou et al., 2009), but levels of adiponectin have not been associated with depressive symptoms during either pregnancy or postpartum when studied cross-sectionally (Rebelo et al., 2016). Future studies investigating the role of leptin and leptin resistance in perinatal depression pathophysiology are needed to draw firm conclusions.

Insulin and Gestational Diabetes

The pancreas, located behind the abdomen, secretes insulin and is the key organ in diabetes mellitus. Diabetes has been associated with depression outside the perinatal period (Farooqi et al., 2022; Yu et al., 2015). During pregnancy, 6–9% of women develop gestational diabetes (CDC, *Diabetes During Pregnancy*, 2019). Gestational diabetes has been linked to perinatal mental health disorders (Wilson et al., 2020). However, although some researchers suggest the involvement of the immune system to explain this phenomenon (Laake et al., 2014), the mechanism behind these associations is still unknown.

Melatonin and Circadian Rhythms

The pineal gland, located in the brain, secretes melatonin that regulates the circadian rhythms and thereby sleep. Melatonin levels increase during pregnancy in women who are healthy, whereas this increase has not been observed for women with postpartum depression, suggesting alterations in systems affecting melatonin synthesis in depressed women (Parry et al., 2008). As reduced sleep deprivation is an important preventive measure to be considered for both perinatal depression and postpartum psychosis (Ross et al., 2005), the role of melatonin in the pathophysiology of these diseases is thought to be important.

Summary

There are studies implicating most of the different endocrine systems described here, but their relative importance in the pathophysiology at the individual level is still unclear. One of the most prominent risk factors for perinatal depression is premenstrual syndrome (Gastaldon et al., 2022), characterized by exacerbation of mood symptoms following fluctuations in sex hormones during the menstrual cycle, similar to the fluctuations seen during the transition from pregnancy to postpartum (Chrousos et al., 1998). As these hormonal fluctuations are inherent to the natural processes of menstruation and childbirth, the reason why some women develop depression and others do not might lay in individual sensitivity, or imbalance in other systems that are impacted by sex hormone changes. Currently, the most investigated endocrine factors as therapeutic targets are estrogen, oxytocin, and allopregnanolone. On the other side, other prominent risk factors impacting many women, such as history of mental disorders and partner violence, might be more related to chronic stress and the HPA axis reactivity, which interact with the reproductive system (Chrousos et al., 1998). On that front, limiting earlier traumatic experiences before pregnancy could have a favorable effect in relation to mental health during and after pregnancy. Future studies assessing all systems at once should be encouraged, to understand possibly different biological pathways to perinatal depression and thus suggest individualized treatments.

The Immune System

The immune system, the body's defense system against pathogenic infections and toxic substances, is affected by alterations in hormone levels (Robinson & Klein, 2012) and undergoes major adaptations throughout the perinatal period. A successful pregnancy requires the maternal body to maintain protection against pathogens and at the same time not reject the semiallogenic fetus (La Rocca et al., 2014). During the past decades, evidence for the role of the immune system in the pathophysiology of depression has increased, with studies reporting elevated levels of primarily proinflammatory biomarkers in patients with major depression (Osimo et al., 2020). Similarities in symptomatology between inflammatory diseases and depression, and the increased risk of developing depression in patients treated with interferon treatment for hepatitis C (Raison, 2006), further support an association. Moreover, there is evidence of immunological effects on the activity of enzymes involved in the synthesis and metabolism of neurotransmitters, such as the enzyme indoleamine pyrrole 2,3-dioxygenase (IDO) and monoamineoxidase-A (Meyer et al., 2009; Sacher et al., 2011).

The IDO enzyme favors the metabolic pathway of L-tryptophan, which as described earlier is the precursor of serotonin, into the kynurenine pathway, which leads to both decreased levels of serotonin synthesis and increased neurodegeneration and oxidative stress, both associated with depression (Wichers et al., 2005; Wichers & Maes, 2004). Furthermore, studies investigating the activity of IDO by measuring the kynurenine/tryptophan ratio in both humans and animals, are debating its effect on mood (Bradley et al., 2015; Mo et al., 2014; Souza et al., 2017). The activity of IDO is thought to be modulated by proinflammatory cytokines such as interleukin (IL)-6, TNF-α, IL-1β, interferon (IFN)-γ, and IL-18, but the results are inconclusive (Duan et al., 2018). Monoamineoxidase-A enzyme is modified by IL-4 and IL-13. IL-4 has been found to be associated with comorbidity of anxiety and depression during pregnancy (Leff Gelman et al., 2019), whereas no association has been found for IL-13 (Fransson et al., 2012). The HPA axis is also modified by molecules involved in the immune system, such as IL-1β, IL-6, IL-10, tumor necrosis factor-α, and IFN-α. IL-10 levels have been associated with depression during pregnancy (Simpson et al., 2016) but not postpartum (Groer & Davis, 2006). Moreover, some studies have investigated the IL-8/IL-10 ratio in relation to cortisol levels and found it as a good predictor of postpartum depression (Corwin et al., 2015), and while IFN-α treatment has proven to be efficient in depression outside the perinatal period in women with hepatitis C (Lotrich, 2009), no association has been found in prenatal depression (Edvinsson et al., 2017).

The activation of the IDO enzyme to reduce L-tryptophan is believed to be a defense mechanism as many pathogenic infections rely on tryptophan metabolism for survival (Kaur et al., 2019). Evolutionarily, depression following an infection or trauma might have served the purpose of minimizing the risk of death; depressive behavior, such as isolation, could have decreased the risk of further infections or attacks from predators at a weak stage, which would contribute to survival chances and further reproductive opportunities. Researchers argue that psychoneuroimmunology – the link between the immune system, the endocrine system, and the central and peripheral nervous systems – has a key role in mental health during the perinatal period (Fransson, 2021).

Growth Factors/BDNF

BDNF is a neurotransmitter modulator involved in neuronal plasticity and has been found low in patients with major depression. Electroconvulsive therapy (ECT) has been shown to increase BDNF levels in depressed patients outside the perinatal period (Luan et al., 2020). During pregnancy, BDNF levels decrease as a consequence of consumption of BDNF by the fetus and the placenta (Christian et al., 2016), but the association with perinatal depression is still unclear and probably has a temporal pattern.

Vitamins, Minerals, and Fatty Acids

Vitamins are essential micronutrients, found in fruits, dietary products, meat, and fish, and some can be produced through sunlight exposure. Some studies suggest lower levels of vitamin B9, folate, in depressed patients (Bender et al., 2017). Folate, together with vitamin B12, has been investigated as a supplement for depressed patients, but results suggest that it does not seem to decrease depression severity (Almeida et al., 2015). Studies have mainly focused on vitamin D deficiency in relation to perinatal depression and mostly found lowered levels in depressed women (Accortt et al., 2016; Amini et al., 2019; Murphy et al., 2010). Moreover, although the vitamin D supply is greatest in the summer, seasonal variation in perinatal depression has not been confirmed (Henriksson et al., 2017).

Some of the most important minerals for body function include iron, zinc, copper, iodine, calcium, magnesium, and phosphorus. During pregnancy, iron requirements increase; iron deficiency and subsequent anemia are, thus, common during and after pregnancy. This can be further accentuated by the loss of blood during childbirth. Anemia has been associated with a higher risk of depression (Maeda et al., 2019), making its treatment paramount to prevent depression. Iron-deficiency anemia and malnutrition are also the most common causes of the eating disorder pica (Borgna-Pignatti & Zanella, 2016), a disorder affecting pregnant women in which the patients have cravings for nonedible items. Pica has also been associated with low levels of zinc (Miao et al., 2015). Both zinc and copper have antioxidative properties, and oxidative stress has been linked to depression, as described in the next section). Furthermore, iodine is required for thyroid function and, in the case of malfunction, there is an increased risk for depression. Iodine supplements during pregnancy have not proven to have an effect on thyroid function or the prevalence of perinatal depression (Wang et al., 2020) and, as both iodine excess and a deficiency during pregnancy can affect the development of the fetus, supplements should be taken with caution. Furthermore, in conjunction with fetal skeleton mineralization during late pregnancy, calcium requirements increase. Calcium is believed to have sedative effects, and to absorb calcium vitamin D and magnesium are needed. Phosphorus, on the other hand, binds to calcium and reduces the availability of calcium. Low levels of both calcium and magnesium have been suggested to increase depression, and dietary intake of magnesium, but not calcium, does seem to reduce depression outside of the perinatal period (Li et al., 2017).

Deficiencies in fatty acids, such as polyunsaturated fatty acids and omega-3, have been associated with mental health disorders, such as depression, anxiety, and bipolar disorders. The requirement for fatty acids gets higher during pregnancy. Fatty acids have also been investigated in relation to perinatal depression, with mixed results and no strong evidence for effect in preventing or treating perinatal depression (Suradom et al., 2021).

Nonetheless, although associations between vitamin D, iron, zinc, copper, iodine, calcium, magnesium, phosphor, polyunsaturated fatty acids, and omega-3 and perinatal depression are present, the effects of nutritional supplements during and after pregnancy in perinatal depression remain unclear (Sparling et al., 2017).

Oxidative Stress

Oxidative stress is an imbalance of the formation of reactive oxidative species, or free radicals, and degradation of these by antioxidants, where excess free radicals cause damage to cells and organs. This imbalance can be of multiple causes, where diet, sun radiation, air pollution, microbes, and habits such as smoking are some plausible causes. Although oxidative stress has been shown to be concurrently associated with multiple reproduction and pregnancy related conditions, such as infertility, miscarriage, preeclampsia, preterm birth and fetal growth restriction, there is little evidence that antioxidant supplements can reduce these adverse effects (Duhig et al., 2016). Outside the perinatal period, an association between both depression (Black et al., 2015; Liu et al., 2015) and obsessive-compulsive disorder (Maia et al., 2019) with oxidative stress parameters has been suggested. Prenatal depression has been linked to increased oxidative stress markers (Venkatesh et al., 2019) and metabolomic analyses also find an association with postpartum depression (Bränn et al., 2021; Papadopoulou et al., 2019). Furthermore, some models associate both oxidative stress and nitrosative stress (i.e., the formation of reactive nitrogen species) with perinatal depression (Roomruangwong et al., 2018). It remains to be investigated if oxidative stress is important in the etiology of perinatal mental health disorders or if it is its consequence.

Preeclampsia is a condition in which pregnant women develop high blood pressure and protein in the urine. Preeclampsia is potentially lethal and has been linked to perinatal depression (Caropreso et al., 2020). It is still unknown whether the association between preeclampsia and perinatal depression is driven by other obstetric complications associated with preeclampsia, such as premature delivery and adverse pregnancy outcomes, or a psychological stress response because of increased worrying in the mother. Some studies suggest preeclampsia to be related to inflammation (Matthiesen et al., 2005; Yang et al.,

2014), oxidative stress (Afrose et al., 2022), metabolomic alterations (Bahado-Singh et al., 2012; Odibo et al., 2011), or alterations in the microbiota (P. Li et al., 2022), all also related to perinatal depression.

The Microbiome

The gut–brain axis consists of the bacteria in the gut, the central nervous system, and neuroendocrine/immune markers, which all impact one another. Both gestational diabetes and preeclampsia have been linked to changes in the microbiota during pregnancy (Ding et al., 2021; Huang et al., 2021), and both of these diseases are linked to depressive mood (Caropreso et al., 2020; Wilson et al., 2020). The microbiome composition is highly regulated by the immune system as well as the HPA axis (Redpath et al., 2019,) but how this complex interaction affects mood is still unknown. Many studies on the role of the microbiota in perinatal mental health are ongoing, but the number of randomized controlled clinical trials for probiotic supplementation is still low. A meta-analysis investigating probiotic supplementation with *Lactobacillus* and *Bifidobacterium lactis* in pregnancy found limited evidence of the effectiveness of probiotics in the reduction of postpartum anxiety and depression (Desai et al., 2021). However, this meta-analysis only included three studies, and more research in this promising area is warranted.

The Metabolome

The metabolome includes all the small molecules that are produced in the chemical reactions in the cells. Metabolic profiling is a method of analyzing pathways of metabolites and their intermediates, and are thought to be the method that best reflects the phenotype. Pregnancy requires an increased basal metabolism (Prentice et al., 1996), and differences between the levels of metabolites in nonpregnant and early pregnant women, and between early pregnant and mid-pregnant (weeks 8–16) women, have been observed (Handelman et al., 2019). Studies analyzing single metabolites or metabolomics to address pregnancy complications such as preeclampsia (Bahado-Singh et al., 2012; Kenny et al., 2010; Odibo et al., 2011), fetal malformations, and chromosomal disorders (Diaz et al., 2011) and risk of being born small for gestational age (Horgan et al., 2011) have been performed, but the literature in mental health during pregnancy is limited. Outside the perinatal period, lower levels of metabolites such as glycerol, fatty acids, and GABA (Paige et al., 2007), and increased levels of branched-chain amino acids (Baranyi et al., 2016) and lipids metabolites (Bot et al., 2020) have been associated with depression. For perinatal depression, only a few studies have been conducted, where lower levels of branched-chain amino acids, and betaine, citrulline, C5 and C5:1 carnitine, and higher levels of three triacylglycerol metabolites have been found in women with prenatal depression (Henriksson et al., 2019; Mitro et al., 2020), whereas women with postpartum depression show alterations in 4-hydroxyhippuric acid, homocysteine, and tyrosine and formate, succinate, 1-methylhistidine, α-glucose, and dimethylamine (Lin et al., 2017; L. Zhang et al., 2019). Furthermore, metabolically different subgroups of postpartum depressed women have been observed with associations to kidney function and metabolic syndrome (Bränn et al., 2021), perhaps with oxidative stress being the common link (Bränn et al., 2021; Papadopoulou et al., 2019). In general, a link has been suggested between obesity (metabolic dysfunction, diabetes phenotype), chronic inflammation, and depression, which might underlie the above findings (Milaneschi et al., 2019).

Pharmacological and Noninvasive Neurostimulation Treatments

The main treatments used for perinatal depression are psychotherapy and antidepressants. Among antidepressants, selective serotonin reuptake inhibitors (SSRIs) are the first-line treatment, having an efficacy of up to 64% (Cipriani et al., 2018; Hirschfeld, 1999). It is nevertheless important with a psychiatric assessment, as SSRIs should not be widely used among patients with bipolar disorder, who could have a high risk for mania. Although SSRIs are widely used to treat depression even during the perinatal period, it is important to increase the dose to correspond to the increased blood volume (Hostetter et al., 2000).

In line with the estrogen depletion hypothesis of perinatal depression, small randomized controlled trials have shown positive effects of estrogen therapy (Q. Zhang et al., 2022). In moderate doses, no significant amount is secreted into breastmilk, and no significant effect on milk production is expected. Nonetheless, transdermal preparations are suggested, to counteract a risk for venous thromboembolism postpartum. With long-term use, endometrial hyperplasia and vaginal bleeding are expected. Studies looking at gestagen use have shown either neutral or negative effects on postpartum mood. Estrogen therapy is not widely clinically used at this point.

The newest pharmacological treatment for postpartum depression is brexanolone, a formulation of the progesterone metabolite allopregnanolone, thus an allosteric modulator of the GABA receptor, which has a fast-acting but long-lasting antidepressant effect in the postpartum period. Both the normalization of allopregnanolone levels by SSRI treatment for perinatal depression, as well as the efficacy of brexanolone, implicates this last substance and/or GABA receptors in the pathophysiology of perinatal depression (Ali et al., 2021; Leader et al., 2019; Meltzer-Brody et al., 2018; Morrison et al., 2019; Zheng et al., 2019). The administration of brexanolone is, unfortunately, demanding as it requires the patient to be monitored throughout treatment due to the risk of unconsciousness. Brexanolone can be administered only to postpartum depressed patients and, not prenatally, as animal studies have shown negative impact on the fetus from similarly acting substances (Manent et al., 2007). Its efficacy during pregnancy is also uncertain, as the hormonally profiled depression potentially mainly applies to postpartum depressed patients who respond to the drastic hormonal drop after the delivery.

Furthermore, noninvasive neurostimulation treatments include repetitive transcranial magnetic stimulation, transcranial direct current stimulation, transcranial alternating current stimulation, trigeminal nerve stimulation, and transcutaneous vagus nerve stimulation (Cole et al., 2019; Marangell et al., 2007). Few studies, and especially few randomized controlled trials, have further investigated promising results from case reports and uncontrolled trials, but these are in line with these first results (Konstantinou et al., 2020).

Conclusion

The understanding of underlying pathophysiological mechanisms behind perinatal mental ill health is of crucial importance, as it can lead to the identification of new therapeutic or preventive targets. Thus far, studies point to traumatic experiences, premenstrual syndrome, unplanned pregnancy and genetic polymorphisms in the serotonin transporter gene as major risk factors (Gastaldon et al., 2022). It is important, nevertheless, to remember that the biological systems in the body work in multidirectional pathways and that perinatal mental disorders are highly heterogenous diseases; different subgroups that might need individualized treatment options are described (Putnam et al., 2017; Wikman et al., 2020). It is very probable that different biological systems interact with environmental stressors and psychosocial and sociocultural factors and are differentially affected in various subgroups of women presenting with mental ill health perinatally; deep phenotyping could be crucial if biomarkers are to be discovered. A holistic approach is important for individualized assessment, prevention, and treatment.

References

Accortt, E. E., Schetter, C. D., Peters, R. M., & Cassidy-Bushrow, A. E. (2016). Lower prenatal vitamin D status and postpartum depressive symptomatology in African American women: Preliminary evidence for moderation by inflammatory cytokines. *Archives of Women's Mental Health*, *19*(2), 373–383. https://doi.org/10.1007/s00737-015-0585-1

Afrose, D., Chen, H., Ranashinghe, A., Liu, C.-C., Henessy, A., Hansbro, P. M., & McClements, L. (2022). The diagnostic potential of oxidative stress biomarkers for preeclampsia: Systematic review and meta-analysis. *Biology of Sex Differences*, *13*(1), 26. https://doi.org/10.1186/s13293-022-00436-0

Ahokas, A., Kaukoranta, J., Wahlbeck, K., & Aito, M. (2001). Estrogen deficiency in severe postpartum depression: Successful treatment with sublingual physiologic 17beta-estradiol: A preliminary study. *Journal of Clinical Psychiatry*, *62*(5), 332–336. https://doi.org/10.4088/jcp.v62n0504

Ali, M., Aamir, A., Diwan, M. N., Awan, H. A., Ullah, I., Irfan, M., & De Berardis, D. (2021). Treating postpartum depression: What do we know about brexanolone? *Diseases (Basel, Switzerland)*, *9*(3), 52. https://doi.org/10.3390/diseases9030052

Almeida, O. P., Ford, A. H., & Flicker, L. (2015). Systematic review and meta-analysis of randomized placebo-controlled trials of folate and vitamin B12 for depression. *International Psychogeriatrics*, *27*(5), 727–737. https://doi.org/10.1017/S1041610215000046

Amini, S., Jafarirad, S., & Amani, R. (2019). Postpartum depression and vitamin D: A systematic review. *Critical Reviews in Food Science and Nutrition*, *59*(9), 1514–1520. https://doi.org/10.1080/10408398.2017.1423276

Bahado-Singh, R. O., Akolekar, R., Mandal, R., Dong, E., Xia, J., Kruger, M., . . . Nicolaides, K. (2012). Metabolomics and first-trimester prediction of early-onset preeclampsia. *The Journal of Maternal-Fetal and Neonatal Medicine*, *25*(10), 1840–1847. https://doi.org/10.3109/14767058.2012.680254

Baranyi, A., Amouzadeh-Ghadikolai, O., von Lewinski, D., Rothenhausler, H. B., Theokas, S., Robier, C., . . . Meinitzer, A. (2016). Branched-chain amino acids as new biomarkers of major depression – A novel neurobiology of mood disorder. *PLoS One*, *11*(8), e0160542. https://doi.org/10.1371/journal.pone.0160542

Bender, A., Hagan, K. E., & Kingston, N. (2017). The association of folate and depression: A meta-analysis. *Journal of Psychiatric Research*, *95*, 9–18. https://doi.org/10.1016/j.jpsychires.2017.07.019

Black, C. N., Bot, M., Scheffer, P. G., Cuijpers, P., & Penninx, B. W. J. H. (2015). Is depression associated with increased oxidative stress? A systematic review and meta-analysis. *Psychoneuroendocrinology*, *51*, 164–175. https://doi.org/10.1016/j.psyneuen.2014.09.025

Borgna-Pignatti, C., & Zanella, S. (2016). Pica as a manifestation of iron deficiency. *Expert Review of Hematology*, *9*(11), 1075–1080. https://doi.org/10.1080/17474086.2016.1245136

Borra, C., Iacovou, M., & Sevilla, A. (2015). New evidence on breastfeeding and postpartum depression: The importance of understanding women's intentions. *Maternal and Child Health Journal*, *19*(4), 897–907. https://doi.org/10.1007/s10995-014-1591-z

Bot, M., Milaneschi, Y., Al-Shehri, T., Amin, N., Garmaeva, S., Onderwater, G. L. J., . . . Consortium, B.-N. M. (2020). Metabolomics profile in depression: A pooled analysis of 230 metabolic markers in 5283 cases with depression and 10,145 controls. *Biological Psychiatry*, *87*(5), 409–418. https://doi.org/10.1016/j.biopsych.2019.08.016

Boulenger, J. P., & Uhde, T. W. (1982). Biological peripheral correlates of anxiety. *L'Encephale*, *8*(2), 119–130.

Bradley, K. A., Case, J. A., Khan, O., Ricart, T., Hanna, A., Alonso, C. M., & Gabbay, V. (2015). The role of the kynurenine pathway in suicidality in adolescent major depressive disorder. *Psychiatry Research*, *227*(2–3), 206–212. https://doi.org/10.1016/j.psychres.2015.03.031

Bränn, E., Malavaki, C., Fransson, E., Ioannidi, M. K., Henriksson, H. E., Papadopoulos, F. C., . . . Skalkidou, A. (2021). Metabolic profiling indicates diversity in the metabolic physiologies associated with maternal postpartum depressive symptoms. *Frontiers in Psychiatry, 12*(862), 685656. https://doi.org/10.3389/fpsyt.2021.685656

Caropreso, L., de Azevedo Cardoso, T., Eltayebani, M., & Frey, B. N. (2020). Preeclampsia as a risk factor for postpartum depression and psychosis: A systematic review and meta-analysis. *Archives of Women's Mental Health, 23*(4), 493–505. https://doi.org/10.1007/s00737-019-01010-1

Carvalho, A. F., Rocha, D. Q. C., McIntyre, R. S., Mesquita, L. M., Köhler, C. A., Hyphantis, T. N., . . . Berk, M. (2014). Adipokines as emerging depression biomarkers: A systematic review and meta-analysis. *Journal of Psychiatric Research, 59*, 28–37. https://doi.org/10.1016/j.jpsychires.2014.08.002

Cato, K., Sylven, S. M., Georgakis, M. K., Kollia, N., Rubertsson, C., & Skalkidou, A. (2019). Antenatal depressive symptoms and early initiation of breastfeeding in association with exclusive breastfeeding six weeks postpartum: A longitudinal population-based study. *BMC Pregnancy Childbirth, 19*(1), 49. https://doi.org/10.1186/s12884-019-2195-9

Cato, K., Sylven, S. M., Lindback, J., Skalkidou, A., & Rubertsson, C. (2017). Risk factors for exclusive breastfeeding lasting less than two months-identifying women in need of targeted breastfeeding support. *PLoS One, 12*(6), e0179402. https://doi.org/10.1371/journal.pone.0179402

CDC, diabetes during pregnancy. (2019, January 16). www.cdc.gov/reproductivehealth/maternalinfanthealth/diabetes-during-pregnancy.htm

Christian, L. M., Mitchell, A. M., Gillespie, S. L., & Palettas, M. (2016). Serum brain-derived neurotrophic factor (BDNF) across pregnancy and postpartum: Associations with race, depressive symptoms, and low birth weight. *Psychoneuroendocrinology, 74*, 69–76. https://doi.org/10.1016/j.psyneuen.2016.08.025

Chrousos, G. P., Torpy, D. J., & Gold, P. W. (1998). Interactions between the hypothalamic-pituitary-adrenal axis and the female reproductive system: Clinical implications. *Annals of Internal Medicine, 129*(3), 229–240. https://doi.org/10.7326/0003-4819-129-3-199808010-00012

Cipriani, A., Furukawa, T. A., Salanti, G., Chaimani, A., Atkinson, L. Z., Ogawa, Y., . . . Geddes, J. R. (2018). Comparative efficacy and acceptability of 21 antidepressant drugs for the acute treatment of adults with major depressive disorder: A systematic review and network meta-analysis. *The Lancet (London, England), 391*(10128), 1357–1366. https://doi.org/10.1016/S0140-6736(17)32802-7

Cole, J., Bright, K., Gagnon, L., & McGirr, A. (2019). A systematic review of the safety and effectiveness of repetitive transcranial magnetic stimulation in the treatment of peripartum depression. *Journal of Psychiatric Research, 115*, 142–150. https://doi.org/10.1016/j.jpsychires.2019.05.015

Corwin, E. J., Pajer, K., Paul, S., Lowe, N., Weber, M., & McCarthy, D. O. (2015). Bidirectional psychoneuroimmune interactions in the early postpartum period influence risk of postpartum depression. *Brain, Behavior, & Immunity, 49*, 86–93. https://doi.org/10.1016/j.bbi.2015.04.012

De Cagna, F., Fusar-Poli, L., Damiani, S., Rocchetti, M., Giovanna, G., Mori, A., . . . Brondino, N. (2019). The role of intranasal oxytocin in anxiety and depressive disorders: A systematic review of randomized controlled trials. *Clinical Psychopharmacology and Neuroscience, 17*(1), 1–11. https://doi.org/10.9758/cpn.2019.17.1.1

Desai, V., Kozyrskyj, A. L., Lau, S., Sanni, O., Dennett, L., Walter, J., & Ospina, M. B. (2021). Effectiveness of probiotic, prebiotic, and synbiotic supplementation to improve perinatal mental health in mothers: A systematic review and meta-analysis. *Frontiers in Psychiatry, 12*, 622181. https://doi.org/10.3389/fpsyt.2021.622181

Diaz, S. O., Pinto, J., Graça, G., Duarte, I. F., Barros, A. S., Galhano, E., . . . Gil, A. M. (2011). Metabolic biomarkers of prenatal disorders: An exploratory NMR metabonomics study of second trimester maternal urine and blood plasma. *Journal of Proteome Research, 10*(8), 3732–3742. https://doi.org/10.1021/pr200352m

Ding, Q., Hu, Y., Fu, Y., & Qian, L. (2021). Systematic review and meta-analysis of the correlation between intestinal flora and gestational diabetes mellitus. *Annals of Palliative Medicine, 10*(9), 9752–9764. https://doi.org/10.21037/apm-21-2061

Doornbos, B., Dijck-Brouwer, D. A., Kema, I. P., Tanke, M. A., van Goor, S. A., Muskiet, F. A., & Korf, J. (2009). The development of peripartum depressive symptoms is associated with gene polymorphisms of MAOA, 5-HTT and COMT. *Prog Neuropsychopharmacol Biological Psychiatry, 33*(7), 1250–1254. https://doi.org/10.1016/j.pnpbp.2009.07.013

Douma, S. L., Husband, C., O'Donnell, M. E., Barwin, B. N., & Woodend, A. K. (2005). Estrogen-related mood disorders: Reproductive life cycle factors. *ANS Advances in Nursing Science*, 28(4), 364–375. https://doi.org/10.1097/00012272-200510000-00008

DSM-5-TRTM classification. (n.d.). Retrieved January 3, 2023, from www.psychiatry.org:443/psychiatrists/practice/dsm

Duan, K. M., Ma, J. H., Wang, S. Y., Huang, Z., Zhou, Y., & Yu, H. (2018). The role of tryptophan metabolism in postpartum depression. *Metabolism Brain Disease*, 33(3), 647–660. https://doi.org/10.1007/s11011-017-0178-y

Duhig, K., Chappell, L. C., & Shennan, A. H. (2016). Oxidative stress in pregnancy and reproduction. *Obstetric Medicine*, 9(3), 113–116. https://doi.org/10.1177/1753495x16648495

Edvinsson, A., Bränn, E., Hellgren, C., Freyhult, E., White, R., Kamali-Moghaddam, M., . . . Sundstrom-Poromaa, I. (2017). Lower inflammatory markers in women with antenatal depression brings the M1/M2 balance into focus from a new direction. *Psychoneuroendocrinology*, 80, 15–25. https://doi.org/10.1016/j.psyneuen.2017.02.027

Eng, L., & Lam, L. (2020). Thyroid function during the fetal and neonatal periods. *NeoReviews*, 21(1), e30–e36. https://doi.org/10.1542/neo.21-1-e30

Farooqi, A., Gillies, C., Sathanapally, H., Abner, S., Seidu, S., Davies, M. J., . . . Khunti, K. (2022). A systematic review and meta-analysis to compare the prevalence of depression between people with and without Type 1 and Type 2 diabetes. *Primary Care Diabetes*, 16(1), 1–10. https://doi.org/10.1016/j.pcd.2021.11.001

Ferguson, E. H., Di Florio, A., Pearson, B., Putnam, K. T., Girdler, S., Rubinow, D. R., & Meltzer-Brody, S. (2017). HPA axis reactivity to pharmacologic and psychological stressors in euthymic women with histories of postpartum versus major depression. *Archives of Women's Mental Health*, 20(3), 411–420. https://doi.org/10.1007/s00737-017-0716-y

Fransson, E. (2021). Psychoneuroimmunology in the context of perinatal depression – Tools for improved clinical practice. *Brain, Behavior, & Immunity – Health*, 17, 100332. https://doi.org/10.1016/j.bbih.2021.100332

Fransson, E., Dubicke, A., Bystrom, B., Ekman-Ordeberg, G., Hjelmstedt, A., & Lekander, M. (2012). Negative emotions and cytokines in maternal and cord serum at preterm birth. *American Journal of Reproductive Immunology*, 67(6), 506–514. https://doi.org/10.1111/j.1600-0897.2011.01081.x

Gastaldon, C., Solmi, M., Correll, C. U., Barbui, C., & Schoretsanitis, G. (2022). Risk factors of postpartum depression and depressive symptoms: Umbrella review of current evidence from systematic reviews and meta-analyses of observational studies. *The British Journal of Psychiatry: The Journal of Mental Science*, 1–12. https://doi.org/10.1192/bjp.2021.222

Giannakopoulou, O., Lin, K., Meng, X., Su, M.-H., Kuo, P.-H., Peterson, R. E., . . . 23andMe Research Team, China Kadoorie Biobank Collaborative Group, and Major Depressive Disorder Working Group of the Psychiatric Genomics Consortium. (2021). The genetic architecture of depression in individuals of East Asian ancestry: A genome-wide association study. *JAMA Psychiatry*, 78(11), 1258–1269. https://doi.org/10.1001/jamapsychiatry.2021.2099

Groer, M. W., & Davis, M. W. (2006). Cytokines, infections, stress, and dysphoric moods in breast-feeders and formula feeders. *Journal of Obstetric, Gynecologic, and Neonatal Nursing*, 35(5), 599–607. https://doi.org/10.1111/j.1552-6909.2006.00083.x

Guintivano, J., Arad, M., Gould, T. D., Payne, J. L., & Kaminsky, Z. A. (2014). Antenatal prediction of postpartum depression with blood DNA methylation biomarkers. *Molecular Psychiatry*, 19(5), 560–567. https://doi.org/10.1038/mp.2013.62

Haga, S. M., Ulleberg, P., Slinning, K., Kraft, P., Steen, T. B., & Staff, A. (2012). A longitudinal study of postpartum depressive symptoms: Multilevel growth curve analyses of emotion regulation strategies, breastfeeding self-efficacy, and social support. *Archives of Women's Mental Health*, 15(3), 175–184. https://doi.org/10.1007/s00737-012-0274-2

Hage, M. P., & Azar, S. T. (2012). The link between thyroid function and depression. *Journal of Thyroid Research*, 2012, 590648. https://doi.org/10.1155/2012/590648

Handelman, S. K., Romero, R., Tarca, A. L., Pacora, P., Ingram, B., Maymon, E., . . . Erez, O. (2019). The plasma metabolome of women in early pregnancy differs from that of non-pregnant women. *PloS One*, 14(11), e0224682–e0224682. PubMed. https://doi.org/10.1371/journal.pone.0224682

Hannerfors, A. K., Hellgren, C., Schijven, D., Iliadis, S. I., Comasco, E., Skalkidou, A., . . . Sundstrom-Poromaa, I. (2015). Treatment with serotonin reuptake inhibitors during pregnancy is associated with elevated corticotropin-releasing hormone levels. *Psychoneuroendocrinology, 58*, 104–113. https://doi.org/10.1016/j.psyneuen.2015.04.009

Harris, B., Johns, S., Fung, H., Thomas, R., Walker, R., Read, G., & Riad-Fahmy, D. (1989). The hormonal environment of post-natal depression. *British Journal of Psychiatry, 154*, 660–667. https://doi.org/10.1192/bjp.154.5.660

Hellgren, C., Akerud, H., Skalkidou, A., Backstrom, T., & Sundstrom-Poromaa, I. (2014). Low serum allopregnanolone is associated with symptoms of depression in late pregnancy. *Neuropsychobiology, 69*(3), 147–153. https://doi.org/10.1159/000358838

Heninger, G. R., & Charney, D. S. (1988). Monoamine receptor systems and anxiety disorders. *The Psychiatric Clinics of North America, 11*(2), 309–326.

Henriksson, H. E., Malavaki, C., Bränn, E., Drainas, V., Lager, S., Iliadis, S. I., . . . Skalkidou, A. (2019). Blood plasma metabolic profiling of pregnant women with antenatal depressive symptoms. *Translational Psychiatry, 9*(1), 204. https://doi.org/10.1038/s41398-019-0546-y

Henriksson, H. E., Sylven, S. M., Kallak, T. K., Papadopoulos, F. C., & Skalkidou, A. (2017). Seasonal patterns in self-reported peripartum depressive symptoms. *European Psychiatry, 43*, 99–108. https://doi.org/10.1016/j.eurpsy.2017.03.001

Hirschfeld, R. M. (1999). Efficacy of SSRIs and newer antidepressants in severe depression: Comparison with TCAs. *The Journal of Clinical Psychiatry, 60*(5), 326–335. https://doi.org/10.4088/jcp.v60n0511

Hoertel, N., Cipel, H., Blanco, C., Oquendo, M. A., Ellul, P., Leaune, E., . . . Costemale-Lacoste, J.-F. (2021). Cerebrospinal fluid levels of monoamines among suicide attempters: A systematic review and random-effects meta-analysis. *Journal of Psychiatric Research, 136*, 224–235. https://doi.org/10.1016/j.jpsychires.2021.01.045

Horgan, R. P., Broadhurst, D. I., Walsh, S. K., Dunn, W. B., Brown, M., Roberts, C. T., . . . Kenny, L. C. (2011). Metabolic profiling uncovers a phenotypic signature of small for gestational age in early pregnancy. *Journal of Proteome Research, 10*(8), 3660–3673. https://doi.org/10.1021/pr2002897

Hostetter, A., Stowe, Z. N., Strader, J. R., McLaughlin, E., & Llewellyn, A. (2000). Dose of selective serotonin uptake inhibitors across pregnancy: Clinical implications. *Depression and Anxiety, 11*(2), 51–57.

Howard, D. M., Adams, M. J., Clarke, T.-K., Hafferty, J. D., Gibson, J., Shirali, M., . . . McIntosh, A. M. (2019). Genome-wide meta-analysis of depression identifies 102 independent variants and highlights the importance of the prefrontal brain regions. *Nature Neuroscience, 22*(3), 343–352. https://doi.org/10.1038/s41593-018-0326-7

Huang, L., Cai, M., Li, L., Zhang, X., Xu, Y., Xiao, J., . . . Yang, W. (2021). Gut microbiota changes in preeclampsia, abnormal placental growth and healthy pregnant women. *BMC Microbiology, 21*(1), 265. https://doi.org/10.1186/s12866-021-02327-7

Iliadis, S. I., Comasco, E., Sylven, S., Hellgren, C., Sundstrom Poromaa, I., & Skalkidou, A. (2015a). Prenatal and postpartum evening salivary cortisol levels in association with peripartum depressive symptoms. *PLoS One, 10*(8), e0135471. https://doi.org/10.1371/journal.pone.0135471

Iliadis, S. I., Sylvén, S., Jocelien, O., Hellgren, C., Hannefors, A.-K., Elfström, D., . . . Skalkidou, A. (2015b). Corticotropin-releasing hormone and postpartum depression: A longitudinal study. *Psychoneuroendocrinology, 61*, 61. https://doi.org/10.1016/j.psyneuen.2015.07.556

Jolley, S. N., Elmore, S., Barnard, K. E., & Carr, D. B. (2007). Dysregulation of the hypothalamic-pituitary-adrenal axis in postpartum depression. *Biological Research for Nursing, 8*(3), 210–222. https://doi.org/10.1177/1099800406294598

Kammerer, M., Taylor, A., & Glover, V. (2006). The HPA axis and perinatal depression: A hypothesis. *Archive of Women's Mental Health, 9*(4), 187–196. https://doi.org/10.1007/s00737-006-0131-2

Katz, E. R., Stowe, Z. N., Newport, D. J., Kelley, M. E., Pace, T. W., Cubells, J. F., & Binder, E. B. (2012). Regulation of mRNA expression encoding chaperone and co-chaperone proteins of the glucocorticoid receptor in peripheral blood: Association with depressive symptoms during pregnancy. *Psychological Medicine, 42*(5), 943–956. https://doi.org/10.1017/S0033291711002121

Kaur, H., Bose, C., & Mande, S. S. (2019). Tryptophan metabolism by gut microbiome and gut-brain-axis: An in silico analysis. *Frontiers in Neuroscience, 13*. www.frontiersin.org/articles/10.3389/fnins.2019.01365

Kenny, L. C., Broadhurst, D. I., Dunn, W., Brown, M., North, R. A., McCowan, L., . . . Baker, P. N. (2010). Robust early pregnancy prediction of later preeclampsia using metabolomic biomarkers. *Hypertension, 56*(4), 741–749. https://doi.org/10.1161/hypertensionaha.110.157297

Kettunen, P., Koistinen, E., Hintikka, J., & Perheentupa, A. (2021). Oestrogen therapy for postpartum depression: Efficacy and adverse effects: A double-blind, randomized, placebo-controlled pilot study. *Nordic Journal of Psychiatry*, 1–10. https://doi.org/10.1080/08039488.2021.1974556

Klier, C. M., Muzik, M., Dervic, K., Mossaheb, N., Benesch, T., Ulm, B., & Zeller, M. (2007). The role of estrogen and progesterone in depression after birth. *Journal of Psychiatric Research*, 41(3–4), 273–279. https://doi.org/10.1016/j.jpsychires.2006.09.002

Konstantakou, P., Chalarakis, N., Valsamakis, G., Sakkas, E. G., Vousoura, E., Gryparis, A., . . . Mastorakos, G. (2021). Associations of thyroid hormones profile during normal pregnancy and postpartum with anxiety, depression, and obsessive/compulsive disorder scores in euthyroid women. *Frontiers in Neuroscience*, 15, 663348. https://doi.org/10.3389/fnins.2021.663348

Konstantinou, G. N., Vigod, S. N., Mehta, S., Daskalakis, Z. J., & Blumberger, D. M. (2020). A systematic review of non-invasive neurostimulation for the treatment of depression during pregnancy. *Journal of Affective Disorders*, 272, 259–268. https://doi.org/10.1016/j.jad.2020.03.151

Kurita, M. (2016). Noradrenaline plays a critical role in the switch to a manic episode and treatment of a depressive episode. *Neuropsychiatric Disease and Treatment*, 12, 2373–2380. https://doi.org/10.2147/NDT.S109835

Laake, J.-P. S., Stahl, D., Amiel, S. A., Petrak, F., Sherwood, R. A., Pickup, J. C., & Ismail, K. (2014). The association between depressive symptoms and systemic inflammation in people with type 2 diabetes: Findings from the South London diabetes study. *Diabetes Care*, 37(8), 2186–2192. https://doi.org/10.2337/dc13-2522

Lara-Cinisomo, S., Grewen, K. M., Girdler, S. S., Wood, J., & Meltzer-Brody, S. (2017). Perinatal depression, adverse life events, and hypothalamic-adrenal-pituitary axis response to cold pressor stress in Latinas: An exploratory study. *Women's Health Issues*, 27(6), 673–682. https://doi.org/10.1016/j.whi.2017.06.004

La Rocca, C., Carbone, F., Longobardi, S., & Matarese, G. (2014). The immunology of pregnancy: Regulatory T cells control maternal immune tolerance toward the fetus. *Immunology Letters*, 162(1 Pt A), 41–48. https://doi.org/10.1016/j.imlet.2014.06.013

Leader, L. D., O'Connell, M., & VandenBerg, A. (2019). Brexanolone for postpartum depression: Clinical evidence and practical considerations. *Pharmacotherapy*, 39(11), 1105–1112. https://doi.org/10.1002/phar.2331

Leff Gelman, P., Mancilla-Herrera, I., Flores-Ramos, M., Saravia Takashima, M. F., Cruz Coronel, F. M., Cruz Fuentes, C., . . . Camacho-Arroyo, I. (2019). The cytokine profile of women with severe anxiety and depression during pregnancy. *BMC Psychiatry*, 19(1), 104. https://doi.org/10.1186/s12888-019-2087-6

Li, B., Lv, J., Wang, W., & Zhang, D. (2017). Dietary magnesium and calcium intake and risk of depression in the general population: A meta-analysis. *The Australian and New Zealand Journal of Psychiatry*, 51(3), 219–229. https://doi.org/10.1177/0004867416676895

Li, H. J., Martinez, P. E., Li, X., Schenkel, L. A., Nieman, L. K., Rubinow, D. R., & Schmidt, P. J. (2020). Transdermal estradiol for postpartum depression: Results from a pilot randomized, double-blind, placebo-controlled study. *Archives of Women's Mental Health*, 23(3), 401–412. https://doi.org/10.1007/s00737-019-00991-3

Li, P., Wang, H., Guo, L., Gou, X., Chen, G., Lin, D., Fan, D., Guo, X., & Liu, Z. (2022). Association between gut microbiota and preeclampsia-eclampsia: A two-sample mendelian randomization study. *BMC Medicine*, 20(1), 443. https://doi.org/10.1186/s12916-022-02657-x

Lin, L., Chen, X. M., & Liu, R. H. (2017). Novel urinary metabolite signature for diagnosing postpartum depression. *Neuropsychiatric Disease and Treatment*, 13, 1263–1270. https://doi.org/10.2147/NDT.S135190

Liu, T., Zhong, S., Liao, X., Chen, J., He, T., Lai, S., & Jia, Y. (2015). A meta-analysis of oxidative stress markers in depression. *PloS One*, 10(10), e0138904. https://doi.org/10.1371/journal.pone.0138904

Lotrich, F. E. (2009). Major depression during interferon-alpha treatment: Vulnerability and prevention. *Dialogues in Clinical Neuroscience*, 11(4), 417–425.

Luan, S., Zhou, B., Wu, Q., Wan, H., & Li, H. (2020). Brain-derived neurotrophic factor blood levels after electroconvulsive therapy in patients with major depressive disorder: A systematic review and meta-analysis. *Asian Journal of Psychiatry*, 51, 101983. https://doi.org/10.1016/j.ajp.2020.101983

Maeda, Y., Ogawa, K., Morisaki, N., Tachibana, Y., Horikawa, R., & Sago, H. (2019). Association between perinatal anemia and postpartum depression: A prospective cohort study of Japanese women. *International Journal of Gynecology & Obstetrics*, 148(1), 48–52. https://doi.org/10.1002/ijgo.12982

Maia, A., Oliveira, J., Lajnef, M., Mallet, L., Tamouza, R., Leboyer, M., & Oliveira-Maia, A. J. (2019). Oxidative and nitrosative stress markers in obsessive-compulsive disorder: A systematic review and meta-analysis. *Acta Psychiatrica Scandinavica*, 139(5), 420–433. https://doi.org/10.1111/acps.13026

Manent, J.-B., Jorquera, I., Mazzucchelli, I., Depaulis, A., Perucca, E., Ben-Ari, Y., & Represa, A. (2007). Fetal exposure to GABA-acting antiepileptic drugs generates hippocampal and cortical dysplasias. *Epilepsia*, 48(4), 684–693. https://doi.org/10.1111/j.1528-1167.2007.01056.x

Marangell, L. B., Martinez, M., Jurdi, R. A., & Zboyan, H. (2007). Neurostimulation therapies in depression: A review of new modalities. *Acta Psychiatrica Scandinavica*, 116(3), 174–181. https://doi.org/10.1111/j.1600-0447.2007.01033.x

Matthiesen, L., Berg, G., Ernerudh, J., Ekerfelt, C., Jonsson, Y., & Sharma, S. (2005). Immunology of preeclampsia. *Chemical Immunology and Allergy*, 89, 49–61. https://doi.org/10.1159/000087912

Mehta, D., Newport, D. J., Frishman, G., Kraus, L., Rex-Haffner, M., Ritchie, J. C., . . . Binder, E. B. (2014). Early predictive biomarkers for postpartum depression point to a role for estrogen receptor signaling. *Psychological Medicine*, 44(11), 2309–2322. https://doi.org/10.1017/S0033291713002231

Meltzer-Brody, S., Colquhoun, H., Riesenberg, R., Epperson, C. N., Deligiannidis, K. M., Rubinow, D. R., . . . Kanes, S. (2018). Brexanolone injection in post-partum depression: Two multicentre, double-blind, randomised, placebo-controlled, phase 3 trials. *The Lancet*, 392(10152), 1058–1070. https://doi.org/10.1016/S0140-6736(18)31551-4

Meltzer-Brody, S., Stuebe, A., Dole, N., Savitz, D., Rubinow, D., & Thorp, J. (2011). Elevated corticotropin releasing hormone (CRH) during pregnancy and risk of postpartum depression (PPD). *Journal of Clinical Endocrinology and Metabolism*, 96(1), E40–47. https://doi.org/10.1210/jc.2010-0978

Meyer, J. H., Wilson, A. A., Sagrati, S., Miler, L., Rusjan, P., Bloomfield, P. M., . . . Houle, S. (2009). Brain monoamine oxidase A binding in major depressive disorder: Relationship to selective serotonin reuptake inhibitor treatment, recovery, and recurrence. *Archives of General Psychiatry*, 66(12), 1304–1312. https://doi.org/10.1001/archgenpsychiatry.2009.156

Miao, D., Young, S. L., & Golden, C. D. (2015). A meta-analysis of pica and micronutrient status. *American Journal of Human Biology*, 27(1), 84–93. https://doi.org/10.1002/ajhb.22598

Milaneschi, Y., Simmons, W. K., van Rossum, E. F. C., & Penninx, B. W. (2019). Depression and obesity: Evidence of shared biological mechanisms. *Molecular Psychiatry*, 24(1), 18–33. https://doi.org/10.1038/s41380-018-0017-5

Mitro, S. D., Larrabure-Torrealva, G. T., Sanchez, S. E., Molsberry, S. A., Williams, M. A., Clish, C., & Gelaye, B. (2020). Metabolomic markers of antepartum depression and suicidal ideation. *Journal of Affective Disorders*, 262, 422–428. https://doi.org/10.1016/j.jad.2019.11.061

Mo, X., Pi, L., Yang, J., Xiang, Z., & Tang, A. (2014). Serum indoleamine 2,3-dioxygenase and kynurenine aminotransferase enzyme activity in patients with ischemic stroke. *Journal of Clinical Neuroscience*, 21(3), 482–486. https://doi.org/10.1016/j.jocn.2013.08.020

Montoya, A., Bruins, R., Katzman, M. A., & Blier, P. (2016). The noradrenergic paradox: Implications in the management of depression and anxiety. *Neuropsychiatric Disease and Treatment*, 12, 541–557. https://doi.org/10.2147/NDT.S91311

Moret, C., & Briley, M. (2011). The importance of norepinephrine in depression. *Neuropsychiatric Disease and Treatment*, 7(Suppl 1), 9–13. https://doi.org/10.2147/NDT.S19619

Morrison, K. E., Cole, A. B., Thompson, S. M., & Bale, T. L. (2019). Brexanolone for the treatment of patients with postpartum depression. *Drugs Today (Barc)*, 55(9), 537–544. https://doi.org/10.1358/dot.2019.55.9.3040864

Moses-Kolko, E. L., Berga, S. L., Kalro, B., Sit, D. K., & Wisner, K. L. (2009). Transdermal estradiol for postpartum depression: A promising treatment option. *Clinical Obstetrics and Gynecology*, 52(3), 516–529. https://doi.org/10.1097/GRF.0b013e3181b5a395

Munn, D. H., Shafizadeh, E., Attwood, J. T., Bondarev, I., Pashine, A., & Mellor, A. L. (1999). Inhibition of T cell proliferation by macrophage tryptophan catabolism. *Journal of Experimental Medicine*, 189(9), 1363–1372. https://doi.org/10.1084/jem.189.9.1363

Murphy, P. K., Mueller, M., Hulsey, T. C., Ebeling, M. D., & Wagner, C. L. (2010). An exploratory study of postpartum depression and vitamin D. *Journal of the American Psychiatric Nurses Association*, 16(3), 170–177. https://doi.org/10.1177/1078390310370476

Myoraku, A., Robakis, T., & Rasgon, N. (2018). Estrogen-based hormone therapy for depression related to reproductive events. *Current Treatment Options in Psychiatry*, 5(4), 416–424.

Odibo, A. O., Goetzinger, K. R., Odibo, L., Cahill, A. G., Macones, G. A., Nelson, D. M., & Dietzen, D. J. (2011). First-trimester prediction of preeclampsia using metabolomic biomarkers: A discovery phase study. *Prenatal Diagnosis*, 31(10), 990–994. https://doi.org/10.1002/pd.2822

Orta, O. R., Gelaye, B., Bain, P. A., & Williams, M. A. (2018). The association between maternal cortisol and depression during pregnancy, a systematic review. *Archives of Women's Mental Health*, 21(1), 43–53. https://doi.org/10.1007/s00737-017-0777-y

Osborne, L., Clive, M., Kimmel, M., Gispen, F., Guintivano, J., Brown, T., . . . Kaminsky, Z. (2016). Replication of epigenetic postpartum depression biomarkers and variation with hormone levels. *Neuropsychopharmacology*, 41(6), 1648–1658. https://doi.org/10.1038/npp.2015.333

Osimo, E. F., Pillinger, T., Rodriguez, I. M., Khandaker, G. M., Pariante, C. M., & Howes, O. D. (2020). Inflammatory markers in depression: A meta-analysis of mean differences and variability in 5,166 patients and 5,083 controls. *Brain, Behavior, & Immunity*, 87, 901–909. https://doi.org/10.1016/j.bbi.2020.02.010

Paige, L. A., Mitchell, M. W., Krishnan, K. R., Kaddurah-Daouk, R., & Steffens, D. C. (2007). A preliminary metabolomic analysis of older adults with and without depression. *International Journal of Geriatric Psychiatry*, 22(5), 418–423. https://doi.org/10.1002/gps.1690

Papadopoulou, Z., Vlaikou, A.-M., Theodoridou, D., Komini, C., Chalkiadaki, G., Vafeiadi, M., . . . Filiou, M. D. (2019). Unraveling the serum metabolomic profile of post-partum depression. *Frontiers in Neuroscience*, 13, 833. https://doi.org/10.3389/fnins.2019.00833

Parry, B. L., Meliska, C. J., Sorenson, D. L., Lopez, A. M., Martinez, L. F., Nowakowski, S., . . . Kripke, D. F. (2008). Plasma melatonin circadian rhythm disturbances during pregnancy and post-partum in depressed women and women with personal or family histories of depression. *American Journal of Psychiatry*, 165(12), 1551–1558. https://doi.org/10.1176/appi.ajp.2008.08050709

Parry, B. L., Sorenson, D. L., Meliska, C. J., Basavaraj, N., Zirpoli, G. G., Gamst, A., & Hauger, R. (2003). Hormonal basis of mood and postpartum disorders. *Current Women's Health Reports*, 3(3), 230–235.

Paul, S., & Corwin, E. J. (2019). Identifying clusters from multidimensional symptom trajectories in postpartum women. *Research in Nursing & Health*, 42(2), 119–127. https://doi.org/10.1002/nur.21935

Prentice, A. M., Spaaij, C. J., Goldberg, G. R., Poppitt, S. D., van Raaij, J. M., Totton, M., . . . Black, A. E. (1996). Energy requirements of pregnant and lactating women. *European Journal of Clinical Nutrition*, 50(Suppl 1), S82–110; discussion S10–1.

Putnam, K. T., Wilcox, M., Robertson-Blackmore, E., Sharkey, K., Bergink, V., Munk-Olsen, T., . . . Treatment, C. (2017). Clinical phenotypes of perinatal depression and time of symptom onset: Analysis of data from an international consortium. *Lancet Psychiatry*, 4(6), 477–485. https://doi.org/10.1016/S2215-0366(17)30136-0

Raison, C. (2006). The effects of hepatitis C and its treatment on mental health. *Focus*, 21(5), 4–6.

Rebelo, F., Farias, D. R., Struchiner, C. J., & Kac, G. (2016). Plasma adiponectin and depressive symptoms during pregnancy and the postpartum period: A prospective cohort study. *Journal of Affective Disorders*, 194, 171–179. https://doi.org/10.1016/j.jad.2016.01.012

Redpath, N., Rackers, H. S., & Kimmel, M. C. (2019). The relationship between perinatal mental health and stress: A review of the microbiome. *Current Psychiatry Reports*, 21(3), 18. https://doi.org/10.1007/s11920-019-0998-z

Robinson, D. P., & Klein, S. L. (2012). Pregnancy and pregnancy-associated hormones alter immune responses and disease pathogenesis. *Hormones and Behavior*, 62(3), 263–271. https://doi.org/10.1016/j.yhbeh.2012.02.023

Roomruangwong, C., Anderson, G., Berk, M., Stoyanov, D., Carvalho, A. F., & Maes, M. (2018). A neuro-immune, neuro-oxidative and neuro-nitrosative model of prenatal and postpartum depression. *Progress in Neuro-Psychopharmacology and Biological Psychiatry*, 81, 262–274. https://doi.org/10.1016/j.pnpbp.2017.09.015

Ross, L. E., Murray, B. J., & Steiner, M. (2005). Sleep and perinatal mood disorders: A critical review. *Journal of Psychiatry and Neuroscience*, 30(4), 247–256.

Sacher, J., Houle, S., Parkes, J., Rusjan, P., Sagrati, S., Wilson, A. A., & Meyer, J. H. (2011). Mono-amine oxidase A inhibitor occupancy during treatment of major depressive episodes with moclobe-mide or St. John's wort: An [11C]-harmine PET study. *Journal of Psychiatry and Neuroscience*, *36*(6), 375–382. https://doi.org/10.1503/jpn.100117

Sanjuan, J., Martin-Santos, R., Garcia-Esteve, L., Carot, J. M., Guillamat, R., Gutierrez-Zotes, A., . . . de Frutos, R. (2008). Mood changes after delivery: Role of the serotonin transporter gene. *British Journal of Psychiatry*, *193*(5), 383–388. https://doi.org/10.1192/bjp.bp.107.045427

Schrocksnadel, K., Widner, B., Bergant, A., Neurauter, G., Schrocksnadel, H., & Fuchs, D. (2003). Tryptophan degradation during and after gestation. *Advances in Experimental Medicine and Biology*, *527*, 77–83. https://doi.org/10.1007/978-1-4615-0135-0_8

Shetty, D. N., & Pathak, S. S. (2002). Correlation between plasma neurotransmitters and memory loss in pregnancy. *Journal of Reproductive Medicine*, *47*(6), 494–496.

Simpson, W., Steiner, M., Coote, M., & Frey, B. N. (2016). Relationship between inflammatory biomarkers and depressive symptoms during late pregnancy and the early postpartum period: A longitudinal study. *Brazilian Journal of Psychiatry*, *38*(3), 190–196. https://doi.org/10.1590/1516-4446-2015-1899

Skalkidou, A., Sylven, S. M., Papadopoulos, F. C., Olovsson, M., Larsson, A., & Sundstrom-Poromaa, I. (2009). Risk of postpartum depression in association with serum leptin and interleukin-6 levels at delivery: A nested case-control study within the UPPSAT cohort. *Psychoneuroendocrinology*, *34*(9), 1329–1337. https://doi.org/10.1016/j.psyneuen.2009.04.003

Slattery, D. A., & Neumann, I. D. (2010). Oxytocin and major depressive disorder: Experimental and clinical evidence for links to aetiology and possible treatment. *Pharmaceuticals (Basel)*, *3*(3), 702–724. https://doi.org/10.3390/ph3030702

Souza, L. C., Jesse, C. R., de Gomes, M. G., Del Fabbro, L., Goes, A. T. R., Donato, F., & Boeira, S. P. (2017). Activation of brain indoleamine-2,3-dioxygenase contributes to depressive-like behavior induced by an intracerebroventricular injection of streptozotocin in mice. *Neurochemical Research*, *42*(10), 2982–2995. https://doi.org/10.1007/s11064-017-2329-2

Sparling, T. M., Henschke, N., Nesbitt, R. C., & Gabrysch, S. (2017). The role of diet and nutritional supplementation in perinatal depression: A systematic review. *Maternal & Child Nutrition*, *13*(1). https://doi.org/10.1111/mcn.12235

Sundström Poromaa, I., Comasco, E., Bäckström, T., Bixo, M., Jensen, P., & Frokjaer, V. G. (2018). Negative association between allopregnanolone and cerebral serotonin transporter binding in healthy women of fertile age. *Frontiers in Psychology*, *9*, 2767. https://doi.org/10.3389/fpsyg.2018.02767

Suradom, C., Suttajit, S., Oon-arom, A., Maneeton, B., & Srisurapanont, M. (2021). Omega-3 polyunsaturated fatty acid (n-3 PUFA) supplementation for prevention and treatment of perinatal depression: A systematic review and meta-analysis of randomized-controlled trials. *Nordic Journal of Psychiatry*, *75*(4), 239–246. https://doi.org/10.1080/08039488.2020.1843710

Sylvén, S. M., Elenis, E., Michelakos, T., Larsson, A., Olovsson, M., Poromaa, I. S., & Skalkidou, A. (2013). Thyroid function tests at delivery and risk for postpartum depressive symptoms. *Psychoneuroendocrinology*, *38*(7), 1007–1013. https://doi.org/10.1016/j.psyneuen.2012.10.004

Szpunar, M. J., & Parry, B. L. (2018). A systematic review of cortisol, thyroid-stimulating hormone, and prolactin in peripartum women with major depression. *Archives of Women's Mental Health*, *21*(2), 149–161. https://doi.org/10.1007/s00737-017-0787-9

Tessier, D. R., Ferraro, Z. M., & Gruslin, A. (2013). Role of leptin in pregnancy: Consequences of maternal obesity. *Placenta*, *34*(3), 205–211. https://doi.org/10.1016/j.placenta.2012.11.035

Thomson, M. (2013). The physiological roles of placental corticotropin releasing hormone in pregnancy and childbirth. *Journal of Physiology and Biochemistry*, *69*(3), 559–573. https://doi.org/10.1007/s13105-012-0227-2

Venkatesh, K. K., Meeker, J. D., Cantonwine, D. E., McElrath, T. F., & Ferguson, K. K. (2019). Association of antenatal depression with oxidative stress and impact on spontaneous preterm birth. *Journal of Perinatology*, *39*(4), 554–562. https://doi.org/10.1038/s41372-019-0317-x

Viktorin, A., Meltzer-Brody, S., Kuja-Halkola, R., Sullivan, P. F., Landén, M., Lichtenstein, P., & Magnusson, P. K. (2016). Heritability of perinatal depression and genetic overlap with nonperinatal depression. *American Journal of Psychiatry*, *173*(2), 158–165. https://doi.org/10.1176/appi.ajp.2015.15010085

Wang, Z., Li, C., Teng, Y., Guan, Y., Zhang, L., Jia, X., . . . Guan, H. (2020). The effect of iodine-containing vitamin supplementation during pregnancy on thyroid function in late pregnancy and postpartum depression in an iodine-sufficient area. *Biological Trace Element Research, 198*(1), 1–7. https://doi.org/10.1007/s12011-020-02032-y

Watkins, S., Meltzer-Brody, S., Zolnoun, D., & Stuebe, A. (2011). Early breastfeeding experiences and postpartum depression. *Obstetrics & Gynecology, 118*(2 Pt 1), 214–221. https://doi.org/10.1097/AOG.0b013e3182260a2d

Wesseloo, R., Kamperman, A. M., Munk-Olsen, T., Pop, V. J., Kushner, S. A., & Bergink, V. (2016). Risk of postpartum relapse in bipolar disorder and postpartum psychosis: A systematic review and meta-analysis. *American Journal of Psychiatry, 173*(2), 117–127. https://doi.org/10.1176/appi.ajp.2015.15010124

Wichers, M. C., Koek, G. H., Robaeys, G., Verkerk, R., Scharpe, S., & Maes, M. (2005). IDO and interferon-alpha-induced depressive symptoms: A shift in hypothesis from tryptophan depletion to neurotoxicity. *Molecular Psychiatry, 10*(6), 538–544. https://doi.org/10.1038/sj.mp.4001600

Wichers, M. C., & Maes, M. (2004). The role of indoleamine 2,3-dioxygenase (IDO) in the pathophysiology of interferon-alpha-induced depression. *Journal of Psychiatry and Neuroscience, 29*(1), 11–17.

Wikman, A., Axfors, C., Iliadis, S. I., Cox, J., Fransson, E., & Skalkidou, A. (2020). Characteristics of women with different perinatal depression trajectories. *Journal of Neuroscience Research, 98*(7), 1268–1282. https://doi.org/10.1002/jnr.24390

Wilson, C. A., Newham, J., Rankin, J., Ismail, K., Simonoff, E., Reynolds, R. M., Stoll, N., & Howard, L. M. (2020). Is there an increased risk of perinatal mental disorder in women with gestational diabetes? A systematic review and meta-analysis. *Diabetic Medicine, 37*(4), 602–622. https://doi.org/10.1111/dme.14170

Wisner, K. L., Sit, D. K., Moses-Kolko, E. L., Driscoll, K. E., Prairie, B. A., Stika, C. S., . . . Wisniewski, S. R. (2015). Transdermal estradiol treatment for postpartum depression: A pilot, randomized trial. *Journal of Clinical Psychopharmacoly, 35*(4), 389–395. https://doi.org/10.1097/jcp.0000000000000351

Witteveen, A. B., Stramrood, C. A. I., Henrichs, J., Flanagan, J. C., van Pampus, M. G., & Olff, M. (2020). The oxytocinergic system in PTSD following traumatic childbirth: Endogenous and exogenous oxytocin in the peripartum period. *Archives of Women's Mental Health, 23*(3), 317–329. https://doi.org/10.1007/s00737-019-00994-0

Yang, Y., Su, X., Xu, W., & Zhou, R. (2014). Interleukin-18 and interferon gamma levels in preeclampsia: A systematic review and meta-analysis. *American Journal of Reproductive Immunology, 72*(5), 504–514. https://doi.org/10.1111/aji.12298

Ystrom, E. (2012). Breastfeeding cessation and symptoms of anxiety and depression: A longitudinal cohort study. *BMC Pregnancy Childbirth, 12*, 36. https://doi.org/10.1186/1471-2393-12-36

Yu, M., Zhang, X., Lu, F., & Fang, L. (2015). Depression and risk for diabetes: A meta-analysis. *Canadian Journal of Diabetes, 39*(4), 266–272. https://doi.org/10.1016/j.jcjd.2014.11.006

Yu, Y., Liang, H.-F., Chen, J., Li, Z.-B., Han, Y.-S., Chen, J.-X., & Li, J.-C. (2021). Postpartum depression: Current status and possible identification using biomarkers. *Frontiers in Psychiatry, 12*. www.frontiersin.org/article/10.3389/fpsyt.2021.620371

Zarrouf, F. A., Artz, S., Griffith, J., Sirbu, C., & Kommor, M. (2009). Testosterone and depression: Systematic review and meta-analysis. *Journal of Psychiatric Practice, 15*(4), 289–305. https://doi.org/10.1097/01.pra.0000358315.88931.fc

Zhang, L., Zou, W., Huang, Y., Wen, X., Huang, J., Wang, Y., & Sheng, X. (2019). A preliminary study of uric metabolomic alteration for postpartum depression based on liquid chromatography coupled to quadrupole time-of-flight mass spectrometry. *Disease Markers, 2019*, 4264803. https://doi.org/10.1155/2019/4264803

Zhang, Q., Dai, X., & Li, W. (2022). Comparative efficacy and acceptability of pharmacotherapies for postpartum depression: A systematic review and network meta-analysis. *Frontiers in Pharmacology, 13*, 950004. https://doi.org/10.3389/fphar.2022.950004

Zheng, W., Cai, D.-B., Zheng, W., Sim, K., Ungvari, G. S., Peng, X.-J., . . . Xiang, Y.-T. (2019). Brexanolone for postpartum depression: A meta-analysis of randomized controlled studies. *Psychiatry Research, 279*, 83–89. https://doi.org/10.1016/j.psychres.2019.07.006

4

RELATIONSHIP AND SEXUAL FUNCTIONING DURING THE TRANSITION TO PARENTHOOD

Mylène Lachance-Grzela, Mylène Ross-Plourde, and Catherine Hunt

The literature on the transition to parenthood characterizes this normative transition as a transformative time for both mothers and fathers, as well as for their romantic relationship. Welcoming a child necessitates the reorganization of life, reevaluation of priorities, and juggling of many repetitive and seemingly never-ending housework and childcare tasks. The demands of parenting, often coupled with a lack of sleep and with questioning about the new role of being a parent, can be overwhelming. Given the new responsibilities and challenges that accompany the transition to parenthood, it is viewed as a time of critical importance for adult psychological, sexual, and relational health. With the birth of a first child, the focus changes from the role of partner to that of parent (Huss & Pollmann-Schult, 2020). All these adjustments mean that fewer resources are available for the maintenance of the relationship. Thus, it is not surprising that research has shown the transition to parenthood to take a toll on couples' relationship quality and sexual satisfaction. Recent literature has documented that the romantic relationship can act as either a protective or risk factor when parents try to adapt to this major life transition. In the past decade, research using a dyadic perspective has multiplied. More than ever, researchers have considered the notion of interdependence in their research and examined how one partner's attitudes, behaviors, and functioning during the transition to parenthood influence the experience of the other partner and vice versa. Many longitudinal studies examining how the birth of a child alters the trajectory of a couple's relationship functioning have also been published recently.

This chapter presents a review of the literature published in the past decade on relationship and sexual satisfaction during the transition to parenthood. The aims are to document the trajectories of change that occur in terms of romantic and sexual relationship satisfaction with the transition to parenthood and to shed light on the factors and processes that are associated with relationship and sexual satisfaction across the transition to parenthood. Understanding how and when relationship quality is influenced by the arrival of a first child is important considering that how well partners are satisfied by their relationship represents a key predictor of separation and divorce (Tach & Halpern-Meekin, 2012) and because it is related to the personal and relational well-being of partners, children, and the family (Redshaw & Martin, 2014). In research on the transition to parenthood, relationship functioning is usually defined as encompassing the perceptions of quality and satisfaction

DOI: 10.4324/9781003206903-6

with the romantic relationship, whereas sexual functioning usually refers to factors such as satisfaction with one's sexual life, sexual desire and sexual arousal, capacity to achieve orgasm, and absence of pain or physiological dysfunction during sexual activity (Opperman et al., 2013).

Trajectories of Change

In the past, several cross-sectional studies have suggested that parents experience lower levels of marital satisfaction than do nonparents (see Twenge et al., 2004 for a meta-analysis of 97 studies comparing parents to childless individuals). More recently, researchers have generally moved away from these methodologies when trying to draw conclusions about the impact of the transition to parenthood on the basis that (a) a cross-sectional design cannot uncover trajectories of change, and (b) these two groups of individuals are likely to be different even before the pregnancy, thus making comparisons between them unreliable. As Doss and Rhoades (2017) have argued, longitudinal studies that examine the life course of couples welcoming a first child are likely to be more informative. As previously documented extensively in the literature (see Mitnick et al., 2009, for a meta-analysis of 37 studies), recent research has generally supported the idea that, on average, new parents experience declines in relationship satisfaction with the transition to parenthood (e.g., Bäckström et al., 2018; Keizer & Schenk, 2012; Leonhardt et al., 2022; Trillingsgaard et al., 2014; see also ter Kuile et al., 2021, for contradicting results suggesting an absence of change in relationship satisfaction from pregnancy to one year postpartum).

In a 12-year longitudinal study based on a large sample of British parents, Keizer and Schenk (2012) documented a *U*-shaped pattern of change in relationship satisfaction after parents welcomed a first child. In comparison to couples who remained childless, parents experienced sharper declines in relationship satisfaction during the first seven years after the arrival of their first child, but their relationship satisfaction returned to levels similar to those of childless couples about ten years after birth.

In the past decade, researchers have argued that focusing on the average experience of new parents paints an incomplete picture of the transition to parenthood because it does not reveal the different trajectories of change that can occur with the arrival of a first child (Don & Mickelson, 2014; Leonhardt et al., 2022). To fill this gap, they have used class-based approaches to examine unique group trajectories among new parents. Their results contrast with the previous narrative of relational declines during the transition to parenthood, instead documenting that many parents' relationship satisfaction remained relatively stable during the transition to parenthood, with average declines being mostly driven by a minority of couples.

Based on a low-risk sample of new-parent couples in the United States, interviewed from pregnancy to nine months postpartum, Don and Mickelson (2014) found that among new mothers, about 80% reported high relationship satisfaction during the pregnancy and moderate declines of satisfaction during the first nine months postpartum (8% decrease from pregnancy levels). The other 20% of mothers reported moderate levels of relationship satisfaction during pregnancy and experienced steep declines following the birth of their child (25% decrease from pregnancy levels). Among new fathers, about half reported high relationship satisfaction during pregnancy and experienced moderate postpartum declines (7% decrease from pregnancy), about 40% started with high levels and experienced steep declines (17% decrease from pregnancy), and about 10% started with moderate levels and experienced steep declines (25% decrease from pregnancy). Their dyadic data analyses also revealed that the relationship satisfaction of both parents tended to evolve in tandem (see also Keizer & Schenk, 2012, for similar results).

These results were corroborated by the study by ter Kuile et al. (2021) based on a Dutch sample of 440 first-time parents (210 couples) who were followed from pregnancy to one year postpartum. Their findings also indicated that most new parents had high relationship satisfaction during pregnancy and that this tended to remain stable during the postpartum period. Among mothers, one out of four reported moderate relationship satisfaction during pregnancy and no changes in the year following the arrival of the child, but a small sub-group of mothers who were also moderately satisfied with their relationship during their pregnancy experienced declines in relationship satisfaction that stabilized in the postpartum period and slowly got back to prebirth levels around the child's first birthday. Among fathers, one out of three experienced a moderate decline in relationship satisfaction across the transition to parenthood and another small subgroup reported lower relationship satisfaction during pregnancy and abrupt declines early postpartum, which improved gradually afterward but had not regained prenatal levels one year after the birth of the child.

Similar results were obtained in a dyadic study by Leonhardt et al. (2022) based on a sample of 203 couples (most of whom were Canadian) transitioning from pregnancy through the first year of the child. Their results revealed that 47% of couples reported being highly satisfied and 38% reported relatively high levels of satisfaction throughout the transition. They found that it was only among a minority of couples (about 15%) that the parental transition was accompanied by significant decreases in relationship satisfaction. A longitudinal study (Le et al., 2016) has suggested that stability in relationship quality persists beyond the first year postpartum. Specifically, this study found that new mothers' and fathers' levels of marital satisfaction at six months postpartum correlated with those they reported three years postpartum.

With regard to sexual functioning, many researchers have attempted to understand how the various aspects of couples' sexual relationships evolve throughout the prenatal and postpartum periods. Khalesi et al. (2018) have demonstrated that, during pregnancy, changes to future mothers' sexual functioning tend to occur mostly during the third trimester, with a decrease in many domains of sexual functioning, such as desire and overall satisfaction. However, contrasting results have also been obtained, where sexual functioning remained stable during pregnancy (Sagiv-Reiss et al., 2012). In this particular study, even if the global sexual functioning of couples did not change, future mothers' sexual pleasure and feelings of being loved during sexual activities with their partners decreased toward the end of pregnancy. Taken together, these results indicate that changes in the sexual life of future parents could be more related to their experience of sexuality and not their perception of relationship quality or global sexual satisfaction. The authors also concluded that these results could indicate diverging trends among different couples that cannot be revealed by studying the means of a sample.

To better understand how couples can experience different trajectories of change in their sexual functioning during the transition to parenthood, Rosen et al. (2021) used latent class growth analysis and dyadic latent class growth analysis with new parents from the second trimester of pregnancy through the first year postpartum. Unsurprisingly, the frequency of sexual activities tended to decrease for all couples, independent of their level of frequency, meaning that both couples who frequently engaged and couples who less frequently engaged in sexual activities experienced a decline in sexual frequency during the transition to parenthood. In both classes, parents reported fewer sexual activities at the end of the pregnancy and at three months postpartum, after which frequency tended to increase, while remaining lower than in the second trimester of pregnancy. Sexual desire followed a similar pattern for mothers, but not fathers, with fathers' sexual desire remaining stable throughout the transition to parenthood, regardless of class membership. Interestingly, sexual satisfaction tended to remain stable regardless of parents' prenatal levels on this variable, with the exception of fathers with low sexual satisfaction in the second trimester of pregnancy, who experienced a further decrease in the early postpartum period. These results were also consistent with those of another study indicating that new mothers' sexual pleasure generally increased from 3 to 18 months postpartum (McDonald et al., 2017). The sexual experience of couples becoming parents has also been studied in relation to its consequences for relational and sexual satisfaction. In a cross-sectional study of new parents, Rosen et al. (2018) observed that more frequent sexual activities in new parents were associated with fathers' greater sexual satisfaction, but no significant link to mothers' sexual satisfaction was found. However, the frequency of sexual activities was not related to either parent's relationship satisfaction. Sexual satisfaction also correlated positively with child age for both parents, meaning that mothers and fathers of older infants tended to experience greater sexual satisfaction. These authors also considered how a discrepancy between partners' desires could be associated with sexual and relational satisfaction, finding that parents reporting a greater gap in sexual desire reported being less sexually satisfied. Nonetheless, couples with similar levels of desire were no more satisfied with their relationship than couples who experienced a desire discrepancy (Rosen et al., 2018).

Qualitative data are a valuable way to provide more details about how couples experience the transition to parenthood and to further understand the quantitative results obtained in other studies. Generally, qualitative results are consistent with those reported in quantitative studies. In a qualitative study of new parents with a child aged between 6 and 12 months, Lévesque et al. (2021) revealed that parents linked the lower frequency of sexual activities to reduced occasions to engage in sex. New mothers and fathers, unsurprisingly, identified feeling exhausted and lacking energy as partly explaining the reduction in occasions to be intimate, as well as the importance placed on the baby and their needs. Understandably, couples reported putting their parental roles first, which meant that their roles as partners and lovers were often put aside. Consistent with the quantitative studies previously summarized, mothers reported a decline in sexual desire after the birth of their child. Nonetheless, couples reported being sexually satisfied and expecting this change in their sexual relationship. This could be explained by what new parents identified as a redefinition of their sexuality. Mothers and fathers found different means of expressing their love and affection for one another and felt that their sexual activities were more satisfying and of greater quality, which helped balance the fact that they occurred less frequently. Converging results have also been obtained in another qualitative study of new fathers. MacAdam et al. (2011) found that fathers also identified new ways to express their sexuality, through showing appreciation and affection for their partner, and explained that parenthood had brought a new understanding of their relationship as a couple.

In brief, recent research has suggested that most parents experience little change in relationship and sexual satisfaction following the arrival of their first child but that small subgroups of parents experience large declines. Therefore, it appears appropriate to conclude that average decreases previously documented are largely explained by the minority of parents for whom the parental transition is accompanied by significant decreases in their relationship satisfaction. A key question in the research on relationship and sexual satisfaction across the transition to parenthood is which factors and processes account for the stability or declines in relationship functioning during this period.

Factors and Processes Related to Relationship and Sexual Satisfaction Across the Transition to Parenthood

Personal Characteristics

Sociodemographic characteristics, such as gender and length of relationship, have been linked to adjustment through the transition to parenthood. Fillo et al. (2015) reported that, when they reported making relatively high contributions to childcare, new fathers experienced steeper declines in relationship satisfaction compared to new fathers who make lower contributions to childcare. In contrast, new mothers' relationship satisfaction was less influenced by the amount of childcare they reported completing. However, in general, research revealed that new mothers tended to perceive the first year postpartum as a greater source of relationship conflict than did new fathers (Newkirk et al., 2017). Evidence also indicates that couples who had been in a relationship for longer at the time when they welcomed their first child were more likely to experience increases in relationship satisfaction during the first 30 months postpartum compared to couples with shorter length of relationship (Trillingsgaard et al., 2014).

Well-Being and Mental Health

Given the challenges couples face when becoming parents – namely, lack of sleep, less time for oneself and leisure activities, and uncertainties about how to raise a child – new parents' well-being and mental health can be impaired. Even before these challenges become the new reality for couples, the well-being of both parents before birth is likely to affect their experience of this life period. More precisely, psychological well-being variables have been consistently identified throughout the transition to parenthood as contributing to relationship satisfaction (e.g., Baldoni et al., 2020; Don et al., 2022; Garthus-Niegel et al., 2018; Trillingsgaard et al., 2014) and sexual satisfaction (e.g., Maas McDaniel et al., 2018; Rosen et al., 2018; Vannier et al., 2018).

Positive Affect

The transition to parenthood brings about a mix of positive and negative emotions, yet the positive side does more than simply compensate for the negative one. Indeed, in two dyadic longitudinal studies of positive affect and relationship satisfaction across the transition to parenthood, Don et al. (2022) demonstrated that the contribution of positive emotions to relationship satisfaction appeared to go above and beyond that of other variables included, such as negative affect, stress, and role satisfaction. More specifically, for fathers, more positive emotions at a given point in time predicted greater relationship satisfaction, when controlling for previous levels of relationship satisfaction. This association was present from the third trimester of pregnancy to nine months postpartum and was replicated in a second study spanning from pregnancy to 24 months after the birth of the child. For mothers, greater positive emotions were associated with more relationship satisfaction (in the second study only; Don et al., 2022). The authors concluded that positive emotions should not be considered to *demonstrate* a better adjustment to this life transition but rather to *contribute* to this adjustment. These results have shown that positive relationships were fostered not only by limiting negative emotions and experiences but also by maximizing positive couple experiences and emotions (Don et al., 2022).

Depression and Anxiety

The joy of welcoming a first child is sometimes obscured by mental health difficulties, such as symptoms of anxiety or depression. These symptoms can become severe, with postpartum depression (PPD) affecting as many as one in seven mothers (American Psychological Association [APA], 2022). It is estimated that around 50% of women with PPD have been experiencing depressive symptoms in the prenatal period, and first-time mothers are generally more likely to present PPD (APA, 2022). Men can also experience depressive symptoms following the birth of their child, with about one in ten fathers reporting such symptoms (Garfield et al., 2022). Many studies have investigated how depressive and anxiety symptoms in first-time parents are associated with relationship satisfaction. A longitudinal study spanning from the third month of pregnancy to 30 months postpartum and using dyadic data found that, in both parents, fewer depressive and anxiety symptoms in early pregnancy were associated with increased relationship satisfaction a year and a half after the birth of the baby (Trillingsgaard et al., 2014). These authors concluded that the early assessment of mental health could be helpful in preventing relationship difficulties in the postpartum period. A cross-sectional study concentrating on the postpartum period also showed that mothers' greater depressive symptoms were associated with their and their partners' lower relationship satisfaction (Rosen et al., 2018).

Similarly, in a longitudinal study covering the first trimester of pregnancy to 30 months postpartum, negative interactions were associated with both parents' depressive symptoms (Figueiredo et al., 2018). Negative interactions between partners were related to increases in depressive and anxiety symptoms during the postpartum period, but depressive and anxiety symptoms were not associated with changes in negative interactions during this same period. This could indicate that couple interactions are not solely a consequence of depressive and anxiety symptoms. Relationship satisfaction was also shown to be negatively associated with paternal (but not maternal) PPD in a cross-sectional study with a relatively small sample size ($N = 73$ couples; Cohen et al., 2019). A study of change in relationship satisfaction through the transition to parenthood supported these results; the depressive symptoms of future mothers and fathers were also significantly associated with a change in their own or their partners' relationship satisfaction (Don & Mickelson, 2014). Nonetheless, further studies are needed to clarify the association between depressive symptoms and relationship functioning.

Additionally, some evidence has shown that anxiety symptoms could negatively impact relationship satisfaction, particularly for mothers. In a study employing a longitudinal dyadic design, paternal symptoms of anxiety in the last trimester of pregnancy were a predictor of a sharp decline in relationship satisfaction for new mothers during the first nine months after delivery (Don & Mickelson, 2014). No such partner effect was demonstrated for fathers' relationship satisfaction.

Depressive symptoms have also been associated with sexual satisfaction. Mothers exhibiting greater depression symptomatology tend to be less sexually satisfied, a trend that has been demonstrated both in a postpartum cross-sectional design (Rosen et al., 2018) and in a longitudinal study from pregnancy to 12 months postpartum (Vannier et al., 2018). Fathers' depressive symptoms have also been associated with their own sexual concerns, with more depressive symptoms being related to more sexual concerns (Dawson et al., 2022). There is also evidence of a partner effect, with mothers' depressive symptoms associated with lower sexual satisfaction in fathers (Rosen et al., 2018). In a study examining the changes in PPD and sexual functioning from 3 to 12 months after the birth of a first child, Dawson et al. (2022) found further evidence of a partner effect by which mothers' symptoms affected fathers' sexual functioning. When mothers felt more depressed at three months postpartum, their partners tended to report more sexual worries or concerns, such as concerns regarding the frequency of intercourse, the impact of child-rearing duties on time for sexual activity, and their own or their partner's body image. However, longitudinal associations showed that mothers' depressive symptoms three months after childbirth were also related to a more pronounced decline in fathers' sexual concerns over the first year postpartum (Dawson et al., 2022). This partner effect was not demonstrated in the other direction. It appears that fathers' depressive symptoms were not significantly associated with mothers' sexual concerns or their evolution over the first year postpartum.

Stress

Stress and the presence of stressors during the transition to parenthood have also been studied in relation to relationship and sexual functioning. A cross-sectional dyadic study of future parents has indicated that stress during pregnancy was indirectly associated with prenatal relationship satisfaction, through depressive symptoms, at both the individual and partner levels (Baldoni et al., 2020). Future mothers and fathers with higher perceived stress tended to report more depressive symptoms, which in turn were associated with lower relationship satisfaction in the prenatal period. A dyadic pattern was also demonstrated in this study, as future mothers' higher stress was related to future fathers' higher depressive symptoms, thus decreasing fathers' relationship satisfaction (Baldoni et al., 2020). In another study using longitudinal dyadic data, parents' stress was not a significant predictor of change in mothers' relationship satisfaction from late pregnancy to nine months postpartum (Don & Mickelson, 2014). However, when mothers reported higher stress prenatally, fathers were more likely to experience a sharp decline in relationship satisfaction after the birth of the baby.

With regard to sexual functioning, a postpartum longitudinal study considered how parents' stress and feelings of being overwhelmed by the various roles and responsibilities they had to fulfill, termed "role overload," were associated with sexual satisfaction in both parents (Maas et al., 2018). Mothers coping with more stress at six months postpartum also tended to be less satisfied with their sexuality at 12 months postpartum, although this association was not present for fathers. Additionally, when both parents reported more role overload when their child was six months old, they also described being less satisfied with certain aspects of their sex life, such as passion and cuddling frequency. Feeling stressed and overwhelmed by the demands and responsibilities of their various roles could imply that parents are left with little energy and resources to invest in their sexual relationship (Maas et al., 2018).

Childbirth-Related Posttraumatic Stress

Childbirth is an intense experience, where an unexpected turn of events is never excluded and the mother's and baby's lives are sometimes at risk. It is, therefore, understandable that some women will develop posttraumatic stress disorder (PTSD) after this pivotal event. It is estimated that 3% of women in community samples meet diagnostic criteria for postpartum PTSD (Grekin & O'Hara, 2014). A few studies have looked at how PTSD relates to relationship functioning. In a quantitative longitudinal study, women experiencing symptoms of posttraumatic stress in the early postpartum period tended to report lower relationship satisfaction two years after the birth, even when also considering prenatal PTSD symptoms, prenatal adverse life events, and postpartum infant temperament (Garthus-Niegel et al., 2018). However, depressive symptoms are thought to explain this association between postpartum PTSD symptomatology and relationship satisfaction. Therefore, it appears that posttraumatic stress after a difficult childbirth led to more depressive symptoms, which contributed to poorer satisfaction (Garthus-Niegel et al., 2018). Posttraumatic symptoms following a traumatic birthing experience are likely to cause women to hold negative beliefs about themselves and their relationship exacerbating depressive symptoms. In turn, these biased cognitions could impact the relationship or, at least, its perception by mothers (Garthus-Niegel et al., 2018).

A review of qualitative studies examining the association between posttraumatic stress following childbirth and couples' relationships also exposed consistent negative effects of these symptoms on couples, sometimes leading to feelings of strain, decreased closeness between partners, and even separation (Delicate et al., 2017). Nonetheless, the review also highlighted a few qualitative studies suggesting that, for some couples, going through this difficult experience and its aftermath could also make their relationship stronger. More quantitative studies are needed to better understand the specific characteristics of couples going down these opposite roads.

Summary

In short, well-being and mental health variables have been associated with relationship functioning and generally indicate, as could be expected, that better mental health during the transition to parenthood is related to greater relationship satisfaction and fewer negative interactions between partners. Depressive symptoms, both during pregnancy and after the birth of the baby, have a significant impact on the relationship between new mothers and fathers. Taken together, these results clearly indicate that the mental well-being of future mothers and fathers should be monitored in the prenatal period. Interventions targeting these early symptoms could help prevent deterioration of new parents' well-being and evolution toward a clinical diagnosis. It should be noted that positive affect is also significant in predicting relationship functioning, underscoring the necessity of considering both the reduction of negative feelings and the fostering of positive couple experiences and emotions. Relatedly, more research is needed to better understand how some couples are able to face traumatic and difficult events in the perinatal period in a constructive way, leading to a strengthened relationship.

Relational Context and Partner Predictors

Multiple researchers have examined how various relationship factors play a role in the adjustment to parenthood. They have documented that the way partners perceive one another and interact with one another influences their adjustment to their new role as parents.

Couple Support

Different variables related to how couple members support each other and perceive the support offered by their partner have been associated with relational and sexual functioning. For instance, during pregnancy, higher relational intimacy and support in the relationship (both offered and received) have been associated with future parents' sexual satisfaction (Gagné et al., 2021). Additionally, emotional satisfaction has been identified as an important predictor of the postpartum sexual pleasure of new mothers (McDonald et al., 2017).

In a cross-sectional study of couples after the birth of their first child, Muise et al. (2017) studied how sexual communal strength, namely, the motivation to respond to a partner's desire or absence of desire to engage in sexual activities, related to sexual and relationship satisfaction. Their dyadic analyses showed an actor effect, such that mothers and fathers with a higher motivation to react to their partner's sexual desire also experienced higher sexual and relationship satisfaction. A partner effect was also discovered. Parents whose partner was higher in sexual communal strength for having sex reported being more satisfied with both their relationship and their sexuality. Interestingly, these authors also considered the sexual communal strength for not having sex, in other words, the motivation to comply with a partner's desire not to engage in sexual activities. Their results indicated that when fathers were sensitive to their partner's absence of sexual desire, their partner was generally more satisfied with their relationship and more sexually satisfied. Moreover, these fathers also reported higher relationship and sexual satisfaction, underscoring the positive effect that being understanding of a partner's desires had on the couple and the sexual relationship for both members (Muise et al., 2017). These dyadic effects were also significant when considering dyadic empathy as a covariate, further demonstrating the importance of being attentive and responsive to a partner's sexual needs in the transition to parenthood. This concept is akin to perceptions of partner responsiveness, which has also been studied in relation to relationship and sexual functioning.

Recent research has revealed that partners' responsiveness – that is, how they understand, validate, and care for one another (Reis & Clark, 2013) – influences global relationship satisfaction across time during the transition to parenthood. Smallen, Eller, Rholes, and Simpson's study (2022), conducted among new parents during the first two years of the transition to parenthood, suggested that, when partners were responsive toward one another, it tended to alleviate the stresses that accompanied this transition and to protect their romantic relationship. Lower levels of both perceived provision and receipt of responsiveness were generally associated with decreases in relationship satisfaction. When parental stress was low, both greater perceived provision and greater receipt of responsiveness predicted greater relationship satisfaction. However, partners did not always benefit from increased partner responsiveness, as this was linked to decreased relationship satisfaction when a highly responsive provider experienced heightened levels of parental stress. These contrasting results correspond to those of a previous study (ter Kuile et al., 2017), which revealed that being the recipient and being the provider of responsiveness did not lead to the same trajectories. On the one hand, ter Kuile et al. (2017) found that higher levels of perceived responsiveness experienced even years prior to the pregnancy could act as a buffer against the challenges that came with the transition to parenthood; on the other hand, providing above-average levels of responsiveness before the pregnancy was associated with poorer adaptation to parenthood over the transition. Overall, it seems that providing high levels of understanding, validation, and care to a partner during the transition to parenthood may put a strain on the responsive partner by draining them of their personal resources, in turn leading them to feel less satisfied in their relationship.

Additionally, in a study of perceived partner responsiveness relative to couples' sexual relationship, Rosen et al. (2020) found that, when mothers reported greater partner responsiveness in the postpartum period, they also tended to be more satisfied with both their sexuality and their relationship. This association was present from 3 to 12 months postpartum. These authors also considered how disclosing concerns about sexuality could contribute to mothers' sexual and relationship satisfaction, but this variable did not significantly contribute to explaining satisfaction. Therefore, mothers feeling validated and understood by their partners in the context of their sexual relationship appear to be more important than sexual disclosure in predicting both their sexual and relationship satisfaction.

Dyadic empathy is another related interpersonal predictor of relationship adjustment that, in the past decade, has attracted the attention of researchers focusing on the transition to parenthood. It refers to the partners' ability to understand one another's point of view and feel concern in response to one another's experience. The empathy expressed by new parents toward one another was shown to protect and facilitate their sexual and relationship quality. Rosen et al. (2017) found that new mothers and fathers reported higher sexual and relationship satisfaction when they and their partners also reported greater dyadic empathy. The results were more nuanced in terms of sexual desire specifically, as new mothers tended to report higher sexual desire when they felt greater dyadic empathy but lower sexual desire when they had more empathic partners (men's sexual desire was not found to be related to their provision of empathy toward their partner or to their experience of empathy from their partner). The associations found remained over and above the effects of other variables such as fatigue, breastfeeding, and pain during intercourse. Similarly, Muise et al. (2017) have also observed that greater dyadic empathy in new parents was related to higher relationship satisfaction and higher sexual satisfaction.

Division of Household Labor and Perception of Unfairness

Considering the significant increase in workload and responsibilities that accompany the arrival of a child, it is not surprising that researchers want to understand the impact of how partners share household labor and childcare. As some authors have argued, the changes that come with the parenting transition are of such magnitude that they may even crystallize gender performances in the family for years to come (Yavorsky et al., 2015). Large-scale longitudinal research with pre- and post-pregnancy data collection has suggested that a traditionalization of housework division occurs across parenthood transitions. For instance, with a nationally representative and prospective study, Hiekel and Ivanova (2022) found that half the parents reported that the unequal division of household labor that existed prior to the arrival of a new child persisted after the birth, and an extra third of them reported an increasingly gendered division of labor in their home after the birth of a child. In both cases, partners agreed that it was the mother who was carrying the lion's share of household responsibilities. A longitudinal study based on a large sample of new parents documented that across the first two years of parenthood, new mothers reported completing about 70% of childcare and men reported completing approximately 30% of childcare (Fillo et al., 2015). Using longitudinal time diaries from a sample of dual-earner couples in which both parents were working when the child was nine months old, Yavorsky et al. (2015) found that when they became mothers, U.S. women in dual-earner couples generally experienced a more pronounced increase in their workload (including paid and unpaid work) compared to their male counterparts. This disparity in workload between new mothers and new fathers is not without consequences for couples' relationships. Cohen et al. (2019) found that, early on after the arrival of a child, both the mother and the father tended to wish the father to be more involved in household, childcare, and family decision-making tasks. Dyadic analyses revealed that a woman's satisfaction with her role as a mother predicted not only her own but also her partner's relationship adjustment in the first months postpartum.

Fillo et al.'s (2015) results based on a large sample of first-time parents across the first two years of parenthood revealed that contributions to childcare continued to be related to relationship satisfaction – and particularly so for fathers – two years after the arrival of the child. Men who reported contributing a greater share of childcare compared to average men experienced greater declines in relationship satisfaction during the first two years of their child's life. Women's changes in relationship satisfaction were not as closely related to the time they spent on childcare. In addition, perceptions of childcare self-efficacy – that is, feeling competent and fulfilled when completing childcare tasks – appeared to protect the relationship satisfaction trajectory for new parents regardless of their level of involvement in childcare per se. On the other hand, experiencing greater work-family conflicts had the opposite effect, especially for men who reported completing a greater proportion of childcare.

Unsurprisingly, research has also revealed that partners' perception of fairness in the division of household labor and childcare was associated with how satisfied they were with their relationship during the transition to parenthood (Chong & Mickelson, 2016; Cohen et al., 2019; Hiekel & Ivanova, 2022). Cross-sectional and longitudinal findings from Chong and Mickelson (2016) revealed that mothers' perceived unfairness of household labor and childcare at one month and nine months postpartum were related to lower levels of perceived emotional spousal support, which was in turn associated with lower levels of relationship satisfaction at nine months postpartum. The authors found no indication of similar mediation for fathers in the cross-sectional analyses of data at nine months postpartum. However, the longitudinal analyses revealed that the more fathers felt that their share of household labor was fair to them one month after the birth of their child, the less satisfied their partner tended to be with their marital relationship when the child reached 9 months of age. Taken together, these results suggest that the division of household labor and childcare early after the arrival of the first child may have a long-lasting impact on the couple's relationship. Similarly, Hiekel and Ivanova's recent results (2022) found that mothers who perceived that the division of household labor was fair both before and after the arrival of their child were the most likely to maintain high relationship satisfaction across a parenthood transition. The opposite was true for women who perceived a persistent unfair division; they experienced the sharpest declines in relationship satisfaction across the transition. In contrast, fathers' perceived fairness of the division of household labor was not related to the variations in their own relationship satisfaction. The authors argued that this was probably because fathers were generally the ones to be advantaged in an unfair division of labor. In some cases, such as when men considered the division of household labor to remain fair throughout the transition and when women found that the division became fairer between the pregnancy and the postpartum period, endorsing non-egalitarian gender roles acted as a risk factor increasing the chances of experiencing steep drops in relationship satisfaction. The authors concluded that, when a discrepancy between the desired and the lived realities occurs, dissatisfaction set in and could have more serious consequences than the division of household labor per se.

Satisfaction with the division of household labor has also been associated with sexual functioning, particularly for mothers. When mothers reported being more satisfied with the division of household tasks six months after the birth of their child, they tended to be more satisfied with their sexual relationship at 12 months postpartum (Maas et al., 2018). In contrast, fathers' satisfaction with the division of labor when their child was six months old was only associated with their satisfaction with the frequency of romance in their relationship when their child was a year old and was not related to other components of their sexual satisfaction (i.e., frequency of sex, cuddling and touching, passion and excitement; Maas et al., 2018). A longitudinal study of postpartum mothers found that, when mothers were satisfied with the division of household tasks with their partner, they also reported being more satisfied emotionally and experienced more sexual pleasure (McDonald et al., 2017). Similarly, when mothers had more time for themselves in a given week, they also tended to be more satisfied emotionally and sexually. These authors also considered two models with multiple variables potentially explaining emotional satisfaction and sexual pleasure, including breastfeeding and reports of sexual health problems. It appeared that mothers' satisfaction with the division of household tasks was an important predictor of emotional satisfaction, and emotional satisfaction in turn was the most important predictor of mothers' sexual pleasure. Although these authors did not examine these variables in a mediation model, it is possible that satisfaction with the division of household labor could be associated with mothers' sexual pleasure through emotional satisfaction.

Conflict Management and Communication

Researchers have tried to understand the way partners navigate challenges and deal with disagreements when they arise in the relationship and how this influences their relationship functioning. Their work has revealed that effective communication and conflict management skills can protect against declines in relationship satisfaction across the transition to parenthood (Ramsdell et al., 2020; Trillingsgaard et al., 2014). During pregnancy, couples who argue more frequently and express more negative affect during conflicts tend to be less satisfied with their relationship (Ramsdell et al., 2020). Similar patterns of results were observed later in the transition to parenthood. In a longitudinal study, Trillingsgaard et al. (2014) found that the patterns of communication that future parents self-reported at 6 months postpartum (i.e., whether they engaged in or avoided discussion and shared their feelings and whether each of them proposed solutions or compromised) were even more reliable predictors of changes in relationship satisfaction at 30 months postpartum than other well-documented predictors of relationship functioning, such as depressive and anxiety symptoms and short length of relationship. In fact, their results support the idea that these predictors of change in relationship satisfaction most likely work additively to influence relationship functioning.

In a qualitative study of the changes in sexual functioning experienced by new fathers, MacAdam et al. (2011) showed that some men, during the postpartum period, felt a growing discrepancy between their and their partner's sexual desire, but these particular men also reported showing understanding and acceptance toward their partner and did not associate this discrepancy with more conflicts. Indeed, new fathers in this study underscored the importance of open communication to prevent potential relationship problems and felt that communication helped improve their sexual satisfaction (MacAdam et al., 2011).

Parenting-Specific Variables

Bäckström et al.'s prospective study (2018) revealed that future mothers who believed that their partners experienced more positive feelings about fatherhood during pregnancy reported higher relationship satisfaction in the postpartum period. Similarly, Gallegos et al. (2020) found that mothers who perceived their partner's parenting as more positive when the baby reached eight months experienced lower levels of hostility in their relationship by the child's second birthday. Mothers' evaluation of the couple's coparenting quality has also been associated with various domains of sexual satisfaction, such as romance, passion, and global sexual satisfaction, meaning that when mothers reported a more positive coparenting relationship with their partner, they also tended to be more satisfied sexually (Maas et al., 2018).

Greater parental self-efficacy – that is, a sense of being competent in the role of parent, feeling self-fulfilled as a parent, and deriving self-worth from caring for a child – was generally found to protect parents' relational dynamics and stability during the transition to parenthood. Fillo et al. (2015) found that, in general, higher levels of childcare self-efficacy shielded new parents from experiencing a decrease in relationship satisfaction during the first two years of parenthood, and that this was independent from parents' relative contribution to childcare. On the contrary, deriving lower self-efficacy from childcare was associated with a greater decline in relationship satisfaction during that same period, and this effect was particularly strong among new fathers with a high contribution to childcare.

Advances, Limitations, and Future Research

Over the past decade, interest in fathers' experience and adjustment to the transition to parenthood has continued to grow. More research than ever has been conducted on both partners' relationship satisfaction across the transition to parenthood, which has helped provide a better understanding of fathers' experiences and of the interrelationships between maternal and paternal relational dimensions. However, research on sexual functioning specifically continues to be dominated by maternal literature. Despite the experience of fathers and dyadic dimensions slowly gaining more attention in that area of research, more consideration is needed to better understand how the transition to parenthood influences their sexual functioning and the mutual influences that occur within the couple.

The literature on the transition to parenthood also remains largely dominated by studies conducted on heterosexual individuals and couples. As in other domains in psychology and in research in general, studies in this area have mainly been conducted in the United States and other high-income Western countries with samples of participants who mainly identify as White and whose primary language is English. Similarly, despite the fact that a growing number of individuals are forming families outside the traditional boundaries of marriage, most research is based on samples of married biological parents. This lack of diversity among research participants limits the generalization of study results, thus impeding the social and clinical implications of research and preventing some groups of individuals from benefiting from knowledge that comes from this research. Therefore, researchers should aim to update their methods of recruitment to enroll participants who reflect the diversity of populations, notably in terms of racial and ethnic backgrounds, gender identity, and sexual orientations.

Although it is widely acknowledged that relationship and sexual functioning are closely related, the two research domains remain largely distinct. However, a number of studies that include both sexual and relational satisfaction have been published in recent decades. This practice should be maintained and reinforced in the future.

Research on relationship and sexual functioning across the transition to parenthood focuses almost exclusively on individual-level or couple-level characteristics. However, it can be argued that the cultural context in which the partners evolve and negotiate the arrival of a firstborn could play a role in their adaptation process. Cultural values, social norms, and the availability of various publicly funded programs vary greatly among countries. These macrolevel characteristics could very well influence how partners negotiate the transition to parenthood. However, we know little about how political, economic, and cultural contexts can influence new parents' transitions. Studies with a cross-national scope that compare the relationship and sexual functioning of samples from different countries could help increase our knowledge of how macrolevel mechanisms influence microlevel functioning during one of the most critical life changes.

Conclusion

Relationship and sexual satisfaction are not stable over time and evolve with life circumstances and events. It is widely acknowledged that the transition to parenthood is one of the most significant and life-changing events for both women and men. However, a paradox emerges with the arrival of a first child, as it brings joy and feelings of accomplishment and pride but also a host of new challenges that can be detrimental to the balance of the new parents' relationship. As documented in the reviewed literature, the transition to parenthood can present a challenge to relationship and sexual satisfaction. In the past decade, efforts have been made to dig deeper and investigate the well-established finding that, on average, new parents experience declines in relationship satisfaction with the transition to parenthood. It has been found that relationship functioning remained relatively stable for most couples and that average declines were driven by a minority of mothers and fathers who experienced steeper declines. Researchers have tried to identify who experiences greater declines and which personal and relational characteristics act as protective or risk factors during this period. They have documented multiple cross-domain factors related to relationship trajectories across the transition period, including personal and partner characteristics, relational context, and parenting-specific variables. It can be argued that couples who cumulate multiple risk factors are more likely not only to experience relational challenges across the transition to parenthood but also to lead more vulnerable families.

In sum, welcoming a first child represents a unique developmental phase within the life cycle of a family, which holds the power to change relationship dynamics among couples. However, because of considerable individual differences in terms of how new parents experience this transition, it would be misleading to define it as a major universal stressor. Despite the fact that the research conducted in the past decade has greatly advanced our general understanding of romantic relationships during this crucial period of development, significant work is still needed to understand how the transition to parenthood is experienced among a diversified population of new parents.

References

American Psychological Association. (2022). *Postpartum depression: Causes, symptoms, risk factors, and treatment options*. Retrieved December 21, 2022, from www.apa.org/topics/women-girls/postpartum-depression

Bäckström, C., Kåreholt, I., Thorstensson, S., Golsäter, M., & Mårtensson, L. B. (2018). Quality of couple relationship among first-time mothers and partners, during pregnancy and the first six months of parenthood. *Sexual & Reproductive Healthcare, 17*, 56–64. https://doi.org/10.1016/j.srhc.2018.07.001

Baldoni, F., Giannotti, M., Casu, G., Luperini, V., & Spelzini, F. (2020). A dyadic study on perceived stress and couple adjustment during pregnancy: The mediating role of depressive symptoms. *Journal of Family Issues, 41*(11), 1935–1955. https://doi.org/10.1177/0192513X20934834

Chong, A., & Mickelson, K. D. (2016). Perceived fairness and relationship satisfaction during the transition to parenthood: The mediating role of spousal support. *Journal of Family Issues, 37*(1), 3–28. https://doi.org/10.1177/0192513X13516764

Cohen, M. J., Pentel, K. Z., Boeding, S. E., & Baucom, D. H. (2019). Postpartum role satisfaction in couples: Associations with individual and relationship well-being. *Journal of Family Issues, 40*(9), 1181–1200. https://doi.org/10.1177/0192513X19835866

Dawson, S. J., Strickland, N. J., & Rosen, N. O. (2022). Longitudinal associations between depressive symptoms and postpartum sexual concerns among first-time parent couples. *The Journal of Sex Research, 59*(2), 150–159. https://doi.org/10.1080/00224499.2020.1836114

Delicate, A., Ayers, S., Easter, A., & McMullen, S. (2018). The impact of childbirth-related post-traumatic stress on a couple's relationship: A systematic review and meta-synthesis. *Journal of Reproductive and Infant Psychology, 36*(1), 102–115. https://doi.org/10.1080/02646838.2017.1397270

Don, B. P., Eller, J., Simpson, J. A., Fredrickson, B. L., Algoe, S. B., Rholes, W. S., & Mickelson, K. D. (2022). New parental positivity: The role of positive emotions in promoting relational adjustment during the transition to parenthood. *Journal of Personality and Social Psychology, 123*, 84–106. https://doi.org/10.1037/pspi0000371

Don, B. P., & Mickelson, K. D. (2014). Relationship satisfaction trajectories across the transition to parenthood among low-risk parents. *Journal of Marriage and Family, 76*(3), 677–692. https://doi.org/10.1111/jomf.12111

Doss, B. D., & Rhoades, G. K. (2017). The transition to parenthood: Impact on couples' romantic relationships. *Current Opinion in Psychology, 13*, 25–28. https://doi.org/10.1016/j.copsyc.2016.04.003

Figueiredo, B., Canário, C., Tendais, I., Pinto, T. M., Kenny, D. A., & Field, T. (2018). Couples' relationship affects mothers' and fathers' anxiety and depression trajectories over the transition to parenthood. *Journal of Affective Disorders, 238*, 204–212. https://doi.org/10.1016/j.jad.2018.05.064

Fillo, J., Simpson, J. A., Rholes, W. S., & Kohn, J. L. (2015). Dads doing diapers: Individual and relational outcomes associated with the division of childcare across the transition to parenthood. *Journal of Personality and Social Psychology, 108*(2), 298–316. https://doi.org/10.1037/a0038572

Gagné, A.-L., Brassard, A., Bécotte, K., Lessard, I., Lafontaine, M.-F., & Péloquin, K. (2021). Associations between romantic attachment and sexual satisfaction through intimacy and couple support among pregnant couples. *European Review of Applied Psychology, 71*(3), 100622. https://doi.org/10.1016/j.erap.2020.100622

Gallegos, M. I., Jacobvitz, D. B., & Hazen, N. L. (2020). Marital interaction quality over the transition to parenthood: The role of parents' perceptions of spouses' parenting. *Journal of Family Psychology, 34*(6), 766–772. https://doi.org/10.1037/fam0000656

Garfield, C. F., Simon, C. D., Stephens, F., Castro Román, P., Bryan, M., et al. (2022). Pregnancy risk assessment monitoring system for dads: A piloted randomized trial of public health surveillance of recent fathers' behaviors before and after infant birth. *PLoS One, 17*(1), e0262366. https://doi.org/10.1371/journal.pone.0262366

Garthus-Niegel, S., Horsch, A., Handtke, E., von Soest, T., Ayers, S., Weidner, K., & Eberhard-Gran, M. (2018). The impact of postpartum posttraumatic stress and depression symptoms on couples' relationship satisfaction: A population-based prospective study. *Frontiers in Psychology, 9*. www.frontiersin.org/article/10.3389/fpsyg.2018.01728

Grekin, R., & O'Hara, M. W. (2014). Prevalence and risk factors of postpartum posttraumatic stress disorder: A meta-analysis. *Clinical Psychology Review, 34*, 389–401. http://dx.doi.org/10.1016/j.cpr.2014.05.003

Hiekel, N., & Ivanova, K. (2022). Changes in perceived fairness of division of household labor across parenthood transitions: Whose relationship Satisfaction is impacted? *Journal of Family Issues, 44*(4), 1046–1073. https://doi.org/10.1177/0192513X211055119

Huss, B., & Pollmann-Schult, M. (2020). Relationship satisfaction across the transition to parenthood: The impact of conflict behavior. *Journal of Family Issues, 41*(3), 383–411. https://doi.org/10.1177/0192513X19876084

Keizer, R., & Schenk, N. (2012). Becoming a parent and relationship satisfaction: A longitudinal dyadic perspective. *Journal of Marriage and Family*, 74(4), 759–773. https://doi.org/10.1111/j.1741-3737.2012.00991.x

Khalesi, Z. B., Bokaie, M., & Attari, S. M. (2018). Effect of pregnancy on sexual function of couples. *African Health Sciences*, 18(2), 227–234. https://doi.org/10.4314/ahs.v18i2.5

Le, Y., McDaniel, B. T., Leavitt, C. E., & Feinberg, M. E. (2016). Longitudinal associations between relationship quality and coparenting across the transition to parenthood: A dyadic perspective. *Journal of Family Psychology*, 30(8), 918–926. https://doi.org/10.1037/fam0000217

Leonhardt, N. D., Rosen, N. O., Dawson, S. J., Kim, J. J., Johnson, M. D., & Impett, E. A. (2022). Relationship satisfaction and commitment in the transition to parenthood: A couple-centered approach. *Journal of Marriage and Family*, 84(1), 80–100. https://doi.org/10.1111/jomf.12785

Lévesque, S., Bisson, V., Fernet, M., & Charton, L. (2021). A study of the transition to parenthood: New parents' perspectives on their sexual intimacy during the perinatal period. *Sexual and Relationship Therapy*, 36(2–3), 238-255. https://doi.org/10.1080/14681994.2019.1675870

Maas, M. K., McDaniel, B. T., Feinberg, M. E., & Jones, D. E. (2018). Division of labor and multiple domains of sexual satisfaction among first-time parents. *Journal of Family Issues*, 39(1), 104–127. https://doi.org/10.1177/0192513X15604343

MacAdam, R., Huuva, E., & Berterö, C. (2011). Fathers' experiences after having a child: Sexuality becomes tailored according to circumstances. *Midwifery*, 27(5), e149–e155. https://doi.org/10.1016/j.midw.2009.12.007

McDonald, E., Woolhouse, H., & Brown, S. J. (2017). Sexual pleasure and emotional satisfaction in the first 18 months after childbirth | Elsevier Enhanced Reader. *Midwifery*, 55, 60–66. http://doi.org/10.1016/j.midw.2017.09.002

Mitnick, D., Heyman, R., & Slep, A. (2009). Changes in relationship satisfaction across the transition to parenthood : A meta-analysis. *Journal of Family Psychology*, 23, 848-852. https://doi.org/10.1037/a0017004

Muise, A., Kim, J. J., Impett, E. A., & Rosen, N. O. (2017). Understanding when a partner is not in the mood: Sexual communal strength in couples transitioning to parenthood. *Archives of Sexual Behavior*, 46(7), 1993–2006. https://doi.org/10.1007/s10508-016-0920-2

Newkirk, K., Perry-Jenkins, M., & Sayer, A. G. (2017). Division of household and childcare labor and relationship conflict among low-income new parents. *Sex Roles*, 76(5–6), 319–333. https://doi.org/10.1007/s11199-016-0604-3

Opperman, E., Benson, L., & Milhausen, R. (2013). Confirmatory factor analysis of the female sexual function index. *The Journal of Sex Research*, 50(1), 29–36. https://doi.org/10.1080/00224499.2011.628423

Ramsdell, E. L., Franz, M., & Brock, R. L. (2020). A multifaceted and dyadic examination of intimate relationship quality during pregnancy: Implications for global relationship satisfaction. *Family Process*, 59(2), 556–570. https://doi.org/10.1111/famp.12424

Redshaw, M., & Martin, C. (2014). The couple relationship before and during transition to parenthood. *Journal of Reproductive and Infant Psychology*, 32(2), 109–111. https://doi.org/10.1080/02646838.2014.896146

Reis, H. T., & Clark, M. S. (2013). Responsiveness. In J. A. Simpson & L. Campbell (Eds.), *The Oxford handbook of close relationships*. Oxford Academic. https://doi.org/10.1093/oxfordhb/9780195398694.013.0018

Rosen, N. O., Bailey, K., & Muise, A. (2018). Degree and direction of sexual desire discrepancy are linked to sexual and relationship satisfaction in couples transitioning to parenthood. *The Journal of Sex Research*, 55(2), 214-225. https://doi.org/10.1080/00224499.2017.1321732

Rosen, N. O., Dawson, S. J., Leonhardt, N. D., Vannier, S. A., & Impett, E. A. (2021). Trajectories of sexual well-being among couples in the transition to parenthood. *Journal of Family Psychology*, 35(4), 523-533. https://doi.org/10.1037/fam0000689

Rosen, N. O., Mooney, K., & Muise, A. (2017). Dyadic empathy predicts sexual and relationship well-being in couples transitioning to parenthood. *Journal of Sex & Marital Therapy*, 43, 543–559. https://doi.org/10.1080/0092623X.2016.1208698

Rosen, N. O., Williams, L., Vannier, S. A., & Mackinnon, S. P. (2020). Sexual intimacy in first-time mothers: Associations with sexual and relationship satisfaction across three waves. *Archives of Sexual Behavior*, 49(8), 2849–2861. https://doi.org/10.1007/s10508-020-01667-1

Sagiv-Reiss, D. M., Birnbaum, G. E., & Safir, M. P. (2012). Changes in sexual experiences and relationship quality during pregnancy. *Archives of Sexual Behavior*, 41(5), 1241–1251. https://doi.org/10.1007/s10508-011-9839-9

Smallen, D., Eller, J., Rholes, W. S., & Simpson, J. A. (2022). Perceptions of partner responsiveness across the transition to parenthood. *Journal of Family Psychology*, 36(4), 618–629. https://doi.org/10.1037/fam0000907

Tach, L. M., & Halpern-Meekin, S. (2012). Marital quality and divorce decisions: How do premarital cohabitation and nonmarital childbearing matter? *Family Relations*, 61(4), 571–585. https://doi.org/10.1111/j.1741-3729.2012.00724.x

Ter Kuile, H., Kluwer, E. S., Finkenauer, C., & Van Der Lippe, T. (2017). Predicting adaptation to parenthood: The role of responsiveness, gratitude, and trust. *Personal Relationships*, 24(3), 663–682. https://doi.org/10.1111/pere.12202

Ter Kuile, H., van der Lippe, T., & Kluwer, E. S. (2021). Relational processes as predictors of relationship satisfaction trajectories across the transition to parenthood. *Family Relations*, 70(4), 1238–1252. https://doi.org/10.1111/fare.12546

Trillingsgaard, T., Baucom, K. J. W., & Heyman, R. E. (2014). Predictors of change in relationship satisfaction during the transition to parenthood. *Family Relations*, 63(5), 667–679. https://doi.org/10.1111/fare.12089

Twenge, J., Campbell, W. K., & Foster, C. (2004). Parenthood and marital satisfaction: A meta-analytic review. *Journal of Marriage and Family*, 65, 574-583. https://doi.org/10.1111/j.1741-3737.2003.00574.x

Vannier, S. A., Adare, K. E., & Rosen, N. O. (2018). Is it me or you? First-time mothers' attributions for postpartum sexual concerns are associated with sexual and relationship satisfaction in the transition to parenthood. *Journal of Social and Personal Relationships*, 35(4), 577-599. https://doi.org/10.1177/0265407517743086

Yavorsky, J. E., Kamp Dush, C. M., & Schoppe-Sullivan, S. J. (2015). The production of inequality: The gender division of labor across the transition to parenthood. *Journal of Marriage and Family*, 77(3), 662–679. https://doi.org/10.1111/jomf.12189

5

BREASTFEEDING AND PERINATAL MENTAL HEALTH

Kathleen Kendall-Tackett

This chapter summarizes research showing the complex interplay between breastfeeding and mothers' mental health. Breastfeeding is far more than a method of feeding; it is a complex relational system that alters mothers' physiology. When breastfeeding is going well, it protects their physical and mental health. This chapter provides a rationale for why breastfeeding should be part of postpartum mental health care and offers suggestions on how mental health providers can support mothers who want to continue breastfeeding while they are being treated.

Key Findings Regarding Breastfeeding and Postpartum Mental Health

Breastfeeding is usually described solely as a method of feeding babies with "superior" food. That statement is true but incomplete; breastfeeding is far more than a way to feed babies. It triggers a complex matrix of hormones in the mother and the baby that other methods of feeding do not provide. Some of these effects can be replicated by formula-feeding babies skin-to-skin. Researchers studying Kangaroo Mother Care, for example, have found that, when mothers and babies are in skin-to-skin contact after birth, mothers' and babies' stress hormones immediately drop (Handlin et al., 2009). The downside is that interventions such as Kangaroo Care must be consciously applied (as opposed to built into breastfeeding) and cannot completely mimic the oxytocin release that mothers and babies experience when babies suckle at the breast.

Every breastfeeding session lowers mothers' stress levels and helps them cope with the demands of new motherhood (Heinrichs et al., 2001; Uvnas-Moberg et al., 2020). Over time, repeated breastfeeding, and its stress-lowering effects, leads to a lifetime lower risk for heart disease and diabetes (Schwartz et al., 2009). These same physiological processes also affect mental health. In short, breastfeeding mothers and babies are an integral unit, and things that are good for babies are also good for mothers and help, rather than harm, their mental health. Although one can mimic some of the effects of breastfeeding, and that is a good thing to do, I make the case that breastfeeding is worth preserving in mothers seen in clinical settings. It is possible to support both breastfeeding and mothers' mental health. The following are three key points regarding breastfeeding and mental health that frame the discussion in this chapter.

DOI: 10.4324/9781003206903-7

It Is Important to Respect Mothers' Breastfeeding Goals

Mental health providers often tell mothers to stop breastfeeding to "protect their mental health," with the rationale being that breastfeeding causes too much stress. Mental health providers may not directly tell mothers to wean, but they will give advice that, if followed, will lead to early weaning (example: telling mothers not to breastfeed at night). Unfortunately, although this advice is well-intentioned, telling mothers to wean, or to "cut back," is counterproductive and increases the risk of the very mental health problems they seek to avoid. When mothers do not meet their breastfeeding goals, they are more likely to become depressed. In the Avon Longitudinal Study of Parents and Children (ALSPAC) study of 14,541 pregnancies in the United Kingdom, women who intended to breastfeed and did had the lowest rates of depression. Conversely, *women who wanted to breastfeed and did not, or stopped early, had the highest rates* (Borra et al., 2015).

These findings parallel population studies showing that early breastfeeding cessation increased the risk of depression. For example, a study using U.S. PRAMS[1] data from 31 sites (N = 32,659) found that women with the highest rate of depression were those who breastfed for less than eight weeks (15.6%), compared to those who never breastfed (14%) and those who breastfed more than eight weeks (11.8%) (Bauman et al., 2020). A study of 1,037 women from Crete also found that breastfeeding for less than eight weeks was associated with an increased risk of depression (Koutra et al., 2018).

According to Brown (2019), mental health providers often miss the significance of mothers' desire to breastfeed and what happens when they are not able to do it. If mothers wanted to breastfeed and could not, they often experienced significant grief and depression. Brown (2018) found that women's negative feelings were not because others told them to breastfeed and made them feel guilty. Rather, women's negative feelings were because they had wanted to breastfeed, and for whatever reason (e.g., bad advice, lack of support, a physical problem), they were not able to do so.

Breastfeeding Protects Mental Health

Beyond mothers' goals and desires, breastfeeding triggers a physiological response that protects women's mental health. Mothers who exclusively breastfeed are less likely to get depressed, and, if they do get depressed, it is often less severe relative to women who do not (Figueiredo et al., 2021; Hahn-Holbrook et al., 2013; Oyentunji & Chandra, 2020). Some have asked me how can we know that it is *breastfeeding*, and not something else, that lowers the risk of depression. One argument that breastfeeding only appears to lower rates of depression is because people who are depressed are less likely to breastfeed and have self-selected into a nonbreastfeeding group. That is a valid point that must be addressed by the research design in studies. With a cross-sectional survey, one cannot tell whether breastfeeding protects maternal mental health. Only a prospective study can answer that question.

With a prospective design, researchers measure depression before the study begins, ensuring that nondepressed mothers are in both breastfeeding and bottle-feeding groups. By time 2, if mothers in the bottle-feeding group are more depressed than those in the breastfeeding group, researchers can conclude that the feeding method did indeed influence mothers' mental health over time. Three prospective studies on feeding methods and mental health demonstrate that breastfeeding lowers the risk of depression or lessens symptoms in mothers who are already depressed.

The first study included 2,072 mothers in Sabah, Malaysia. Using the *Edinburgh Postnatal Depression Scale* (EPDS; Cox et al., 1987), the researchers measured depression at 36 to 38 weeks' gestation and 3 months postpartum (Yusuff et al., 2016). At 3 months postpartum, exclusively breastfeeding mothers had significantly lower EPDS scores than nonbreastfeeding mothers. Second, a California study included 205 new mothers who were assessed prenatally and at 3, 6, 12, and 24 months postpartum (Hahn-Holbrook et al., 2013). Women breastfeeding nine times a day at 3 months (exclusive breastfeeding) had significantly lower depression at 24 months than those who breastfed four times a day (mixed feeding). Finally, a prospective study of 334 mothers from Portugal included 70 mothers who were depressed during their pregnancies and 264 mothers who were not depressed (Figueiredo et al., 2021). The mothers were assessed in the third trimester of pregnancy and at 3 to 6 months postpartum. If women were depressed during pregnancy, exclusive breastfeeding lessened their symptoms and led to lower rates of depression between 3 and 6 months postpartum. However, exclusive breastfeeding did not lower the risk of depression for the 197 women who were not depressed when the study began.

All three studies found that only *exclusive* breastfeeding protected mental health. Partial or mixed breastfeeding provides short-term benefits for mothers and babies (Handlin et al., 2009; Heinrichs et al., 2001; Uvnas-Moberg et al., 2020), but, *in terms of mental health protection,* mixed feeding does not differ significantly from formula-feeding (Kendall-Tackett et al., 2011, 2018b). Similar findings come from the sleep literature. These studies also found that exclusive breastfeeding protects mental health, whereas mixed feeding does not (Dorheim et al., 2009a; Kendall-Tackett et al., 2011). Taken together, these studies suggest that there is something physiologically unique about exclusive breastfeeding compared to mixed- or partial breastfeeding.

Depression, Anxiety, and Posttraumatic Stress Disorder Are Direct Threats to Breastfeeding

Whereas breastfeeding lowers the risk of mental health issues, women's mental health issues can cause women to wean early or never start.

Depression and Breastfeeding Cessation

Hahn-Holbrook et al. (2013) found that mothers who were depressed during their pregnancies were less likely to breastfeed and weaned an average of 2.3 months earlier than nondepressed mothers. Similarly, a prospective cohort study of first-time mothers from Australia found that when mothers were depressed at 3 months postpartum, they were significantly less likely to be breastfeeding at 6 months compared to nondepressed mothers (49% vs. 61%) (Woolhouse et al., 2016). In a study of 34 Latinas, those who had postpartum depression and anxiety, and prenatal depression, were more likely to stop breastfeeding by 8 weeks than the nondepressed women (Lara-Cinisomo et al., 2017). These researchers found lower oxytocin levels in the women who were depressed and stopped breastfeeding by 8 weeks, relative to nondepressed women.

Anxiety and Breastfeeding Cessation

Women with depression and anxiety introduced formula and stopped breastfeeding earlier than women without symptoms in another recent study (Stuebe et al., 2019). The sample included 222 mother–infant dyads in late pregnancy, 87 women with current depression or anxiety, 64 women with a history of depression or anxiety, and 71 with no psychiatric history. A systematic review of 33 studies found that women with postpartum anxiety were less likely to initiate breastfeeding and more likely to supplement in the hospital than women without postpartum anxiety (Fallon et al., 2016). Anxiety also reduced breastfeeding self-efficacy, which predicts the duration of breastfeeding.

Two more recent studies had similar findings. Using data from a sample of 412 women who participated in a longitudinal pregnancy cohort study, researchers found that for every one-unit increase in pregnancy-specific anxiety in the first or third trimester of pregnancy, there was a 5% to 6% reduction in the odds of exclusive breastfeeding at 6 to 8 weeks postpartum (Horsely et al., 2019). A prospective study of 229 women from Chile found that depression during pregnancy was associated with nonexclusive breastfeeding at 3 months postpartum (Coo et al., 2020). However, women who were exclusively breastfeeding at 3 months were more likely to still be breastfeeding at 6 months relative to women who were not exclusively breastfeeding.

Posttraumatic Stress Disorder and Breastfeeding Cessation

Traumatic childbirth and posttraumatic stress disorder (PTSD) lowered breastfeeding self-efficacy at 3 months postpartum in a prospective longitudinal study of 102 Turkish women (Turkmen et al., 2020). In a sample of 1,480 women from the Akershus Birth Cohort study, women with postpartum PTSD were 6 times less likely to initiate breastfeeding and continue for 12 months compared to women without postpartum PTSD (Garthus-Niegel, Horsch, Ayers, et al., 2018). The authors emphasized the importance of screening new mothers for PTSD, which is usually not done. A systematic review of 26 samples found that maternal PTSD is associated with lower rates of breastfeeding and a negative impact on mother–infant interaction compared to women without PTSD (Cook et al., 2018).

A survey of 1,611 mothers who gave birth during COVID restrictions was compared with a matched control group of 640 women who gave birth prior to COVID (Mayopoulos et al., 2021). The mothers were matched on demographic factors and prior mental health issues or trauma. The goal was to determine the unique contribution of COVID to their experiences. The researchers found more acute stress in the COVID group, with significantly more childbirth-related PTSD, less mother–infant bonding, and more breastfeeding difficulties.

Inflammation: The Underlying Physiology of Depression, Anxiety, and PTSD

Many practitioners do not understand why breastfeeding provides many health benefits for mothers. We usually only describe the "benefits of breastfeeding" in terms of babies' health so that we think that there are no effects beyond the psychosocial ones (i.e., able to call themselves "breastfeeding mothers"). Psychosocial effects are important, but there is so much more. Breastfeeding protects women's physical and mental health because it directly acts on the stress system. The stress response is the physiological reaction that underlies depression and most other mental health conditions (Bergink et al., 2014; Kendall-Tackett, 2007; Kiecolt-Glaser et al., 2015). Breastfeeding helps because it dampers the stress response.

The Stress Response

The stress response is designed to protect us when we are physically or psychologically threatened. It is meant to be an acute response but causes problems when it is chronically activated. The stress response has three main components (Kendall-Tackett, 2023; Kim & Ahn, 2015).

Catecholamine Response

The catecholamine response triggers the sympathetic nervous system and causes the fight-or-flight response. As the name implies, it is designed to help a person flee danger or fight their way out of it. In response to threat or danger, three neurotransmitters— norepinephrine, epinephrine, and dopamine—are released. The neurotransmitter most people associate with the stress response is epinephrine, which is also known as adrenaline.

HPA Axis

The hypothalamic–pituitary–adrenal (HPA) axis also responds to threats with a cascade response between three systems. The hypothalamus starts this process by releasing corticotrophin-releasing hormone/factor (CRH/F), which causes the pituitary to release adrenocorticotrophin hormone (ACTH), which then causes the adrenal cortex to release cortisol, a glucocorticoid. CRH, ACTH, and cortisol are all considered stress hormones.

Inflammatory Response System

In response to threats, our bodies also increase inflammation via molecules called proinflammatory cytokines. Cytokines are proteins that regulate immune response. If our bodies anticipate that we might be wounded, they increase inflammation because proinflammatory cytokines have two important functions: fighting infection and healing wounds.

The role of inflammation in depression is well-established (Kiecolt-Glaser, 2009; Maes, 2001; Maes & Smith, 1998). Inflammation causes depression (i.e., when there are high levels of proinflammatory cytokines, people are more likely to get depressed), and depression increases inflammation. Inflammation is also the physiological process underlying anxiety, PTSD, and other psychiatric conditions, such as bipolar disorders and postpartum psychosis (Bergink et al., 2014; Beurel et al., 2020; Kohler et al., 2016). The proinflammatory cytokines that researchers identified most consistently as being elevated in depression are interleukin-1β (IL-1), interleukin-6 (IL-6), and tumor necrosis factor-alpha (TNFα) (Kiecolt-Glaser et al., 2015; Maes et al., 2009).

Inflammation levels can be 40% to 50% higher in depressed people than in their non-depressed counterparts (Berk et al., 2013). One recent study found that increased inflammation is caused by increases in the rates of depression, anxiety, obsessive-compulsive symptoms, and insomnia (Mazza et al., 2020).

All types of physical and psychological stressors increase inflammation (Finy & Christian, 2018; Kiecolt-Glaser et al., 2015). Although the sources and types of stressors vary, the underlying physiological response to these stressors is the same: an activation of the stress response, including increasing inflammation (Kiecolt-Glaser et al., 2015). The perinatal period is an especially vulnerable time because inflammation levels normally rise significantly during the last trimester of pregnancy, which is also the time when women are at highest risk for depression (Kendall-Tackett, 2017). Moreover, common experiences of new parenthood, such as sleep disturbance, postpartum pain, and psychological trauma, also increase inflammation.

The Anti-Inflammatory Effects of Oxytocin

The hormone oxytocin is necessary for breastfeeding, and breastfeeding increases circulating oxytocin. Oxytocin causes milk ejection and facilitates mother–infant bonding. It is often referred to as "the love hormone." Oxytocin also specifically downregulates the stress response (Uvnas-Moberg et al., 2020) including ACTH, cortisol (Handlin et al., 2009; Heinrichs et al., 2001; Uvnas-Moberg et al., 2020), and inflammation (Ahn & Corwin, 2015; Groer & Kendall-Tackett, 2011). In other words, breastfeeding protects mothers' mental health because it upregulates oxytocin, which downregulates the stress system. Groer et al. noted that breastfeeding's downregulation of the stress response is a survival advantage because it facilitates milk production, energy conservation, and attachment to the baby (Groer et al., 2002).

Unfortunately, stress can downregulate oxytocin, which increases mothers' risk of both breastfeeding and mental health problems. In the next section, I describe some common stressors that occur in the postpartum period. Interestingly, research on some of these stressors provides further insights into why breastfeeding protects mental health.

Risk Factors for Depression and Their Relation to Breastfeeding

Stressors that increase inflammation, and therefore the risk of mental health disorders, can be physical or psychological. Three categories of stressors are particularly common for new mothers: sleep disturbance, pain, and psychological trauma.

Sleep Disturbance

Disturbed sleep is perhaps the most daunting challenge for new parents. Not surprisingly, depression and sleep are intimately related, and the association is bidirectional: sleep disturbances can cause depression, and depression causes sleep disturbances (Bhatti & Richards, 2015; Saxbe et al., 2016). A systematic review of 13 studies found a strong association between sleep disturbance and postpartum depression (Bhatti & Richards, 2015). A longitudinal study of 711 low-income, racially diverse couples clearly showed the bidirectional relationship between sleep and depression, with their examination of causal pathways linking sleep to postpartum depression over the first year (Saxbe et al., 2016). They found that depressive symptoms at 1-month postpartum predicted sleep problems at 6 months, which predicted depressive symptoms at 6 to 12 months. Anxiety and PTSD also impair sleep, although studies with postpartum women are lacking. Sleep disruptions can increase inflammation in postpartum women. In a study of 479 new mothers, 5 hours of sleep or less per night at 1 year postpartum was associated with higher IL-6 at 3 years postpartum (Taveras et al., 2011).

Exclusive Breastfeeding Protects Sleep

Like many people, I once assumed that mothers who exclusively breastfeed got less sleep and were more tired than their mixed- or formula-feeding counterparts. In fact, in one article, I openly wondered why exclusively breastfeeding mothers were at lower risk for depression considering they got less sleep (Kendall-Tackett, 2007). It did not make sense to me. Subsequent research addressed this conundrum, and it surprised many of us. Exclusively breastfeeding mothers actually get more sleep, and all the other measures of well-being, including daily fatigue and depression, were consistent with what they reported (Doan et al., 2007; Dorheim et al., 2009a; Kendall-Tackett et al., 2011).

Exclusive breastfeeding helps even immediately after birth. A study of 30 women at 48 hours postpartum examined their total sleep time while in the hospital (Hughes et al., 2018). Overall, the mothers slept an average of 9.7 hours in the first 48 hours postpartum. Exclusively breastfeeding mothers slept 2.6 hours longer than those who bottle-fed. The authors concluded that exclusive breastfeeding promotes maternal sleep, even in challenging circumstances.

Trauma survivors also benefit from the effects of exclusive breastfeeding on sleep. In our sample of 6,410 new mothers, 994 women reported that they had been raped (Kendall-Tackett et al., 2013). Not surprisingly, when sexual assault was examined by itself, it had a pervasive negative effect on all sleep variables. However, when sexual assault status was combined with the feeding method (exclusive vs. nonexclusive), exclusively breastfeeding mothers reported more total sleep time and fewer minutes to get to sleep than assaulted mothers who were mixed- or formula-feeding. Sexual assault still affected them, but, for those who were exclusively breastfeeding, the effects were significantly lessened.

Sleep Parameters and Mental Health

To understand why exclusive breastfeeding makes a difference, it is instructive to look at two sleep parameters that predict postpartum depression: self-reported total sleep time and minutes to get to sleep (Dorheim et al., 2009b). Mothers who have shorter self-reported total sleep time and/or take more than 25 minutes to fall asleep are at higher risk for depression relative to women who go to sleep in 20 minutes or less. The feeding method influences both. Mothers who exclusively breastfeed take fewer minutes to get to sleep, which likely results in a longer total sleep time. That lowers their risk of depression (Doan et al., 2007; Dorheim et al., 2009a; Kendall-Tackett et al., 2011).

Feeding and sleep are so intertwined that mother–infant sleep researcher, Dr. James McKenna, coined a new word: *breastsleeping* to describe an intimate relationship between sleep and breastfeeding (McKenna, 2020). Breastsleeping includes a whole constellation of behaviors. When breastfeeding and sleeping near each other, mothers' and babies' sleep cycles synchronize. When sleeping, breastfeeding mothers form a protective C-shape with their bodies around their babies and they sleep facing each other. When formula feeding, mothers do not sync with their babies in the same way. They do not form the protective C, nor do they always face their babies (Ball, 2006; McKenna et al., 2007). McKenna stated that breastfeeding and sleep are so intrinsically related that is impossible to make recommendations about sleep without knowing how that baby is fed.

Sleep location is another important sleep parameter that influences mental health. We found that where a baby sleeps directly influenced depression, anxiety, and anger/irritability. We examined the interaction of the feeding method by sleep location (bed-sharing vs. in another room) (Kendall-Tackett et al., 2018a). Mothers who exclusively breastfed had lower depressive symptoms regardless of the baby's sleep location. However, bedsharing when mothers were not exclusively breastfeeding turned out to be a very bad idea. Mothers who were bedsharing but not exclusively breastfeeding had the *highest* levels of anxiety and anger/irritability. In contrast, mothers who were bedsharing and exclusively breastfeeding had the lowest levels of both anxiety and anger/irritability.

Supplementation Can Harm Rather Than Help Mothers' Sleep

It is important to note that *all* the mothers in our study, regardless of feeding method, were tired. The postpartum period is challenging, and breastfeeding does not change that. However, does supplementing make mothers less fatigued? No, as mothers who supplement report even more fatigue than those who breastfeed exclusively. In other words, advising mothers to supplement so that they can "get some rest" actually increases their fatigue, which increases their risk of depression. Doan et al. (2007) noted the following:

> Using supplementation as a coping strategy for minimizing sleep loss can actually be detrimental . . . maintenance of breastfeeding, as well as deep restorative sleep stages, may be greatly compromised for new mothers who cope with infant feeding by supplementing in an effort to get more sleep time.
>
> *(p. 201)*

As practitioners, we can work with rather than against the feeding method. If an exclusively breastfeeding mother is very fatigued, we can address that without resorting to supplementing. They may be tired because they have no help, they have anemia or a low-grade infection, or they have developed postpartum hypothyroidism. One mother with whom I worked had her baby sleep clearly across her room. Every time the baby woke, she needed to get completely out of bed to get to her baby. It was exhausting for her and was easily fixed by moving the baby to be closer to her bed. Providers should not assume that the problem is always due to breastfeeding, but, instead, they should ask some questions about why she is tired and where her baby is sleeping. There may be other changes that she can make that will help, or there may be a medical issue that needs to be addressed. Furthermore, if she is bedsharing when not exclusively breastfeeding, she should consider having the baby near but not sharing a bed.

Pain

Pain is another risk factor for depression and other mental health issues because it activates the stress system; the body believes it is being attacked. That is a normal response. Pain indicates that something is wrong.

Breastfeeding Pain

Unfortunately, breast and nipple pain is shockingly common for mothers in the early weeks of breastfeeding. (These numbers shock me because nipple pain is usually easy to address.

I am amazed when practitioners ignore it.) In two studies, more than half of new mothers reported nipple pain at 5 weeks (McGovern et al., 2006) and 2 months postpartum (Ansara et al., 2005). Not surprisingly, nipple pain can also cause postpartum depression. In a study of 2,586 women in the United States, nipple pain at day 1, week 1, and week 2 was associated with depression at 2 months postpartum (Watkins et al., 2011).

When it comes to breast and nipple pain, some of my colleagues can be quite blasé. Mothers have told me that practitioners have said, "that should get better in a few weeks." That is quite negligent. Although postpartum pain, such as breast and nipple pain, is *common* (i.e., it happens a lot), it is *not normal* and should never be ignored. If breasts or nipples are painful, we need to figure out why and address it quickly to protect the mother's physical and mental well-being.

Interestingly, in the Watkins et al. (2011) study, if the mothers received breastfeeding help, that help protected mothers' mental health, even when they had moderate to severe pain. The anti-inflammatory effect of oxytocin explains this finding. A recent meta-analysis found that social support is anti-inflammatory (Uchino et al., 2018), and we know that social support increases oxytocin (Uvnas-Moberg, 2013, 2015). This suggests that breastfeeding support increased oxytocin and downregulated stress, which lowered the risk of depression (Uvnas-Moberg et al., 2020).

A study of 229 women from Melbourne, Australia, examined whether the high burden of breastfeeding problems (i.e., two or more problems with nipple pain, mastitis, frequent expressing, and over/undersupply) and high burden of physical health problems (i.e., two or more problems with cesarean/perineal pain, back pain, constipation, hemorrhoids, or urinary/bowel incontinence) impacted maternal mental health (Cooklin et al., 2018). They found that, when women experienced breastfeeding problems alone or with comorbid physical health problems, they were more likely to be depressed at 8 weeks. Body pain can also cause depression.

Bodily Pain and Depression

Several studies have examined the link between postpartum body pain and depression. In a study of 1,288 new mothers, mode of delivery (vaginal vs. cesearean) was not related to depression. It was severity of pain: the more severe the pain, the higher the risk of depression. Women's acute pain following birth increased their risk of depression by three times (Eisenach et al., 2008).

An observational study of 72 women assessed during their third trimester and at 3 months postpartum found that women's pain scores at during labor and at 6 weeks predicted depression was scores at 3 months (Lim et al., 2020). For vulnerable women in the sample, the combination of prenatal, labor, and postpartum pain increased the risk of depression at 6 weeks even when the women were satisfied with the labor support and pain management they received. In addition, a study of 645 Danish new mothers demonstrated the co-occurrence of pain and depression. If mothers had pain before pregnancy, they were 3.7 times more likely to have persistent pain by 8 weeks postpartum (Rosseland et al., 2020). Negative birth experiences, mothers' history of depression, and mothers' history of pre-pregnancy pain increased the risk of depression by two to four times at 8 weeks.

Psychological Trauma and Its Relation to Breastfeeding

In general conversation, many people use the term "traumatic" to refer to any negative event. In the clinical sense, however, a traumatic event is defined by the "event criteria"

(Criterion A) in the diagnosis for PTSD in the *Diagnostic and Statistical Manual*, 5th ed-TR (APA, 2022). According to the PTSD criteria from the DSM-5, traumatic events include death or threatened death, actual or threatened serious injury, or actual or threatened sexual violation. The event can be experienced directly, witnessed, or happened to a close friend or relative.

To meet full criteria for PTSD, the person must also have symptoms in four clusters: reexperiencing, avoidance, negative changes in belief or mood, and changes in arousal or reactivity. The symptoms must last for at least for at least one month and cause significant impairment in daily life (American Psychiatric Association, 2013, 2022). A trauma survivor can have symptoms of PTSD without meeting the full criteria for a diagnosis. In addition, PTSD is only one sequela of trauma, but others are more common, including depression, anxiety, insomnia, and somatic complaints (Mazza et al., 2020).

Although mothers can experience a range of traumatic events, the three types that you are most likely to encounter are adverse childhood experiences (ACEs), intimate partner violence (IPV), and birth trauma.

Childhood Abuse and ACEs

ACEs include a range of adversities in childhood: physical and sexual abuse; emotional abuse; neglect (physical and emotional); and witnessing parental IPV, parental mental illness, substance abuse, and criminal activity. These effects are additive. The more types of experiences people have had in childhood, the higher their ACE score, which can lead to potentially worse outcomes as adults (Anda et al., 2009).

ACEs were first conceptualized as a construct in the Adverse Childhood Experiences Study, a study of more than 17,000 patients in the Kaiser Permanente system, a health maintenance organization in San Diego, California. The authors believed that, to truly understand the impact of childhood adversity, all the different types needed to be included in the same model rather than studying one type at a time. In this middle-class, middle-age sample, 51% of patients had experienced at least one ACE (Felitti et al., 1998). Participants who had experienced four or more ACEs had an increased risk of serious diseases, such as cardiovascular disease, diabetes, cancer, and overall premature mortality. Subsequent studies have linked ACEs to many other conditions, such as sleep disturbances and chronic pain syndromes (Sachs-Ericsson et al., 2009).

ACEs also increase chronic inflammation in ACE survivors, which is relevant for both physical and mental health. Data from the Collaborative Perinatal Project, which enrolled pregnant women from 1959 to 1972, found that both prenatal and childhood adversity increased inflammation in the offspring at the mean age of 42 (Slopen et al., 2015). In fact, prenatal adversity increased inflammation (C-reactive protein) in the adult offspring by three times. In the Dunedin Multidisciplinary Health and Development Study, a birth cohort study from Dunedin, New Zealand, childhood maltreatment was related to increased inflammation (C-reactive protein) 20 years later. There was a dose–response effect: the more severe the abuse, the higher the inflammation (Danese et al., 2007). At the 32-year assessment in this same study, those who experienced childhood adversities (low socioeconomic status, maltreatment, or social isolation) had higher rates of major depression, systemic inflammation, and at least three metabolic risk markers (Danese et al., 2009). All the sequelae are related to increased inflammation.

Sequelae of Childhood Abuse in the Perinatal Period

Depression is the most common sequela of childhood abuse in the perinatal period, but abuse also increases the risk of anxiety and PTSD. A review of 43 studies found that women who were either abused as children, or by their partners, had more lifetime depression and depression during pregnancy and postpartum. When women experienced both child abuse and partner violence, they had more severe depression (Alvarez-Segura et al., 2014). Seng et al.'s (2013) study of the association between abuse and mental health included 566 pregnant women. There were three groups: those who currently had PTSD, those who were trauma-exposed but had no symptoms (resilient), and those with no trauma exposure. They found that mothers who had experienced childhood physical or sexual abuse were the ones most likely to have PTSD. PTSD combined with postpartum depression made it difficult for mothers to interact with their babies, and it impaired mother–infant bonding.

The Impact of ACEs on Breastfeeding Initiation and Duration

Findings are mixed regarding whether ACEs influence breastfeeding initiation or duration. Two studies demonstrated that women who had histories of childhood sexual abuse had *higher* rates of intention to breastfeed relative to women who did not have histories of childhood sexual abuse. The first sample included low-income Black women in Baltimore (Benedict et al., 1994), and the second was a nationally representative sample of U.S. mothers of children under the age of 3 (Prentice et al., 2002). In our study, we found that sexual assault survivors exclusively breastfed at the same rate as nonassaulted women (both at 78%) (Kendall-Tackett et al., 2013).

A study of 3,778 women from the 1973–1978 cohort of the Australian Longitudinal Study on Women's Health found that 15.5% reported a history of child sexual abuse (Coles et al., 2016). Their initial analysis found that sexual abuse survivors were less likely to breastfeed than those who had not experienced sexual abuse. However, once they controlled for demographic factors, they found no difference between the groups. The authors concluded that the rates were similar for the abused women versus non-abused women.

A study of women from the 2011–2012 Canadian Community Health Survey ($n = 697$ and $n = 633$) found that ACEs were not related to breastfeeding initiation after controlling for educational level (Ukah et al., 2016). The authors did find, however, that women with histories of ACEs were less likely to exclusively breastfeed relative to women without histories of ACEs.

The largest sample was from the Norwegian Mother and Child Cohort Study ($N = 53,934$) (Sorbo et al., 2015). In this sample, 19% reported adult abuse, and 18% reported childhood abuse. Their study outcome variable was breastfeeding cessation before 4 months. The authors found that breastfeeding cessation was strongly associated with both childhood and adult abuse. Breastfeeding cessation was 22% more likely if women experienced childhood sexual violence, 41% more likely if they experienced one or more types of violence, 40% more likely if they experienced violence in the past 12 months, and 28% more likely if the perpetrator is known to them.

In summarizing these findings, I believe that they suggest that it is *not abuse per se* that lowers breastfeeding rates but the *sequelae of abuse*, such as depression and PTSD. When abuse sequelae are treated, breastfeeding rates will likely improve in populations of women who have experienced ACEs.

Intimate Partner Violence

IPV is abuse by a partner that can be physical, emotional, sexual, or financial. The partner does not have to live with the victim for it to be considered IPV. Not surprisingly, women who have experienced IPV have higher rates of depression than women who have not experienced IPV. For example, a study of Latina women in the United States included 92 who reported IPV and 118 who did not; 44% met the criteria for depression. The women were assessed during pregnancy and at 3, 7, and 13 months postpartum (Valentine et al., 2011). IPV was a better predictor of postpartum depression than depression during pregnancy, which has traditionally been viewed as the strongest risk factor for postpartum depression. Furthermore, a study of 5,162 pregnant women in Montreal found that 15% reported IPV, which was most common for lower-income women (Miszkurka et al., 2012). The combination of immigrant status and IPV increased the risk of depression by seven times. IPV also impacted the mental health status of native-born women and increased their risk of depression by almost five times.

IPV and Breastfeeding

The findings on IPV and breastfeeding initiation and duration have also been mixed. One of the original studies found no difference in initiation or duration of breastfeeding between the IPV and no-IPV groups (Bair-Merritt et al., 2006). However, the sample size for both groups was small (*n* = 10 vs. *n* = 11). A larger study replicated these results. In a sample of 2,621 women from Melbourne, Australia, 6.3% reported IPV (James et al., 2014). Breastfeeding rates did not significantly differ between IPV and non-IPV groups.

Unfortunately, more recent studies are less positive and have found that IPV is a significant barrier to breastfeeding. For example, a large population study from 51 low- to middle-income countries, which included between 95,320 and 102,318 mother–infant dyads, found that 33% had experienced IPV (28% physical violence, 8% sexual violence, and 16% emotional violence). Mothers exposed to any type of IPV were less likely to initiate breastfeeding early and breastfeed exclusively for the first 6 months (Caleyachetty et al., 2019). In addition, a study of 2,000 mothers from Bangladesh found that 50% had experienced violence in the previous 12 months and that 28% had high levels of common mental disorders (Tran et al., 2020). Women who experienced IPV were 2 to 2.3 times more likely to have "common mental health disorders" and 28% to 34% less likely to breastfeed exclusively. The authors noted a direct path between violence and breastfeeding cessation and an indirect path via mental health disorders.

Conclusions drawn by scholars who have conducted systematic reviews also reflect the mixed state of this literature. For example, a recent systematic of 12 studies found that partner violence led to lower rates of breastfeeding (Mezzavilla et al., 2018). Another recent review of 16 studies also found that partner violence lowered breastfeeding, but not all studies were consistent (Normann et al., 2020). The authors indicated that many of these studies were of fair to poor quality. They found that four of seven studies found that IPV lowered breastfeeding duration, five of ten found that IPV led to early termination of exclusive breastfeeding, and two of six studies found that IPV reduced breastfeeding initiation. The lack of agreement between these studies suggests that other factors are involved.

Culture also appears to play a role. A study of 760 low-income women from upstate New York found that a history of violence led to breastfeeding cessation for White women but had the opposite effect for Black women. Violence increased the likelihood of a breastfeeding plan and initiation for Black women (Holland et al., 2018). One possible explanation is that they were trying to protect their babies from a highly toxic situation. Breastfeeding also calmed them. Moreover, for any new mother, breastfeeding may become a way to protect their babies and themselves. A White mother once told me that she had left a 30+-year abusive marriage. She breastfed all four children and said that it "saved them." Breastfeeding may be a strategy whereby mothers and their children can survive an abusive relationship, but there are many barriers to its success.

Breastfeeding's Positive Effects for Violence Survivors

Even in the face of violence, breastfeeding has some surprising benefits that will be particularly helpful for trauma survivors. The first potential benefit is the lessening of trauma symptoms. This effect is likely due to breastfeeding's downregulation of the stress system. As I described earlier in our sample of rape survivors, sexual assault negatively affected every sleep variable we studied. The same was true for all the measures of well-being (Kendall-Tackett et al., 2011, 2013). However, exclusive breastfeeding attenuated trauma's effects on depression, anxiety, and self-reported health. The most striking finding was for anger and irritability, which were dramatically lower for women who were exclusively breastfeeding relative to those who were not. The rate was like that of nonassaulted women. We concluded that exclusive breastfeeding did not eliminate the sequelae of trauma, but it lessened its effects for every variable that was studied, particularly anger and irritability.

The second benefit is that breastfeeding lessens the risk that mothers will abuse their children. Abuse and trauma survivors often worry about passing trauma to their children. Strathearn et al. (2009) conducted a 15-year longitudinal study that included 7,223 Australian mother–infant dyads. There were 500 documented (by child protection) cases of maternal-perpetrated physical abuse and neglect. They found that mothers who breastfed for at least 4 months were 3.8 times less likely to neglect their children and 2.6 times less likely to physically abuse them. The authors attributed their findings to breastfeeding's effects on oxytocin and increased mother–infant bonding. Based on our findings with sexual assault survivors (Kendall-Tackett et al., 2013), oxytocin may have also reduced anger and irritability, which would also lower the risk of abuse.

Birth Trauma

The third type of trauma that providers are likely to encounter is birth trauma. Childbirth-related PTSD is a worldwide problem and is so common that the World Health Organization issued a statement indicating that women deserve respectful and nonabusive care while in labor (World Health Organization, 2014). Giving birth in a wealthy country does not automatically lower the rate of birth trauma. It is, unfortunately, also common in affluent and industrialized nations.

Incidence

In the U.S. Listening to Mothers II Survey, 9% of mothers met the full criteria for PTSD, and an additional 18% in the entire sample scored above the cutoff for posttraumatic stress symptoms following birth (Beck et al., 2011). The percentage was even higher for African American mothers: 28% of whom had trauma symptoms (Declercq et al., 2008). When considering the percentage of women who met the full criteria for PTSD, 9% may not seem particularly high, so it is helpful to compare it to another number. In the months following the September 11 terrorist attacks, 7.5% of residents in lower Manhattan, New York, met the full criteria for PTSD (Galea et al., 2003). The rate of birth trauma in the United States was higher than it was following a terrorist attack.

Some argue that birth trauma is inevitable because birth is difficult. It is, but they do not account for the model of care (midwifery vs. obstetric). We can examine the effect of the model of care by looking at studies of women in countries where birth is treated as a normal event and who have continuous labor support (midwifery model). In these studies, women have lower rates of PTSD relative to women born in countries with an obstetric care model. Two countries that have a midwifery model of care are Sweden and the Netherlands, and this is reflected in their birth trauma statistics. For example, a prospective study of 1,224 women in Sweden found that 1.3% had birth-related PTSD, and 9% described their births as traumatic (Soderquist et al., 2009). Similarly, a study of 907 women in the Netherlands found that 1.2% of women had birth-related PTSD and 9% identified their births as traumatic (Stramrood et al., 2011). Interestingly, providers (obstetricians and midwives) also had lower rates of secondary trauma related to birth in these same countries, which suggests that the model of care also influences providers' experiences (Kendall-Tackett & Beck, 2022).

Conversely, in countries, such as the United States, where the obstetric model predominates, the rate of birth trauma is much higher (Beck et al., 2011). In addition, women who give birth in countries where the status of women is generally low have even higher rates of birth trauma than women giving birth in the United States. A study from Iran of 400 women found that 55% of participants reported traumatic births at 6 to 8 weeks postpartum and 20% had postpartum PTSD (Modarres et al., 2012).

Risk Factors for Birth Trauma

Providers sometimes say that birth trauma happens because of patients' "unrealistic expectations" or that their personalities cause them to be unhappy about their births. Researchers have identified several risk factors for traumatic births. Three recent studies have found that *the strongest predictor of birth trauma was the relationship with their providers.* A positive relationship protected women, but a negative relationship, where the provider was cold or harsh, increased their risk (Dikmen-Yildiz et al., 2017; Garthus-Niegel, Horsch, Handtke, et al., 2018; Simpson & Catling, 2016).

A systematic review of 21 articles published in the past 5 years also found that, in addition to the patient–provider relationship, previous mental health disorders, obstetric emergencies, and neonatal complications were also risk factors for birth trauma (Simpson & Catling, 2016). A study from Montreal found that anxiety in pregnancy and a history of sexual trauma increased mothers' vulnerability to birth trauma (Verreault et al., 2012). In their sample of 308 women at 25 to 40 weeks' gestation, 4 to 6 weeks, and 3 and 6 months postpartum, 6% met full criteria for PTSD and 12% met partial criteria. PTSD was three times more common in sexual assault survivors.

Birth's Impact on Breastfeeding and Mental Health

Beck et al.'s qualitative studies of birth trauma and breastfeeding are some of the few that have addressed this relation. They found two prominent themes among the mothers who experienced birth trauma. Either the mothers were too overwhelmed to breastfeed and found it triggering, or they felt that breastfeeding helped heal their trauma and "prove their success" as mothers (Beck, 2008, 2011; Beck & Watson, 2008).

Birth interventions by themselves do not, necessarily, lead to birth trauma. However, because they interfere with the oxytocin system, birth interventions can cause downstream negative effects on both breastfeeding and mental health. For example, in our study, mothers who had unassisted vaginal births had the highest rates of exclusive breastfeeding (83%) compared to 69% to 71% for all other types of birth (Kendall-Tackett et al., 2015). A study of 5,332 mothers in the United Kingdom found more breastfeeding problems at three months postpartum following forceps-assisted and unplanned cesarean births (Rowlands & Redshaw, 2012).

Epidurals have also been a source of controversy, with some providers insisting that they have no negative effects, and others noting both breastfeeding difficulties and increased risk of depression. The data regarding this issue are mixed. For example, a prospective study of 1,280 Australian mothers found that epidurals were associated with breastfeeding difficulties at one week postpartum and cessation at three months (Torvaldsen et al., 2006). In our study of 6,410 new mothers, bivariate analyses indicated significantly higher depressive symptoms in women who had epidurals than those who did not. However, we realized that epidurals may simply be markers for complications (such as overwhelming pain), which often lead to other birth interventions. To account for this possibility, we controlled for birth interventions and other factors that we knew increased the risk of depression (history of depression or sexual assault, low income or education level, anxiety, and anger/irritability) (Kendall-Tackett et al., 2015). After controlling for all these variables, three variables were related to depressive symptoms: postpartum hemorrhage, postpartum surgery, and epidurals. Some studies with small samples, however, have not found that epidurals increased breastfeeding problems (Hiltunen et al., 2004) or depression (Ding et al., 2014).

Traumatic births can also suppress another hormone necessary for breastfeeding: prolactin. A study from Guatemala found that a highly stressful birth delayed lactogenesis II (when milk becomes more abundant around days 3 to 4) because high cortisol levels suppress prolactin (Grajeda & Perez-Escamilla, 2002). In addition, the sequelae of a traumatic birth, such as depression, anxiety, or PTSD, can cause breastfeeding cessation as described previously.

For both partner violence and birth trauma, the impact on breastfeeding may be more directly related to hormonal changes that happen in the wake of these traumas. For a more distal stressor, such as childhood abuse, the impact on breastfeeding is likely to be indirect, via sequelae of abuse, such as depression, anxiety, and PTSD.

Summary

The mental health needs of breastfeeding mothers are similar to those who are not breastfeeding, but there are some unique considerations. When working with breastfeeding mothers, it is critical that mental health providers find out about mothers' breastfeeding goals and support them. This also means not giving advice that will lead to premature weaning. To reiterate, breastfeeding is more than simply a way to feed babies. Yes, a mother can feed babies with formula, but formula feeding does not cause the physiological changes between mothers and babies that breastfeeding does. The stress-lowering effect lessens (but not eliminates) mothers' risk of depression and other mental health conditions. Recommending that mothers wean to "protect their mental health" will likely be counterproductive and lead to more symptoms.

However, although breastfeeding lowers the risk of mental health issues, the relation between breastfeeding and maternal mental health is complex and bidirectional. Women who are depressed, anxious, or have PTSD are less likely to initiate breastfeeding and are more likely to stop prematurely. Furthermore, early cessation also increases the risk of depression. For example, mothers in a U.S. sample who stopped breastfeeding before 8 weeks have the highest rates of depression compared to mothers who breastfed longer than 8 weeks or those who never breastfed. In addition to suppressing the stress response, breastfeeding modifies mothers' sleep by increasing the total sleep time and reducing the number of minutes to get to sleep, two of the key sleep parameters that predict postpartum depression. Finally, breastfeeding lowers the risk of maternal-perpetrated abuse and neglect, and it attenuates trauma symptoms, which will be particularly important for mothers who have experienced trauma.

Collaborating With Lactation Consultants

It can be particularly helpful for mental health providers to work with lactation consultants to support new mothers in their care. So, for example, if mothers worry about a low milk supply, a lactation consultant can determine whether it is actually low (and address that) or the mother is worrying about something that has not happened. If a mother has pain, refer her to someone who can address it rather than simply telling her to stop. Nipple pain can cause serious mental health issues if ignored but can usually be quickly addressed by a skilled lactation provider. (And if one lactation provider ignores it, get a second opinion.)

Another example of collaborative care is when mothers have severe fatigue. An initial question can be about where the baby is sleeping. The goal is to have the baby near enough so that mothers do not need to completely wake. Mental health or lactation providers might suggest adjustments to make nighttime care easier. Mothers might also look into some "breastfeeding hacks" that can help when babies are on and off all night (e.g., using breast compressions can get more fatty milk into the baby who might fall asleep before they have a complete feed). Lactation providers can help with that. Mobilizing mothers' social support so that they can get more rest can also help. These are just a few examples of how mental health and lactation providers can work together. I believe that collaboration can provide optimum care for breastfeeding mothers seeking mental health services, and mothers and their families will benefit greatly from these collaborative efforts made on their behalf.

Note

1 Pregnancy Risk Assessment Monitoring System (from the Centers for Disease Control and Prevention).

References

Ahn, S., & Corwin, E. J. (2015). The association between breastfeeding, the stress response, inflammation, and postpartum depression during the postpartum period: Prospective cohort study. *International Journal of Nursing Studies, 52*, 1582–1590.

Alvarez-Segura, M., Garcia-Esteve, L., Torres, A., Plaza, A., Imaz, M. L., Hermida-Barros, L., . . . Burtchen, N. (2014). Are women with a history of abuse more vulnerable to perinatal depressive symptoms? A systematic review. *Archives of Women's Mental Health, 17*, 343–357.

American Psychiatric Association. (2013). *Diagnostic and statistical manual-5*. American Psychiatric Association.

American Psychiatric Association. (2022). *Diagnostic and statistical manual* (5th ed., text rev.). American Psychiatric Association.

Anda, R. F., Dong, M., Brown, D. W., Felitti, V. J., Giles, W. H., Perry, G. S., . . . Dube, S. R. (2009). The relationship of adverse childhood experiences to a history of premature death of family members. *BMC Public Health, 9*, 106. https://doi.org/10.1186/1471-2458-9-106

Ansara, D., Cohen, M. M., Gallop, R., Kung, R., Kung, R., & Schei, B. (2005). Predictors of women's physical health problems after childbirth. *Journal of Psychosomatic Obstetrics & Gynecology, 26*, 115–125.

Bair-Merritt, M. H., Blackstone, M., & Feudtner, C. (2006). Physical health outcomes of childhood exposure to intimate partner violence: A systematic review. *Pediatrics, 117*, 278–290.

Ball, H. L. (2006). Parent-infant bed-sharing behavior: Effects of feeding type and presence of father. *Human Nature, 17*(3), 301–308.

Bauman, B. L., Ko, J. Y., Cox, S., D'Angelo, D. V., Warner, L., Folger, S., . . . Barfield, W. D. (2020). Postpartum depressive symptoms and provider discussions about perinatal depression: United States 2018. *Morbidity & Mortality Weekly Report, 69*(19), 575–581.

Beck, C. T. (2008). Impact of birth trauma on breastfeeding: A tale of two pathways. *Nursing Research, 57*(4), 229–236.

Beck, C. T. (2011). A metaethnography of traumatic childbirth and its aftermath: Amplifying causal looping. *Qualitative Health Research, 21*, 301–311. https://doi.org/10.1177/1049732310390698

Beck, C. T., Gable, R. K., Sakala, C., & Declercq, E. R. (2011). Posttraumatic stress disorder in new mothers: Results from a two-stage U.S. national survey. *Birth, 38*(3), 216–227.

Beck, C. T., & Watson, S. (2008). Impact of birth trauma on breast-feeding. *Nursing Research, 57*(4), 228–236.

Benedict, M. I., Paine, L., & Paine, L. (1994). *Long-term effects of child sexual abuse on functioning in pregnancy and pregnancy outcomes (final report)*. National Center of Child Abuse & Neglect.

Bergink, V., Gibney, S. M., & Drexhage, H. A. (2014). Autoimmunity, inflammation, and psychosis: A search for peripheral markers. *Biological Psychiatry, 75*, 324–331.

Berk, M., Williams, L. J., Jacka, F. N., O'Neil, A., Pasco, J. A., Moylan, S., . . . Maes, M. (2013). So depression is an inflammatory disease, but where does the inflammation come from? *BMC Medicine, 11*, 200. www.biomedcentral.com/1741-7015/11/200

Beurel, E., Toups, M., & Nemeroff, C. B. (2020). The bidirection relationship of depression and inflammation: Double trouble. *Neuron, 107*(2), 234–256. https://doi.org/10.1016/j.neuron.2020.06.002

Bhatti, S., & Richards, K. (2015). A systematic review of the relationship between postpartum sleep disturbance and postpartum depression. *Journal of Obstetric, Gynecologic, and Neonatal Nursing, 44*(3), 350–357. https://doi.org/10.1111/1552-6909.12562

Borra, C., Iacovou, M., & Sevilla, A. (2015). New evidence on breastfeeding and postpartum depression: The importance of understanding women's intentions. *Maternal & Child Health Journal, 19*(4), 897–907.

Brown, A. E. (2018). What do women lose if they are prevented from meeting their breastfeeding goals? *Clinical Lactation, 9*(4), 200–207.

Brown, A. E. (2019). *Why breastfeeding grief and trauma matter*. Pinter and Martin.

Caleyachetty, R., Uthman, O. A., Bekele, H. N., Martin-Canavate, R., Marais, D., Coles, J., . . . Koniz-Booher, P. (2019). Maternal exposure to intimate partner violence and breastfeeding practices in 51 low-income and middle-income countries: A population-based cross-sectional study. *PLoS Medicine, 16*(10), e1002921. https://doi.org/10.1371/journal.pmed.1002921

Coles, J., Anderson, A., & Loxton, D. (2016). Breastfeeding duration after childhood sexual abuse: An Australian cohort study. *Journal of Human Lactation, 32*(3), NP28–35.

Coo, S., Garcia, M. I., Mira, A., & Valdes, V. (2020). The role of perinatal anxiety and depression in breast-feeding practices. *Breastfeeding Medicine, 15*(8), 495–500. https://doi.org/10.1089/bfm.2020.0091

Cook, N., Ayers, S., & Horsch, A. (2018). Maternal posttraumatic stress disorder during the perinatal period and child outcomes: A systematic review. *Journal of Affective Disorders, 225,* 18–31. https://doi.org/10.1016/j.jad.2017.07.045

Cooklin, A. R., Amir, L. H., Nguyen, C. D., Buck, M. L., Cullinane, M., Fisher, J. R. W., . . . CASTLE Study Team. (2018). Physical health, breastfeeding problems and maternal mood in the early post-partum: A prospective cohort study. *Archives of Women's Mental Health, 21*(3), 365–374. https://doi.org/10.1007/s00737-017-0805-y

Cox, J. L., Holden, J. M., & Sagovsky, R. (1987). Detection of postnatal depression: Development of the 10-item Edinburgh Postnatal Depression Scale. *British Journal of Psychiatry, 150,* 782–786.

Danese, A., Moffitt, T. E., Harrington, H., Milne, B. J., Polanczyk, G., Pariante, C. M., & Caspi, A. (2009). Adverse childhood experiences and adult risk factors for age-related disease: Depression, inflammation, and clustering of metabolic risk factors. *Archives of Pediatric and Adolescent Medicine, 163*(12), 1135–1143.

Danese, A., Pariante, C. M., Caspi, A., Taylor, A., & Poulton, R. (2007). Childhood maltreatment predicts adult inflammation in a life-course study. *Proceedings of the National Academy of Sciences U S A, 104*(4), 1319–1324. https://doi.org/10.1073/pnas.0610362104

Declercq, E. R., Sakala, C., Corry, M. P., & Applebaum, S. (2008). *New mothers speak out: National survey results highlight women's postpartum experiences.* Childbirth Connection.

Dikmen-Yildiz, P., Ayers, S., & Phillips, L. (2017). The prevalence of posttraumatic stress disorder in pregnancy and after birth: A systematic review and meta-analysis. *Journal of Affective Disorders, 208,* 634–645.

Ding, T., Wang, D. X., Chen, Q., & Zhu, S. N. (2014). Epidural labor analgesia is associated with a decreased risk of postpartum depression: A prospecitive cohort study. *Anesthesia & Analgesia, 119*(2), 383–392. https://doi.org/10.1213/ANE.0000000000000107

Doan, T., Gardiner, A., Gay, C. L., & Lee, K. A. (2007). Breastfeeding increases sleep duration of new parents. *Journal of Perinatal & Neonatal Nursing, 21*(3), 200–206.

Dorheim, S. K., Bondevik, G. T., Eberhard-Gran, M., & Bjorvatn, B. (2009a). Sleep and depression in postpartum women: A population-based study. *Sleep, 32*(7), 847–855.

Dorheim, S. K., Bondevik, G. T., Eberhard-Gran, M., & Bjorvatn, B. (2009b). Subjective and objective sleep among depressed and non-depressed postnatal women. *Acta Psychiatrica Scandinavia, 119,* 128–136.

Eisenach, J. C., Pan, P. H., Smiley, R., Lavand'homme, P., Landau, R., & Houle, T. T. (2008). Severity of acute pain after childbirth, but not type of delivery, predicts persistent pain and postpartum depression. *Pain, 140,* 87–94.

Fallon, V., Groves, R., Halford, J. C. G., Bennett, K. M., & Harrold, J. A. (2016). Postpartum anxiety and infant-feeding outcomes. *Journal of Human Lactation, 32*(4), 740–758. https://doi.org/10.1177/0890334416662241

Felitti, V. J., Anda, R. F., Nordenberg, D., Williamson, D. F., Spitz, A. M., Edwards, V., . . . Marks, J. S. (1998). Relationship of childhood abuse and household dysfunction to many of the leading causes of death in adults: The Adverse Childhood Experiences (ACE) study. *American Journal of Preventive Medicine, 14*(4), 245–258. https://doi.org/10.1016/S0749379798000178

Figueiredo, B., Pinto, T. M., & Costa, R. (2021). Exclusive breastfeeding moderates the association between prenatal and postpartum depression. *Journal of Human Lactation, 37,* 784–794. https://doi.org/10.1177/0890334421991051

Finy, M. S., & Christian, L. (2018). Pathways linking childhood abuse history and current socioeconomic status to inflammation during pregnancy. *Brain, Behavior & Immunity, 74,* 231–240.

Galea, S., Vlahov, D., Resnick, H., Ahern, J., Susser, E., Gold, J., . . . Kilpatrick, D. (2003). Trends of probable post-traumatic stress disorder in New York City after the September 11 terrorist attacks. *American Journal of Epidemiology, 158,* 514–524.

Garthus-Niegel, S., Horsch, A., Ayers, S., Junge-Hoffmeister, J., Weidner, K., & Eberhard-Gran, M. (2018). The influence of postpartum PTSD on breastfeeding: A longitudinal population-based study. *Birth, 45*(2), 193–201.

Garthus-Niegel, S., Horsch, A., Handtke, E., Von Soest, T., Ayers, S., Weidner, K., & Eberhard-Gran, M. (2018). The impact of postpartum posttraumatic stress and depression symptoms on couples' relationship satisfaction: A population-based prospective study. *Frontiers in Psychology, 9.*

Grajeda, R., & Perez-Escamilla, R. (2002). Stress during labor and delivery is associated with delayed onset of lactation among urban Guatemalan women. *Journal of Nutrition, 132,* 3055–3060.

Groer, M. W., Davis, M. W., & Hemphill, J. (2002). Postpartum stress: Current concepts and the possible protective role of breastfeeding. *Journal of Obstetric, Gynecologic, & Neonatal Nursing, 31*(4), 411–417. www.ncbi.nlm.nih.gov/entrez/query.fcgi?cmd=Retrieve&db=PubMed&dopt=Cit ation&list_uids=12146930

Groer, M. W., & Kendall-Tackett, K. A. (2011). *How breastfeeding protects women's health throughout the lifespan: The psychoneuroimmunology of human lactation.* Hale Publishing.

Hahn-Holbrook, J., Haselton, M. G., Schetter, C. D., & Glynn, L. M. (2013). Does breastfeeding offer protection against maternal depressive symptomatology? A prospective study from pregnancy to 2 years after birth. *Archives of Women's Mental Health, 16,* 411–422.

Handlin, L., Jonas, W., Pettersson, M., Ejdeback, M., Ransjo-Arvidson, A.-B., Nissen, A., & Uvnas-Moberg, K. (2009). Effects of sucking and skin-to-skin contact on maternal ACTH and cortisol levels during the second day postpartum – Influences of epidural analgesia and oxytocin in the perinatal period. *Breastfeeding Medicine, 4*(4), 207–220.

Heinrichs, M., Meinlschmidt, G., Neumann, I., Wagner, S., Kirschbaum, C., Ehlert, U., & Hellhammer, D. H. (2001). Effects of suckling on hypothalamic-pituitary-adrenal axis responses to psychosocial stress in postpartum lactating women. *Journal of Clinical Endocrinology & Metabolism, 86,* 4798–4804.

Hiltunen, P., Raudaskoski, T., Ebeling, H., & Moilanen, I. (2004). Does pain relief during delivery decrease the risk of postnatal depression? *Acta Obstetrica Gynecologica Scandanavica, 83*(3), 257–261.

Holland, M. L., Thevenent-Morrison, K., Mittal, M., Nelson, A., & Dozier, A. M. (2018). Breastfeeding and exposure to past, current, and neighborhood violence. *Maternal & Child Health Journal, 22,* 82091. https://doi.org/10.1007/s10995-017-2357-1

Horsely, K., Nguyen, T.-V., Ditto, B., & Da Costa, D. (2019). The association between pregnancy-specific anxiety and exclusive breastfeeding status early in the postpartum period. *Journal of Human Lactation, 35*(4), 729–736. https://doi.org/10.1177/0890334419838482

Hughes, O., Mohamed, M. M., Doyle, P., & Burke, G. (2018). The significance of breastfeedding on sleep patterns during the first 48 hours postpartum for first time mothers. *Journal of Obstetrics & Gynaecology, 38*(3), 316–320. https://doi.org/10.1080/01443615.2017.1353594

James, J. P., Taft, A., Amir, L. H., & Agius, P. (2014). Does intimate partner violence impact on women's initiation and duration of breastfeeding? *Breastfeeding Review, 22*(2), 11–19.

Kendall-Tackett, K. A. (2007). A new paradigm for depression in new mothers: The central role of inflammation and how breastfeeding and anti-inflammatory treatments protect maternal mental health. *International Breastfeeding Journal, 2*(6). https://doi.org/doi:10.1186/1746-4358-2-6

Kendall-Tackett, K. A. (2023). *Depression in new mothers* Vol I (4th ed.). Routledge.

Kendall-Tackett, K. A., & Beck, C. T. (2022). Secondary traumatic stress and moral injury in maternity care providers: A narrative and exploratory review. *Frontiers in Global Women's Health, 3.*

Kendall-Tackett, K. A., Cong, Z., & Hale, T. W. (2011). The effect of feeding method on sleep duration, maternal well-being, and postpartum depression. *Clinical Lactation, 2*(2), 22–26.

Kendall-Tackett, K. A., Cong, Z., & Hale, T. W. (2013). Depression, sleep quality, and maternal well-being in postpartum women with a history of sexual assault: A comparison of breastfeeding, mixed-feeding, and formula-feeding mothers *Breastfeeding Medicine, 8*(1), 16–22.

Kendall-Tackett, K. A., Cong, Z., & Hale, T. W. (2015). Birth interventions related to lower rates of exclusive breastfeeding and increased risk of postpartum depression in a large sample. *Clinical Lactation, 6*(3), 87–97.

Kendall-Tackett, K. A., Cong, Z., & Hale, T. W. (2018a). The impact of feeding method and infant sleep location on mother and infant sleep, maternal depression, and mothers' well-being. *Clinical Lactation, 9*(3). https://doi.org/10.1891/2158-0782.9.3

Kendall-Tackett, K. A., Cong, Z., & Hale, T. W. (2018b). The impact of feeding method and infant sleep location on mother/infant sleep, maternal depression, and mothers' well-being. *Clinical Lactation, 9*(3), 117–124. https://doi.org/10.1891/2158-0782.9.3.117

Kiecolt-Glaser, J. K. (2009). Psychoneuroimmunology psychology's gateway to the biomedical future. *Perspectives in Psychological Science, 4*(4), 367–369. https://doi.org/doi:10.1111/j.1745-6924.2009.01139.x

Kiecolt-Glaser, J. K., Derry, H. M., & Fagundes, C. P. (2015). Inflammation: Depression fans the flames and feasts on the heat. *American Journal of Psychiatry, 172*(11), 1075–1091. https://doi.org/10.1176/appi.ajp.2015.15020152

Kim, Y., & Ahn, S. (2015). A review of postpartum depression: Focused on psychoneuroimmunological interaction. *Korean Women's Health Nursing, 21*(2), 106–114.

Kohler, O., Kroph, J., Mors, O., & Benros, M. E. (2016). Inflammation in depression and the potential for anti-inflammatory treatment. *Current Neuroparmacology, 14*(7), 732–742. https://doi.org /10.2174/1570159x14666151208113700

Koutra, K., Vassilaki, M., Georgiou, V., Koutis, A., Bitsios, P., Kogevinas, M., & Chatzi, L. (2018). Pregnancy, perinatal, and postpartum complications as determinants of postpartum depression: The Rhea mother-child cohort in Crete, Greece. *Epidemiology and Psychiatric Sciences, 27*(3), 244–255. https://doi.org/10.1017/S2045796016001062

Lara-Cinisomo, S., McKenney, K., DiFlorio, A., & Meltzer-Brody, S. (2017). Associations between postpartum depression, breastfeeding, and oxytocin levels in Latina mothers. *Breastfeeding Medicine, 12*(7), 436–442. https://doi.org/10.1089/bfm.2016.0213

Lim, G., LaSorda, K. R., Farrell, L. M., McCarthy, A. M., Facco, F., & Wasan, A. D. (2020). Obstetric pain correlates with postpartum depression symptoms: A pilot prospective observational study. *BMC Pregnancy and Childbirth, 20*(1), 240. https://doi.org/10.1186/s12884-020-02943-7

Maes, M. (2001). Psychological stress and the inflammatory response system. *Clinical Science, 101*, 193–194.

Maes, M., & Smith, R. S. (1998). Fatty acids, cytokines, and major depression. *Biological Psychiatry, 43*, 313–314.

Maes, M., Yirmyia, R., Noraberg, J., Brene, S., Hibblen, J., Perini, G., . . . Maj, M. (2009). The inflammatory & neurodegenerative (I&ND) hypothesis of depression: Leads for future research and new drug development. *Metabolic Brain Disease, 24*, 27–53.

Mayopoulos, G. A., Ein-Dor, T., Dishy, G., Nandru, R., Chan, S. J., Hanley, L. E., . . . Dekel, S. (2021). COVID-19 is associated with traumatic childbirth and subsequent mother-infant bonding problems. *Journal of Affective Disorders, 282*, 122–125. https://doi.org/10.1016/j. jad.2020.12.101

Mazza, M. G., DeLorenzo, R., Conte, C., Poletti, S., Vai, B., Bollettini, I., . . . Benedetti, F. (2020). Anxiety and depression in COVID-19 survivors: Role of inflammatory and clinical predictors. *Brain, Behavior & Immunity, 89*, 594–600. https://doi.org/10.1016/j.bbi.2020.07.037

McGovern, P., Dowd, B. E., Gjerdingen, D., Gross, C. R., Kenney, S., Ukestad, L., . . . Lundberg, U. (2006). Postpartum health of employed mothers 5 weeks after childbirth. *Annals of Family Medicine, 4*(2), 159–167.

McKenna, J. J. (2020). *Safe infant sleep: Expert answers to your cosleeping questions.* Platypus Media.

McKenna, J. J., Ball, H. L., & Gettler, L. T. (2007). Mother-infant cosleeping, breastfeeding, and Sudden Infant Death Syndrome: What biological anthropology has discovered about normal infant sleep and pediatric sleep medicine. *Yearbook of Physical Anthropology, 50*, 133–161.

Mezzavilla, R. D. S., Ferreira, M. D. F., Curloni, C. C., Lindsay, A. C., & Hasselman, M. H. (2018). Intimate partner violence and breastfeeding practices: A systematic review of observational studies. *Jornal de Pediatria, 94*, 226–237. https://doi.org/10.1016/j.jped.2017.07.007

Miszkurka, M., Zuzunegui, M. V., & Goulet, L. (2012). Immigrant status, antenatal depressive symptoms, and frequency and source of violence: What's the relationship. *Archives of Women's Mental Health, 15*, 387–396.

Modarres, M., Afrasiabi, S., Rahnama, P., & Montazeri, A. (2012). Prevalence and risk factors of childbirth-related post-traumatic stress symptoms. *BMC Pregnancy and Childbirth, 12*, 88. www. biomedcentral.com/1471-2393/12/88

Normann, A. K., Bakiewicz, A., Madsen, F. K., Khan, K. S., Rasch, V., & Linde, D. S. (2020). Intimate partner violence and breastfeeding: A systematic review. *BMJ Open, 10*(10), e034153. https://doi. org/10.1136/bmjopen-2019-034153

Oyentunji, A., & Chandra, P. (2020). Postpartum stress and infant outcome: A review of current literature. *Psychiatric Research, 284*, 112769. https://doi.org/10.1016/j.psychres.2020.112769

Prentice, J. C., Lu, M. C., Lange, L., & Halfon, N. (2002). The association between reported childhood sexual abuse and breastfeeding initiation. *Journal of Human Lactation, 18*, 291–226.

Rosseland, L. A., Reme, S. E., Simonsen, T. B., Thoresen, M., Nielsen, C. V., & Gran, M. E. (2020). Are labor pain and birth experience associated with persistent pain and postpartum depression? A prospective cohort study. *Scandinavian Journal of Pain, 20*(3), 591–602. https://doi.org/10.1515/ sjpain-2020-0025

Rowlands, I. J., & Redshaw, M. (2012). Mode of birth and women's psychological and physical wellbeing in the postnatal period. *BMC Pregnancy and Childbirth*, 12, 138. www.biomedcentral. com/1471-2393/12/138

Sachs-Ericsson, N., Cromer, K., Hernandez, A., & Kendall-Tackett, K. A. (2009). Childhood abuse, health and pain-related problems: The role of psychiatric disorders and current life stress. *Journal of Trauma & Dissociation*, 10, 170–188.

Saxbe, D. E., Schetter, C. D., Guardino, C. M., Ramey, S. L., Shalowitz, M. U., Thorp, J., . . . National Institute of Child Human Development Community Child Health, N. (2016). Sleep quality predicts persistence of parental postpartum depressive symptoms and transmission of depressive symptoms from mothers to fathers. *Annals of Behavioral Medicine*, 50(6), 862–875. https://doi. org/10.1007/s12160-016-9815-7

Schwartz, E. B., Ray, R. M., Stuebe, A. M., Allison, M. A., Ness, R. B., Freiberg, M. S., & Cauley, J. A. (2009). Duration of lactation and risk factors for maternal cardiovascular disease. *Obstetrics & Gynecology*, 113(5), 974–982.

Seng, J. S., Sperlich, M. A., Low, L. K., Ronis, D. L., Muzik, M., & Liberzon, I. (2013). Childhood abuse history, posttraumatic stress disorder, postpartum mental health, and bonding: A prospective cohort study. *Journal of Midwifery and Women's Health*, 58(1), 57–68.

Simpson, M., & Catling, C. (2016). Understanding psychological traumatic birth: A literature review. *Women & Birth*, 29, 203–207.

Slopen, N., Loucks, E. B., Appleton, A. A., Kawachi, I., Kubzansky, L. D., Non, A. L., . . . Gilman, S. E. (2015). Early origins of inflammation: An examination of prenatal and childhood social adversity in a prospective cohort study. *Psychoneuroendocrinology*, 51, 403–413.

Soderquist, I., Wijma, B., Thorbert, G., & Wijma, K. (2009). Risk factors in pregnancy for post-traumatic stress and depression after childbirth. *British Journal of Obstetrics & Gynecology*, 116, 672–680.

Sorbo, M. F., Lukasse, M., Brantsaeter, A. L., & Grimstad, H. (2015). Past and recent abuse is associated with early cesation of breast feeding: Results from a large prospective cohort in Norway. *BMJ Open*, 5(12), 009240.

Stramrood, C. A., Paarlberg, K. M., Velt, E. M. H. I. T., Berger, L. W. A. R., Vingerhoets, A. J. J. M., Schultz, W. C. M. W., & Van Pampus, M. G. (2011). Posttraumatic stress following childbirth in homelike- and hospital settings. *Journal of Psychosomatic Obstetrics & Gynecology*, 32(2), 88–97.

Strathearn, L., Mamun, A. A., Najman, J. M., & O'Callaghan, M. J. (2009). Does breastfeeding protect against substantiated child abuse and neglect? A 15-year cohort study. *Pediatrics*, 123(2), 483–493. https://doi.org/123/2/483 [pii]10.1542/peds.2007-3546

Stuebe, A. M., Meltzer-Brody, S., Propper, C., Pearson, B., Beiler, P., Elam, M., . . . Grewen, K. (2019). The mood, mother, and infant study: Association between maternal mood in pregnancy and breastfeeding outcome. *Breastfeeding Medicine*, 14(8), 551–559. https://doi.org/10.1089/ bfm.2019.0079

Taveras, E. M., Rifas-Shiman, S. L., Rich-Edwards, J. W., & Mantzoros, C. S. (2011). Maternal short sleep duration associated with increased levels of inflammatory markers at 3 years postpartum. *Metabolism*, 60(7), 982–986.

Torvaldsen, S., Roberts, C. L., Simpson, J. M., Thompson, J. F., & Ellwood, D. A. (2006). Intrapartum epidural analgesia and breastfeeding: A prospective cohort study. *International Breastfeeding Journal*, 1(1), 24 https://doi.org/10.1186/1746-4358-1-24

Tran, L. M., Nguyen, P. H., Naved, R. T., & Menon, P. (2020). Intimate partner violence is associated with poorer mental health and breastfeeding practices in Bangladesh. *Health Policy & Planning*, 35(Supplement_1), i19–i29. https://doi.org/10.1093/heapol/czaa106

Turkmen, H., Dilcen, H. Y., & Akin, B. (2020). The effect of labor comfort on traumatic childbirth perception, posttraumatic stress disorder, and breastfeeding. *Breastfeeding Medicine*, 15(12), 779–788. https://doi.org/10.1089/bfm.2020.0138

Uchino, B. N., Trettevik, R., Kent de Grey, R. G., Cronan, S., Hogan, J., & Baucom, B. R. W. (2018). Social support, social integration, and inflammatory cytokines: A meta-analysis. *Health Psychology*, 37(5), 462–471.

Ukah, U. V., Adu, P. A., De Silva, D. A., & von Dadelzen, P. (2016). The impact of history of adverse childhood experiences on breastfeeding initiation and exclusivity: Findings from a National Population Health Survey. *Breastfeeding Medicine*, 11, 544–550. https://doi.org/10.1089/ bfm.2016.0053

Uvnas-Moberg, K. (2013). *The hormone of closeness: The role of oxytocin in relationships*. Pinter and Martin.

Uvnas-Moberg, K. (2015). *Oxytocin: The biological guide to motherhood*. Praeclarus Press.

Uvnas-Moberg, K., Ekstrom-Bergstrom, A., Buckley, S., Massarotti, C., Pajalic, Z., Luegmair, K., . . . Dencker, A. (2020). Maternal plasma levels of oxytocin during breastfeeding. *PLoS One, 15*(8), e0235806. https://doi.org/10.1371/journal.pone.0235806

Valentine, J. M., Rodriguez, M. A., Lapeyrouse, L. M., & Zhang, M. (2011). Recent intimate partner violence as a prenatal predictor of maternal depression in the first year postpartum among Latinas. *Archives of Women's Mental Health, 14*, 135–143.

Verreault, N., Da Costa, D., Marchand, A., Ireland, K., Banack, H., Dritsa, M., & Khalife, S. (2012). PTSD following childbirth: A prospective study of incidence and risk factors in Canadian women. *Journal of Psychosomatic Research, 73*, 257–263.

Watkins, S., Meltzer-Brody, S., Zolnoun, D., & Stuebe, A. M. (2011). Early breastfeeding experiences and postpartum depression. *Obstetrics & Gynecology, 118*(2), 214–221.

Woolhouse, H., James, J., Gartland, D., McDonald, E., & Brown, S. J. (2016). Maternal depressive symptoms at three months postpartum and breastfeeding rates at six months postpartum: Implications for primary care in a prospective cohort study of primiparous women in Australia. *Women & Birth, 29*(4), 381–387. https://doi.org/10.1016/j.wombi.2016.05.008

World Health Organization. (2014). *The prevention and elimination of disrespect and abuse during facility-based childbirth*. http://apps.who.int/iris/bitstream/10665/134588/1/WHO_RHR_14.23_eng.pdf?ua=1&ua=1

Yusuff, A. S. M., Tang, L., Binns, C. W., & Lee, A. H. (2016). Breastfeeding and postnatal depression: A prospective cohort study in Sabah, Malaysia. *Journal of Human Lactation, 32*(2), 277–281.

6

PERINATAL MATERNAL MENTAL HEALTH AND CHILD DEVELOPMENT

Kelli K. MacMillan, Josephine Power,
Katherine Sevar, and Megan Galbally

The period from conception to the end of the first postpartum year is one of significant development and vulnerability for a child (Fox et al., 2010). The effects of exposure to adverse experiences during this time may have implications on an individual's capacity to contribute to society across a lifetime (Georgieff et al., 2018). This may be seen in the continuing impact of long-term outcomes such as employment, medical costs, and incarceration rates. Identification of potential risk factors for mother and child is, therefore, necessary to facilitate optimal developmental outcomes. Increasing research proposes that perinatal mental health disorders may have negative implications for child development (Gutman & Feinstein, 2010; Stein et al., 2014); however, the study findings are not consistent with the methodological differences observed.

Women with perinatal mental health disorders experience significant challenges; consequently, it is important not to add to their burden with misinformation on possible associated risks to their infants. Similarly for healthcare providers, the allocation of funding to evidence-based interventions is reliant upon the accurate translation of research findings. It is, therefore, necessary to apply a critical framework to the literature that proposes an association between perinatal mental health and child development to understand how any reported effects may translate to developmental outcomes. The question then is: where there is an association, what is the magnitude of that association, and why does an association exist for some individuals and not for others? This may be explained by other coexisting risk factors (e.g., maternal trauma, maternal education, maternal and infant nutrition).

To address this question, we divide this chapter into four parts:

1. Part I provides an overview of the current findings examining the relationship between perinatal mental health and child development by defining each of the terms, identifying the methodological challenges of the research, the proposed mode of potential transmission of risk from mother to child, and other maternal and infant factors that might influence developmental outcomes.
2. Part II critically appraises the evidence regarding perinatal mental health disorders and child developmental outcomes. We examine perinatal depression and anxiety, bipolar

DOI: 10.4324/9781003206903-8

disorder, borderline personality disorder, eating disorders, schizophrenia, and maternal trauma.
3. Part III provides the clinical context and the translation of research findings regarding perinatal mental health and child developmental outcomes.
4. Part IV provides a summary of the key points of the chapter.

The Role of Child Development in the Context of Perinatal Mental Health

Perinatal mental health disorders are the most common complication of the perinatal period and are typically defined as disorders occurring in pregnancy and across the first year (Howard & Khalifeh, 2020). The occurrence of perinatal mental health disorders is in the presence of a developing fetus, and, with early life, a critical period for later child development, perinatal mental health has been secured as a major public health concern (Hadi et al., 2019). The emergence of evidence documenting the adverse effects of perinatal mental health disorders on child outcomes has increased public interest and investment (Aktar et al., 2019; Vigod et al., 2014), though the focus has been on the most prevalent perinatal depression and anxiety, with a growing evidence base for other disorders (Howard et al., 2014; Meltzer-Brody et al., 2018).

In addition, understanding child development can facilitate optimal outcomes and, in the context of perinatal mental health, can be applied to inform service structure so that vulnerable children are identified for early intervention. Child development is a complex and varied subject, with no one theory that can account for it in its entirety. Broadly speaking for this chapter, we can separate child development into four domains. This classification of child developmental categories is reflected in Table 6.1 (Black et al., 2015).

Methodological Challenges in Perinatal Mental Health Research

It is recommended that consumers of research consider the methodological issues in perinatal mental health research as a framework when interpreting and applying study findings.

Longitudinal Study of Child Development to Understand Risk Factors

The Kauai Longitudinal Study in 1955 provided our first longitudinal evidence of the biological, psychosocial, and environmental factors that might interact to influence child

Table 6.1 Broad Domains of Child Development

Domain	Definition
Cognitive	Intelligence; perception; attention; language; problem solving; reasoning; memory; conceptual understanding; executive functioning
Social emotional	Emotional understanding and expression; relationships with family and peers and others; self-understanding
Motor	Process of learning how to use the muscles to move; includes fine motor (movement of muscles in hands and wrists) and gross motor (whole body movement that requires core stabilizing muscles to perform everyday tasks)

development (Werner, 1995). Since that time, perinatal mental health has emerged with its own research base, and longitudinal studies have facilitated the investigation of factors present from conception.

For example, the Norwegian Arkershus Birth Cohort Study (ABC), a prospective pregnancy cohort study that collected information at trimesters two and three of pregnancy, and postpartum at eight weeks (Osnes et al., 2019). This indicated the chronicity of maternal mental health with symptomatic measurement at multiple time points. Similarly, the Australian Mercy Pregnancy and Emotional Wellbeing Study (MPEWS; Galbally et al., 2017) is a selected cohort design that collects data across the perinatal period (i.e., early pregnancy, late pregnancy; at childbirth; and at 6 and 12 months) and is continuing today into middle childhood (e.g., Galbally, Watson, Keelan, et al., 2020; Galbally, Watson, van IJzendoorn, et al., 2021; Galbally, Watson, van Rossum, et al., 2020). MPEWS repeated measures longitudinal design facilitates the analysis of risk factors from early pregnancy that might influence child outcomes and the inclusion of data collection across the perinatal period can inform the optimal time for clinical intervention.

However, longitudinal research is not without its challenges, including attrition rates and the labor, resources, expense, and time involved in conducting research over an extended period (Saiepour et al., 2019). Although a longitudinal design provides the best opportunity to understand the accumulation of risk in the context of child development from conception.

Inconsistency in Research Findings Regarding Perinatal Mental Health and Child Development

The current evidence is conflicting regarding the association between perinatal mental health and child development. This is demonstrated by systematic review of the association between postpartum maternal depression and child cognitive development (Aoyagi & Tsuchiya, 2019). Of the 11 studies identified, only 6 studies showed any adverse effect (i.e., Ali et al., 2013; Azak, 2012; Cogill et al., 1986; Conroy et al., 2012; Koutra et al., 2013; Smith-Nielsen et al., 2016). Though among the six studies, the findings are not convincing. For instance, Smith-Nielsen et al. (2016) reported developmental differences on the *Bayley Scale of Infant and Toddler Development* (the *Bayley Scales*; Bayley, 2006a) for infants of mothers with postpartum depression at four months compared to the control group. Yet no differences in Bayley scores were maintained between the groups postnatally by 13 months.

Consideration of sample size facilitates the assessment of the quality and translatability of the research. However, between studies that have assessed the association between maternal depression and child development, the sample sizes relied upon vary. For example, Ali et al. (2013) and Koutra et al. (2013) used samples of 420 and 470 women, respectively, compared to Cogill et al. (1986) that relied upon a sample of 94 mother–child dyads, and Azak (2012) only using 50 mother–infant dyads.

Differential susceptibility is another issue raised in the developmental literature but not yet captured empirically. Not all children are equally susceptible to both the adverse and beneficial effects of parenting and other contextual factors (Belsky et al., 2007). Yet most of the research focuses on the equal application of parenting effects to children, struggling to capture whether and how much the child's temperament or other individual characteristics may influence the interaction between parenting, temperament, and child outcomes (Ellis & Boyce, 2011).

Methodological Challenges for Child Development Research

The methodological challenges in child development research are evident in the inconsistency of findings, with the use of multimodal assessment with subjective and objective measurement recommended. This was highlighted in the meta-analysis by Grove et al. (2018), who assigned differences in the effect sizes of the 18 studies to differences in researcher reliance on objective measurement (i.e., standardized measures of motor development) versus brief parent or clinician self-report measure. Subsequent researchers identify this need for multimodal assessment (e.g., child motor development; Fitton et al., 2020; Galbally, Watson, Spigset, et al., 2021). Further extension of the issue is demonstrated by a recent review regarding the association between maternal perinatal depression and child executive functioning. Power et al. (2021) noted that the only validated measure of executive functioning is the one subtask in the NEPSY-II, with a paucity of research studies applying measurement using this tool, particularly in early childhood. An eagerness to detect dysfunction early in life may lead to measures being applied in younger ages where the tool is not validated, and the capacity in question has not yet emerged. Consideration of the type of measurement tool applied by a researcher is necessary to prevent the inaccurate application of study findings that either overemphasize or underemphasize any risk factor to optimal child developmental outcomes.

Caution Regarding the Predictive Validity of Early Childhood Assessment

Some research highlights the poor predictive validity of early child development of later child outcomes. Of 330 infants assessed at 20 months and 8 years, the *Bayley Scales* showed poor predictive validity of cognitive function (Hack et al., 2005), a finding reflected by other researchers (Group, 1991; Kitchen et al., 1989; Koller et al., 1997; Ment et al., 2003). This reinforces the complex interaction of biopsychosocial factors that contribute to child outcomes with differences in performance between early and late childhood reflective of possible exposure to other factors (e.g., maternal education; socioeconomic status; nutrition; trauma; home environment).

The Interrelatedness of Child Developmental Domains

The interrelatedness of child developmental domains is demonstrated by Table 6.2 in which child developmental measures are identified, with overlapping domains. Higher-order cognitive capabilities such as executive function (EF) depend on intact perception, motor function, and language to administer most available tests. This means that no developmental domain is usefully examined in isolation.

Other Co-Occurring Maternal and Child Factors

Child developmental outcomes are the result of a dynamic and complex interaction of biopsychosocial risk and protective factors (Aktar et al., 2019). Investigations that fail to account for these other factors may be limited in their application (e.g., perinatal depression and child development; Nix et al., 2021). Other maternal factors may include maternal education, alcohol and substance use, poverty, trauma, family violence, and social support (Maselko et al., 2015), with child factors such as the home environment, child nutrition, and child trauma.

Table 6.2 Selection of Commonly Cited Measurement Tools in Child Development

Type of measurement	Child development domain	Measurement tool	Time to administer	Training required	Validity and reliability
Individually administered ability test; 6–16 years	Cognitive	*Wechsler Intelligence Scale for Children-Third Edition* (WISC-V; Wechsler, 2014)	60 minutes	Administration by psychologists; clinical psychologists; neuropsychologists	Valid and reliable; (Wechsler, 2014)
Individual administered assessment for 1 month to 42 months	Cognitive, social emotional, motor	*The Bayley Scale of Infant and Toddler Development* (Bayley, 2006a)	30–60 minutes	Occupational therapist; psychologist; speech pathologist; physiotherapist; or fully qualified neonatologist or developmental pediatrician with at least 6–12 months experience with the *Bayley Scales*	Valid and reliable; (Bayley, 2006b)
Individually administered assessment; two forms ages 3–4 years, and 5–16 years	Cognitive; social emotional	*Developmental Neuropsychological Assessment* (NEPSY; Korkman et al., 1998)	Preschool age: 90 minutes; school ages: 2–3 hours	School psychologists; neuropsychologists; research psychologists	Valid and reliable; (Korkman et al., 1998)
Parent/primary caregiver report structured diagnostic interview two to five years	Cognitive; social emotional; basic motor	*Preschool Age Psychiatric Assessment* (Egger & Angold, 2004)	60–90 minutes	Formal training that is estimated to take around four days	Validity and reliability supported in a sample of parent–child dyads (Egger et al., 2006)
Parent/caregiver structured interview 9–17 years	Cognitive; social emotional; basic motor	*Child and Adolescent Psychiatric Assessment* (Angold & Costello, 1995)	60–90 minutes	Formal training is required by the trainer, and takes around four days	Validity and reliability supported in sample of 9–17 years (Angold & Costello, 1995)
Self-report teacher or parent/caregiver; CBCL/2 for ages 2–3 years; and CBCL/4–18 years	Social emotional	*Child Behavior Checklist* (CBCL; Achenbach & Edelbrock, 1983)	10–15 minutes (Achenbach & Ruffle, 2000)	None	(Döpfner et al., 1994)
Self-report teacher or caregiver	Social emotional	*Strength and Difficulties Questionnaire* (Goodman, 1997)	10–15 minutes	None	Valid and reliable; (Stone et al., 2015)

Sociodemographic Factors

Maternal factors may include the home environment that can provide the safety, stimulation, and organization that is required for optimal child development (Bradley et al., 2001). Similarly, given that child nutrition is at the foundation of optimal development (Hanson et al., 2016; Sayer et al., 1998), and appetite changes can be a symptom of maternal mental health disorders (e.g., depression, anxiety), maternal or child nutrition may also be a factor in the context of child development. Consideration of maternal social support is supported by the perinatal literature (Li et al., 2017), though findings on its influence on child development are mixed (McDonald et al., 2016; Milgrom et al., 2019). Other factors include maternal education (e.g., Carneiro et al., 2013; Dollaghan et al., 1999; Jeong et al., 2017; Magnuson et al., 2009) and breastfeeding (Horta et al., 2015; Straub et al., 2019), with caution required not to overstate the effect size in the breastfeeding studies. Childhood socioeconomic status (SES) has attracted focus as both a risk and protective factor (Lawson et al., 2018), as has the potential role that fathers can also play in the context of perinatal mental health disorders (Cardenas et al., 2022).

Maternal Intergenerational Trauma and Child Trauma

Trauma across generations, such as a history of maternal childhood trauma (i.e., intergenerational trauma), can be an additional risk factor over and above any risk of perinatal mental health (Hesse & Main, 2000). Consideration of intergenerational trauma and its possible impact on child development (e.g., child social emotional development; Folger et al., 2017), is necessary when analyzing maternal perinatal mental health because of the comorbidity of mental health and trauma (Giovanelli et al., 2016). Similarly, with an estimated one-third of children experiencing childhood adversity, childhood trauma may be another co-occurring factor to explain differences in individual outcomes for children in the presence of maternal perinatal mental health (Kessler et al., 2010).

Theoretical Pathways for the Transfer of Maternal
Risk From Mental Health to Child Developmental Outcomes

A mechanism that explains how maternal mental health may influence child developmental outcomes is required. Mechanisms through which this may occur include biological pathways in pregnancy, impairment of the mother–infant relationship, or impact on the family system. There are also potential moderators—risk or protective factors—of the association (e.g., socioeconomic context, maternal social support) and mediators (e.g., chronic exposure, parenting) that influence its strength (Stein et al., 2014).

Biological

The fetal programming hypothesis (Swanson & Wadhwa, 2008) has been posited to explain the relationship between pregnancy exposures and later experience of psychopathology or disease (Lewis et al., 2015). Mechanisms such as epigenetic changes might account for the long-term effects of the pregnancy environment on later behavioral phenotypes (Aktar et al., 2019). Maternal lifestyle and health behaviors can also be altered in the presence of mental health, with higher rates of prenatal alcohol, tobacco, and substance use; less utilization of prenatal care; and exposure to psychotropic medications, all of which may directly impact fetal development. However, understanding the risk of specific environmental exposures has occurred in the context of infant and child mental health (Lyons-Ruth et al., 2017), and not child development, as is the focus of this chapter.

The Mother–Infant Dyad

Children exist within their social and environmental systems. Child development is therefore inextricably connected to the child's caregiving experiences, starting with the mother–infant relationship (Clark et al., 2020). The mother–infant relationship is frequently cited as a mechanism through which the risk of maternal mental disorder may influence the infant and later the child (Goodman & Gotlib, 1999; Howard & Challacombe, 2018). Parenting quality is a possible mediator between maternal mental health and child outcomes (Stein et al., 2014), just as the mother–infant relationship may enhance specific child outcomes. If the quality of mother–infant interactions is reduced by maternal mental health, there may be detrimental effects on the child. However, research understanding the exact association between perinatal mental health and the mother–infant relationship is conflicting.

Women with depression have been reported to show a reduction in maternal sensitivity, positive affect and verbal input, and an increase in irritability and hostility during mother–infant interactions (Bernard et al., 2018; Ierardi et al., 2019; Milgrom et al., 2004). Similarly, women with generalized anxiety symptoms have been reported to exhibit increased intrusiveness (Möller et al., 2015), and women with schizophrenia are documented as less sensitive and responsive (Wan et al., 2008). Yet, other studies have not reflected the same outcomes with women still able to engage sensitively with their infants in the context of perinatal mental health disorders (Cicchetti et al., 1999). Findings suggest that reduced relationship quality may not be the inevitable outcome (Fonseca et al., 2010; MacMillan et al., 2020), and instead it is the combination of maternal perinatal depression with other risk factors that can lead to mother–infant relationship difficulties (e.g., Kluczniok et al., 2016; MacMillan et al., 2021).

Cultural Considerations

Culture shapes child development, and although the developmental process is similar across cultures, progression may vary as children acquire culture-specific skills (Black et al., 2017). Although cultural status and immigration are often confounded in developmental research (e.g., Tseng, 2006), the separation of these factors is recommended (Quintana et al., 2006). This requires the identification of two distinct experiences in the literature; women in culturally and linguistically diverse (CaLD) groups who live in a new country because of migration (i.e., forced or elected) and women living in low- and middle-income countries (LMIC). There may also be limitations around the application of research findings to women from diverse cultural groups living in their country of origin. Developmental measures may require modification to capture these differences.

Culturally Appropriate Child Development Measures in LMIC

Access to culturally appropriate child development assessment measures is necessary. This was addressed by the WHO through the development and standardization of culturally appropriate individual scales of psychosocial development for children aged 0–6 years

(Lansdown et al., 1996). Since this study, the World Bank has published Examining Early Child Development in Low-Income Countries: A Toolkit for the Assessment of Children in the First Five Years of Life (Fernald et al., 2017), which is a comprehensive framework for the utilization of child development measures across LMIC. There are very few studies examining child development in infants from CaLD groups who have migrated, with unique methodological challenges involved. This is demonstrated by a recent study in the United Kingdom, which investigated prelinguistic and early language development in 59 infants from CaLD backgrounds (Cameron-Faulkner et al., 2021).

Cultural Considerations When Examining the Evidence between Perinatal Mental Health Disorders and Child Development

Women from CaLD backgrounds have been shown to have both a higher (Fellmeth et al., 2017) and lower (Anderson et al., 2017) prevalence of perinatal mental health disorders; however, there is considerable methodological and study population heterogeneity observed in these studies. There is also a paucity of research examining the association between perinatal mental health disorders and child development in women from CaLD backgrounds, with women from CaLD backgrounds more likely to experience barriers in their access to medical and mental health services, leading to potential delays in diagnosis and treatment (e.g., Byrow et al., 2020).

While children in LMIC are at greater risk of not fulfilling their developmental potential, there is only limited evidence of perinatal depression as a risk factor (Walker et al., 2011). There is a putative relationship between perinatal mental health disorders acting indirectly on child development through mechanisms mediated by proven risk factors. For example, poor maternal nutrition; higher rates of unemployment increasing the risk of poverty; or self-medication for untreated perinatal mental health disorders with substance or alcohol use, which, depending on the timing, as well as the frequency and duration of the exposure, can have adverse effects on fetal and child development (Georgieff et al., 2018; Hoyme et al., 2005).

Examination of Perinatal Mental Health Disorders and Child Development Outcomes: Critical Analysis of the Evidence

Maternal Perinatal Depression and Child Developmental Outcomes

Of the different types of perinatal psychopathology, depression is the most prevalent and estimated in 10– 25% of women (Elisei et al., 2013; Gotlib et al., 1989; O'Hara & Swain, 1996), although perinatal anxiety is estimated in 10–24% of women (Field, 2018). Other serious perinatal mental illnesses may include maternal bipolar disorder, schizophrenia, eating disorder, borderline personality disorder, maternal trauma, and alcohol and substance use. Our focus in this chapter is on perinatal depression, which has the greatest volume of research on perinatal disorders.

Child Cognitive Development

Findings are mixed regarding an association between maternal perinatal depression and child cognitive outcomes. Some researchers suggest a relation between maternal perinatal depression and poorer child cognitive development (e.g., Bluett-Duncan et al., 2021), citing systematic and meta-analytic reviews in support (Grace et al., 2003; Kingston et al., 2015; Kingston et al., 2012; Liu et al., 2017). However, methodological variation between these studies reduces the certainty of this association.

The conceptualization of perinatal depression and the timing of its measurement is important in the interpretation of findings. This is demonstrated by Lyons-Ruth et al. (1986), who concluded that perinatal depression may have a profound impact on infant cognitive development. Yet, maternal depression was assessed using symptomatic measurement only at two time points, one of which was childbirth, and the other was postnatally at 18 months, after the conclusion of the perinatal period. Data in this study may represent women with increased depressive symptoms at childbirth, a time of physical and emotional change, but not capture women with perinatal depressive disorder.

In contrast, other studies may rely on symptomatic and diagnostic measurements of perinatal depression but conceptualize child cognitive development differently. For instance, Murray (1992) administered the EPDS postnatally at six weeks, followed by diagnostic assessment at two to three months. Their sample included 56 women who had experienced an episode of postpartum depression in the first three months. Although significant differences were observed between the infants of depressed and nondepressed mothers on the object permanence and the object concept tasks, no differences were recorded for the *Bayley Scales* or the *Reynell Scales of Language Development* (Reynell & Huntley, 1985). Whether this study supports deficits in "child cognitive development" is questionable, with any conclusion regarding cognitive child development requiring performance in Piaget's task to be contextualized more broadly.

It is also necessary to separate studies that examine the impact of perinatal depression on child development from those that capture exposure to chronic maternal depression across childhood. Hay et al. (2001) examined postpartum depression at three months using diagnostic and symptomatic measurement of depression and child cognitive development at 11 years using the Wechsler. Significant differences were recorded between the IQ of children of mothers who did not have depression at three months who scored around the population mean ($M = 103$), and those whose mothers did have depression who scored lower ($M = 89.3$). However, there were only 29 women comprising the depressed sample, and it is possible that at least some of those women had experienced subsequent episodes after the perinatal period and not a single episode of postpartum depression at three months. This means the impact on child cognitive development may be attributed to repeated exposure to maternal depression across the first 11 years rather than specifically to perinatal depression.

Chronic or recurrent maternal depression may be more likely to impact child development (e.g., Petterson & Albers, 2001), as well as how severe and prolonged the depression is, and the presence of other maternal or child factors (e.g., education, poverty, trauma). Children of mothers who experienced depressive disorder in the first postpartum year scored significantly lower on the General Cognitive Index at age four years than children of mothers without depression (Cogill et al., 1986). However, when Hay and Kumar (1995) revisited these data, they identified that the lower cognitive performance was for children of mothers with low educational attainment and a history of perinatal depressive disorder. Similarly, in a meta-analysis of the relationship between postpartum depression and child cognitive development (Grace et al., 2003), of the seven studies identified, small effects of postpartum depression on infant performance on cognitive tasks were reported, with that effect mainly isolated to boys (e.g., Murray, 1992) and thereby at least in part attributable to gender differences.

Other studies have reported no association between perinatal depression and child cognitive performance (e.g., Murray et al., 1996). Most recently, a robust methodological design employed by Nix et al. (2021) found no relation between perinatal depression and child cognitive development. Women were categorized into three groups (i.e., current major depressive episode in pregnancy; history of major depressive disorder; and control), according to diagnostic assessment in pregnancy with chronicity of postpartum depressive symptoms measured at 2, 5, and 12 months. Child development was assessed using the *Neonatal Behavioral Assessment Scale* (Brazelton & Nugent, 1995) at 2 and 6 months and the *Bayley Scales* at 12 months. No significant correlations between maternal prenatal or current depression scores and child cognitive development were reported. Nix noted their findings did not replicate other studies (i.e., Murray et al., 1996; Koutra et al., 2013), with differences possibly reflecting the variation in methodological approaches across this literature.

A recent meta-analysis by Rogers et al. (2020) reported a small association between perinatal depression, memory, and language ($r = -.14, .21$, respectively), with a larger association with IQ ($r = -.57$; Hay & Kumar, 1995; Milgrom et al., 2004). The issue with reliance on these findings is related to the limitations of meta-analytic research. Included in the composition of the effect size to quantify the relationship between perinatal depression and memory or language are studies with different methodological designs, maternal perinatal depression measured symptomatically, diagnostically, and at single and multiple time points.

A specific cognitive outcome potentially affected by perinatal depression is child EF. The most widely accepted definition of EF is that it is a set of cognitive skills related to self-regulation (Miyake et al., 2000), and is itself a predictor of psychosocial outcomes over the lifespan. As such, EF may represent an adverse developmental pathway in children exposed to maternal depression. A meta-analysis suggested there was a small association ($r = .07$; Power et al., 2021), but the interpretation is tempered by variability in the measurement of exposure to maternal depression, and the lack of validated measures of child EF used. This analysis also suggested that maternal depressive symptoms occurring after the perinatal period may be important for EF development, highlighting the consideration that different cognitive capacities may have different critical windows or that chronicity of symptoms is a key variable.

Child Social Emotional Development

Child social emotional development is important and predictive of relationship functioning and attachment; school performance; and mental health (Denham et al., 2009). Some evidence suggests that perinatal mental health may adversely influence these outcomes. In a sample of 1,235 women, a three to fourfold increase in child social emotional issues at two years was reported for children of mothers with depressive symptoms at 32 weeks' gestation or postnatally at eight weeks (Junge et al., 2017). These results replicated other research that applied a similar conceptualization and measurement of perinatal depression (Koutra et al., 2013).

Despite these findings, the association between perinatal maternal depression and child social and emotional development is not to be overstated. There are methodological differences in the conceptualization of child social emotional development. Waxler et al.'s (2011) review applied the construct of attachment to measure child social emotional development. In contrast, other longitudinal research has relied upon the *Strengths and Difficulties Questionnaire* (Niclasen et al., 2012); the *Ages and Stages Questionnaire* (Squires et al., 1997);

and the *Bayley Scales* (Bayley, 1969; Sikander et al., 2019). To ensure accurate translation of research findings, it is necessary to distinguish the methodology of each study.

Motor Development

Infant motor development is central to adaptive functioning and predictive of child cognitive outcomes as well as neurodevelopmental disorders (Marrus et al., 2018). Investigation of any association between perinatal maternal depression and infant motor development is important to identify infants that may require early intervention. However, research findings are mixed regarding the relationship between perinatal depression and child gross and fine motor development (Slomian et al., 2019).

For instance, a significant difference is observed between infant motor development at six months for infants of mothers with prenatal depression diagnosis, compared to infants whose mothers did not have prenatal depression diagnosis (O'Leary et al., 2019). Though with only 57 women in the depression group, a small effect size, and differences not maintained at 12 months, this evidence has limited application. Similarly, motor development delay was reported for infants of mothers with depressive symptoms compared to those without depressive symptoms, but depression was captured using symptomatic measurement at a single time point at the end of pregnancy, when maternal mood can fluctuate in the context of significant physical and biological changes (Zhang et al., 2019). There are also other studies (e.g., Piteo et al., 2012; Sutter-Dallay et al., 2011) that do not demonstrate any association, indicating that adverse infant motor development is by no means an inevitable outcome of exposure to perinatal depression.

Maternal Perinatal Anxiety and Child Developmental Outcomes

Maternal perinatal anxiety is common and often comorbid with depression (Goodman et al., 2016; Skouteris et al., 2009). Identification of perinatal anxiety may be more challenging with issues around the failure to access treatment for this disorder (e.g., Smith et al., 2009). This may be because there is no validated and reliable gold standard screening measure for perinatal anxiety (Furtado et al., 2018).

Child Cognitive Development

The evidence regarding perinatal anxiety and child cognitive development lacks agreement. Some studies conceptualize perinatal anxiety as symptoms of panic disorder and somatic anxiety, whereas others define it as trait anxiety (e.g., Bolea-Alamañac et al., 2018; Mennes et al., 2009). Given the psychopathology and symptoms of different anxiety disorders are unique, it is necessary to exercise caution in the application of findings to other studies with comparable conceptualization.

Bolea-Alamañac et al. (2018) examined prenatal maternal anxiety and child inattention at eight and a half years using data from the Avon Longitudinal Study of Parents and Children (ALSPC), a population-based cohort from the United Kingdom. Perinatal maternal anxiety was assessed at 18 and 32 weeks' gestation and encompassed symptoms of panic disorder and somatic anxiety using the Crown Crisp Experiential Index (Crown & Crisp, 1966) to form a factor researchers labeled "somatic anxiety in pregnancy." No evidence of an association between somatic anxiety in pregnancy and cognitive tasks (i.e., sky search;

sky search dual task or opposite words) was reported from the Test of Everyday Attention for Children (TEA-Ch; Heaton et al., 2001).

In contrast, other studies support an association between perinatal anxiety and child cognitive outcomes. For example, Mennes et al. (2009) reported a relation between prenatal anxiety measured using the *State-Trait Anxiety Inventory* (STAI; Spielberger, 1983), and cognitive performance defined as a gambling paradigm testing endogenous cognitive control at 17 years of age. However, with only eight boys in the sample of higher anxiety, this provides limited evidence. The findings build on those by Van den Bergh et al. (2005), who also measured perinatal anxiety using the STAI, and reported increased impulsivity in an encoding task at age 15 years for children of mothers in the high anxiety group, though there was no effect of exposure to high perinatal anxiety on any of the other cognitive tasks. Examining the research applying anxiety disorder diagnosis, Reck et al. (2018) observed a significantly lower performance on language tasks for infants of mothers diagnosed with anxiety disorder, but with 34 women in their clinical sample, their findings are not to be over generalized.

Social Emotional Development

There are mixed findings regarding the relation between maternal perinatal anxiety and child social emotional development with some of the existing research relying on maternal self-report measurement. As outlined in the first section of this chapter, maternal self-report may be subject to bias and not necessarily representative of child functioning. Particularly in the context of maternal anxiety, researchers have observed negative cognitions and perceptions associated with maternal anxiety can influence the experience of the infant, response to the infant's signals (Kaitz & Maytal, 2005), and even the memory of different events (e.g., night waking; Morrell & Steele, 2003). We would seek research that measures child social emotional development by both subjective and objective measurement.

Evidence using only subjective measurement to assess child development is seen in the population-based studies. A Norwegian study reported that children exposed prenatally to increased anxiety symptoms were two times more likely to experience infant difficulties postnatally at six months as assessed by the *Infant Characteristics Questionnaire* and the CBCL (Bekkhus et al., 2018). This study replicated findings from another Netherlands population-based study (Henrichs et al., 2009), in which high maternal anxiety symptoms prenatally at 20 weeks' gestation and postnatally at six months predicted increased perceived infant temperamental difficulties (i.e., increased infant activity level, distress at limitations, and sadness measured using the *Infant Behavior Questionnaire*). These studies both rely on maternal self-report only, so application of their findings requires awareness of this bias and its possible impact on the results.

Other studies rely upon multiple sources of self-report (e.g., parent and teacher). Loomans et al. (2011), based on teacher and maternal report, observed an association between prenatal maternal state-trait anxiety and child emotional problems, peer problems and prosocial behavior at age five years. Interestingly, there were only weak to moderate cross-informant correlations between maternal and teacher report, a finding reflective of other studies (Lambert et al., 1998). The strongest support for the association between maternal perinatal anxiety and the child outcome was with the maternal report of the child's behavior. It is possible that these findings capture the association between maternal anxiety and the endorsement of child problem behaviors (Kroes et al., 2003; Najman et al., 2000), rather than maternal anxiety and child developmental outcomes.

Motor Development

Recent meta-analysis reported a medium to large association between postpartum anxiety and motor development ($r = -.31$; Rogers et al., 2020), with two studies cited in support. The first study used the same measure to assess depressive and anxious symptoms; the *Zung Depression and Anxiety Scale*; (Zung, 1971), with researchers extracting those items related to perinatal maternal anxiety (Galler et al., 2000). The data may, therefore, only represent those somatic and psychological symptoms of anxiety included in the scale. The second study measured maternal perinatal anxiety using diagnostic measurement (i.e., the MINI International Neuropsychiatric Interview; Sheehan et al., 1998), with the *Alberta Infant Motor Scale* to assess child motor development (Pinheiro et al., 2014). However, although the sample included 152 women, only 20 women were identified as having perinatal maternal anxiety, so findings provide a starting point for further investigation.

Serious Mental Illness and Child Development

We assess the current evidence regarding maternal bipolar disorder, schizophrenia, eating disorders, borderline personality disorder, maternal trauma, alcohol and substance use, and child development.

Maternal Bipolar Disorder

With an age of onset estimated before 25 years (Vieta et al., 2018), women with bipolar disorder are required to consider their pregnancy and the postpartum period in the context of their mental health disorder. Yet there is no clear research regarding maternal bipolar disorder and child developmental outcomes. Related research has tried to understand perinatal risk factors for these women, but the findings are not consistent; sample sizes vary, as well as differences in the categorization of perinatal risk, and the interpretation of findings (Rusner et al., 2016).

Population-based studies have examined cognitive outcomes using databases for children of women with bipolar disorder. In the United States, Ranning et al. (2016) reported children of parents with diagnosed bipolar disorder were 1.6 times more likely not to graduate primary school then other children. However, unlike some studies (Duffy et al., 2007; Ranning et al., 2016), children of mothers with bipolar disorder did not show different grades, a finding which replicates other research (Jundong et al., 2012; Lin et al., 2016). Similar data is reflected in a West Australian study of 6,303 women, in which children with an intellectual disability were 3.1 times more likely to have a mother with bipolar disorder (Morgan et al., 2008). However, findings from these population-based studies do not provide insight into the association between the psychopathology of bipolar disorder and child cognitive outcomes, with rates of intellectual disability a possible reflection of an interaction of other comorbid factors for women with this disorder.

Maternal Schizophrenia

For women with schizophrenia, there can be associated disability that is of particular relevance to understanding the impact of this mental disorder in the perinatal period (Taylor et al., 2020). The overrepresentation of women with schizophrenia experiencing a loss of custody of their child, the involvement of social work, or single parenting (Howard et al.,

2004; Ranning et al., 2016; Seeman, 2012), highlights the need for specialized treatment. Although evidence regarding child developmental outcomes for children of parents with schizophrenia has been examined by Hameed and Lewis' (2016) systematic review, the studies cited in the context of child cognitive, perceptual, and motor outcomes are at least 20 years old, with the majority published between 1977 and 1987 (Hameed & Lewis, 2016). There is a need for current longitudinal research capable of testing these relationships by employing a robust methodological approach.

Existing study findings may also not be as conclusive as some researchers may suggest. For instance, no differences between children at high risk of schizophrenia and controls have been reported on a range of cognitive tests (i.e., *Wechsler Intelligence Scale for Children Verbal Scale*; *Bender Gestalt Test*; *Taylor Closure Test*; *Draw a Man Test*; *Roscharch Test*; and *Thematic Apperception Test*), though specific differences were observed including arithmetic proficiency; perceptual motor functioning and some verbalization patterns (Sohlberg, 1985). In contrast, infants of parents with schizophrenia have demonstrated reduced motor and sensorimotor in the first year (Marcus et al., 1981), as well as reduced social competence and IQ (Goodman, 1987). Similarly, Di Prinzio et al. (2018) reported that children with intellectual disability were 3.8 times more likely to have a mother with schizophrenia. Notably, documented adverse outcomes for children of a mother with schizophrenia may reflect a culmination of other risk factors that can be comorbid with the disorder but which may impact on child development, including maternal substance use, homelessness, poverty, and poor self-care and nutrition (Ayano et al., 2019; Westermeyer, 2006).

Maternal Eating Disorders

With a physical and mental health component to the disorder, eating disorders present unique challenges for obstetric and psychopathological treatment. Prevalence rates estimate that 10% of women experience an eating disorder (Fogarty et al., 2018), though obtaining accuracy is challenging given the level of concealment and denial associated with the disorder. High rates of comorbid anxiety and depression exist (Swinbourne & Touyz, 2007), with the impact of pregnancy on eating disorder symptoms not consistent. Some studies document the protection of pregnancy (Lacey & Smith, 1987). Other studies demonstrate a reduction in eating disordered behaviors but not a cessation, and then there are women that experience either a worsening of symptoms or the maintenance of pre-pregnancy levels (Bulik et al., 2007; Tierney et al., 2011).

Growing literature examines the effect of perinatal eating disorder on child development, though results are not conclusive (see Watson et al., 2018, for a review). The variation in study methodology makes the development of an evidence base difficult, as diversity is observed in the conceptualization and measurement of maternal eating disorders. Kothari et al. (2014) investigated early cognitive development for "children at high risk of developing an eating disorder." Eating disorder was measured by maternal self-report of history of anorexia nervosa or bulimia nervosa. The difficulty of exclusive reliance on self-report is that only low to moderate agreement has been observed between self-report of eating disorder symptoms and objective measurement using eating disorder diagnosis and clinical assessment (Wolk et al., 2005).

In contrast, Sadeh-Sharvit et al. (2016) recruited women with a perinatal eating disorder diagnosis from a psychiatrist applying DSM-IV criteria (American Psychiatric Association, 2000), with chronicity of current symptoms also assessed with the *Eating Disorders*

Inventory (Garner et al., 1982). Researchers reported maternal eating disorder symptom severity as the strongest predictor of mental and psychomotor child development at 18–42 months using the *Bayley Scales*; however, with only 29 women in the sample, further investigation is required.

Barona et al. (2017) provided this opportunity in their prospective study of 137 women recruited in the first or second trimester of pregnancy. Based on diagnostic assessment, women were categorized into three groups: women diagnosed with current eating disorders ($n = 37$), women with a history of eating disorders ($n = 39$); and healthy controls ($n = 61$). Chronicity of eating disorder symptoms was assessed in the third trimester of pregnancy, and the *Bayley Scales* was administered to assess infant development at 12 months of age. Results showed significant differences between women with a history of eating disorders and healthy controls for language composite and language receptive, as well as fine motor, gross motor, and motor composite scale. There was increased likelihood of language issues and gross motor development for infants of mothers with lifetime anorexia nervosa compared to healthy controls. Similarly, overall lower cognitive development, language and motor development was noted for infants of mothers with a history of bulimia nervosa compared to healthy controls. Notably, there were 20 women in the sample with anorexia and 15 women with bulimia history, so again, any association is a starting point. That said, the potential risk of maternal eating disorder replicates other study findings (Micali et al., 2014).

Maternal Borderline Personality Disorder

There is little research regarding maternal borderline personality disorder (BPD) in the context of the perinatal period, a concern given the stability of personality traits, which unlike depressive symptoms, do not fluctuate and have the same consistent influence on a child (Fajkowska & Kreitler, 2018). This is why personality disorder may have increased influence over parenting style (Raine et al., 2019), and has been suggested as a stronger predictor of adverse child outcomes than parental psychopathology (Rutter, 1984).

Research regarding the developmental effects of BPD on offspring identify the increased risk of child psychopathology (Barnow et al., 2006), attentional and behavioral disorders (Weiss et al., 1996), reduced quality mother–infant interactions (Newman et al., 2007), and increased likelihood of adverse events including removal from home, exposure to parental substance abuse, or frequent school change (Macfie, 2009). It is difficult to locate research that assesses the developmental perspective by measuring cognitive, motor, or social emotional outcomes for children of mothers with BPD. Given the known impact of BPD on difficulties with self-regulation, suicidal ideation, substance use and other self-destructive behaviors, coupled with prevalence estimates (Lieb et al., 2004), the potential impact for offspring of women with BPD on experiencing an environment capable of supporting optimal child development is concerning (Blankley et al., 2015; Lewis et al., 2015; Stepp et al., 2012).

Maternal Trauma

Many women worldwide experience trauma; armed conflict, sexual, physical, or emotional abuse or neglect, or exposure to a traumatic event (e.g., cancer diagnosis; car accident; death or bereavement). It has been estimated that two billion people are living in areas exposed to armed conflict (Garry & Checchi, 2020) and at higher risk of mental disorders (Rozanov et al., 2019), with prevalence rates telling us that physical, sexual and emotional abuse and neglect are experienced by a not insignificant proportion of our female population (Dworkin et al., 2021). Research findings regarding maternal trauma and child development are mixed, though this may reflect the variation in types of maternal trauma that women can experience (e.g., health trauma vs. armed conflict vs. intimate partner violence; IPV).

A study regarding the impact of cancer diagnosis in pregnancy on child development did not evidence any differences between child cognitive, language, or motor scores (measured using the *Bayley Scales*) at 6 to 42 months (Betchen et al., 2020). In contrast, among 502 Palestinian mothers and infants exposed to traumatic war events in pregnancy, structural equation modeling revealed that maternal trauma exposure was associated with increased postpartum maternal mental health issues at six months, and reduced infant motor, cognitive and social emotional development at 18 months (measured using the *Bayley Scales*; Qouta et al., 2021). Similarly, substantial evidence documents the increased rates of women experiencing posttraumatic stress disorder in the context of IPV (Nathanson et al., 2012; Norwood & Murphy, 2012), as well as the impact on maternal parenting capacity.

IPV is conceptualized as intimate partner violence that may involve physical, sexual, emotional, or psychological abuse. Increased parenting stress that occurs in the context of IPV is associated with a reduction in positive parenting practices (e.g., maternal sensitivity, positive reinforcement), reduced consistency, increased likelihood of physical discipline, and increased permissiveness (Levendosky et al., 2006; Rossman & Rea, 2005). There is also evidence of the social emotional consequences of IPV exposure in early childhood, including emotional dysregulation at 24 months (Hibel et al., 2011), as well as emotional insecurity (El-Sheikh et al., 2008). For instance, six-month-old infants showed reduced emotional regulation (measured by the *Bayley Scales*) where they were exposed to marital conflict compared to infants that were not exposed to marital conflict (Porter et al., 2003).

Maternal Substance and Alcohol Use

Given the prevalence rates of alcohol and substance use and their comorbidity with perinatal mental health disorders (Glantz et al., 2020), as well as the possible implications for child development, it is necessary to examine both in the context of this chapter.

Alcohol use estimates in pregnancy range widely from 20% to 80% (O'Keeffe et al., 2015). Other estimates among pregnant women in the United States indicate that 3.1% report binge drinking, with 10.1% reporting alcohol use, and one in ten women noting they had consumed alcohol in the past 30 days (Tan et al., 2015). Concerns about alcohol use in pregnancy stem from alcohol fetal syndrome, a fetal condition caused by high levels of exposure to intermittent or chronic maternal perinatal alcohol use (Hoyme et al., 2005). The effect of alcohol exposure varies between individual children and can be influenced by the timing in the gestation of exposure, the quantity and frequency of the exposure, and other maternal factors including genetic predisposition, other drug use, maternal age, and SES (O'Leary, 2004). Whereas evidence is undisputed regarding the risk of high levels of alcohol intake on child development, the position regarding lower rates of alcohol consumption is mixed, with some evidence that low to moderate alcohol use may not be associated with adverse child outcomes (Robinson et al., 2010).

An estimated 27 million women in the United States report the use of prescription or illicit opioids routinely (Goettsche et al., 2014). Prevalence is likely to be even higher than this, with substance use generally underreported because of the stigma it attracts (Van Boekel et al., 2013), a stigma that is heightened in pregnancy (Nichols et al., 2021). One study compared maternal self-report to the objective assessment of substance use using an analysis of meconium (Messinger et al., 2004). There was 66% agreement between positive meconium report and maternal self-reported drug use, with 38% of women who tested positive for cocaine or opiate use, denying any substance use. Significantly, the use of different substances was also common with only 2% of women using cocaine alone.

Although there is convincing evidence regarding the adverse obstetric and neonatal outcomes associated with substance use in pregnancy, the research regarding the direct effect of that use on child developmental outcomes is less clear (Baldacchino et al., 2014). Again, the timing of the exposure to the substance, as well as the frequency and duration of that exposure, is important when considering the child developmental outcomes (Georgieff et al., 2018). If exposure is only short term, then long-term developmental effects may be avoided (Georgieff et al., 2018).

In the U.S. Maternal Lifestyle Study of 11,800 women, participant drug use was self-reported and objectively assessed, and child developmental outcomes were assessed at one, two, and three years of age using the *Bayley Scales*. Results showed that infants exposed to cocaine were 1.6 points lower on the mental developmental index than infants without exposure (Messinger et al., 2004). Infants exposed to opiates were 3.8 points lower in psychomotor development. Significant differences in IQ for children exposed to cocaine increased over time, with 1.45 points difference at three years of age and 4.4 points at four and seven years of age. Children exposed to cocaine use prenatally were also 1.56 times more likely to be referred to special education than children without exposure. For opiate-exposed infants, although psychomotor developmental scores were lower at age three years, by age ten years there were no significant differences in cognitive outcomes; however, there did remain a significant difference in children's ability to understand complex sentences (Bauer et al., 2020).

Although the cognitive effects of substance use in pregnancy on child cognitive outcomes were not the size one might anticipate, even these small effects could adversely impact the functional capacity of those individual children (Shankaran et al., 2007). Given the comorbidity of maternal substance use and other risk factors including parental quality, child abuse, and trauma (Appleyard et al., 2011; Yoon et al., 2021), it is likely an interaction of these factors that contributes to this group of children not reaching their developmental potential rather than the exclusive direct effects of the substance itself.

Clinical Application

Prompt identification and service access are required for perinatal mental health problems for the individual woman as well as attention to the potential impact on the mother–infant relationship and the developing fetus and child (England et al., 2018). Despite differences in the association observed between perinatal mental health and child developmental outcomes, there is sufficient evidence to establish perinatal mental health as a potential risk factor that may influence child outcomes, particularly in the context of other adverse maternal or infant factors (e.g., maternal education, social support, maternal or child trauma, maternal substance, or alcohol use). It is this interaction of different factors that shapes maternal and infant outcomes and supports the establishment of an integrated perinatal service. An integrated approach to perinatal mental health services could facilitate multidisciplinary service access, as well as the capacity to support the mother and the infant to maximize both maternal and infant outcomes (Judd et al., 2018; Lomonaco-Haycraft et al., 2019; Myors et al., 2013).

Application of child developmental considerations into a perinatal mental health service requires consideration of how to incorporate child developmental screening into perinatal mental health treatment given that perinatal mental health services are usually limited in most jurisdictions to conception to 12 months. Seminal work by Goldberg and Huxley (1980) proposed a tiered mental healthcare system. The first tier encompasses subthreshold symptoms and involves recommended self-help and lifestyle changes (e.g., voluntary community groups and mothers' groups). The second tier includes access to outpatient care for individuals with mild to moderate symptoms. The third tier provides access to specialist perinatal mental health services delivered by an expert multidisciplinary team, with specialized prenatal and postpartum mental health assessment and treatment, as well as preconception care to women with complex or severe mental health disorders who are considering pregnancy. The final tier is reserved for complex or severe mental health problems with treatment in an inpatient setting at a mother–baby unit, which may encompass the final trimester of pregnancy and, for most units includes from birth up to 12 months (Galbally et al., 2019). Child developmental screening could occur at the third or fourth tier.

Incorporation of Infant Developmental Considerations Into an Integrated Perinatal Mental Health Service

By providing another primary care medium of surveillance for infant development, an integrated perinatal service would have the capability for early identification of infants that may demonstrate developmental delay, with early intervention a well-established requirement to optimize child outcomes (Case-Smith et al., 2013; Namasivayam et al., 2021). For those mothers with perinatal mental health problems, the application of developmental screening could facilitate their own mental health treatment, with evidence to challenge maternal cognitions or beliefs that their own mental health has adversely impacted their infant's development. In the case where there may be developmental concerns, the woman might be supported in early identification and access to treatment intervention. This integration of infant developmental considerations into a perinatal service could occur through either screening or referral.

Screening of Infant/Child Development Within a Perinatal Service

There could be two options available to incorporate infant/child developmental screening for a perinatal mental health service. First, clinicians could administer a self-report measure for the mother to complete. The benefit of this is that it is time-limited and achievable within a service setting, with no specialist qualifications required. In contrast, an objective measure is often administered by a specialist (e.g., psychologist, speech therapist, occupational therapist, physiotherapist, or pediatrician) and generally requires more time for administration. The inclusion of developmental screening could form a part of the embedded collaborative process established with developmental specialists, which would acknowledge the presence of the infant and the possibility that some infants may experience developmental delay particularly when there are other comorbid risk factors.

Alternatively, the service could embed an assessment of infant development within the mother's individual psychotherapy assessment. Clinicians in perinatal mental health have as part of their training observational assessment skills and the theoretical framework to identify developmental concerns. The challenge for perinatal services is to provide the framework to support clinicians to deliver a service that is inclusive of the needs of the infant while still being able to deliver evidence-based and specialized perinatal mental health treatment to the mother. The demarcation between the role of the perinatal service in providing developmental screening, with referral to specialized child developmental services where the infant is identified as either being at risk of nonoptimal outcomes, does not involve the integration of perinatal services with child developmental services but collaboration between the bodies. Collaboration and not integration could also protect against the blurring from the woman as the focus in the delivery of care in a perinatal service.

Referral to Specialized Infant and Child Developmental Services

If the establishment of an integrated perinatal service is not possible, then the referral process to other child developmental services by the perinatal provider is critical. If this is provided as a process with a framework of steps for clinicians and training in how to engage in the referral process, it could facilitate women at risk of reduced developmental outcomes for their child accessing multidisciplinary support. Referral rates can present challenges. For instance, a referral rate of only 61% for children who had failed screens (King et al., 2010). The difficulties involved in screening highlights the benefit of an integrated service where the referral process requires less management since the patient can be linked to the specialist through the processes they are already engaged with at the practice.

Key Messages

The following are key messages from this chapter regarding child development and perinatal mental health:

- Child developmental considerations are required in the context of perinatal mental health research, treatment, and services.
- Child developmental outcomes are a complex interaction of different biopsychosocial factors, so overemphasis on any one factor including perinatal mental health does not reflect the evidence in the developmental literature.
- Accurate interpretation and translation of research findings regarding the size of any risk associated with perinatal mental health disorders for child development is critical to protect against stigma or additional distress that could otherwise be experienced by women with perinatal mental health disorders.
- Methodological challenges including differences in the conceptualization and measurement of perinatal mental health disorders and child developmental outcomes limit the applicability of existing findings.
- Existing studies that demonstrate an adverse effect of perinatal mental health on child developmental outcomes generally show small effect sizes, so the impact is not to be overstated.
- The focus in the literature is predominantly on maternal perinatal depression and anxiety, with less known about other serious perinatal mental illness and child development.
- Sociodemographic factors, as well as other maternal factors including poverty, poor nutrition, alcohol or substance use exposure, social support, trauma, or breastfeeding, may either increase or decrease any adverse effect of perinatal mental health on child development.

- Awareness of how infant/child developmental concerns may present in the context of treatment for women with perinatal mental health disorders is necessary for perinatal service providers.
- Incorporation of infant developmental considerations into integrated perinatal mental health services is necessary to provide early intervention and service access to infants that may be at risk.

References

Achenbach, T. M., & Edelbrock, C. (1983). *Manual for the child behaviour checklist and revised child behaviour profile*. Department of Psychiatry, University of Vermont.

Achenbach, T. M., & Ruffle, T. M. (2000). The Child Behavior Checklist and related forms for assessing behavioral/emotional problems and competencies. *Pediatrics in Review, 21*(8), 265–271.

Aktar, E., Qu, J., Lawrence, P. J., Tollenaar, M. S., Elzinga, B. M., & Bögels, S. M. (2019). Fetal and infant outcomes in the offspring of parents with perinatal mental disorders: Earliest influences. *Frontiers in Psychiatry, 10*, 391.

Ali, N. S., Mahmud, S., Khan, A., & Ali, B. S. (2013). Impact of postpartum anxiety and depression on child's mental development from two peri-urban communities of Karachi, Pakistan: A quasi-experimental study. *BMC Psychiatry, 13*(1), 1–12.

American Psychiatric Association. (2000). *Diagnostic and statistical manual of mental disorders* (4th ed., text rev.). Author.

Anderson, F. M., Hatch, S. L., Comacchio, C., & Howard, L. M. (2017). Prevalence and risk of mental disorders in the perinatal period among migrant women: A systematic review and meta-analysis. *Archives of Women's Mental Health, 20*(3), 449–462.

Angold, A., & Costello, E. J. (1995). A test – retest reliability study of child-reported psychiatric symptoms and diagnoses using the Child and Adolescent Psychiatric Assessment (CAPA-C). *Psychological Medicine, 25*(4), 755–762.

Aoyagi, S. S., & Tsuchiya, K. J. (2019). Does maternal postpartum depression affect children's developmental outcomes? *Journal of Obstetrics and Gynaecology Research, 45*(9), 1809–1820.

Appleyard, K., Berlin, L. J., Rosanbalm, K. D., & Dodge, K. A. (2011). Preventing early child maltreatment: Implications from a longitudinal study of maternal abuse history, substance use problems, and offspring victimization. *Prevention Science, 12*(2), 139–149.

Ayano, G., Tesfaw, G., & Shumet, S. (2019). The prevalence of schizophrenia and other psychotic disorders among homeless people: A systematic review and meta-analysis. *BMC Psychiatry, 19*(1), 1–14.

Azak, S. (2012). Maternal depression and sex differences shape the infants' trajectories of cognitive development. *Infant Behavior and Development, 35*(4), 803–814.

Baldacchino, A., Arbuckle, K., Petrie, D. J., & McCowan, C. (2014). Neurobehavioral consequences of chronic intrauterine opioid exposure in infants and preschool children: A systematic review and meta-analysis. *BMC Psychiatry, 14*(1), 1–12.

Barnow, S., Spitzer, C., Grabe, H. J., Kessler, C., & Freyberger, H. J. (2006). Individual characteristics, familial experience, and psychopathology in children of mothers with borderline personality disorder. *Journal of the American Academy of Child & Adolescent Psychiatry, 45*(8), 965–972.

Barona, M., Taborelli, E., Corfield, F., Pawlby, S., Easter, A., Schmidt, U., . . . Micali, N. (2017). Neurobehavioural and cognitive development in infants born to mothers with eating disorders. *Journal of Child Psychology and Psychiatry, 58*(8), 931–938.

Bauer, C. R., Langer, J., Lambert-Brown, B., Shankaran, S., Bada, H. S., Lester, B., . . . Hammond, J. (2020). Association of prenatal opiate exposure with youth outcomes assessed from infancy through adolescence. *Journal of Perinatology, 40*(7), 1056–1065.

Bayley, N. (2006a). *Bayley scales of infant development: Bayley-III*. Harcourt Assessment.

Bayley, N. (2006b). *Manual for the Bayley scales of infant and toddler development*. NCS Pearson.

Bekkhus, M., Lee, Y., Nordhagen, R., Magnus, P., Samuelsen, S. O., & Borge, A. I. (2018). Re-examining the link between prenatal maternal anxiety and child emotional difficulties, using a sibling design. *International Journal of Epidemiology, 47*(1), 156–165.

Belsky, J., Bakermans-Kranenburg, M. J., & Van IJzendoorn, M. H. (2007). For better and for worse: Differential susceptibility to environmental influences. *Current Directions in Psychological Science*, 16(6), 300–304.

Bernard, K., Nissim, G., Vaccaro, S., Harris, J. L., & Lindhiem, O. (2018). Association between maternal depression and maternal sensitivity from birth to 12 months: A meta-analysis. *Attachment & Human Development*, 20(6), 578–599.

Betchen, M., Grunberg, V. A., Gringlas, M., & Cardonick, E. (2020). Being a mother after a cancer diagnosis during pregnancy: Maternal psychosocial functioning and child cognitive development and behavior. *Psycho-Oncology*, 29(7), 1148–1155.

Black, M. M., Pérez-Escamilla, R., & Fernandez Rao, S. (2015). Integrating nutrition and child development interventions: Scientific basis, evidence of impact, and implementation considerations. *Advances in Nutrition*, 6(6), 852–859.

Black, M. M., Walker, S. P., Fernald, L. C., Andersen, C. T., DiGirolamo, A. M., Lu, C., . . . Shiffman, J. (2017). Early childhood development coming of age: Science through the life course. *The Lancet*, 389(10064), 77–90.

Blankley, G., Galbally, M., Snellen, M., Power, J., & Lewis, A. J. (2015). Borderline personality disorder in the perinatal period: Early infant and maternal outcomes. *Australasian Psychiatry*, 23(6), 688–692.

Bluett-Duncan, M., Kishore, M. T., Patil, D. M., Satyanarayana, V. A., & Sharp, H. (2021). A systematic review of the association between perinatal depression and cognitive development in infancy in low and middle-income countries. *PloS One*, 16(6), e0253790.

Bolea-Alamañac, B., Davies, S. J., Evans, J., Joinson, C., Pearson, R., Skapinakis, P., & Emond, A. (2018). Do mothers who are anxious during pregnancy have inattentive children? *Journal of Affective Disorders*, 236, 120–126.

Bradley, R. H., Corwyn, R. F., McAdoo, H. P., & García Coll, C. (2001). The home environments of children in the United States part I: Variations by age, ethnicity, and poverty status. *Child Development*, 72(6), 1844–1867.

Brazelton, T. B., & Nugent, J. K. (1995). *Neonatal behavioral assessment scale* (No. 137). Cambridge University Press.

Bulik, C. M., Von Holle, A., Hamer, R., Berg, C. K., Torgersen, L., Magnus, P., . . . Reichborn-Kjennerud, T. (2007). Patterns of remission, continuation and incidence of broadly defined eating disorders during early pregnancy in the Norwegian Mother and Child Cohort Study (MoBa). *Psychological Medicine*, 37(8), 1109–1118.

Byrow, Y., Pajak, R., Specker, P., & Nickerson, A. (2020). Perceptions of mental health and perceived barriers to mental health help-seeking amongst refugees: A systematic review. *Clinical Psychology Review*, 75, 101812.

Cameron-Faulkner, T., Malik, N., Steele, C., Coretta, S., Serratrice, L., & Lieven, E. (2021). A cross-cultural analysis of early prelinguistic gesture development and its relationship to language development. *Child Development*, 92(1), 273–290.

Cardenas, S. I., Morris, A. R., Marshall, N., Aviv, E. C., Martínez García, M., Sellery, P., & Saxbe, D. E. (2022). Fathers matter from the start: The role of expectant fathers in child development. *Child Development Perspectives*, 16, 54–59.

Carneiro, P., Meghir, C., & Parey, M. (2013). Maternal education, home environments, and the development of children and adolescents. *Journal of the European Economic Association*, 11(suppl_1), 123–160.

Case-Smith, J., Frolek Clark, G. J., & Schlabach, T. L. (2013). Systematic review of interventions used in occupational therapy to promote motor performance for children ages birth – 5 years. *The American Journal of Occupational Therapy*, 67(4), 413–424.

Cicchetti, D., Toth, S. L., & Rogosch, F. A. (1999). The efficacy of toddler-parent psychotherapy to increase attachment security in offspring of depressed mothers. *Attachment & Human Development*, 1(1), 34–66.

Clark, H., Coll-Seck, A. M., Banerjee, A., Peterson, S., Dalglish, S. L., Ameratunga, S., . . . Borrazzo, J. (2020). A future for the world's children? A WHO – UNICEF – Lancet commission. *The Lancet*, 395(10224), 605–658.

Cogill, S., Caplan, H., Alexandra, H., Robson, K. M., & Kumar, R. (1986). Impact of maternal postnatal depression on cognitive development of young children. *British Medical Journal (Clinical Research Ed)*, 292(6529), 1165–1167.

Conroy, S., Pariante, C. M., Marks, M. N., Davies, H. A., Farrelly, S., Schacht, R., & Moran, P. (2012). Maternal psychopathology and infant development at 18 months: The impact of maternal personality disorder and depression. *Journal of the American Academy of Child & Adolescent Psychiatry, 51*(1), 51–61.

Crown, S., & Crisp, A. (1966). A short clinical diagnostic self-rating scale for psychoneurotic patients: The Middlesex Hospital Questionnaire (MHQ). *British Journal of Psychiatry, 112*(490), 917–923.

Denham, S. A., Wyatt, T., Bassett, H. H., Echeverria, D., & Knox, S. (2009). Assessing social-emotional development in children from a longitudinal perspective. *Journal of Epidemiology & Community Health, 63*(Suppl 1), i37–i52.

Di Prinzio, P., Morgan, V. A., Björk, J., Croft, M., Lin, A., Jablensky, A., & McNeil, T. F. (2018). Intellectual disability and psychotic disorders in children: Association with maternal severe mental illness and exposure to obstetric complications in a whole-population cohort. *American Journal of Psychiatry, 175*(12), 1232–1242.

Dollaghan, C. A., Campbell, T. F., Paradise, J. L., Feldman, H. M., Janosky, J. E., Pitcairn, D. N., & Kurs-Lasky, M. (1999). Maternal education and measures of early speech and language. *Journal of Speech, Language, and Hearing Research, 42*(6), 1432–1443.

Döpfner, M., Schmeck, K., Berner, W., Lehmkuhl, G., & Poustka, F. (1994). Reliability and factorial validity of the Child Behavior Checklist – an analysis of a clinical and field sample. *Zeitschrift fur Kinder-und Jugendpsychiatrie, 22*(3), 189–205.

Duffy, A., Alda, M., Crawford, L., Milin, R., & Grof, P. (2007). The early manifestations of bipolar disorder: A longitudinal prospective study of the offspring of bipolar parents. *Bipolar Disorders, 9*(8), 828–838.

Dworkin, E. R., Krahé, B., & Zinzow, H. (2021). The global prevalence of sexual assault: A systematic review of international research since 2010. *Psychology of Violence, 11*(5), 497.

Egger, H. L., & Angold, A. (2004). The preschool age psychiatric assessment (PAPA): A structured parent interview for diagnosing psychiatric disorders in preschool children. In R. DelCarmen-Wiggins & A. Carter (Eds.), *Handbook of infant, toddler and preschool mental assessment* (pp. 223–243). Oxford University Press.

Egger, H. L., Erkanli, A., Keeler, G., Potts, E., Walter, B. K., & Angold, A. (2006). Test-retest reliability of the preschool age psychiatric assessment (PAPA). *Journal of the American Academy of Child & Adolescent Psychiatry, 45*(5), 538–549.

Elisei, S., Lucarini, E., Murgia, N., Ferranti, L., & Attademo, L. (2013). Perinatal depression: A study of prevalence and of risk and protective factors. *Psychiatrica Danubina, 25*(Suppl 2), S258–S262.

Ellis, B. J., & Boyce, W. T. (2011). Differential susceptibility to the environment: Toward an understanding of sensitivity to developmental experiences and context. *Development and Psychopathology, 23*(1), 1–5.

El-Sheikh, M., Cummings, E. M., Kouros, C. D., Elmore-Staton, L., & Buckhalt, J. (2008). Marital psychological and physical aggression and children's mental and physical health: Direct, mediated, and moderated effects. *Journal of Consulting and Clinical Psychology, 76*(1), 138.

England, N., Improvement, N., & Health, N. C. C. F. M. (2018). *The perinatal mental health care pathways*. NHS England.

Fajkowska, M., & Kreitler, S. (2018). Status of the trait concept in contemporary personality psychology: Are the old questions still the burning questions? *Journal of Personality, 86*(1), 5–11.

Fellmeth, G., Fazel, M., & Plugge, E. (2017). Migration and perinatal mental health in women from low-and middle-income countries: A systematic review and meta-analysis. *BJOG: An International Journal of Obstetrics & Gynaecology, 124*(5), 742–752.

Fernald, L. C., Prado, E., Kariger, P., & Raikes, A. (2017). *A toolkit for measuring early childhood development in low and middle-income countries*. https://openknowledge.worldbank.org/entities/publication/deb106bb-7361-55c3-9c3d-edb33986a1e6

Field, T. (2018). Postnatal anxiety prevalence, predictors and effects on development: A narrative review. *Infant Behavior and Development, 51*, 24–32.

Fitton, C., Steiner, M., Aucott, L., Pell, J., Mackay, D., Fleming, M., & McLay, J. (2020). In utero exposure to antidepressant medication and neonatal and child outcomes: A systematic review. *Acta Psychiatrica Scandinavica, 141*(1), 21–33.

Fogarty, S., Elmir, R., Hay, P., & Schmied, V. (2018). The experience of women with an eating disorder in the perinatal period: A meta-ethnographic study. *BMC Pregnancy and Childbirth, 18*(1), 1–18.

Folger, A. T., Putnam, K. T., Putnam, F. W., Peugh, J. L., Eismann, E. A., Sa, T., . . . Ammerman, R. T. (2017). Maternal interpersonal trauma and child social-emotional development: An intergenerational effect. *Paediatric and Perinatal Epidemiology, 31*(2), 99–107.

Fonseca, V. R. J., Silva, G. A. D., & Otta, E. (2010). The relationship between postpartum depression and maternal emotional availability. *Cadernos de Saúde Pública, 26*(4), 738–746.

Fox, S. E., Levitt, P., & Nelson, III, C. A. (2010). How the timing and quality of early experiences influence the development of brain architecture. *Child Development, 81*(1), 28–40.

Furtado, M., Chow, C. H., Owais, S., Frey, B. N., & Van Lieshout, R. J. (2018). Risk factors of new onset anxiety and anxiety exacerbation in the perinatal period: A systematic review and meta-analysis. *Journal of Affective Disorders, 238*, 626–635.

Galbally, M., Sved-Williams, A., Kristianopulos, D., Mercuri, K., Brown, P., & Buist, A. (2019). Comparison of public mother – baby psychiatric units in Australia: Similarities, strengths and recommendations. *Australasian Psychiatry, 27*(2), 112–116.

Galbally, M., van IJzendoorn, M., Permezel, M., Saffery, R., Lappas, M., Ryan, J., . . . Lewis, A. J. (2017). Mercy Pregnancy and Emotional Well-being Study (MPEWS): Understanding maternal mental health, fetal programming and child development: Study design and cohort profile. *International Journal of Methods in Psychiatric Research, 26*(4), e1558.

Galbally, M., Watson, S. J., Keelan, J., MacMillan, K. K., Power, J., van IJzendoorn, M., & Lewis, A. J. (2020). Maternal perinatal depression, circulating oxytocin levels and childhood emotional disorders at 4 years of age: The importance of psychosocial context. *Journal of Psychiatric Research, 130*, 247–253.

Galbally, M., Watson, S. J., Spigset, O., Boyce, P., Oberlander, T. F., & Lewis, A. J. (2021). Antidepressant exposure in pregnancy and child sensorimotor and visuospatial development. *Journal of Psychiatric Research, 143*, 485–491.

Galbally, M., Watson, S. J., van IJzendoorn, M. H., Tharner, A., Luijk, M., de Kloet, E. R., . . . Lewis, A. J. (2021). Prenatal predictors of childhood anxiety disorders: An exploratory study of the role of attachment organization. *Development and Psychopathology*, 1–12.

Galbally, M., Watson, S. J., van Rossum, E. F., Chen, W., De Kloet, E. R., & Lewis, A. J. (2020). The perinatal origins of childhood anxiety disorders and the role of early-life maternal predictors. *Psychological Medicine*, 1–9.

Galler, J. R., Harrison, R. H., Ramsey, F., Forde, V., & Butler, S. C. (2000). Maternal depressive symptoms affect infant cognitive development in Barbados. *The Journal of Child Psychology and Psychiatry and Allied Disciplines, 41*(6), 747–757.

Garner, D. M., Olmsted, M. P., Bohr, Y., & Garfinkel, P. E. (1982). The eating attitudes test: Psychometric features and clinical correlates. *Psychological Medicine, 12*(4), 871–878.

Garry, S., & Checchi, F. (2020). Armed conflict and public health: Into the 21st century. *Journal of Public Health, 42*(3), e287–e298.

Georgieff, M. K., Tran, P. V., & Carlson, E. S. (2018). Atypical fetal development: Fetal alcohol syndrome, nutritional deprivation, teratogens, and risk for neurodevelopmental disorders and psychopathology. *Development and Psychopathology, 30*(3), 1063–1086.

Giovanelli, A., Reynolds, A. J., Mondi, C. F., & Ou, S.-R. (2016). Adverse childhood experiences and adult well-being in a low-income, urban cohort. *Pediatrics, 137*(4), e2–154016.

Glantz, M. D., Bharat, C., Degenhardt, L., Sampson, N. A., Scott, K. M., Lim, C. C., . . . Cardoso, G. (2020). The epidemiology of alcohol use disorders cross-nationally: Findings from the World Mental Health Surveys. *Addictive Behaviors, 102*, 106128.

Goettsche, E., Griep, T., & Mattson, M. (2014). *Behavioral health research reports on substance abuse and mental health among women and girls, published from 2001–2014*. Center for Behavioral Health Statistics and Quality, SAMHSA, HHS.

Goldberg, D., & Huxley, P. (1980). *Mental health in the community: The pathways to psychiatric care*. Tavistock Publications.

Goodman, J. H., Watson, G. R., & Stubbs, B. (2016). Anxiety disorders in postpartum women: A systematic review and meta-analysis. *Journal of Affective Disorders, 203*, 292–331.

Goodman, R. (1997). The strength and difficulties questionnaire: A research note. *Journal of Child Psychology and Psychiatry, 38*, 581–586.

Goodman, S. H. (1987). Emory University project on children of disturbed parents. *Schizophrenia Bulletin, 13*(3), 411–423.

Goodman, S. H., & Gotlib, I. H. (1999). Risk for psychopathology in the children of depressed mothers: A developmental model for understanding mechanisms of transmission. *Psychological Review, 106*(3), 458–490.

Gotlib, I. H., Whiffen, V. E., Mount, J. H., Milne, K., & Cordy, N. I. (1989). Prevalence rates and demographic characteristics associated with depression in pregnancy and the postpartum. *Journal of Consulting and Clinical Psychology, 57*(2), 269–274.

Grace, S. L., Evindar, A., & Stewart, D. (2003). The effect of postpartum depression on child cognitive development and behavior: A review and critical analysis of the literature. *Archives of Women's Mental Health, 6*(4), 263–274.

Group, V. I. C. S. (1991). Eight-year outcome in infants with birth weight of 500 to 999 grams: Continuing regional study of 1979 and 1980 births. *The Journal of Pediatrics, 118*(5), 761–767.

Grove, K., Lewis, A. J., & Galbally, M. (2018). Prenatal antidepressant exposure and child motor development: A meta-analysis. *Pediatrics, 142*(1), e20180356.

Gutman, L. M., & Feinstein, L. (2010). Parenting behaviours and children's development from infancy to early childhood: Changes, continuities and contributions. *Early Child Development and Care, 180*(4), 535–556.

Hack, M., Taylor, H. G., Drotar, D., Schluchter, M., Cartar, L., Wilson-Costello, D., . . . Morrow, M. (2005). Poor predictive validity of the Bayley Scales of Infant Development for cognitive function of extremely low birth weight children at school age. *Pediatrics, 116*(2), 333–341.

Hadi, F., Shirazi, E., & Soraya, S. (2019). Perinatal mental health: A public health concern. *International Journal of Fertility & Sterility, 13*(1), 86.

Hameed, M. A., & Lewis, A. J. (2016). Offspring of parents with schizophrenia: A systematic review of developmental features across childhood. *Harvard Review of Psychiatry, 24*(2), 104–117.

Hanson, M., Cooper, C., Aihie Sayer, A., Eendebak, R., Clough, G., & Beard, J. (2016). Developmental aspects of a life course approach to healthy ageing. *The Journal of Physiology, 594*(8), 2147–2160.

Hay, D. F., Asten, P., Mills, A., Kumar, R., Pawlby, S., & Sharp, D. (2001). Intellectual problems shown by 11-year-old children whose mothers had postnatal depression. *The Journal of Child Psychology and Psychiatry and Allied Disciplines, 42*(7), 871–889.

Hay, D. F., & Kumar, R. (1995). Interpreting the effects of mothers' postnatal depression on children's intelligence: A critique and re-analysis. *Child Psychiatry and Human Development, 25*(3), 165–181.

Heaton, S. C., Reader, S. K., Preston, A. S., Fennell, E. B., Puyana, O. E., Gill, N., & Johnson, J. H. (2001). The Test of Everyday Attention for Children (TEA-Ch): Patterns of performance in children with ADHD and clinical controls. *Child Neuropsychology, 7*(4), 251–264.

Henrichs, J., Schenk, J. J., Schmidt, H. G., Velders, F. P., Hofman, A., Jaddoe, V. W., . . . Tiemeier, H. (2009). Maternal pre- and postnatal anxiety and infant temperament: The generation R study. *Infant and Child Development: An International Journal of Research and Practice, 18*(6), 556–572.

Hesse, E., & Main, M. (2000). Disorganized infant, child, and adult attachment: Collapse in behavioral and attentional strategies. *Journal of the American Psychoanalytic Association, 48*(4), 1097–1127.

Hibel, L. C., Granger, D. A., Blair, C., Cox, M. J., & Investigators, F. L. P. K. (2011). Maternal sensitivity buffers the adrenocortical implications of intimate partner violence exposure during early childhood. *Development and Psychopathology, 23*(2), 689–701.

Horta, B. L., Loret de Mola, C., & Victora, C. G. (2015). Breastfeeding and intelligence: A systematic review and meta-analysis. *Acta Paediatrica, 104*, 14–19.

Howard, L. M., & Challacombe, F. (2018). Effective treatment of postnatal depression is associated with normal child development. *The Lancet Psychiatry, 5*(2), 95–97.

Howard, L. M., & Khalifeh, H. (2020). Perinatal mental health: A review of progress and challenges. *World Psychiatry, 19*(3), 313–327.

Howard, L. M., Molyneaux, E., Dennis, C.-L., Rochat, T., Stein, A., & Milgrom, J. (2014). Non-psychotic mental disorders in the perinatal period. *The Lancet, 384*(9956), 1775–1788.

Howard, L. M., Thornicroft, G., Salmon, M., & Appleby, L. (2004). Predictors of parenting outcome in women with psychotic disorders discharged from mother and baby units. *Acta Psychiatrica Scandinavica, 110*(5), 347–355.

Hoyme, H. E., May, P. A., Kalberg, W. O., Kodituwakku, P., Gossage, J. P., Trujillo, P. M., . . . Khaole, N. (2005). A practical clinical approach to diagnosis of fetal alcohol spectrum disorders: Clarification of the 1996 institute of medicine criteria. *Pediatrics, 115*(1), 39–47.

Ierardi, E., Ferro, V., Trovato, A., Tambelli, R., & Riva Crugnola, C. (2019). Maternal and paternal depression and anxiety: Their relationship with mother-infant interactions at 3 months. *Archives of Women's Mental Health*, 22(4), 527–533.

Jeong, J., McCoy, D. C., & Fink, G. (2017). Pathways between paternal and maternal education, caregivers' support for learning, and early child development in 44 low-and middle-income countries. *Early Childhood Research Quarterly*, 41, 136–148.

Judd, F., Newman, L. K., & Komiti, A. A. (2018). Time for a new zeitgeist in perinatal mental health. *Australian & New Zealand Journal of Psychiatry*, 52(2), 112–116.

Jundong, J., Kuja-Halkola, R., Hultman, C., Långström, N., D'Onofrio, B. M., & Lichtenstein, P. (2012). Poor school performance in offspring of patients with schizophrenia: What are the mechanisms? *Psychological Medicine*, 42(1), 111–123.

Junge, C., Garthus-Niegel, S., Slinning, K., Polte, C., Simonsen, T. B., & Eberhard-Gran, M. (2017). The impact of perinatal depression on children's social-emotional development: A longitudinal study. *Maternal and Child Health Journal*, 21(3), 607–615.

Kaitz, M., & Maytal, H. (2005). Interactions between anxious mothers and their infants: An integration of theory and research findings. *Infant Mental Health Journal*, 26(6), 570–597.

Kessler, R. C., McLaughlin, K. A., Green, J. G., Gruber, M. J., Sampson, N. A., Zaslavsky, A. M., . . . Angermeyer, M. (2010). Childhood adversities and adult psychopathology in the WHO World Mental Health Surveys. *The British Journal of Psychiatry*, 197(5), 378–385.

King, T. M., Tandon, S. D., Macias, M. M., Healy, J. A., Duncan, P. M., Swigonski, N. L., . . . Lipkin, P. H. (2010). Implementing developmental screening and referrals: Lessons learned from a national project. *Pediatrics*, 125(2), 350–360.

Kingston, D., McDonald, S., Austin, M.-P., & Tough, S. (2015). Association between prenatal and postnatal psychological distress and toddler cognitive development: A systematic review. *PloS One*, 10(5), e0126929.

Kingston, D., Tough, S., & Whitfield, H. (2012). Prenatal and postpartum maternal psychological distress and infant development: A systematic review. *Child Psychiatry & Human Development*, 43(5), 683–714.

Kitchen, W., Rickards, A., Ford, G., Doyle, L., Kelly, E., & Ryan, M. (1989). Selective improvement in cognitive test scores of extremely low birthweight infants aged between 2 and 5 years. *Journal of Paediatrics and Child Health*, 25(5), 288–291.

Kluczniok, D., Boedeker, K., Fuchs, A., Hindi Attar, C., Fydrich, T., Fuehrer, D., . . . Heinz, A. (2016). Emotional availability in mother – child interaction: The effects of maternal depression in remission and additional history of childhood abuse. *Depression and Anxiety*, 33(7), 648–657.

Koller, H., Lawson, K., Rose, S. A., Wallace, I., & McCarton, C. (1997). Patterns of cognitive development in very low birth weight children during the first six years of life. *Pediatrics*, 99(3), 383–389.

Korkman, M., Kirk, U., & Kemp, S. (1998). *NEPSY developmental neuropsychological assessment*. Psychological Corporation.

Kothari, R., Rosinska, M., Treasure, J., & Micali, N. (2014). The early cognitive development of children at high risk of developing an eating disorder. *European Eating Disorders Review*, 22(2), 152–156.

Koutra, K., Chatzi, L., Bagkeris, M., Vassilaki, M., Bitsios, P., & Kogevinas, M. (2013). Antenatal and postnatal maternal mental health as determinants of infant neurodevelopment at 18 months of age in a mother – child cohort (Rhea Study) in Crete, Greece. *Social Psychiatry and Psychiatric Epidemiology*, 48(8), 1335–1345.

Kroes, G., Veerman, J. W., & De Bruyn, E. E. (2003). Bias in parental reports? Maternal psychopathology and the reporting of problem behavior in clinic-referred children. *European Journal of Psychological Assessment*, 19(3), 195.

Lacey, J. H., & Smith, G. (1987). Bulimia nervosa: The impact of pregnancy on mother and baby. *The British Journal of Psychiatry*, 150(6), 777–781.

Lambert, M. C., Lyubansky, M., & Achenbach, T. M. (1998). Behavioral and emotional problems among adolescents of Jamaica and the United States: Parent, teacher, and self-reports for ages 12 to 18. *Journal of Emotional and Behavioral Disorders*, 6(3), 180–187.

Lansdown, R. G., Goldstein, H., Shah, P. M., Orley, J. H., Di, G., Kaul, K. K., . . . Reddy, V. (1996). Culturally appropriate measures for monitoring child development at family and community level: A WHO collaborative study. *Bulletin of the World Health Organization*, 74(3), 283–290.

Lawson, G. M., Hook, C. J., & Farah, M. J. (2018). A meta-analysis of the relationship between socioeconomic status and executive function performance among children. *Developmental Science, 21*(2), e12529.

Levendosky, A. A., Leahy, K. L., Bogat, G. A., Davidson, W. S., & Von Eye, A. (2006). Domestic violence, maternal parenting, maternal mental health, and infant externalizing behavior. *Journal of Family Psychology, 20*(4), 544–552.

Lewis, A. J., Austin, E., Knapp, R., Vaiano, T., & Galbally, M. (2015). *Perinatal maternal mental health, fetal programming and child development.* Healthcare.

Li, Y., Long, Z., Cao, D., & Cao, F. (2017). Social support and depression across the perinatal period: A longitudinal study. *Journal of Clinical Nursing, 26*(17–18), 2776–2783.

Lieb, K., Zanarini, M. C., Schmahl, C., Linehan, M. M., & Bohus, M. (2004). Borderline personality disorder. *The Lancet, 364*(9432), 453–461.

Lin, A., Di Prinzio, P., Young, D., Jacoby, P., Whitehouse, A., Waters, F., . . . Morgan, V. A. (2016). Academic performance in children of mothers with schizophrenia and other severe mental illness, and risk for subsequent development of psychosis: A population-based study. *Schizophrenia Bulletin, 43*(1), 205–213.

Liu, Y., Kaaya, S., Chai, J., McCoy, D., Surkan, P., Black, M., . . . Smith-Fawzi, M. (2017). Maternal depressive symptoms and early childhood cognitive development: A meta-analysis. *Psychological Medicine, 47*(4), 680–689.

Lomonaco-Haycraft, K. C., Hyer, J., Tibbits, B., Grote, J., Stainback-Tracy, K., Ulrickson, C., . . . Hoffman, M. C. (2019). Integrated perinatal mental health care: A national model of perinatal primary care in vulnerable populations. *Primary Health Care Research & Development, 20*, e77.

Loomans, E. M., van der Stelt, O., van Eijsden, M., Gemke, R., Vrijkotte, T., & Van den Bergh, B. (2011). Antenatal maternal anxiety is associated with problem behaviour at age five. *Early Human Development, 87*(8), 565–570.

Lyons-Ruth, K., Todd Manly, J., Von Klitzing, K., Tamminen, T., Emde, R., Fitzgerald, H., . . . Foley, M. (2017). The worldwide burden of infant mental and emotional disorder: Report of the task force of the world association for infant mental health. *Infant Mental Health Journal, 38*(6), 695–705.

Lyons-Ruth, K., Zoll, D., Connell, D., & Grunebaum, H. U. (1986). The depressed mother and her one-year-old infant: Environment, interaction, attachment, and infant development. *New Directions for Child and Adolescent Development, 1986*(34), 61–82.

Macfie, J. (2009). Development in children and adolescents whose mothers have borderline personality disorder. *Child Development Perspectives, 3*(1), 66–71.

MacMillan, K. K., Lewis, A. J., Watson, S. J., & Galbally, M. (2020). Maternal depression and the emotional availability of mothers at six months postpartum: Findings from the Mercy Pregnancy and Emotional Wellbeing Study (MPEWS) pregnancy cohort. *Journal of Affective Disorders, 266*, 678–685.

MacMillan, K. K., Lewis, A. J., Watson, S. J., Jansen, B., & Galbally, M. (2021). Maternal trauma and emotional availability in early mother-infant interaction: Findings from the Mercy Pregnancy and Emotional Well-being Study (MPEWS) cohort. *Attachment & Human Development, 23*(6), 853–875.

Magnuson, K. A., Sexton, H. R., Davis-Kean, P. E., & Huston, A. C. (2009). Increases in maternal education and young children's language skills. *Merrill-Palmer Quarterly (1982–)*, 319–350.

Marcus, J., Auerbach, J., Wilkinson, L., & Burack, C. M. (1981). Infants at risk for schizophrenia: The Jerusalem infant development study. *Archives of General Psychiatry, 38*(6), 703–713.

Marrus, N., Eggebrecht, A. T., Todorov, A., Elison, J. T., Wolff, J. J., Cole, L., . . . Swanson, M. R. (2018). Walking, gross motor development, and brain functional connectivity in infants and toddlers. *Cerebral Cortex, 28*(2), 750–763.

Maselko, J., Sikander, S., Bhalotra, S., Bangash, O., Ganga, N., Mukherjee, S., . . . Liaqat, R. (2015). Effect of an early perinatal depression intervention on long-term child development outcomes: Follow-up of the Thinking Healthy Programme randomised controlled trial. *The Lancet Psychiatry, 2*(7), 609–617.

McDonald, S., Kehler, H., Bayrampour, H., Fraser-Lee, N., & Tough, S. (2016). Risk and protective factors in early child development: Results from the All Our Babies (AOB) pregnancy cohort. *Research in Developmental Disabilities, 58*, 20–30.

Meltzer-Brody, S., Howard, L. M., Bergink, V., Vigod, S., Jones, I., Munk-Olsen, T., . . . Milgrom, J. (2018). Postpartum psychiatric disorders. *Nature Reviews Disease Primers, 4*(1), 1–18.

Mennes, M., Van den Bergh, B., Lagae, L., & Stiers, P. (2009). Developmental brain alterations in 17 year old boys are related to antenatal maternal anxiety. *Clinical Neurophysiology, 120*(6), 1116–1122.

Ment, L. R., Vohr, B., Allan, W., Katz, K. H., Schneider, K. C., Westerveld, M., . . . Makuch, R. W. (2003). Change in cognitive function over time in very low-birth-weight infants. *JAMA, 289*(6), 705–711.

Messinger, D. S., Bauer, C. R., Das, A., Seifer, R., Lester, B. M., Lagasse, L. L., . . . Smeriglio, V. L. (2004). The maternal lifestyle study: Cognitive, motor, and behavioral outcomes of cocaine-exposed and opiate-exposed infants through three years of age. *Pediatrics, 113*(6), 1677–1685.

Micali, N., De Stavola, B., Ploubidis, G. B., Simonoff, E., & Treasure, J. (2014). The effects of maternal eating disorders on offspring childhood and early adolescent psychiatric disorders. *International Journal of Eating Disorders, 47*(4), 385–393.

Milgrom, J., Hirshler, Y., Reece, J., Holt, C., & Gemmill, A. W. (2019). Social support – a protective factor for depressed perinatal women? *International Journal of Environmental Research and Public Health, 16*(8), 1426.

Milgrom, J., Westley, D. T., & Gemmill, A. W. (2004). The mediating role of maternal responsiveness in some longer term effects of postnatal depression on infant development. *Infant Behavior and Development, 27*(4), 443–454.

Miyake, A., Friedman, N. P., Emerson, M. J., Witzki, A. H., Howerter, A., & Wager, T. D. (2000). The unity and diversity of executive functions and their contributions to complex "frontal lobe" tasks: A latent variable analysis. *Cognitive Psychology, 41*(1), 49–100.

Möller, E. L., Majdandžić, M., & Bögels, S. M. (2015). Parental anxiety, parenting behavior, and infant anxiety: Differential associations for fathers and mothers. *Journal of Child and Family Studies, 24*(9), 2626–2637.

Morgan, V. A., Leonard, H., Bourke, J., & Jablensky, A. (2008). Intellectual disability co-occurring with schizophrenia and other psychiatric illness: Population-based study. *The British Journal of Psychiatry, 193*(5), 364–372.

Morrell, J., & Steele, H. (2003). The role of attachment security, temperament, maternal perception, and care-giving behavior in persistent infant sleeping problems. *Infant Mental Health Journal, 24*(5), 447–468.

Murray, L. (1992). The impact of postnatal depression on infant development. *Journal of Child Psychology and Psychiatry, 33*(3), 543–561.

Murray, L., Hipwell, A., Hooper, R., Stein, A., & Cooper, P. (1996). The cognitive development of 5-year-old children of postnatally depressed mothers. *Journal of Child Psychology and Psychiatry, 37*(8), 927–935.

Myors, K. A., Schmied, V., Johnson, M., & Cleary, M. (2013). Collaboration and integrated services for perinatal mental health: An integrative review. *Child and Adolescent Mental Health, 18*(1), 1–10.

Najman, J. M., Williams, G. M., Nikles, J., Spence, S., Bor, W., O'Callaghan, M., . . . Andersen, M. J. (2000). Mothers' mental illness and child behavior problems: Cause-effect association or observation bias? *Journal of the American Academy of Child & Adolescent Psychiatry, 39*(5), 592–602.

Namasivayam, A. K., Huynh, A., Granata, F., Law, V., & van Lieshout, P. (2021). PROMPT intervention for children with severe speech motor delay: A randomized control trial. *Pediatric Research, 89*(3), 613–621.

Nathanson, A. M., Shorey, R. C., Tirone, V., & Rhatigan, D. L. (2012). The prevalence of mental health disorders in a community sample of female victims of intimate partner violence. *Partner Abuse, 3*(1), 59–75.

Newman, L. K., Stevenson, C. S., Bergman, L. R., & Boyce, P. (2007). Borderline personality disorder, mother – infant interaction and parenting perceptions: Preliminary findings. *Australian & New Zealand Journal of Psychiatry, 41*(7), 598–605.

Nichols, T. R., Welborn, A., Gringle, M. R., & Lee, A. (2021). Social stigma and perinatal substance use services: Recognizing the power of the good mother ideal. *Contemporary Drug Problems, 48*(1), 19–37.

Niclasen, J., Teasdale, T. W., Andersen, A.-M. N., Skovgaard, A. M., Elberling, H., & Obel, C. (2012). Psychometric properties of the Danish Strength and difficulties questionnaire: The SDQ assessed for more than 70,000 raters in four different cohorts. *PloS One, 7*(2), e32025.

Nix, L., Nixon, E., Quigley, J., & O'Keane, V. (2021). Perinatal depression and children's developmental outcomes at 2 years postpartum. *Early Human Development, 156*, 105346.

Norwood, A., & Murphy, C. (2012). What forms of abuse correlate with PTSD symptoms in partners of men being treated for intimate partner violence? *Psychological Trauma: Theory, Research, Practice, and Policy, 4*(6), 596–604.

O'hara, M. W., & Swain, A. M. (1996). Rates and risk of postpartum depression – a meta-analysis. *International Review of Psychiatry, 8*(1), 37–54.

O'Keeffe, L. M., Kearney, P. M., McCarthy, F. P., Khashan, A. S., Greene, R. A., North, R. A., . . . Dekker, G. A. (2015). Prevalence and predictors of alcohol use during pregnancy: Findings from international multicentre cohort studies. *BMJ Open, 5*(7), e006323.

O'Leary, C. M. (2004). Fetal alcohol syndrome: Diagnosis, epidemiology, and developmental outcomes. *Journal of Paediatrics and Child Health, 40*(1–2), 2–7.

O'Leary, N., Jairaj, C., Molloy, E. J., McAuliffe, F. M., Nixon, E., & O'Keane, V. (2019). Antenatal depression and the impact on infant cognitive, language and motor development at six and twelve months postpartum. *Early Human Development, 134*, 41–46.

Osnes, R. S., Roaldset, J. O., Follestad, T., & Eberhard-Gran, M. (2019). Insomnia late in pregnancy is associated with perinatal anxiety: A longitudinal cohort study. *Journal of Affective Disorders, 248*, 155–165.

Petterson, S. M., & Albers, A. B. (2001). Effects of poverty and maternal depression on early child development. *Child Development, 72*(6), 1794–1813.

Pinheiro, K. A. T., Pinheiro, R. T., Coelho, F. M. D. C., da Silva, R. A., Quevedo, L. A., Schwanz, C. C., . . . Lucion, A. B. (2014). Serum NGF, BDNF and IL-6 levels in postpartum mothers as predictors of infant development: The influence of affective disorders. *PloS One, 9*(4), e94581.

Piteo, A. M., Yelland, L. N., & Makrides, M. (2012). Does maternal depression predict developmental outcome in 18 month old infants? *Early Human Development, 88*(8), 651–655.

Porter, C. L., Wouden-Miller, M., Silva, S. S., & Porter, A. E. (2003). Marital harmony and conflict: Links to infants' emotional regulation and cardiac vagal tone. *Infancy, 4*(2), 297–307.

Power, J., van IJzendoorn, M., Lewis, A. J., Chen, W., & Galbally, M. (2021). Maternal perinatal depression and child executive function: A systematic review and meta-analysis. *Journal of Affective Disorders, 291*, 218–234.

Qouta, S. R., Vänskä, M., Diab, S. Y., & Punamäki, R.-L. (2021). War trauma and infant motor, cognitive, and socioemotional development: Maternal mental health and dyadic interaction as explanatory processes. *Infant Behavior and Development, 63*, 101532.

Quintana, S. M., Aboud, F. E., Chao, R. K., Contreras-Grau, J., Cross, W. E., Hudley, C., . . . Vietze, D. L. (2006). Race, ethnicity, and culture in child development: Contemporary research and future directions. *Child Development, 77*(5), 1129–1141.

Raine, K. H., Cockshaw, W., Boyce, P., & Thorpe, K. (2019). Prenatal maternal personality as an early predictor of vulnerable parenting style. *Archives of Women's Mental Health, 22*(6), 799–807.

Ranning, A., Laursen, T. M., Thorup, A., Hjorthøj, C., & Nordentoft, M. (2016). Children of parents with serious mental illness: With whom do they grow up? A prospective, population-based study. *Journal of the American Academy of Child & Adolescent Psychiatry, 55*(11), 953–961.

Reck, C., Tietz, A., Müller, M., Seibold, K., & Tronick, E. (2018). The impact of maternal anxiety disorder on mother-infant interaction in the postpartum period. *PloS One, 13*(5), e0194763.

Reynell, J. K., & Huntley, M. (1985). *Reynell developmental language scales* (2nd ed.). NFER-Nelson.

Robinson, M., Oddy, W., McLean, N., Jacoby, P., Pennell, C., De Klerk, N., . . . Newnham, J. (2010). Low–moderate prenatal alcohol exposure and risk to child behavioural development: A prospective cohort study. *BJOG: An International Journal of Obstetrics & Gynaecology, 117*(9), 1139–1152.

Rogers, A., Obst, S., Teague, S. J., Rossen, L., Spry, E. A., Macdonald, J. A., . . . Hutchinson, D. (2020). Association between maternal perinatal depression and anxiety and child and adolescent development: A meta-analysis. *JAMA Pediatrics, 174*(11), 1082–1092.

Rossman, B., & Rea, J. G. (2005). The relation of parenting styles and inconsistencies to adaptive functioning for children in conflictual and violent families. *Journal of Family Violence, 20*(5), 261–277.

Rozanov, V., Frančišković, T., Marinić, I., Macarenco, M.-M., Letica-Crepulja, M., Mužinić, L., . . . Wiederhold, B. (2019). Mental health consequences of war conflicts. In *Advances in psychiatry* (pp. 281–304). Springer.

Rusner, M., Berg, M., & Begley, C. (2016). Bipolar disorder in pregnancy and childbirth: A systematic review of outcomes. *BMC Pregnancy and Childbirth*, 16(1), 1–18.

Rutter, M. (1984). Psychopathology and development: I. Childhood antecedents of adult psychiatric disorder. *Australian and New Zealand Journal of Psychiatry*, 18(3), 225–234.

Sadeh-Sharvit, S., Levy-Shiff, R., & Lock, J. D. (2016). Maternal eating disorder history and toddlers' neurodevelopmental outcomes: A brief report. *Eating Disorders*, 24(2), 198–205.

Saiepour, N., Najman, J., Ware, R., Baker, P., Clavarino, A., & Williams, G. (2019). Does attrition affect estimates of association: A longitudinal study. *Journal of Psychiatric Research*, 110, 127–142.

Sayer, A. A., Cooper, C., Evans, J. R., Rauf, A., Wormald, R. P. L., Osmond, C., & Barker, D. J. P. (1998). Are rates of ageing determined in utero? *Age and Ageing*, 27(5), 579–583.

Seeman, M. V. (2012). Intervention to prevent child custody loss in mothers with schizophrenia. *Schizophrenia Research and Treatment*, 2012, 796763.

Shankaran, S., Lester, B. M., Das, A., Bauer, C. R., Bada, H. S., Lagasse, L., & Higgins, R. (2007). Impact of maternal substance use during pregnancy on childhood outcome. *Seminars in Fetal and Neonatal Medicine*, 12, 143–150.

Sheehan, D. V., Lecrubier, Y., Sheehan, K. H., Amorim, P., Janavs, J., Weiller, E., . . . Dunbar, G. C. (1998). The Mini-International Neuropsychiatric Interview (MINI): The development and validation of a structured diagnostic psychiatric interview for DSM-IV and ICD-10. *Journal of Clinical Psychiatry*, 59(20), 22–33.

Sikander, S., Ahmad, I., Bates, L. M., Gallis, J., Hagaman, A., O'Donnell, K., . . . Maselko, J. (2019). Cohort profile: Perinatal depression and child socioemotional development; the Bachpan cohort study from rural Pakistan. *BMJ Open*, 9(5), e025644.

Skouteris, H., Wertheim, E. H., Rallis, S., Milgrom, J., & Paxton, S. J. (2009). Depression and anxiety through pregnancy and the early postpartum: An examination of prospective relationships. *Journal of Affective Disorders*, 113(3), 303–308.

Slomian, J., Honvo, G., Emonts, P., Reginster, J.-Y., & Bruyère, O. (2019). Consequences of maternal postpartum depression: A systematic review of maternal and infant outcomes. *Women's Health*, 15, 1745506519844044.

Smith, M. V., Shao, L., Howell, H., Wang, H., Poschman, K., & Yonkers, K. A. (2009). Success of mental health referral among pregnant and postpartum women with psychiatric distress. *General Hospital Psychiatry*, 31(2), 155–162.

Smith-Nielsen, J., Tharner, A., Krogh, M. T., & Vaever, M. S. (2016). Effects of maternal postpartum depression in a well-resourced sample: Early concurrent and long-term effects on infant cognitive, language, and motor development. *Scandinavian Journal of Psychology*, 57(6), 571–583.

Sohlberg, S. C. (1985). Personality and neuropsychological performance of high-risk children. *Schizophrenia Bulletin*, 11(1), 48–60.

Spielberger, C. D. (1983). *State-trait anxiety inventory for adults. Bibliography* (2nd ed.). Consulting Psychologists Press.

Squires, J., Bricker, D., & Potter, L. (1997). Revision of a parent-completed developmental screening tool: Ages and stages questionnaires. *Journal of Pediatric Psychology*, 22(3), 313–328.

Stein, A., Pearson, R. M., Goodman, S. H., Rapa, E., Rahman, A., McCallum, M., . . . Pariante, C. M. (2014). Effects of perinatal mental disorders on the fetus and child. *The Lancet*, 384(9956), 1800–1819.

Stepp, S. D., Whalen, D. J., Pilkonis, P. A., Hipwell, A. E., & Levine, M. D. (2012). Children of mothers with borderline personality disorder: Identifying parenting behaviors as potential targets for intervention. *Personality Disorders: Theory, Research, and Treatment*, 3(1), 76–91.

Stone, L. L., Janssens, J. M., Vermulst, A. A., Van Der Maten, M., Engels, R. C., & Otten, R. (2015). The strengths and difficulties questionnaire: Psychometric properties of the parent and teacher version in children aged 4–7. *BMC Psychology*, 3, 1–12.

Straub, N., Grunert, P., Northstone, K., & Emmett, P. (2019). Economic impact of breast-feeding-associated improvements of childhood cognitive development, based on data from the ALSPAC. *British Journal of Nutrition*, 122(s1), S16–S21.

Sutter-Dallay, A.-L., Murray, L., Dequae-Merchadou, L., Glatigny-Dallay, E., Bourgeois, M.-L., & Verdoux, H. (2011). A prospective longitudinal study of the impact of early postnatal vs. chronic maternal depressive symptoms on child development. *European Psychiatry*, 26(8), 484–489.

Swanson, J. D., & Wadhwa, P. M. (2008). Developmental origins of child mental health disorders. *Journal of Child Psychology and Psychiatry, and Allied Disciplines*, 49(10), 1009–1019.

Swinbourne, J. M., & Touyz, S. W. (2007). The co-morbidity of eating disorders and anxiety disorders: A review. *European Eating Disorders Review*, 15(4), 253–274.

Tan, C. H., Denny, C. H., Cheal, N. E., Sniezek, J. E., & Kanny, D. (2015). Alcohol use and binge drinking among women of childbearing age – United States, 2011–2013. *Morbidity and Mortality Weekly Report*, 64(37), 1042–1046.

Taylor, C. L., Munk-Olsen, T., Howard, L. M., & Vigod, S. N. (2020). Schizophrenia around the time of pregnancy: Leveraging population-based health data and electronic health record data to fill knowledge gaps. *BJPsych Open*, 6(5).

Tierney, S., Fox, J., Butterfield, C., Stringer, E., & Furber, C. (2011). Treading the tightrope between motherhood and an eating disorder: A qualitative study. *International Journal of Nursing Studies*, 48(10), 1223–1233.

Tseng, V. (2006). Unpacking immigration in youths' academic and occupational pathways. *Child Development*, 77(5), 1434–1445.

Van Boekel, L. C., Brouwers, E. P., Van Weeghel, J., & Garretsen, H. F. (2013). Stigma among health professionals towards patients with substance use disorders and its consequences for healthcare delivery: Systematic review. *Drug and Alcohol Dependence*, 131(1–2), 23–35.

Van den Bergh, B. R., Mulder, E. J., Mennes, M., & Glover, V. (2005). Antenatal maternal anxiety and stress and the neurobehavioural development of the fetus and child: Links and possible mechanisms: A review. *Neuroscience & Biobehavioral Reviews*, 29(2), 237–258.

Vieta, E., Berk, M., Schulze, T. G., Carvalho, A. F., Suppes, T., Calabrese, J. R., . . . Grande, I. (2018). Bipolar disorders. *Nature Reviews Disease Primers*, 4(1), 1–16.

Vigod, S., Kurdyak, P., Dennis, C., Gruneir, A., Newman, A., Seeman, M., . . . Ray, J. (2014). Maternal and newborn outcomes among women with schizophrenia: A retrospective population-based cohort study. *BJOG: An International Journal of Obstetrics & Gynaecology*, 121(5), 566–574.

Walker, S. P., Wachs, T. D., Grantham-McGregor, S., Black, M. M., Nelson, C. A., Huffman, S. L., . . . Lozoff, B. (2011). Inequality in early childhood: Risk and protective factors for early child development. *The Lancet*, 378(9799), 1325–1338.

Wan, M. W., Warren, K., Salmon, M. P., & Abel, K. M. (2008). Patterns of maternal responding in postpartum mothers with schizophrenia. *Infant Behavior and Development*, 31(3), 532–538.

Watson, H. J., O'Brien, A., & Sadeh-Sharvit, S. (2018). Children of parents with eating disorders. *Current Psychiatry Reports*, 20(11), 1–11.

Waxler, E., Thelen, K., & Muzik, M. (2011). Maternal perinatal depression-impact on infant and child development. *European Psychiatry Review*, 4(1), 41–47.

Wechsler, D. (2014). *Wechsler intelligence scale for children, fifth edition (WISC-V)*. Pearson.

Weiss, M., Zelkowitz, P., Feldman, R. B., Vogel, J., Heyman, M., & Paris, J. (1996). Psychopathology in offspring of mothers with borderline personality disorder: A pilot study. *The Canadian Journal of Psychiatry*, 41(5), 285–290.

Werner, E. E. (1995). Resilience in development. *Current Directions in Psychological Science*, 4(3), 81–84.

Westermeyer, J. (2006). Comorbid schizophrenia and substance abuse: A review of epidemiology and course. *American Journal on Addictions*, 15(5), 345–355.

Wolk, S. L., Loeb, K. L., & Walsh, B. T. (2005). Assessment of patients with anorexia nervosa: Interview versus self-report. *International Journal of Eating Disorders*, 37(2), 92–99.

Yoon, S., Coxe, K., Bunger, A., Freisthler, B., Dellor, E., Langaigne, A., & Millisor, J. (2021). Feasibility of engaging child welfare-involved parents with substance use disorders in research: Key challenges and lessons learned. *Journal of Public Child Welfare*, 1–19.

Zhang, H., Liu, S., Si, Y., Zhang, S., Tian, Y., Liu, Y., Li, H., & Zhu, Z. (2019). Natural sunlight plus vitamin D supplementation ameliorate delayed early motor development in newborn infants from maternal perinatal depression. *Journal of Affective Disorders*, 257, 241–249.

Zung, W. W. (1971). A rating instrument for anxiety disorders. *Psychosomatics: Journal of Consultation and Liaison Psychiatry*, 12(6), 371–379.

PART II

Prenatal Mental Health Disorders

7

PRENATAL DEPRESSION

Elizabeth H. Eustis, Maya Nauphal,
Grace E. DeCost, and Cynthia L. Battle

Prenatal depression, or antenatal depression, refers to depression that occurs during pregnancy up to the point of birth. Major and subthreshold episodes of depression can occur during this time. Major episodes of depression are consistent with the diagnostic criteria for major depressive disorder (MDD) in the 5th edition of the *Diagnostic and Statistical Manual of Mental Disorders* (DSM-5) classification system used in the United States and refer to the presence of five or more symptoms of depression, one of which is depressed mood or loss of interest in activities, for at least two weeks with significant associated impairment (American Psychiatric Association [APA], 2013). The DSM-5 includes the specifier "with peripartum onset" for a diagnosis of MDD, which indicates that the onset of mood symptoms occurred during pregnancy or in the first four weeks after delivery. The *International Classification of Diseases*, Tenth Revision (ICD-10) includes a code for postpartum depression, and prenatal depression can be captured under a code for "other mental disorders complicating pregnancy" (WHO, 2022). Subthreshold prenatal depression, which may encompass cases of minor depression (i.e., having two to four symptoms of depression over the past two weeks) or other depressive symptom elevations, is also frequently referenced in the perinatal mental health literature and refers to experiences of depressive symptoms that are clinically relevant yet do not meet full criteria for a major depressive episode (Marchesi et al., 2009). Symptoms of depression during pregnancy are generally consistent with symptoms experienced outside the prenatal period and include depressed or low mood; loss of interest in activities; a sense of worthlessness, hopelessness, and guilt; changes in sleep and eating patterns; fatigue; difficulty with concentration; feeling restless or slowed down; and thoughts about death (APA, 2013). Negative thinking patterns that are common in prenatal depression may include themes and thoughts focused on the experience of pregnancy or the role of being a parent. Some symptoms may be harder to detect as they overlap with common experiences during pregnancy, including changes in energy, sleep, appetite, and libido (ACOG, 2018). In addition, many people who experience prenatal depression also report symptoms of anxiety (e.g., Heron et al., 2004; Pampaka et al., 2018).

DOI: 10.4324/9781003206903-10

In this chapter, we describe the case of Karina. Karina is a 38-year-old White European-American woman who is 24 weeks pregnant. She is cisgender and identifies as queer in terms of her sexual orientation. She has experienced several episodes of depression as a teenager and an adult, most recently in her early thirties. Karina and her wife, Maria, have been married for five years. Becoming parents is very important to both of them. Karina had one previous pregnancy that ended in a miscarriage at eight weeks' gestation last year. Due to the ongoing COVID-19 pandemic, Karina has spent more time at home during the current pregnancy and has avoided crowded places. She is worried about getting sick with COVID-19 and how that would impact the baby. Her wife has not been able to come to the prenatal ultrasound visits due to COVID-19 protocols, and she is worried about what delivery will be like if there is another surge in cases in her area. She started feeling depressed around 12 weeks' gestation. Specifically, she noticed feeling down, needing to push herself to get things done throughout the day and, at times, views herself as a failure. She is experiencing significant fatigue, and it has been hard for her to know if that is due to the pregnancy or potentially related to the depression. Given the challenges Karina has experienced in becoming pregnant, she feels guilty that she does not feel happy. She often thinks, "What's wrong with me, I should be happy," and "I'm already a bad mother." Her wife, Maria, is supportive but has to work long hours and is not home as much as she used to be. In addition, Karina has been experiencing pelvic pain that has made it harder to go on long walks, which is something she usually finds helpful when she is feeling down.

Prevalence

Although the true global prevalence of prenatal depression is difficult to determine, available estimates from international surveys indicate that prenatal depression, as defined either by depression symptom elevations or by clinical diagnosis, is common, with reported rates ranging from 14.6% to 34% (Fekadu Dadi et al., 2020; Okagbue et al., 2019; Tomfohr-Madsen et al., 2021; Woody et al., 2017; Yin et al., 2021). Prevalence rates of prenatal depression as determined by scoring above a clinical cutoff on a self-report screening measure are typically higher than rates of a major depression diagnosis as assessed via structured clinical interview (e.g., 20.7% vs. 15%; Yin et al., 2021). In addition to differential rates depending on assessment strategy, the variability across studies can be explained by other factors, including sampling methods, stage of pregnancy, culture, and country of origin (Ashley et al., 2016). In terms of geographic variation, systematic reviews, and meta-analyses indicate that prevalence rates for prenatal depression are higher in low- and middle-income countries relative to high-income countries (Fekadu Dadi et al., 2020; Woody et al., 2017; Yin et al., 2021), with rates of symptom elevations as high as 50% in some countries (e.g., Ghana; Kugbey et al., 2021).

Within the United States, prevalence rates of prenatal depression based on clinical symptoms or diagnosis are consistent with global estimates, ranging between 10% and 30% (Ashley et al., 2016; Benatar et al., 2020; Mukherjee et al., 2016). Some evidence suggests that rates of major depression are similar among pregnant and nonpregnant people but that rates of subthreshold depression (i.e., the presence of symptoms of depression that do not meet DSM-5 criteria for major depression) are higher among pregnant people relative to their nonpregnant counterparts (Ashley et al., 2016). Similar to global estimates, there is substantial heterogeneity in prevalence estimates across subgroups of individuals in the United States. For example, higher rates of prenatal depression symptoms have been reported among people living in rural areas (Nidey et al., 2020) and people who identify as non-Hispanic Black and Hispanic (Mukherjee et al., 2016).

In addition to the concerningly high rates of prenatal depression globally, some reports indicate that rates of prenatal depression might be increasing over time (e.g., Berthelot et al., 2020; Pearson et al., 2018; Vacaru et al., 2021). For example, a two-generational cohort study found higher rates of high depressive symptoms, defined as scoring 13 or higher on the *Edinburgh Postnatal Depression Scale* (EPDS; Cox et al., 1987), among young pregnant women between the ages of 19 and 24 living in southwest England surveyed in 2010 (25%) compared to women surveyed in the 1990s (17%; Pearson et al., 2018). Furthermore, rates of depression among pregnant women have increased over the course of the recent COVID-19 global pandemic. In several cohort studies comparing depressive symptoms in pregnant women before and after the start of the pandemic, reports indicate that rates of depressive symptoms were significantly higher (almost double in one sample) among women surveyed after the start of the pandemic (Berthelot et al., 2020; Vacaru et al., 2021).

Correlates and Risk Factors

A sizeable body of research has identified factors associated with an increased risk for, or higher rates of, prenatal depression. Although a majority of studies are correlational in nature (thus limiting our ability to infer causal relationships), an overview of common risk factors associated with prenatal depression allows for a better understanding of who might be most at risk for adverse outcomes. This literature can be summarized into broad categories of risk factors or correlates of prenatal depression, including sociodemographic characteristics; experiences of stressful life events; pregnancy-related experiences and stressors; access to care; relationship, family, and interpersonal factors; and physical and mental health.

Sociodemographic Characteristics

Sociodemographic characteristics associated with an increased risk for prenatal depression include the individual's race, ethnicity, income, employment status, education level, sexual orientation, and immigration status. Non-Hispanic Black and Hispanic people report higher levels of prenatal depression relative to White people in the United States (Benatar et al., 2020; Mukherjee et al., 2016), and this increased risk can largely be explained by experiences of racial discrimination (Noroña-Zhou et al., 2022) as well as limited access to prenatal care (Wong et al., 2020) among pregnant people of color. Among pregnant sexual minority women in the United States and abroad, experiences of discrimination and higher concealment motivation (i.e., the desire or need to conceal aspects of one's identity) are also associated with higher symptoms of prenatal depression (Marsland et al., 2022). Furthermore, lower levels of education, economic difficulties, lower income levels, and unemployment are also associated with an increased risk for prenatal depression (Cena et al., 2021; Fekadu Dadi et al., 2020; Okagbue et al., 2019; van de Loo et al., 2018; Yin et al., 2021). In the context of the COVID-19 pandemic specifically, financial strain was associated with a greater likelihood of clinically significant depression, even after controlling for education and income (Thayer

& Gildner, 2021). Finally, immigration status appears to differentially impact rates of prenatal depression depending on the country where studies are conducted (e.g., Anderson et al., 2017). Therefore, an "intersectional" lens that considers how various aspects of identity interact (e.g., race, gender, sexual orientation, social class; Crenshaw, 1989) is necessary when considering the influence of sociodemographic factors and identities on the risk for prenatal depression, as individuals with multiple intersecting marginalized identities will likely experience heightened risk for prenatal depression (e.g., Hankivsky et al., 2010).

Stressful Life Events

Experiences of stressful life events during pregnancy, including work-related stress and high global perceived stress, are associated with increased risk for prenatal depression (Biaggi et al., 2016; Kaiyo-Utete et al., 2020; Khan et al., 2021; Okagbue et al., 2019). Additionally, experiences of abuse or neglect early in life, as well as exposure to any kind of violence, are associated with high rates of prenatal depression (Fekadu Dadi et al., 2020; Gross et al., 2020; Shamblaw et al., 2019). Within this literature, substantial evidence supports the association between experiences of intimate partner violence and risk for both prenatal depression and suicidal thoughts and behaviors among pregnant people (Benatar et al., 2020; Biaggi et al., 2016; Kaiyo-Utete et al., 2020; Khan et al., 2021; Yin et al., 2021).

Pregnancy-Related Stressors and Access to Care

Pregnancy-related stressors, such as pregnancy-related unwanted physical symptoms (e.g., nausea, vomiting, extreme fatigue) and pregnancy-related complications, put pregnant people at greater risk for prenatal depression, with rates of prenatal depression up to 44.2% among those with obstetric complications (Biaggi et al., 2016; Fekadu Dadi et al., 2020; Tsakiridis et al., 2019; van de Loo et al., 2018). Other pregnancy-related risk factors include unplanned pregnancies (Benatar et al., 2020; Biaggi et al., 2016; Okagbue et al., 2019; van de Loo et al., 2018; Yin et al., 2021), having previous pregnancies or other children (Benatar et al., 2020; Cena et al., 2021), as well as a history of miscarriages or pregnancy loss (Koleva et al., 2011). Finally, some evidence suggests that the risk for prenatal depression might vary based on the pregnancy stage, with some data indicating that rates of prenatal depression are highest during later trimesters (Fekadu Dadi et al., 2020; Okagbue et al., 2019; van de Loo et al., 2018); however, other studies report no differences in rates across trimesters (e.g., Yin et al., 2021). Relatedly, limited access to prenatal care is associated with an increased risk for prenatal depression (e.g., Benatar et al., 2020). On average, Black people in the United States, in particular, are more likely to initiate prenatal care later than they want to due to a number of barriers to accessing care (Wong et al., 2020), which may in turn increase risk for prenatal depression.

Relationship, Family, and Interpersonal Factors

The availability of social support plays an important role in the context of prenatal depression just as it does with postpartum depression. Substantial evidence supports the association between lack of social support and symptoms of depression and other mental health concerns during pregnancy (Biaggi et al., 2016; Fekadu Dadi et al., 2020; Khan et al., 2021; Okagbue et al., 2019; Yin et al., 2021). In the context of minoritized and marginalized communities, some evidence suggests that a lack of social support mediates the relationship between experiences of discrimination, identity concealment, and prenatal depressive symptoms (e.g.,

Marsland et al., 2022). Lack of support or interpersonal conflict in the context of romantic relationships, including high levels of relationship distress, as well as not having a partner or spouse, also puts pregnant people at greater risk for depressive symptoms (Benatar et al., 2020; Fekadu Dadi et al., 2020; Kaiyo-Utete et al., 2020; Yin et al., 2021).

Physical and Mental Health

A range of markers of mental and physical health appears to put pregnant people at risk for prenatal depression. Among these, a history of mental health concerns—in particular depression—is associated with an increased risk for prenatal depression (Biaggi et al., 2016; Fekadu Dadi et al., 2020; van de Loo et al., 2018; Yin et al., 2021). Additionally, rates of substance use, including cannabis use (e.g., Goodwin et al., 2020) and tobacco use (e.g., Jones et al., 2020), are higher among pregnant people with prenatal depression relative to pregnant people without depression. Regarding physical health, physical inactivity during pregnancy (Sánchez-Polán et al., 2021; van de Loo et al., 2018), poor sleep (Tsai et al., 2021), poor diet quality (Avalos et al., 2020; Khan et al., 2020), and a diagnosis of gestational diabetes (e.g., Miller et al., 2021) are all associated with greater risk for prenatal depression. The impact of these mental and physical health markers is further complicated by the fact that people with prenatal depression are less likely to engage with routine medical care for nonpsychiatric concerns and to use urgent care services, and these odds are further exacerbated by lack of insurance coverage (Masters et al., 2020). Finally, many studies document that prenatal depression puts people at significantly greater risk for developing postpartum depression (Underwood et al., 2016).

At the start of Karina's pregnancy, she was already at risk for prenatal depression given her history of depression, in addition to her history of pregnancy loss. Karina often felt that she needed to hide her sexual orientation from healthcare providers to avoid unwanted bias or judgment and had experienced discrimination during medical appointments before. She often felt anxious during prenatal appointments as she anticipated having to correct staff about her partner's gender and feared negative reactions from staff. Medical providers had asked her about her "husband" during fertility appointments, and the paperwork she had to fill out often used heteronormative language. In addition, Karina worried about finances in part related to COVID-19. As a public high school teacher, Karina decided to take a medical leave during part of her pregnancy to limit her risk of exposure to COVID-19. In addition, due to COVID-19 restrictions, her wife was not able to attend any prenatal or ultrasound appointments and she worried about whether there would be other impacts on her pregnancy if COVID-19 cases continued increasing and what things would be like when the baby was born. Furthermore, Karina felt nauseous and tired most days, and this, combined with persistent pelvic pain, made it hard to get out and walk or stay active.

Effects on the Partner Relationship, Children, and Other Family Members

In addition to the detrimental impact prenatal depression has on the pregnant individual, perinatal depression frequently impacts children, partners, and family systems.

With regard to child-related outcomes, prenatal depression is associated with a host of negative developmental outcomes for children from birth through adolescence. Prenatal depression is associated with preterm labor and delivery, lower baby weight at birth (e.g., Nylen et al., 2013), and a greater risk of infant hospitalization in the first year of life (Jacques et al., 2019). Furthermore, prenatal depression is associated with poorer child and adolescent socioemotional, cognitive, and behavioral development (Kingston & Tough, 2014; Madigan et al., 2018; Rogers et al., 2020). In one meta-analysis of 71 studies of the impact of prenatal depression and anxiety on the socioemotional development of children up to 18 years of age, the odds of having children with behavioral difficulties were between 1.5 and 2 times greater among people who experienced prenatal depression, and the association between depressive symptoms and behavioral problems was strongest for people with more severe depression (Madigan et al., 2018). In addition to negative developmental outcomes, prenatal depression seems to impact interactions between parents and their children. In a longitudinal study of 900 mother–child dyads, Pearson et al. (2012) document that women with prenatal depression demonstrated a 30% increased risk for low maternal responsiveness (i.e., a mother's ability to engage with, and respond to, her child's communications) when the children were 12 months old relative to mothers without a history of prenatal depression.

Consistent with the evidence referenced earlier, some research suggests that social support might play a role in buffering the association between prenatal depression and negative outcomes for children. In a prospective study, pregnant women who rated their partners as less supportive were more likely to experience negative birth outcomes relative to women who reported higher levels of perceived partner support (Nylen et al., 2013). Additionally, several hypothesized mechanisms have been proposed to explain the association between prenatal depression and child brain and behavioral development. For example, increased cortisol levels among pregnant people with depression could impact fetal brain development or increased exposure to pregnancy hormones due to difficulties in the placenta's ability to perform its regulatory role in fetal development (e.g., Madigan et al., 2018).

In addition to being associated with negative child-related outcomes, prenatal depression is associated with increased mental health concerns among partners and nonbirthing parents. Of note, the vast majority of this literature focuses on heteronormative couples (i.e., pregnant cisgender women and male partners) and the exclusion of LGBTQ+ individuals should be considered a significant limitation of the existing literature. Within this literature, substantial evidence supports the association between maternal prenatal depression and paternal prenatal and postpartum depression. In a meta-analysis, the prevalence rate of prenatal depression in fathers was 9.76% across all trimesters (Rao et al., 2020). Systematic reviews and meta-analyses document that prenatal maternal depression is a significant risk factor for paternal prenatal depression, postpartum depression, and perinatal anxiety (Chhabra et al., 2020; Paulson & Bazemore, 2010; Thiel et al., 2020). However, in one systematic review of the association between maternal and paternal perinatal depression, Wang et al. (2021) found that maternal postpartum depression, but not prenatal depression, was associated with paternal postpartum depression.

Karina and Maria generally have a strong relationship and are supportive of one another. Maria has had a hard time, understandably, managing her own emotions related to their experiences of infertility, pregnancy loss, and the current pregnancy. She has tried to be extra supportive of Karina, but it seems like Karina has been pulling away from her. Recently, Maria has been feeling anxious about whether Karina is going to become even more depressed, and she is worried that something bad might happen to the baby. Maria keeps having thoughts about the last miscarriage they experienced. Lately, these worries have been making it harder for her to fall asleep at night. She wants to be there for Karina and the baby but feels like she is becoming more and more worn out trying to balance everything. Karina noticed that they have gotten into more arguments lately. Usually, Karina would spend more time with her extended family and friends, especially when things felt strained in her relationship with her wife, but she has not been seeing them in person much due to COVID-19, and it seems like everyone is managing their own busy lives and stressors.

Assessment

Given the estimated prevalence of prenatal depression, combined with the host of negative outcomes associated with it, there is a need to screen for depression during pregnancy to identify individuals at risk for negative outcomes and connect them to appropriate services. However, there is disagreement about whether universal screening should be implemented (Thombs et al., 2017). Both the American College of Obstetricians and Gynecologists (ACOG) and the U.S. Preventive Services Task Force recommend universal screening during the perinatal period (ACOG, 2018; Siu et al., 2016). ACOG recommends screening for depression with a validated instrument at minimum once during the perinatal period (ACOG committee opinion No. 757, 2018). However, the most recent (2019) recommendation from the United Kingdom National Screening Committee (UK NSC) does not recommend universal screening for prenatal or postpartum mental health problems due to concerns about the lack of evidence about effective screening tools and lack of ability to make treatment recommendations based on existing evidence (Hamel et al., 2019, UK NSC, 2019). The Marcé International Society has suggested that decisions regarding the appropriateness of universal depression screening should be made locally based on resources and models of care (Austin & Marcé Society Position Statement Advisory Committee, 2014).

Data on actual screening rates across health systems remain limited. One study conducted in a large U.S. health system found that 65.1% of pregnant patients were screened for depression during pregnancy (Sidebottom et al., 2021). Research has documented higher screening rates in public versus private clinics and disparities in screening such that English-speaking individuals were more likely to be screened (Boland et al., 2020). Avalos et al. (2016) found that a universal screening program can significantly increase the percentage of patients who are screened for depression.

The most commonly used form of assessment for prenatal depression is self-report questionnaires. Out of these, the EPDS is the most widely used in both research and clinical settings to assess perinatal depression. A cutoff score of ≥12 or 13 was found to be suggestive of clinically significant depression (Cox et al., 1987). The ACOG opinion (2018) indicates that the EPDS offers advantages over other screening tools in part because it is available in 50+ languages, includes questions about symptoms of anxiety that are common in prenatal depression (e.g., feeling anxious or worried for no good reason, feeling scared or panicky for no good reason), and does not include questions about symptoms that overlap significantly with expected changes that occur during pregnancy, such as changes in sleep (ACOG, 2018). Although it was originally developed to assess postpartum depression, research has validated the EPDS for use during pregnancy (Bergink et al., 2011; Bunevicius et al., 2009). A lower cutoff score during pregnancy has been recommended compared to postpartum, and some experts have suggested using different cutoff scores depending on the trimester of pregnancy. For example, a cutoff score of ≥11 or 12 has been recommended in the first trimester and ≥10 or 11 in the second and third trimesters (Bergink et al., 2011; Bunevicius et al., 2009). A recent systematic review and meta-analysis found an EPDS cutoff of 11 maximized both sensitivity and specificity during the perinatal period, while a cutoff of 13 was less sensitive but more specific (Levis et al., 2020).

Other depression measures are also used to identify prenatal depression. Specifically, the *Patient Health Questionnaire-9* (PHQ-9; Spitzer et al., 1999) is the most widely used measure globally to assess depressive symptoms generally (i.e., not specifically during pregnancy). Similar to the EPDS, it is shorter than other available self-report measures, and, given its wide use, it is already integrated into many electronic health records and healthcare systems. It has also been validated for assessing prenatal depression specifically with a suggested cutoff score of 10 (Sidebottom et al., 2012; Wang et al., 2021) and was found to perform similarly to the EPDS in a recent meta-analysis (Wang et al., 2021). Additional self-report measures (e.g., *the Beck Depression Inventory-II*; Beck et al., 1996; the *Center for Epidemiologic Studies Depression Scale*; Radloff, 1977) have been described as acceptable to use during the perinatal period (ACOG, 2015; Kendig et al., 2017). Some research suggests that there may be differences between scores when measures are self-administered versus administered by a clinician (Badiya et al., 2021).

Depressive symptoms can also be assessed through clinician-rated measures (e.g., the *Quick Inventory of Depressive Symptomatology*, clinician rating [QIDS-C]; Rush et al., 2003) and semistructured diagnostic interviews (e.g., the *Structured Clinical Interview for DSM-5*; First et al., 2015; the *Mini-International Neuropsychiatric Interview* [MINI]; Sheehan et al., 1998). These instruments require more training, resources, and time, and, therefore, are not feasible to use in most real-world settings. However, they can more fully assess the criteria for a diagnosis of depression, including distress and interference related to symptoms.

Research has documented cultural differences in the experience of depressive symptoms, symptom presentations, and stigma and that perinatal assessment tools may yield different results with various populations (e.g., Halbreich & Karkun, 2006). This highlights the need for cultural considerations in the assessment of prenatal depression, including consideration of the symptoms examined, language used, and cutoff scores (Halbreich & Karkun, 2006). For example, Tsai et al. (2013) identified that a cutoff score of ≥ 10 on the EPDS performed better in a sample of individuals from sub-Saharan Africa, compared to the cutoff of ≥ 12 or 13 typically used in the United States and Europe. Furthermore, research has documented that pregnant people of color and those with lower education levels are more likely to be underdiagnosed with prenatal depression (e.g., Faisal-Cury et al., 2021; Prady et al., 2016), underscoring the need for cultural considerations in the assessment of prenatal depression, culturally validated assessment measures, and the role of provider bias.

Karina received a message asking her to complete the EPDS in her patient portal before her upcoming prenatal visit with her obstetrician (OB). She knew she had been feeling depressed. She had tried to go for more walks since that helped in the past, but it was hard to do because she felt tired every day and she was experiencing worsening pelvic pain. Although she knew she was feeling depressed and that it was not getting better, she did not really want to admit this to anyone else. She worried about what it might mean to have this information permanently in her medical record. On top of this, it already felt hard enough navigating her appointments as a queer woman, and she wondered if this would impact how her providers thought about her parenting abilities. She thought about not filling out the depression screener but figured she would probably have to complete it in the waiting room if she did not complete it before the appointment. She reminded herself that while she had negative interactions with some providers and staff, she genuinely felt that her OB cared about her. She read the questions and decided to endorse the depression symptoms she was experiencing.

Treatment

Despite guidelines emphasizing the importance of screening being followed by treatment and mental health referrals as appropriate (ACOG, 2015; Kendig et al., 2017), less than one-fifth of people with prenatal depression receive adequate treatment (Byatt et al., 2016). Important work is being done to identify ways to help implement guideline recommendations for treatment (Kendig et al., 2017). Available treatments include psychotherapy, including cognitive behavioral therapy (CBT), interpersonal psychotherapy (IPT), and pharmacotherapy. Research has found that many pregnant people have a preference for nonpharmacological treatment related to a number of concerns with pharmacological treatment, including potential adverse effects on the developing baby and feelings of shame and guilt associated with medication use (Battle et al., 2013; Goodman, 2009). For example, one study examining treatment preferences among pregnant people found that individual psychotherapy was the first-choice preference for depression treatment for 72.5% of participants, whereas medication was only the first-choice preference for 7.3% of participants (Goodman, 2009). Research has also examined a range of complementary health practices (e.g., yoga and physical activity; Eustis et al., 2019). Existing guidelines indicate psychosocial interventions, including psychotherapy, may be adequate for mild to moderate depression, whereas high-intensity psychological interventions, like CBT, and treatment with antidepressant medication is recommended for people who experience moderate to severe depression, taking into account the individual's history of depression, level of symptoms, and preferences (National Institute for Health and Care Excellence [NICE], 2014; Yonkers et al., 2009, reaffirmed in 2014). Notably, prior research with clinically depressed populations (DeRubeis et al., 2005) has found that psychotherapy alone can be efficacious in treating even moderate to severe cases of depression; although this research did not include perinatal women, the implications may be particularly relevant to individuals wishing to avoid pharmacologic interventions.

Cognitive Behavioral Therapy

Research suggests CBT is effective for prenatal depression (Li et al., 2020; Shortis et al., 2020). Shortis et al. (2020) conducted a systematic review of five randomized controlled trials (RCTs) conducted with pregnant women that examined CBTs compared to treatment as usual or an alternative intervention that used a validated measure of depression at pre- and post-intervention. Results indicated that participants generally found CBT to be acceptable. In addition, participants who received CBT reported significant reductions in depressive symptoms that were greater than participants in comparison conditions. Three of these five studies did not report effect sizes. However, one study reported a large effect size between the CBT and treatment as usual condition (Hedge's g = 1.21; Forsell et al., 2017), and another reported a moderate effect size between CBT and treatment as usual (Cohen's d = 0.53; Milgrom et al., 2015). CBT interventions were delivered in individual and group formats, and one study examined an Internet-based treatment. In the three studies that included follow-up assessments, which ranged from the early postpartum period to nine months postpartum, gains were maintained. Meta-analysis was not possible due to variation across studies.

Li et al. (2020) conducted a systematic review and meta-analysis of RCTs examining CBTs for perinatal depression in people who were pregnant or within 12 months of birth compared to usual care, supportive consultation, or no intervention. The majority of the 13 RCTs included examined prenatal populations; however, at least one study included participants during the post-partum period. Results indicated that participants in CBT conditions reported significantly lower symptoms of depression at post-treatment and during the early postpartum period (i.e., < four months) compared to comparison conditions, but there were no differences between conditions later in the postpartum period (i.e., > four months). Because the studies included used different measures to assess depression, the standardized mean difference (SMD) was used to report effect sizes. At post-treatment, differences between CBT and comparison conditions were moderate in magnitude (SMD = –0.52), and during the early postpartum period they were small to moderate in magnitude (SMD = –0.41). Qualitative research has suggested specific modifications to CBT during the perinatal period, including a focus on cultural beliefs about motherhood, the theme of self-sacrifice, and interpersonal support (O'Mahen et al., 2012). Research has also begun to examine mindfulness and acceptance-based CBTs, such as acceptance and commitment therapy for the treatment of perinatal depression in both inpatient and outpatient settings (e.g., Bonacquisti et al., 2017; Waters et al., 2020) and has found these approaches to generally be acceptable and effective, though less research is available on these approaches than traditional CBTs.

Research has also examined CBT-based prevention programs for prenatal depression. In a recent systematic review and meta-analysis, Yasuma et al. (2020) examined 18 studies and found a significant effect of prenatal intervention on prenatal depression across studies. In addition, they found a significant effect that was moderate in magnitude (Cohen's d = 0.53) when examining a subgroup of four studies that were identified as CBT-based preventions. Of note, research has also examined CBTs including mindfulness-based cognitive therapy, for the prevention of prenatal depression in people with a history of depression and found them to be effective in reducing depressive symptoms (e.g., Dimidjian et al., 2015).

Interpersonal Psychotherapy

Research also indicates that IPT, a time-limited intervention that focuses on attachment and interpersonal relationships and is effective for depression in the general population (Weissman et al., 2000), is also effective for perinatal depression (Grote et al., 2009; Sockol et al., 2011; Sockol, 2018), with some evidence indicating IPT may result in better outcomes compared to CBT. For example, in a meta-analysis of 27 studies, including open trials, quasi-randomized trials, and RCTs, Sockol et al. (2011) reported significant reductions in depression across pharmacotherapy, CBT, and IPT interventions that were large in magnitude, after controlling for outliers (Hedge's g = 1.61). In addition, results indicated that studies that included an IPT intervention yielded significantly larger effect sizes for depression (Hedge's g = 0.96, n = 5) than studies that included a CBT intervention (Hedge's g = 0.40; n = 6). Another meta-analysis and systematic review of 28 studies examining IPT during the perinatal period found IPT to be effective in decreasing depressive symptoms and the prevalence of depressive episodes as a preventive intervention and effective as a treatment in reducing symptoms of depression (Sockol, 2018). After removing outliers, the overall within (Hedge's g = 1.41) and between condition (Hedge's g = 1.05) effect sizes for reductions in depressive symptoms in treatment studies of IPT were large in magnitude. Although this meta-analysis and systematic review focused on the perinatal period, the authors note that the majority of studies included IPT beginning during pregnancy. The IPT interventions were delivered in individual and group formats, and some interventions included involvement from a partner.

Pharmacotherapy

Pharmacotherapy, such as sertraline and other types of antidepressant medication, has been found to be effective in treating prenatal and perinatal depression (Lusskin et al., 2018; Molenaar et al., 2018; NICE, 2014; Yonkers et al., 2014). Expert guidelines recommend psychological and behavioral interventions as frontline treatment for mild to moderate prenatal depression, with pharmacotherapy approaches recommended for more severe cases. Given ethical challenges in research on pharmacotherapy treatments for prenatal depression, the evidence base for the efficacy and safety of prenatal antidepressant use comes from cohort and case control studies, as RCTs are typically not conducted. Another challenge in this area of research, in terms of examining potential adverse medication effects, is that both prenatal depression and exposure to antidepressants have been associated with changes in fetal growth and shorter gestation (Yonkers et al., 2014). However, measurement of these exposures can be difficult for a variety of reasons, and studies examining antidepressant effects often do not adequately take into account the effects and risks associated with prenatal depression itself (Lusskin et al., 2018; Yonkers et al., 2014). As a result, while there is a large literature addressing the safety of prenatal antidepressant use, interpreting this literature can be challenging, and decisions regarding care may be difficult to make (Meltzer-Brody & Jones, 2015). The complexity of decision-making regarding prenatal antidepressant use has led to the development and evaluation of patient decision aids (Khalifeh et al., 2019; Vigod et al., 2019), and recommendations for clinicians to have supportive decision-making conversations with patients, factoring in current symptoms and impairment, prior history, and patient preferences for care (Kimmel et al., 2018).

In general, the most common medications used to treat prenatal depression are selective serotonin reuptake inhibitors (SSRIs), and clinical guidelines indicate a preference for the use of sertraline during the perinatal period (Molenaar et al., 2018). Data suggest that prenatal SSRI use has become substantially more common in recent years (Meltzer-Brody & Jones, 2015), with rates of use in the United States typically higher than in Europe and other parts of the world (Molenaar et al., 2020). Although some of the literature is mixed, many studies do not show significant increases in long-term risks associated with prenatal use of SSRIs, serotonin–norepinephrine reuptake inhibitors (SNRIs), or tricyclic antidepressants (Lusskin et al., 2018; Prady et al., 2018; Ross et al., 2013). However, due to the complexities of conducting research on antidepressant use during pregnancy, additional studies of high quality are needed to clarify their efficacy and safety to assist pregnant individuals and their providers in making decisions about starting a new antidepressant during pregnancy, as well as decisions regarding continuation versus discontinuation of antidepressants upon learning of pregnancy for individuals who were already taking antidepressants before pregnancy. In response to concerns about fetal exposure, research suggests that some pregnant individuals will abruptly discontinue the use of antidepressants during pregnancy, and others may reduce the dose of antidepressants while pregnant. Unfortunately, sudden discontinuation (particularly in the absence of other forms of care) can lead to increases in symptoms, and taking a reduced dose of one's antidepressant can also increase the risk for the fetus to be exposed to both the effects of the medication and the undertreated depressive symptoms. As such, it is important that mental health and prenatal care providers who work with pregnant individuals are familiar with these issues and can help women with decisions about medication use or facilitate referrals to providers with sufficient training in this area. Because many pregnant people may prefer nonpharmacological interventions (Battle et al., 2013; Goodman, 2009), it is also important for providers to facilitate referrals to other forms of care to prevent women from becoming disengaged from treatment during the perinatal period.

Complementary Health Practices

Yoga and physical activity-based interventions have been found to be acceptable to women during the perinatal period, and the available literature indicates these interventions can be effective in reducing symptoms of depression (e.g., Battle et al., 2015; Eustis et al., 2019). For example, Battle et al. (2015) conducted an open trial of a ten-week prenatal yoga intervention, consistent with prenatal yoga classes available in the community, for women between 12 and 26 weeks' gestation. Participants reported significant reductions in depression from pre- to post-intervention that were large in magnitude. Next, Battle and her colleagues tested this intervention in the context of a small pilot RCT (Uebelacker et al., 2016). Results supported the acceptability and feasibility of the intervention. Although there were no significant differences between the yoga and comparison condition (perinatal health education), perhaps due to sample size, the nonsignificant condition results favored the yoga condition. Currently, this intervention is being tested in a fully powered RCT (ClinicalTrials.gov: NCT02738216). Some studies on yoga and physical activity-based intervention have not found significant differences compared to control conditions and long-term follow-up data are lacking. Still, these types of interventions have the potential to reach many people and may address some barriers to traditional face-to-face treatment (e.g., concerns about mental health stigma, cost, and schedule conflicts).

Additional complementary health practices have also been examined. High-quality and well-powered studies are lacking, but available evidence supports the potential of omega-3 fatty acids, folate, and vitamin D as natural products that may be able to reduce prenatal depression (Reza et al., 2018).

Novel Delivery Formats

Recent years have seen an increase in digital mental health interventions that are delivered via the Internet typically through smartphone applications or computer-based programs. Many programs that are commercially available have not been tested in research studies. However, there is a strong research base that supports the efficacy of these smartphone and computer-based interventions for depression in the general population (e.g., Andrews et al., 2018; Cuijpers et al., 2019; Firth et al., 2017; Wright et al., 2019). Research has also begun to examine these interventions for the perinatal period as they may be able to increase access to care and address some barriers to traditional face-to-face treatments (e.g.,

Bright et al., 2022; Forsell et al., 2017; Heller et al., 2020), including in low- and middle-income countries that tend to report higher rates of perinatal depression, though additional research is needed in this area (Dosani et al., 2020).

> At her prenatal appointment, Karina's obstetrician (OB) asked how she had been feeling lately. Karina shared that she had been feeling depressed, overwhelmed, and not sure what to do about it. Her OB reviewed her answers to the questionnaire, and they talked about some of the symptoms together. Her OB suggested she meet with the integrated behavioral health therapist in their office that day after their appointment. Initially, Karina was not sure how she felt about this, but, ultimately, she felt that it was nice that the therapist was on site and could meet her that same day. It seemed easier to not have to make a separate appointment (and in fact, Karina was not sure she would have followed through if she had to return on a different day). Ultimately, the therapist offered to see her several times over the coming weeks and provided referrals for outpatient therapists she could work with beyond that timeframe. The therapist provided information about how common depression during pregnancy is, which made Karina feel better and gave her the sense that it was not her fault. She also talked about how important it is to get support and how certain skills can be helpful in managing thoughts and behaviors. Karina received CBT in the past, and much of what the therapist talked about seemed familiar. She also thought that getting more support from other people would be important now and for when the baby arrived. Although she still felt depressed, Karina left the office feeling less alone and like she had a plan and support for getting better.

Cultural Considerations

Pregnancy is a significant life event that, like other life events, is influenced by the sociocultural context. Expecting a child may have a particular meaning to individuals based on their culture, societal expectations, family traditions, and values, which can impact the overall experience of pregnancy and birth. Therefore, as mentioned in some prior sections, cultural considerations are needed with regard to understanding the prevalence and presentation of prenatal depression, its correlates and risk factors, its impact on relationships, and culturally responsive assessment and treatment (Onoye et al., 2016). Despite the documented importance of culture, a major limitation of the current literature on prenatal and perinatal depression is that it predominately focuses on people from North American and European cultures and is largely based on samples who are predominantly White, European/European American, and middle class.

Racism, and other forms of discrimination, broadly speaking and enacted by healthcare providers specifically, have been found to increase the risk of perinatal depression (Bécares & Atatoa-Carr, 2016; Segre et al., 2021). Mistrust of providers or fear of potential negative outcomes following interactions with providers might limit certain individuals from seeking help for prenatal depression until symptoms are more severe or might reduce their willingness to disclose certain information to providers (e.g., marital discord among LGBTQ+ couples). Structural and societal changes are needed to address racism and discrimination. In addition, healthcare providers should receive training in cultural responsiveness and the language and terms in questionnaires and forms should be inclusive (e.g., asking if the patient has a partner or spouse vs. using heteronormative language such as "husband" or making assumptions about the gender of a pregnant person or their partner).

Additional research is needed on how to deliver culturally responsive interventions during the prenatal period. Limited research has examined cultural adaptations of CBT for specific populations during the perinatal period. One example of a cross-cultural adaptation of a CBT program comes from Nisar et al. (2020), who adapted a CBT-based program, originally developed in Pakistan, for pregnant people in China. Examples of adaptations included adding common Chinese proverbs, the Chinese traditional model of the body, updating examples to convey social norms including a family with one child, and healthy local activities (e.g., tai chi). Fourteen out of the 15 participants found the program to be culturally relevant. Ward et al. (2022) collaborated with stakeholders from tribal communities in the United States to adapt a perinatal depression prevention program, based on CBT and attachment theory, for use in tribal communities in the United States. Surface-level adaptations, such as revising illustrations, were made, along with deep-level adaptations to include relevant spiritual elements, ancestral teachings, and cultural values.

Existing research on cultural responsivity for treatment with the general population should also be used to inform culturally responsive treatment during the prenatal period (e.g., Graham et al., 2013; Hays, 2016; Pantalone et al., 2009). For example, during the intake or early sessions, providers should ask about patients' identities, personal and cultural beliefs about pregnancy and parenting, and experiences of racism and discrimination that may be relevant to treatment, without making assumptions about individuals' lived experiences. For CBT, providers should be careful with cognitive restructuring to not challenge the validity of thoughts related to experiences of racism or discrimination (Graham et al., 2013). Instead, providers should validate these experiences and any associated emotions. Subsequently, it may be helpful to reframe thoughts related to the internalization of these experiences (e.g., I am not valuable or worthy; I am bad at my job).

Karina attributed part of the pressure she put on herself to be a "good mother" to the model her mother and grandmother provided. To her, it seemed like they always had things under control and sacrificed a great deal to provide for their families. Karina wanted to provide the same stability and support for her child. Although family was an important value for Karina, she often found it unhelpful when she used this value to set unattainable expectations for herself. Karina received support from friends in the LGBTQ+ community during her pregnancy and found it helpful to be immersed in a supportive, feminist community, where people affirmed her individual choices. She also found her conversations with other queer women navigating pregnancy and parenting transitions to be validating and noticed that they often helped her to take some of the pressure off herself to be a "perfect" parent. Karina's identity as a queer woman also impacted her experience of pregnancy and birth in some more challenging ways. She experienced frequent microaggressions as healthcare providers often asked about her "husband." These experiences made Karina hesitant initially to seek out therapy during her pregnancy, for fear that her providers might invalidate her experiences or judge her negatively. However, the therapist she was referred to asked inclusive questions about her life and identity, and this helped Karina feel like she could open up and trust this therapist.

Conclusion and Future Directions

In summary, prenatal depression is a common experience associated with a range of negative outcomes for individuals as well as children, partners, and other family members. Risk factors include sociodemographic variables, stressful life events, pregnancy-related stressors, limited access to care, low social support, and physical and mental health conditions. Prenatal depression is most often assessed in real-world settings via self-report questionnaires, but questions remain about the best way to assess prenatal depression. Some clinical guidelines recommend universal screening, whereas others do not, citing concerns about available assessment methods and the ability to make treatment recommendations based on the existing literature. Psychotherapy, including CBT and IPT, and pharmacotherapy are the most common treatments and are effective for prenatal depression. Some research has also begun to examine complementary health practices, such as prenatal yoga, for prenatal depression as both adjunctive interventions and stand-alone interventions, but more research is needed. Culture and identities can impact the experience of and expectations for pregnancy, presentation of symptoms of depression during pregnancy, and prevalence rates of prenatal depression and need to be thoughtfully considered in both assessment and treatment.

Much of the available literature focuses on depression during the perinatal period broadly defined, which includes pregnancy and the 12-month period following birth. Additional research is needed to examine the prevalence, assessment, and treatment of depression during the prenatal period specifically. Future studies should also examine the biological mechanisms that play a role in prenatal depression, such as maternal inflammation (Sawyer, 2021). There is also a need for studies on best practices for assessing prenatal depression in culturally responsive ways that can be utilized in real-world settings and how to ensure that assessment leads to connection with resources and referrals. Implementation science research and frameworks should be utilized to determine how to implement and sustain effective assessment and treatment approaches in real-world settings, including how to best train providers.

In terms of treatment, additional fully powered, methodologically rigorous RCTs with follow-up periods are needed to examine the treatment effects of psychotherapy. Given the barriers to accessing traditional mental health treatments during the prenatal period, research is also needed on how to best use technology to increase access to care. This includes research on digital mental health interventions, such as computer-based approaches and smartphone applications, as well as the use of telehealth. With regard to computer-based programs and smartphone applications, existing research indicates that programs that include some type of human support, often delivered via asynchronous written messages within a portal or via text messages, yield higher engagement and larger effect sizes on outcomes compared to programs without support (e.g., Cuijpers et al., 2019; Richards & Richardson, 2012; Wright et al., 2019). Research is needed to examine how to best provide support for these programs specifically during the prenatal period.

In addition, given the salience of family, partners, and social support to prenatal and perinatal depression, future research should consider how treatments can better incorporate family members and partners in the treatment process (Battle et al., 2021; Cohen & Schiller, 2017). Future research should also seek to understand the experiences and treatment needs of pregnant people with co-occurring conditions that may put them at higher risk for depression and poor physical health outcomes, including history of a substance use disorder (Reddy et al., 2017), people with physical disabilities (Smeltzer et al., 2016), those with multiple gestation pregnancies (Wenze & Battle, 2018), and other health conditions (e.g., obesity, Molyneaux et al., 2016; diabetes, Wilson et al., 2020).

References

American college of obstetricians and gynecologists committee opinion no. 630: Screening for perinatal depression. (2015). *Obstetrics & Gynecology, 125*(5), 1268–1271. https://doi.org/10.1097/01.AOG.0000465192.34779.dc

American college of obstetricians and gynecologists committee opinion no. 757: Screening for perinatal depression. (2018). *Obstetrics & Gynecology, 132*(5), e208–e212. https://doi.org/10.1097/AOG.0000000000002927

American Psychiatric Association. (2013). *Diagnostic and statistical manual of mental disorders* (5th ed.). https://doi.org/10.1176/appi.books.9780890425596

Anderson, F. M., Hatch, S. L., Comacchio, C., & Howard, L. M. (2017). Prevalence and risk of mental disorders in the perinatal period among migrant women: A systematic review and meta-analysis. *Archives of Women's Mental Health, 20*(3), 449–462. https://doi.org/10.1007/s00737-017-0723-z

Andrews, G., Basu, A., Cuijpers, P., Craske, M. G., McEvoy, P., English, C. L., & Newby, J. M. (2018). Computer therapy for the anxiety and depression disorders is effective, acceptable and practical health care: An updated meta-analysis. *Journal of Anxiety Disorders, 55*, 70–78. https://doi.org/10.1016/j.janxdis.2018.01.001

Ashley, J. M., Harper, B. D., Arms-Chavez, C. J., & LoBello, S. G. (2016). Estimated prevalence of antenatal depression in the US population. *Archives of Women's Mental Health, 19*(2), 395–400. https://doi.org/10.1007/s00737-015-0593-1

Austin, M. P., & Marcé Society Position Statement Advisory Committee. (2014). Marcé International Society position statement on psychosocial assessment and depression screening in perinatal women. *Best Practice & Research: Clinical Obstetrics & Gynaecology, 28*(1), 179–187. https://doi.org/10.1016/j.bpobgyn.2013.08.016

Avalos, L. A., Caan, B., Nance, N., Zhu, Y., Li, D. K., Quesenberry, C., . . . Hedderson, M. M. (2020). Prenatal depression and diet quality during pregnancy. *Journal of the Academy of Nutrition and Dietetics, 120*(6), 972–984. https://doi.org/10.1016/j.jand.2019.12.011

Avalos, L. A., Raine-Bennett, T., Chen, H., Adams, A. S., & Flanagan, T. (2016). Improved perinatal depression screening, treatment, and outcomes with a universal obstetric program. *Obstetrics and Gynecology, 127*(5), 917–925. https://doi.org/10.1097/AOG.0000000000001403

Badiya, P. K., Siddabattuni, S., Dey, D., Hiremath, A. C., Nalam, R. L., Srinivasan, V., . . . Ramamurthy, S. S. (2021). Effect of mode of administration on Edinburgh Postnatal Depression Scale in the south Indian population: A comparative study on self-administered and interviewer-administered scores. *Asian Journal of Psychiatry, 66*, 102890. https://doi.org/10.1016/j.ajp.2021.102890

Battle, C. L., Londono Tobon, A., Howard, M., & Miller, I. W. (2021). Father's perspectives on family relationships and mental health treatment participation in the context of maternal postpartum depression. *Frontiers in Psychology, 12*, 705655. https://doi.org/10.3389/fpsyg.2021.705655

Battle, C. L., Salisbury, A. L., Schofield, C. A., & Ortiz-Hernandez, S. (2013). Perinatal antidepressant use: Understanding women's preferences and concerns. *Journal of Psychiatric Practice, 19*(6), 443–453. https://doi.org/10.1097/01.pra.0000438183.74359.46

Battle, C. L., Uebelacker, L. A., Magee, S. R., Sutton, K. A., & Miller, I. W. (2015). Potential for prenatal yoga to serve as an intervention to treat depression during pregnancy. *Women's Health Issues: Official Publication of the Jacobs Institute of Women's Health, 25*(2), 134–141. https://doi.org/10.1016/j.whi.2014.12.003

Bécares, L., & Atatoa-Carr, P. (2016). The association between maternal and partner experienced racial discrimination and prenatal perceived stress, prenatal and postnatal depression: Findings from the growing up in New Zealand cohort study. *International Journal for Equity in Health, 15*(1), 155. https://doi.org/10.1186/s12939-016-0443-4

Beck, A. T., Steer, R. A., & Brown, G. K. (1996). *Manual for the Beck depression inventory-II.* The Psychological Corporation.

Benatar, S., Cross-Barnet, C., Johnston, E., & Hill, I. (2020). Prenatal depression: Assessment and outcomes among Medicaid participants. *The Journal of Behavioral Health Services & Research, 47*(3), 409–423. https://doi.org/10.1007/s11414-020-09689-2

Bergink, V., Kooistra, L., Lambregtse-van den Berg, M. P., Wijnen, H., Bunevicius, R., van Baar, A., & Pop, V. (2011). Validation of the Edinburgh depression scale during pregnancy. *Journal of Psychosomatic Research, 70*(4), 385–389. https://doi.org/10.1016/j.jpsychores.2010.07.008

Berthelot, N., Lemieux, R., Garon-Bissonnette, J., Drouin-Maziade, C., Martel, É., & Maziade, M. (2020). Uptrend in distress and psychiatric symptomatology in pregnant women during the coronavirus disease 2019 pandemic. *Acta Obstetricia et Gynecologica Scandinavica*, 99(7), 848–855. https://doi.org/10.1111/aogs.13925

Biaggi, A., Conroy, S., Pawlby, S., & Pariante, C. M. (2016). Identifying the women at risk of antenatal anxiety and depression: A systematic review. *Journal of Affective Disorders*, 191, 62–77. https://doi.org/10.1016/j.jad.2015.11.014

Boland, J. H., Schenhals, E., Grant, A., Tyler, L., & Carlson, L. (2020). 448: Disparities in prenatal depression screening and referral: A retrospective cohort study. *American Journal of Obstetrics and Gynecology*, 222(1). https://doi.org/10.1016/j.ajog.2019.11.464

Bonacquisti, A., Cohen, M. J., & Schiller, C. E. (2017). Acceptance and commitment therapy for perinatal mood and anxiety disorders: Development of an inpatient group intervention. *Archives of Women's Mental Health*, 20(5), 645–654. https://doi.org/10.1007/s00737-017-0735-8

Bright, K. S., Stuart, S., Mcneil, D. A., Murray, L., & Kingston, D. E. (2022). Feasibility and acceptability of Internet-based interpersonal psychotherapy for stress, anxiety, and depression in prenatal women: Thematic analysis. *JMIR Formative Research*, 6(6), e23879. https://doi.org/10.2196/23879

Bunevicius, A., Kusminskas, L., Pop, V. J., Pedersen, C. A., & Bunevicius, R. (2009). Screening for antenatal depression with the Edinburgh depression scale. *Journal of Psychosomatic Obstetrics and Gynaecology*, 30(4), 238–243. https://doi.org/10.3109/01674820903230708

Byatt, N., Xiao, R. S., Dinh, K. H., & Waring, M. E. (2016). Mental health care use in relation to depressive symptoms among pregnant women in the USA. *Archives of Women's Mental Health*, 19(1), 187–191. https://doi.org/10.1007/s00737-015-0524-1

Cena, L., Mirabella, F., Palumbo, G., Gigantesco, A., Trainini, A., & Stefana, A. (2021). Prevalence of maternal antenatal and postnatal depression and their association with sociodemographic and socioeconomic factors: A multicentre study in Italy. *Journal of Affective Disorders*, 279, 217–221. https://doi.org/10.1016/j.jad.2020.09.136

Chhabra, J., McDermott, B., & Li, W. (2020). Risk factors for paternal perinatal depression and anxiety: A systematic review and meta-analysis. *Psychology of Men & Masculinities*, 21(4), 593–611. https://doi.org/10.1037/men0000259

Cohen, M. J., & Schiller, C. E. (2017). A theoretical framework for treating perinatal depression using couple-based interventions. *Psychotherapy (Chicago, Ill.)*, 54(4), 406–415. https://doi.org/10.1037/pst0000151

Cox, J. L., Holden, J. M., & Sagovsky, R. (1987). Detection of postnatal depression: Development of the 10-item Edinburgh Postnatal Depression Scale. *British Journal of Psychiatry*, 150, 782–786. https://doi.org/10.1192/bjp.150.6.782

Crenshaw, K. (1989). Demarginalizing the intersection of race and sex: A Black feminist critique of antidiscrimination doctrine, feminist theory and antiracist politics. *University of Chicago Legal Forum*, 1989(1), 139–167.

Cuijpers, P., Noma, H., Karyotaki, E., Cipriani, A., & Furukawa, T. A. (2019). Effectiveness and acceptability of cognitive behavior therapy delivery formats in adults with depression: A network meta-analysis. *JAMA Psychiatry*, 76(7), 700–707. https://doi.org/10.1001/jamapsychiatry.2019.0268

DeRubeis, R. J., Hollon, S. D., Amsterdam, J. D., Shelton, R. C., Young, P. R., Salomon, R. M., . . . Gallop, R. (2005). Cognitive therapy vs medications in the treatment of moderate to severe depression. *Archives of General Psychiatry*, 62(4), 409–416. https://doi.org/10.1001/archpsyc.62.4.409

Dimidjian, S., Goodman, S. H., Felder, J. N., Gallop, R., Brown, A. P., & Beck, A. (2015). An open trial of mindfulness-based cognitive therapy for the prevention of perinatal depressive relapse/recurrence. *Archives of Women's Mental Health*, 18(1), 85–94. https://doi.org/10.1007/s00737-014-0468-x

Dosani, A., Arora, H., & Mazmudar, S. (2020). mHealth and perinatal depression in low-and middle-income countries: A scoping review of the literature. *International Journal of Environmental Research and Public Health*, 17(20), 7679. https://doi.org/10.3390/ijerph17207679

Eustis, E. H., Ernst, S., Sutton, K., & Battle, C. L. (2019). Innovations in the treatment of perinatal depression: The role of yoga and physical activity interventions during pregnancy and postpartum. *Current Psychiatry Reports*, 21(12), 133. https://doi.org/10.1007/s11920-019-1121-1

Faisal-Cury, A., Levy, R. B., Azeredo, C. M., & Matijasevich, A. (2021). Prevalence and associated risk factors of prenatal depression underdiagnosis: A population-based study. *International Journal of Gynaecology and Obstetrics*, 153(3), 469–475. https://doi.org/10.1002/ijgo.13593

Fekadu Dadi, A., Miller, E. R., & Mwanri, L. (2020). Antenatal depression and its association with adverse birth outcomes in low and middle-income countries: A systematic review and meta-analysis. *PloS One, 15*(1), e0227323. https://doi.org/10.1371/journal.pone.0227323

First, M. B., Williams, J. B. W., Karg, R. S., & Spitzer, R. L. (2015). *Structured clinical interview for DSM-5 – research version (SCID-5 for DSM-5, research version; SCID-5-RV).* American Psychiatric Association.

Firth, J., Torous, J., Nicholas, J., Carney, R., Pratap, A., Rosenbaum, S., & Sarris, J. (2017). The efficacy of smartphone-based mental health interventions for depressive symptoms: A meta-analysis of randomized controlled trials. *World Psychiatry, 16*(3), 287–298. https://doi.org/10.1002/wps.20472

Forsell, E., Bendix, M., Holländare, F., Szymanska von Schultz, B., Nasiell, J., Blomdahl-Wetterholm, M., . . . Kaldo, V. (2017). Internet delivered cognitive behavior therapy for antenatal depression: A randomised controlled trial. *Journal of Affective Disorders, 221*, 56–64. https://doi.org/10.1016/j.jad.2017.06.013

Goodman, J. H. (2009). Women's attitudes, preferences, and perceived barriers to treatment for perinatal depression. *Birth, 36*(1), 60–69. https://doi.org/10.1111/j.1523536X.2008.00296.x

Goodwin, R. D., Zhu, J., Heisler, Z., Metz, T. D., Wyka, K., Wu, M., & Das Eiden, R. (2020). Cannabis use during pregnancy in the United States: The role of depression. *Drug and Alcohol Dependence, 210*, 107881. https://doi.org/10.1016/j.drugalcdep.2020.107881

Graham, J. R., Sorenson, S., & Hayes-Skelton, S. A. (2013). Enhancing the cultural sensitivity of cognitive behavioral interventions for anxiety in diverse populations. *The Behavior Therapist, 36*(5), 101–108.

Gross, G. M., Kroll-Desrosiers, A., & Mattocks, K. (2020). A longitudinal investigation of military sexual trauma and perinatal depression. *Journal of Women's Health, 29*(1), 38–45. https://doi.org/10.1089/jwh.2018.7628

Grote, N. K., Swartz, H. A., Geibel, S. L., Zuckoff, A., Houck, P. R., & Frank, E. (2009). A randomized controlled trial of culturally relevant, brief interpersonal psychotherapy for perinatal depression. *Psychiatric Services, 60*(3), 313–321. https://doi.org/10.1176/appi.ps.60.3.313

Halbreich, U., & Karkun, S. (2006). Cross-cultural and social diversity of prevalence of postpartum depression and depressive symptoms. *Journal of Affective Disorders, 91*(2–3), 97–111. https://doi.org/10.1016/j.jad.2005.12.051

Hamel, C., Lang, E., Morissette, K., Beck, A., Stevens, A., Skidmore, B., . . . Moher, D. (2019). Screening for depression in women during pregnancy or the first year postpartum and in the general adult population: A protocol for two systematic reviews to update a guideline of the Canadian task force on preventive health care. *Systematic Reviews, 8*(1), 27. https://doi.org/10.1186/s13643-018-0930-3

Hankivsky, O., Reid, C., Cormier, R., Varcoe, C., Clark, N., Benoit, C., & Brotman, S. (2010). Exploring the promises of intersectionality for advancing women's health research. *International Journal for Equity in Health, 9*(5). https://doi.org/10.1186/1475-9276-9-5

Hays, P. A. (2016). *Addressing cultural complexities in practice: Assessment, diagnosis, and therapy* (3rd ed.). American Psychological Association. https://doi.org/10.1037/14801-000

Heller, H. M., Hoogendoorn, A. W., Honig, A., Broekman, B. F., & van Straten, A. (2020). The effectiveness of a guided Internet-based tool for the treatment of depression and anxiety in pregnancy (MamaKits Online): Randomized controlled trial. *Journal of Medical Internet Research, 22*(3), e15172. https://doi.org/10.2196/15172

Heron, J., O'Connor, T. G., Evans, J., Golding, J., Glover, V., & ALSPAC Study Team (2004). The course of anxiety and depression through pregnancy and the postpartum in a community sample. *Journal of Affective Disorders, 80*(1), 65–73. https://doi.org/10.1016/j.jad.2003.08.004

Jacques, N., de Mola, C. L., Joseph, G., Mesenburg, M. A., & da Silveira, M. F. (2019). Prenatal and postnatal maternal depression and infant hospitalization and mortality in the first year of life: A systematic review and meta-analysis. *Journal of Affective Disorders, 243*, 201–208. https://doi.org/10.1016/j.jad.2018.09.055

Jones, A. M., Carter-Harris, L., Stiffler, D., Macy, J. T., Staten, L. K., & Shieh, C. (2020). Smoking status and symptoms of depression during and after pregnancy among low-income women. *Journal of Obstetric, Gynecologic, and Neonatal Nursing: JOGNN, 49*(4), 361–372. https://doi.org/10.1016/j.jogn.2020.05.006

Kaiyo-Utete, M., Dambi, J. M., Chingono, A., Mazhandu, F., Madziro-Ruwizhu, T. B., Henderson, C., . . . Chirenje, Z. M. (2020). Antenatal depression: An examination of prevalence and its associated factors among pregnant women attending Harare polyclinics. *BMC Pregnancy and Childbirth, 20*(1), 197. https://doi.org/10.1186/s12884-020-02887-y

Kendig, S., Keats, J. P., Hoffman, M. C., Kay, L. B., Miller, E. S., Moore Simas, T. A., . . . Lemieux, L. A. (2017). Consensus bundle on maternal mental health: Perinatal depression and anxiety. *Obstetrics & Gynecology, 129*(3), 422–430. https://doi.org/10.1097/AOG.0000000000001902

Khalifeh, H., Molyneaux, E., Brauer, R., Vigod, S., & Howard, L. M. (2019). Patient decision aids for antidepressant use in pregnancy: A pilot randomised controlled trial in the UK. *BJGP Open, 3*(4). Advance online publication. https://doi.org/10.3399/bjgpopen19X101666

Khan, R., Waqas, A., Bilal, A., Mustehsan, Z. H., Omar, J., & Rahman, A. (2020). Association of maternal depression with diet: A systematic review. *Asian Journal of Psychiatry, 52*, 102098. https://doi.org/10.1016/j.ajp.2020.102098

Khan, R., Waqas, A., Mustehsan, Z. H., Khan, A. S., Sikander, S., Ahmad, I., Jamil, A., Sharif, M., Bilal, S., Zulfiqar, S., Bibi, A., & Rahman, A. (2021). Predictors of prenatal depression: A cross-sectional study in rural Pakistan. *Frontiers in Psychiatry, 12*, 584287. https://doi.org/10.3389/fpsyt.2021.584287

Kimmel, M. C., Cox, E., Schiller, C., Gettes, E., & Meltzer-Brody, S. (2018). Pharmacologic treatment of perinatal depression. *Obstetrics and Gynecology Clinics of North America, 45*(3), 419–440. https://doi.org/10.1016/j.ogc.2018.04.007

Kingston, D., & Tough, S. (2014). Prenatal and postnatal maternal mental health and school-age child development: A systematic review. *Maternal and Child Health Journal, 18*(7), 1728–1741. https://doi.org/10.1007/s10995-013-1418-3

Koleva, H., Stuart, S., O'Hara, M. W., & Bowman-Reif, J. (2011). Risk factors for depressive symptoms during pregnancy. *Archives of Women's Mental Health, 14*(2), 99–105. https://doi.org/10.1007/s00737-010-0184-0

Kugbey, N., Ayanore, M., Doegah, P., Chirwa, M., Bartels, S. A., Davison, C. M., & Purkey, E. (2021). Prevalence and correlates of prenatal depression, anxiety and suicidal behaviours in the Volta Region of Ghana. *International Journal of Environmental Research and Public Health, 18*(11), 5857. https://doi.org/10.3390/ijerph18115857

Levis, B., Negeri, Z., Sun, Y., Benedetti, A., & Thombs, B. D. (2020). Accuracy of the Edinburgh Postnatal Depression Scale (EPDS) for screening to detect major depression among pregnant and postpartum women: Systematic review and meta-analysis of individual participant data. *British Medical Journal, 371*, 4022. https://doi.org/10.1136/bmj.m4022

Li, Z., Liu, Y., Wang, J., Liu, J., Zhang, C., & Liu, Y. (2020). Effectiveness of cognitive behavioural therapy for perinatal depression: A systematic review and meta-analysis. *Journal of Clinical Nursing, 29*, 3170–3182. https://doi.org/10.1111/jocn.15378

Lusskin, S. I., Khan, S. J., Ernst, C., Habib, S., Fersh, M. E., & Albertini, E. S. (2018). Pharmacotherapy for perinatal depression. *Clinical Obstetrics and Gynecology, 61*(3), 544–561. https://doi.org/10.1097/GRF.0000000000000365

Madigan, S., Oatley, H., Racine, N., Fearon, R., Schumacher, L., Akbari, E., . . . Tarabulsy, G. M. (2018). A meta-analysis of maternal prenatal depression and anxiety on child socioemotional development. *Journal of the American Academy of Child and Adolescent Psychiatry, 57*(9), 645–657.e8. https://doi.org/10.1016/j.jaac.2018.06.012

Marchesi, C., Bertoni, S., & Maggini, C. (2009). Major and minor depression in pregnancy. *Obstetrics & Gynecology, 113*(6), 1292–1298. https://doi.org/10.1097/AOG.0b013e3181a45e90

Marsland, S., Treyvaud, K., & Pepping, C. A. (2022). Prevalence and risk factors associated with perinatal depression in sexual minority women. *Clinical Psychology & Psychotherapy, 29*(2), 611–621. https://doi.org/10.1002/cpp.2653

Masters, G. A., Li, N., Lapane, K. L., Liu, S. H., Person, S. D., & Byatt, N. (2020). Utilization of health care among perinatal women in the United States: The role of depression. *Journal of Women's Health (2002), 29*(7), 944–951. https://doi.org/10.1089/jwh.2019.7903

Meltzer-Brody, S., & Jones, I. (2015). Optimizing the treatment of mood disorders in the perinatal period. *Dialogues in Clinical Neuroscience, 17*(2), 207–218. https://doi.org/10.31887/DCNS.2015.17.2/smeltzerbrody

Milgrom, J., Holt, C., Holt, C. J., Ross, J., Ericksen, J., & Gemmill, A. W. (2015). Feasibility study and pilot randomised trial of an antenatal depression treatment with infant follow-up. *Archives of Women's Mental Health*, 18(5), 717–730. https://doi.org/10.1007/s00737-015-0512-5

Miller, N. E., Curry, E., Laabs, S. B., Manhas, M., & Angstman, K. (2021). Impact of gestational diabetes diagnosis on concurrent depression in pregnancy. *Journal of Psychosomatic Obstetrics and Gynaecology*, 42(3), 190–193. https://doi.org/10.1080/0167482X.2019.1709816

Molenaar, N. M., Bais, B., Lambregtse-van den Berg, M. P., Mulder, C. L., Howell, E. A., Fox, N. S., . . . Kamperman, A. M. (2020). The international prevalence of antidepressant use before, during, and after pregnancy: A systematic review and meta-analysis of timing, type of prescriptions and geographical variability. *Journal of Affective Disorders*, 264, 82–89. https://doi.org/10.1016/j.jad.2019.12.014

Molenaar, N. M., Kamperman, A. M., Boyce, P., & Bergink, V. (2018). Guidelines on treatment of perinatal depression with antidepressants: An international review. *Australian and New Zealand Journal of Psychiatry*, 52(4), 320–327. https://doi.org/10.1177/0004867418762057

Molyneaux, E., Poston, L., Khondoker, M., & Howard, L. M. (2016). Obesity, antenatal depression, diet and gestational weight gain in a population cohort study. *Archives of Women's Mental Health*, 19(5), 899–907. https://doi.org/10.1007/s00737-016-0635-3

Mukherjee, S., Trepka, M. J., Pierre-Victor, D., Bahelah, R., & Avent, T. (2016). Racial/ethnic disparities in antenatal depression in the United States: A systematic review. *Maternal and Child Health Journal*, 20(9), 1780–1797. https://doi.org/10.1007/s10995-016-1989-x

National Institute for Health and Care Excellence (NICE). (2014). *Antenatal and postnatal mental health: Clinical management and service guidance* [CG192]. Retrieved April 26, 2022, from www.nice.org.uk/guidance/cg192/chapter/1-Recommendations#treatment-decisions-advice-and-monitoring-for-women-who-are-planning-a-pregnancy-pregnant-or-in-2

Nidey, N., Tabb, K. M., Carter, K. D., Bao, W., Strathearn, L., Rohlman, D. S., . . . Ryckman, K. (2020). Rurality and risk of perinatal depression among women in the United States. *Journal of Rural Health*, 36(1), 9–16. https://doi.org/10.1111/jrh.12401

Nisar, A., Yin, J., Yiping, N., Lanting, H., Zhang, J., Wang, D., . . . Li, X. (2020). Making therapies culturally relevant: Translation, cultural adaptation and field-testing of the thinking healthy programme for perinatal depression in China. *BMC Pregnancy Childbirth*, 20(368). https://doi.org/10.1186/s12884-020-03044-1

Noroña-Zhou, A., Aran, Ö., Garcia, S. E., Haraden, D., Perzow, S., Demers, C. H., . . . Davis, E. P. (2022). Experiences of discrimination and depression trajectories over pregnancy. *Women's Health Issues*, 32(2), 147–155. https://doi.org/10.1016/j.whi.2021.10.002

Nylen, K. J., O'Hara, M. W., & Engeldinger, J. (2013). Perceived social support interacts with prenatal depression to predict birth outcomes. *Journal of Behavioral Medicine*, 36(4), 427–440. https://doi.org/10.1007/s10865-012-9436-y

Okagbue, H. I., Adamu, P. I., Bishop, S. A., Oguntunde, P. E., Opanuga, A. A., & Akhmetshin, E. M. (2019). Systematic review of prevalence of antepartum depression during the trimesters of pregnancy. *Open Access Macedonian Journal of Medical Sciences*, 7(9), 1555–1560. https://doi.org/10.3889/oamjms.2019.270

O'Mahen, H., Fedock, G., Henshaw, E., Himle, J. A., Forman, J., & Flynn, H. A. (2012). Modifying CBT for perinatal depression: What do women want?: A qualitative study. *Cognitive and Behavioral Practice*, 19(2), 359–371. https://doi.org/10.1016/j.cbpra.2011.05.005.

Onoye, J. M., Goebert, D. A., & Morland, L. A. (2016). Cross-cultural differences in adjustment to pregnancy and the postpartum period. In A. Wenzel (Ed.), *The Oxford handbook of perinatal psychology* (pp. 632–662). Oxford University Press. https://10.1093/oxfordhb/9780199778072.013.31

Pampaka, D., Papatheodorou, S. I., AlSeaidan, M., Al Wotayan, R., Wright, R. J., Buring, J. E., . . . Christophi, C. A. (2018). Depressive symptoms and comorbid problems in pregnancy – results from a population based study. *Journal of Psychosomatic Research*, 112, 53–58. https://doi.org/10.1016/j.jpsychores.2018.06.011

Pantalone, D. W., Iwamasa, G. Y., & Martell, C. R. (2009). Cognitive-behavioral therapy with diverse populations. In Dobson (Ed.), *Handbook of cognitive-behavioral therapies* (pp. 445–464). Guilford Press.

Paulson, J. F., & Bazemore, S. D. (2010). Prenatal and postpartum depression in fathers and its association with maternal depression: A meta-analysis. *Journal of the American Medical Association*, 303(19), 1961–1969. https://doi.org/10.1001/jama.2010.605

Pearson, R. M., Carnegie, R. E., Cree, C., Rollings, C., Rena-Jones, L., Evans, J., Stein, A., Tilling, K., Lewcock, M., & Lawlor, D. A. (2018). Prevalence of prenatal depression symptoms among 2 generations of pregnant mothers: The Avon longitudinal study of parents and children. *JAMA Network Open, 1*(3), e180725. https://doi.org/10.1001/jamanetworkopen.2018.0725

Pearson, R. M., Melotti, R., Heron, J., Joinson, C., Stein, A., Ramchandani, P. G., & Evans, J. (2012). Disruption to the development of maternal responsiveness? The impact of renatal depression on mother-infant interactions. *Infant Behavior & Development, 35*(4), 613–626. https://doi.org/10.1016/j.infbeh.2012.07.020

Prady, S. L., Hanlon, I., Fraser, L. K., & Mikocka-Walus, A. (2018). A systematic review of maternal antidepressant use in pregnancy and short- and long-term offspring's outcomes. *Archives of Women's Mental Health, 21*(2), 127–140. https://doi.org/10.1007/s00737-017-0780-3

Prady, S. L., Pickett, K. E., Petherick, E. S., Gilbody, S., Croudace, T., Mason, D., . . . Wright, J. (2016). Evaluation of ethnic disparities in detection of depression and anxiety in primary care during the maternal period: Combined analysis of routine and cohort data. *British Journal of Psychiatry, 208*(5), 453–461. https://doi.org/10.1192/bjp.bp.114.158832

Radloff, L. S. (1977). The CES-D scale: A self-report depression scale for research in the general population. *Applied Psychological Measurement, 1*(3), 385–401. https://doi.org/10.1177/014662167700100306

Rao, W. W., Zhu, X. M., Zong, Q. Q., Zhang, Q., Hall, B. J., Ungvari, G. S., & Xiang, Y. T. (2020). Prevalence of prenatal and postpartum depression in fathers: A comprehensive meta-analysis of observational surveys. *Journal of Affective Disorders, 263*, 491–499. https://doi.org/10.1016/j.jad.2019.10.030

Reddy, U. M., Davis, J. M., Ren, Z., Greene, M. F., & Opioid Use in Pregnancy, Neonatal Abstinence Syndrome, and Childhood Outcomes Workshop Invited Speakers. (2017). Opioid use in pregnancy, neonatal abstinence syndrome, and childhood outcomes: Executive summary of a joint workshop by the Eunice Kennedy Shriver National Institute of Child Health and Human Development, American College of Obstetricians and Gynecologists, American Academy of Pediatrics, Society for Maternal-Fetal Medicine, Centers for Disease Control and Prevention, and the March of Dimes Foundation. *Obstetrics & Gynecology, 130*(1), 10–28. https://doi.org/10.1097/AOG.0000000000002054

Reza, N., Deligiannidis, K. M., Eustis, E. H., & Battle, C. L. (2018). Complementary health practices for treating perinatal depression. *Obstetrics and Gynecology Clinics of North America, 45*(3), 441–454. https://doi.org/10.1016/j.ogc.2018.04.002

Richards, D., & Richardson, T. (2012). Computer-based psychological treatments for depression: A systematic review and meta-analysis. *Clinical Psychology Review, 32*(4), 329–342. https://doi.org/10.1016/j.cpr.2012.02.004

Rogers, A., Obst, S., Teague, S. J., Rossen, L., Spry, E. A., Macdonald, J. A., . . . Hutchinson, D. (2020). Association between maternal perinatal depression and anxiety and child and adolescent development: A meta-analysis. *JAMA Pediatrics, 174*(11), 1082–1092. https://doi.org/10.1001/jamapediatrics.2020.2910

Ross, L. E., Grigoriadis, S., Mamisashvili, L., Vonderporten, E. H., Roerecke, M., Rehm, J., . . . Cheung, A. (2013). Selected pregnancy and delivery outcomes after exposure to antidepressant medication: A systematic review and meta-analysis. *JAMA Psychiatry, 70*(4), 436–443. https://doi.org/10.1001/jamapsychiatry.2013.684

Rush, A. J., Trivedi, M. H., Ibrahim, H. M., Carmody, T. J., Arnow, B., Klein, D. N., . . . Keller, M. B. (2003). The 16-item quick inventory of depressive symptomatology (QIDS), clinician rating (QIDS-C), and self-report (QIDS-SR): A psychometric evaluation in patients with chronic major depression. *Biological Psychiatry, 54*(5), 573–583. https://doi.org/10.1016/s0006-3223(02)01866-8

Sánchez-Polán, M., Franco, E., Silva-José, C., Gil-Ares, J., Pérez-Tejero, J., Barakat, R., & Refoyo, I. (2021). Exercise during pregnancy and prenatal depression: A systematic review and meta-analysis. *Frontiers in Physiology, 12*, 640024. https://doi.org/10.3389/fphys.2021.640024

Sawyer, K. M. (2021). The role of inflammation in the pathogenesis of perinatal depression and offspring outcomes. *Brain, Behavior, & Immunity – Health, 18*, 100390. https://doi.org/10.1016/j.bbih.2021.100390

Segre, L. S., Mehner, B. T., & Brock, R. L. (2021). Perceived racial discrimination and depressed mood in perinatal women: An extension of the domain specific stress index. *Women's Health Issues, 31*(3), 254–262. https://doi.org/10.1016/j.whi.2020.12.008

Shamblaw, A. L., Cardy, R. E., Prost, E., & Harkness, K. L. (2019). Abuse as a risk factor for prenatal depressive symptoms: A meta-analysis. *Archives of Women's Mental Health*, 22(2), 199–213. https://doi.org/10.1007/s00737-018-0900-8

Sheehan, D. V., Lecrubier, Y., Sheehan, K. H., Amorim, P., Janavs, J., Weiller, E., . . . Dunbar, G. C. (1998). The mini-international neuropsychiatric interview (M.I.N.I.): The development and validation of a structured diagnostic psychiatric interview for DSM-IV and ICD-10. *Journal of Clinical Psychiatry*, 59(Suppl 20), 22–57.

Shortis, E., Warrington, D., & Whittaker, P. (2020). The efficacy of cognitive behavioral therapy for the treatment of antenatal depression: A systematic review. *Journal of Affective Disorders*, 272, 485–495. https://doi.org/10.1016/j.jad.2020.03.067

Sidebottom, A., Vacquier, M., LaRusso, E., Erickson, D., & Hardeman, R. (2021). Perinatal depression screening practices in a large health system: Identifying current state and assessing opportunities to provide more equitable care. *Archives of Women's Mental Health*, 24(1), 133–144. https://doi.org/10.1007/s00737-020-01035-x

Sidebottom, A. C., Harrison, P. A., Godecker, A., & Kim, H. (2012). Validation of the Patient Health Questionnaire (PHQ)-9 for prenatal depression screening. *Archives of Women's Mental Health*, 15, 367–374. https://doi.org/10.1007/s00737-012-0295-x

Siu, A. L., US Preventive Services Task Force (USPSTF), Bibbins-Domingo, K., Grossman, D. C., Baumann, L. C., Davidson, K. W., . . . Pignone, M. P. (2016). Screening for depression in adults: US preventive services task force recommendation Statement. *JAMA*, 315(4), 380–387. https://doi.org/10.1001/jama.2015.18392

Smeltzer, S. C., Mitra, M., Iezzoni, L. I., Long-Bellil, L., & Smith, L. D. (2016). Perinatal experiences of women with physical disabilities and their recommendations for clinicians. *Journal of Obstetric, Gynecologic, and Neonatal Nursing: JOGNN*, 45(6), 781–789. https://doi.org/10.1016/j.jogn.2016.07.007

Sockol, L. E. (2018). A systematic review and meta-analysis of interpersonal psychotherapy for perinatal women. *Journal of Affective Disorders*, 232, 316–328. https://doi.org/10.1016/j.jad.2018.01.018

Sockol, L. E., Epperson, C. N., & Barber, J. P. (2011). A meta-analysis of treatments for perinatal depression. *Clinical Psychology Review*, 31(5), 839–849. https://doi.org/10.1016/j.cpr.2011.03.009

Spitzer, R. L., Kroenke, K., Williams, J. B. W., & the Patient Health Questionnaire Primary Care Study Group. (1999). Validation and utility of a self-report version of PRIME-MD: The PHQ primary care study. *JAMA*, 282(18), 1737–1744. https://doi.org/10.1001/jama.282.18.1737

Thayer, Z. M., & Gildner, T. E. (2021). COVID-19-related financial stress associated with higher likelihood of depression among pregnant women living in the United States. *American Journal of Human Biology*, 33(3), e23508. https://doi.org/10.1002/ajhb.23508

Thiel, F., Pittelkow, M. M., Wittchen, H. U., & Garthus-Niegel, S. (2020). The relationship between paternal and maternal depression during the perinatal period: A systematic review and meta-analysis. *Frontiers in Psychiatry*, 11, 563287. https://doi.org/10.3389/fpsyt.2020.563287

Thombs, B. D., Saadat, N., Riehm, K. E., Karter, J. M., Vaswani, A., Andrews, B. K., . . . Cosgrove, L. (2017). Consistency and sources of divergence in recommendations on screening with questionnaires for presently experienced health problems or symptoms: A comparison of recommendations from the Canadian Task Force on Preventive Health Care, UK National Screening Committee, and US Preventive Services Task Force. *BMC Medicine*, 15(1), 150. https://doi.org/10.1186/s12916-017-0903-8

Tomfohr-Madsen, L. M., Racine, N., Giesbrecht, G. F., Lebel, C., & Madigan, S. (2021). Depression and anxiety in pregnancy during COVID-19: A rapid review and meta-analysis. *Psychiatry Research*, 300, 113912. https://doi.org/10.1016/j.psychres.2021.113912

Tsai, A. C., Scott, J. A., Hung, K. J., Zhu, J. Q., Matthews, L. T., Psaros, C., & Tomlinson, M. (2013). Reliability and validity of instruments for assessing perinatal depression in African settings: Systematic review and meta-analysis. *PLoS ONE*, 8(12), e82521. https://doi.org/10.1371/journal.pone.0082521

Tsai, S. Y., Lee, P. L., Gordon, C., Cayanan, E., & Lee, C. N. (2021). Objective sleep efficiency but not subjective sleep quality is associated with longitudinal risk of depression in pregnant women: A prospective observational cohort study. *International Journal of Nursing Studies*, 120, 103966. https://doi.org/10.1016/j.ijnurstu.2021.103966

Tsakiridis, I., Bousi, V., Dagklis, T., Sardeli, C., Nikolopoulou, V., & Papazisis, G. (2019). Epidemiology of antenatal depression among women with high-risk pregnancies due to obstetric complications: A scoping review. *Archives of Gynecology and Obstetrics, 300*(4), 849–859. https://doi.org/10.1007/s00404-019-05270-1

Uebelacker, L. A., Battle, C. L., Sutton, K. A., Magee, S. R., & Miller, I. W. (2016). A pilot randomized controlled trial comparing prenatal yoga to perinatal health education for antenatal depression. *Archives of Women's Mental Health, 19*(3), 543–547. https://doi.org/10.1007/s00737-015-0571-7

Underwood, L., Waldie, K., D'Souza, S., Peterson, E. R., & Morton, S. (2016). A review of longitudinal studies on antenatal and postnatal depression. *Archives of Women's Mental Health, 19*(5), 711–720. https://doi.org/10.1007/s00737-016-0629-1

United Kingdom National Screening Committee. (2019). *Antenatal screening programme postnatal depression.* Retrieved April 26, 2022, from https://view-health-screening-recommendations.service.gov.uk/postnatal-depression/

Vacaru, S., Beijers, R., Browne, P. D., Cloin, M., van Bakel, H., van den Heuvel, M. I., & de Weerth, C. (2021). The risk and protective factors of heightened prenatal anxiety and depression during the COVID-19 lockdown. *Scientific Reports, 11*(1), 20261. https://doi.org/10.1038/s41598-021-99662-6

van de Loo, K., Vlenterie, R., Nikkels, S. J., Merkus, P., Roukema, J., Verhaak, C. M., . . . van Gelder, M. (2018). Depression and anxiety during pregnancy: The influence of maternal characteristics. *Birth (Berkeley, Calif.), 45*(4), 478–489. https://doi.org/10.1111/birt.12343

Vigod, S. N., Hussain-Shamsy, N., Stewart, D. E., Grigoriadis, S., Metcalfe, K., Oberlander, T. F., . . . Dennis, C. L. (2019). A patient decision aid for antidepressant use in pregnancy: Pilot randomized controlled trial. *Journal of Affective Disorders, 251*, 91–99. https://doi.org/10.1016/j.jad.2019.01.051

Wang, L., Kroenke, K., Stump, T. E., & Monahan, P. O. (2021). Screening for perinatal depression with the patient health questionnaire depression scale (PHQ-9): A systematic review and meta-analysis. *General Hospital Psychiatry, 68*, 74–82.

Ward, E. A., Iron Cloud-Two Dogs, E., Gier, E. E., Littlefield, L., & Tandon, S. D. (2022). Cultural adaptation of the Mothers and Babies Intervention for use in tribal communities. *Frontiers in Psychiatry, 13*, 807432. https://doi.org/10.3389/fpsyt.2022.807432

Waters, C. S., Annear, B., Flockhart, G., Jones, I., Simmonds, J. R., Smith, S., . . . Williams, J. F. (2020). Acceptance and commitment therapy for perinatal mood and anxiety disorders: A feasibility and proof of concept study. *British Journal of Clinical Psychology, 59*(4), 461–479. https://doi.org/10.1111/bjc.12261

Weissman, M. M., Markowitz, J. C., & Klerman, G. L. (2000). *Comprehensive guide to interpersonal psychotherapy.* Basic Books.

Wenze, S. J., & Battle, C. L. (2018). Perinatal mental health treatment needs, preferences, and barriers in parents of multiples. *Journal of Psychiatric Practice, 24*(3), 158–168. https://doi.org/10.1097/PRA.0000000000000299

Wilson, C. A., Newham, J., Rankin, J., Ismail, K., Simonoff, E., Reynolds, R. M., . . . Howard, L. M. (2020). Is there an increased risk of perinatal mental disorder in women with gestational diabetes? A systematic review and meta-analysis. *Diabetic Medicine: A Journal of the British Diabetic Association, 37*(4), 602–622. https://doi.org/10.1111/dme.14170

Wong, A. C., Rengers, B., Nowak, A. L., Schoeppner, S., Price, M., Zhang, L., . . . Giurgescu, C. (2020). Timing of prenatal care initiation and psychological wellbeing in Black women: MCN. *American Journal of Maternal Child Nursing, 45*(6), 344–350. https://doi.org/10.1097/NMC.0000000000000661

Woody, C. A., Ferrari, A. J., Siskind, D. J., Whiteford, H. A., & Harris, M. G. (2017). A systematic review and meta-regression of the prevalence and incidence of perinatal depression. *Journal of Affective Disorders, 219*, 86–92. https://doi.org/10.1016/j.jad.2017.05.003

World Health Organization. (2022, February). *6E20 mental or behavioural disorders associated with pregnancy, childbirth or the puerperium, without psychotic symptoms.* World Health Organization ICD-11 for Mortality and Morbidity Statistics. Retrieved July 11, 2022, from https://icd.who.int/browse11/l-m/en#/http://id.who.int/icd/entity/1124422593

Wright, J. H., Owen, J. J., Richards, D., Eells, T. D., Richardson, T., Brown, G. K., . . . Thase, M. E. (2019). Computer-assisted cognitive-behavior therapy for depression: A systematic review and meta-analysis. *Journal of Clinical Psychiatry, 80*(2), 18r12188. https://doi.org/10.4088/JCP.18r12188

Yasuma, N., Narita, Z., Sasaki, N., Obikane, E., Sekiya, J., Inagawa, T., . . . Nishi, D. (2020). Antenatal psychological intervention for universal prevention of antenatal and postnatal depression: A systematic review and meta-analysis. *Journal of Affective Disorders, 273*, 231–239. https://doi.org/10.1016/j.jad.2020.04.063

Yin, X., Sun, N., Jiang, N., Xu, X., Gan, Y., Zhang, J., . . . Gong, Y. (2021). Prevalence and associated factors of antenatal depression: Systematic reviews and meta-analyses. *Clinical Psychology Review, 83*, 101932. https://doi.org/10.1016/j.cpr.2020.101932

Yonkers, K. A., Blackwell, K. A., Glover, J., & Forray, A. (2014). Antidepressant use in pregnant and postpartum women. *Annual Review of Clinical Psychology, 10*, 369–392. https://doi.org/10.1146/annurev-clinpsy-032813-153626

Yonkers, K. A., Wisner, K. L., Stewart, D. E., Oberlander, T. F., Dell, D. L., Stotland, N., . . . Lockwood, C. (2009). The management of depression during pregnancy: A report from the American Psychiatric Association and the American College of Obstetricians and Gynecologists. *General Hospital Psychiatry, 31*(5), 403–413. https://doi.org/10.1016/j.genhosppsych.2009.04.003

8

PRENATAL ANXIETY

Pamela S. Wiegartz, Polina Teslyar, Kylie M. Steinhilber,
Natalie Feldman, Gali Hashmonay, and Leena Mittal

Pregnancy, along with dramatic biological and physical transformation, brings significant relationship and role changes, social and lifestyle adjustments, and associated environmental stressors. Some degree of anxiety during pregnancy is nearly universal, and these worries often do not
rise to the level of clinical diagnosis. For many women, however, this anxiety becomes highly
distressing, severe, or debilitating—it becomes an anxiety *disorder*. Despite anxiety disorders
during pregnancy being quite common, with some estimates nearing 15% (Dennis et al., 2017),
only in recent years has attention shifted to elevate anxiety alongside depression in the discussion of perinatal mental health. Although the research literature remains relatively sparse by
comparison, awareness is growing and, with it, our understanding of prenatal anxiety.

Anna is a 32-year-old cisgender Latina woman mid-way through the second trimester of her
first pregnancy. A lifelong worrier, her anxiety was manageable before but has been slowly
escalating over the course of her pregnancy. What was previously minor and periodic preoccupation with the health of family members, relationships, and work performance has shifted
to nearly constant fear that she will miscarry, that the baby will be born with a serious birth
defect, or that delivery will go awry and she or the baby (or both) will die. She often feels
tense and nervous and has difficulty falling asleep due to racing thoughts and "what if?"
scenarios running through her mind. In the waiting room, prior to her 20-week ultrasound,
Anna's anxiety became unbearable—with her heart racing, palms sweating, and stomach in
knots, she rushed outside and called her husband, who was parking the car, to come and pick
her up. Anna and her husband have been married for three years, but her relationship with
him has been strained over the past months—he doesn't understand her need for repeated
reassurance about the baby and her irritability when he doesn't answer her calls immediately
or is not convincing enough in his quelling of her worries. They moved across the country
together to pursue busy professional careers, but Anna is now in danger of losing her job
as she is missing deadlines, often feeling distracted and spending hours at her desk searching the Internet for pregnancy-related information, messaging questions to her obstetrician's
(OB's) office, and scrolling through pregnancy discussion boards. After some bleeding in her

DOI: 10.4324/9781003206903-11

first trimester, she stopped attending the exercise classes she once enjoyed and spent most evenings "taking it easy" to ensure she didn't do anything to harm the baby or threaten the pregnancy.

For women who develop significant anxiety during pregnancy, this can mean an escalation or shifting of pre-existing symptoms, as for Anna, whereas others may experience onset for the first time during pregnancy. In fact, this is a time of great vulnerability for the development of anxiety disorders due to myriad interactions between normal pregnancy-related changes and underlying genetic, biological, and psychological factors. Anxiety disorders in pregnancy can be difficult to characterize, as symptoms span from worry, to obsessive-compulsive, to panic attacks, to phobic fear of childbirth. Furthermore, authors have made a valid contrast between anxiety and *pregnancy-related anxiety* (PRA) (e.g., Brunton et al., 2019), making interpretation of the extant research literature even more complex. Synthesizing findings requires some acceptance of the imprecision in definition and measurement, with distinction when possible, to understand what we know and how much we have left to discover.

Prevalence and Salient Features

The true prevalence of prenatal anxiety has been difficult to assess due to its frequent comorbidity with depression, lack of studies that focus exclusively on pregnancy rather than the perinatal period, varied assessment timing and methodology (e.g., self-report vs. clinical interview), and lack of distinction between anxiety *symptoms* and anxiety *disorders*. Meta-analytic studies have calculated clinical diagnosis of an anxiety disorder during pregnancy at around 15% (Dennis et al., 2017) and the likelihood of at least one anxiety disorder during pregnancy *or* postpartum at 20.7%, with a trend toward greater prevalence in pregnancy (Fawcett et al., 2019). Rates of self-reported prenatal anxiety symptoms range from 18.2% to 24.6% across trimesters (Dennis et al., 2017). When examining only studies conducted during the COVID-19 pandemic, meta-analyses found 37% to 40% of pregnant women reporting anxiety symptoms across Asia, Europe, North America, and South America (Yan et al., 2020; Shorey et al., 2021), with rates of prenatal anxiety exceeding those of depression.

Generalized Anxiety Disorder

Perhaps the most common prenatal anxiety disorder, generalized anxiety disorder (GAD) was found to have an overall pooled prevalence rate of 2.0% across studies in a recent meta-analysis (Fawcett et al., 2019). However, rates based on DSM-IV-TR criteria have been reported as high as 10.5% in some samples (Adewuya et al., 2006) and as low as 1.7% in others (Usuda et al., 2016), illustrating the wide variability of findings. Of note, women in the first study were late in their pregnancies (>32 weeks), whereas the latter focused on gestational age of 12 to 24 weeks, pointing to problems in comparing results gathered in different trimesters, as well as when adhering strictly to time-based diagnostic criteria in a time-limited phenomenon like pregnancy. Studies suspending the time criterion of six months of excessive worry for GAD diagnosis, using instead the past month, in women in their second trimester have found rates similar to the Adewuya study at 11.0% (Matthey & Ross-Hamid, 2011).

Since Anna's long-standing worry never interfered with her functioning and relationships before, she would likely not have been diagnosed with an anxiety disorder previously. Now the primary content of her worries has shifted to focus on the pregnancy and outcomes, and, though her worries about relationships and family health remain, they are minor by comparison. Though her anxiety is now prominent, pervasive, and disruptive, her worries do not significantly encompass a range of life circumstances and she would not technically meet DSM time criteria for GAD, illustrating how difficult it can be to characterize prenatal anxiety.

As in Anna's case, worries during pregnancy tend to fall into a few broad categories: fears of labor and delivery, concerns about the baby's health or viability, concerns about parenting or motherhood, and the negative impact of having a baby on marriage, work, or social functioning. But, for pregnant women with GAD, these worries can span a number of life areas, including those unrelated to pregnancy (e.g., work performance or routine minor matters) and, because it is hard to control these thoughts, sleep is often disrupted and relaxation is difficult. Irritability, fatigue, and overthinking make it challenging to stay present in the moment and it can seem impossible to concentrate on tasks or make decisions.

Panic Disorder

Rates of panic disorder in pregnancy seem to reflect those of nonpregnant populations, with pooled averages of around 1.6% in meta-analytic studies (Fawcett et al., 2019). Marchesi et al. (2014) diagnosed 7.5% of pregnant women in their sample with panic disorder, whereas Sutter-Dallay et al. (2004) only 1.4%, identifying a much smaller cohort and, again, reflecting the wide discrepancies found in the literature. One explanation is the broad overlap between normal physical changes in pregnancy and DSM criteria for panic, such as shortness of breath, increased heart rate, nausea, and sweating. In fact, some researchers have found rates of panic drop when normal pregnancy-related physical symptoms are excluded from the diagnosis (Matthey & Ross-Hamid, 2011).

For instance, uncomfortable somatic sensations during pregnancy due to the crowding of the diaphragm by the growing baby and the adaptation of the respiratory system to allow large amounts of oxygen to be carried to the placenta can lead women to chronic hyperventilation. For some women, particularly those with somatic sensitivity, symptoms associated with hyperventilation may leave them vulnerable to the onset or worsening of pre-existing panic. When misinterpretations occur (e.g., "these sensations mean something is wrong with me/the baby") or avoidance begins (e.g., "it may be unsafe to stay home alone"), symptoms can quickly escalate to panic disorder.

Obsessive-Compulsive Disorder

Meta-analytic data estimate around 2% of pregnant women meet the criteria for obsessive-compulsive disorder (OCD) compared to around 1% in the general female population (Russell et al., 2013). Although some studies have found as many as 5.2% of their sample met OCD criteria (Adewuya et al, 2006), more recent reports fall closer to those pooled estimates at 2.9% (Fairbrother et al., 2021). Of note, the Fairbrother study found a steady increase in diagnostic rates through late pregnancy that peaked at approximately eight weeks after delivery, indicating the rising risk for the development of OCD in the third trimester and early postpartum period. During the COVID-19 pandemic, some studies found that a whopping 7% of pregnant participants self-reported clinically significant OC symptoms (Mahaffey et al., 2022).

Obsessions (recurrent unwanted thoughts and impulses) are the hallmark of OCD. Different from worry, obsessions are experienced as distressing and out of character. In an effort to decrease the anxiety or distress associated with obsessions, compulsions or rituals are typically performed. Compulsions can be repetitive behavior—as in repeatedly checking for evidence of environmental teratogens like lead paint—or mental acts, like repeating a certain phrase the "right" number of times to protect against an intrusive thought of stillbirth. Avoiding contact with all household cleaners and other chemicals, choosing only the safest of foods, repeatedly checking for fetal movement, or excessively researching and gathering information are common symptoms of prenatal OCD.

Though Anna's reassurance-seeking questions to her husband and repeated messages to her OB could be mistaken for compulsions, these types of behaviors are also commonly associated with worry. The differential between obsessions and worries can be similarly complex, though worry content tends to be about everyday situations, more realistic and probable, and more aligned with the person's character or values. Obsessions are experienced as intrusive or unexpected, tend to be less realistic or probable, and are ego-dystonic (inconsistent with one's personality, values, or beliefs). Anna's thoughts fall into the worry category.

Though more prominent in postpartum, pregnant women are also vulnerable to ego-dystonic thoughts of harm, particularly to the unborn baby—for instance, images or urges to throw oneself down the stairs or stab one's growing belly. Though researchers have found intrusive thoughts of harm to be exceedingly common in new moms (e.g., Fairbrother & Woody, 2008), they are frightening and easy to misinterpret, leaving women reluctant to disclose them for fear they will be considered "crazy" or that their baby or other children will be taken away. Direct questions and psychoeducation about the normative nature of intrusive thoughts can increase accurate identification and referral to treatment for women struggling with OCD.

Provider:	Can you tell me a little about the kinds of worries you're having?
Patient:	I feel anxious all the time and can't stop thinking about bad things happening. No matter how hard I try to push the thoughts away, I just keep thinking the worst.
Provider:	It sounds like these thoughts keep coming back even though you're trying not to think about them. Do the thoughts feel like they don't make sense to you?
Patient:	Yeah, they don't make any sense. It's like my brain is thinking the exact opposite of what I want it to, of things I would *never* do.
Provider:	That sounds frustrating, but you should know that *all* brains work that way. The more we try to *not* think about something, the more we tend to think about it.

> Do you ever need to do anything in response to these thoughts, like performing a behavior or repeating something in your head to "fix" things or lower your anxiety?
>
> *Patient:* Well, I have a prayer that I say whenever a bad thought comes in. But sometimes I can't get it just right and then have to start over and be sure to clasp my hands just the right way and make sure I'm not distracted and that I'm concentrating fully on the words.
>
> *Provider:* I know it may be difficult to tell me the thoughts that you are having, so I first want you to know that it's very common for women during pregnancy and postpartum to have intrusive thoughts that are very distressing—these can be thoughts of harming others, including your baby, or images of terrible outcomes, or even urges to do something that makes no sense. Because these thoughts are so scary and upsetting, it's easy to misinterpret their significance and fear that they mean something awful. But when we avoid these thoughts or keep them a secret, they tend to get worse, as you've noticed. Do you think you could tell me more about some of the thoughts you've been having?

Phobias and Trauma

Pooled prevalence rates for specific phobias have been noted at 6% during pregnancy (Viswasam et al., 2019), encompassing studies including all categories of phobic disorders. Specific fears of childbirth—like labor pain or health complications for self/baby—are common during pregnancy, but clinically significant childbirth phobias (i.e., tokophobia) account for a smaller subset of women at around 2% (e.g., Brockington et al., 2006). Untreated, these fears can put women at risk for traumatic delivery experiences and the development of posttraumatic stress disorder (PTSD). Estimates of PTSD during pregnancy vary greatly, ranging from 0% in some samples (Usuda et al., 2016) to 16% in others (Morland et al., 2007), with pool analyses estimating overall prevalence at 3% (Viswasam et al., 2019). Considering prior pregnancy loss may impact rates with some studies finding up to 12.5% of their pregnant subjects with a history of pregnancy complications (e.g., miscarriage, ectopic pregnancy, and termination) met the criteria for PTSD (Forray et al., 2009).

Pregnancy-Related Anxiety

Though not yet a DSM diagnosis, PRA is becoming increasingly acknowledged as a unique form of prenatal anxiety. Specific worries focusing on childbirth, the health of the baby, fear of loss, and appearance-related concerns are key features (Brunton et al., 2019; Bayrampour et al., 2016), falling into two distinct factors: concerns about the child's health and concerns about the birth (Blackmore et al., 2016). Several studies have distinguished PRA from general, trait or state anxiety, depression, and the DSM-diagnosed anxiety disorders described earlier (Blackmore et al., 2016; Anderson et al., 2019). Studies show that measures of PRA (i.e., *Pregnancy-Related Anxiety Questionnaire-Revised* [PRAQ-R]; Huizink et al., 2004a) and *Pregnancy-Related Anxiety Questionnaire-Revised* [PRAQ-R2]; Huizink et al., 2016) share little variance with general measures of anxiety and depression, supporting PRA as distinct (Anderson et al., 2019; Brunton et al., 2019) and raising the concern that the use of standard assessments may be underestimating true prevalence rates. Highlighted during the pandemic, reports of COVID-19-related stressors correlated with higher PRA (Moyer et al., 2020).

Anna's situation is a good example of the overlap and distinction between typical anxiety disorders and the presentation of pregnancy-related anxiety. Prior to pregnancy, Anna reported worry about a number of life areas, but it was not impairing. Currently, her anxiety symptoms are significantly distressing and interfering with her functioning but are quite focused on one arena: her pregnancy. She worries about having a miscarriage and doing something to harm the baby and that something will go wrong during delivery. She feels guilty that she is not enjoying the pregnancy more and fears that she will not be a good mother. She worries about the impact of the pregnancy on her marriage and how she will cope with her parents living so far away from their first grandchild. Often tense and unable to sleep, she is afraid that her anxiety will be damaging to her baby—she even worries about her worry and feels stuck in an endless loop of "what ifs?"

Risk Factors and Correlates

Many studies report on correlates of anxiety during pregnancy, though it is more complicated to determine whether these variables are *causal* in the development of prenatal anxiety. To our knowledge, large-scale prospective studies are not available to determine factors that exist *prior* to pregnancy and then follow subjects to predict the development of prenatal symptoms. Despite limitations, reviewing correlates and potential risk factors may be helpful, however, in identifying women with an increased likelihood of prenatal anxiety and the potential for adverse outcomes. These correlates span biopsychosocial domains—cutting across environmental, genetic/biological, and psychological realms—and can be broadly categorized into sociodemographic and health, pregnancy-related experiences, relationship and life stressors, and mental health history.

Sociodemographic Characteristic and Health Behaviors

In some studies, factors such as age (Chan et al., 2013), smoking (Soto-Balbuena et al., 2018; Chan et al., 2013), educational level (Nasreen et al., 2011; Chan et al., 2013), and body mass index (Holton et al., 2019) have been linked to prenatal anxiety with those who are younger, smoke, have less education, or are classified as obese more likely to report anxiety during pregnancy, though these findings are inconsistent (Furtado et al., 2018). Scholl et al. (2022), for example, found no differences in the prevalence of anxiety disorders between teen and adult samples, despite significant differences between the groups in education, socioeconomic status, and employment. Furthermore, it is difficult to disentangle health-related factors, for instance, smoking or obesity, from their impact on pregnancy complications like gestational diabetes and preeclampsia (Stubert et al., 2018), which more consistently correlate with prenatal anxiety.

Pregnancy-Related Experiences and Complications

Medical and pregnancy complications do appear to increase women's risk for prenatal anxiety (Bayrampour et al., 2018; Biaggi et al., 2016). Compared to those with low-risk pregnancies, the incidence of anxiety disorders during pregnancy was over five times higher in those classified with high-risk pregnancies (Fairbrother et al., 2017). History of miscarriage or conception after in vitro fertilization is also associated with anxiety and worry (Gourounti et al., 2013). Interestingly, although lower educational attainment or unwanted/unplanned pregnancy have been linked to prenatal anxiety in some studies (e.g., Chan et al., 2013), despite the complex interplay of these variables in engagement with or access to prenatal care, medical risk and history seem to predict anxiety above and beyond those factors (e.g., Gourounti et al., 2013; Fairbrother et al., 2017).

Relationships, Social Support, and Stress

History of childhood abuse (Bayrampour et al., 2018), trauma (Martini et al., 2015), and intimate partner violence (Insan et al., 2022) have been associated with increased prenatal anxiety. Additionally, low marital or partner satisfaction (Chan et al., 2013; Martini et al., 2015), having a partner who struggles with alcoholism or drug addiction (Soto-Balbuena et al., 2018), and perceived lack of social support (Chan et al., 2013; Martini et al., 2015; Soto-Balbuena et al., 2018) have been linked to anxiety during pregnancy, with some studies showing a sevenfold increase in anxiety for pregnant women with low affectionate support or low positive social interaction (Bedaso et al., 2021). For women pregnant during the COVID-19 pandemic, perceived social support was lower (Goyal et al., 2022), and a third reported increased stress and relationship conflict, with increases in PRA related to COVID-19 stressors (Moyer et al., 2020).

Mental Health and Psychological Vulnerabilities

A history of mental health problems has been associated with increased prenatal anxiety (Bayrampour et al., 2018; Biaggi et al., 2016). In fact, a history of anxiety or depression is one of the strongest predictors of anxiety during pregnancy (e.g., Martini et al., 2015). As in the general population, family history of OCD is much higher in pregnant women with OCD (Uguz et al., 2007), suggesting a potential genetic predisposition. Preliminary findings exist that biomarker models associated with epigenetic variation in gonadal hormone sensitivity were able to predict OCD symptoms during pregnancy (Kaminsky et al., 2020), suggesting a link between genetic and biological risk factors for prenatal anxiety. On the nurture side, childhood experience with a maternal parenting style low in affection and high in control represents an environmental contribution leading to a sixfold greater likelihood of prenatal anxiety (Grant et al., 2012). Parental self-efficacy may further predict PRA in expectant mothers (Brunton et al., 2020).

The psychological variables that underlie anxiety disorders in the general population may also play a role in the development of prenatal anxiety (Wenzel, 2011). For instance, *intolerance of uncertainty* (i.e., a dispositional characteristic that results from a set of negative beliefs about uncertainty and its implications) has been associated with worry (Buhr et al., 2009). In a perinatal, predominantly pregnant, sample, intolerance of uncertainty was associated with increased depression and anxiety (Sbrilli et al., 2021) and has been linked to separation anxiety in pregnancy as well (Degirmenci et al., 2020). Models for perinatal OCD suggest an important role for *overestimation of responsibility* in the development and maintenance of obsessive-compulsive symptoms. In fact, studies have supported the predictive validity of heightened baby-related responsibility beliefs (Barrett et al., 2016) and both prenatal experiential avoidance and misinterpretation of intrusive thoughts in obsessive-compulsive symptoms postpartum (Ojalehto et al., 2021). Finally, *anxiety sensitivity*, or the fear of anxiety-related sensations arising from beliefs that these sensations have harmful somatic, psychological, or social consequences, has been associated with panic and agoraphobic avoidance in general populations (Taylor, 1995) and women who are sensitive to somatic sensations may be more vulnerable to prenatal anxiety. In fact, scores on anxiety sensitivity (physical concerns factor) have been found to predict elevated fears of childbirth in pregnant women (Spice et al., 2009; Jokić-Begić et al., 2014) and are correlated with the amplification of somatosensory symptoms (Koc et al., 2021).

Reduced social support, stress at work, and conflict with her husband may, in part, have contributed to Anna's risk for anxiety during pregnancy. In a new city, away from her support system, she is relying more heavily on her husband, adding to marital tension. Her worries about "overdoing" it and harming the baby keep her home most nights, so she is no longer connecting with coworkers or friends from the gym. Anna's behavioral avoidance of the situations and activities that make her anxious may have further put her at risk by eliminating her typical coping strategies. A high achiever with a demanding career, Anna is unaccustomed to not "having the answers." This pregnancy feels out of her control, and it bothers her to not know exactly how things are developing and how it will turn out. Her discomfort with the unknown, or intolerance of uncertainty, has her seeking information and reassurance and striving for guaranteed pregnancy outcomes, inadvertently resulting in even higher anxiety.

Impact of Prenatal Anxiety

Research suggests that the impact of heightened anxiety during pregnancy may be associated with negative effects on maternal, obstetric, and infant/child outcomes. From a biological perspective, prenatal anxiety has been shown to increase cortisol levels during pregnancy, as well as pro-inflammatory cytokines (Field, 2017). Cortisol levels have been found to be increased in highly anxious pregnant women (Leff-Gelman et al., 2020). Stress hormones, such as cortisol, are transmitted across the placenta and into the fetal bloodstream, and this has been shown to impact the fetus in terms of fetal heart rate and movement (Van den Bergh, 1992). One hypothesis suggests that an increase in maternal catecholamines related to stress decreases blood flow to the fetus and therefore limits oxygen and nutrients (Lobel et al., 1992). During sensitive periods of development, these changes in the uterine environment may underlie the impacts of prenatal anxiety by causing lasting changes in infant brain structure and function, including to the hypothalamic–pituitary–adrenal axis (e.g., Glover et al., 2010).

However, it is also difficult to separate the role of environment from biology when considering impact because anxiety in pregnancy is associated with anxiety postpartum (Heron et al., 2004), as well as a threefold increase in postpartum depression (Sutter-Dallay et al., 2004). The resultant impact of maternal mental health on attachment and caregiving may also contribute to neonatal and childhood outcomes. Biological, psychological, and environmental factors likely interact to result in the relatively consistent findings that prenatal anxiety increases risk for obstetrical complications, poorer postpartum maternal mental health, disrupted mother–child attachment, and longer-term emotional and behavioral impairment for children.

Pregnancy and Obstetric Outcomes

Prenatal anxiety has been associated with an increased risk of preeclampsia (Kurki et al., 2000) as well as adverse perinatal outcomes such as preterm birth and lower birth weight (Grigoriadis et al., 2018; Lilliecreutz et al., 2011; Orr et al., 2007), though here again results are inconsistent (Littleton et al., 2007; Grigoriadis et al., 2018). Higher anxiety during pregnancy has also been associated with lower Apgar scores in some studies (Berle et al., 2005). Recent work has distinguished general prenatal anxiety and worry from specific PRA (e.g., Huizink et al., 2004b; Brunton et al., 2019), with some finding that the latter significantly predicted birth weight and gestational age, independent of general measures (Blackmore et al., 2016).

Infant and Child Outcomes

Prenatal anxiety not only impacts the pregnancy itself—maternal anxiety experienced during this period has been shown to have long-term deleterious effects on infant and child development. Although, again, it is difficult to separate the effects of prenatal anxiety from postpartum maternal mental health on child development, infant studies report that prenatal anxiety predicts distress to novelty and limitations, lower attention span, lessened positive affect, and more difficulty soothing at three months (Coplan et al., 2005). Heightened behavioral reactivity has been found in four-month-old infants of mothers with anxiety and depression during pregnancy (Davis et al., 2004) and twofold odds of "difficult" temperament at four to six months (Austin et al., 2005). Predictors of infant temperament and development may differ when considering general prenatal anxiety versus pregnancy-specific anxiety. Some studies have found that pregnancy-specific anxiety predicted higher levels of infant activity, fearfulness, and sadness while general prenatal anxiety was associated with infant distress to limitations at six months (Henrichs et al., 2009), suggesting similar, yet distinct, constructs and impacts. Relatedly, pregnancy-specific anxiety, not general distress, was found to predict lower infant development scores at 12 months (Davis & Sandman, 2010). PRA in particular, apart from depression or state anxiety, contributes to issues with inhibitory control in females (Buss et al., 2010), a common symptom of attention-deficit hyperactivity disorder (ADHD). In children aged 8 to 9 years, maternal prenatal anxiety during weeks 12 to 22 gestation (though not during weeks 32 to 40) was an independent predictor of ADHD and self-reported anxiety (Van den Bergh & Marcoen, 2004). Adolescents with prenatal exposure to maternal anxiety during the same gestational period showed flattened cortisol response and associated depressive symptoms in females (Ven den Bergh et al., 2008).

Attachment and Relationships

With prenatal anxiety associated with postpartum anxiety and depression, this means that both directly and via impact on postpartum mental health anxiety during pregnancy may result in disruption in attachment, caregiving, and relationships. Higher levels of prenatal anxiety have been related to less optimal maternal–fetal attachment and more negative attitudes toward motherhood, as well as a negative view of self as a mother (Hart & McMahon, 2006). More recently, COVID-19 anxiety has shown a negative correlation with prenatal attachment as well (Karaca et al., 2022). This has significant implications as prenatal attachment between mother and unborn baby is a good predictor of the early mother–infant relationship and mothers with higher prenatal attachment show more involvement with and more effective means of stimulating their babies during those interactions (Siddiqui & Hägglöf, 2000).

In fact, elevated prenatal anxiety may lead to mothers showing more unpredictability in maternal care, leading to inconsistent sensory signals in caregiving and less secure attachment postpartum (Holmberg et al., 2020). Of note, these unpredictable caregiving signals have been associated with poorer cognitive functioning in children (Davis et al., 2017), as well as poorer executive functioning as measured by effortful control tasks (Davis et al.,

2019), perhaps combining with the biological effects of prenatal anxiety to explain infant and childhood outcomes (Davis et al., 2017, 2019; Parfitt et al., 2013). Prenatal mental health, particularly anxiety, has been associated with postpartum parenting to an even greater extent than postpartum mental health in some studies (Parfitt et al., 2013), correlating with negative parenting behaviors such as maternal intrusiveness (Hakanen et al., 2019). Notably, some researchers have found prenatal anxiety disorders to be associated with higher *perceived* bonding impairment, not with observed mother–infant interaction quality (Nath et al., 2019). This introduces the possibility that anxiety may play a role in mothers' experience of connection and competence, distinct from actual parenting quality, and underscores the importance of psychoeducation and effective intervention during pregnancy.

Perceptions of support and relationship satisfaction may also be influenced by anxiety. Compared to women without anxiety and depressive disorders prior to pregnancy, women with comorbid anxiety and depressive disorders reported less perceived support during pregnancy and postpartum, lower satisfaction, and overall partnership quality as well as decreases in communication and increases in quarreling from pre- to postpartum (Asselmann et al., 2016).

From a clinical perspective, supporting an individual who is experiencing anxiety during pregnancy can often be an experience of helplessness for the family. Watching their pregnant partner struggle can lead to frustration or anxiety when feeling there is little that they can do. At other times, partners may inadvertently exacerbate symptoms of anxiety by participating in reassurance-seeking, checking, and other worry behaviors or compulsions. In attempts to assuage their pregnant partner's fears, the assurances provided or behavioral accommodations made may actually contribute to the maintenance and escalation of anxiety via negative reinforcement and feedback loops.

In Anna's case, her husband has become frustrated with her repeated phone calls and questions. No matter how many times he reassures her that the baby will be fine, it does not seem to make her any less anxious. As a result, he admits that he sometimes lets her calls go straight to voicemail, especially if he is busy at work. Anna shares that her anxiety rises sharply when she is not able to reach him. She begins to worry that something bad might have happened to him, leaving her to raise a baby on her own without her primary support, alone in an unfamiliar city. So she calls and texts repeatedly, or contacts his administrative assistant to find out where he is. This anxious loop continues until she reaches him and gets reassurance from him that addresses her latest worry. She feels relieved for the moment, making it more likely that she will pursue the same path in the future—despite the negative impact on her marriage.

Screening and Assessment

While a previous study found only 20% of obstetrics-gynecology physicians screen for anxiety during pregnancy (Coleman et al., 2008), strides have since been made in recognizing the importance of detecting prenatal anxiety. Both the U.K. National Institute for Health and Care Excellence and the American College of Obstetricians and Gynecologists (ACOG) have now recommended screening for anxiety in pregnancy and postpartum (NICE, 2014; Committee on Obstetric Practice, 2018), and the Women's Preventive

Services Initiative (WPSI) suggests screening for anxiety in *all* women aged 13 and over, including pregnant and postpartum women (Women's Preventive Services Initiative [WPSI], 2018; www.womenspreventivehealth.org). Awareness is growing that early recognition is key in improving outcomes, though the question remains of how to best identify prenatal anxiety and incorporate screening into standard prenatal care.

Screening Measures

The most commonly used screening tools are anxiety scales validated in the general population, for instance, the Generalized Anxiety Disorder-7 (GAD-7; Spitzer et al., 2006; Löwe et al., 2008) or *State-Trait Anxiety Inventory* (STAI; Spielberger et al., 1970). However, these may not be ideal for assessing prenatal anxiety in part due to the tendency to focus on physiological symptoms of anxiety or more general worry. Questions that ask about physical symptoms of anxiety may be confounded by common symptoms of pregnancy (such as shortness of breath, palpitations, or sleep disturbance), resulting in artificially inflated scores. Worries frequently seen during pregnancy (such as specific pregnancy-related concerns about outcomes or motherhood), or other prominent prenatal symptom presentations like OCD, may not be captured well by these general anxiety questionnaires, leading to under-recognition. Few studies have evaluated anxiety scales in perinatal populations, fewer still have validated measures against a "gold standard" reference like diagnostic interviews in pregnant populations alone (Sinesi et al., 2019). For instance, the Sinesi et al. (2019) review identified only one methodologically sound study (Zhong et al., 2015) examining the psychometric properties of the GAD-7 in a pregnant population, and there a cutoff score of seven (rather than the general population cutoff of ten) yielded moderately good sensitivity/specificity.

In the perinatal period, the *Edinburgh Postnatal Depression Scale* (EPDS) is a frequently used screener (Cox et al., 1987). Although originally developed to detect postpartum depression, a subscale of the EPDS can be used to screen for anxiety as well (Matthey, 2007). Three items comprise this anxiety subscale (EPDS-3A; items 3, 4, and 5) and relate to self-blame, worry, and feelings of fear/panic. When used to identify pregnant women with a DSM-diagnosed anxiety disorder, the EPDS-3A outperformed both a general screening tool (*Hospital Anxiety and Depression Scale*, anxiety subscale—HADS-A) and pregnancy-specific scale (PRAQ-R) in one study (Matthey et al., 2013). Similarly, in a group of pregnant women in the third trimester, researchers noted empirical support for the screening use of the EPDS-3A (not the GAD-7), though the diagnostic reference standard used here was also a self-report measure (Austin et al., 2022). Other authors, however, have found *both* the EPDS-3A and the GAD-7 lacking, finding neither correctly classified postpartum women (when compared to diagnostic interview) with enough accuracy to be a clinically useful screening measure (Fairbrother et al., 2019).

Measures like the *Cambridge Worry Scale* (Green et al., 2003), PRAQ-R2 (Huizink et al., 2016), and *Wijma Delivery Expectancy/Experience Questionnaire* (W-DEQ; Wijma et al., 1998) represent efforts to capture important symptoms unique to pregnancy. While helpful in identifying PRA, in contrast to more general measures using these as screeners may overlook women with symptoms that do *not* directly relate to pregnancy or motherhood. To effectively screen, scales must be broad enough to capture a wide range of symptoms but also sensitive to how anxiety presents during the perinatal period.

One promising option is the *Perinatal Anxiety Screening Scale* (PASS; Somerville et al., 2014), created specifically to screen for a broad range of anxiety symptoms during pregnancy and postpartum. Four categories of anxiety are addressed by the PASS, including (a) acute anxiety and adjustment; (b) general worry and specific fears; (c) perfectionism, control, and trauma; and (d) social anxiety. As a screening tool, the PASS was found to identify 68% of perinatal women with a diagnosed anxiety disorder (compared to EPDS-3A which detected only 36%) (Somerville et al., 2014). The severity of perinatal anxiety symptoms can also be measured by the PASS, using established cutoffs for minimal, mild-moderate, and severe anxiety (Somerville et al., 2015), adding utility in triaging more urgent cases for referral to care. Studies comparing the PASS to the PRAQ-R2 again found support for PRA as a distinct construct (with the PRAQ-R2 sharing little variance with general measures of anxiety and depression) and concluded that the PASS may be better suited for comprehensive screening for prenatal anxiety disorders but, given its overlap with other measures of anxiety, potentially less useful (than the PRAQ-R2) in assessing the specific construct of PRA (Anderson et al., 2019).

In fact, it is interesting that Anna's symptoms may have been easily overlooked by EPDS 3A questions due to the qualifying wording of both the worry and panic questions ("for no good reason"). Anna believes that there is plenty of "good reason" for her anxiety, as the health of her baby is the utmost priority. The PRAQ-R2 would likely pick up her worry about delivery and the health of her baby but miss any general worries, as well as the repetitive behaviors, avoidance, and disruption in functioning captured by the PASS.

Clinically, in addition to formal screening, providers may take note of both verbal and nonverbal signs of anxiety present either at or between appointments. For instance, frequent calls or messages from patients—particularly with repetition of questions or reassurance-seeking around catastrophic "what if?" scenarios—may indicate the presence of OCD or generalized anxiety. Restlessness and physical arousal, or even avoidance of appointments altogether, may be signs of anxiety, panic, or prior trauma. Although self-report screening measures can provide the opportunity for women to express their concerns, there is often a reluctance to disclose symptoms due to fears of negative evaluation by providers or misperceptions of the meaning of symptoms and/or the consequences of disclosure. An open dialogue helps to decrease mental health stigma and establish trust, encouraging women to share concerns.

Provider: I noticed that you've been messaging with questions about some of the physical symptoms you've been experiencing. Do you have any concerns today that I can help with?

Patient: I don't know. I just don't feel like myself. It feels like something bad is going to happen at any moment.

Provider: Do you have any physical symptoms when you feel like that? Like shortness of breath, nausea, or dizziness or chest tightness?

Patient: No, but I feel my heart racing and get sweaty.

Provider: Anything else?

Patient: Well . . . I feel weird, like I'm watching things happening but I'm not really there. And I get restless, like I want to jump out of my skin. I can hardly stand it.

Provider:	Would it reassure you to know that many women feel this way during pregnancy? There are a lot of physical and hormonal changes happening for you and, combined with managing the stress and worry of this new experience, it can lead to some really uncomfortable sensations.
Patient:	Really? I've never felt like this before. I was afraid to tell you, of what you'd think of me. I was really worried I was losing my mind.

Of note, despite the high prevalence of prenatal anxiety, attributing symptoms to anxiety without ruling out underlying medical explanations can have grave consequences. In one large study, mistaking medical conditions for anxiety was the most common misdiagnosis in cases of pregnancy-related deaths from cardiovascular disease (VanOtterloo et al., 2019). Furthermore, when clinically significant anxiety has been established, detection is only the first step on a long road to accessing care. Extrapolating from prenatal depression screening and treatment studies, we know that screening rates often do not reflect rates of referral to treatment or receipt of adequate treatment (Cox et al., 2016). Making women aware of effective, evidence-based treatments available for anxiety, referring them for care, and working to remove obstacles to engagement are all crucial to improving outcomes.

Treatment

Broadly, the treatment of prenatal anxiety disorders follows that of anxiety disorders in the general population, and clinical support can be found for both pharmacological and psychological interventions. However, there is extensive discussion around the use of medication in pregnancy, and conflicting opinions/reports can contribute to decisional conflict for women in need of care. This conflict can lead not only to emotional distress but also to delayed or ineffective treatment decisions. For instance, among pregnant women considering antidepressant use, difficulties weighing maternal versus infant health, lack of high-quality information, negative external influences, and emotional factors have been found to contribute to challenges with decision-making (Walton et al., 2014). Interpersonal support and accessible subspecialty care can positively impact care decisions; however, many do not have access to specialized women's mental health services. Ultimately, treatment decisions are multifactorial and based on both available data and personal preference, with consideration of factors like symptom severity, comorbid conditions, mental health history, and previous treatment response.

Psychological Treatments

For mild to moderate symptoms, there is strong evidence for the use of psychological treatments in anxiety disorders. Furthermore, given the reluctance of many women to engage in pharmacological treatment during pregnancy, psychotherapy represents an important and effective option for care. The two most studied therapies in perinatal patients include cognitive behavioral therapy (CBT) and interpersonal psychotherapy (IPT). Although there are a limited number of high-quality, randomized controlled trials (and studies often tend to include both pregnant and postpartum women or women with anxiety *and* depression), we can draw some conclusions regarding effectiveness in prenatal anxiety.

Cognitive Behavioral Therapy

CBT is widely considered a first-line treatment for anxiety disorders in the general population and an effective treatment for anxiety in pregnant women (USPSTF, 2019). CBT is a short-term, skills-based approach focusing on the association between thoughts, feelings, and behaviors. In CBT, patients learn to identify and modify distorted thinking, like catastrophizing, leading to better management of anxiety, as well as to break feedback loops caused by problematic behaviors, such as avoidance. Psychoeducation is often included in CBT protocols, which may prove particularly important in addressing stigma and misperceptions of anxiety symptoms during this time period. Although large-scale prospective studies remain lacking, CBT has been shown to benefit prenatal anxiety. For instance, in pregnant women diagnosed with GAD who received CBT consisting of psychoeducation, relaxation strategies, and cognitive therapy, significant reductions were found in *Hamilton Rating Scale for Anxiety Scores* (HAM-A; Hamilton, 1959) from baseline to the eighth week of treatment (15.12(6.03) to 6.96(2.75)), with 60.9% of the patients treated with CBT showing at least a 50% reduction in HAM-A scores (Uguz & Ak, 2021).

For anxiety disorders in the general population, CBT often includes an exposure therapy component essential in addressing fear and avoidance. Large-scale RCTs directly examining the use of exposure-based treatment for anxiety during pregnancy are lacking, perhaps due to concerns for adverse impact on the fetus. Acceptability studies, however, show that both pregnant and nonpregnant women report a preference for exposure-based CBT over pharmacologic treatment (Arch, 2014). Moreover, at least one exposure-based group treatment study of blood-injury-injection phobia during pregnancy reported no adverse events, no patient attrition, and significant reductions in phobic anxiety from pre- to post-treatment, with gains maintained postpartum (Lilliecreutz et al., 2010). More research is needed to define effects of exposure-based treatment in this group, but some have suggested that potential risks are unlikely, particularly when weighed against the impact of untreated anxiety disorders (Arch et al., 2012). Arch et al. also provide recommendations for the use of exposure in clinical practice that include use of heart rate-based guidelines to gauge safe parameters during exposure work and potential modifications to maximize tolerability in pregnant patients, particularly with interoceptive exposures.

In clinical practice, CBT is often delivered in a group format for prenatal anxiety and may include at least discussion of exposure-based elements, like behavioral experiments. Cognitive behavioral group therapy (CBGT) studies in perinatal populations have shown promising results in reduction of anxiety and worry compared to waitlist controls. For instance, Green et al. (2020) found perinatal women (pregnant n = 16, postpartum n = 28) completing CBGT reported significantly greater reductions in anxiety on the *State-Trait Inventory* for Cognitive and Somatic Anxiety, Trait version (STICSA; Grös et al., 2007) at six weeks post-baseline, as well as significantly lower anxiety symptoms on that measure compared to waitlist participants (48.60 [12.03] to 41.59 [10.94] vs. 46.21 [9.08] to 47.19 [10.76]). In this study, clinician-rated anxiety (HAM-A scores) also reflected a significantly greater reduction in anxiety symptoms in the CBGT group relative to waitlist (16.18 [7.47] to 11.31 [6.12] vs. 16.90 [6.58] to 16.48 [7.11]). With recent modifications to CBGT protocols addressing COVID-19-related anxiety by targeting intolerance of uncertainty in pregnant women, statistically significant reductions in GAD symptoms from pre- to post-CBGT treatment (as measured by GAD-7 scores; 11.64 [4.89] to 4.29 [5.01]) have also been found (Green et al., 2022).

Studies of mindfulness-based cognitive therapy groups for pregnant women similarly found statistically and clinically significant improvements in worry (as measured by the *Penn State Worry Questionnaire* [PSWQ]; Meyer et al., 1990) in 69.6% (16/23) of women who completed the treatment, with 93.8% (15/16) women who met diagnostic criteria for GAD at baseline no longer meeting criteria post-intervention (Goodman et al., 2014). More recently, brief mindfulness-based interventions delivered electronically (eMBI) to women with high-risk pregnancies, showed statistically significant reductions in general anxiety (as measured by STAI state scores) after completing the 1-week course of mindfulness. Participants with higher engagement with the app also had significantly lower PRAQ-R scores (18.74 [4.49] vs. 22.54 [6.90]), reflecting lower specific PRA (Goetz et al., 2020).

CBT may serve a preventive role for women at risk for prenatal anxiety or with vulnerabilities to the development or exacerbation of perinatal anxiety. For instance, reductions in anxiety in women screening positive for fetal chromosomal disorders have been found with a brief CBT intervention. In this randomized controlled trial, following four sessions of individual CBT, pregnant women showed a statistically significant decrease in STAI state scores from baseline (63.63 [6.13] vs. 40.2 [11.05]) and significant differences between intervention and control groups (partial eta square .63) (Bayat et al., 2021). Timpano et al. (2011) found in a prospective, randomized controlled trial that six weeks of a cognitive behavioral prevention program for pregnant participants identified as vulnerable to OCD (based on high scores on the *Obsessive Beliefs Questionnaire* [OBQ]; OCCWG, 2005) resulted in significantly lower levels of obsessive-compulsive symptoms (measured by the *Yale-Brown Obsessive-Compulsive Scale* [Y-BOCS]; Goodman et al., 1989a, 1989b) postpartum than a credible childbirth education program control. This held true at one month, three months, and six months postpartum (d = .41, d = .68, d = .73, respectively) after controlling for baseline symptoms. Similarly, in pregnant women with high levels of perfectionism (measured by the *Frost Multidimensional Perfectionism Scale*; Frost et al., 1990), a guided CBT self-help intervention over four weeks in the third trimester showed significant reductions in perfectionism post-treatment compared to waitlist controls (d = .59). An indirect effect of the intervention via changes in perfectionism also accounted for noted improvements in anxiety (measured by the EPDS-3A) in this study (Lowndes et al., 2019).

Interpersonal Psychotherapy

IPT is a time-limited psychotherapy initially developed to treat depression (Klerman et al., 1984). In IPT, the clinician and patient work together to identify issues in relationships and improve interpersonal functioning. This therapy may be well-suited for the perinatal population with its focus on the interpersonal context in which symptoms develop, given that problems such as low social support and emotional disconnect in relationships are strongly associated with symptoms of anxiety in this population (Pilkington et al., 2015). Because pregnancy and motherhood present challenging role transitions, the goals of IPT align well with likely problem areas. Most research on IPT has centered on depression, with some studies finding significantly reduced depressive symptoms on the EPDS in pregnant women following IPT, compared to a parenting education control group (Spinelli & Endicott, 2003). Recent meta-analyses have reported a significant reduction in symptoms of anxiety as well among depressed participants receiving IPT and moderate effect sizes (Hedge's g = .60) (Sockol, 2018).

For Anna, one could make the case for IPT given the relationship strife in her marriage. However, given the role of her anxiety and worry behaviors in contributing to marital tension and the effectiveness of CBT in addressing both cognitive and behavioral symptoms, it makes sense to start there. Cognitive behavioral treatment for Anna would likely focus on improving awareness of thoughts that are leading to anxiety and identifying any ways in which these thoughts might be distorted or erroneous. Learning strategies to step back from these thoughts and evaluate them more accurately, as well as recognizing the aspects that are unknowable or uncontrollable, would likely improve Anna's ability to sit with the discomfort of uncertainty. Addressing her reassurance and checking behaviors that feel helpful at the moment but ultimately serve to maintain and reinforce fears would be critical. Staying off Internet discussion boards, restricting information flow to one trusted resource, and limiting nonurgent phone calls and messages to her OB may help to break the established anxiety cycle. Including her husband in some sessions would be helpful in developing a plan for alternative ways to respond to Anna's reassurance-seeking and bolster good communication.

Pharmacological Management

For moderate to severe anxiety, pharmacological therapies may be indicated and are first-line treatment for severe, persistent, or relapsing anxiety disorders. Although there are no medications with a specific indication for treatment during pregnancy and lactation, there is a large evidence base for the use of these medications among pregnant and lactating individuals. The most commonly prescribed medications for the management of anxiety in the perinatal period are the selective serotonin reuptake inhibitors/serotonin-norepinephrine reuptake inhibitors (SSRI/SNRIs), as they have demonstrated a wide evidence base for use in pregnancy. Tricyclic antidepressants are effective as well but often carry higher side effect burden than SSRIs (Misri & Kendrick, 2007). Monoamine oxidase inhibitors are generally avoided in pregnant individuals as they are associated with fetal growth restriction (Briggs et al., 2012). Generally, pharmacotherapy for anxiety is divided into prevention (SSRI/SNRI, buspirone) and anxiolysis (benzodiazepines [BZDs] and antihistamines) (Shyken et al., 2019). Anxiolytics are very effective at stopping anxiety symptoms; however, they should not be used as monotherapy as they do not prevent the development of anxiety symptoms and carry risks of sedation, intoxication, dependence, and/or overdose (Shyken et al., 2019).

SSRIs have been widely used to manage mood and anxiety disorders, including in pregnancy, since the 1980s. A review of safety literature often gives conflicting outcomes, highlighting the difficulty in studying this patient population. There are no available randomized controlled trials of pregnant patients taking SSRIs, and all studies must control for confounding variables, such as the illness under treatment (e.g., anxiety) and its effects. Large meta-analytic studies of SSRI use in pregnancy did not find an increased risk of major or minor malformations or cardiovascular malformations with first-trimester exposure—they did, however, note an increased risk of early spontaneous abortion (Rahimi et al., 2006). Studies evaluating the neurocognitive development of infants exposed to SSRI in utero have found no difference in IQ, language, or behavioral development (Nulman et al., 1997). Neonatal adaptation syndrome (NAS) is reported in about 30% of neonates exposed to SSRI in utero, whereas the syndrome is reported to occur in 6–9% of neonates with no exposure, and additionally NAS is associated with the severity of maternal illness (Levison-Castiel et al., 2006; Oberlander et al., 2004; Misri et al., 2004). In some studies, there is a small increased risk of persistent pulmonary hypertension of the newborn with exposure to SSRI in the later half of pregnancy (Chambers et al., 1996). The choice of medication should be primarily driven by the patient's history, with the preference for the use of medication that has been shown to be effective in the past. If no prior history is available, sertraline is usually the first-line agent given its low levels of transmission across the placental barrier and into breastmilk. Paroxetine has been found to be associated with a higher risk of malformations (in particular increased risk of ventricular septal defects) and is generally not recommended for use in pregnancy (GlaxoSmithKline, 2005).

SNRIs, which include venlafaxine, duloxetine, and desvenlafaxine, have fewer studies on their safety in pregnancy. Research that does exist reflects data in line with the SSRIs and appears reassuring (Einarson et al., 2001). Although data are limited, there also does not appear to be an increased risk of malformations with mirtazapine and trazodone, which are often used to help with insomnia during pregnancy (Kesim et al., 2002; Einarson et al., 2003) or with buspirone, which carries FDA indication for the management of generalized anxiety (Shyken et al., 2019; Thorsness et al., 2018).

BZDs are anxiolytic medications that work via their gamma-aminobutyric acid type A (GABA-A) receptor binding properties. Short-term effects include a feeling of relaxation, lethargy, sedation, and fatigue. Higher doses can lead to temporary confusion, dizziness, vertigo, suppressed respiration, or euphoria. BZDs can contribute to falls, and long-term use can lead to physiological and behavioral dependence, amnesia, low mood, memory loss, cognitive impairments, and tolerance (Shyken et al., 2019). BZDs are very effective for the management of anxiety in the short term as their short onset of action brings rapid relief compared to SSRIs, which can take weeks to take full effect. However, daily use can lead to tolerance, loss of efficacy, and dependence, as well as risk for life-threatening seizures and withdrawal. Thus, this class of medications should be reserved only for short treatment courses or for rare use, such as when managing specific phobia or panic disorder.

If BZDs are prescribed in pregnancy, lorazepam, temazepam, and oxazepam are preferred due to their hepatic metabolism to inactive metabolites (Shyken et al., 2019). Although some early studies raised concern that prenatal BZD use may increase the risk of facial cleft and skeletal anomalies in animals (Miller & Becker, 1975), subsequent prospective studies in humans failed to show increased risk of malformations after BZD use (Addis et al., 2000). There does appear to be an association between BZD use and preterm delivery; however, this is also true for anxiety disorders (Shyken et al., 2019). The use of BZD at the end of pregnancy has been consistently found to be a risk factor for admission to neonatal intensive care, as the use at near delivery is associated with decreased neonatal muscle tone, poor feeding, drowsiness, delayed feeding, and poor respiration (Shyken et al., 2019), and studies are insufficient to evaluate development beyond the newborn period. Abrupt discontinuation of BZDs can lead to dangerous withdrawal, but successful tapering can be done during pregnancy without major maternal or neonatal side effects by using a slow taper on a long-acting agent (Shyken et al., 2019).

Treatment Decisions in Prenatal Anxiety

Weighing the risks and benefits of treatment versus the impact of untreated anxiety can be difficult for women during pregnancy. Choices are further complicated by the availability of treatment options and access to specialty care. Promising efforts are underway to develop patient decision aids that reduce decisional conflict and assist in clarifying these complex options in pregnancy (Hussain-Shamsy et al., 2022; Vigod et al., 2019), preventing delayed or declined treatment. When direct expert care is unavailable to provide thoughtful discussion of the pros and cons of available treatment options and risks of ongoing anxiety, consultative services from trained women's mental health psychiatrists are available to help frontline providers identify and address concerns, as well as for women to access resources and support (e.g., Postpartum Support International; www.postpartum.net).

Cultural Considerations

Anxiety during pregnancy is a ubiquitous phenomenon, but presentation may be less universal when taking into account racial, ethnic, and cultural factors—and this has important implications for how we should best screen, assess, and treat prenatal anxiety. Stigma and psychosocial stressors, as well as cultural influences, may prevent access to care or reduce treatment-seeking behaviors for many women from marginalized groups. Though we know decreased access to resources, racism, trauma, and cultural barriers can impede appropriate mental healthcare for pregnant women from minoritized racial or ethnic groups, data on how to best address these variables remain sparse in the literature on prenatal anxiety.

Large multisite studies have found approximately a third of non-Hispanic Black and Latina women in the United States report elevated anxiety during pregnancy (Grobman et al., 2016). In Canada, over a quarter of pregnant Black and Latina women report symptoms of anxiety (as well as increased stress and inadequate social support), significantly more than the White "reference" group (Robinson et al., 2016). Varying patterns of anxiety throughout pregnancy (Wenzel et al., 2021) may have implications for screening, in that questions posed at the incorrect time potentially miss the opportunity to identify women in need of services.

Great disparities exist in mental healthcare for Black women and Latinas. Significantly lower rates of perinatal healthcare utilization have been noted (e.g., Declercq et al., 2022), particularly addressing mental health. In fact, in one study around half as many low-income Black and Latina women received counseling or medication for depression postpartum, compared to low-income White women (Kozhimannil et al., 2011). The impact of systemic racism and other forms of discrimination may discourage treatment-seeking behaviors and interact with certain cultural beliefs to provide obstacles to care (Lara-Cinisomo et al., 2018).

Awareness of cultural impact on Anna's risk for anxiety as well as factors that may impact her perspective on and participation in treatment would be advisable. As a Latina woman valuing close family relationships, relocating across the country may have disrupted the support system she relied on. Family engagement can be an important cultural source of resilience during pregnancy for Latinas (Campos et al., 2008), and its absence may have contributed to the risk of anxiety for Anna. Beliefs that her needs are less important than those of her growing baby may also be, in part, culturally congruent (Lara-Cinisomo et al., 2018). While abandoning enjoyable and healthy coping activities is certainly escalating her social isolation and anxiety symptoms, making changes to this pattern would require careful consideration of the beliefs that underlie this decision and the cultural context in which they developed.

Though meta-analytic studies have reported culturally adapted CBT interventions for depression and anxiety to be efficacious in general populations (Arundell et al., 2021), how this specifically plays out in prenatal anxiety is unclear. There is only a handful of treatment studies directly examining prenatal anxiety in minority populations (Ponting et al., 2022) and even fewer with mention of cultural adaptations. Encouragingly, one study in low-income Latina women in their first trimester found significant reductions in prenatal anxiety following a culturally adapted CBT intervention based on problem-solving and acceptance-based therapies (Ruiz et al., 2019). Plans to extend this protocol (Mastery Lifestyle Intervention or MLI) as a prospective RCT have been reported, including both pregnant Latina and Black/African-American women, with integration of care into regular prenatal clinics (Ruiz et al., 2022).

The model of including interventions in standard prenatal care is a promising vehicle for improving access to treatment for women from marginalized groups (Gennaro et al., 2020). Linking mental healthcare with regular OB or primary care visits and including education on what is "normal" in pregnancy may help to reduce stigma and provide a gateway to improved outcomes. The success of culturally adapted interventions for prenatal depression and anxiety (e.g., Ruiz et al., 2019; Grote et al., 2009) holds promise, though much work remains to improve and test interventions that highlight relevant cultural values.

Conclusions and Future Directions

Pregnancy is a challenging time—bringing significant hormonal and physical changes, relationship and role transitions, social and lifestyle adjustments, and associated environmental stressors. Over the past decade or so, deserved attention has finally been paid to the anxiety that so often accompanies pregnancy. With prenatal anxiety outpacing rates of depression in some studies and associated with overuse of obstetric resources (Peress et al., 2018), the need for screening with standardized, validated tools is now recognized (Committee on Obstetric Practice, 2018). Although full consensus is lacking on which measures best accomplish this task, we now have at least a few to choose from. Despite this progress, we have much left to learn—from the intersection of anxiety and cultural or ethnic factors, the interplay of biological, genetic, and psychological vulnerabilities to the effectiveness of treatment interventions in pregnant populations, and the distinction between DSM disorders and specific PRA. As the knowledge base continues to expand, we are poised to build on this foundation and improve our screening, prevention, and treatment for *all* women struggling with anxiety during pregnancy.

Research examining the construct of PRA as distinct from DSM-diagnosed anxiety disorders or self-reported anxiety may hold promise for better understanding the conflicting findings often seen in the literature. Better articulation of the definition of "prenatal anxiety" as we move forward would allow the interpretation of risk factors and correlates unique to PRA and those associated with anxiety disorders occurring or exacerbated during pregnancy. Future studies comparing these groups at different time points throughout pregnancy may also shed light on the trajectory of anxiety symptoms across trimesters and important associated variables in this population.

Continued efforts are needed to understand the interplay between genetic predisposition, biological sensitivities, and psychological variables that may place women at risk for prenatal anxiety. Although exciting preliminary findings suggest we may be closer to understanding the role of these factors in the development of anxiety during pregnancy, replication and expansion of this research is needed before we can confidently identify high-risk groups and target them for screening and treatment.

Despite consensus on its importance, little research has addressed the impact of racial, ethnic, and cultural variables on the presentation, prevalence, assessment, or treatment of anxiety in pregnant women. Although existing studies seem to indicate elevated rates of prenatal anxiety, we have little information to contextualize the experience for minority women. Assessment measures used in most studies may not be culturally appropriate or relevant across the board and standard psychological treatments may not consider important cultural components. While some limited findings suggest that culturally adapted protocols of evidence-based treatments are effective at reducing prenatal anxiety symptoms, this area remains glaringly inadequate. Identifying accurate assessment and treatment delivery, addressing barriers and stigma, and improving access to care should be high on the collective research agenda.

Although we have come a long way in recognizing the presence of anxiety during pregnancy, providers remain relatively unaware of the unique features that can present during this time. In a recent study, nearly 70% of perinatal health practitioners did not accurately identify obsessive-compulsive symptoms in a hypothetical case vignette and the majority endorsed at least one *contraindicated* clinical management strategy (Mulcahy et al., 2020). Programs informing providers of the frequency of anxiety in this population and familiarizing them with common features and treatment options are critical. Similarly, education for both clinicians and mothers about "normal" anxiety during pregnancy may help prevent misinterpretation of symptoms and stigma and promote referral to and engagement in effective treatments. With many anxious women turning to the Internet for information and support, creating perinatal websites with higher-quality health information and clear, evidence-based information on managing anxiety is needed (Kirby et al., 2018). Digital interventions and self-guided programs may provide the flexibility needed for pregnant women to access treatment, especially in low-income or rural populations.

References

Addis, A., Dolovich, L. R., Einarson, T. R., & Koren, G. (2000). Can we use anxiolytics during pregnancy without anxiety? *Canadian Family Physician, 46*, 549–551.

Adewuya, A. O., Ola, B. A., Aloba, O. O., & Mapayi, B. M. (2006). Anxiety disorders among Nigerian women in late pregnancy: A controlled study. *Archives of Women's Mental Health, 9*, 325–328.

Anderson, C. M., Brunton, R. J., & Dryer, R. (2019). Pregnancy-related anxiety: Re-examining its distinctiveness. *Australian Psychologist, 54*, 132–142. https://doi.org/10.1111/ap.12365

Arch, J. (2014). Cognitive behavioral therapy and pharmacotherapy for anxiety: Treatment preferences and credibility among pregnant and non-pregnant women. *Behaviour Research and Therapy, 52*, 53–60.

Arch, J., Dimidjian, S., & Chessick, C. (2012). Are exposure-based cognitive behavioral therapies safe during pregnancy? *Archives of Women's Mental Health, 15*, 445–457.

Arundell, L. L., Barnett, P., Buckman, J. E. J., Saunders, R., & Pilling, S. (2021). The effectiveness of adapted psychological interventions for people from ethnic minority groups: A systematic review and conceptual typology. *Clinical Psychology Review, 88*, 102063. https://doi.org/10.1016/j.cpr.2021.102063.

Asselmann, E., Wittchen, H. U., Erler, L., & Martini, J. (2016). Peripartum changes in social support among women with and without anxiety and depressive disorders prior to pregnancy: A prospective-longitudinal study. *Archives of Women's Mental Health, 19*, 943–952. https://doi.org/10.1007/s00737-016-0608-6

Austin, M. P. V., Hadzi-Pavlovic, D., Leader, L., Saint, K., & Parker, G. (2005). Maternal trait anxiety, depression and life event stress in pregnancy: Relationships with infant temperament. *Early Human Development*, *81*(2), 183–190. https://doi.org/10.1016/j.earlhumdev.2004.07.001

Austin, M. P. V., Mule, V., Hadzi-Pavlovic, D., & Reilly, N. (2022). Screening for anxiety disorders in third trimester pregnancy: A comparison of four brief measures. *Archives of Women's Mental Health*, *25*, 389–397. https://doi.org/10.1007/s00737-021-01166-9

Barrett, R., Wroe, A., & Challacombe, F. (2016). Context is everything: An investigation of responsibility beliefs and interpretations and the relationship with obsessive-compulsive symptomatology across the perinatal period. *Behavioural and Cognitive Psychotherapy*, *44*(3), 318–330. https://doi.org/10.1017/S1352465815000545

Bayat, A., Amiri-Farahani, L., Soleimani, M., Eshraghi, N., & Haghani, S. (2021). Effect of short-term psychological intervention on anxiety of pregnant women with positive screening results for chromosomal disorders: A randomized controlled trial. *BMC Pregnancy Childbirth*, *21*(1), 757. https://doi.org/10.1186/s12884-021-04206-5

Bayrampour, H., Ali, E., McNeil, D. A., Benzies, K., MacQueen, G., & Tough, S. (2016). Pregnancy-related anxiety: A concept analysis. *International Journal of Nursing Studies*, *55*, 115–130.

Bayrampour, H., Vinturache, A., Hetherington, E., Lorenzetti, D. L., & Tough, S. (2018). Risk factors for antenatal anxiety: A systematic review of the literature. *Journal of Reproductive and Infant Psychology*, *36*(5), 476–503. https://doi.org/10.1080/02646838.2018.1492097

Bedaso, A., Adams, J., Peng, W., & Sibbritt, D. (2021). The association between social support and antenatal depressive and anxiety symptoms among Australian women. *BMC Pregnancy Childbirth*, *21*(1), 708. https://doi.org/10.1186/s12884-021-04188-4

Berle, J. Ø., Mykletun, A., Daltveit, A. K., Rasmussen, S., Holsten, F., & Dahl, A. A. (2005). Neonatal outcomes in offspring of women with anxiety and depression during pregnancy: A linkage study from The Nord-Trøndelag Health Study (HUNT) and Medical Birth Registry of Norway. *Archives of Women's Mental Health*, *8*(3), 181–189. https://doi.org/10.1007/s00737-005-0090-z

Biaggi, A., Conroy, S., Pawlby, S., & Pariante, C. M. (2016). Identifying the women at risk of antenatal anxiety and depression: A systematic review. *Journal of Affective Disorders*, *191*, 62–77. https://doi.org/10.1016/j.jad.2015.11.014

Blackmore, E. R., Gustafsson, H., Gilchrist, M., Wyman, C., & O'Connor, T. G. (2016). Pregnancy-related anxiety: Evidence of distinct clinical significance from a prospective longitudinal study. *Journal of Affective Disorders*, *197*, 251–258. https://doi.org/10.1016/j.jad.2016.03.008

Briggs, G. G., Freeman, R. K., & Yaffe, S. J. (2012). *Drugs in pregnancy and lactation: A reference guide to fetal and neonatal risk*. Lippincott Williams & Wilkins.

Brockington, I. F., Macdonald, E., & Wainscott, G. (2006). Anxiety, obsessions and morbid preoccupations in pregnancy and the puerperium. *Archives of Women's Mental Health*, *9*(5), 253–263. https://doi.org/10.1007/s00737-006-0134-z

Brunton, R. J., Dryer, R., Saliba, A., & Kohlhoff, J. (2019). Re-examining pregnancy-related anxiety: A replication study. *Women and Birth*, *32*(1), e131–e137. https://doi.org/10.1016/j.wombi.2018.04.013

Brunton, R. J., Simpson, N., & Dryer, R. (2020). Pregnancy-related anxiety, perceived parental self-efficacy and the influence of parity and age. *International Journal of Environmental Research and Public Health*, *17*(18), 6709. https://doi.org/10.3390/ijerph17186709

Buhr, K., & Dugas, M. J. (2009). The role of fear of anxiety and intolerance of uncertainty in worry: An experimental manipulation. *Behaviour Research and Therapy*, *47*(3), 215–223. https://doi.org/10.1016/j.brat.2008.12.004

Buss, C., Davis, E. P., Muftuler, L. T., Head, K., & Sandman, C. A. (2010). High pregnancy anxiety during mid-gestation is associated with decreased gray matter density in 6–9-year-old children. *Psychoneuroendocrinology*, *35*(1), 141–153. https://doi.org/10.1016/j.psyneuen.2009.07.010

Campos, B., Schetter, C. D., Abdou, C. M., Hobel, C. J., Glynn, L. M., & Sandman, C. A. (2008). Familialism, social support, and stress: Positive implications for pregnant Latinas. *Cultural Diversity and Ethnic Minority Psychology*, *14*(2), 155–162. https://doi.org/10.1037/1099-9809.14.2.155

Chambers, C. D., Johnson, K. A., Dick, L. M., Felix, R. J., & Jones, K. L. (1996). Birth outcomes in pregnant women taking fluoxetine. *New England Journal of Medicine*, *335*(14), 1010–1015. https://doi.org/10.1056/NEJM199610033351402

Chan, C., Lee, A., Lam, S., Lee, C., Leung, K., Koh, Y., & Tang, C. (2013). Antenatal anxiety in the first trimester: Risk factors and effects on anxiety and depression in the third trimester and 6-week postpartum. *Open Journal of Psychiatry*, 3, 301–310. https://doi.org/10.4236/ojpsych.2013.33030

Coleman, V. H., Carter, M. M., Morgan, M. A., & Schulkin, J. (2008). Obstetrician-gynecologists' screening patterns for anxiety during pregnancy. *Depression and Anxiety*, 25, 114–123. https://doi.org/10.1002/da.20278

Committee on Obstetric Practice. (2018). Screening for perinatal depression: ACOG committee opinion no. 757: American college of obstetricians and gynecologists. *Obstetrics & Gynecology*, 32, e208–e212.

Coplan, R. J., O'Neil, K., & Arbeau, K. A. (2005). Maternal anxiety during and after pregnancy and infant temperament at three months of age. *Journal of Prenatal & Perinatal Psychology & Health*, 19(3), 199–215. www.proquest.com/scholarly-journals/maternal-anxiety-during-after-pregnancy-infant/docview/198689185/se-2

Cox, E. Q., Sowa, N. A., Meltzer-Brody, S. E., & Gaynes, B. N. (2016). The perinatal depression treatment cascade: Baby steps toward improving outcomes. *Journal of Clinical Psychiatry*, 77(9), 1189–1200. https://doi.org/10.4088/JCP.15r10174

Cox, J. L., Holden, J. M., & Sagovsky, R. (1987). Detection of postnatal depression: Development of the 10-item Edinburgh Postnatal Depression Scale. *British Journal of Psychiatry*, 150, 782–786. https://doi.org/10.1192/bjp.150.6.782. PMID: 3651732.

Davis, E. P., Korja, R., Karlsson, L., Glynn, L. M., & Sandman, C. A., Vegetabile, B., . . . Baram, T. Z. (2019). Across continents and demographics, unpredictable maternal signals are associated with children's cognitive function. *EBioMedicine*, 46, 256–263. https://doi.org/10.1016/j.ebiom.2019.07.025

Davis, E. P., & Sandman, C. A. (2010). The timing of prenatal exposure to maternal cortisol and psychosocial stress is associated with human infant cognitive development. *Child Development*, 81(1), 131–148. https://doi.org/10.1111/j.1467-8624.2009.01385.x

Davis, E. P., Snidman, N., Wadhwa, P. D., Glynn, L. M., Dunkel-Schetter, C., & Sandman, C. A. (2004). Prenatal maternal anxiety and depression predict negative behavioral reactivity in infancy. *Infancy*, 6, 319–331.

Davis, E. P., Stout, S. A., Molet, J., Vegetabile, B., Glynn, L. M., Sandman, C. A., . . . Baram, T. Z. (2017). Exposure to unpredictable maternal sensory signals influences cognitive development across species. *Proceedings of the National Academy of Science U S A*, 114(39), 10390–10395. https://doi.org/10.1073/pnas.1703444114

Declercq, E., Feinberg, E., & Belanoff, C. (2022). Racial inequities in the course of treating perinatal mental health challenges: Results from listening to mothers in California. *Birth*, 49, 132–140. https://doi.org/10.1111/birt.12584

Degirmenci, S., Kosger, F., Altinoz, A. E., Essizoglu, A., & Aksaray, G. (2020). The relationship between separation anxiety and intolerance of uncertainty in pregnant women. *Journal of Maternal and Fetal Neonatal Medicine*, 33(17), 2927–2932. https://doi.org/10.1080/14767058.2018.1564030

Dennis, C. L., Falah-Hassani, K., & Shiri, R. (2017). Prevalence of antenatal and postnatal anxiety: Systematic review and meta-analysis. *British Journal of Psychiatry*, 210(5), 315–323. https://doi.org/10.1192/bjp.bp.116.187179

Einarson, A., Bonari, L., Voyer-Lavigne, S., et al. (2003). A multicentre prospective controlled study to determine the safety of trazodone and nefazodone use during pregnancy. *Canadian Journal of Psychiatry*, 48(2), 106–110. https://doi.org/10.1177/070674370304800207

Einarson, A., Fatoye, B., Sarkar, M., et al. (2001). Pregnancy outcome following gestational exposure to venlafaxine: A multicenter prospective controlled study. *American Journal of Psychiatry*, 158(10), 1728–1730. https://doi.org/10.1176/appi.ajp.158.10.1728

Fairbrother, N., Collardeau, F., Albert, A. Y. K., Challacombe, F. L., Thordarson, D. S., Woody, S. R., & Janssen, P. A. (2021). High prevalence and incidence of obsessive-compulsive disorder among women across pregnancy and the postpartum. *Journal of Clinical Psychiatry*, 82(2), 20m13398. https://doi.org/10.4088/JCP.20m13398

Fairbrother, N., Corbyn, B., Thordarson, D. S., Ma, A., & Surm, D. (2019). Screening for perinatal anxiety disorders: Room to grow. *Journal of Affective Disorders*, 250, 363–370. https://doi.org/10.1016/j.jad.2019.03.052

Fairbrother, N., & Woody, S. R. (2008). New mothers' thoughts of harm related to the newborn. *Archives of Women's Mental Health, 11*(3), 221–229. https://doi.org/10.1007/s00737-008-0016-7

Fairbrother, N., Young, A. H., Zhang, A., Janssen, P., & Antony, M. M. (2017). The prevalence and incidence of perinatal anxiety disorders among women experiencing a medically complicated pregnancy. *Archives of Women's Mental Health, 20*(2), 311–319. https://doi.org/10.1007/s00737-016-0704-7

Fawcett, E. J., Fairbrother, N., Cox, M. L., White, I. R., & Fawcett, J. M. (2019). The prevalence of anxiety disorders during pregnancy and the postpartum period: A multivariate Bayesian meta-analysis. *The Journal of Clinical Psychiatry, 80*(4), 18r12527. https://doi.org/10.4088/JCP.18r12527

Field, T. (2017). Prenatal anxiety effects: A review. *Infant Behavior and Development, 49*, 120–128. https://doi.org/10.1016/j.infbeh.2017.08.008

Forray, A., Mayes, L. C., Magriples, U., & Epperson, C. N. (2009). Prevalence of post-traumatic stress disorder in pregnant women with prior pregnancy complications. *Journal of Maternal-Fetal & Neonatal Medicine, 22*(6), 522–527. https://doi.org/10.1080/14767050902801686

Frost, R. O., Marten, P., Lahart, C., & Rosenblate, R. (1990). The dimensions of perfectionism. *Cognitive Therapy and Research, 14*, 449–468.

Furtado, M., Chow, C. H. T., Owais, S., Frey, B. N., & Van Lieshout, R. J. (2018). Risk factors of new onset anxiety and anxiety exacerbation in the perinatal period: A systematic review and meta-analysis. *Journal of Affective Disorders, 238*, 626–635. https://doi.org/10.1016/j.jad.2018.05.073

Gennaro, S., O'Connor, C., McKay, E. A., Gibeau, A., Aviles, M., Hoying, J., & Melnyk, B. M. (2020). Perinatal anxiety and depression in minority women. *MCN American Journal of Maternal and Child Nursing, 45*(3), 138–144. https://doi.org/10.1097/NMC.0000000000000611

GlaxoSmithKline. (2005). Preliminary report on bupropion in pregnancy and the occurrence of cardiovascular and major congenital malformation. *Data on File. Glaxo Smith Kline, UK*. www.cmaj.ca/content/cmaj/suppl/2006/03/27/173.11.1320.DC1/epip0831.pdf

Glover, V., O'Connor, T. G., & O'Donnell, K. (2010). Prenatal stress and the programming of the HPA axis. *Neuroscience and Biobehavioral Reviews, 35*(1), 17–22. https://doi.org/10.1016/j.neubiorev.2009.11.008

Goetz, M., Schiele, C., Müller, M., Matthies, L. M., Deutsch, T. M., Spano, C., . . . Wallwiener, S. (2020). Effects of a brief electronic mindfulness-based intervention on relieving prenatal depression and anxiety in hospitalized high-risk pregnant women: Exploratory pilot study. *Journal of Medical Internet Research, 22*(8), e17593. https://doi.org/10.2196/17593

Goodman, J. H., Guarino, A., Chenausky, K., Klein, L., Prager, J., Petersen, R., . . . Freeman, M. (2014). CALM pregnancy: Results of a pilot study of mindfulness-based cognitive therapy for perinatal anxiety. *Archives of Women's Mental Health, 17*(5), 373–387. https://doi.org/10.1007/s00737-013-0402-7

Goodman, W. K., Price, L. H., Rasmussen, S. A., & Mazure, C. (1989a). The Yale-Brown obsessive compulsive scale: I. Development, use, and reliability. *Archives of General Psychiatry, 46*, 1006–1011.

Goodman, W. K., Price, L. H., Rasmussen, S. A., Mazure, C., Delgado, P., Henninger, G. R., & Charney, D. S. (1989b). The Yale-Brown obsessive compulsive scale: II. Validity. *Archives of General Psychiatry, 46*, 1012–1016.

Gourounti, K., Anagnostopoulos, F., & Lykeridou, K. (2013). Coping strategies as psychological risk factor for antenatal anxiety, worries, and depression among Greek women. *Archives Women's Mental Health, 16*(5), 353–361. https://doi.org/10.1007/s00737-013-0338-y

Goyal, D., Rosa, L., Mittal, L., Erdei, C., & Liu, C. H. (2022). Unmet prenatal expectations during the COVID-19 pandemic. *MCN American Journal of Maternal and Child Nursing, 47*(2), 66–70. https://doi.org/10.1097/NMC.0000000000000801

Grant, K. A., Bautovich, A., McMahon, C., Reilly, N., & Austin, M. P. (2012). Parental care and control during childhood: Associations with maternal perinatal mood disturbance and parenting stress. *Archives of Women's Mental Health, 15*, 297–305. https://doi.org/10.1007/s00737-012-0292-0

Green, J. M., Kafetsios, K., Statham, H. E., & Snowdon, C. M. (2003). Factor structure, validity and reliability of the Cambridge Worry Scale in a pregnant population. *Journal of Health Psychology, 8*(6), 753–764. https://doi.org/10.1177/13591053030086008

Green, S. M., Donegan, E., McCabe, R. E., Streiner, D. L., Agako, A., & Frey, B. N. (2020). Cognitive behavioral therapy for perinatal anxiety: A randomized controlled trial. *Australian & New Zealand Journal of Psychiatry, 54*(4), 423–432. https://doi.org/10.1177/0004867419898528

Green, S. M., Inness, B., Furtado, M., McCabe, R. E., & Frey, B. N. (2022). Evaluation of an augmented cognitive behavioural group therapy for perinatal generalized anxiety disorder (GAD) during the COVID-19 pandemic. *Journal of Clinical Medicine, 11*(1), 209. https://doi.org/10.3390/jcm11010209

Grigoriadis, S., Graves, L., Peer, M., Mamisashvili, L., Tomlinson, G., Vigod, S., . . . Richter, M. (2018). Maternal anxiety during pregnancy and the association with adverse perinatal outcomes: Systemic review and meta-analysis. *Journal of Clinical Psychiatry, 79*(5), 17r12011. https://doi.org/10.1016/S0029-7844(99)00602-X

Grobman, W. A., Parker, C., Wadhwa, P. D., Willinger, M., Simhan, H., Silver, B., . . . Reddy, U. M. (2016). Racial/ethnic disparities in measures of self-reported psychosocial states and traits during pregnancy. *American Journal of Perinatology, 33*(14), 1426–1432. https://doi.org/10.1055/s-0036-1586510

Grös, D. F., Antony, M. M., Simms, L. J, & McCabe, R. E. (2007). Psychometric properties of the State-Trait Inventory for Cognitive and Somatic Anxiety (STICSA): Comparison to the State-Trait Anxiety Inventory (STAI). *Psychological Assessment, 19*, 369–381.

Grote, N. K., Swartz, H. A., Geibel, S. L., Zuckoff, A., Houck, P. R., & Frank, E. (2009). A randomized controlled trial of culturally relevant, brief interpersonal psychotherapy for perinatal depression. *Psychiatric Services, 60*(3), 313–321. https://doi.org/10.1176/ps.2009.60.3.313

Hakanen, H., Flykt, M., Sinervä, E., Nolvi, S., Kataja, E. L., Pelto, J., . . . Korja, R. (2019). How maternal pre- and postnatal symptoms of depression and anxiety affect early mother-infant interaction? *Journal of Affective Disorders, 257*, 83–90. https://doi.org/10.1016/j.jad.2019.06.048

Hamilton, M. (1959). The assessment of anxiety states by rating. *British Journal of Medical Psychology, 32*, 50–55.

Hart, R., & McMahon, C. A. (2006). Mood state and psychological adjustment to pregnancy. *Archives of Women's Mental Health, 9*, 329–337. https://doi.org/10.1007/s00737-006-0141-0

Henrichs, J., Schenk, J. J., Schmidt, H. G., Velders, F. P., Hofman, A., Jaddoe, V. W. V., . . . Tiemeier, H. (2009). Maternal pre- and postnatal anxiety and infant temperament: The generation R study. *Infant and Child Development, 18*, 556–572. https://doi.org/10.1002/icd.639

Heron, J., O'Connor, T. G., Evans, J., Golding, J., & Glover, V. (2004). The course of anxiety and depression through pregnancy and the postpartum in a community sample. *Journal of Affective Disorders, 80*(1), 65–73. https://doi.org/10.1016/j.jad.2003.08.004

Holmberg, E., Teppola, T., Pajulo, M., Davis, E. P., Nolvi, S., Kataja, E.-L., . . . Korja, R. (2020). Maternal anxiety symptoms and self-regulation capacity are associated with the unpredictability of maternal sensory signals in caregiving behavior. *Frontiers in Psychology, 11*, 564158. https://doi.org/10.3389/fpsyg.2020.564158

Holton, S., Fisher, J., Nguyen, H., Brown, W. J., & Tran, T. (2019). Pre-pregnancy body mass index and the risk of antenatal depression and anxiety. *Women Birth, 32*(6), e508–e514. https://doi.org/10.1016/j.wombi.2019.01.007

Huizink, A. C., Delforterie, M. J., Scheinin, N. M., Tolvanen, M., Karlsson, L., & Karlsson, H. (2016). Adaption of pregnancy anxiety questionnaire–revised for all pregnant women regardless of parity: PRAQ-R2. *Archives of Women's Mental Health, 19*, 125–132. https://doi.org/10.1007/s00737-015-0531-2

Huizink, A. C., Mulder, E. J., Robles de Medina, P. G., Visser, G. H., & Buitelaar, J. K. (2004a). Is pregnancy anxiety a distinctive syndrome? *Early Human Development, 79*(2), 81–91. https://doi.org/10.1016/j.earlhumdev.2004.-4.014

Huizink, A. C., Mulder, E. J. H., & Buitelaar, J. K. (2004b). Prenatal stress and risk for psychopathology: Specific effects or induction of general susceptibility? *Psychological Bulletin, 130*(1), 115–142. https://doi.org/10.1037/0033-2909.130.1.115.

Hussain-Shamsy, N., Somerton, S., Stewart, D. E., Grigoriadis, S., Metcalfe, K., Oberlander, T. F., . . . Vigod, S. N. (2022). The development of a patient decision aid to reduce decisional conflict about antidepressant use in pregnancy. *BMC Medical Informatics and Decision Making, 22*, 130. https://doi.org/10.1186/s12911-022-01870-1

Insan, N., Weke, A., Forrest, S., & Rankin, J. (2022). Social determinants of antenatal depression and anxiety among women in South Asia: A systematic review & meta-analysis. *PLoS ONE, 17*(2), e0263760. https://doi.org/10.1371/journal.pone.0263760

Jokić-Begić, N., Žigić, L., & Radoš, S. N. (2014). Anxiety and anxiety sensitivity as predictors of fear of childbirth: Different patterns for nulliparous and parous women. *Journal of Psychosomatic Obstetrics & Gynecology, 35*(1), 22–28. https://doi.org/10.3109/0167482X.2013.866647

Kaminsky, Z. A., Osborne, L. M., Guglielmi, V., Jones, I., Grenier, W., Clark, K., . . . Nestadt, G. (2020). Postpartum depression biomarkers predict exacerbation of OCD symptoms during pregnancy. *Psychiatry Research*, *293*, 113332. https://doi.org/10.1016/j.psychres.2020.113332

Karaca, P. P., Koyucu, R. G., & Aksu, S. C. (2022). The relationship between pregnant women's anxiety levels about coronavirus and prenatal attachment. *Archives of Psychiatric Nursing*, *36*, 78–84. https://doi.org/10.1016/j.apnu.2021.12.001

Kesim, M., Yaris, F., Kadioglu, M., et al. (2002). Mirtazapine use in two pregnant women: Is it safe? *Teratology*, *66*(5), 204–204. https://doi.org/10.1002/tera.10095

Kirby, P. L., Reynolds, K. A., Walker, J. R., Furer, P., & Pryor, T. A. M. (2018). Evaluating the quality of perinatal anxiety information available online. *Archives of Women's Mental Health*, *21*, 813–820. https://doi.org/10.1007/s00737-018-0875-5

Klerman, G. L., Weissman, M. M., Rounsaville, B. J., & Chevron, E. (1984). *Interpersonal psychotherapy of depression*. Basic Books.

Koc, A. E., Colak, S., Colak, G. V., Pusuroglu, M., & Hocaoglu, C. (2021). Investigating fear of childbirth in pregnant women and its relationship between anxiety sensitivity and somatosensory amplification. *Journal of Obstetrics and Gynaecology*, *41*(2), 217–223. https://doi.org/10.1080/0 1443615.2020.1732894

Kozhimannil, K. B., Trinacty, C. M., Busch, A. B., Huskamp, H. A., & Adams, A. S. (2011). Racial and ethnic disparities in postpartum depression care among low-income women. *Psychiatric Services*, *62*(6), 619–625. https://doi.org/10.1176/ps.62.6.pss6206_0619

Kurki, T., Hiilesmaa, V., Raitasalo, R., Mattila, H., & Ylikorkala, O. (2000). Depression and anxiety in early pregnancy and risk for preeclampsia. *Obstetrics & Gynecology*, *95*(4), 487–490. https://doi.org/10.1016/S0029-7844(99)00602-X

Lara-Cinisomo, S., Clark, C. T., & Wood, J. (2018). Increasing diagnosis and treatment of perinatal depression in Latinas and African American women: Addressing stigma is not enough. *Women's Health Issues*, *28*(3), 201–204. https://doi.org/10.1016/j.whi.2018.01.003

Leff-Gelman, P., Flores-Ramos, M., Carrasco, A. E. Á., Martínez, M. L., Takashima, M. F. S., Coronel, F. M. C., . . . Camacho-Arroyo, I. (2020). Cortisol and DHEA-S levels in pregnant women with severe anxiety. *BMC Psychiatry*, *20*, 393. https://doi.org/10.1186/s12888-020-02788-6

Levison-Castiel, R., Merlob, P., Linder, N., Sirota, L., & Klinger, G. (2006). Neonatal abstinence syndrome after in utero exposure to selective serotonin reuptake inhibitors in term infants. *Archives of Pediatric and Adolescent Medicine*, *160*(2), 173–176. https://doi.org/10.1001/archpedi.160.2.173

Lilliecreutz, C., Josefsson, A., & Sydsjö, G. (2010). An open trial with cognitive behavioral therapy for blood- and injection phobia in pregnant women – a group intervention program. *Archives of Women's Mental Health*, *13*, 259–265.

Lilliecreutz, C., Sydsjö, G., & Josefsson, A. (2011). Obstetric and perinatal outcomes among women with blood- and injection phobia during pregnancy. *Journal of Affective Disorders*, *129*(1–3), 289–295. https://doi.org/10.1016/j.jad.2010.08.013

Littleton, H. L., Breitkopf, C. R., & Berenson, A. B. (2007). Correlates of anxiety symptoms during pregnancy and association with perinatal outcomes: A meta-analysis. *American Journal of Obstetrics and Gynecology*, *196*(5), 424–432. https://doi.org/10.1016/j.ajog.2007.03.042

Lobel, M., Dunkel-Schetter, C., & Scrimshaw, S. C. M. (1992). Prenatal maternal stress and prematurity: A prospective study of socioeconomically disadvantaged women. *Health Psychology*, *11*(1), 32–40.

Löwe, B., Decker, O., Müller, S., Brähler, E., Schellberg, D., Herzog, W., & Herzberg, P. Y. (2008). Validation and standardization of the Generalized Anxiety Disorder Screener (GAD-7) in the general population. *Medical Care*, *46*(3), 266–274. https://doi.org/10.1097/MLR.0b013e318160d093

Lowndes, T. A., Egan, S. J., & McEvoy, P. M. (2019). Efficacy of brief guided self-help cognitive behavioral treatment for perfectionism in reducing perinatal depression and anxiety: A randomized controlled trial. *Cognitive Behaviour Therapy*, *48*(2), 106–120. https://doi.org/10.1080/16506073.201 8.1490810

Mahaffey, B. L., Levinson, A., Preis, H., & Lobel, M. (2022). Elevated risk for obsessive-compulsive symptoms in women pregnant during the COVID-19 pandemic. *Archives of Women's Mental Health*, *25*(2), 367–376. https://doi.org/10.1007/s00737-021-01157

Marchesi, C., Ampollini, P., Paraggio, C., Giaracuni, G., Ossola, P., De Panfilis, C., . . . Viviani, D. (2014). Risk factors for panic disorder in pregnancy: A cohort study. *Journal of Affective Disorders, 156*, 134–138. https://doi.org/10.1016/j.jad.2013.12.006

Martini, J., Petzoldt, J., Einsle, F., Beesdo-Baum, K., Höfler, M., & Wittchen, H. U. (2015). Risk factors and course patterns of anxiety and depressive disorders during pregnancy and after delivery: A prospective-longitudinal study. *Journal of Affective Disorders, 175*, 385–395. https://doi.org/10.1016/j.jad.2015.01.012

Matthey, S. (2007). Using the Edinburgh Postnatal Depression Scale to screen for anxiety disorders. *Depression and Anxiety, 25*(11), 926–931. https://doi.org/10.1002/da.20415

Matthey, S., & Ross-Hamid, C. (2011). The validity of DSM symptoms for depression and anxiety disorders during pregnancy. *Journal of Affective Disorders, 133*(3), 546–552. https://doi.org/10.1016/j.jad.2011.05.004

Matthey, S., Valenti, B., Souter, K., & Ross-Hamid, C. (2013). Comparison of four self-report measures and a generic mood question to screen for anxiety during pregnancy in English-speaking women. *Journal of Affective Disorders, 148*(2–3), 347–351. https://doi.org/10.1016/j.jad.2012.12.022

Meyer, T. J., Miller, M. L., Metzger, R. L., & Borkovec, T. D. (1990). Development and validation of the Penn State Worry Questionnaire. *Behavior Research and Therapy, 28*, 487–495.

Miller, R. P., & Becker, B. A. (1975). Teratogenicity of oral diazepam and diphenylhy-dantoin in mice. *Toxicology and Applied Pharmacology, 132*, 53–61. https://doi.org/10.1016/0041-008X(75)90194-5

Misri, S., & Kendrick, K. (2007). Treatment of perinatal mood and anxiety disorders: A review. *Canadian Journal of Psychiatry, 52*(8), 489–498. https://doi.org/10.1177/070674370705200803

Misri, S., Oberlander, T. F., Fairbrother, N., Cartner, D., Ryan, D., Kuan, A., & Reebye, P. (2004). Relation between prenatal maternal mood and anxiety and neonatal health. *Canadian Journal of Psychiatry, 49*(10), 684–689. https://doi.org/10.1177/070674370404901006.

Morland, L., Goebert, D., Onoye, J., Frattarelli, L., Derauf, C., Herbst, M., Matsu, C., & Friedman, M. (2007). Posttraumatic stress disorder and pregnancy health: Preliminary update and implications. *Psychosomatics, 48*(4), 304–308. https://doi.org/10.1176/appi.psy.48.4.304

Moyer, C. A., Compton, S. D., Kaselitz, E., & Muzik, M. (2020). Pregnancy-related anxiety during COVID-19: A nationwide survey of 2740 pregnant women. *Archives of Women's Mental Health, 23*(6), 757–765. https://doi.org/10.1007/s00737-020-01073-5

Mulcahy, M., Rees, C., Galbally, M., & Anderson, R. (2020). Health practitioners' recognition and management of postpartum obsessive-compulsive thoughts of infant harm. *Archives of Women's Mental Health, 23*(5), 719–726. https://doi.org/10.1007/s00737-020-01026-y

Nasreen, H. E., Kabir, Z. N., Forsell, Y., & Edhburg, M. (2011). Prevalence and associated factors of depressive and anxiety symptoms during pregnancy: A population-based study in rural Bangladesh. *BMC Women's Health, 11*, 22. https://doi.org/10.1186/1472-6874-11-22

Nath, S., Pearson, R. M., Moran, P., Pawlby, S., Molyneaux, E., Challacombe, F. L., & Howard, L. M. (2019). The association between prenatal maternal anxiety disorders and postpartum perceived and observed mother-infant relationship quality. *Journal of Anxiety Disorders, 68*, 102148. https://doi.org/10.1016/j.janxdis.2019.102148

National Institute for Health and Care Excellence. (2014). *Antenatal and postnatal mental health: Clinical management and service guidance* (CG192). www.nice.org.uk/guidance/cg192

Nulman, I., Rovet, J., Stewart, D. E., Wolpin, J., Gardner, A., Theis, J. G. W., . . . Koren, G. (1997). Neurodevelopment of children exposed in utero to antidepressant drugs. *New England Journal of Medicine, 336*(4), 258–262. https://doi.org/10.1056/NEJM199701233360404

Oberlander, T. F., Misri, S., Fitzgerald, C. E., Kostaras, X., Rark, D., & Riggs, W. (2004). Pharmacologic factors associated with transient neonatal symptoms following prenatal psychotropic medication exposure. *Journal of Clinical Psychiatry, 65*(2), 230–237.

Obsessive Compulsive Cognitions Working Group. (2005). Psychometric validation of the obsessive belief questionnaire and interpretation of intrusions inventory. *Behaviour Research and Therapy, 43*, 1527–1542.

Ojalehto, H. J., Hellberg, S. N., Butcher, M. W., Buchholz, J. L., Timpano, K. R., & Abramowitz, J. S. (2021). Experiential avoidance and the misinterpretation of intrusions as prospective predictors of postpartum obsessive-compulsive symptoms in first-time parents. *Journal of Contextual Behavioral Science, 20*, 137–143. https://doi.org/10.1016/j.jcbs.2021.04.003

Orr, S. T., Reiter, J. P., Blazer, D. G., & James, S. A. (2007). Maternal prenatal pregnancy-related anxiety and spontaneous preterm birth in Baltimore, Maryland. *Psychosomatic Medicine*, 69(6), 566–570. https://doi.org/10.1097/PSY.0b013e3180cac25d

Parfitt, Y., Pike, A., & Ayers, S. (2013). The impact of parents' mental health on parent-baby interaction: A prospective study. *Infant Behavior and Development*, 36(4), 599–608. https://doi.org/10.1016/j.infbeh.2013.06.003

Peress, D. A., Elovitz, M. A., & Downes, K. L. (2018). Pregnant women who screen positive for depression or anxiety are more likely to overutilize an obstetrical triage unit. *American Journal of Obstetrics and Gynecology*, 218(1), S518–S519. https://doi.org/10.1016/j.ajog.2017.11.407

Pilkington, P. D., Whelan, T. A., & Milne, L. C. (2015). A review of partner-inclusive interventions for preventing postnatal depression and anxiety. *Clinical Psychologist*, 19(2), 63–75. https://doi.org/10.1111/cp.12054

Ponting, C., Urizar, Jr., G. G., & Schetter, C. D. (2022). Psychological interventions for prenatal anxiety in Latinas and Black women: A scoping review and recommendations. *Front Psychiatry*, 13, 820343. https://doi.org/10.3389/fpsyt.2022.820343

Rahimi, R., Nikfar, S., & Abdollahi, M. (2006). Pregnancy outcomes following exposure to serotonin reuptake inhibitors: A meta-analysis of clinical trials. *Reproductive Toxicology*, 22(4), 571–575. https://doi.org/10.1016/j.reprotox.2006.03.019

Robinson, A. M., Benzies, K. M., Cairns, S. L., Fung, T., & Tough, S. C. (2016). Who is distressed? A comparison of psychosocial stress in pregnancy across seven ethnicities. *BMC Pregnancy Childbirth*, 16(215). https://doi.org/10.1186/s12884-016-1015-8

Ruiz, R. J., Grimes, K., Spurlock, E., Stotts, A., Northrup, T. F., Villarreal, Y., . . . Pickler, R. H. (2022). The mastery lifestyle intervention to reduce biopsychosocial risks for pregnant Latinas and African Americans and their infants: Protocol for a randomized controlled trial. *BMC Pregnancy and Childbirth*, 22, 979. https://doi.org/10.1186/s12884-022-05284-9

Ruiz, R. J., Newman, M., Records, K., Wommack, J. C., Stowe, R. P., & Pasillas, R. M. (2019). Pilot study of the lifestyle intervention. *Nursing Research*, 68(6), 494–500. https://doi.org/10.1097/NNR.0000000000000384

Russell, E. J., Fawcett, J. M., & Mazmanian, D. (2013). Risk of obsessive-compulsive disorder in pregnant and postpartum women: A meta-analysis. *Journal of Clinical Psychiatry*, 74(4), 377–385. https://doi.org/10.4088/JCP.12r07917. PMID: 23656845.

Sbrilli, M. D., Haigler, K., & Laurent, H. K. (2021). The indirect effect of parental intolerance of uncertainty on perinatal mental health via mindfulness during COVID-19. *Mindfulness*, 12(8), 1999–2008. https://doi.org/10.1007/s12671-021-01657-x

Scholl, C. C., Trettim, J. P., Böhm, D. M., Molina, M. L., Soares, M. C., Dias, N. D. C., . . . Quevedo, L. A. (2022). Are adolescents more likely to have antenatal anxiety disorders than adult women? A comparison between two samples. *Journal of Affective Disorders*, 316, 50–55. https://doi.org/10.1016/j.jad.2022.07.071

Shorey, S. Y., Ng, E. D., & Chee, C. Y. I. (2021). Anxiety and depressive symptoms of women in the perinatal period during the COVID-19 pandemic: A systematic review and meta-analysis. *Scandinavian Journal of Public Health*, 49(7), 730–740. https://doi.org/10.1177/14034948211011793

Shyken, J. M., Babbar, S., Babbar, S., & Forinash, A. (2019). Benzodiazepines in pregnancy. *Clinical Obstetrics and Gynecology*, 62(1), 156–167.

Siddiqui, A., & Hägglöf, B. (2000). Does maternal prenatal attachment predict postnatal mother – infant interaction? *Early Human Development*, 59(1), 13–25. https://doi.org/10.1016/S0378-3782(00)00076-1

Sinesi, A., Maxwell, M., O'Carroll, R., & Cheyne, H. (2019). Anxiety scales used in pregnancy: Systematic review. *British Journal of Psychiatry Open*, 5(1), E5. https://doi.org/10.1192/bjo.2018.75

Sockol, L. E. (2018). A systematic review and meta-analysis of interpersonal psychotherapy for perinatal women. *Journal of Affective Disorders*, 232, 316–328. https://doi.org/10.1016/j.jad.2018.01.018

Somerville, S., Byrne, S. L., Dedman, K., Hagan, R., Coo, S., Oxnam, E., . . . Page, A. C. (2015). Detecting the severity of perinatal anxiety with the Perinatal Anxiety Screening Scale (PASS). *Journal of Affective Disorders*, 186, 18–25. https://doi.org/10.1016/j.jad.2015.07.012

Somerville, S., Dedman, K., Hagan, R., Oxnam, E., Wettinger, M., Byrne, S., . . . Page, A. C. (2014). The perinatal anxiety screening scale: Development and preliminary validation. *Archives of Women's Mental Health*, 17(5), 443–454. https://doi.org/10.1007/s00737-014-0425-8

Soto-Balbuena, C., Rodríguez, M. F., Gomis, A. I. E., Barriendos, F. J. F., Le, H. N., & Pmb-Huca, G. (2018). Incidence, prevalence and risk factors related to anxiety symptoms during pregnancy. *Psicothema*, *30*(3), 257–263. https://doi.org/10.7334/psicothema2017.379.

Spice, K., Jones, S. L., Hadjistavropoulos, H. D., Kowalyk, K., & Stewart, S. H. (2009). Prenatal fear of childbirth and anxiety sensitivity. *Journal of Psychosomatic Obstetrics & Gynecology*, *30*(3), 168–174. https://doi.org/10.1080/01674820902950538

Spielberger, C. D., Gorsuch, R. L., & Lushene, R. E. (1970). *Manual for the state-trait anxiety inventory*. Consulting Psychologists Press.

Spinelli, M. G., & Endicott, J. (2003). Controlled clinical trial of interpersonal psychotherapy versus parenting education program for depressed pregnant women. *American Journal of Psychiatry*, *160*(3), 555–562. https://doi.org/10.1176/appi.ajp.160.3.555

Spitzer, R. L., Kroenke, K., Williams, J. B. W., & Löwe, B. (2006). A brief measure for assessing generalized anxiety disorder: The GAD-7. *Archives of Internal Medicine*, *166*(10), 1092–1097. https://doi.org/10.1001/archinte.166.10.1092

Stubert, J., Reister, F., Hartmann, S., & Janni, W. (2018). The risks associated with obesity in pregnancy. *Deutsches Arzteblatt International*, *15*(16), 276–283. https://doi.org/10.3238/arztebl.2018.0276

Sutter-Dallay, A. L., Giaconne-Marcesche, V., Glatigny-Dallay, E., & Verdoux, H. (2004). Women with anxiety disorders during pregnancy are at increased risk of intense postnatal depressive symptoms: A prospective survey of the MATQUID cohort. *European Psychiatry*, *19*(8), 459–463. https://doi.org/10.1016/j.eurpsy.2004.09.025. PMID: 15589703.

Taylor, S. (1995). Anxiety sensitivity: Theoretical perspectives and recent findings. *Behaviour Research and Therapy*, *33*(3), 243–258.

Thorsness, K. R., Watson, C., & LaRusso, E. M. (2018). Perinatal anxiety: Approach to diagnosis and management in the obstetric setting. *American Journal of Obstetrics and Gynecology*, *219*(4), 326–345. https://doi.org/10.1016/j.ajog.2018.05.017

Timpano, K. R., Abramowitz, J. S., Mahaffey, B. L., Mitchell, M. A., & Schmidt, N. B. (2011). Efficacy of a prevention program for postpartum obsessive-compulsive symptoms. *Journal of Psychiatric Research*, *45*(11), 1511–1517. https://doi.org/10.1016/j.jpsychires.2011.06.015

Uguz, F., & Ak, M. (2021). Cognitive-behavioral therapy in pregnant women with generalized anxiety disorder: A retrospective cohort study on therapeutic efficacy, gestational age and birth weight. *Brazilian Journal of Psychiatry*, *43*(1), 61–64. https://doi.org/10.1590/1516-4446-2019-0792

Uguz, F., Gezginc, K., Zeytinci, I. E., Karatayli, S., Askin, R., Guler, O., ... Gecici, O. (2007). Course of obsessive-compulsive disorder during early postpartum period: A prospective analysis of 16 cases. *Comprehensive Psychiatry*, *48*(6), 558–561. https://doi.org/10.1016/j.comppsych.2007.05.010

U.S. Preventive Services Task Force. (2019). Perinatal depression: Preventive Interventions. *UPSTF*. www.uspreventiveservicestaskforce.org/uspstf/recommendation/perinatal-depression-preventive-interventions

Usuda, K., Nishi, D., Makino, M., Tachimori, H., Matsuoka, Y., Sano, Y., ... Takeshima, T. (2016). Prevalence and related factors of common mental disorders during pregnancy in Japan: A cross-sectional study. *Biopsychosocial Medicine*, *10*, 17. https://doi.org/10.1186/s13030-016-0069-1

Van den Bergh, B. R. H. (1992). Maternal emotions during pregnancy and fetal and neonatal behaviour. In J. G. Nijhuis (Ed.), *Fetal behaviour: Developmental and perinatal aspects* (pp. 157–178). Oxford University Press.

Van den Bergh, B. R. H., & Marcoen, A. (2004). High antenatal maternal anxiety is related to ADHD symptoms, externalizing problems, and anxiety in 8-and 9-year-olds. *Child Development*, *75*(4), 1085–1097. https://doi.org/10.1111/j.1467-8624.2004.00727.x

Van den Bergh, B. R. H., Van Calster, B., Smits, T., Van Huffel, S., & Lagae, L. (2008). Antenatal maternal anxiety is related to HPA-axis dysregulation and self-reported depressive symptoms in adolescence: A prospective study on the fetal origins of depressed mood. *Neuropsychopharmacology*, *33*, 536–545. https://doi.org/10.1038/sj.npp.1301450

VanOtterloo, L. R., Morton, C. H., Seacrist, M. J., & Main, E. K. (2019). Quality improvement opportunities identified through case review of pregnancy-related deaths from cardiovascular disease. *Journal of Obstetric, Gynecologic, and Neonatal Nursing*, *48*(3), 263–274. https://doi.org/10.1016/j.jogn.2019.03.001

Vigod, S. N., Hussain-Shamsy, N., Stewart, D. E., Grigoriadis, S., Metcalfe, K., Oberlander, T. F., . . . Dennis, C. L. (2019). A patient decision aid for antidepressant use in pregnancy: Pilot randomized controlled trial. *Journal of Affective Disorders, 251,* 91–99. https://doi.org/10.1016/j.jad.2019.01.051

Viswasam, K., Eslick, G. D., & Starcevic, V. (2019). Prevalence, onset and course of anxiety disorders during pregnancy: A systematic review and meta analysis. *Journal of Affective Disorders, 255,* 27–40. https://doi.org/10.1016/j.jad.2019.05.016

Walton, G. D., Ross, L. E., Stewart, D. E., Grigoriadis, S., Dennis, C. L., & Vigod, S. (2014). Decisional conflict among women considering antidepressant medication use in pregnancy. *Archives of Women's Mental Health, 17*(6), 493–501.

Wenzel, A. (2011). *Anxiety in childbearing women: Diagnosis and treatment.* American Psychological Association. https://doi.org/10.1037/12302-000

Wenzel, E. S., Gibbons, R. D., O'Hara, M. W., Duffecy, J., & Maki, P. M. (2021). Depression and anxiety symptoms across pregnancy and the postpartum in low-income Black and Latina women. *Archives of Women's Mental Health, 24,* 979–986. https://doi.org/10.1007/s00737-021-01139-y

Wijma, K., Wijma, B., & Zar, M. (1998). Psychometric aspects of the W-DEQ: A new questionnaire for the measurement of fear of childbirth. *Journal of Psychosomatic Obstetrics and Gynecology, 19,* 84–97.

Women's Preventive Services Initiative (WPSI). (2018). *Screening for anxiety.* ACOG Foundation. www.womenspreventivehealth.org/recommendations/screening-for-anxiety/

Yan, H., Ding, Y., & Guo, W. (2020). Mental health of pregnant and postpartum women during the coronavirus disease 2019 pandemic: A systematic review and meta-analysis. *Frontiers in Psychology, 11,* 617001. https://doi.org/10.3389/fpsyg.2020.617001

Zhong, Q. Y., Gelaye, B., Zaslavsky, A. M., Fann, J. R., Rondon, M. B., Sánchez, S. E., & Williams, M. A (2015). Diagnostic validity of the Generalized Anxiety Disorder – 7 (GAD-7) among pregnant women. *PLoS One, 10*(4), e0125096. https://doi.org/10.1371/journal.pone.0125096

9

PRENATAL EATING DISORDERS AND BODY IMAGE DISTURBANCE

Alyssa M. Minnick, Molly Moore,
Nathaniel Holmes, and Kelly C. Allison

Description and Salient Features

Body Image Disturbances During Pregnancy

Body image is a multifaceted construct that encompasses "a person's perceptions, thoughts, and feelings about his or her body" (Grogan, 2021, p. 4). This definition includes psychological experiences of the body, both negative and positive perceptions, as well as thoughts and feelings related to physical aspects of the body. Pregnancy is a major life transition and involves changes to bodily anatomy, appearance, and sensations.

Women have differing reactions to bodily changes during pregnancy, with some having positive experiences of their changing bodies. One study of women in Kenya (Barasa & Kinuthia, 2018) found an association between positive emotions with pregnancy and awareness of the expected bodily changes. Women in this study subsequently chose to wear more fitting and comfortable maternity clothing to "maintain their body image" during pregnancy (Barasa & Kinuthia, 2018, p. 52). Other women in Australia reported that focusing on their growing fetus, such as feeling the baby kick, hearing the fetal heartbeat, and having their partner rub and talk to their pregnant stomach, improved their ability to adapt to their changing pregnant body (Clark et al., 2009). Women from multiple countries indicated that they placed the health and development of their babies above the priority to adhere to societal ideals for thinness (Clark et al., 2009) and saw body changes as a sign of fertility (Barasa & Kinuthia, 2018) and the baby's development (Chang et al., 2006). Women have also described a sense of sharing their body with the fetus, which provides comfort during pregnancy (Hodgkinson et al., 2014).

Many other pregnant people, however, experience body image disturbances. Some women indicated that pregnancy felt like the fetus was invading their bodies (Hodgkinson et al., 2014), perhaps, in part, due to the uncontrollable changes to the body. Women from Kenya reported that negative emotions during pregnancy were associated with being unhappy with pregnancy-related body changes and not being ready to lose their pre-pregnancy body shape and size (Barasa & Kinuthia, 2018). In addition, women have reported that negative body image is related to undesirable changes to their bodies during pregnancy,

DOI: 10.4324/9781003206903-12

including fluid retention, larger or leaking breasts, alterations of nipple color, dry facial skin, varicose veins, skin rashes, acne, and loss of muscle tone; however, the most common complaint was excess weight gain (Clark et al., 2009).

Weight gain during pregnancy is necessary for healthy fetal growth and development. Weight gain recommendations for singleton pregnancies from the U.S. Institute of Medicine by body mass classification are as follows: underweight (body mass index [BMI] < 18.5) 28–40 lb; normal weight (BMI of 18.5–24.9) 25–25 lb; overweight (BMI of 25–29.9) 15–25 lb; and obesity (BMI ≥ 30) 11–20 lb (Centers for Disease Control and Prevention [CDC], 2022). Data from U.S. women indicated that 32% gain weight within these recommended ranges, whereas 48% gain weight above and 21% gain weight below the recommendations (CDC, 2022).

Gestational weight gain was the most salient experience related to body image disturbances. In a qualitative, interview-based study, two (out of 20) Australian women who had negative feelings about their bodily changes indicated that they perceived "too much" weight gain in their legs, thighs, and buttocks; they also indicated being focused on their body shape, weight, and size pre-pregnancy (Clark et al., 2009). Pregnant women were also concerned about how their weight gain was perceived by others and by society in general (Chang et al., 2006). They expressed concerns about appearing "fat" (Earle, 2003) and wanted it to be apparent that their weight was due to pregnancy (e.g., from their baby bump) rather than a gain in fat mass (Clark et al., 2009). Messages related to gaining "too much" weight, looking bigger than their gestational age, or being asked if they were carrying twins were identified as contributors to negative mood and body image during the prenatal period (Clark et al., 2009).

Eating Disorders during Pregnancy

Body image disturbances have been theorized to contribute to increased risk for and development of eating disorders (EDs). According to the dual-pathway model, the pursuit of the thin ideal promotes body image concerns that result in negative affect and dieting, which both increase the risk for compensatory weight control behaviors and/or binge eating (Stice, 2001). Given that pregnancy may negatively influence body image, it is important to assess and address disordered eating behaviors (EDs), whether these behaviors were present preconception or developed during the gestational period. ED behaviors can present across the continuum of eating, from restricting caloric intake to binge-eating behaviors to compensatory behaviors after eating used to control weight (Soares et al., 2009; Martínez-Olcina et al., 2020). These behaviors, in any form or frequency, should be addressed with pregnant patients, and a clinical diagnosis is considered when symptoms interfere with daily functioning and/or cause significant distress.

The *Diagnostic and Statistical Manual*, 5th edition (DSM 5; American Psychiatric Association, 2013) includes several feeding and EDs that could present during pregnancy. Anorexia nervosa (AN) includes restriction of energy intake that results in significantly lower body weight than is expected for age, sex, developmental period, and physical health. The diagnosis also requires an intense fear of gaining weight or being "fat," as well as body weight or shape having an excessive influence on self-evaluation and/or disturbance in how the person perceives their body weight or shape. Clinicians should specify if the AN is a restricting or binge-eating/purging subtype.

Bulimia nervosa (BN) includes recurrent episodes of binge eating, which is defined as eating an unusually large amount of food in a discrete period of time (i.e., two hours) with an accompanying sense of loss of control overeating (i.e., termed "objective binge episode"). The person also engages in recurrent inappropriate compensatory behaviors after eating to prevent weight gain, such as self-induced vomiting, excessive use of laxatives, diuretics or other diet pills, fasting, or excessive exercise. These episodes of binge eating and compensatory behaviors must occur, on average, at least once per week for three months to meet diagnostic criteria. In BN, self-worth and self-evaluation are also heavily influenced by body weight and shape.

Binge eating disorder (BED) is the most common ED. Similar to BN, recurrent episodes of binge eating must occur, on average, once per week for three months; however, no compensatory behaviors are employed. The OBEs must be associated with at least three of the following experiences: (a) eating more rapidly than usual; (b) being uncomfortably full after eating; (c) eating large amounts of food despite lack of physical hunger; (d) eating alone due to feeling embarrassed by the amount of food consumed; and (e) negative feelings about oneself after eating (e.g., disgust, depressed, or very guilty). Women may also be diagnosed with an Other Specified Feeding or Eating Disorder (OSFED) (formerly known as Eating Disorder Not Otherwise Specified [ED-NOS in DSM-IV]; American Psychiatric Association, 1994) if they present with significantly disordered EDs but do not meet full criteria for the other EDs. This diagnosis also includes syndromes that have not yet been designated as a clinical diagnosis, such as night eating syndrome (NES) and purging disorder (American Psychiatric Association, 2013).

Finally, pica is a feeding disorder that presents as the persistent ingestion of nonnutritive, nonfood substances for at least one month (American Psychiatric Association, 2013). Pregnant women may ingest one specific substance or multiple types of substances, including ice, freezer frost, corn starch, laundry starch, or clay dirt, among other substances (Corbett et al., 2003). Anemia, which may be caused by a nutritional deficiency, has been positively associated with pica during pregnancy (Fawcett et al., 2016), although it is yet unclear if there is a causal relationship between these two conditions (Young, 2010).

Pre-Existing EDs and Pregnancy

Qualitative data provide important insights into the experience of being pregnant and having a past or current ED. Claydon et al. (2018) identified several themes among women who were pregnant, planning for pregnancy, or had decided against pregnancy. In a theme of "control," pregnancy was distressing because women had less or limited control over changes to their body. The lack of control was particularly upsetting because disordered eating strategies used prior to pregnancy (i.e., controlling weight and caloric intake and tracking calories) were strategies used to cope with or manage stress in life. Therefore, women described difficulties with modifying their strict tracking of weight and/or calories prenatally.

Another important theme reflected gestational weight and body concerns (Claydon et al., 2018). Women reported understanding that weight gain was needed for the health of the baby; however, the fear of weight gain that is central to AN and BN interfered. Some women also identified an "ideal" pregnant body with concerns about conforming to this ideal (Claydon et al., 2018). In particular, women perceived that they "should" only gain weight in their "baby bump" area but not in other areas (Vanderkruik et al., 2022). This may be particularly pronounced because pregnant women with EDs reported that their body defines them as a person and is one of the most important factors in judging their self-worth (Tierney et al., 2013). There were also specific concerns about weight checks at the obstetrics/gynecology office, as well as the way information regarding weight gain would be delivered by their provider (Claydon et al., 2018). Due to these concerns, some women requested to not be weighed (although this may not be possible for medical monitoring of the pregnancy) or weighed blindly (e.g., the patient turned backward so the weight was not seen; Claydon et al., 2018).

Furthermore, women described their ED (current or lifetime history) as "a secret" that either no one else or only few people knew about prior to pregnancy (Claydon et al., 2018). Women were concerned about feeling isolated from their partner or others in their lives if they disclosed a past or current ED diagnosis. These concerns were particularly pronounced, and even mixed among women in the study, when deciding whether or not to disclose ED information to a medical provider, such as their obstetrician or gynecologist (OB/GYN). They cited that not wanting ED treatment or thoughts that their provider could not help them with the ED as contributors to this decision. Challenges when disclosing also included a lack of communication between maternity and psychiatric providers.

One of the most prominent themes detailed a "battle" between pregnancy and ED (Claydon et al., 2018). Some women reported adopting a "mama bear" mentality that motivated them to change behaviors, whereas other women described a conflict between being pregnant and having an ED (even past history). Women stated that pregnancy-related symptoms, such as nausea, were sometimes used as an excuse to engage in ED behaviors, including vomiting (Claydon et al., 2018; Tierney et al., 2013). Women indicated feeling guilty if they were unable to stop all ED symptoms during pregnancy and experienced high anticipation of their baby's birth, so they could resume disordered behaviors (e.g., caloric restriction) without the possible direct impact on the baby (Claydon et al., 2018). Other research indicated that women thought (preconception) that being pregnant would effectively cure their ED but were distressed when disordered EDs continued (Tierney et al., 2013).

Development of EDs During Pregnancy

There is less research examining the onset of EDs during pregnancy (relative to the presence of pre-existing EDs), and its incidence seems rare for most disorders, with more frequent occurrences of BED (Knoph et al., 2013). Previous research has indicated multiple psychological, social, and health-related correlates of developing BED in pregnancy. A lifetime history of sexual or physical abuse or major depression, low life satisfaction, low self-esteem, and low satisfaction with partner relationships were related to BED incidence during the first half of pregnancy; concerns about pregnancy-related weight gain were also associated with BED onset (Knoph Berg et al., 2011). The body's adaptation to pregnancy may also contribute to increased food intake during pregnancy in that the body becomes leptin-resistant and produces progesterone during pregnancy than in other times in life, both of which are hormones that contribute to increased appetite, food intake, and fat storage needed to support a growing fetus and prepare for lactation postpartum (Brunton & Russell, 2008). These physiological changes could lead to increased hunger and BEDs during pregnancy.

Pica may also develop prenatally, perhaps in part due to nutritional deficiencies in pregnancy (e.g., iron), although pica is also seen in other populations, including children (Lacey, 1990). A meta-analysis of the worldwide prevalence of pica in pregnant women found that increased risk for pica was associated with living in Africa, low educational attainment, identifying as African American, and reporting anemia (Fawcett et al., 2016). Furthermore, among pregnant women in Ghana, those with pica perceived white clay or ice to be nutritious had a craving for these substances and/or felt the scent or taste of the substance(s) reduced nausea and vomiting during pregnancy (Konlan et al., 2020). Pregnant Kurdish women in Iraq indicated similar reasons for pica in that nonnutritive substances were consumed to reduce nausea, stress, and hunger (Galali, 2020). Pica may develop for multiple reasons, and it is important to assess for this feeding disorder, particularly to ensure that women are not ingesting harmful substances.

Introduction to the Case

Emily is 28 years old and identifies as a second-generation Mexican-American woman. She has a history of BN. She first experienced body image concerns when she was on the high school soccer team and felt social pressure to have a "fit" body shape and size. To achieve this ideal, she dieted during the day but then became hungry after soccer practice and would lose control over her eating. She ate large portions at dinner with her family and felt a sense of loss of control overeating. At times, she also experienced binge-eating episodes after dinnertime while she was alone. Emily would often make herself vomit after binge-eating episodes, attempting to avoid gaining weight. BN continued into college, although she did not continue playing soccer, but she was able to hide the behaviors from her roommate and friends. BN remitted during her junior year of college when she first met her future husband, but she periodically engaged in binge eating and self-induced vomiting during stressful situations, such as when she started her first full-time job.

After college, Emily settled at a BMI of 27 kg/m2 (within the overweight range) and was working on accepting the changes to her body in adulthood. As she and her husband discussed starting a family, Emily became worried about how pregnancy would affect her body weight, shape, and size, as well as her binge-eating and compensatory behaviors. She is now 15 weeks pregnant with her first child, and her BN-related behaviors have re-emerged. She has been experiencing daytime nausea since early pregnancy, which reduced her food intake, but, in the evening, her hunger increases, and she often has binge-eating episodes. She continues to have nausea after these episodes, so she often vomits after eating to alleviate this bodily sensation but also to avoid weight gain. Emily expressed being particularly worried about staying within the recommended weight gain range of 15–25 lb during pregnancy. She has been increasingly uncomfortable in her body, particularly since she started wearing maternity clothing. She tried to hide her behaviors, but her husband discovered her relapse and was concerned.

Prevalence

Several large epidemiological studies have examined the prevalence of EDs during pregnancy, along with several smaller cohort studies, most using DSM-IV criteria. In the United Kingdom, the Avon Longitudinal Study of Parents and Children examined cross-sectional estimates of EDs during pregnancy based on surveys administered at 12 weeks' gestation. Among 10,137 women, 4.1% had any ED, with 1.4% having AN, 1.8% having BN, and 0.1 having "mixed AN and BN symptoms" (Micali et al., 2012). Prevalence of BED was not reported. Similarly, in Norway, a large, community-based cohort was followed in the

Mother and Child Cohort Study (MoBa). They also used a self-report questionnaire to study ED symptoms retrospectively six months' preconception and a current estimate at 19 weeks' gestation among 37,307 women (Dellava et al., 2011). They found that 6.3% reported any ED, 0.09% had AN, 0.9% had BN, 5.2% had BED, and 0.1% had ED-NOS-Purging. Easter et al. (2013) reported similar numbers in the United Kingdom, showing the following prevalence estimates of EDs: 7.5% for any ED, 0.5% with AN, 0.1% with BN, 1.8% with BED, 0.1% with ED-NOS-Purging, and 5% with other ED-NOS. From a symptom perspective, OBEs were present in 8.8% and regular inappropriate compensatory behaviors occurred in 2.3%. Finally, 23.4% endorsed elevated weight and shape concerns.

Other studies have found higher estimates of EDs, including Koubaa et al. (2015) in Sweden, who interviewed 96 women using DSM-IV diagnostic criteria and a medical record review. They reported that 38.5% had any ED, including 8% active AN, 12.5% past AN, 1% current BN, and 16.7% past BN. Furthermore, Linna et al. (2014) used physician-based diagnoses with 4,299 Finnish women and found that 15.3% reported any ED, including 4.2% with AN, 10.1% with BN, and just 0.9% with BED. In the only South American cohort study found, ED pathology was high among the sample of 712 low-income women at pregestation and lower during pregnancy, respectively: OBEs in 27.6% and 19.2%, vomiting in 6.8% and 1.4%, laxative misuse in 6.3% and 0%, diuretic misuse in 3.3% and 0%, and excessive exercise in 0% and 1.6% (this was the only compensatory behavior that increased during pregnancy; Angélica Nunes et al., 2014).

Two studies used surveys from women in the MoBa cohort to examine lifetime as compared to current ED symptoms (Siega-Riz et al., 2008; Knoph et al., 2013). They reported a lifetime prevalence estimate of 6.1% for any ED: 4.6% for any active ED; 0.2% having BN prepregnancy and during pregnancy, 0.2% reporting BN prepregnancy and then BED during pregnancy, 2% for those with BED prepregnancy and during pregnancy, and 2% who reported no ED before pregnancy but developed BED during pregnancy. There were no cases of women developing AN during pregnancy, and <0.1% developed ED-NOS. One further analysis of the MoBa cohort reported the proportions of women remitting from their ED during pregnancy were 78% ED-NOS, 40% purging BN, 39% BED, 34% BED any type, and 29% BN nonpurging (Bulik et al., 2007).

Most studies showed that ED symptoms improved during pregnancy but returned to baseline levels during the postpartum period (Dörsam et al., 2019; Micali et al., 2012). Crow et al. (2008) examined the course of ED symptoms in a cohort of 42 women with EDs prior to pregnancy in the McKnight Longitudinal Study of Eating Disorders in the United States. They reported that prepregnancy, they endorsed having 8.7 OBEs in the past 28 days, but this improved to 2.9 OBEs in the past 28 days during pregnancy. Morgan et al. (1999) also reported improvements in OBEs with each successive trimester and with others showing complete cessation of OBEs by the third trimester in 75% (Lacey & Smith, 1987). Finally, in a sample of 43 women with EDs, among those with restriction, 65% improved nutrition or stopped restricting, and 7% ceased restricting during pregnancy (Lemberg & Phillips, 1989). Among those with OBEs, 56% improved, 18.6% worsened, and 14% reported complete cessation (Lemberg & Phillips, 1989).

Of a sample of women who had recovered from an ED, 25 (21 BN and 4 AN) women participated in a qualitative study with interviews every two weeks during pregnancy (Makino et al., 2020). They reported that 67% relapsed with ED symptoms during the first trimester (all with a history of AN and 48% of those with BN), but all improved over the course of the pregnancy with counseling.

The prevalence of pica was not often reported in studies of ED during pregnancy. Its assessment varies widely, as do its prevalence estimates. One meta-analysis that included 70 studies showed an aggregate prevalence estimate of 27.8%, which is very high (Fawcett et al., 2016).

Finally, estimates of night eating were reported in one study of 120 Black women with obesity during pregnancy, showing 4% screening positive for NES, with 32% consuming at least 25% of their daily caloric intake after dinner (evening hyperphagia) (Allison et al., 2012). Sixty-four percent reported awakening during the night more than once per week, and 9.4% reported eating during the night at least half of the time they awoke (nocturnal ingestions). None of these women met the criteria for BED, with 4% reporting occasional OBEs. No cases of BN were endorsed.

Correlates and Risk Factors

Depression and Anxiety

Depression and anxiety are common comorbidities of EDs, including among pregnant individuals, and research has shown that depression and anxiety are risk factors for developing EDs during pregnancy. Past depression diagnosis and symptoms of both depression and anxiety during pregnancy are related to the incidence of BED during pregnancy (*Relative risk [RR]* = 2.47, $p < .001$ and $RR = 2.30$, $p < .001$, respectively; Knoph Berg et al., 2011). Specifically, individuals with major depression were found to be more than two times at risk of developing BED prenatally than those without major depression (Knoph Berg et al., 2011). The incidence of BN during pregnancy is related to both anxiety and mood symptomology ($RR = 3.99$, $p < .001$; Knoph Berg et al., 2008). In a population of Chinese women, disordered eating during pregnancy was associated with both anxiety and depression at each of the three trimesters, even after controlling for prepregnancy disordered eating, BMI (including change during pregnancy), and other factors (e.g., self-esteem, social support, and marital satisfaction) within each trimester (all relationships $p < .0001$, except between depressive symptoms and disordered eating in early pregnancy, which is $p < .05$; Chan et al., 2019).

A current or lifetime history of ED also represents a risk factor for developing anxiety and depression during pregnancy. Individuals with a current or past ED had higher depression and anxiety (trait and state) across the perinatal period than individuals in a non-ED, healthy control group (Easter et al., 2015). Additionally, women with EDs are at similar risk for developing depression during pregnancy as women with a history of major depressive disorder (Mazzeo et al., 2006). In a U.K. sample, individuals with both ED symptoms during pregnancy and a history of depression preconception had the highest risk for developing depression and anxiety in the perinatal period ($OR = 5.7$, $p < 0.0001$); however, in this sample, a history of ED before pregnancy alone did not increase the risk of developing depression while pregnant ($OR = 1.3$, $p =$ ns; Micali et al., 2011). It, therefore, appears that ED symptoms may exacerbate an individual's previous pathologies and result in a heightened risk of mental illness during the perinatal period. More research is needed to establish these associations, which also appear to be bidirectional in nature.

Body Image Concerns

Women may become increasingly concerned with their body image throughout pregnancy. Negative body image is a predictor of dysfunctional eating in the third trimester among pregnant Portuguese individuals (Gonçalves et al., 2015). Body image concerns can be a risk factor for ED development during pregnancy as women may deviate from gestational nutritional recommendations in an attempt to prescribe to societal norms around weight loss (Dryer et al., 2020). In Australian individuals, body dissatisfaction predicted pregnancy-related anxiety and symptoms of both depression and EDs (Dryer et al., 2020). Furthermore, "fat talk," or making negative or disparaging comments about one's own body weight, shape, or size or of others' bodies, partially mediated the relation between body dissatisfaction and symptoms of depression, EDs, and pregnancy-related anxiety (Dryer et al., 2020). These findings indicate that body image disturbance is related to internal and external body-related dialogue that may influence pathology, particularly during pregnancy when women have little control over their changing bodies.

Media consumption can also put pregnant individuals at risk for EDs or body image issues as media often portray unrealistic beauty standards (Holland & Tiggemann, 2016; Mingoia et al., 2017; Rollero, 2015). In a Lebanese sample of pregnant individuals, posting on social media ($r = 0.16$, $p = 0.04$) and anxiety/dependence on technology ($r = 0.30$, $p < 0.001$) were related to poor body image and competitiveness about their bodies during pregnancy (Zeeni et al., 2021). However, social media posting ($r = 0.17$, $p = 0.03$) and social media usage (viewing; $r = 0.15$, $p = 0.049$) were also correlated with healthy eating in pregnant individuals (Zeeni et al., 2021). The authors noted that they did not assess the reasons for healthy eating, which they speculated could be due to multiple factors such as the health of the unborn baby or a form of dieting. Although some aspects of social media (i.e., usage and posting) can inspire healthy eating, other aspects (i.e., posting and technological dependence) can harm body image. The combination of these social media facets likely contributes to EDs in pregnant women (Zeeni et al., 2021). Furthermore, pregnant individuals expressed poorer body image after exposure to magazine media portraying pregnant and postpartum celebrities, in comparison to a control group of pregnant women exposed to a home improvement magazine (t [102] = 1.99, $p < .05$, $d = .39$; Coyne et al., 2018). Therefore, it may not be simply social media usage or posting, but the specific content that is potentially harmful to body image and eating behaviors during pregnancy.

In an Iranian sample of pregnant women, researchers examined the relation between EDs, body image, and "maladaptive perfectionism," defined as self-critical behavior and having extremely high standards for oneself (Kiani-Sheikhabadi et al., 2019). This type of perfectionism was positively correlated with current symptoms of AN ($r = 0.45$, $p < 0.05$), ED symptoms ($r = 0.34$, $p < 0.05$), and nervous longing to eat ($r = 0.38$, $p < 0.05$). Women who were critical with themselves were more likely to inaccurately view their pregnancy weight and appearance and were at an increased risk of compensatory ED behaviors (Kiani-Sheikhabadi et al., 2019).

Body Weight and Diet

The research on the influence of weight and BMI on body image and eating behaviors during pregnancy is mixed. In a Chinese sample, disordered eating in all three trimesters was unrelated to BMI or BMI change from prepregnancy weight (Chan et al., 2019). However, in Portuguese individuals, it was established that higher BMI before pregnancy and increased weight gain during the pregnancy period were risk factors for dysfunctional eating in the third trimester (Gonçalves et al., 2015). Furthermore, others found that BED during pregnancy was associated with overevaluation of weight ($RR = 2.77$, $p < .001$) and thoughts of having overweight prior to pregnancy ($RR = 1.35$, $p < .001$) and, most significantly, worrying about gestational weight gain ($RR = 3.51$, $p < .001$; Knoph Berg et al., 2011). Perhaps it is not solely the physical weight changes that a pregnant individual undergoes prenatally but also the perception of their weight and body image that increases the risk of developing an ED.

Obesity is also a risk factor for body dissatisfaction, as individuals with obesity tend to diet ($OR = 3.4$, $p < .001$), have a desire to lose weight ($OR = 2.1$, $p < .001$), and be dissatisfied with weight gain during the prenatal period ($OR = 1.2$, $p < .01$) in comparison to a control group without obesity (Micali et al., 2007). However, it should be noted that these individuals with obesity had lower concerns with their weight and shape during pregnancy compared to the prepregnancy period. Women with obesity were also significantly less likely to engage in compensatory behaviors (i.e., laxative use, self-induced vomiting) during pregnancy compared to women with a recent ED (Micali et al., 2007). Additionally, individuals with high pregravid BMI who desire to be thinner had less risk of gaining weight above the Institute of Medicine's recommendations (Mehta et al., 2011). Whereas women with average weight may be at risk for excessive weight gain during pregnancy due to a loosening of standards around their body image (i.e., they are expected to gain weight during pregnancy), women with a high BMI might be more careful about pregnancy weight gain due to their already high weight and desire for thinness (Mehta et al., 2011).

Diet quality is another predictor of body satisfaction during pregnancy, as one study found that the strength of healthy eating habits (e.g., "eating a variety of vegetables, fruits, and whole grains is something that I do automatically") in the second trimester of pregnancy predicted higher body satisfaction at the end of pregnancy (Pullmer et al., 2018). Thus, more automatic healthy eating habits may be a protective factor that can help buffer women from the negative perspectives on body image that emerge during this time (Pullmer et al., 2018). The authors speculated that eating healthy may be out of concern for the growing fetus, and, therefore, may lead individuals to place less attention on their body and weight (Pullmer et al., 2018). However, it should be noted that dieting, or restricting daily caloric intake and/ or certain food groups, is often regarded as an ED symptom and has been linked to pregnant individuals with a recent ED (Micali et al., 2007). Specifically, a healthy diet is linked to mothers who have a past history of ED (Nguyen et al., 2017), including an increased rate of vegetarianism in those with an ED history (Dörsam et al., 2019). Therefore, the reasons for healthy eating should be assessed, particularly if the individual has an ED history.

History of EDs

Pregnancy may predispose women to a relapse of ED symptoms. Research has linked pregravid disordered eating as a risk factor for disordered eating at each of the three trimesters of pregnancy in a Chinese sample (Chan et al., 2019). Furthermore, British individuals with a recent ED were at risk for many ED symptoms during pregnancy, including ED cognitions, dieting, laxative use, self-induced vomiting, overexercising, and high weight and shape concerns (Micali et al., 2007). Individuals with a past history of EDs were also at an increased risk of displaying these symptoms during pregnancy compared to controls without a lifetime history of EDs, although not to the extent of the group with a more recent ED (Micali et al., 2007). In a Danish population that had ED remission for at least six months pregravid, one quarter had an ED relapse, and two-thirds occurred during the first 20 weeks of pregnancy (Sollid et al., 2021), demonstrating that, during pregnancy, women may become susceptible to ED behaviors once again.

Abuse

Physical and sexual abuse are also correlates of EDs during pregnancy. Individuals with AN and BN during the perinatal period reported more instances of trauma (i.e., physical and sexual abuse) than women with perinatal depression but no ED history (Meltzer-Brody et al., 2011). Interestingly, no relation between BED and history of abuse was found in this American sample (Meltzer-Brody et al., 2011). However, in one Norwegian study, an abuse history (i.e., lifetime physical and sexual abuse) was related to an increased risk of developing BED during pregnancy ($RR = 1.68$, $p < .001$; $RR = 1.57$, $p < .001$, respectively; Knoph Berg et al., 2011). Thus, there seems to be a relationship between abuse and ED symptoms during pregnancy, but more research is needed to clarify the relationship between abuse and specific EDs.

Fetal Health and Birth Complications

Individuals with EDs throughout the prenatal period can have birth complications such as premature birth, caesarian sections, and/or a miscarriage, along with many other possible difficulties and abnormalities (Arnold et al., 2019). Complications vary depending on the ED symptoms. BED during pregnancy was correlated with having a large-for-gestational-age infant, whereas women with AN and BN were more likely to have a low-weight infant (Linna et al., 2014; Sebastiani et al., 2020). Other health issues such as slow fetal growth, premature contractions, very premature birth, anemia, and perinatal death can occur in mothers specifically with AN due to undernutrition (Linna et al., 2014). Mothers with a current ED had an increased risk of birth complications compared to women with a past ED (Charbonneau & Seabrook, 2019).

Sleep

Sleep is an important factor to consider in relation to EDs during pregnancy. During the first 18 weeks of pregnancy, Ulman et al. (2012) showed that all pregnant individuals had an increase in sleep problems. However, women with a history of and current BED had more issues with their sleep as compared to individuals not reporting BED symptoms. Given that sleep issues are common, yet variable, in pregnancy (Allison et al., 2012), it is important to assess how they may influence disordered eating behaviors during its course.

Therapist: What are some of your triggers for binge-eating episodes or vomiting?

Emily: I'm not really sure. It feels like an automatic thing since it's been happening off and on since I was a teenager.

T: Yes, I know it can be difficult to pinpoint what is going on in these situations, especially when we are in the moment. Let's talk about the last time a binge episode happened during this past week. Would that be okay?

E: Sure. It was earlier this week, and just like every day during this pregnancy, I felt so sick and nauseous all day. I can barely stand the smell of certain foods, like chicken or meat, so I tend to just not eat or just nibble throughout the day on fruit or crackers or chew gum. But then by dinnertime, I am pretty hungry, even though

I still feel pretty nauseous. On that day, I ate dinner, and, it was okay, but then later that night, I was still hungry and just kept going back to the cabinet for more snacks. Afterward, I felt gross, because I was still nauseous, and I knew that I had really messed up and would gain too much weight. I told my husband that I wasn't feeling well and said I was going to lie down for a bit, but, instead, I went into the bathroom and threw up. I felt better for maybe a minute but then worried about if I was taking nutrition away from the baby, so I felt bad about myself.

T: I appreciate all of that detail. It seems like the pregnancy-related nausea is really affecting you.

E: Yeah, it has been such an unpleasant and unexpected experience with the pregnancy. None of the other women in my family experienced it, so I thought I might avoid it. It is so emotionally draining to feel sick all the time, while also trying to still work, be a wife, do house things, and everything else.

T: It sounds like the nausea is affecting you in a lot of different ways. From what you said, it is also influencing your eating?

E: Yes, definitely. A lot of time, I can't even stand the thought of eating, or I can only tolerate light foods, bread, crackers, or sweet things. It's hard, too, because some of the foods are the ones I tend to binge on.

T: Tell me more about that and what you've noticed in your pregnancy.

E: The nausea has basically sent me back into my pattern of not eating so much during the day and then having binge eating at night. I also sometimes justify throwing up after eating because I do feel nauseous.

T: You said "justify" the purging. What do you mean by that?

E: I guess, if I'm being honest, it's kind of an excuse. Yes, I do feel better briefly after throwing up, like physically not nauseous, but I know the nausea is not going to go away after I do it. I'm also very focused on how what I just ate will make me gain weight. Then I feel bad about my body because it's not fully apparent yet that I'm pregnant, so I just look fat. I hate that people probably just look at me and think that I have belly fat or look bloated.

Effects on Relationships

Social Support and Partner Relationship

Social support is crucial for individuals suffering from EDs, as it can act as a protective factor and buffer the effects of EDs and body image issues. This is particularly true in pregnancy, with a significant correlation found between low social support and the incidence of BED ($RR = 0.60$, $p < .001$; Knoph Berg et al., 2011). The quality of the relationship between the mother and their partner can have a particularly important influence on the mother's ED. In individuals in the third trimester of pregnancy, poor marital relationships were significantly correlated with dysfunctional eating ($r = .23$, $p = .019$; Gonçalves et al., 2015). One aspect of body image issues, a drive for thinness, was associated with poor spousal support in a Chinese sample ($r = -.14$, $p < .05$;

Lai et al., 2005). Furthermore, BED incidence during pregnancy was associated with low partner relationship satisfaction among the Norwegian population ($RR = 0.70$, $p < .001$; Knoph Berg et al., 2011). Satisfaction within the relationship is likely bidirectional in that a poor relationship can contribute to a woman's ED as a means of gaining control of her situation. On the other hand, an ED can put a strain on the relationship due to the stress of these disorders and the impact they can have on the health of both the mother and the baby.

Social support may also influence body image concerns and disordered eating behaviors among women without a history of an ED. In particular, high relationship satisfaction and social support in early pregnancy were associated with lower shape concerns between early-mid and mid-late pregnancy (Baskin et al., 2021). It is important to note that, in this study, anxiety played an interesting role. In early pregnancy, individuals with low anxiety and high relationship satisfaction reported decreased dietary restraint from early-mid to mid-late pregnancy. However, among individuals with high levels of anxiety, elevated relationship satisfaction in early-mid-pregnancy was actually associated with increased dietary restraint throughout pregnancy (Baskin et al., 2021). Some supportive partners may try to avoid conflict by ignoring the symptoms of disordered eating in their pregnant partner, which could lead to an increase in disordered eating (Baskin et al., 2021).

Furthermore, sociocultural pressure not just from the media but also from an individual's peers and family is related to both ED symptoms and pregnancy-related anxiety (Dryer et al., 2020). Fat talk partially mediates the relation between these variables, indicating that pressure from a pregnant woman's support system is intensified via the negative comments an individual makes about their own or others' bodies (Dryer et al., 2020). Overall, social support, partner support, and relationship satisfaction have been shown to be important to the health of pregnant individuals. With a supportive social environment, the stressors of pregnancy may be buffered; thus, EDs may be less likely to develop or worsen.

Relationship With the Fetus

A pregnant individual's relationship, attitudes, and attachment toward their developing fetus may affect the development of an ED. Gonçalves et al. (2015) established that poor attitudes toward the baby and pregnancy were both associated with higher levels of disordered eating ($r = .32$, $p = .001$). Similarly, pregnant Taiwanese individuals with a negative body image pregravid and in the third trimester scored lower in maternal–fetal attachment ($r = -0.20$, $p < 0.01$, for both relationships; Huang et al., 2004). Negative attitudes toward pregnancy were associated with an increase in disordered eating in early to mid-pregnancy (Baskin et al., 2020). In mid- to late pregnancy, maladaptive and negative attitudes toward motherhood were related to disordered eating via both depression and anxiety as mediators (Baskin et al., 2020). Pregnant individuals who struggle to create a connection with their developing baby may also struggle with their eating habits because they may have less acceptance of the necessity for weight gain during this critical period. Furthermore, women may use disordered eating as a means to cope with and regulate negative effects arising from a lack of connection with their growing fetus (Baskin et al., 2020). This is likely a bidirectional association, as disordered eating behaviors can leave women feeling less connected to the baby because there is a conflict between the pregnancy and the ED.

Therapist: How has the binge eating and purging affected your relationship with your partner?

Emily: It makes me feel more distant from my husband because I was trying to hide it from him. He realized what was going on when he came into the bedroom a few times in a week after I told him I was lying down to help with the nausea.

T: What did he do or say when he noticed what was happening?

E: He was trying to be really supportive. He knows that I had an eating disorder in high school and kind of in college.

T: What does he do to support you?

E: He tries to be kind when he sees me getting dressed in the morning—when it feels like nothing fits right now and I just feel fat. He asks how he can help me do something else after eating, so I don't go into the bathroom. But sometimes, I still feel judged by him. He doesn't say it, but I bet he does.

T: What does he do or say to indicate that?

E: He doesn't do anything overt, but I should be able to just stop binge eating and throwing up. I feel like I'm letting him down as a wife and the mother of our child. But it does help to know that he's trying his best to support me.

Assessment

There are a few existing guidelines for assessing EDs during pregnancy. Past research shows that the majority of OB/GYNs do not ask their patients directly about past or current history of disordered eating (Bannatyne et al., 2018). There are several barriers to assessing EDs during pregnancy. First, patients often feel uncomfortable disclosing ED symptoms to their providers. This could be for many reasons, including fear of stigmatization or because they may not want to engage in treatment. Furthermore, providers often do not feel comfortable bringing up the topic due to their own lack of training in EDs and poor existing resources for referrals if treatment is needed for their patients. Finally, there are no fully validated ED screening questionnaires for use during pregnancy, and the existing surveys may not be appropriate for use during this time due to symptom overlap between pregnancy and EDs, such as hyperemesis and vomiting as an inappropriate compensatory behavior after eating.

There has been debate about whether all pregnant individuals should be screened for EDs or if only those at the highest risk should be queried (Franko & Spurrell, 2000; Hawkins & Gottlieb, 2013; Dörsam et al., 2022). There are several warning signs that have been identified as possible flags for ED screening. These include history of an ED prior to pregnancy, lack of weight gain in two consecutive OB visits in the second trimester, hyperemesis gravidarum (particularly past the first trimester), signs of depression, and signs of dieting (Franko & Spurrell, 2000; Hawkins & Gottlieb, 2013). However, a more recent Delphi study found expert consensus that all pregnant persons should be screened for EDs at the beginning of their obstetric care (Bannatyne et al., 2018).

The field is less united around what ED screening measure(s) to use. The most common measure utilized in research for this population has been the Eating Disorder Examination (EDE), which is available as a questionnaire, EDE-Q (Fairburn & Beglin, 1994), or an interview (Fairburn et al., 2008). The EDE assesses both ED attitudes and behaviors, including items to diagnose AN, BN, BED, and several forms of OSFED. It also assesses four subscales of ED attitudes: restraint, eating concern, shape concern, and weight concern. The EDE-Q has not been validated specifically for pregnancy, and it is too long, with 28 items, to act as a brief ED screener in clinical practice. The EDE in its interview form has been validated for use in pregnancy (EDE-PV) among a sample of women with overweight or obesity (Emery et al., 2017). So, for research purposes, either the EDE in a questionnaire or interview form seems to be the most desirable, although more validation of these measures is needed.

The most commonly used clinical screening ED instrument is the SCOFF, a five-item questionnaire (the abbreviation letter corresponds to the symptom assessed in each item) designed to screen for AN and BN (Morgan et al., 1999). It contains the following items: (a) Do you make yourself Sick (vomit) because you feel uncomfortably full? (b) Do you worry that you have lost Control over how much you eat? (c) Have you lost more than One stone (15 lb) in a 3-month period? (d) Do you believe yourself to be Fat when others say you are too thin? and (e) Would you say that Food dominates your life? Historically, the SCOFF was recommended for use in pregnant persons as nothing else was available (Hawkins & Gottlieb, 2013), but it is evident that these items might not be appropriate during pregnancy. The first item may be denied in women with BN, as they could hide their symptoms behind hyperemesis gravidarum. Also, they may not be gaining sufficient weight but not losing, which would be worrisome. A modified six-item SCOFF was devised to address these issues (Dörsam et al., 2022). It broadens the reasons for vomiting and changes item 3 to focus on concerns about gestation weight gain. It also assesses recent low weight and history of purging behaviors. The current version, however, has low sensitivity and positive predictive value and needs further work for widespread use.

Finally, Claydon et al. (2022) are currently developing the Prenatal Eating Behaviors Screening (PEBS) tool. This is a 12-item screener developed from items from the EDE, SCOFF, and other validated ED surveys to assess for the presence of AN, BN, or BED. They validated the PEBS in subsamples in all three trimesters against the patients' self-report of lifetime or current ED diagnosis with acceptable sensitivity and specificity. Women who scored a total of 39 points or more on the PEBS were about 16 times more likely to have an ED diagnosis than women who scored lower. However, validation against a diagnostic interview or tool is needed as a next step.

OB/GYN: Emily, thank you for completing the paperwork for today's visit. Can we discuss your answers to these questions?

Emily: Sure, that's fine.

O: It seems here from your responses that you may have had a history of an ED? Perhaps bulimia?

E: Yes, it started in high school, and it's been kind of off and on during my life.

O: Okay, I appreciate that you told me that. It's important for me to know about your history to help me provide you with the best care during your pregnancy.

E: Sure. I don't really like to talk about it. Other doctors seem to judge me.

O: I understand that it is hard to discuss. It looks like from your answers here that you may have recently experienced some binge episodes, vomiting, and concerns about weight gain during pregnancy.

E:	Well, I do feel nauseous most of the day but then get hungry at night and overeat. I sometimes feel nauseous again afterward and vomit to get rid of that feeling. I also don't want to gain too much weight, especially over the recommendations we talked about in our last appointment.
O:	Yes, the nausea can be difficult to manage throughout the day. Can we talk about options to help you manage these behaviors and thoughts?
E:	Okay, I'm open to it.

Treatment

There are limited treatments that have been specifically developed to target body dissatisfaction and disordered eating behaviors in pregnant women. The management of these pathologies, therefore, may be more difficult in clinical settings. Researchers found that medical providers, such as OBGYN and fertility specialists, may not feel these behaviors lie within their clinical responsibility or expertise (Paslakis & de Zwaan, 2019). There are treatments, however, that can be considered when addressing body image and EDs during pregnancy.

Cognitive behavioral therapy (CBT) is the first-line treatment for many EDs. Fairburn's enhanced CBT (CBT-E) has shown superiority over interpersonal therapy for EDs (Fairburn et al., 2015). To our knowledge, no trials of CBT-E for pregnant women with EDs have been published. However, the premise that low self-esteem and body dissatisfaction can lead to restriction/dieting, promoting AN, or causing binge eating and purging in the case of BN can apply to EDs during pregnancy. This active, present-focused therapy would target the ED attitudes and beliefs while also establishing improved eating behaviors to prevent restriction, OBEs, and compensatory behaviors. Examples of Socratic questioning, an essential therapeutic method in CBT, are embedded in the case example dialogues.

The Body Project (Stice et al., 2000) is an intervention based on the dual-pathway model of EDs (Stice, 1994). According to this model, sociocultural pressures to be thin lead to thin-ideal internationalization, thus resulting in increased body dissatisfaction, unhealthy weight control behaviors, and negative affect. The Body Project uses a dissonance-based approach to explore the negative consequences of following the thin ideal with verbal, written, and behavioral exercises (Becker & Stice, 2017). By engaging in these exercises, participants generate ideas, attitudes, and behaviors counter to the thin ideal, which decreases its internalization. It is based on the principle that one's thoughts and behaviors must align, and, if they do not, one aspect (i.e., either thoughts or behaviors) must shift to meet the other. Therefore, when participants in the Body Project start to think counter to the thin ideal in the exercises, then their behaviors will start to align with this new way of thinking. The intervention has evolved over time from being a researcher-led program into a peer-led treatment that has adopted a "train the trainer" approach to increase dissemination. The Body Project intervention has also been implemented internationally, including in the United States, Canada, Mexico, and Latin America (Becker & Stice, 2017).

One study aimed to understand the best ways to adapt the Body Project intervention for women in the perinatal and postpartum periods (Vanderkruik et al., 2022). Participants in their study were either pregnant or within one year postpartum, and 55% of the sample reported dissatisfaction with their body image during and/or after their pregnancy. Approximately 80% of the sample indicated that they would have appreciated the opportunity to participate in a program focused on body acceptance or expectations of body changes in pregnancy or postpartum, which suggests a high need. These women identified themes that would be helpful in an intervention, including (a) "help accepting body changes," (b) "focus on nutrition/healthy living," (c) "peer support," (d) "learning what changes to expect," and (e) "education." They also reported themes or topics that would have likely assisted them in accepting or being more comfortable with body changes in pregnancy and postpartum: (a) "more realistic perinatal bodies in the media," (b) "setting realistic expectations," (c) "placing less pressure on appearance," (d) "normalizing different sizes and body changes," and (e) "celebrating pregnancy." The authors of this study indicated that many of these themes overlap or are already central in the Body Project, which makes it a viable option to adapt this intervention for perinatal and postpartum women.

Another pilot study aimed to use a self-compassion-based intervention to improve body image during the perinatal and postpartum periods (Papini et al., 2022). The three-week self-compassion meditation program focused on improving body shame, body dissatisfaction, body appreciation, and self-compassion, compared to a waitlist control group. The authors found that the intervention group reported significantly reduced body shame and body dissatisfaction, as well as significantly improved body appreciation and self-compassion, relative to women in the control group. Of note, however, most participants identified as White women, indicating that research is needed in diverse samples. Attrition was roughly 39%, and women who reported higher body dissatisfaction and lower physical activity at baseline were more likely to drop out as compared to participants with lower body dissatisfaction and higher physical activity at baseline. Factors for this attrition were not clear; additional research is required to demonstrate that a self-compassion meditation-based treatment is effective for pregnant women.

Clinical recommendations for providers who are working with pregnant or fertility clinic patients who have an ED have also been proposed (Paslakis & de Zwaan, 2019). First, they emphasize the need for improved medical training for these providers to increase awareness of and ability to assess ED symptoms. This training would allow for more open discussions about EDs and behaviors with women who identify any history (either acute or lifetime). The recommendations also challenged providers to assess their own attitudes toward weight, BMI, and EDs to reflect upon if/how these experiences may influence communication about these topics with patients.

Recommendations from other sources suggest that more frequent visits, particularly up to 16 weeks, may be warranted due to the increased risk for hyperemesis (Harris, 2010). These visits can be used to monitor disordered eating behaviors and provide psychoeducation about pregnancy-related symptoms that may overlap with an ED, such as nausea and vomiting, and discuss plans to reduce the risk of triggering ED symptoms (Harris, 2010). Other topics may include increasing awareness of bodily sensations, given that women with EDs may have learned to ignore certain cues such as hunger; education about the relationship between nutrition and bodily functioning; meal planning for adequate nutrition; the utility of food records (and discussion if it will facilitate meeting nutritional needs or trigger disordered eating); risk and appropriate treatment for constipation among women with a history of excessive laxative use; assessment of the use of herbal or over-the-counter weight loss supplements, which have largely not been tested in pregnant people; and signs of preterm labor due to the greater risk in the ED population (Harris, 2010).

Researchers have also emphasized the importance of building a multidisciplinary team that involves mental health professionals for consultation, assessment, and treatment needs during the peripartum period. This type of treatment team not only can benefit those with clinical diagnoses of an ED but may also provide support to all women who experience body image disturbance, stress, and/or emotional changes during this major life transition.

Therapist: You've said previously that the changes to your body that you've experienced during pregnancy have been really distressing and tied to your binge eating and purging.

Emily: Yes, it almost consumes my day since I can't get away from my body. My clothes are no longer fitting, especially my pants, so I have to wear maternity pants now. This experience of having a big stomach that I can't control was like my worst nightmare when I was younger.

T: You said it was your worst nightmare when you were younger; how about now?

E: Well, I don't like that my stomach is getting bigger, and my pants are uncomfortable—and I'm just starting to show, so my grandmother just says I just look like I'm getting a belly—but I know it's my growing baby, so it makes it a little better.

T: When you notice your belly or that your pants are uncomfortable, what are you thinking about?

E: I think that people view me as lazy, or I can't control myself. That others are judging me and won't accept me.

The treatment of pica must also incorporate any medical or psychological comorbidities, including complications from persistent digestion of toxic substances. The role of culture must be considered with pica given that, in certain cultures, ingestion of substances, such as clay, may be viewed as related to fertility and reproductivity (Bhatia & Kaur, 2014). Women can be counseled on the effects of consuming nonfood substances. Previous authors have emphasized the importance of using nonjudgmental language when assessing and treating pica. Women whose pica may be associated with a nutritional deficiency, such as iron (anemia), could be treated with iron supplements, if clinically appropriate, which may resolve the cravings (Corbett et al., 2003).

T: Okay, I wonder if we can try an exercise together to reshape these thoughts about your pregnant body and the thoughts of what your body says about you as a person. Would that be okay?

E: Sure.

T: When you have this internal dialogue—and most times these thoughts might be automatic for us—what feelings or emotions does it bring up?

E: I feel unattractive, incapable, like a bad person, and that I don't know why my husband is with me if I look this way.

T: It sounds like it doesn't feel good.

E: No definitely not. I feel really bad when these negative thoughts about my body come up, and it makes me want to purge after my next meal or maybe not eat as much.

T: So there is a cost to "buying into" these thoughts about yourself?

E: Yeah, I guess there's a big consequence to focusing on these thoughts.

T: Okay, so maybe let's write down these thoughts that you have about yourself when you think about your pregnant body or have trouble with your clothing.

E: Okay.

T: Right, so let's imagine that you have a friend who is also 15 weeks pregnant. Do you think that you would think those thoughts about her or say those things to her?

E: Absolutely not!

T: Why not?

E: Because it would make her feel bad, and I don't think I would have those thoughts about a friend. Her body is literally growing a baby, which is quite amazing.

T: So why be so harsh on yourself if you're in the same situation?

E: I don't know. It's so automatic, and I know others are probably thinking those negative things about me.

T: If you wouldn't say those statements to your friend, what would you tell her if she confided in you that she's having trouble with her body changes?

E: I think I would tell her I completely understand and also that she doesn't have control over her body right now—her body is growing a little human being. I would probably ask if I can help or support her in some way.

T: And what if she pushed back and said "No, you're just trying to be nice. You have to say those nice things to me. People just think I'm lazy and can't control myself. Have you seen the pictures of mothers in the maternity stores and online, looking so cute? I don't look like that at all."

E: I would tell her, "I don't think that about you, and I don't think others do either. Plus, I'm almost positive that those pictures in the stores are photoshopped—those women might not even be pregnant! The store wants us to feel bad about ourselves so we think that buying their products and clothes will magically make us feel better."

T: When you have negative thoughts about your body, have you ever pushed back on these thoughts like this? Or questioned the messages you're getting from society, like the advertisements or social media posts, like you would do with your friend?

E: No. I guess I never thought to.

T: After challenging those negative thoughts in your friend's situation, what are you thinking about or feeling?

E: I'm thinking that maybe I'm not alone in feeling this way, if other women might be feeling that too, and that the media puts our unrealistic images of what pregnancy "should" look like. I feel a bit less pressure on myself to look that way.

Cultural Considerations

There is a clear dearth in the literature focusing specifically on the cultural aspects in the prenatal period that may influence disordered eating and disturbed body image. Research has indicated, however, that multiple identity factors may influence these pathologies.

This section reviews salient cultural considerations for EDs, including racial and ethnic background, socioeconomic status (SES), and cultural aspects specifically related to pica. Failing to consider these factors then would impact assessment, treatment, and prevention efforts.

Racial and Ethnic Background

There is limited research examining racial and ethnic differences in eating pathology and body image disturbances in the perinatal period. In the general (nonperinatal) literature, there are studies that show larger body ideals among Black/African American women compared to White women ($p = .005$; Gluck & Geliebter, 2002), which may influence body image during pregnancy. ED symptom presentation may also vary by racial and/or ethnic background. Some research has found more frequent binge-eating episodes among Black individuals than among Whites and Latinos, whereas others have found that White women indicated an earlier age of onset for binge-eating and dieting behaviors compared to Black women (Rodgers et al., 2018). Research has also indicated that symptom distress and/or impairment was highest among Latino and Native American participants (compared to other groups), but Latino and Native Americans were less likely to be referred for further evaluation as compared to their White counterparts (Latino: $OR = .603$, $p = .0035$; Native American: $OR = .54$, $p = .04$; Becker et al., 2003). Acculturative stress experienced in minority populations may also contribute to disordered eating (Rodgers et al., 2018).

Socioeconomic Status

Disparities between high and low SES can affect the manifestation of disturbed body image and disordered eating, although there is limited research in pregnancy. "Downward social trajectory" in multiparous women was associated with experiencing body dissatisfaction, whereas researchers did not find any significant results regarding SES in relation to body satisfaction for primiparous women (Henriques et al., 2015). Among adolescents, body dissatisfaction was related to almost a threefold greater risk of developing binge eating in a high-SES group, whereas body dissatisfaction was not significantly associated with binge eating in a low-SES comparison group ($RR = 2.6$, $RR = 1.0$, respectively, interaction $p < .01$; West et al., 2019). Food insecurity, however, was related to BEDs in these low-SES adolescents ($RR = 1.4$). Food insecurity is consistently associated (in cross-sectional studies) with binge eating, compensatory behaviors, BED, and BN (Hazzard et al., 2020). Food assistance programs that aim to increase food access, or experiences of living paycheck-to-paycheck, may actually exacerbate eating disturbances. The benefits provide a month's worth of food at the beginning of the month and/or larger amounts of food are purchased when a paycheck is received, which may increase food consumption in the earlier parts of the month. This pattern subsequently results in food restriction by the end of the month after the food supply has been consumed (Hazzard et al., 2020). In pregnant populations, food insecurity can lead to a multitude of negative health outcomes including disordered eating (Laraia et al., 2015) and thinness or malnutrition when at higher levels of severity (Demétrio et al., 2020). Few interventions targeted for food insecurity during pregnancy exist (McKay et al., 2022; Merchant et al., 2023).

Pica

Pica appears to have a heightened prevalence in certain communities, affecting Latinx and African populations most commonly (Fawcett et al., 2016; Lin et al., 2014). Research regarding perceptions of pica is mixed. Some research stresses the necessity of prevention and treatment due to potential negative health outcomes (Jackson et al., 2020; Traugott et al., 2019), whereas other research highlights the cultural aspects of pica (Bhatia & Kaur, 2014; Huebl et al., 2016). In certain cultures, pica is viewed as a custom or culturally appropriate practice rather than a form of psychopathology (Bhatia & Kaur, 2014). For instance, in some rural areas of India, mud, clay, and ash, among other substances, are thought to be positive for health and spiritual practice (Bhatia & Kaur, 2014). Some places in Northern India use cravings for substances to predict the sex of the baby, with women who crave ash believed to be pregnant with a girl and those who want dust will have a boy (Bhatia & Kaur, 2014). Among "Chagga" women in Africa, consumption of soil is related to fertility and reproduction, and eating mud is believed to increase blood flow to the fetus. Women who do not adhere to these cultural traditions may be viewed negatively by their community (Bhatia & Kaur, 2014). It is important, therefore, to be sensitive to the cultural factors that may be influencing pica and include questions related to cultural customs and expectations during assessment. Treatment should aim to reduce potential harm to the fetus (if indicated by the substance(s) ingested) while allowing women to honor their cultural practices. Overall, it is encouraged that investigators consider the ways in which individuals' multifaceted backgrounds affect ED and negative body image pathology in prenatal populations.

T: How do your family's views about pregnancy influence your thoughts and feelings about your body?

E: My mother and grandmother encourage me to eat enough "for two" and this feels overwhelming. I see how they want me to eat foods that they consider comfort foods, such as tortillas, rice, and beans, but I am worried that I will gain too much weight if I have them regularly.

T: How do you respond when they make these comments?

E: I usually just try to get out of eating them by distracting them or bringing my own food. Then I feel guilty.

T: Do you like these foods? Would you want to eat them if you did not fear weight gain?

E: Yes.

T: How might you consider eating them in moderation, if you like them and they are providing some nutritional value? Is there something in between "eating for two" and avoiding them altogether?

E: I suppose that depriving myself of them might be setting me up to want them more later in the day when I end up losing control over my eating. I could try having them in a reasonable portion at a meal so that I can feel more "normal" and not have to restrict myself.

Conclusion and Future Directions

Body image and EDs are essential to address during pregnancy. These disordered thoughts and behaviors can significantly impact the woman and fetus, as well as other relationships in her life. It is important for providers to have knowledge about the risk factors that may predispose women to these disordered experiences, as well as correlates that may exacerbate psychopathology. Even women without a clinical diagnosis of an ED can be affected by poor body image and disordered eating behaviors. Therefore, assessment and treatment are essential to support women during pregnancy, with consideration of salient cultural considerations to improve patient–provider interactions and outcomes.

Although there is research to indicate the importance of body image and EDs to pregnancy experiences, future research is urgently needed in multiple domains specifically within pregnant populations. Studies should continue to clarify the risk factors and correlates of body image and EDs in pregnancy, such as examining the distinct relationships between depression, anxiety, and EDs, investigating BMI and physical activity in relation to EDs and body image, and clarifying the associations between abuse and specific EDs.

Findings from these future investigations will inform the improvement of prevention and treatment programs. There are very few evidence-based and widely available treatments for body image disturbance and EDs during pregnancy. Researchers should focus attention on this special population given that effective treatment would likely improve the short- and long-term health and well-being of not only the mother but also the baby and their relationships. Researchers have considered options for adapting the Body Project for pregnant women or using a self-compassion-based meditation intervention; however, future validation of these treatments is needed, including among diverse racial/ethnic populations. Additional training of medical providers is needed to improve the assessment and care of pregnant patients with body image and/or eating disturbances. Providers are encouraged to reflect on their own opinions and views regarding BMI, EDs, and disordered body image and perhaps to question or reshape these perceptions, especially when they interfere with providing proper care and treatment.

Lastly, it is imperative for future research to investigate cultural factors influencing EDs and body image disturbance during the prenatal period. This line of research will provide a better understanding of the multitude of factors that contribute to the development and/or maintenance of pathology. Intersectionality of identities should also be considered given that many women may have multiple minority statuses, and each person's combination of identities requires a personalized care approach.

References

Allison, K. C., Wrotniak, B. H., Paré, E., & Sarwer, D. B. (2012). Psychosocial characteristics and gestational weight change among overweight. *African American Pregnant Women: Obstetrics and Gynecology International, 2012*, 1–9. https://doi.org/10.1155/2012/878607

American Psychiatric Association. (1994). *Diagnostic and statistical manual of mental disorders – Fourth edition*. American Psychiatric Association.

American Psychiatric Association. (2013). *Diagnostic and statistical manual of mental disorders – Fifth edition*. American Psychiatric Association. https://doi.org/10.1176/appi.books.9780890425596

Angélica Nunes, M., Poyastro Pinheiro, A., Feliciati Hoffmann, J., & Inês Schmidt, M. (2014). Eating disorders symptoms in pregnancy and postpartum: A prospective study in a disadvantaged population in Brazil. *International Journal of Eating Disorders, 47*(4), 426–430. https://doi.org/10.1002/eat.22236

Arnold, C., Johnson, H., Mahon, C., & Agius, M. (2019). The effects of eating disorders in pregnancy on mother and baby: A review. *Psychiatria Danubina, 31*(Suppl 3), 615–618.

Bannatyne, A. J., Hughes, R., Stapleton, P., Watt, B., & MacKenzie-Shalders, K. (2018). Consensus on the assessment of disordered eating in pregnancy: An international Delphi study. *Archives of Women's Mental Health, 21*(4), 383–390. https://doi.org/10.1007/s00737-017-0806-x

Barasa, N., & Kinuthia, D. L. N. (2018). Views of young expectant women aged 16–35 years regarding their psychological body changes during pregnancy and their influence on -maternity wear selection. *International Journal of Sciences, 42*(3), 47–55.

Baskin, R., Meyer, D., & Galligan, R. (2020). Psychosocial factors, mental health symptoms, and disordered eating during pregnancy. *International Journal of Eating Disorders*, *53*(6), 873–882. https://doi.org/10.1002/eat.23264

Baskin, R., Meyer, D., & Galligan, R. (2021). Predicting the change in perinatal disordered eating symptoms: An examination of psychosocial factors. *Body Image*, *37*, 162–171. https://doi.org/10.1016/j.bodyim.2021.02.002

Becker, A. E., Franko, D. L., Speck, A., & Herzog, D. B. (2003). Ethnicity and differential access to care for eating disorder symptoms. *International Journal of Eating Disorders*, *33*(2), 205–212. https://doi.org/10.1002/eat.10129

Becker, C. B., & Stice, E. (2017). From efficacy to effectiveness to broad implementation: Evolution of the body project. *Journal of Consulting and Clinical Psychology*, *85*(8), 767–782. https://doi.org/10.1037/ccp0000204

Bhatia, M. S., & Kaur, J. (2014). Pica as a culture bound syndrome. *Delhi Psychiatry Journal*, *17*(1), 144–147.

Brunton, P. J., & Russell, J. A. (2008). The expectant brain: Adapting for motherhood. *Nature Reviews Neuroscience*, *9*(1), Article 1. https://doi.org/10.1038/nrn2280

Bulik, C. M., Von Holle, A., Hamer, R., Knoph Berg, C., Torgersen, L., Magnus, P., . . . Reichborn-Kjennerud, T. (2007). Patterns of remission, continuation and incidence of broadly defined eating disorders during early pregnancy in the Norwegian Mother and Child Cohort Study (MoBa). *Psychological Medicine*, *37*(8), 1109–1118. https://doi.org/10.1017/S0033291707000724

Centers for Disease Control and Prevention. (2022, June 13). *Weight gain during pregnancy*. www.cdc.gov/reproductivehealth/maternalinfanthealth/pregnancy-weight-gain.htm

Chan, C. Y., Lee, A. M., Koh, Y. W., Lam, S. K., Lee, C. P., Leung, K. Y., & Tang, C. S. K. (2019). Course, risk factors, and adverse outcomes of disordered eating in pregnancy. *International Journal of Eating Disorders*, *52*(6), 652–658. https://doi.org/10.1002/eat.23065

Chang, S. R., Chao, Y. M., & Kenney, N. J. (2006). I am a woman and I'm pregnant: Body image of women in Taiwan during the third trimester of pregnancy. *Birth*, *33*(2), 147–153. https://doi.org/10.1111/j.0730-7659.2006.00087.x

Charbonneau, K. D., & Seabrook, J. A. (2019). Adverse birth outcomes associated with types of eating disorders: A review. *Canadian Journal of Dietetic Practice and Research*, *80*(3), 131–136. https://doi.org/10.3148/cjdpr-2018-044\

Clark, A., Skouteris, H., Wertheim, E. H., Paxton, S. J., & Milgrom, J. (2009). My baby body: A qualitative insight into women's body-related experiences and mood during pregnancy and the postpartum. *Journal of Reproductive and Infant Psychology*, *27*(4), 330–345. https://doi.org/10.1080/02646830903190904

Claydon, E. A., Davidov, D. M., Zullig, K. J., Lilly, C. L., Cottrell, L., & Zerwas, S. C. (2018). Waking up every day in a body that is not yours: A qualitative research inquiry into the intersection between eating disorders and pregnancy. *BMC Pregnancy and Childbirth*, *18*(1), 463. https://doi.org/10.1186/s12884-018-2105-6

Claydon, E. A., Lilly, C. L., Ceglar, J. X., & Dueñas-Garcia, O. F. (2022). Development and validation across trimester of the prenatal eating behaviors screening tool. *Archives of Women's Mental Health*, *25*(4), 705–716. https://doi.org/10.1007/s00737-022-01230-y

Corbett, R. W., Ryan, C., & Weinrich, S. P. (2003). Pica in pregnancy: Does it affect pregnancy outcomes? *MCN: The American Journal of Maternal/Child Nursing*, *28*(3), 183.

Coyne, S. M., Liechty, T., Collier, K. M., Sharp, A. D., Davis, E. J., & Kroff, S. L. (2018). The effect of media on body image in pregnant and postpartum women. *Health Communication*, *33*(7), 793–799. https://doi.org/10.1080/10410236.2017.1314853

Crow, S. J., Agras, W. S., Crosby, R., Halmi, K., & Mitchell, J. E. (2008). Eating disorder symptoms in pregnancy: A prospective study. *International Journal of Eating Disorders*, *41*(3), 277–279. https://doi.org/10.1002/eat.20496

Dellava, J. E., Von Holle, A., Torgersen, L., Reichborn-Kjennerud, T., Haugen, M., Meltzer, H. M., & Bulik, C. M. (2011). Dietary supplement use immediately before and during pregnancy in Norwegian women with eating disorders. *International Journal of Eating Disorders*, *44*(4), 325–332. https://doi.org/10.1002/eat.20831

Demétrio, F., Teles, C. A. D. S., Santos, D. B. D., & Pereira, M. (2020). Food insecurity in pregnant women is associated with social determinants and nutritional outcomes: A systematic review and meta-analysis. *Ciência & Saúde Coletiva*, *25*, 2663–2676. https://doi.org/10.1590/1413-81232020257.24202018

Dörsam, A. F., Bye, A., Graf, J., Howard, L. M., Throm, J. K., Müller, M., . . . Giel, K. E. (2022). Screening instruments for eating disorders in pregnancy: Current evidence, challenges, and future directions. *International Journal of Eating Disorders, 55*(9), 1208–1218. https://doi.org/10.1002/eat.23780

Dörsam, A. F., Preißl, H., Micali, N., Lörcher, S. B., Zipfel, S., & Giel, K. E. (2019). The impact of maternal eating disorders on dietary intake and eating patterns during pregnancy: A systematic review. *Nutrients, 11*(4), 840. https://doi.org/10.3390/nu11040840

Dryer, R., Graefin von der Schulenburg, I., & Brunton, R. (2020). Body dissatisfaction and fat talk during pregnancy: Predictors of distress. *Journal of Affective Disorders, 267*, 289–296. https://doi.org/10.1016/j.jad.2020.02.031

Earle, S. (2003). "Bumps and boobs": Fatness and women's experiences of pregnancy. *Women's Studies International Forum, 26*(3), 245–252. https://doi.org/10.1016/S0277-5395(03)00054-2

Easter, A., Bye, A., Taborelli, E., Corfield, F., Schmidt, U., Treasure, J., & Micali, N. (2013). Recognising the symptoms: How common are eating disorders in pregnancy? *European Eating Disorders Review, 21*(4), 340–344. https://doi.org/10.1002/erv.2229

Easter, A., Solmi, F., Bye, A., Taborelli, E., Corfield, F., Schmidt, U., Treasure, J., & Micali, N. (2015). Antenatal and postnatal psychopathology among women with current and past eating disorders: Longitudinal patterns. *European Eating Disorders Review, 23*(1), 19–27. https://doi.org/10.1002/erv.2328

Emery, R. L., Grace, J. L., Kolko, R. P., & Levine, M. D. (2017). Adapting the eating disorder examination for use during pregnancy: Preliminary results from a community sample of women with overweight and obesity. *International Journal of Eating Disorders, 50*(5), 597–601. https://doi.org/10.1002/eat.22646

Fairburn, C. G., Bailey-Straebler, S., Basden, S., Doll, H. A., Jones, R., Murphy, R., . . . Cooper, Z. (2015). A transdiagnostic comparison of enhanced Cognitive Behaviour Therapy (CBT-E) and interpersonal psychotherapy in the treatment of eating disorders. *Behaviour Research and Therapy, 70*, 64–71.

Fairburn, C. G., & Beglin, S. J. (1994). Assessment of eating disorders: Interview or self-report questionnaire? *International Journal of Eating Disorders, 16*(4), 363–370. https://doi.org/10.1002/1098-108X(199412)16:4<363::AID-EAT2260160405>3.0.CO;2-#

Fairburn, C. G., Cooper, Z., & O'Connor, M. (2008). Eating disorder examination (Edition 16.0 D). *Cognitive Behavior Therapy and Eating Disorders*, 265–308.

Fawcett, E. J., Fawcett, J. M., & Mazmanian, D. (2016). A meta-analysis of the worldwide prevalence of pica during pregnancy and the postpartum period. *International Journal of Gynecology & Obstetrics, 133*(3), 277–283. https://doi.org/10.1016/j.ijgo.2015.10.012

Franko, D. L., & Spurrell, E. B. (2000). Detection and management of eating disorders during pregnancy. *Obstetrics & Gynecology, 95*(6, Part 1), 942–946. https://doi.org/10.1016/S0029-7844(00)00792-4

Galali, Y. M. (2020). Study the prevalence, characteristics of mothers and associated risk factors of pica eating among pregnant women. *Cihan University-Erbil Scientific Journal, 4*(2), Article 2. https://doi.org/10.24086/cuesj.v4n2y2020.pp19-24

Gluck, M. E., & Geliebter, A. (2002). Racial/ethnic differences in body image and eating behaviors. *Eating Behaviors, 3*(2), 143–151. https://doi.org/10.1016/S1471-0153(01)00052-6

Gonçalves, S., Freitas, F., Freitas-Rosa, M. A., & Machado, B. C. (2015). Dysfunctional eating behaviour, psychological well-being and adaptation to pregnancy: A study with women in the third trimester of pregnancy. *Journal of Health Psychology, 20*(5), 535–542. https://doi.org/10.1177/1359105315573432

Grogan, S. (2021). *Understanding body dissatisfaction in men, women and children* (4th ed.). Routledge. https://doi.org/10.4324/9781003100041

Harris, A. A. (2010). Practical advice for caring for women with eating disorders during the perinatal period. *Journal of Midwifery & Women's Health, 55*(6), 579–586. https://doi.org/10.1016/j.jmwh.2010.07.008

Hawkins, L. K., & Gottlieb, B. R. (2013). Screening for eating disorders in pregnancy: How uniform screening during a high-risk period could minimize under-recognition. *Journal of Women's Health, 22*(4), 390–392. https://doi.org/10.1089/jwh.2013.4313

Hazzard, V. M., Loth, K. A., Hooper, L., & Becker, C. B. (2020). Food insecurity and eating disorders: A review of emerging evidence. *Current Psychiatry Reports, 22*(12), 74. https://doi.org/10.1007/s11920-020-01200-0

Henriques, A., Alves, L., Alves, E., Silva, S., Barros, H., & Azevedo, A. (2015). Social trajectory and body image satisfaction in childbearing women. *Maternal and Child Health Journal*, *19*(6), 1237–1244. https://doi.org/10.1007/s10995-014-1629-2

Hodgkinson, E. L., Smith, D. M., & Wittkowski, A. (2014). Women's experiences of their pregnancy and postpartum body image: A systematic review and meta-synthesis. *BMC Pregnancy and Childbirth*, *14*, 330. https://doi.org/10.1186/1471-2393-14-330

Holland, G., & Tiggemann, M. (2016). A systematic review of the impact of the use of social networking sites on body image and disordered eating outcomes. *Body Image*, *17*, 100–110. https://doi.org/10.1016/j.bodyim.2016.02.008

Huang, H.-C., Wang, S.-Y., & Chen, C.-H. (2004). Body image, maternal-fetal attachment, and choice of infant feeding method: A study in Taiwan. *Birth*, *31*(3), 183–188. https://doi.org/10.1111/j.0730-7659.2004.00303.x

Huebl, L., Leick, S., Guettl, L., Akello, G., & Kutalek, R. (2016). Geophagy in northern Uganda: Perspectives from consumers and clinicians. *American Journal of Tropical Medicine and Hygiene*, *95*(6), 1440–1449. https://doi.org/10.4269/ajtmh.15-0579

Jackson, M. S., Adedoyin, A. C., & Winnick, S. N. (2020). Pica disorder among African American women: A call for action and further research. *Social Work in Public Health*, *35*(5), 261–270. https://doi.org/10.1080/19371918.2020.1791778

Kiani-Sheikhabadi, M., Beigi, M., & Mohebbi-Dehnavi, Z. (2019). The relationship between perfectionism and body image with eating disorder in pregnancy. *Journal of Education and Health Promotion*, *8*, 242. https://doi.org/10.4103/jehp.jehp_58_19

Knoph Berg, C., Bulik, C. M., Von Holle, A., Torgersen, L., Hamer, R., Sullivan, P., & Reichborn-Kjennerud, T. (2008). Psychosocial factors associated with broadly defined bulimia nervosa during early pregnancy: Findings from the Norwegian mother and child cohort study. *Australian & New Zealand Journal of Psychiatry*, *42*(5), 396–404. https://doi.org/10.1080/00048670801961149

Knoph Berg, C., Torgersen, L., Von Holle, A., Hamer, R. M., Bulik, C. M., & Reichborn-Kjennerud, T. (2011). Factors associated with binge eating disorder in pregnancy. *International Journal of Eating Disorders*, *44*(2), 124–133. https://doi.org/10.1002/eat.20797

Knoph, C., Von Holle, A., Zerwas, S., Torgersen, L., Tambs, K., Stoltenberg, C., . . . Reichborn-Kjennerud, T. (2013). Course and predictors of maternal eating disorders in the postpartum period. *International Journal of Eating Disorders*, *46*(4), 355–368. https://doi.org/10.1002/eat.22088

Konlan, K. D., Abdulai, J. A., Konlan, K. D., Amoah, R. M., & Doat, A. (2020). Practices of pica among pregnant women in a tertiary healthcare facility in Ghana. *Nursing Open*, *7*(3), 783–792. https://doi.org/10.1002/nop2.451

Koubaa, S., Hällström, T., Brismar, K., Hellström, P. M., & Hirschberg, A. L. (2015). Biomarkers of nutrition and stress in pregnant women with a history of eating disorders in relation to head circumference and neurocognitive function of the offspring. *BMC Pregnancy and Childbirth*, *15*, 318. https://doi.org/10.1186/s12884-015-0741-7

Lacey, E. P. (1990). Broadening the perspective of pica: Literature review. *Public Health Reports*, *105*(1), 29–35.

Lacey, J. H., & Smith, G. (1987). Bulimia nervosa: The impact of pregnancy on mother and baby. *British Journal of Psychiatry*, *150*(6), 777–781. https://doi.org/10.1192/bjp.150.6.777

Lai, B.-Y., Tang, C.-K., & Tse, W.-L. (2005). Prevalence and psychosocial correlates of disordered eating among Chinese pregnant women in Hong Kong. *Eating Disorders*, *13*(2), 171–186. https://doi.org/10.1080/10640260590918991

Laraia, B., Vinikoor-Imler, L. C., & Siega-Riz, A. M. (2015). Food insecurity during pregnancy leads to stress, disordered eating, and greater postpartum weight among overweight women. *Obesity*, *23*(6), 1303–1311. https://doi.org/10.1002/oby.21075

Lemberg, R., & Phillips, J. (1989). The impact of pregnancy on anorexia nervosa and bulimia. *International Journal of Eating Disorders*, *8*(3), 285–295. https://doi.org/10.1002/1098-108X(198905)8:3<285::AID-EAT2260080304>3.0.CO;2-P

Lin, J. W., Temple, L., Trujillo, C., Mejia-Rodriquez, F., Rosas, L. G., Fernald, L., & Young, S. L. (2014). Pica during pregnancy among Mexican-born women: A formative study. *Maternal & Child Nutrition*, *11*(4), 550–558. https://doi.org/10.1111/mcn.12120

Linna, M. S., Raevuori, A., Haukka, J., Suvisaari, J. M., Suokas, J. T., & Gissler, M. (2014). Pregnancy, obstetric, and perinatal health outcomes in eating disorders. *American Journal of Obstetrics and Gynecology*, 211(4), 392.e1–392.e8. https://doi.org/10.1016/j.ajog.2014.03.067

Makino, M., Yasushi, M., & Tsutsui, S. (2020). The risk of eating disorder relapse during pregnancy and after delivery and postpartum depression among women recovered from eating disorders. *BMC Pregnancy and Childbirth*, 20(1), 323. https://doi.org/10.1186/s12884-020-03006-7

Martínez-Olcina, M., Rubio-Arias, J. A., Reche-García, C., Leyva-Vela, B., Hernández-García, M., Hernández-Morante, J. J., & Martínez-Rodríguez, A. (2020). Eating disorders in pregnant and breastfeeding women: A systematic review. *Medicina*, 56(7), 352.

Mazzeo, S. E., Slof-Op't Landt, M. C. T., Jones, I., Mitchell, K., Kendler, K. S., Neale, M. C., . . . Bulik, C. M. (2006). Associations among postpartum depression, eating disorders, and perfectionism in a population-based sample of adult women. *International Journal of Eating Disorders*, 39(3), 202–211. https://doi.org/10.1002/eat.20243

McKay, F. H., Spiteri, S., Zinga, J., Sulemani, K., Jacobs, S. E., Ranjan, N., . . . van der Pligt, P. (2022). Systematic review of interventions addressing food insecurity in pregnant women and new mothers. *Current Nutrition Reports*, 11(3), 486–499. https://doi.org/10.1007/s13668-022-00418-z

Mehta, U. J., Siega-Riz, A. M., & Herring, A. H. (2011). Effect of body image on pregnancy weight gain. *Maternal and Child Health Journal*, 15(3), 324–332. https://doi.org/10.1007/s10995-010-0578-7

Meltzer-Brody, S., Zerwas, S., Leserman, J., Holle, A. V., Regis, T., & Bulik, C. (2011). Eating disorders and trauma history in women with perinatal depression. *Journal of Women's Health*, 20(6), 863–870. https://doi.org/10.1089/jwh.2010.2360

Merchant, T., Soyemi, E., Roytman, M. V., DiTosto, J. D., Beestrum, M., Niznik, C. M., & Yee, L. M. (2023). Healthcare-based interventions to address food insecurity during pregnancy: A systematic review. *American Journal of Obstetrics & Gynecology MFM*, 5(5), 100884. https://doi.org/10.1016/j.ajogmf.2023.100884

Micali, N., Northstone, K., Emmett, P., Naumann, U., & Treasure, J. L. (2012). Nutritional intake and dietary patterns in pregnancy: A longitudinal study of women with lifetime eating disorders. *British Journal of Nutrition*, 108(11), 2093–2099. https://doi.org/10.1017/S0007114512000256

Micali, N., Simonoff, E., & Treasure, J. (2011). Pregnancy and post-partum depression and anxiety in a longitudinal general population cohort: The effect of eating disorders and past depression. *Journal of Affective Disorders*, 131(1), 150–157. https://doi.org/10.1016/j.jad.2010.09.034

Micali, N., Treasure, J., & Simonoff, E. (2007). Eating disorders symptoms in pregnancy: A longitudinal study of women with recent and past eating disorders and obesity. *Journal of Psychosomatic Research*, 63(3), 297–303. https://doi.org/10.1016/j.jpsychores.2007.05.003

Mingoia, J., Hutchinson, A. D., Wilson, C., & Gleaves, D. H. (2017). The relationship between social networking site use and the internalization of a thin ideal in females: A meta-analytic review. *Frontiers in Psychology*, 8. www.frontiersin.org/articles/10.3389/fpsyg.2017.0135

Morgan, J. F., Lacey, J. H., & Sedgwick, P. M. (1999). Impact of pregnancy on bulimia nervosa. *British Journal of Psychiatry*, 174, 135–140. https://doi.org/10.1192/bjp.174.2.135

Morgan, J. F., Reid, F., & Lacey, J. H. (1999). The SCOFF questionnaire: Assessment of a new screening tool for eating disorders. *British Medical Journal*, 319(7223), 1467–1468.

Nguyen, A. N., de Barse, L. M., Tiemeier, H., Jaddoe, V. W. V., Franco, O. H., Jansen, P. W., & Voortman, T. (2017). Maternal history of eating disorders: Diet quality during pregnancy and infant feeding. *Appetite*, 109, 108–114. https://doi.org/10.1016/j.appet.2016.11.030

Papini, N. M., Mason, T. B., Herrmann, S. D., & Lopez, N. V. (2022). Self-compassion and body image in pregnancy and postpartum: A randomized pilot trial of a brief self-compassion meditation intervention. *Body Image*, 43, 264–274. https://doi.org/10.1016/j.bodyim.2022.09.010

Paslakis, G., & de Zwaan, M. (2019). Clinical management of females seeking fertility treatment and of pregnant females with eating disorders. *European Eating Disorders Review*, 27(3), 215–223. https://doi.org/10.1002/erv.2667

Pullmer, R., Zaitsoff, S., & Cobb, R. (2018). Body satisfaction during pregnancy: The role of health-related habit strength. *Maternal and Child Health Journal*, 22(3), 391–400. https://doi.org/10.1007/s10995-017-2406-9

Rodgers, R. F., Berry, R., & Franko, D. L. (2018). Eating disorders in ethnic minorities: An update. *Current Psychiatry Reports*, 20(10), 90. https://doi.org/10.1007/s11920-018-0938-3

Rollero, C. (2015). "I know you are not real": Salience of photo retouching reduces the negative effects of media exposure via internalization. *Studia Psychologica, 57,* 195–202.

Sebastiani, G., Andreu-Fernández, V., Herranz Barbero, A., Aldecoa-Bilbao, V., Miracle, X., Meler Barrabes, E., . . . García-Algar, O. (2020). Eating disorders during gestation: Implications for mother's health, fetal outcomes, and epigenetic changes. *Frontiers in Pediatrics, 8.* www.frontiersin.org/articles/10.3389/fped.2020.00587

Siega-Riz, A. M., Haugen, M., Meltzer, H. M., Von Holle, A., Hamer, R., Torgersen, L., . . . Bulik, C. M. (2008). Nutrient and food group intakes of women with and without bulimia nervosa and binge eating disorder during pregnancy. *American Journal of Clinical Nutrition, 87*(5), 1346–1355.

Soares, R. M., Nunes, M. A., Schmidt, M. I., Giacomello, A., Manzolli, P., Camey, S., . . . Duncan, B. B. (2009). Inappropriate eating behaviors during pregnancy: Prevalence and associated factors among pregnant women attending primary care in southern Brazil. *International Journal of Eating Disorders, 42*(5), 387–393. https://doi.org/10.1002/eat.20643

Sollid, C., Clausen, L., & Maimburg, R. D. (2021). The first 20 weeks of pregnancy is a high-risk period for eating disorder relapse. *International Journal of Eating Disorders, 54*(12), 2132–2142. https://doi.org/10.1002/eat.23620

Stice, E. (1994). Review of the evidence for a sociocultural model of bulimia nervosa and an exploration of the mechanisms of action. *Clinical Psychology Review, 14*(7), 633–661. https://doi.org/10.1016/0272-7358(94)90002-7

Stice, E. (2001). A prospective test of the dual-pathway model of bulimic pathology: Mediating effects of dieting and negative affect. *Journal of Abnormal Psychology, 110*(1), 124–135.

Stice, E., Mazotti, L., Weibel, D., & Agras, W. S. (2000). Dissonance prevention program decreases thin-ideal internalization, body dissatisfaction, dieting, negative affect, and bulimic symptoms: A preliminary experiment. *International Journal of Eating Disorders, 27*(2), 206–217. https://doi.org/10.1002/(SICI)1098-108X(200003)27:2<206::AID-EAT9>3.0.CO;2-D

Tierney, S., McGlone, C., & Furber, C. (2013). What can qualitative studies tell us about the experiences of women who are pregnant that have an eating disorder? *Midwifery, 29*(5), 542–549. https://doi.org/10.1016/j.midw.2012.04.013

Traugott, M. T., Singh, M., Raj, D. K., & Kutalek, R. (2019). Geophagy in India: A qualitative exploratory study on motivation and perception of female consumers. *Transactions of the Royal Society of Tropical Medicine and Hygiene, 113*(3), 123–130. https://doi.org/10.1093/trstmh/try123

Ulman, T. F., Von Holle, A., Torgersen, L., Stoltenberg, C., Reichborn-Kjennerud, T., & Bulik, C. M. (2012). Sleep disturbances and binge eating disorder symptoms during and after pregnancy. *Sleep, 35*(10), 1403–1411. https://doi.org/10.5665/sleep.2124

Vanderkruik, R., Ellison, K., Kanamori, M., Freeman, M. P., Cohen, L. S., & Stice, E. (2022). Body dissatisfaction and disordered eating in the perinatal period: An underrecognized high-risk timeframe and the opportunity to intervene. *Archives of Women's Mental Health, 25*(4), 739–751. https://doi.org/10.1007/s00737-022-01236-6

West, C. E., Goldschmidt, A. B., Mason, S. M., & Neumark-Sztainer, D. (2019). Differences in risk factors for binge eating by socioeconomic status in a community-based sample of adolescents: Findings from project EAT. *International Journal of Eating Disorders, 52*(6), 659–668. https://doi.org/10.1002/eat.23079

Young, S. L. (2010). Pica in pregnancy: New ideas about an old condition. *Annual Review of Nutrition, 30,* 403–422. https://doi.org/10.1146/annurev.nutr.012809.104713

Zeeni, N., Abi Kharma, J., & Mattar, L. (2021). Social media use impacts body image and eating behavior in pregnant women. *Current Psychology.* https://doi.org/10.1007/s12144-021-01848-8

10

PRENATAL ALCOHOL AND DRUG MISUSE

Jacqueline Jacobs, Kelly Elliott, Tracy Moran Vozar, Lauren Gross, and Dakota Staren

"Olivia" began experimenting with substances when she was 12 years old. She started by taking a few pain pills from her mother's cabinet every once and a while before school. Olivia's use continued throughout middle school and high school. Over time, her use escalated to heroin and subsequently methamphetamines. She attempted to stop using at various points in her life, but each stint in treatment and attempt at sobriety left her feeling defeated, lonely, and more distressed. She was 19 years old when she learned she was pregnant. Her motivation to seek treatment was renewed. She was hesitant to reach out for services, fearing the shame, judgment, or legal ramifications she may face. Nonetheless, she decided to try. She reached out to numerous facilities in hopes they could support her in detoxing and enrolling in treatment. However, she struggled to find a facility that would accept her as she was considered "high risk" due to her pregnancy. The very concern that motivated her to seek treatment was the same issue disqualifying her from it. It took her nearly three months of searching and one month of waiting for an opening before she entered treatment.

Prevalence

Olivia's case is only one example of how substance use can occur in the prenatal period. In the United States and around the globe, prenatal substance use represents a public health crisis. In the United States between 2018 and 2020, 13.5% of pregnant people reported current drinking of alcohol, whereas 5.2% reported binge drinking in the past 30 days (Gosdin et al., 2022). These numbers represent slight increases from an earlier Centers for Disease Control and Prevention (CDC) dataset, spanning 2015 to 2017. In contrast, a systematic meta-analysis estimates that about 9.8% of pregnant people worldwide consume alcohol (in any amount) during their pregnancy (Popova et al., 2017). These researchers found that Europe had the highest rates of prenatal alcohol use (25.2%), followed by the Americas (11.2%), Africa (10.0%), and the Western Pacific region (8.6%). The lowest rates of alcohol use were in the Southeast Asian region (1.8%) and the Eastern Mediterranean region (0.2%).

DOI: 10.4324/9781003206903-13

Tobacco is another commonly used substance during pregnancy. In a 2016 U.S. sample, 7.2% of people who gave birth reported smoking cigarettes during pregnancy (Drake et al., 2018). In Australia, data from two public hospitals suggest that about 18.5% of pregnant people use tobacco during their pregnancy (Hotham et al., 2008). In 2018, England's National Health Service estimated that 10.4% of pregnant women were known smokers at the time of delivery (NHS, 2018). A study examining substance use in sub-Saharan Africa found that rates of prenatal tobacco use fluctuated greatly (Yaya et al., 2018). The highest rate of use was found in Madagascar (11%), whereas the lowest rates were in Zimbabwe, Cameroon, Ghana, Nigeria, and Togo (0.3%).

Cannabis use during pregnancy varies widely. In the United States, the use of cannabis overall has increased, as more states legalize its use for adults (Chang, 2020). CDC data from eight states found that 4.2% of the sample continued to use cannabis during pregnancy (Ko et al., 2020). However, there is considerable variability across states—the rate of continued use in Maine was 12.1%, whereas New York was 2.6%. Studies conducted in Australia, Canada, and France found rates of cannabis use ranged from 0.45% to 4.5% (Betts et al., 2022; Corsi et al., 2018; Hotham et al., 2008; Saurel-Cubizolles et al., 2014).

By examining hospital discharge data, the CDC found that rates of opioid use disorders in pregnant women have quadrupled between 1999 and 2014, from 1.5 per 1,000 delivery hospitalizations to 6.5 (Haight et al., 2018). In the 28 states with available data, rates of prenatal opioid use are rising; however, the speed of increase varies between states. Similarly, rates of opioid exposure were found to increase over time in a Canadian sample (Zhao et al., 2021). In 1998, fetuses in 3.6% of pregnancies were exposed to opioids, compared to 5.1% in 2011. A Spanish study found that 6.3% of infants tested positive for opiate metabolites (Pichini et al., 2005). In this study, the use of opiates was also associated with smoking tobacco, higher amounts of tobacco use, and using cannabis.

The use of stimulants (including cocaine, ecstasy, methamphetamines, and prescription stimulants) is also on the rise in the United States—among adults the lifetime prevalence rate is 29.2% (Smid et al., 2019). As rates of substance misuse rise nationally, similar patterns are seen in the pregnant population. In 2015, 3.4% of pregnant women reported using cocaine in the past month. Between 1988 and 2004, the number of pregnant women who were hospitalized for amphetamine doubled. A study examining the rates of exposure to illicit substances in newborns in Spain found that 3.1% of samples tested positive for cocaine, whereas 0.1% tested positive for methylenedioxymethamphetamine (MDMA; Pichini et al., 2005).

Understanding the rates of substance use in the prenatal population, both in the United States and internationally, presents a challenge for researchers for several reasons. First, methodological differences across studies often make it difficult to make accurate and appropriate comparisons. For example, some data are from large, population-based surveillance systems (e.g., Denny et al., 2019; Ko et al., 2020), whereas others sample specific groups. In addition, some studies are interested in the amount of substance use (e.g., distinguishing between light, moderate, and heavy alcohol consumption), whereas others ask if any amount of the substance has been used.

Moreover, the stigma around prenatal substance use poses another major barrier. Research has demonstrated that pregnant women consistently underreport substance use frequency and related concerns (Chang, 2020; Pichini et al., 2005). Bakhireva et al. (2021), suggested that the formatting and language used in screening questions may contribute to inconsistent reporting. For example, they found that targeted questions about the maximum number of drinks in a 24-hour period and the total number of drinks in the most recent drinking episode yielded higher estimates of alcohol use than more in-depth interviews. Although questions about the timing and frequency of alcohol use provide researchers with valuable data, they may also lead to overall underestimates of use, particularly binge use.

The reluctance to accurately report substance use is multiplied in areas where prenatal substance use has been criminalized (Chang, 2020). As of November 1, 2022, 24 states and the District of Colombia have laws that consider substance use during pregnancy to be child abuse, which can be used to push for termination of parental rights (Guttmacher Institute, 2022). In three states (i.e., Minnesota, South Dakota, and Wisconsin), prenatal substance use can be used as grounds for civil commitment, including involuntary admission for inpatient treatment. In 25 states and the District of Columbia, healthcare professionals are required by law to report any suspected substance use by a pregnant person. In eight of those states, there is an additional mandate to test for prenatal drug exposure in suspected cases. Concerns about legal ramifications discourage both pregnant people from disclosing substance use and physicians or researchers from asking. These types of laws not only make it difficult to accurately understand the scope of the problem but also frequently keep pregnant people who are using substances from prenatal and/or substance use care (Hui et al., 2017).

In addition, research on prenatal substance use is heavily skewed toward U.S. samples. Even in work that examines rates of prenatal substance use across countries, the United States is disproportionately represented. For example, in Singh et al.'s (2020) study examining the prevalence of prenatal cannabis use in high-income countries, 29 of the 41 studies were conducted in the United States. The next two best-represented nations were Australia and Canada, with three studies each. Little research on prenatal substance use has been conducted outside of Western, English-speaking countries. The research that does exist is a patchwork of studies that vary by substance and country, which makes it challenging to paint a full picture of how prenatal substance use varies around the world.

Correlates and Risk Factors

Olivia was primarily raised by her mother and maternal grandmother who both had substance use concerns. Olivia's childhood was steeped in chaos. She felt loved by her mother and grandmother, but their active substance abuse prevented them from caring for her in the way she needed. She recalled early memories of sitting on the floor of their shared bedroom playing, as they sat half asleep on the bed beside her. She developed symptoms of both anxiety and depression early in life. She recalled memories of meeting with a school counselor in the third grade due to their concerns about her well-being and mental health. Olivia started experimenting with substances when she was just 12 years old. She could not recall why she took her first pill. Was it to manage her anxiety and sadness, or did it just seem like what her family was doing around her?

Although it is challenging to accurately estimate prevalence rates across various substances and geographic regions, the literature shows moderate overlap across risk factors of prenatal substance use and correlates for mental health. However, the literature does not differentiate between risk factors (i.e., predictors) of substance use and correlates (i.e., co-occurring stressors) of substance use. Often, risk factor variables are retrospectively accounted for, and the same variables are interchangeably described as both risk factors and correlates across research

(Brown et al., 2019; Kennare et al., 2005; Vythilingum et al., 2012; Chasnoff et al., 2001; Havens et al., 2009; Hutchins & DiPietro, 1997; Jorda et al., 2021). Further complicating factors across research include the inclusion of some but not all types of substances used. The most common substances discussed in the literature include alcohol, tobacco, and cannabis (Brown et al., 2019; Kennare et al., 2005; Vythilingum et al., 2012; Chasnoff et al., 2001; Havens et al., 2009; Jorda et al., 2021). More research (including international samples) is needed to comprehensively assess risk factors across multiple time points for several substances. Given the limited research and international focus available on this topic, this review is a good-faith effort to provide information on precipitating and co-occurring factors of prenatal substance use.

A combination of psychiatric, social, and demographic factors often co-occur with alcohol, tobacco, cannabis, and illicit drug use during pregnancy. Across samples in Canada, Australia, South Africa, the United States, and Tribal Nations in the United States, psychiatric conditions, specifically depression, were found to be one of the strongest, if not the strongest, associated correlates of prenatal substance use (Brown et al., 2019; Kennare et al., 2005; Vythilingum et al., 2012; Chasnoff et al., 2001; Havens et al., 2009; Hutchins & DiPietro, 1997; Jorda et al., 2021). Anxiety also correlates positively with substance use during pregnancy (Brown et al., 2019). Accompanying prenatal mental health screening tools with substance use screeners may provide a more comprehensive screening approach in healthcare and mental health settings.

In addition, several social and demographic factors are associated with prenatal substance use across samples in Canada, Australia, the United States, and Tribal Nations in the United States, including young age, single or nonmarital status, living with someone or having a family member with substance use issues, less education low income, homelessness, residing in a metropolitan area, unstable housing, and inconsistent healthcare (Brown et al., 2019; Kennare et al., 2005; Chasnoff et al., 2001; Havens et al., 2009; Hutchins & DiPietro, 1997; Jorda et al., 2021). It is also important to note that prenatal substance use is related to use prior to pregnancy (e.g., periconceptual substance use) (Chasnoff et al., 2001; Vythilingum et al., 2012). Being aware of social and demographic correlates of prenatal substance use may provide opportunities to develop preventive and early intervention supports for individuals who may be at increased risk.

Racial and Ethnic Disparities: The Intersection Between Structural Racism and Prenatal Substance Use in the United States

Olivia identifies as a cis-gender, heterosexual, Latinx woman. Her mother and grandmother's substance abuse went unnoticed for the early years of Olivia's life. However, when Olivia was three years old, her mother's doctor reported the family to Child Protective Services (CPS) due to concerns for substance abuse and neglect. This was the first of many CPS reports. She described how her mother, and/or grandmother, would maintain their sobriety just long enough for Olivia to return home prior to relapsing and ultimately triggering a subsequent CPS report. Throughout her childhood and adolescence, she spent a total of six and a half years in foster care. When Olivia learned she was pregnant, she told her mother she wanted to seek out treatment. Her mother urged her to attempt to stop using on her own, warning her the system would take her child away from her once he was born.

Prenatal substance use exacerbates the already stifling racial inequities related to maternal and infant health outcomes (Le & Coombs, 2021). Although providers may mistakenly believe that they know who of their patients is at greatest risk for substance use during pregnancy, the perinatal substance use literature is clear that pregnant women across income levels and racial, and ethnic groups are susceptible to substance use (Wallman et al., 2011). These findings highlight the need for universal screening of all pregnant women. Universal screening, discussed later in the chapter, limits provider bias based on racial, ethnic, income, and other subjectivities, which has plagued substance use screening and prevention practices in the past (Garg et al., 2015; Le & Coombs, 2021).

Despite no documented greater risk for developing a substance use disorder (SUD), pregnant women of color face significantly more challenges in receiving appropriate diagnosis and/ or accessing adequate treatment/care in the United States and elsewhere (Garg et al., 2015). Historical precedents of mistreatment of individuals of color in the healthcare system curate a present-day sense of distrust and discouragement (Le & Coombs, 2021). The hesitancy and fear are intensified for pregnant women of color due to the widespread shame and stigma associated with prenatal substance use (Le & Coombs, 2021). Moreover, Black women, followed by women of color more generally, are significantly more likely to (a) be screened for substance use concerns, (b) be reported to child welfare authorities for their drug use, and (c) subsequently lose custody of their child(ren) than White women (Garg et al., 2015; Le & Coombs, 2021). More specifically, one study found that Black women are 1.5 times more likely to be screened for illicit drug use compared to non-Black counterparts (Kunnis et al., 2007). The increased likelihood of screening for women of color may be responsible for the arbitrarily inflated prevalence rates of prenatal substance use and disorders for women of color (Stone, 2015).

In sum, particularly in the United States, structural racism and persistent racial inequities result in a lower standard of care for pregnant women of color with SUDs. The cumulative consequences of bias screening, inadequate treatment, higher child custody loss, and more reinforce intergenerational patterns of colonialism, displacement, trauma, and psychological pain (Garg et al., 2015; Le & Coombs, 2021).

Consequences of Prenatal Substance Use

Prevention and early identification of prenatal substance use have numerous implications on maternal, fetal, and familial outcomes. Extensive research demonstrates the harmful physical health effects on developing infants of maternal substance use during pregnancy. As a brief overview, infants exposed to alcohol in utero are at risk for fetal alcohol spectrum disorders (FASD) with associated concerns including developmental delays, intellectual disabilities, attention difficulties, and mental health concerns (Mattson et al., 2019). It is unclear what dosage or timing of alcohol use is linked to FASD, causing some providers to err on the side of caution, stating that no amount of alcohol use during pregnancy is "safe." Although about 1 in 10 pregnant people drink alcohol, worldwide, it is estimated that approximately 7.7 out of every 1,000 children have FASD (Popova et al., 2017).

Illicit substance use has similar effects to alcohol and depending on the substance(s) used, dosage, and timing of use; additional impacts on the health of the pregnancy and the developing fetus can occur including serious health concerns such as low birth weight, difficulty breathing, prematurity, and risks for long-term disabilities (Forray, 2016). Infants prenatally exposed to opiates can experience neonatal opioid withdrawal syndrome (NOWS), which often requires hospitalization to treat symptoms such as irritability, tremors, and fever (American Academy of Pediatrics, n.d.). In 2014, approximately 8 per 1,000 infants born in hospitals in the United

States had symptoms of NOWS (Weller et al., 2021). True prevention of these deleterious effects must start with providing knowledge to all women of childbearing age as many women are unaware they are pregnant until several months into pregnancy. Although ceasing substance use is the main goal, any diminished use of substances and improvement of nutrition and lifestyle factors is beneficial during pregnancy (Virginia Department of Social Services, 2017).

A limited number of studies have examined the impact of partner substance use on perinatal women in a romantic relationship. Partners smoking tobacco, drinking alcohol, using cocaine, and/or other drugs predicted maternal use of the same substance(s) during the perinatal period (Gaysina et al., 2013; Hoyme, May, & Kalberg et al., 2005; DiFranza et al., 2004; Herrmann et al., 2008; Hofhuis, 2003). For young mothers (i.e., adolescents through young adults) in relationships, substance use in the partner is related to postpartum substance use in the mothers. For instance, examining partners' cigarette and cannabis use during pregnancy predicts mothers' use at six months postpartum. This predictive relation continues into the postpartum period for cannabis as examining partners' use at 6 months postpartum predicts mothers' use at 12 months postpartum. The literature suggests two theoretical mechanisms that may explain partner substance use correlations (Rhule-Louie & McMahon, 2007): (a) assortative mating (i.e., selecting partners like themselves in this case regarding substance use and/or substance use attitudes) and (b) behavior contagion (i.e., a process in which the partner's use influences substance use behaviors in the mother). For example, mothers whose partners smoke may also smoke to increase sociability and compatibility. Mothers' motivation to enhance sociability and compatibility with their partners may be enhanced during the postpartum period in the context of the additional social isolation, as well as emotional and financial vulnerability that can accompany caring for an infant, resulting in their additional susceptibility to behavior contagion influences. Mothers who have abstained from substances throughout their pregnancy but have been exposed to drug cues via their partners' use may experience an increased likelihood of resuming substances in the postpartum period. Further research is needed to better understand the importance of partners on maternal substance use during pregnancy.

Screening and Assessment

Out of concern about being reported to CPS, Olivia avoided screening at prenatal care appointments, often not completing the paperwork attached to the clipboard. When a provider would follow up and request she complete the screening questions, she did not endorse symptoms, resulting in a score of 0. Olivia noted that substance use was not addressed on the screening tool her practice used, the Edinburgh Postnatal Depression Scale, and realized she was rarely asked about any potential use of substances. When she was asked, the provider often stated the question in a close-ended manner, such as "You're not using any alcohol or other substances, right?" This style of questioning made Olivia reluctant to disclose her use and increased her fears of judgment and the potential ramifications of disclosing her use. She decided to remain quiet at her prenatal care appointments unless a provider seemed more open to discussing substance use with her in a caring, nonjudgmental, and empathic manner.

Early screening and detection of substance use is essential for psychoeducation, support, and services provision (Polak et al., 2019). To understand the scope of prenatal substance

Table 10.1 Screening Tools for Perinatal Substance Use

Measure Name	Constructs Assessed	Items	Clinical Threshold	Citation
Perinatal Specific Tools				
4P's Plus	Triggers for substance use/abuse, follow-up for quantity	7 plus follow up	Affirmative response to any of the last four items	Chasnoff et al. (2007)
5P's	Substance use by women's parents, peers, and partners, during her pregnancy and in her past	5 plus follow up	Affirmative response to any item suggests follow-up needed	Kennedy et al. (2004)
SURP-P	Cannabis and alcohol use; desire to cut down	3 items	One affirmative response = moderate risk, 2–3 affirmative responses = high-risk for substance use	Yonkers et al. (2010)
Substance Use Tools Non-specific to Perinatal Period				
CAGE	Heavy alcohol use; modified to include drug use (CAGE-AID)	4 items	Score of two or greater	Ewing (1984)
TWEAK	Harmful drinking habits in pregnant women	5 items	Score of two or greater	Chan et al. (1993)
T-ACE	Identifiers of risky and harmful alcohol use	4 items	Score of two or greater	Chang et al. (2010)
AUDIT-C	Identifiers of risky alcohol use	3 items	Score of three or greater	Bush (1998)
NIDA-ASSIST	Use of alcohol, tobacco products, nonmedical need-based prescription drugs, illegal drugs; frequency and impairment related to use	2 parts, 4 items, and 8 items	Lower risk (scores 0–3), moderate risk (scores 4–26), or high risk (scores 27 or higher)	National Institute on Drug Abuse (2011)

use and, therefore, plan for treatment needs, an effectively implemented, universal screening system is needed. Follow-up assessment and treatment planning from trained professionals are also required for women with positive screens to be connected with the services needed to address their substance use.

Table 10.1 lists commonly reported tools used to screen for perinatal substance use and substance use with a general population. This list is not intended to be exhaustive but instead to provide a starting point for selecting screening tools. Notably, three of the measures included in the table (i.e., 4P's Plus, SURP-P, and NIDA-ASSIST) are listed by the World Health Organization (2013) as being brief and validated to promote screening of multiple substances, though not consistent with perinatal populations. Coleman-Cowger et al. (2019) examined the utility of screening perinatal women with three tools, the SURP-P (Yonkers et al., 2010), 4P's Plus (Chasnoff et al., 2007), and NIDA Quick Screen-ASSIST (National Institute on Drug Abuse, 2011). The authors found the first two to have preferable validity for the perinatal population and suggested a preference for their use over the NIDA Quick Screen-ASSIST.

As briefly discussed, the biased practices in screening and assessment of perinatal substance use in communities of color exacerbate the already-overwhelming racial inequities related to maternal and infant health and well-being (Le & Coombs, 2021). Women across income levels and racial/ethnic groups are equally susceptible to developing a SUD, yet disparities exist in screening, assessment, and reporting practices (Benoit et al., 2014; Wallman et al., 2011). Pregnant women of color are more frequently screened for perinatal substance use and more often reported to CPS than their White counterparts (Benoit et al., 2014; Garg et al., 2015; Le & Coombs, 2021). Racially inequitable screening and reporting procedures contribute to longstanding criminalization and reinforce intergenerational trauma and emotional pain for women of color (Garg et al., 2015; Le & Coombs, 2021; Maralit, 2022). Even when Black perinatal women receive substance use treatment, their Black infants are more likely to be removed to receive care from the child welfare system (Roberts & Nuru-Jeter, 2012), demonstrating one of numerous structural disparities that disproportionately harm Black families. In addition, in areas with universal screening protocols, there is a four times greater likelihood for Black women to be reported to CPS compared to their White counterparts (Roberts & Nuru-Jeter, 2012). Biased screening and reporting practices arbitrarily inflate prenatal substance use prevalence for women of color, reinforcing racist beliefs regarding rates of substance misuse in communities of color (Stone, 2015). Furthermore, oppressive healthcare system policies and procedures perpetuate mistrust in seeking care for women of color, thereby resulting in reduced quantity and quality of care for women of color with perinatal substance use (Le & Coombs, 2021) and contributing to the heightened rates of maternal morbidity and mortality seen in the United States for perinatal women of color.

Universal screenings (i.e., screening all patients in a practice) are the "gold standard" for screening substance use, intimate partner violence, and mental health difficulties during pregnancy (Wright et al., 2016; Cook et al., 2017). Universal screening results in increased positive screens and increased referrals for services (Ulrich et al., 2021; Wallman et al., 2011). Repeated universal screenings provide multiple opportunities to identify pregnant women currently using or at risk for substance abuse. In the case of a positive screen, providers can take the opportunity to discuss options for caring for the woman and developing the baby (e.g., promoting prenatal vitamin use, exercise, and nutrition) as well as to diminish or cease their substance consumption during pregnancy. Ulrich et al. (2021) found the implementation of universal screening to be feasible and effective in promoting the screening of most patients within an outpatient prenatal clinic in a tertiary care hospital. They noted that protocols for promoting successful referrals to treatment were lacking and needed as next steps.

Wright et al. (2016) summarized findings from a 2012 CDC-convened Expert Meeting on Perinatal Illicit Drug Abuse on best practices in Screening, Brief Intervention, and Referral to Treatment (SBIRT) specific to pregnancy. Universal screening promotes the classification of women into risk groups according to the pattern of use. Women deemed low risk should receive brief advice, women at moderate risk should engage in brief intervention, and women deemed high risk require specialty care. In SBIRT terms, a brief intervention for substance use is patient-centered counseling involving motivational interviewing practices (Wright et al., 2016). Early identification in pregnancy can provide enhanced motivation to diminish or cease using substances, as most women want to prioritize what is healthy for their infant (Wallman et al., 2011). Even one interaction with a provider addressing risks of prenatal substance use can promote decreased or ceased use, with additional research suggesting that screening at multiple time points throughout pregnancy can increase the sensitivity of screening.

Treatment Considerations

Despite the barriers and judgment that she experienced; Olivia persevered in her search for help. As she entered her third trimester, she finally found a provider who asked her open-ended questions about her possible use of substances. The nurse practitioner at her medical practice asked, "I realize we haven't spoken much about use of substances. Are you using any alcohol, tobacco, or other drugs at this time? I'm asking so we can share important information about your health and your baby's development and help you in finding treatment if you are using." Olivia felt relieved to open up to this caring professional. Following their discussion, she was referred to a residential treatment facility that worked with prenatal and postpartum women. They functioned as a multidisciplinary team with physicians and psychiatrists on board with specialized training in medication provision to substance-using mothers. Even more exciting to Olivia, this facility offered the ability to remain in residential treatment with her infant following labor and delivery. Her service provision team worked to support her in strengthening her relationship with her son as she progressed through treatment. She and her primary clinician explored how, in part, her patterns of substance misuse were rooted in her difficulty with emotion regulation and her family's intergenerational substance use models. As Olivia's capacity for supporting her son's distress strengthened, she found herself more capable of nurturing her own needs.

Specialized and effective treatment options for pregnant women with problematic substance use patterns are lacking (Cioffi et al., 2019; Clark et al., 2001; Sahker et al., 2015). Many pregnant women considering starting treatment report feelings of hesitancy in light of their previous negative, and failed, experiences (Clark et al., 2001). Sahker et al. (2015) analyzed the retrospective outcome data of pregnant and nonpregnant women in substance use treatment. They suggested that, for pregnant women entering substance use treatment, a significant discrepancy existed between the treatment placement setting and the treatment settings associated with the greatest success when compared to nonpregnant women. For instance, approximately 65% of nonpregnant women were found to successfully complete detox-ambulatory services, whereas only 30% of pregnant women successfully completed treatment. The significant differences they found suggest that treatment planning, referral, and support of pregnant women with SUDs must be thoughtfully planned and tailored to their unique presentation.

Pregnant women face numerous barriers that impede their ability to access effective mental health treatment (Lavin et al., 2021). Substance misuse only exacerbates the difficulties faced when seeking services. To be effective, treatment should be modified and tailored to fit prenatal client's individualized needs by implementing flexible modalities, women-focused programming, wrap-around services (i.e., services in which providers from numerous disciplines collaborate to provide holistic care in which a client can get all their needs met within on setting or clinic, such as mental health, community support, and medical needs), and centering the parent–child relationship as a mechanism for change (Hand et al., 2017; Cioffi et al., 2019; Staudt, 2018; Krans et al., 2018; Sarkola et al., 2012).

Gender-specific treatment has been shown to be significantly more effective when compared to mixed-gendered treatment options for prenatal clients with SUDs (Staudt, 2018; Krans et al., 2018; Lander et al., 2015). For example, Krans et al. (2018) found that women in gender-specific programming were significantly more likely to initiate services and engage in postpartum visits when compared to women in non-gender-specific programming (81.4% vs. 44.2%; 67.9% vs. 52.6%). Furthermore, perinatal clients struggling with substance misuse present with unique etiological considerations, comorbidities, and psychosocial stressors. For instance, women, generally, require smaller doses of a drug across a smaller period prior to entering a disease and/or addicted state (Bezrutczyk, 2021). SUDs in women are associated with higher rates of domestic violence and higher rates of anxiety and depression. Women-centered programming allows for gender-responsive service provision focusing on substance use treatment as well as pregnancy-related concerns such as safe detoxification while pregnant, family planning, infant feeding, parenting, housing/resource instance, prenatal and postpartum care, and trauma-informed care (Krans et al., 2018). Women in gender-specific programming found the treatment to be more relevant to their needs, developed a stronger sense of community with their peers, and were less likely to relapse after completing treatment (Lander et al., 2015). Moreover, women in gender-specific programming were shown to have significantly higher retention rates than those in programs that were not gender-specific. This effect was even higher when women were allowed to retain custody of their infants following labor and delivery (Staudt, 2018).

The benefits of women-centered programming are increased when paired with integrated care and services aimed at supporting holistic prenatal well-being (Staudt, 2018; Tarasoff et al., 2018). It is essential that patterns of substance misuse be conceptualized, and treated, within the context of an individual's environment (Grant et al., 2005). This is particularly imperative when considering prenatal substance use treatment. Women with SUDs have co-occurring mental health difficulties, histories of trauma, inadequate prenatal care, low social support, financial difficulty, involvement in child welfare, and other legal difficulties (Tarasoff et al., 2018). Treatment that is thoughtfully designed to broadly address the vast needs prenatal SUD clients may face has been demonstrated to be associated with higher levels of success (Grant et al., 2005; Tarasoff et al., 2018; Crane et al., 2019). Specifically, integrated treatment programs with wrap-around service provision have been shown to be correlated with increased program adherence, positive substance use treatment outcomes, positive psychosocial outcomes, and positive parenting-related outcomes (Grant et al., 2005; Tarasoff et al., 2018).

It is important to discuss specific considerations related to prenatal clients with opioid use disorder. It is paramount that clinical staff (behavioral health, medical, and otherwise) partner with women and empower them to understand the variety of ways in which they can manage their opioid use disorder throughout pregnancy and delivery. Medication for opioid use disorder has been the standard of care for individuals with opioid addiction since the 1970s (Howard & Freeman, 2020). Methadone is commonly prescribed for individuals with moderate to severe opioid use disorder. In 2002, buprenorphine was approved as an alternative medication option and can be utilized for clients with mild to severe opioid use disorders, as well as with clients who are on multiple medications (Howard & Freeman, 2020; Mattocks et al., 2017). Whereas methadone requires daily visits to a federally funded clinic (typically accompanied by significant stigma, shame, and logistical stress), buprenorphine is available in prescription form that can be administered at home (Mattocks et al., 2017).

The American College of Obstetricians and Gynecologists (ACOG) recommends utilization of medication services for prenatal clients with opioid use disorders. When administered in a supportive and stigma-free environment, medication has been shown to be associated with improved prenatal care, better perinatal outcomes, improved maternal nutrition, improved neonatal birth weight, reduced risk of relapse, decreased rates of unhealthy substance-related behaviors, and higher retention in treatment programs (Preis et al., 2020; Mattocks et al., 2017; Macife et al., 2020).

There is some debate regarding the effect of medication services on infant well-being due to its documented correlation with NOWS. NOWS occurs when an infant has become dependent on opioids. In the United States, the incidence of NOWS increased by 433% between 2004 and 2014 during the opioid epidemic, and the prevalence of NOWS continues to be on the rise (Weller et al., 2021). Due to NOWS's clear association with long-term health effects, providers are determined to work toward decreasing NOWS rates and increasing infant well-being. As such, there can be hesitancy from healthcare providers to support the utilization of medication services during pregnancy. However, research suggests that opioid detox on its own (i.e., without the support of medication services) may leave women more vulnerable to relapse and in turn may leave infants more vulnerable to harm and distress (Macife et al., 2020). Additionally, medication services throughout the prenatal and postpartum periods are associated with increased prenatal care and increased engagement in behavioral health services, which in turn decreased the adverse health effects of prenatal substance use on maternal and infant well-being (Jones et al., 2012; Mittal, 2020). Moreover, breastfeeding while on medication for opioid use disorder has been shown to further decrease the negative impacts of opioid use on infant well-being (Reece-Stremtan & Marinelli, 2015).

Despite its well-documented efficacy, it is challenging for clients to locate physicians with specialized training in prenatal substance use and/or medication service provision (Hand et al., 2017; Mattocks et al., 2017). Women face significant challenges in finding qualified obstetricians with experience in treating pregnant women using medication (Mattocks et al., 2017). Guilt, shame, and fear regarding their pregnancy and potential ramifications (legal and physical) play a prominent role in the decision of whether to seek out medication services (Mattocks et al., 2017). Prenatal substance use treatment programs that integrate wrap-around services provide a much-needed pathway for women with opioid use disorder to access specialized medication services in a reduced-stigma environment (Mattocks et al., 2017; Kissin et al., 2004; Hand et al., 2017).

Centering the Parent–Child Relationship: Attachment Considerations

Postrecovery from substance use, Olivia refers to her son as her greatest inspiration. She feels her pregnancy was a major factor in her seeking and sticking with treatment. She recalls what it was like being a young child who was cared for by a mother using substances and remembers how alone, confused, and sometimes scared she felt. She describes wanting to be a "different kind of mom" to her son and wanting him to know he is loved and well cared for. She wants to "break the cycle" of substances for women in her family and plans to remain sober from substances into the future.

The association between addiction and attachment insecurity is well-documented (Parolin & Simonelli, 2016). Our attachment style is intertwined with our regulatory system; it is through our relationship with our primary caregivers that we learn to cope, manage, and regulate our distress. An insecure attachment history may hinder an individual's ability to cope with and understand their emotions independently (Lyden & Suchman, 2013; Khantzian et al., 2014). Substances effectively, and often quickly, manage and quiet internal distress. Thus, they replace the regulatory deficits resulting from an insecure attachment. Prenatal substance use treatment offers a prime opportunity to both treat the SUD and to promote attachment security for both the mother herself and the future parent–child dyad.

Women with SUDs are likely to seek out treatment during pregnancy sooner than they otherwise may have (Kissin et al., 2004). Pregnant women report feeling motivated by their pregnancy and desire to care for their infant. Given the increased role community health agencies play in a woman's life during pregnancy, prenatal women with SUDs are more likely to receive referrals to substance use treatment than women with SUDs who are not pregnant. These combined factors render the prenatal period an opportune time for intervention and support.

Prenatal substance use treatment that integrates the parent–child relationship and works to promote a secure dyadic relationship is associated with better maternal SUD outcomes (Pajulo et al., 2016; Lyden & Suchman, 2013). For instance, a randomized clinical pilot trial of an attachment-based treatment program for maternal SUD, *The Mothers and Toddlers Program*, found that mothers in the attachment-based program showed higher levels of reflective functioning, higher levels of caregiving behaviors, and fewer symptoms of depression and psychiatric distress (Suchman et al., 2011). Lyden and Suchman (2013) discussed how maladaptive internal working models (i.e., insecure attachment systems) are highly transmissible across generations. Prenatal substance use treatment offers an opportunity to both treat the SUD and promote attachment security for both the mother herself and the future parent–child dyad. Parolin and Simonelli (2016) reviewed a variety of attachment-based interventions for perinatal substance use that centered on the parent–child relationship and found that this approach led to increased attachment security and better maternal substance use treatment outcomes. Espinet et al. (2016) examined the impact of an integrated relational and substance use treatment program, *Breaking the Cycle*. They found that women participating in Breaking the Cycle had improved levels of addiction severity, mental health functioning, and relationship capacity when compared to mothers in the standard treatment group (Espinet et al., 2016). Furthermore, they found that relationship functioning quality predicted addiction severity to a greater degree than abstinence, social support, or mental health, suggesting that focusing on relational functioning may prove to be a highly efficacious means of treating substance misuse (Espinet et al., 2016). It is important to note that attachment-based treatment for prenatal substance use is an emerging approach. As such, studies quantifying the direct impact of attachment and parent–child-based approaches on prenatal substance use are limited. In sum, attachment-based and parent–child focused intervention may allow mothers the opportunity to reflect on both their past and current circumstances that resulted in their problematic substance use patterns (Parolin & Simonelli, 2016; Pajulo et al., 2016).

U.S. Policies Impacting Pregnant Individuals With Substance Abuse Disorder

State-Level Policies

Despite increasing acceptance of SUD as a medical condition rather than a moral failing, stigma against people with SUDs, perhaps especially including pregnant people, remains written into laws and child welfare service policies and dictates how state and federal government officials have historically allocated resources (Weber et al., 2021). In the United States, 24 states, including the District of Columbia, consider substance abuse during pregnancy to be child abuse under civil child welfare statutes (Guttmacher Institute, 2022). Of these states, three consider substance use during pregnancy to be grounds for civil commitment. Additionally, 25 states and the District of Columbia require healthcare professionals to report suspected or confirmed prenatal substance use regardless of patient consent to do so (Guttmacher Institute, 2022). Some states have also elected to include prenatal substance use in their civil child welfare requirements, meaning that substance use even before pregnancy (i.e., prenatal use) can be grounds for terminating parental rights due to child neglect or abuse (Guttmacher Institute, 2022).

As of 2018, 38 states have also implemented additional punitive laws, known as "fetal assault" or "fetal homicide" laws (ACOG, 2018). These laws are often used to limit behaviors during pregnancy that legislators deem harmful to the fetus and are used to punish pregnant people for a wide range of actions (ACOG, 2018). Furthermore, policy experts have found that these laws are associated with increased out-of-state births, which puts both the pregnant individual and the infant at greater risk (Choi et al., 2023).

Legal restrictions and punitive sanctions on pregnant individuals with SUD are further cited to be key driver in treatment gaps (Davis & Carr, 2019). Atkins and Durrance (2020) did not find evidence that punitive prenatal substance use policies reduced maternal narcotic exposure at birth. Instead, evidence showed that punitive policies deterred pregnant women from seeking substance use treatment during pregnancy. Much like the Atkins and Durrance (2020) study, a study of Medicaid beneficiaries also found no association between punitive policies and neonatal abstinence syndrome (Faherty et al., 2022). Reporting policies, however, were associated with decreased odds of neonatal abstinence syndrome, if controlled for all other relevant policies (Faherty et al., 2022).

Policy experts have also explored the impact of state Medicaid expansion on SUD treatment for pregnant individuals. Even though pregnant women were eligible for Medicaid prior to the Affordable Care Act (ACA), the ACA and Medicaid expansion increased coverage for mental health and SUD treatment services for vulnerable populations, including pregnant women. Choi et al. (2021) examined the impact of Medicaid expansion on access to substance use treatment for pregnant individuals. Researchers found that states with Medicaid expansion and without prohibiting laws for substance use treatment in pregnant individuals had higher utilization of care compared to non-expansion, prohibiting states. Evidence concluded that Medicaid expansion was associated with improved access to SUD treatment for pregnant people.

U.S. Federal Efforts

At the federal level in the United States, the Biden Administration has supported efforts to improve access to substance use treatment for pregnant individuals. In a 2022 report on SUDs during pregnancy, the Administration outlined a multi-step policy agenda to improve access to treatment and decrease provider stigma for substance use in pregnancy. The agenda highlighted proposed efforts such as improved data reporting at the state and federal level, increased access to medication for pregnant people with SUD, and federal investment in community-based organizations that serve vulnerable communities.

Additional efforts have been made in Congress, with multiple federal legislators proposing bills that support the care of pregnant parents with SUDs. The bill *Into the Light for Maternal Mental Health and Substance Use Disorders Act of 2022*, proposed and passed within the same fiscal year, reauthorized a program that addresses maternal depression and expands its scope to include mental health and SUDs. Furthermore, the bill also requires the Department of Health and Human Services to maintain a national hotline to provide mental health and SUD resources to perinatal women and their families.

Impact of Current Policies

Evidence shows that policies regarding SUDs for pregnant individuals disproportionally impact historically marginalized communities, including people of color and incarcerated individuals (Bishop et al., 2017; Stone, 2015). These communities have borne a disproportionate share of the misery from the war on drugs and typically perpetuate a vicious cycle, as those who are marginalized and have SUDs often cannot access effective treatments for their conditions (Bishop et al., 2017). Many of these policies are also associated with punitive measures beyond losing custody of the child, such as steep fines, loss of a driver's license, and incarceration.

Even with well-meaning policies in place, pregnant individuals often still experience stigma when seeking care. For example, in a "secret shopper" field experiment, researchers contacted licensed SUD treatment facilities in ten states, some of which had care mandates, to determine if pregnancy was a factor in receiving treatment. Throughout this experiment, individuals posing as pregnant women with a SUD were 17% less likely to be accepted for substance use treatment appointments by outpatient buprenorphine providers compared to nonpregnant women (Davis & Carr, 2019).

Conclusion and Future Directions

Prenatal substance use is a growing epidemic that negatively impacts mothers, their children, their families, and surrounding communities. However, despite its prevalence, adequate information, screening, resources, and treatment options available to pregnant women with substance use concerns are limited. Screening for perinatal substance use as well as comorbid mental health concerns including posttraumatic stress disorder, mood disorders, and anxiety disorders should be a required element of a cost-effective model of integrated medical and mental healthcare. This screening needs to be conducted in an educated, relational, and empathic manner, while meeting the client and other parenting partners' mental health needs at the forefront of the professional's mind. Effective screening needs to be integrated into a variety of settings (obstetrics, pediatrics, WIC [Special Supplemental Nutrition Program for Women, Infants, and Children] offices, occupational health programs, parent–child groups, midwife offices, doulas, and home-visiting program centers), as well as being standardized at hospital discharge from maternity wards and the neonatal intensive care unit.

An expansive training effort is required for professionals to meet the needs of those struggling with perinatal SUDs and comorbid mental health difficulties. Training needs to occur across mental and physical health providers to enhance collaboration and understanding and to reduce stigma. Future research should examine the current knowledge base in an effort to identify specific training deficits. Moreover, our current understanding regarding best practices, treatments, and interventions for prenatal substance use is continuing to develop. Future research is needed to fine-tune our understanding of how to maximize our interventions during this critical period. Specifically, expanded research examining the utility of attachment-based and relational treatment for prenatal substance use is needed.

Efforts should be made to tailor the treatment of prenatal substance use to the unique etiology and presentation of this population. There is a rare opportunity to address, and potentially heal, intergenerational patterns of attachment insecurity and trauma *in addition* to treating substance use concerns within the prenatal period. Treatment should center on the parent–child relationship and utilize attachment-based interventions to optimize outcomes and success. In addition, research suggests that examining the involvement of parenting partners/fathers in psychoeducation and intervention for mothers' prenatal substance use and care is warranted as they may be effective in reducing use and enhancing care during the perinatal period (Desrosiers et al., 2015). Pregnancy may serve as a critical window for reducing substance use in mothers and parenting partners/fathers. Couples' interventions during this critical window may be particularly impactful, given findings of similar patterns of use in romantic partnerships (Desrosiers et al., 2015).

Olivia graduated from the program after a year and a half of participating. She and her son were supported in finding community housing, employment, and outpatient therapy resources. Olivia felt lucky to have found such an understanding and accommodating treatment resource. She knew that many, or even most, are not so lucky.

However, even with the support, her transition out of residential treatment was difficult. Socially, Olivia described feeling like she was "back in middle school." It has been nearly a decade since she had functioned in a social setting without using substances. She worked weekly with her therapist to continue strengthening her sense of self, apart from her addiction. Moreover, her job was a 45-minute drive from her house, making it challenging to drop her son off at daycare and get to work on time. Many days she was forced to take her son to work with her due to traffic or difficult road conditions. Her boss was initially supportive, but over time began to view Olivia's tardiness as noncompliance. She was subsequently put on a "probationary watch" and was warned she was at risk of losing her job. She shared her struggles with her therapist. Thankfully, Olivia's therapist worked as a part of a multidisciplinary team.

She connected Olivia with a social worker who was able to support Olivia in finding a quality childcare provider closer to her place of employment.

As time progressed, Olivia and her son grew accustomed to their new life. Olivia created community and social support through a Moms in Recovery group she had joined. She continued attending weekly individual therapy to work on processing her trauma and early childhood experiences and strengthen her sense of self. As she bolstered her sense of self and strengthened her regulatory capacity, her relationship with her son grew stronger. There continued to be moments when she was overwhelmed by parenting, but she felt confident she had the tools to use them.

References

American Academy of Pediatrics. (n.d.). Neonatal Opioid Withdrawal Syndrome (NOWS): What families need to know. *HealthyChildren.org*. Retrieved December 5, 2022, from www.healthychildren.org/English/ages-stages/prenatal/Pages/Neonatal-Opioid-Withdrawal-Syndrome.aspx

American College of Obstetrics and Gynecologists. (2018). *Opposition to criminalization of individuals during pregnancy and the postpartum period*. www.acog.org/clinical-information/policy-and-position-statements/statements-of-policy/2020/opposition-criminalization-of-individuals-pregnancy-and-postpartum-period

Atkins, D. N., & Durrance, C. P. (2020). State policies that treat prenatal substance use as child abuse or neglect fail to achieve their intended goals. *Health Affairs (Project Hope)*, 39(5), 756–763. https://doi.org/10.1377/hlthaff.2019.00785

Bakhireva, L. N., Leeman, L., Roberts, M., Rodriguez, D. E., & Jacobson, S. W. (2021). You didn't drink during pregnancy, did you? *Alcoholism: Clinical and Experimental Research*, 45(3), 543–547. https://doi.org/10.1111/acer.14545

Benoit, C., Stengel, C., Marcellus, L., Hallgrimsdottir, H., Anderson, J., MacKinnon, K., Phillips, R., Zazueta, P., & Charbonneau, S. (2014). Providers' constructions of pregnant and early parenting women who use substances. *From Health Behaviours to Health Practices*, 95–105. https://doi.org/10.1002/9781118898345.ch9

Betts, K. S., Kisely, S., & Alati, R. (2022). Prenatal cannabis use disorders and offspring primary and secondary educational outcomes. *Addiction*, 117(2), 425–432. https://doi.org/10.1111/add.15629

Bezrutczyk, D. (2021). The differences in addiction between men and women. *Addiction Center*. Retrieved June 24, 2022, from www.addictioncenter.com/addiction/differences-men-women/

Bishop, D., Borkowski, L., Couillard, M., Allina, A., Baruch, S., & Wood, S. (2017). *Bridging the divide white paper: Pregnant women and substance use: Overview of research & policy in the United States*. Jacobs Institute of Women's Health. Paper 5. https://hsrc.himmelfarb.gwu.edu/sphhs_centers_jacobs/5

Brown, D. H., Gilliland, J., & Seabrook, J. A. (2019). Predictors of drug use during pregnancy: The relative effects of socioeconomic, demographic, and mental health risk factors. *Journal of Neonatal-Perinatal Medicine*, 12(2), 179–187.https://doi.org/10.3233/NPM-1814

Bush, K. (1998). The Audit Alcohol Consumption Questions (audit-c): An effective brief screening test for problem drinking. *Archives of Internal Medicine*, 158(16), 1789–1795. https://doi.org/10.1001/archinte.158.16.1789

Chan, A. W., Pristach, E. A., Welte, J. W., & Russell, M. (1993). Use of the tweak test in screening for alcoholism/heavy drinking in three populations. *Alcoholism: Clinical and Experimental Research*, 17(6), 1188–1192. https://doi.org/10.1111/j.1530-0277.1993.tb05226.x

Chang, G. (2020). Maternal substance use: Consequences, identification, and interventions. *Alcohol Research: Current Reviews*, 40(2), 06. https://doi.org/10.35946/arcr.v40.2.06

Chang, G., Fisher, N. D., Hornstein, M. D., Jones, J. A., & Orav, E. J. (2010). Identification of risk drinking women: T-ACE screening tool or the medical record. *Journal of Women's Health*, 19(10), 1933–1939. https://doi.org/10.1089/jwh.2009.1911

Chasnoff, I. J., Neuman, K., Thornton, C., & Callaghan, M. A. (2001). Screening for substance use in pregnancy: A practical approach for the primary care physician. *American Journal of Obstetrics and Gynecology, 184*(4), 752–758. https://doi.org/10.1067/mob.2001.109939

Chasnoff, I. J., Wells, A. M., McGourty, R. F., & Bailey, L. K. (2007). Validation of the 4P's plus© screen for substance use in pregnancy validation of the 4p's plus. *Journal of Perinatology, 27*(12), 744–748. https://doi.org/10.1038/sj.jp.7211823

Choi, S. W., Agbese, E., Cohrs, A. C., Ramos, C., & Leslie, D. L. (2023). The implementation of the Tennessee Fetal Assault Law and its association with out-of-state births among residents of Tennessee. *Women's Health Issues, 33*(1), 3–9. https://doi.org/10.1016/j.whi.2022.09.006

Choi, S. W., Stein, M. D., Raifman, J., Rosenbloom, D., & Clark, J. A. (2021). Estimating the impact on initiating medications for opioid use disorder of state policies expanding Medicaid and prohibiting substance use during pregnancy. *Drug and Alcohol Dependence, 229*(Pt A), 109162. https://doi.org/10.1016/j.drugalcdep.2021.109162

Cioffi, C. C., Leve, L. D., & Seeley, J. R. (2019). Accelerating the pace of science: Improving parenting practices in parents with opioid use disorder. *Parenting, 19*(3), 244–266. https://doi.org/10.1080/15295192.2019.1615801

Clark, K. A., Dee, D. L., Bale, P. L., & Martin, S. L. (2001). Treatment compliance among prenatal care patients with substance abuse problems. *American Journal of Drug and Alcohol Abuse, 27*(1), 121–136. https://doi.org/10.1081/ada-100103122

Coleman-Cowger, V. H., Oga, E. A., Peters, E. N., Trocin, K. E., Koszowski, B., & Mark, K. (2019). Accuracy of three screening tools for prenatal substance use. *Obstetrics & Gynecology, 133*(5), 952–961. https://doi.org/10.1097/aog.0000000000003230

Cook, J. L., Green, C. R., de la Ronde, S., Dell, C. A., Graves, L., Morgan, L., . . . Wong, S. (2017). Screening and management of substance use in pregnancy: A review. *Journal of Obstetrics and Gynaecology Canada, 39*(10), 897–905. https://doi.org/10.1016/j.jogc.2017.07.017

Corsi, D. J., Hsu, H., Weiss, D., Fell, D. B., & Walker, M. (2018). Trends and correlates of cannabis use in pregnancy: A population-based study in Ontario, Canada from 2012 to 2017. *Canadian Journal of Public Health Revue Canadienne de Santé Publique, 110*(1), 76–84. https://doi.org/10.17269/s41997-018-0148-0

Crane, D., Marcotte, M., Applegate, M., Massatti, R., Hurst, M., Menegay, M., . . . Williams, S. (2019). A statewide Quality Improvement (QI) initiative for better health outcomes and family stability among pregnant women with Opioid Use Disorder (OUD) and their infants. *Journal of Substance Abuse Treatment, 102*, 53–59. https://doi.org/10.1016/j.jsat.2019.04.010

Davis, C. S., & Carr, D. H. (2019). Legal and policy changes urgently needed to increase access to opioid agonist therapy in the United States. *International Journal of Drug Policy, 73*, 42–48. https://doi.org/10.1016/j.drugpo.2019.07.006

Denny, C. H., Acero, C. S., Naimi, T. S., & Kim, S. Y. (2019). Consumption of alcohol beverages and binge drinking among pregnant women aged 18–44 years United States, 2015–2017. *MMWR: Morbidity and Mortality Weekly Report, 68*(16), 365–368. https://doi.org/10.15585/mmwr.mm6816a1

Desrosiers, A., Thompson, A., Divney, A., Magriples, U., & Kershaw, T. (2015). Romantic partner influences on prenatal and postnatal substance use in young couples. *Journal of Public Health, 38*(2), 300–307. https://doi.org/10.1093/pubmed/fdv039

DiFranza, J. R., Aligne, C. A., & Weitzman, M. (2004). Prenatal and postnatal environmental tobacco smoke exposure and children's health. *Pediatrics, 113*(Supplement 3), 1007–1015. https://doi.org/10.1542/peds.113.s3.1007

Drake, P., Driscoll, A. K., & Mathews, T. J. (2018). Cigarette smoking during pregnancy: United States, 2016. *NCHS Data Brief, 305*, 1–8.

Espinet, S. D., Motz, M., Jeong, J. J., Jenkins, J. M., & Pepler, D. (2016). "Breaking the cycle" of maternal substance use through relationships: A comparison of integrated approaches, *Addiction Research & Theory, 24*, 5, 375–388. https://doi.org/10.3109/16066359.2016.1140148

Ewing, J. A. (1984). Detecting alcoholism. *JAMA, 252*(14), 1905. https://doi.org/10.1001/jama.1984.03350140051025

Faherty, L. J., Heins, S., Kranz, A. M., Patrick, S. W., & Stein, B. D. (2022). Association between punitive policies and neonatal abstinence syndrome among Medicaid-insured infants in complex policy environments. *Addiction, 117*(1), 162–171. https://doi.org/10.1111/add.15602

Forray, A. (2016). Substance use during pregnancy. *F1000Research*, 5, 887. https://doi.org/10.12688/f1000research.7645.1

Garg, M., Garrison, L., Leeman, L., Hamidovic, A., Borrego, M., Rayburn, W. F., & Bakhireva, L. (2015). Validity of self-reported drug use information among pregnant women. *Maternal and Child Health Journal, 20*(1), 41–47. https://doi.org/10.1007/s10995-015-1799-6

Gaysina, D., Fergusson, D. M., Leve, L. D., Horwood, J., Reiss, D., Shaw, D. S., . . . Harold, G. T. (2013). Maternal smoking during pregnancy and offspring conduct problems. *JAMA Psychiatry, 70*(9), 956–963. https://doi.org/10.1001/jamapsychiatry.2013.127

Grant, T. M., Ernst, C. C., Streissguth, A., & Stark, K. (2005). Preventing alcohol and drug exposed births in Washington State: Intervention findings from three parent-child assistance program sites. *American Journal of Drug and Alcohol Abuse, 31*(3), 471–490. https://doi.org/10.1081/ada-200056813

Gosdin, L. K., Deputy, N. P., Kim, S. Y., Dang, E. P., & Denny, C. H. (2022). Alcohol consumption and binge drinking during pregnancy among adults aged 18–49 years – United States, 2018–2020. *Morbidity and Mortality Weekly Report, 71*(1), 10–13. https://doi.org/10.15585/mmwr.mm7101a2

Guttmacher Institute. (2022). *Substance use during pregnancy.* www.guttmacher.org/state-policy/explore/substance-use-during-pregnancy

Hand, D. J., Short, V. L., & Abatemarco, D. J. (2017). Substance use, treatment, and demographic characteristics of pregnant women entering treatment for opioid use disorder differ by United States census region. *Journal of Substance Abuse Treatment, 76*, 58–63. https://doi.org/10.1016/j.jsat.2017.01.011

Haight, S. C., Ko, J. Y., Tong, V. T., Bohm, M. K., & Callaghan, W. M. (2018). Opioid use disorder documented at delivery hospitalization – United States, 1999–2014. *MMWR Morbidity and Mortality Weekly Report, 67*, 845–849. http://dx.doi.org/10.15585/mmwr.mm6731a1externalicon

Havens, J. R., Simmons, L. A., Shannon, L. M., & Hansen, W. F. (2009). Factors associated with substance use during pregnancy: Results from a national sample. *Drug and Alcohol Dependence, 99*(1–3), 89–95. https://doi.org/10.1016/j.drugalcdep.2008.07.010

Herrmann, M., King, K, & Weitzman, M. (2008). Prenatal tobacco smoke and postnatal secondhand smoke exposure and child neurodevelopment. *Current Opinion in Pediatrics, 20*, 184–190. https://doi.org/10.1097/MOP.0b013e3282f56165

Hofhuis, W. (2003). Adverse health effects of prenatal and postnatal tobacco smoke exposure on children. *Archives of Disease in Childhood, 88*(12), 1086–1090. https://doi.org/10.1136/adc.88.12.1086

Hotham, E., Ali, R., White, J., & Robinson, J. (2008). Pregnancy-related changes in tobacco, alcohol and cannabis use reported by antenatal patients at two public hospitals in South Australia. *Australian and New Zealand Journal of Obstetrics and Gynaecology, 48*(3), 248–254. https://doi.org/10.1111/j.1479-828x.2008.00827.x

Howard, H. G., & Freeman, K. (2020). U.S. survey of factors associated with adherence to standard of care in treating pregnant women with opioid use disorder. *Journal of Psychosomatic Obstetrics & Gynecology, 41*(1), 74–81. https://doi.org/10.1080/0167482x.2019.1634048

Hoyme, H. E., May, P. A., Kalberg, W. O., Kodituwakku, P., Gossage, J. P., Trujillo, P. M., . . . Robinson, L. K. (2005). A practical clinical approach to diagnosis of fetal alcohol spectrum disorders: Clarification of the 1996 institute of medicine criteria. *Pediatrics, 115*(1), 39–47. https://doi.org/10.1542/peds.2004-0259

Hutchins, E., & DiPietro, J. (1997). Psychosocial risk factors associated with cocaine use during pregnancy: A case-control study. *Obstetrics & Gynecology, 90*(1), 142–147. https://doi.org/10.1016/S0029-7844(97)00181-6

Hui, K., Angelotta, C., & Fisher, C. E. (2017). Criminalizing substance use in pregnancy: Misplaced priorities. *Addiction (Abingdon, England), 112*(7), 1123–1125. https://doi.org/10.1111/add.13776

Jones, H. E., Fischer, G., Heil, S. H., Kaltenbach, K., Martin, P. R., Coyle, M. G., . . . Arria, A. M. (2012). Maternal Opioid Treatment: Human Experimental Research (MOTHER) – Approach, issues and lessons learned. *Addiction (Abingdon, England), 107*(Suppl 1, 1), 28–35. https://doi.org/10.1111/j.1360-0443.2012.04036.x

Jorda, M., Conant, B. J., Sandstrom, A., Klug, M. G., Angal, J., & Burd, L. (2021). Protective factors against tobacco and alcohol use among pregnant women from a tribal nation in the Central United States. *PLoS One, 16*(2), e0243924. https://doi.org/10.1371/journal.pone.0243924

Kennare, R., Heard, A., & Chan, A. (2005). Substance use during pregnancy: Risk factors and obstetric and perinatal outcomes in South Australia. *Australian & New Zealand Journal of Obstetrics & Gynaecology, 45*(3), 220–225. https://doi.org/10.1111/j.1479-828X.2005.00379.x

Kennedy, C., Finkelstein, N., Hutchins, E., & Mahoney, J. (2004). Improving screening for alcohol use during pregnancy: The Massachusetts ASAP program. *Maternal and Child Health Journal, 8,* 137–147.

Khantzian, E. J. (2014). The self-medication hypothesis and attachment theory: Pathways for understanding and ameliorating addictive suffering. In R. Gill (Ed.), *Addictions from an attachment perspective: Do broken bonds and early trauma lead to addictive behaviours?* (pp. 33–56). Routledge.

Kissin, W. B., Svikis, D. S., Moylan, P., Haug, N. A., & Stitzer, M. L. (2004). Identifying pregnant women at risk for early attrition from substance abuse treatment. *Journal of Substance Abuse Treatment, 27*(1), 31–38. https://doi.org/10.1016/j.jsat.2004.03.007

Ko, J. Y., Coy, K. C., Haight, S. C., Haegerich, T. M., Williams, L., Cox, S., . . . Grant, A. M. (2020). Characteristics of marijuana use during pregnancy – Eight states, pregnancy risk assessment monitoring system, 2017. *MMWR: Morbidity and Mortality Weekly Report, 69*(32), 1058–1063. https://doi.org/10.15585/mmwr.mm6932a2

Krans, E. E., Bobby, S., England, M., Gedekoh, R. H., Chang, J. C., Maguire, B., . . . English, D. H. (2018). The pregnancy recovery center: A women-centered treatment program for pregnant and postpartum women with opioid use disorder. *Addictive Behaviors, 86,* 124–129. https://doi.org/10.1016/j.addbeh.2018.05.016

Kunnis, H. V., Bellin, E., Chazotte, C., Du, E., & Arnsten, J. H. (2007). The effect of race on provider decisions to test for illicit drug use in the peripartum setting. *Journal of Women's Health, 16*(2), 245–255. https://doi.org/10.1089/jwh.2006.0070

Lander, L. R., Gurka, K. K., Marshalek, P. J., Riffon, M., & Sullivan, C. R. (2015). A comparison of pregnancy-only versus mixed-gender group therapy among pregnant women with opioid use disorder. *Social Work Research, 39*(4), 235–244. https://doi.org/10.1093/swr/svv02

Lavin, K., Jacobs, J., Pinch, S., Hairston Peetz, P., Holmberg, J., Van Arsdale, A., . . . Moran Vozar, T. (2021, August). *Maternal mortality and morbidity: Recognizing perinatal mental health warning signs and connecting women and parenting partners to resources.* [Web article]. www.societyforpsychotherapy.org/maternal-mortality-and-morbidity

Lyden, H. M., & Suchman, N. E. (2013). Transmission of parenting models at the level of representation: Implications for mother-child dyads affected by maternal substance abuse. In N. E. Suchman, M. Pajulo, & L. C. Mayes (Eds.), *Parenting and substance abuse: Developmental approaches to intervention* (pp. 100–125). Oxford University Press. https://doi-org.du.idm.oclc.org/10.1093/med:psych/9780199743100.003.0006

Le, C., & Coombs, S. (2021). *Moms & babies series; substance use disorder hurts moms & babies.* Robert Wood Johnson Foundation.

Macife, J., Towers, C. V., Fortner, K. B., Stuart, G. L., Zvara, B. J., Kurdziel-Adams, G., . . . Cohen, C. T. (2020). Medication-assisted treatment vs. detoxification for women who misuse opioids in pregnancy: Associations with dropout, relapse, Neonatal Opioid Withdrawal Syndrome (NOWS), and childhood sexual abuse. *Addictive Behaviors Reports, 12,* 100315. https://doi.org/10.1016/j.abrep.2020.100315

Maralit, A. M. (2022). Beyond the bump: Ethical and legal considerations for psychologists providing services to pregnant individuals who use substances. *Ethics & Behavior, 33*(2), 89–100. https://doi.org/10.1080/10508422.2022.2093202

Mattocks, K. M., Clark, R., & Weinreb, L. (2017). Initiation and engagement with methadone treatment among pregnant and postpartum women. *Women's Health Issues, 27*(6), 646–651. https://doi.org/10.1016/j.whi.2017.05.002

Mattson, S. N., Bernes, G. A., & Doyle, L. R. (2019). Fetal alcohol spectrum disorders: A review of the neurobehavioral deficits associated with prenatal alcohol exposure. *Alcoholism: Clinical and Experimental Research, 43*(6), 1046–1062. https://doi.org/10.1111/acer.14040

Mittal, L. (2020, July). *Perinatal substance use disorders: Emerging trends in substance use treatment for perinatal women.* Presented at the Virtual Postpartum Support International Annual Conference, Virtual Conference.

National Institute on Drug Abuse (NIDA). (2011). *Screening for drug use in general medical settings: Resource guide.* National Institute of Health.

NHS. (2018, September 6). Statistics on women's smoking status at time of delivery, England -Quarter 1, 2018–19. *NHS Digital*. Retrieved May 9, 2022, from https://digital.nhs.uk/data-and-information/publications/statistical/statistics-on-women-ssmoking-status-at-time-of-delivery-england/statistics-on-womens-smoking-status-at-time-of-delivery-england-quarter-1-april-2018-to-june-2018

Pajulo, H., Pajulo, M., Jussila, H., & Ekholm, E. (2016). Substance-abusing pregnant women: Prenatal intervention using ultrasound consultation and mentalization to enhance the mother-child relationship and reduce substance use. *Infant Mental Health Journal*, 37(4), 317–334. https://doi.org/10.1002/imhj.21574

Parolin, M., & Simonelli, A. (2016). Attachment theory of maternal drug addiction: The contribution to parenting interventions. *Frontiers in Psychiatry*, 7, 152. https://doi.org/10.3389/fpsyt.2016.00152

Polak, K., Kelpin, S., & Terplan, M. (2019). Screening for substance use in pregnancy and the newborn. *Seminars in Fetal and Neonatal Medicine*, 24(2), 90–94. https://doi.org/10.1016/j.siny.2019.01.007

Popova, S., Lange, S., Probst, C., Gmel, G., & Rehm, J. (2017). Estimation of national, regional, and global prevalence of alcohol use during pregnancy and fetal alcohol syndrome: A systematic review and meta-analysis. *The Lancet Global Health*, 5(3), e290–e299. https://doi.org/10.1016/s2214-109x(17)30021-9

Pichini, S., Puig, C., Zuccaro, P., Marchei, E., Pellegrini, M., Murillo, J., . . . García-Algar, Ó. (2005). Assessment of exposure to opiates and cocaine during pregnancy in a Mediterranean city: Preliminary results of the "meconium project". *Forensic Science International*, 153(1), 59–65. https://doi.org/10.1016/j.forsciint.2005.04.013

Preis, H., Inman, E. M., & Lobel, M. (2020). Contributions of psychology to research, treatment, and care of pregnant women with opioid use disorder. *American Psychologist*, 75(6), 853–865. https://doi.org/10.1037/amp0000675

Reece-Stremtan, S., & Marinelli, K. A. (2015). ABM clinical protocol #21: Guidelines for breastfeeding and substance use or substance use disorder, revised 2015. *Breastfeeding Medicine*, 10(3), 135–141. https://doi.org/10.1089/bfm.2015.9992

Rhule-Louie, D. M., & McMahon, R. J. (2007). Problem behavior and romantic relationships: Assortative mating, behavior contagion, and desistance. *Clinical Child and Family Psychology Review*, 10(1), 53–100. https://doi.org/10.1007/s10567-006-0016-y

Roberts, S. C., & Nuru-Jeter, A. (2012). Universal screening for alcohol and drug use and racial disparities in child protective services reporting. *Journal of Behavioral Health Services & Research*, 39(1), 3–16. https://doi.org/10.1007/s11414-011-9247-x

Sahker, E., McCabe, J. E., & Arndt, S. (2015). Differences in successful treatment completion among pregnant and non-pregnant American women. *Archives of Women's Mental Health*, 19(1), 79–86. https://doi.org/10.1007/s00737-015-0520-5

Sarkola, T., Gissler, M., Kahila, H., Autti-Rämö, I., & Halmesmäki, E. (2012). Alcohol and substance abuse identified during pregnancy: Maternal morbidity, child morbidity and welfare interventions. *Acta Paediatrica*, 101(7), 784–790. https://doi.org/10.1111/j.1651-2227.2012.02670.x

Saurel-Cubizolles, M., Prunet, C., & Blondel, B. (2014). Cannabis use during pregnancy in France in 2010. *BJOG*, 121(8), 971–977. https://doi.org/10.1111/1471-0528.12626

Singh, S., Filion, K., Abenhaim, H., & Eisenberg, M. (2020). Prevalence and outcomes of prenatal recreational cannabis use in high-income countries: A scoping review. *BJOG: An International Journal of Obstetrics & Gynaecology*, 127(1), 8–16. https://doi.org/10.1111/1471-0528.15946

Smid, M. C., Metz, T. D., & Gordon, A. J. (2019). Stimulant use in pregnancy: An under-recognized epidemic among pregnant women. *Clinical Obstetrics and Gynecology*, 62(1), 168–184. https://doi.org/10.1097/grf.0000000000000418

Staudt, M. (2018). Best practices for enhancing substance abuse treatment retention by pregnant women. *Best Practices in Mental Health*, 14(2), 48–63.

Stone, R. (2015). Pregnant women and substance use: Fear, stigma, and barriers to care. *Health & Justice*, 3(1). https://doi.org/10.1186/s40352-015-0015-5

Suchman, N. E., Decoste, C., Mcmahon, T. J., Rounsaville, B., & Mayes, L. (2011). The mothers and toddlers program, an attachment-based parenting intervention for substance-using women: Results at 6-week follow-up in a randomized clinical pilot. *Infant Mental Health Journal*, 32(4), 427–449. https://doi.org/10.1002/imhj.20303

Tarasoff, L. A., Milligan, K., Le, T. L., Usher, A. M., & Urbanoski, K. (2018). Integrated treatment programs for pregnant and parenting women with problematic substance use: Service descriptions and client perceptions of care. *Journal of Substance Abuse Treatment, 90*, 9–18. https://doi.org/10.1016/j.jsat.2018.04.008

Ulrich, M., Memmo, E. P., Cruz, A., Heinz, A., & Iverson, R. E. (2021). Implementation of a universal screening process for substance use in pregnancy. *Obstetrics & Gynecology, 137*(4), 695–701. https://doi.org/10.1097/aog.0000000000004305

Virginia Department of Social Services. (2017). *Perinatal substance use: Promoting healthy outcomes.* Virginia Department of General Services.

Vythilingum, B., Roos, A., Faure, S. C., Geerts, L., & Stein, D. J. (2012). Risk factors for substance use in pregnant women in South Africa. *South African Medical Journal, 102*(11), 851. https://doi.org/10.7196/samj.5019

Wallman, C. M., Smith, P. B., & Moore, K. (2011). Implementing a perinatal substance abuse screening tool. *Advances in Neonatal Care, 11*(4), 255–267. https://doi.org/10.1097/anc.0b013e318225a20b

Weber, A., Miskle, B., Lynch, A., Arndt, S., & Acion, L. (2021). Substance use in pregnancy: Identifying stigma and improving care. *Substance Abuse and Rehabilitation, 12*, 105–121. https://doi.org/10.2147/SAR.S319180

Weller, A. E., Crist, R. C., Reiner, B. C., Doyle, G. A., & Berrettini, W. H. (2021). Neonatal Opioid Withdrawal Syndrome (NOWS): A transgenerational echo of the opioid crisis. *Cold Spring Harbor Perspectives in Medicine, 11*(3), a039669. https://doi.org/10.1101/cshperspect.a039669

World Health Organization (WHO). (2013). *WHO recommendations for the prevention and management of tobacco use and second-hand smoke exposure in pregnancy.* World Health Organization.

Wright, T. E., Terplan, M., Ondersma, S. J., Boyce, C., Yonkers, K., Chang, G., & Creanga, A. A. (2016). The role of screening, brief intervention, and referral to treatment in the perinatal period. *American Journal of Obstetrics and Gynecology, 215*(5), 539–547. https://doi.org/10.1016/j.ajog.2016.06.038

Yaya, S., Uthman, O. A., Adjiwanou, V., & Bishwajit, G. (2018). Exposure to tobacco use in pregnancy and its determinants among sub-Saharan Africa women: Analysis of pooled cross-sectional surveys. *Journal of Maternal-Fetal & Neonatal Medicine, 33*(9), 1–231. https://doi.org/10.1080/14767058.2018.1520835

Yonkers, K. A., Gotman, N., Kershaw, T., Forray, A., Howell, H. B., & Rounsaville, B. J. (2010). Screening for prenatal substance use. *Obstetrics & Gynecology, 116*(4), 827–833. https://doi.org/10.1097/aog.0b013e3181ed8290

Zhao, J.-P., Berthod, C., Sheehy, O., Kassaï, B., Gorgui, J., & Bérard, A. (2021). Prevalence and duration of prescribed opioid use during pregnancy: A cohort study from the Quebec Pregnancy cohort. *BMC Pregnancy and Childbirth, 21*(1), 1–12. https://doi.org/10.1186/s12884-021-04270-x

Acknowledgment

The authors would like to acknowledge the ongoing support and contributions to our team's writing from Kim Jacques.

11

PRE-EXISTING SERIOUS MENTAL ILLNESS IN THE PRENATAL PERIOD

Leah A. Millard and Anja Wittkowski

Of women in the perinatal period (i.e., pregnancy and up to one year postpartum), around 10% to 20% experience a mental health condition (NICE, 2020a). Anxiety and/or depression during pregnancy are relatively common, with reported prevalence rates of 15–20% (Howard & Khalifeh, 2020; Yin et al., 2021). However, perinatal mental health conditions can occur across the diagnostic spectrum and differ in terms of their severity (Howard & Khalifeh, 2020). For instance, a much smaller number of women can be susceptible to the onset or the recurrence of a serious mental illness (SMI) in the early postpartum stage, with approximately one to two women in every 1,000 births requiring postpartum psychiatric admission (Howard & Khalifeh, 2020; Jones et al., 2014). According to Public Health England (2018), SMI refers to psychological difficulties that cause significant and debilitating impairment to an individual's everyday functioning. SMIs typically refer to psychosis-related and bipolar-related disorders (Public Health England, 2018). This chapter predominantly focuses on these two SMI conditions.

As will be discussed in this chapter, reviews have identified that women who present with histories of SMIs before their pregnancies (i.e., the prenatal period) are at a particularly high risk of a recurrence of symptoms and/or developing a more severe condition, such as postpartum psychosis (Howard & Khalifeh, 2020; Jones et al., 2014). These conditions will be referred to as pre-existing SMIs throughout this chapter (the authors prefer the term *severe mental health difficulties/problems*, but we have used the more widely used terminology of SMI in this chapter). Experiencing an SMI episode, such as psychosis or bipolar disorder, in the perinatal period may lead to long-term effects on the well-being of the mother, cause disruption in the attachment between the mother and the baby, and elicit future psychosocial difficulties in the child (Jones et al., 2014; Stein et al., 2014). SMIs during pregnancy have been found to have higher levels of adverse postpartum outcomes, such as premature births, low birth weight, and maternal mortality, in comparison to the general population (Easter et al., 2021). Therefore, the following chapter on women with pre-existing SMIs during the prenatal period (the time from conception up until birth) will aim to identify and discuss:[1]

- A brief outline of the criteria for psychosis-related and bipolar-related disorders
- Consequences associated with pre-existing SMIs during the prenatal period

DOI: 10.4324/9781003206903-14

- Assessment of pregnant women presenting with SMIs
- Recommended psychological and psychotropic treatments of SMIs during the prenatal period
- SMIs and the effects on familial relationships during the prenatal period
- Sociocultural considerations associated with SMIs in the prenatal period

Serious Mental Illnesses

Psychosis-Related Disorders

The criteria for psychosis-related disorders, such as schizophrenia, are similar across the World Health Organization's (WHO's) *International Classification of Diseases*, 11th Revision (ICD-11; WHO, 2019) and the American Psychological Association's (APA's) *Diagnostic and Statistical Manual of Mental Disorders*, Fifth Edition (DSM-5; APA, 2013). Psychosis-related disorders are marked by an impairment of reality testing and behavior changes, which can be exhibited through positive symptoms including delusions and hallucinations, negative symptoms including flat affect and lack of motivation, disorganized thinking and/or behavior, and psychomotor dysfunction (APA, 2013; WHO, 2019). There are two age ranges when women are more at risk of psychosis-related onset. The first period of risk is between 20 and 39 years old, and the second is during the early stages of menopause. The prevalence of psychosis in women significantly increases above the age of 40 years (Li et al., 2022). Compared to women, men have only one peak age range for the potential onset of psychosis, between the ages of 20 and 29 years (Li et al., 2022).

In addition to the age of onset, the presentation of psychosis-related disorders is also different for men and women. In their review of 17 studies, Mazza et al. (2021) identified that, during the early stages of psychosis, women tend to present with more mood-related symptoms (e.g., low mood, anxiety) and have better social functioning than men. In consequence, these differences in presentation can lead to a misdiagnosis and/or a delay in the onset of treatment for women. Furthermore, Mazza et al. (2021) suggested that women were much more likely than men to have physical comorbidities and be susceptible to metabolic and endocrine-induced side effects of antipsychotic medications. These differences in presentation are perhaps particularly important when considering prenatal care for women with SMIs.

Although relatively rare, postpartum psychosis, sometimes referred to as puerperal psychosis or psychosis after childbirth, is regarded as the most severe mental health condition that women can experience in the postpartum period (Jones et al., 2014). As will be discussed in this chapter, women with pre-existing SMIs are at a high risk of developing the condition in the postpartum period (Howard & Khalifeh, 2020).

Bipolar-Related Disorders

The WHO (2019) ICD-11 states that bipolar disorders are characterized by a disturbance in mood, which involves elevated mood and an increase in activity and behavior for at least seven days (known as mania) or over a shorter period (hypomania) and a lowering of mood and energy (depression). Bipolar disorders commonly consist of two types: type I and type II. Type I is characterized by at least one episode of mania, which can be accompanied by some depressive episodes. Type II is defined by at least one depressive episode with hypo-manic symptoms. According to NICE guidelines (2020b), the peak age of onset for bipolar disorder is typically 15 to 19 years, with some findings indicating that the onset occurs ear-lier in men than women (Dell'Osso et al., 2021). Women typically experience bipolar type II, alongside episodes of rapid cycling and suicide attempts (Dell'Osso et al., 2021). For women with bipolar disorder, pregnancy and childbirth are periods of high risk of relapse as there is a strong association between these reproductive life events and a severe recur-rence of symptoms (Diflorio & Jones, 2010).

Consequences of Pre-Existing SMIs

In the following section, we examine specific features associated with pre-existing SMIs during pregnancy, including the prevalence of comorbid physical health problems. We also consider how these factors may lead to a higher risk of obstetric and neonatal complica-tions in this group of women.

History of Mental Health Problems

Women with a pre-existing severe mood disorder, such as bipolar-related disorder, have been found to be at an increased risk of having a postpartum relapse (Jones et al., 2014). The majority of women who experience such a relapse in mental health symptoms are most commonly those with a history of mental health problems prenatally, particularly bipolar disorder (Munk-Olsen et al., 2016).

Across 37 studies, Wesseloo et al. (2016) conducted a systematic review of postpar-tum relapse risk (i.e., psychosis, mania, and/or hospitalization) in pregnant women with histories of postpartum psychosis and/or bipolar disorder. From 5,700 deliveries in 4,023 patients, the overall risk for postpartum relapse among this group of women was reported to be 35%. Specifically, 20% of women with pre-existing bipolar disorder experienced a postpartum SMI. However, those with pre-existing bipolar disorder were significantly less likely to experience a severe postpartum episode (17%) in comparison to those who have a history of postpartum psychosis (29%). In addition, relapse rates were higher among women with bipolar disorder who were medication free during pregnancy versus those who took medication (Wesseloo et al., 2016). Similar findings were reported in an earlier review by Jones et al. (2014): women with a history of bipolar disorder were at a high risk of a recurrence of severe bipolar-related symptoms while being at an even higher risk of developing any form of mood disorder in the postpartum period.

As Howard and Khalifeh (2020) identified that women experiencing mental health con-ditions during pregnancy were also at a higher risk of mortality than women without a perinatal mental health condition, it is imperative that optimal care is accessible to women with pre-existing SMIs to prevent such serious outcomes. According to the National Peri-natal Epidemiology Unit's annual audit into maternal deaths and morbidity, known as the *Mothers and Babies: Reducing Risk through Audits and Confidential Enquires across the UK* (MBRRACE-UK) report, suicide was a leading cause of death between 2018 and 2020 in mothers from six weeks to one year postpartum (Knight et al., 2022). Suicide accounted for 18% of maternal deaths during this period. Furthermore, between 2015 and 2017, 28% of pregnant/postpartum women who died had a pre-existing mental health condition (Knight et al., 2019). Specifically, Knight et al. (2019) reported that mental health problems were the cause of death in 21 of 99 women who died before 24 weeks' gestation while pregnant or after their pregnancy ended at less than 24 weeks. Reid et al.'s (2022) comprehensive review of risk factors for perinatal suicide ideation and behavior identified that guilt, shame, and worthlessness were significantly associated with suicidal ideation in perinatal women. Furthermore, abuse experienced recently or during childhood was commonly associated with suicidal ideation, attempts, and death among samples of pregnant women only (Reid et al., 2022). We acknowledge that the current research on perinatal mental health and suicide pertains to all mental health conditions and not specifically bipolar or psychosis, although Moitra et al.'s (2021) review found the risk of suicide to be significantly associated with bipolar disorder and psychosis-related disorders in clinical adult populations. This association was found to be lower in women than men at the level of a statistical trend (Moitra et al., 2021). Extrapolating from these findings, it is important to highlight that suicide is a possible risk factor among pregnant women with pre-existing SMIs.

Comorbid Physical Health Problems

Comorbid physical health difficulties are particularly prevalent among those diagnosed with an SMI across both men and women compared to the general population (Public Health England, 2018). The reasons for this disparity are considered complex and not completely understood, with most of this research derived from the nonperinatal population. These inequalities include rates of obesity, diabetes, coronary heart disease, and asthma being higher in the SMI population (Public Health England, 2018). Consequently, those diagnosed with an SMI have a reduced life expectancy of about 15 to 20 years, compared to those without (Public Health England, 2018). Five modifiable primary risk factors for poor physical health were identified by Firth et al. (2019) among those experiencing mental health difficulties across both genders, which were smoking, alcohol misuse, sleep disturbance, physical inactivity, and dietary risks. During the prenatal period, these physical health inequalities and risk factors among women with SMIs persist. For instance, in the prenatal period, women with pre-existing schizophrenia and bipolar disorder were more likely to smoke, use illicit drugs, and drink alcohol during pregnancy compared to women without either bipolar disorder or psychosis (Judd et al., 2014).

Howard and Khalifeh (2020) explained that, in the United Kingdom, women experiencing an SMI during pregnancy are currently referred to separate services that address specific comorbidity (i.e., smoking cessation and substance misuse service). Although integrative interventions would provide optimal prenatal care for those with SMIs, there are very few interventions have been developed (Howard & Khalifeh, 2020). However, the prevalence of physical comorbidities and their associated risks highlight how integrative services for pregnant women would optimize their care.

Recent statistics revealed that approximately 9% of pregnant women in England were known to be smoking at the time of delivery (NHS Digital, 2023). Compared to the general population, smoking is a lifestyle factor that is more prevalent among men and women with SMIs (Gilbody et al., 2019). Women with mental health difficulties (including both SMIs and other mental health conditions) have been shown to be more likely to continue smoking throughout their pregnancies than those without a psychiatric diagnosis (Howard et al., 2013a). In comparison to women without a mental health difficulty, Vigod et al. (2020) reported that women with schizophrenia were more likely to smoke during pregnancy fourfold. Nevertheless, women with mental health difficulties have been shown to be more motivated to engage in smoking cessation interventions; however, they found it more difficult to stop compared to women without mental health difficulties (Howard et al., 2013a). These findings were attributed to concerns about how smoking cessation might inadvertently lead to a deterioration in mental health, which caused practitioners to overlook smoking cessation programs (Howard et al., 2013a).

Obesity is an additional factor that is a common morbidity in the SMI population, which has been shown to have an increased prevalence among pregnant women with mental health difficulties (Easter et al., 2021). In their systematic review and meta-analysis, Afzal et al. (2021) reported that those with SMIs (including both men and women) were more likely to live with obesity threefold than the general population. Specifically, there was a higher prevalence of obesity in women with schizophrenia than in men, but this gender difference was not observed with bipolar disorder (Afzal et al., 2021). Previous findings derived from the general population have shown that obesity during pregnancy was associated with adverse outcomes including cardiac issues and obstetric embolisms (Easter et al., 2021; Sebire et al., 2001). However, in a historic cohort study of electronic health records among perinatal women with SMIs, Easter et al. (2021) were unable to derive sufficient data on pregnancy weight to determine how obesity may affect birth outcomes in women with SMIs.

Pharmacological interventions may also contribute to the physical health comorbidities in the SMI population. Antipsychotic medication, commonly used in those with SMIs, has been associated with metabolic side effects across both men and women (i.e., increase in blood pressure, weight, and blood sugar levels), which may contribute to physical health conditions, such as obesity, diabetes, and cardiovascular disease (Public Health England, 2018). As previously noted, women are more likely than men to experience the metabolic and endocrine-induced side effects of these medications (Mazza et al., 2021). Due to the ethical issues that would be associated with such trials, there are no published randomized controlled trials on the use of psychotropic medication with pregnant women (Howard & Khalifeh, 2020).

Obstetric and Neonatal Complications

The comorbid physical health problems and associated lifestyle factors mentioned earlier (e.g., smoking, low physical activity, poor diet, and alcohol and substance misuse) can lead to comorbidities that are prevalent in pre-existing SMIs, such as obesity, gestational diabetes, and hypertension, which in turn can precipitate obstetric and neonatal complications (Howard & Khalifeh, 2020; Scott & Happell, 2011). Therefore, comorbid physical health problems may mediate the risk between pre-existing SMIs and adverse obstetric and neonatal outcomes (Howard & Khalifeh, 2020).

Regardless of severity, it has been consistently shown that women experiencing any type of mental health condition are at an increased risk of preterm birth and fetal growth impairments (Howard & Khalifeh, 2020). However, there are also high risks of medical comorbidities such as pre-eclampsia, prenatal and postpartum hemorrhage, placental abruptions, and stillbirth in perinatal women with SMIs (Howard & Khalifeh, 2020). In Australia, a review of 595,792 singleton births showed that women with SMIs (who accounted for 2,046 births) were at an increased likelihood of having gestational diabetes, having an induced labor, an unplanned cesarean section, and/or being admitted to intensive care postpartum (Edvardsson et al., 2022). In terms of infant outcomes, infants of mothers with an

SMI were more likely than mothers without an SMI to have higher rates of preterm birth, low birth weight, a low Apgar score at five minutes, and/or admission to a neonatal unit (Edvardsson et al., 2022).

Women with an SMI during pregnancy may experience higher rates of morbidity compared to women without any mental health history, which may lead to serious consequences during childbirth. Easter et al. (2021) investigated obstetric near misses (i.e., life-threatening obstetric complications) in women with an SMI during pregnancy versus women who had no history of such. Of 100,000 pre-existing SMI births, 884 (0.88%) resulted in an obstetric near miss, compared to 575 (0.58%) births of 100,000 in the general population. The highest rates of life-threatening complications for pre-existing SMIs were acute kidney failure, cardiac arrest, failure or infarction, and obstetric embolism. After accounting for age, ethnicity, and social deprivation, women experiencing pre-existing SMIs were still significantly at more risk of serious obstetric complications (Easter et al., 2021).

The overrepresentation of adverse obstetric outcomes may be attributed to "diagnostic overshadowing" due to the shared characteristics between common obstetric complications and mental illness (Easter et al., 2021, p. 498). Maternal mortalities have previously been shown to be a consequence of obstetric complications being mistakenly associated with the effects of mental illness, which may also precipitate delayed diagnosis and mistreatment (Easter et al., 2021; Knight et al., 2019). A higher incidence of domestic violence is also prevalent among women with any pre-existing mental health condition compared to women without, which is another prominent vulnerability factor for adverse obstetric and neonatal outcomes (Howard & Khalifeh, 2020; Howard et al., 2013b).

As will be elaborated on, this group of women has also shown to have poorer and/or delayed attendance at prenatal care due to the complexities of their conditions (Edvardsson et al., 2022; Frayne et al., 2019; Howard & Khalifeh, 2020). From this evidence, it is apparent that the interplay among variables associated pre-existing SMI is convoluted. However, these findings highlight the need for this group of women to receive frequent maternity care.

Assessment

When pregnant, a woman is usually invited to attend an initial prenatal appointment with a midwife. In the United Kingdom, women typically have this appointment by the tenth week of their pregnancy (NICE, 2021). During this appointment, midwives are advised to gather information on a woman's history, including whether they have any history or current experiences with SMI, any previous or current treatment from specialist mental health services, any current medication, and any SMIs among first-degree relatives, such as their mother or sister (NICE, 2021; Schofield & Kapoor, 2019). In conjunction, the midwife considers whether the woman presents with possible risk factors such as self-neglect, self-harm, suicidal ideation, risk to others (including the infant), smoking, alcohol, or substance misuse, and domestic violence. With permission from the woman, this risk assessment should also include her partner, family, or carer. By gathering this information, clinicians can make an informed decision on a woman's pathway of care (i.e., referral to a specialist perinatal mental health service), as well as whether additional referrals to social care and safeguarding services are required (Schofield & Kapoor, 2019).

In most cases, pregnant women who have a pre-existing SMI require care from specialist perinatal mental health services (McAllister-Williams et al., 2017; Schofield & Kapoor,

2019). Maternity services have a significant role in identifying and referring this group of women to these specialist perinatal mental health services (Schofield & Kapoor, 2019). Communication between maternity services, mental health services, and general practitioners (GPs) is paramount in providing appropriate care for women with an SMI during pregnancy. Maternal deaths have been significantly associated with poor communication between practitioners (i.e., obstetricians, psychiatrists, GPs, health visitors, and midwives); thus, written and oral communication between healthcare professionals throughout a woman's care is vital (Schofield & Kapoor, 2019). To facilitate communication between practitioners and service users, regular prenatal appointments are advised to allow for routine monitoring of their mental health (Schofield & Kapoor, 2019).

Reports by Cantwell et al. (2015, 2018) identified different presentations that determine a woman's referral timeframe to specialist perinatal mental health services (i.e., routine, urgent, or emergency referral). For instance, only a routine referral is required for pregnant women with histories of SMI who are currently well. However, an urgent referral during pregnancy is warranted during a presentation of current SMI symptoms (Cantwell et al., 2015, 2018). An emergency referral would be required when a woman in the early postpartum period has a new onset of symptoms, which may be associated with an SMI (Cantwell et al., 2015). Schofield and Kapoor (2019) outlined four subcategories that can assist in establishing a referral and treatment route, including those who are well and either taking medication or not and those who are deemed not well and either taking medication or not. Regardless of their current presentation, NHS England et al. (2018) have advised that pregnant women with a pre-existing SMI should be referred to a specialist perinatal mental health team for a biopsychosocial assessment. Such an assessment involves a clinician identifying possible biological, psychological, and social factors that may be contributing to the woman's difficulties (National Collaborating Centre for Mental Health, 2018).

Treatment for Pre-Existing SMI During Pregnancy

Optimizing the outcomes of the pregnancy, infant, and the physical and mental well-being of women is the aim of perinatal treatment (Schofield & Kapoor, 2019). From their review of postpartum relapse risk, Wesseloo et al. (2016) proposed individualized relapse prevention plans for women with an SMI during pregnancy. Each plan should include psychotropic medication planning, an obstetric birth plan (e.g., mode of delivery preference), interventions that can be implemented from the first sign of relapse, the assessment of children who have had in utero medication exposure, baby feeding preference, reducing levels of stress, mother–infant bonding, and strategies in helping women maintain sufficient sleep and stable circadian rhythm (Wesseloo et al., 2016).

The NICE guidelines advise that perinatal women are involved in all decisions about their care (NICE, 2020a). In the treatment of pre-existing SMIs, an integrated and individualized care plan should be developed (NICE, 2020a). This plan should outline the care and treatment of the SMI and the role of each clinician that is involved in the woman's care, such as setting out who is responsible for the coordination of the care plan, the schedule of monitoring, and who delivers the interventions and facilitates the outcomes with the woman (NICE, 2018). It should be established whether all clinicians are aware of their responsibilities, that information is shared effectively, that the mental health of the woman is considered during all parts of the care plan, and that it is taken into account how interventions are delivered in accordance with each stage of pregnancy. These NICE

(2020a) recommendations are also reflected in the clinical practice guidance of Australia's Centre of Perinatal Excellence (COPE, 2023) and the American College of Obstetricians and Gynecologists (ACOG, 2023), which similarly emphasize the importance of multidimensional care.

Specialized Prenatal Care

According to WHO (2016), prenatal care has been linked to a reduction in maternal and perinatal morbidity and mortality by identifying risks and preventing and managing pregnancy-related complications and/or medical conditions. Pregnant women with histories of SMI should be under the care of mental health services, ideally a specialized perinatal mental health service (McAllister-Williams et al., 2017).

This population has been shown to have poorer and/or delayed attendance to prenatal care due to the complexities of their conditions when compared to women in the general population (Edvardsson et al., 2022; Frayne et al., 2019). Nevertheless, when comparing a group of pregnant women with and without any psychiatric diagnosis, those with mental health difficulties were at risk of either overusing or underusing the specialized prenatal service (Ben-Sheetrit et al., 2018). Interestingly, the risk across both of these categories was greater in women with anxiety and/or depression than women with an SMI. Women with schizophrenia had a tendency to underuse the prenatal service. Psychosocial factors, such as low levels of motivation, have been suggested as a possible contributor to underusing the prenatal service. In contrast, psychopharmacological treatment was associated with high utilization of prenatal care. High attendance rates may be explained by the demand for high-risk pregnancies in women with pre-existing SMI, particularly if taking psychotropic medication that requires regular monitoring (Ben-Sheetrit et al., 2018).

Offering an integrated obstetric-psychiatric service may improve the utilization and address the complexities of prenatal care among the pre-existing SMI population. Several studies were conducted within a specialized prenatal care clinic in Western Australia for women with pre-existing SMI, which assessed women both obstetrically and psychiatrically (e.g., Hauck et al., 2013; Nguyen et al., 2013; Frayne et al., 2014, 2019). For example, Frayne et al. (2019) conducted a cohort study of 420 completed pregnancy records within the specialized prenatal clinic. Ninety-one percent of the sample displayed high attendance rates, suggesting that specialized care leads to greater engagement with services among this group of women (Frayne et al., 2019). The service also showed good acceptability through qualitative analysis (Hauck et al., 2013). However, studies have not yet compared the outcomes from specialized prenatal care with those from general prenatal services in Australia.

In the United Kingdom, several National Health Service (NHS) services offer combined obstetric and psychiatric care. A quality improvement project was conducted within an NHS perinatal mental health team in London, which ran a combined clinic for women deemed to be at "high risk" of adverse postpartum outcomes (Millard et al., 2020). Known as the joint obstetric-psychiatric clinic, service users were seen by both a consultant perinatal psychiatrist and a consultant specialist obstetrician during the same appointment. Compared with women with moderate mental health conditions (i.e., anxiety, depression, eating disorders), the preliminary findings showed that women with SMI attended significantly more appointments (i.e., had two or more clinic visits). Furthermore, poor attendance at the joint obstetric-psychiatric clinic (had one clinic visit or less) was a predictor of adverse neonatal outcomes (i.e., preterm birth and/or neonatal admission; Millard et al., 2020). It is important to note that these unpublished findings were preliminary and that research into the benefits of specialized prenatal care is still in its infancy.

Psychotropic Medication

Decisions regarding the prescribing of psychotropic medication in pregnant women is an ongoing challenge due to the risks associated with maternal and infant outcomes (McAllister-Williams et al., 2017). When women discover that they are pregnant, it is estimated that around 90% of women with a pre-existing mental health condition will discontinue their psychotropic medication and often without consultation with a healthcare professional (NHS England et al., 2018). The British Association for Psychopharmacology current guidelines advise that discussions between the clinician and the mother should include the risks of exposure both in utero and through breastfeeding on the child, which may increase the risk of birth defects and adversely affect development as well as the possible side effects of changing or discontinuing medication (McAllister-Williams et al., 2017). NICE (2020a) recommends psychotropic medication with the lowest risk profile for the woman, fetus, and baby. Medications must have a well-researched reproductive safety profile. Only one medication should be prescribed, which should be at the minimal effective dose to limit fetus exposure (Raffi et al., 2019). Similar guidance is also reflected in other national perinatal care guidelines, such as guidelines from Australia and the United States. The use of pharmacological intervention for pregnant women with pre-existing SMIs is recommended to help prevent relapse and adverse postpartum outcomes (ACOG, 2023; COPE, 2023).

The primary reason for discontinuation of medication during pregnancy is the avoidance of fetal exposure (Bayrampour et al., 2020). Psychotropic medication crosses the placenta, which exposes the fetal central nervous system and may increase the risk of abnormal organ and/or skeletal development (Galbally et al., 2014; Ornoy et al., 2017). Based on this evidence, it is unsurprising that pregnancy is a strong predictor of the discontinuation of psychotropic medication, which increases the risk of relapse in pregnancy and postpartum (McAllister-Williams et al., 2017; Petersen et al., 2016). In bipolar disorder, the discontinuation of prophylactic mood stabilizers in pregnant women doubled the risk of relapse and shortened the time of its onset (Jones et al., 2014). These findings were also supported by Tosato et al.'s (2017) review, whereby at least 50% of pregnant women with bipolar disorder who discontinued medication became symptomatic. Furthermore, there was a twofold increase in recurrence risk and an increase in the time of illness burden. Moreover, Jones et al.'s (2014) review noted that discontinuation of both typical and atypical antipsychotic medications in pregnancy has been associated with an increased relapse risk. Particularly, a 13-fold relapse risk increase in the discontinuation of typical antipsychotic medication (Tosato et al., 2017). Therefore, women who are receiving psychotropic mediation prenatally are at an increased risk of relapse if medication is discontinued during pregnancy (Jones et al., 2014).

The Royal College of Psychiatrists (RC-Psych) currently states that there is no sufficient evidence to suggest that one specific antipsychotic medication is the safest to use during pregnancy (RC-Psych, 2018). However, a review by Betcher et al. (2019) summarized that most studies did not report a strong association between antipsychotic medication use in pregnancy and major birth defects, but risperidone is a possible exception. Some antipsychotics, such as quetiapine or olanzapine, have been associated with gestational diabetes and larger babies (Heinonen et al., 2022).

Mood stabilizers are typically administered to treat bipolar disorder (NICE, 2014). In the United Kingdom, the NHS (2023) reports that lithium is the most prevalent first-line choice. Although anticonvulsant medications are alternative options, such as sodium valproate, carbamazepine, or lamotrigine, sodium valproate is not recommended to pregnant women due to the evidence base indicating increased risks of birth defects (COPE, 2023; NHS, 2023). For this reason, the use and possible discontinuation of any medication needs to be carefully considered by women and discussed with their clinician. For women with pre-existing SMIs who are planning a pregnancy, NICE (2020a) guidelines suggest that women are referred to preconception counseling within a specialist perinatal mental health team to discuss medication.

Psychotherapeutic Intervention

Psychotherapeutic interventions are recommended to manage the stress associated with pregnancy, particularly if psychotropic medication has been changed or discontinued (NICE, 2020a). The British Psychological Society (BPS, 2019) puts forth that psychotherapeutic interventions can provide women with an understanding of their mental health problems within a wider context via formulation and can empower women to manage their mental health difficulties.

These interventions may also help to manage secondary mental health conditions associated with SMI, such as anxiety and/or depression (COPE, 2023). In the United Kingdom, women with pre-existing SMIs in the perinatal period are likely to receive psychotherapeutic treatment under a specialist perinatal community mental health team. Referrals to these specialist teams can be initiated through a woman's maternity service (e.g., a midwife or health visitor) or their current community mental health team if they have existing mental health difficulties (NHS England et al., 2018).

Although interventions can be offered as a treatment for a range of mental health difficulties, including SMIs (NHS England et al., 2018), it is important for services to adapt evidence-based psychotherapies (e.g., cognitive behavioral therapy [CBT]) for the perinatal period (O'Mahen & Healy, 2021). For women with bipolar depression, it is advised that clinicians consider structured psychotherapies delivered in an individual, group, or family format. These therapies may include CBT, interpersonal psychotherapy (IPT), or behavioral couple's therapy (NICE, 2020b). O'Brien et al.'s (in press) review of clinical psychology guidelines for perinatal mental health reported that CBT or IPT is universally recommended across guidelines. For women with psychosis-related disorders, CBT or family intervention is recommended, which mirrors the guidelines for psychosis-related disorders in the general adult population (NICE, 2014). Psychotherapeutic intervention is particularly pertinent in reducing the risk of relapse in pregnant women who are experiencing stress associated with their pregnancy or have either changed or discontinued their antipsychotic medication (NICE, 2020a). The authors were unable to identify any studies on the efficacy of psychotherapeutic interventions in women with pre-existing SMIs during pregnancy. Howard and Khalifeh (2020) identified several studies on psychotherapeutic interventions for women with mental health difficulties in the perinatal period; however, all these studies focused on anxiety and/or depression.

Sociocultural Considerations

So far, the evidence has highlighted the importance of accessibility to healthcare that addresses the complexities of pre-existing SMI. However, these complexities are further exacerbated by sociocultural factors, which can generate multiple barriers for perinatal women accessing perinatal mental health services in the United Kingdom (Sambrook Smith et al., 2019). The societal expectations of motherhood and the stigma associated with perinatal mental health conditions, which can elicit feelings of guilt and shame, have been attributed to women's reluctance to access mental health services (Sambrook Smith et al., 2019). For instance, some women are concerned about stigma and/or fear of losing custody of children if they disclose perinatal mental health difficulties (Higgins et al., 2016). The fear of custody loss in those with pre-existing SMIs can hinder communication with services and lead to the masking of symptoms (Dolman et al., 2013). Overall, feelings of shame and guilt in women are strengthened by the negative perceptions surrounding perinatal diagnosis and treatment, which becomes a primary barrier for women accessing specialist services (Sambrook Smith et al., 2019).

In people from ethnic minority groups, this stigma is often further exacerbated. Compared with pregnant White women, pregnant women from ethnic minorities in the United Kingdom have significantly lower rates of accessing mental health services and higher levels of involuntary admissions to inpatient psychiatric care (Jankovic et al., 2020). Not specific to perinatal mental health care, there are alarming disparities for women in ethnic minority groups accessing maternity services in the United Kingdom. When comparing maternal mortality rates in the United Kingdom, the difference between ethnic minority groups and White women was four times higher for Black women and two times higher for mixed ethnicity and Asian women (Knight et al., 2021). In response, the *Five x More* (2022) report surveyed 1,340 Black and Black mixed mothers on their maternity care experiences. Despite reporting high levels of self-reported engagement with prenatal services, over a quarter (27%) of the sample rated the care that they received as unsatisfactory (*Five x More*, 2022).

Culturally insensitive attitudes were identified by Sambrook Smith et al. (2019) as a prominent barrier to perinatal women receiving optimal care. Improvements in cultural competency are an integral part of engaging women from ethnic minority groups in perinatal mental health services (Higgins et al., 2018). Social and cultural differences may influence how a pregnant woman engages with prenatal services; therefore, improving sensitivity to the differences and nuances of mental health across cultures is imperative (Higgins et al., 2018). NICE (2020a) guidelines recommend that clinicians provide women with culturally relevant information on perinatal mental health difficulties and provide assurance that they are not uncommon. To improve the cultural competency of services, Higgins et al. (2018) suggested the introduction of culturally sensitive assessment tools and skilled interpreters and having clinicians acknowledge models and theories of mental health within different social and cultural contexts that go beyond Westernized constructs. However, Higgins et al. (2018) also acknowledge that there are organizational barriers that prevent the delivery of effective services such as staff shortages and time constraints.

Pre-Existing SMI and Familial Relationships

Family members can often be an integral part of identifying symptoms of perinatal mental health conditions. However, family members can also impede mothers from disclosing diagnoses due to the perceived stigma associated with mental health difficulties (Sambrook Smith et al., 2019). Nevertheless, women who have experienced an SMI at postpartum emphasized the importance of family being included in treatment and discharge planning processes (Dolman et al., 2013; Forde et al., 2020). In addition, pregnant women with poor social support from a partner were found to be more likely to have prenatal depressive symptoms (Bilszta et al., 2008).

Due to the important role a partner can have during the prenatal period, NICE (2020a) guidelines recommend that partners/family members be involved with all processes of care, with the consent of the woman. Therefore, due to their involvement, it is important to acknowledge the effects that pre-existing SMIs may have on partners and the family network including other offspring in the management of prenatal SMIs (Jones et al., 2014).

Frayne et al. (2014) conducted a cross-sectional survey with male partners (*n* = 40) of women with pre-existing SMIs. These men reported a high rate of psychosocial difficulties including smoking, alcohol and/or drug misuse (60%), a history of domestic violence (18%), and a history of an SMI (12.5%). However, all reported feeling positive about the forthcoming arrival of the infant, and most believed that they were receiving adequate emotional and practical support from their network of family and/or friends. Furthermore, most of the men felt positive about their relationship with their partner and were self-assured in their ability to recognize their partner's psychiatric symptoms. Only 8% had negative feelings toward their partner's mental health (Frayne et al., 2014).

However, there is currently limited research on how pre-existing SMIs may affect members of the family during the prenatal period. Predominantly, the research focuses on the experiences of partners during the postpartum period (i.e., following the onset of postpartum psychosis). Therefore, further evidence is required within the prenatal period to ensure that partners and family members that appropriate support can be integrated into prenatal care.

Conclusion and Future Directions

Complex associations between the various risk factors of pre-existing SMIs (i.e., history of mental health difficulties, physical health, lifestyle behaviors, and sociocultural considerations) mean that pregnant women with SMIs require specialized prenatal care. Pregnant women with a pre-existing SMI who present themselves to prenatal services require comprehensive assessments in an environment where they feel able to disclose their mental health difficulties, and where a detailed treatment plan can be formulated.

This chapter has highlighted future areas of research to optimize the maternity care of this group of women and inform future prenatal care guidance. Such research should involve an investigation into the benefits of providing joint psychiatric-obstetric prenatal care for women with pre-existing SMIs and how services can accommodate their complex needs. A gap in the literature has also been identified in the research on the efficacy of psychological interventions for this group of women in managing their pregnancies and preventing a relapse of symptoms (i.e., randomized controlled trials). Moreover, to reduce the alarming disparities in prenatal care among pregnant ethnic minority women, an examination into their experiences of specialized perinatal mental health care is warranted.

Note

1 This chapter primarily draws on evidence from UK-based perinatal mental health research.

References

Afzal, M., Siddiqi, N., Ahmad, B., Afsheen, N., Aslam, F., Ali, A., . . . G. A. (2021). Prevalence of overweight and obesity in people with severe mental illness: Systematic review and meta-analysis. *Frontiers in Endocrinology, 12.* https://doi.org/10.3389/fendo.2021.769309

American College of Obstetricians and Gynecologists [ACOG]. (2023). Treatment and management of mental health conditions during pregnancy and postpartum. *Clinical Practice Guideline 5*.www.acog.org/programs/perinatal-mental-health/assessment-and-treatment-of-perinatal-mental-health-conditions

American Psychiatric Association [APA]. (2013). *Diagnostic and statistical manual of mental disorders* (5th ed.). American Psychiatric Association. https://doi.org/10.1176/appi.books.9780890425596

Awe, T., Abe, C., Peter, M., & Wheeler, R. (2022). The Black maternity experiences survey: A nationwide study of Black women's experiences of maternity services in the United Kingdom. *Five x More*. https://fivexmore.org/blackmereport

Bayrampour, H., Kapoor, A., Bunka, M., & Ryan, D. (2020). The risk of relapse of depression during pregnancy after discontinuation of antidepressants. *Journal of Clinical Psychiatry, 81*(4), 19r13134. https://doi.org/10.4088/jcp.19r13134

Ben-Sheetrit, J., Huller-Harari, L., Rasner, M., Magen, N., Nacasch, N., & Torena, P. (2018). Psychiatric disorders and compliance with prenatal care: A 10-year retrospective cohort compared to controls. *European Psychiatry, 49*, 23–29. https://doi.org/10.1016/j.eurpsy.2017.11.011

Betcher, H. K., Montiel, C., & Clark, C. T. (2019). Use of antipsychotic drugs during pregnancy. *Current Treatment Options in Psychiatry, 6*, 17–31. https://doi.org/10.1007/s40501-019-0165-5

Bilszta, J. L. C., Tang, M., Meyer, D., Milgrom, J., Ericksen, J., & Buist, A. E. (2008). Single motherhood versus poor partner relationship: Outcomes for antenatal mental health. *Australian & New Zealand Journal of Psychiatry, 42*(1), 56–65. https://doi.org/10.1080/00048670701732731

Cantwell, R., Knight, M., Oates, M., & Shakespeare, J, On Behalf of the MBRRACE-UK Mental Health Chapter Writing Group. (2015). Lessons on maternal mental health. In M. Knight, D. Tuffnell, S. Kenyon, J. Shakespeare, R. Gray, & J. J. Kurinczuk (Eds.), *Saving lives, improving mothers' care – Surveillance of maternal deaths in the UK 2011–13 and lessons learned to inform maternity care from the UK and Ireland confidential enquiries into maternal deaths and morbidity 2009–13* (pp. 22–41). National Perinatal Epidemiology Unit, University of Oxford.

Cantwell, R., Youd, E., & Knight, M, On Behalf of the MBRRACE-UK Mental Health Chapter Writing Group. (2018). Messages for mental health. In M. Knight, K. Bunch, D. Tuffnell, R. Patel, J. Shakespeare, R. Kotnis, S. Kenyon, & J. J. Kurinczuk (Eds.), *Saving lives, improving mothers' care – Lessons learned to inform maternity care from the UK and Ireland confidential enquiries into maternal deaths and morbidity 2014–16* (pp. 42–60). National Perinatal Epidemiology Unit, University of Oxford.

Centre of Perinatal Excellence [COPE]. (2023). *Effective mental health care in the perinatal period: Australian clinical practice guideline.* www.cope.org.au/health-professionals/health-professionals-3/review-of-new-perinatal-mental-health-guidelines/

Dell'Osso, B., Cafaro, R., & Ketter, T. A. (2021). Has bipolar disorder become a predominantly female gender related condition? Analysis of recently published large sample studies. *International Journal of Bipolar Disorders, 9*(1), 3. https://doi.org/10.1186/s40345-020-00207-z

Diflorio, A., & Jones, I. (2010). Is sex important? Gender differences in bipolar disorder. *International Review of Psychiatry, 22*(5), 437–452. https://doi.org/10.3109/09540261.2010.514601

Dolman, C., Jones, I., & Howard, L. M. (2013). Pre-conception to parenting: A systematic review and meta-synthesis of the qualitative literature on motherhood for women with severe mental illness. *Archives of Womens Mental Health, 16*(3), 173–196. https://doi.org/10.1007/s00737-013-0336-0

Easter, A., Sandall, J., & Howard, L. M. (2021). Obstetric near misses among women with serious mental illness: Data linkage cohort study. *British Journal of Psychiatry, 219*(3), 494–500. https://doi.org/10.1192/bjp.2020.250

Edvardsson, K., Hughes, E., Copnell, B., Mogren, I., Vicendese, D., & Gray, R. (2022). Severe mental illness and pregnancy outcomes in Australia: A population-based study of 595 792 singleton births 2009–2016. *PLoS One, 17*(2), e0264512. https://doi.org/10.1371/journal.pone.0264512

Firth, J., Siddiqi, N., Koyanagi, A., Siskind, D., Rosenbaum, S., Galletly, C., . . . Stubbs, B. (2019). The lancet psychiatry commission: A blueprint for protecting physical health in people with mental illness. *The Lancet Psychiatry, 6*(8), 675–712. https://doi.org/10.1016/S2215-0366(19)30132-4

Forde, R., Peters, S., & Wittkowski, A. (2020). Recovery from postpartum psychosis: A systematic review and metasynthesis of women's and families' experiences. *Archives of Women's Mental Health, 23*, 597–612. https://doi.org/10.1007/s00737-020-01025-z

Frayne, J., Brooks, J., Nguyen, T. N., Allen, S., Maclean, M., & Fisher, J. (2014). Characteristics of men accompanying their partners to a specialist antenatal clinic for women with severe mental illness. *Asian Journal of Psychiatry*, 7, 46–51. https://doi.org/10.1016/j.ajp.2013.10.008

Frayne, J., Nguyen, T., Allen, S., Hauck, Y., Liira, H., & Vickery, A. (2019). Obstetric outcomes for women with severe mental illness: 10 years of experience in a tertiary multidisciplinary antenatal clinic. *Archives of Gynecology and Obstetrics*, 300(4), 889–896. https://doi.org/10.1007/s00404-019-05258-x

Galbally, M., Snellen, M., & Power, J. (2014). Antipsychotic drugs in pregnancy: A review of their maternal and fetal effects. *Therapeutic Advances in Drug Safety*, 5(2), 100–109. https://doi.org/10.1177/2042098614522682

Gilbody, S., Peckham, E., Bailey, D., Arundel, C., Heron, P., Crosland, S., . . . Vickers, C. (2019). Smoking cessation for people with severe mental illness (SCIMITAR+): A pragmatic randomised controlled trial. *The Lancet Psychiatry*, 6(5), 379–390. https://doi.org/10.1016/s2215-0366(19)30047-1

Hauck, Y., Allen, S., Ronchi, F., Faulkner, D., Frayne, J., & Nguyen, T. (2013). Pregnancy experiences of Western Australian women attending a specialist childbirth and mental illness antenatal clinic. *Health Care for Women International*, 34(5), 380–394. https://doi.org/10.1080/07399332.2012.736577

Heinonen, E., Forsberg, L., Nörby, U., Wide, K., & Källén, K. (2022). Antipsychotic use during pregnancy and risk for gestational diabetes: A national register-based cohort study in Sweden. *CNS Drugs*, 36(5), 529–539. https://doi.org/10.1007%2Fs40263-022-00908-2

Higgins, A., Downes, C., Monahan, M., Gill, A., Lamb, S. A., & Carroll, M. (2018). Barriers to midwives and nurses addressing mental health issues with women during the perinatal period: The mind mothers study. *Journal of Clinical Nursing*, 27(9–10), 1872–1883. https://doi.org/10.1111/jocn.14252

Higgins, A., Tuohy, T., Murphy, R., & Begley, C. (2016). Mothers with mental health problems: Contrasting experiences of support within maternity services in the Republic of Ireland. *Midwifery*, 36, 28–34. https://doi.org/10.1016/j.midw.2016.02.023

Howard, L. M., Bekele, D., Rowe, M., Demilew, J., Bewley, S., & Marteau, T. M. (2013a). Smoking cessation in pregnant women with mental disorders: A cohort and nested qualitative study. *British Journal of Obstetrics and Gynaecology*, 120(3), 362–370. https://doi.org/10.1111/1471-0528.12059

Howard, L. M., & Khalifeh, H. (2020). Perinatal mental health: A review of progress and challenges. *World Psychiatry*, 19(3), 313–327. https://doi.org/https://doi.org/10.1002/wps.20769

Howard, L. M., Oram, S., Galley, H., Trevillion, K., & Feder, G. (2013b). Domestic violence and perinatal mental disorders: A systematic review and meta-analysis. *PLoS Medicine*, 10(5), e1001452. https://doi.org/10.1371/journal.pmed.1001452

Jankovic, J., Parsons, J., Jovanović, N., Berrisford, G., Copello, A., Fazil, Q., & Priebe, S. (2020). Differences in access and utilisation of mental health services in the perinatal period for women from ethnic minorities – A population-based study. *BMC Medicine*, 18, 245 (2020). https://doi.org/10.1186/s12916-020-01711-w

Jones, I., Chandra, P. S., Dazzan, P., & Howard, L. M. (2014). Bipolar disorder, affective psychosis, and schizophrenia in pregnancy and the post-partum period. *The Lancet*, 384(9956), 1789–1799. https://doi.org/10.1016/s0140-6736(14)61278-2

Judd, F., Komiti, A., Sheehan, P., Newman, L., Castle, D., & Everall, I. (2014). Adverse obstetric and neonatal outcomes in women with severe mental illness: To what extent can they be prevented? *Schizophrenia Research*, 157(1), 305–309. https://doi.org/10.1016/j.schres.2014.05.030

Knight, M., Bunch, K., Patel, R., Shakespeare, J., Kotnis, R., Kenyon, S., & Kurinczuk, J. J, On Behalf of MBRRACE-UK. (2022). *Saving lives, improving mothers' care – core report: Lessons learned to inform maternity care from the UK and Ireland confidential enquiries into maternal deaths and morbidity 2018–20*. National Perinatal Epidemiology Unit, University of Oxford. www.npeu.ox.ac.uk/mbrrace-uk/reports

Knight, M., Bunch, K., Tuffnell, D., Patel, R., Shakespeare, J., Kotnis, R., Kenyon, S., & Kurinczuk, J. J, On Behalf of MBRRACE-UK. (2021). *Saving lives, improving mothers' care – Lessons learned to inform maternity care from the UK and Ireland confidential enquiries into maternal deaths and morbidity 2017–19*. National Perinatal Epidemiology Unit, University of Oxford. www.npeu.ox.ac.uk/mbrrace-uk/reports

Knight, M., Bunch, K., Tuffnell, D., Shakespeare, J., Kotnis, R., Kenyon, S., & Kurinczuk, J. J, On Behalf of MBRRACE-UK. (2019). *Saving lives, improving mothers' care – Lessons learned to inform maternity care from the UK and Ireland confidential enquiries into maternal deaths and morbidity 2015–17*. National Perinatal Epidemiology Unit, University of Oxford. www.npeu.ox.ac.uk/mbrrace-uk/reports

Li, X., Zhou, W., & Yi, Z. (2022). A glimpse of gender differences in schizophrenia. *General Psychiatry, 35*(4), e100823–e100823. https://doi.org/10.1136/gpsych-2022-100823

Mazza, M., Caroppo, E., De Berardis, D., Marano, G., Avallone, C., Kotzalidis, G. D., . . . Sani, G. (2021). Psychosis in women: Time for personalized treatment. *Journal of Personalized Medicine, 11*(12), 1279–1291. https://mdpi-res.com/d_attachment/jpm/jpm-11-01279/article_deploy/jpm-11-01279.pdf?version=1638437989

McAllister-Williams, R. H., Baldwin, D. S., Cantwell, R., Easter, A., Gilvarry, E., Glover, V., . . . Young, A. H. (2017). British association for psychopharmacology consensus guidance on the use of psychotropic medication preconception, in pregnancy and postpartum 2017. *Journal of Psychopharmacology, 31*(5), 519–552. https://doi.org/10.1177/0269881117699361

Millard, L. A., Salice, C., Maimagani, A., Smith, H., Rawat, N., Bano, F., & Fusté, M. (2020, November 3). *Can specialised antenatal care improve maternal and neonatal outcomes? A retrospective cohort study of an NHS joint obstetric-psychiatric clinic*. Royal College of Psychiatrists Faculty of Perinatal Psychiatry Annual Conference. [Poster Presentation].

Moitra, M., Santomauro, D., Degenhardt, L., Collins, P. Y., Whiteford, H., Vos, T., & Ferrari, A. (2021). Estimating the risk of suicide associated with mental disorders: A systematic review and meta-regression analysis. *Journal of Psychiatric Research, 137*, 242–249. https://doi.org/10.1016/j.jpsychires.2021.02.053

Munk-Olsen, T., Maegbaek, M. L., Johannsen, B. M., Liu, X., Howard, L. M., di Florio, A., . . . Meltzer-Brody, S. (2016). Perinatal psychiatric episodes: A population-based study on treatment incidence and prevalence. *Translational Psychiatry, 6*(10), e919. https://doi.org/10.1038/tp.2016.190

National Collaborating Centre for Mental Health. (2018). *The perinatal mental health care pathways: Full implementation guidance*. www.rcpsych.ac.uk/docs/default-source/improving-care/nccmh/perinatal/nccmh-the-perinatal-mental-health-care-pathways-full-implementation-guidance.pdf?sfvrsn=73c19277_4

National Institute for Health and Care Excellence (NICE). (2014). Psychosis and schizophrenia in adults: Prevention and management. *Clinical Guideline [CG178]*. www.nice.org.uk/guidance/cg178/chapter/Recommendations#how-to-deliver-psychological-interventions

National Institute for Health and Care Excellence (NICE). (2020a). Antenatal and postnatal mental health: Clinical management and service guidance. *Clinical Guideline 192*. www.nice.org.uk/guidance/cg192/evidence/full-guideline-pdf-4840896925

National Institute for Health and Care Excellence (NICE). (2020b). Bipolar disorder: Assessment and management. *Clinical Guidance [CG185]*. www.nice.org.uk/guidance/cg185

National Institute for Health and Care Excellence (NICE). (2021). Antenatal care. *NICE Guideline [NG201]*. www.nice.org.uk/guidance/ng201

Nguyen, T. N., Faulkner, D., Frayne, J. S., Allen, S., Hauck, Y. L., Rock, D., & Rampono, J. (2013). Obstetric and neonatal outcomes of pregnant women with severe mental illness at a specialist antenatal clinic. *Medical Journal of Australia, 199*(S3), S26–S29. https://doi.org/10.5694/mja11.11152

NHS. (2023). *Treatment – Bipolar disorder*. www.nhs.uk/mental-health/conditions/bipolar-disorder/treatment/

NHS Digital. (2023). *Statistics on women's smoking status at time of delivery: England, Quarter 3, 2022–23*. https://digital.nhs.uk/data-and information/publications/statistical/statistics-on-women-s-smoking-status-at-time-of-delivery-england/statistics-on-womens-smoking-status-at-time-of-delivery-england-quarter-3-2022-23

NHS England, NHS Improvement, & National Collaborating Centre for Mental Health. (2018). *The perinatal mental health care pathways*. www.england.nhs.uk/wp-content/uploads/2018/05/perinatal-mental-health-care-pathway.pdf

O'Brien, J., Gregg, L., & Wittkowski, A. (in press). A systematic review of clinical psychology guidance for perinatal mental health. *BMC Psychiatry*.

O'Mahen, H., & Healy, S. (2021). *IAPT perinatal competency framework*. www.ucl.ac.uk/pals/sites/pals/files/iapt_perinatal_competancy_framework_final_version_sept_2021-1.pdf

Ornoy, A., Weinstein-Fudim, L., & Ergaz, Z. (2017). Antidepressants, antipsychotics, and mood stabilizers in pregnancy: What do we know and how should we treat pregnant women with depression. *Birth Defects Research, 109*(12), 933–956. https://doi.org/10.1002/bdr2.1079

Petersen, I., McCrea, R. L., Sammon, C. J., Osborn, D. P., Evans, S. J., Cowen, P. J., . . . Nazareth, I. (2016). Risks and benefits of psychotropic medication in pregnancy: Cohort studies based on UK electronic primary care health records. *Health Technology Assessment, 20*(23), 1–176.

Public Health England. (2018, September 27). Severe Mental Illness (SMI) and physical health inequalities: Briefing. *GOV.UK*. www.gov.uk/government/publications/severe-mental-illness-smi-physical-health-inequalities/severe-mental-illness-and-physical-health-inequalities-briefing#fn:1

Raffi, E. R., Nonacs, R., & Cohen, L. S. (2019). Safety of psychotropic medications during pregnancy. *Clinics in Perinatology, 46*(2), 215–234.

Reid, H. E., Pratt, D., Edge, D., & Wittkowski, A. (2022). Maternal suicide ideation and behaviour during pregnancy and the first postpartum year: A systematic review of psychological and psychosocial risk factors. *Frontiers in Psychiatry, 13*, 765118. https://doi.org/10.3389/fpsyt.2022.765118

Royal College of Psychiatrists [RC-Psych]. (2018). *Antipsychotics in pregnancy and breastfeeding.* www.rcpsych.ac.uk/mental-health/treatments-and-wellbeing/antipsychotics-in-pregnancy

Sambrook Smith, M., Lawrence, V., Sadler, E., & Easter, A. (2019). Barriers to accessing mental health services for women with perinatal mental illness: Systematic review and meta-synthesis of qualitative studies in the UK. *BMJ Open, 9*(1), e024803. https://doi.org/10.1136/bmjopen-2018-024803

Schofield, Z., & Kapoor, D. (2019). Pre-existing mental health disorders and pregnancy. *Obstetrics, Gynaecology & Reproductive Medicine, 29*(3), 74–79. https://doi.org/10.1016/j.ogrm.2019.01.005

Scott, D., & Happell, B. (2011). The high prevalence of poor physical health and unhealthy lifestyle behaviours in individuals with severe mental illness. *Issues in Mental Health Nursing, 32*(9), 589–597. https://doi.org/10.3109/01612840.2011.569846

Sebire, N. J., Jolly, M., Harris, J. P., Wadsworth, J., Joffe, M., Beard, R. W., . . . Robinson, S. (2001). Maternal obesity and pregnancy outcome: A study of 287,213 pregnancies in London. *International Journal of Obesity, 25*(8), 1175–1182. https://doi.org/10.1038/sj.ijo.0801670

Stein, A., Pearson, R. M., Goodman, S. H., Rapa, E., Rahman, A., McCallum, M., . . . Pariante, C. M. (2014). Effects of perinatal mental disorders on the fetus and child. *The Lancet, 384*(9956), 1800–1819. https://doi.org/10.1016/S0140-6736(14)61277-0

The British Psychological Society [BPS]. (2019). *Position paper – Perinatal psychology provision in specialist community mental health services.* https://doi.org/10.53841/bpsrep.2019.pp19

Tosato, S., Albert, U., Tomassi, S., Iasevoli, F., Carmassi, C., Ferrari, S., . . . Atti, A. R. (2017). A systematized review of atypical antipsychotics in pregnant women: Balancing between risks of untreated illness and risks of drug-related adverse effects. *Journal of Clinical Psychiatry, 78*(5), e477–e489.

Vigod, S. N., Fung, K., Amartey, A., Bartsch, E., Felemban, R., Saunders, N., . . . Brown, H. K. (2020). Maternal schizophrenia and adverse birth outcomes: What mediates the risk? *Social Psychiatry and Psychiatric Epidemiology, 55*(5), 561–570. https://doi.org/10.1007/s00127-019-01814-7

Wesseloo, R., Kamperman, A. M., Munk-Olsen, T., Pop, V. J. M., Kushner, S. A., & Bergink, V. (2016). Risk of postpartum relapse in bipolar disorder and postpartum psychosis: A systematic review and meta-analysis. *American Journal of Psychiatry, 173*(2), 117–127. https://doi.org/10.1176/appi.ajp.2015.15010124

World Health Organization [WHO]. (2016). *WHO recommendations on antenatal care for a positive pregnancy experience.* www.who.int/publications/i/item/9789241549912

World Health Organization [WHO]. (2019). *International statistical classification of diseases and related health problems* (11th ed.). https://icd.who.int/

Yin, X., Sun, N., Jiang, N., Xu, X., Gan, Y., Zhang, J., . . . Gong, Y. (2021). Prevalence and associated factors of antenatal depression: Systematic reviews and meta-analyses. *Clinical Psychology Review, 83*, 101932. https://doi.org/10.1016/j.cpr.2020.101932

PART III

Postpartum Mental Health Disorders

12

POSTPARTUM DEPRESSION

Elizabeth Cox and Samantha Meltzer-Brody

Postpartum depression (PPD) is one of the most common complications following child-birth and with significant morbidity, yet, it is vastly undertreated and can be devastating for the patient and family, and it can have negative impacts on the economy and public health system at large (Luca, Margiotta, et al., 2020). Throughout this chapter, we describe the pathology, prevalence, correlates and risk factors, and potential consequences on family members and loved ones of PPD, as well as discuss assessment, treatment, and cultural considerations. Please note that nearly all research in PPD to date has been done in cis-gender women; as such, we use "women" in the chapter but acknowledge that future research is needed in gender-diverse populations. Analogously, the data are largely from European, British, American, and Canadian populations, reflecting regional bias; thus, we also acknowledge that more research is needed in geographically diverse populations.

Pathology

Although many symptoms of PPD overlap with those of major depressive disorder (MDD) outside of the perinatal period, the pathology of PPD differs from that of MDD, as it exists within a different biopsychosocial framework. Similar to MDD, the full extent of the pathophysiology of PPD is unknown. Fluctuations in reproductive steroid levels are thought to play a major role in generating symptoms of PPD for many women, and it is postulated that PPD is due to disruptions in the signaling of reproductive hormones (Bloch, Schmidt, et al., 2000; Bloch, Daly, et al., 2003). Estrogen and progesterone levels are 10 and 50 times higher than prepregnancy levels by the third trimester of pregnancy and then abruptly plummet following delivery; at the same time, the hypothalamic–pituitary–adrenal (HPA) axis responds with reciprocal compensatory changes.

Bloch et al. (2000) demonstrated this sensitivity to changes in reproductive steroid levels that many women with PPD experience. In this landmark study, euthymic women with a history of PPD again developed depression when they were blindly exposed to high dosages of estradiol and progesterone, with subsequent rapid withdrawal; this was not seen in women with no history of PPD. In recent years, this finding was replicated by Schiller et al. (2020). Reproductive steroids are known to be involved in the regulation of nearly every neurotransmitter (including serotonin, norepinephrine, glutamate, GABA, and dopamine), as well as the regulation of the HPA axis (Rubinow, Schmidt, et al., 1998). Allopregnanolone is a derivative of progesterone and a powerful activator of GABA receptors, which are needed for neuronal inhibition. An increase in stress reactivity is associated with impairments in GABA networks. Disturbances in GABA pathways may be due to fluctuations in reproductive steroid levels in certain genetically vulnerable populations, as demonstrated by Maguire and Mody (2008) in a mouse model for PPD of mice with genetically induced disturbances of GABA networks. In this study, female mice displayed normative behaviors until delivery; at delivery, activation was shown in the prefrontal cortices and the amygdala as the mothers demonstrated symptoms of stress and depression, all of which were reversed by the administration of allopregnanolone. This study led to the development and use of the first-ever Federal Drug Administration (FDA)-approved treatment for PPD in human mothers—intravenous allopregnanolone (brexanolone [BRX]) has demonstrated rapid and sustained improvement in symptoms of PPD when infused over the course of 60 hours (Meltzer-Brody, Howard, et al., 2018).

The formal diagnosis of PPD is similar to that of MDD but with postpartum onset—symptoms must be present for two weeks or longer and include either low mood or anhedonia, as well as four further symptoms, including low energy, psychomotor retardation or activation, insomnia or hypersomnia, change in appetite or weight, guilt, or suicidal ideation. The symptoms must cause significant distress and impact the patient's ability to function either occupationally or socially and must not be better attributed to a substance use disorder or general medical condition. According to the *Diagnostic and Statistical Manual of Mental Disorders*, 5th edition (DSM-5), the "peripartum" specifier of onset may include during pregnancy or within the first four weeks postpartum (American Psychiatric Association, 2013). According to the ICD-10 criteria, postpartum onset must be within the first six weeks postpartum (Putnam, Wilcox, et al., 2017). However, the World Health Organization and American College of Obstetricians and Gynecologists (ACOG), as well as most experts acknowledge that in clinical practice patients may present any time within the first 12 months following delivery(Gynecologists, 2018); as such, the ICD-11 specifier includes the entirety of the perinatal time period, both prenatal and postpartum onset (O'Hara & Wisner, 2014). Indeed, research has shown that PPD cases typically reach peak frequency two to three months postpartum (O'Hara & Wisner, 2014). Many women may struggle with progressively worsening symptoms before finally reaching out for help later in the postpartum period, and others may not develop symptoms at all until further postpartum, possibly in relation to lactation difficulties or weaning (Stuebe, Grewen, et al., 2012).

Salient features of PPD include overlap with features of anxiety—many women present with an anxious or agitated affect. Common anxieties can include worries about the health of the baby, including worries about feeding the baby and weight gain. Intrusive thoughts of picturing something awful happening to the baby, including breathing issues, can be common and disturbing. Out-of-control anxiety can often lead to issues sleeping and getting rest, even when the baby is sound asleep and the patient has the opportunity to sleep. This can all lead to significant irritability, overwhelm, and a sense of inadequacy in role and expectations of motherhood.

Sarah is a bright and driven 33-year-old woman who has always excelled academically and is now in her career as an attorney. She describes herself as "type A" and "a worrier." Historically, her anxiety has benefited her and led to her staying on top of her studies and the tasks at hand. Looking back, she has had some possible obsessive-compulsive disorder (OCD) traits of counting to 7 when stressed that dates back to childhood; however, she never spent hours of her day on this ritual and denies any other persistent or chronic obsessions or compulsions. She married her husband, Sam, while in law school. They were married for five years before deciding to start a family. Unfortunately, her first pregnancy resulted in a miscarriage at eight weeks, which was devastating for them both. Sarah, in particular, had felt quite bonded and excited and struggled with her grief for several months. She was thankful that she became pregnant a second time not too many months later, although, with this pregnancy, she had difficulties getting excited or feeling attached. She felt guilty for not feeling happier or more excited, as well as quite anxious that something was wrong with the health of her baby and that she might again lose this child. However, she continued to function at work and pushed through without significant difficulties prenatally. She carried a healthy pregnancy to term; however, she ultimately had to deliver her daughter via cesarean secondary to breech positioning. This was a huge disappointment to Sarah, who had been working closely with her doula and midwife with plans to deliver "naturally" and without much medical intervention (including no epidural). Her daughter was beautiful and healthy, though Sarah was left feeling she and her body had somehow "failed." In the days following delivery, Sarah felt her mood declining, she had trouble enjoying her new baby, and she could not quite feel a connection or that her baby was hers. Though her spouse, Sam, was supportive and engaged, she felt somehow alone and isolated. She felt tremendous guilt for not feeling bright, happy and as she pictured she would and "should" feel. She was consumed with anxiety that something was wrong with her daughter, despite reassurances from her pediatrician. She found herself lying awake, watching her daughter's breathing with fear in the middle of the night while the baby and Sam both remained sound asleep. She was determined to breastfeed but found that her milk was not coming in very well, and her daughter was not gaining weight at her pediatrician appointments. his led to further distress, with frequent visits back to the pediatrician for weight checks. When supplementation with formula was recommended, she again viewed herself as a failure. She started to experience hopelessness and worthlessness and began to wonder if her daughter and Sam would be better off without her.

Prevalence

PPD is the most common unrecognized complication of pregnancy (Meltzer-Brody, Howard, et al., 2018). Timing of PPD onset impacts prevalence; at three days postpartum, prevalence is approximated to be 11%, and at three months postpartum, it is approximately roughly 17% (Elisei, Lucarini, et al., 2013). It is estimated that almost 22% of women will meet criteria for PPD within the first 12 months following delivery (Elisei, Lucarini, et al., 2013). Sadly, PPD is often missed; up to 50% of women with PPD go undiagnosed, and upward of 85% do not receive any treatment (Cox, Sowa, et al., 2016). Furthermore, the impact of the COVID-19 pandemic has been associated with worsening perinatal mental health and increased prevalence of symptoms of PPD. Ongoing research is needed to follow the longitudinal impact over time on mothers and mental health (Esscher, Essen, et al., 2016).

Correlates and Risk Factors

PPD is correlated with postpartum weight retention, as well as difficulties with lactation and breastfeeding (Biesmans et al., 2013; Herring et al., 2008). Although breastfeeding is widely recommended by most medical experts, and it is estimated that more than 80% of women in the United Kingdom and the United States attempt to breastfeed, lactation failure has been correlated with PPD. There seems to be a likely shared neuroendocrine association between PPD and issues with breastfeeding (Stuebe, Grewen, et al., 2012). PPD is further correlated with greater numbers of overall adverse life events and stressors, as well as greater perceived stress levels and financial hardships (Vliegen et al., 2013).

Untreated depression during pregnancy is the biggest risk factor for developing PPD (Gaynes, Gavin, et al., 2005; Milgrom, Gemmill, et al., 2008; Meltzer-Brody, Bledsoe-Mansori, et al., 2013). Importantly, untreated PPD is associated with substantial morbidity; in developed countries, suicide is one of the leading causes of death during the first year postpartum (Frautschi, Cerulli, et al., 1994, Austin, Kildea, et al., 2007, Esscher, Essen, et al., 2016). Women with prior mental illness are at higher risk for development of PPD and for perinatal suicide (Lindahl, Pearson, et al., 2005). Up to 30% of patients with a history of MDD may develop PPD, as well as 20% to 50% of those with a history of bipolar affective disorder (BPAD), 14% of those with a history of generalized anxiety disorder, and 35% of those with a history of an eating disorder (Meltzer-Brody, Howard, et al., 2018). Additional risk factors for developing PPD include psychosocial stressors, such as relationship conflict, marital strain, limited support systems, racial disparities, financial discord, unemployment, work-related stressors, and those who are stay-at-home moms (Elisei, Lucarini, et al., 2013). Family history also contributes to risk. Up to 50% of women with a family history of postpartum psychosis (PPP) or a personal history of prior PPP may develop PPD.

Furthermore, trauma or adverse childhood experiences are noteworthy risk factors for the development of PPD. Traumas may include emotional abuse, physical abuse, sexual abuse, systemic racism, intimate partner violence (IPV), or medical traumas, particularly traumatic deliveries where the patient may feel either her own life or the life of her child is in danger. Race and systemic racism must not be overlooked; discrimination in the form of racism unfortunately is still pervasive and can adversely affect the patient's experience of pregnancy, delivery, childbirth, and even motherhood. The symptoms themselves of PPD may make women more susceptible to IPV in particular; approximately one-third of perinatal women are likely to experience IPV (Howard, Oram, et al., 2013). Clinicians must be sure to meet with patients privately, as they must always be screened for IPV. Over and above, clinicians must be aware of local resources to provide to link patients and families with support in local communities. Screening patients to inquire whether there were any pregnancy or delivery complications, including the need for neonatal intensive care unit stay is important for the clinician to also be aware of providing trauma-informed care and further evaluating the patient for trauma-related symptoms, as indicated. Furthermore, women with a history of loss are also at increased risk for PPD; losses may include loss of family of origin, loss of a prior pregnancy, or death of another child.

In addition to stressors, psychiatric history, trauma history, and loss, underlying genetics may play a significant role in the risk for the development of PPD. The Postpartum Depression, Action toward Causes and Treatment (PACT) consortium is a global genome-wide association study currently exploring what genetic differences may be linked with some women being more susceptible to shifts and changes in reproductive hormone levels (Guintivano et al., 2018). These data have found that women who developed symptoms postpartum experienced almost four times more severe illness than those who developed symptoms prenatally (Putnam, Wilcox, et al., 2017).

Sarah's course of PPD is correlated with medical complications, including cesarean section and lactation difficulties. She had risk factors for PPD, placing her at higher risk than others in the general population—a history of loss with a prior miscarriage that also may have been traumatic to her medically, as well as a past psychiatric history of anxiety (though albeit mild historically, but with features of obsessive-compulsive traits). She is also at an advantage with numerous supports—a supportive partner/spouse, employment, and socioeconomic status.

Effects on the Partner Relationship, Children, and Other Family Members

As mentioned previously, untreated PPD is associated with substantial morbidity for the mother. Furthermore, the partner relationship, children, and other family members are significantly affected. For example, PPD is associated with dissatisfaction in the marital relationship (Pahlavan et al., 2020). Additionally, paternal or partner depression has been estimated to have roughly 10% prevalence during the first year postpartum (while roughly 3.8% of men in the general population suffer from depression annually; Meltzer-Brody & Jones, 2015). Thus, partners should also be assessed for depression, particularly when the mother is struggling with PPD, as untreated partner depression can also adversely impact the well-being of the child, other children, and the family unit.

Untreated PPD is associated with damaging and detrimental outcomes for the child and mother–infant dyad. Infants of women with PPD have been shown to gain less weight as opposed to infants of nondepressed mothers and have also shown significant detriments in motor development, cognitive development, and language development (Gress-Smith et al., 2012; Nasreen et al., 2013; Slomian et al., 2019). Furthermore, a significant association has been demonstrated between PPD and overall health concerns in infants (Slomian et al., 2019) The risk of toxic stress associated with untreated maternal depression can lead to disruptions in the development of the infant's brain architecture (Shonkoff, Garner, et al., 2011).

Untreated PPD is further associated with impairments in bonding, which is essential for ideal infant brain development and neuron pruning (Winston & Chicot, 2016). Those children with a history of toxic stress in utero have been shown to have persistent elevated cortisol levels through preschool years, which is associated with an increase in anxiety and a decrease in social inhibition (Shonkoff, Garner, et al., 2011). Children exposed to depression in utero have been found to have an increased risk for behavioral disturbances, emotional developmental delays, as well as increased risk for the development of their own mental health disorders later in life (Earls & Health, 2010; Lahti, Savolainen, et al., 2017; Shonkoff, Garner, et al., 2011). PPD impacts the mother's ability to connect with the child, respond appropriately to the child's cues, and display appropriate, nurturing behaviors (Ashman, Dawson, et al., 2002; Earls & Health, 2010; Warnock, Craig, et al., 2016). This can all have a long-lasting influence on development and behavior and impacts all children in the family unit.

Sarah's partner, Sam, should also be assessed during Sarah's assessment and course of treatment. He is now also at increased risk for depression and, at minimum, would also likely benefit from individual therapy to further support him as Sarah is treated. Should Sam also develop more significant symptoms, medication or other treatment modalities may also be appropriate. Should Sarah not receive appropriate treatment, the bond and connection with her daughter may be adversely affected. If Sarah's symptoms were to go unaddressed, her daughter may be at increased risk for cognitive issues and developmental and emotional issues. Appropriate treatment for Sarah and Sam (if necessary) will be paramount for the well-being of each individual within their family.

Assessment

Though ideally patients would self-disclose and reach out for help when struggling with PPD, this is not always the case. The ACOG mandates screening of pregnant and postpartum women for depression (Gynecologists, 2018). Although a screening tool is not the same as a full assessment and does not convey a diagnosis necessarily, screening is instrumental in identifying women with PPD. The *Edinburgh Postnatal Depression Scale* (EPDS) has been studied at length and is one of the most widely utilized tools around the world for perinatal depression (validated in pregnancy and postpartum) (Levis, Negeri, et al., 2020). The EPDS is a ten-item self-report inventory, where a score of 12 or higher is associated with "a positive screen," and scores 0 to 6 typically correlate with no/minimal depression, 7 to 13 correlate with mild depression, 14 to 19 correlate with moderate depression, and 19 to 30 correlate with severe depression (Cox, Holden, et al., 1987; Levis, Negeri, et al., 2020; McCabe-Beane et al., 2016). Clinicians are recommended to screen patients at the initial prenatal visit, once per trimester while pregnant, and at 6 weeks, 3 months, 6 months, 9 months, and 12 months postpartum. As patients do not typically see their obstetrician at three and nine months postpartum, the clinician who screens the patient is often the pediatrician at those time intervals. It is important to ask more questions if the patient's body language or other signs indicate possible distress or depressive symptomatology, as patients may under-report symptoms; screening tools can never replace direct questioning and assessment.

Interviewing the patient in a private, face-to-face setting is imperative when making a formal diagnostic assessment of PPD. Common postpartum experiences, such as low energy, fatigue, trouble concentrating, and lack of sleep are both "typical" experiences for a sleep-deprived new parent, as well as overlap with more significant symptoms of clinical depression. Clinicians must not necessarily assume these features are depression without further evaluation, but must also not dismiss these as "normal" without closer investigation.

As is the case with MDD, key features of PPD include a total of five symptoms over a two-week period or longer, including the presence of low mood or anhedonia, in addition to change in appetite or weight, change in sleep (hypersomnia or insomnia), psychomotor agitation or retardation, fatigue, sense of worthlessness or inappropriate guilt, trouble concentrating or suicidal thoughts. Symptoms must not be attributed to another underlying medical condition or substance abuse and must significantly impact functioning. Common features unique to PPD that differ from classic MDD outside of the perinatal period include a great overlap with anxiety symptomatology, including OCD traits; there is often excessive irritability, agitation, and ego-dystonic intrusive thoughts. Patients may seem to be either disengaged with a lack of interest in their newborn, or hypervigilant. Data from the PACT Consortium reveal during the first two months postpartum, many women display an anxious anhedonic phenotype that is often severe and can last upward of five months through the postpartum period (Putnam, Wilcox, et al., 2017).

Given this overlap with anxiety symptomatology, comorbid anxiety disorders must also be assessed. It has been estimated that nearly 50% of women with perinatal depression also have a comorbid anxiety disorder; overall postpartum anxiety disorders are estimated to be 12% prevalence overall—roughly 6% prevalence for generalized anxiety disorder and 2% for OCD (Meltzer-Brody, Howard, et al., 2018). As mentioned previously, in addition to specific questions regarding IPV, general trauma should always be screened for, particularly any medical delivery complications, as there is a 3% to 6% prevalence of posttraumatic stress disorder perinatally (Meltzer-Brody, Howard, et al., 2018). Additionally, given the significant overlap with agitation and irritability, BPADs must also be ruled out when diagnosing PPD. Irritability is sensitive for BPAD but not specific; however, astute clinicians will inquire in greater detail about the history of episodes or times of decreased need for sleep with an increase in goal-oriented behaviors and other features of mania or hypomania— past or present. Lastly, clinicians must also screen for other common co-occurring disorders, such as substance use disorders and eating disorders.

Proper assessment also includes blood work to rule out any possible underlying medical etiology for the symptoms or other co-occurring health issues. Postpartum patients should receive the following orders during assessments: pregnancy test, complete blood count, chemistry panel (including glucose), thyroid panel, vitamin D level, vitamin B_{12} level, folic acid level, and toxicology tests (including blood alcohol level). If there are any signs of seizure activity, EEG must be ordered. For individuals with recent brain injury or trauma, change in cognition, any concern for a comorbid neurological disorder, treatment resistance, or new onset psychotic features, neuroimaging is indicated.

Sarah and Sam presented to their pediatrician for another weight check for their daughter. Their clinician noted how anxious and distressed both parents appeared. The EPDS was administered to Sarah, and she scored 18, correlating with moderate depression. The pediatrician used this as an opportunity to have a more in-depth conversation about PPD and anxiety with both Sarah and Sam. During this discussion, the clinician asked more in-depth questions and utilized supportive counseling, normalizing their experience and letting them both know just how common this all can be. The clinician also made a point of asking Sam how things were going for him as a new father, when Sam opened up about also feeling anxious, sad, and disappointed in himself. Thankfully, the pediatrician referred both Sarah and Sam to a local psychiatry practice that was able to see them individually for a proper assessment.

The following week, Sarah was seen by one clinician at that practice and diagnosed with PPD with notable features of obsessive-compulsive traits and some components of trauma (but did not meet the full criteria for OCD or posttraumatic stress disorder). Sarah's symptoms had progressed within the week and her EPDS score was now 25, correlating with severe depression. The thoughts she had been having of wondering if her family would be better off without her had grown. They remained ego-dystonic intrusive thoughts—she described flashes of seeing herself driving the car off the road or harming herself but adamantly denied any desire to act on these thoughts or planning. She very much wanted to live for her daughter and spouse and at the same time wondered if they would be better without her; she also very much wanted to get better and to live. She was plagued by intermittent, overwhelming sensations of hopelessness. Sam was seen by a separate clinician and diagnosed with adjustment disorder with mixed anxiety and depressed mood.

Treatment

As mentioned previously, it has been estimated that nearly 85% of patients who develop depression during pregnancy or postnatally do not receive any treatment (Cox, Sowa et al., 2016). Furthermore, this same analysis found that over 90% of patients with perinatal depression do not receive adequate care (defined as treatment through evidence-based psychotherapy for six weeks or longer or administration of daily antidepressants for six weeks or longer) (Cox, Sowa et al., 2016). These numbers are astounding, particularly given that depression during pregnancy and PPD are very treatable conditions. Clinicians must provide comprehensive care, which includes evidence-based psychotherapies, psychopharmacology when indicated, and alternative approaches to target environmental stressors; the goal is always full symptom remission and helping the patient feel like themselves once more.

For milder symptoms (often correlated with EPDS "subthreshold" symptoms), supportive psychotherapy, problem solving around strategies for sleep and other environmental stressors (i.e., support with any feeding issues or other concerns), and lifestyle changes (i.e., exercise, nutrition) are indicated first-line. Protected sleep for each partner is recommended—ideally each parent gets a total of 8 hours of sleep per 24 hours, which is typically piecemeal in earlier days and months postpartum. When possible, attempting to get one interval of five hours of sleep in a row, uninterrupted, is recommended (Meltzer-Brody & Jones, 2015). This will require a support system in place and is much more difficult for those who lack support. Problem solving around alternative individuals those new mothers can reach out to for help and support, even just watching the baby during a nap during the day, is instrumental. When supports are available at night, staggering hours of who is "on" when during the night for feeds and to be up with the baby can help achieve protected sleep.

Protected sleep is still possible while also supporting breastfeeding. Mothers can either have their support bring the baby into the nurse while they are laying/resting and then remove the baby from the setting, while the mother gets more rest and the support person burps, diaper changes, swaddles, and puts the baby back down in a separate space to continue their shift "on" duty. Alternatively, the support could feed the baby a bottle of pumped milk or supplemented formula while the mother sits up briefly to pump and then lay back down following pumping—the pumped milk has natural antimicrobial properties and can sit out in room air for several hours until the next morning to be stored and pump parts cleaned. For patients with limited support and resources, perinatal clinicians must advocate for and facilitate access to local community resources and programs, particularly for those who face food scarcity. Practices that work with perinatal programs will optimally include case management or licensed clinical social workers who are familiar with local food bank programming, as well as other areas of support, including but not limited to domestic violence resources, lactation support, weight management, and smoking cessation programs. Postpartum Support International is an organization that can be especially helpful in navigating resources throughout the globe for perinatal patients.

For moderate symptoms (typically correlated with an EPDS of 14 or higher score), psychotherapy is considered first-line treatment, and medication management may also be indicated, or alternative treatments are considered (i.e., transcranial magnetic stimulation [TMS]). When symptoms are severe, medication will most always be a part of a complete treatment plan, and other treatment modalities may also be considered (i.e., electroconvulsive therapy [ECT] or BRX). For any patients who answer yes to question 10 on the EPDS (i.e., thoughts of self-harm) or for those whose psychosis is suspected or concerns exist for homicidal ideation, urgent evaluation is required by a perinatal mental health specialist or emergency room or urgent care. For some severe cases, hospitalization may ultimately be required.

As detailed earlier, evidence-based psychotherapy is the first-line treatment for PPD whenever the patient is receptive to this treatment. This option requires the desire from the patient to participate in care and access to therapy. By definition, psychotherapy is a collaborative treatment based on the core doctrines of empathy, acceptance, and genuineness. Therapists set goals with patients to improve both the symptoms of the patient and improve bonding and facilitate the relationship of the mother–infant dyad. An adequate trial of psychotherapy is often defined as at least six or more sessions occurring on a weekly or biweekly schedule. Therapies with solid evidence and efficacy in the perinatal period include interpersonal psychotherapy (IPT; O'Hara, Stuart, et al., 2000), cognitive behavioral therapy (Shortis, Whittaker, et al., 2020), acceptance and commitment therapy (Bonacquisti, Cohen, et al., 2017), and dialectical behavioral therapy (Rabiee, Nazari, et al., 2020).

When psychotropic medications are indicated, collaborative care among psychiatry, obstetrics, and pediatrics is recommended for assurance of providing fully comprehensive and compassionate care. If a patient has previously taken medications, the best option is typically whatever medication was found to be most beneficial (including most tolerable and efficacious) when used previously (Kimmel et al., 2018). However, if no formal trials of psychotropics exist, sertraline is often chosen first for straightforward PPD symptomatology based upon the medication's indication for use, general tolerability, and data for use in the perinatal time period, which includes low transfer into breastmilk should the patient be breastfeeding. Basic principles for prescribing to perinatal patients are similar to that of prescribing in general psychiatry: monotherapy is preferred to polypharmacy, and the lowest therapeutic doses are ideal—one must first attempt to maximize efficacy and minimize side effects by attempting to use fewer psychotropics and in the lowest dose that is fully therapeutic for the patient.

Commonly prescribed psychotropics for PPD include selective serotonin reuptake inhibitors (SSRIs, such as sertraline, citalopram, escitalopram, and fluoxetine), serotonin-norepinephrine reuptake inhibitors (such as duloxetine, venlafaxine), alternative antidepressants (such as mirtazapine and bupropion), tricyclic antidepressants (TCAs) or monoamine oxidase inhibitors (MAOIs) (Kimmel et al., 2018). There is the most substantial data showing the efficacy of SSRIs in treating PPD, as well as some data for venlafaxine and bupropion (Cohen et al., 2001; Nonacs et al., 2005; Stowe et al., 1995; Suri et al., 2005, 2001; Wisner et al., 2006; Yonkers et al., 2008). Before initiating treatment with these commonly prescribed medications, adequate assessment to rule out a history of mania or hypomania is paramount, as antidepressants can trigger mania, and, as such, different pharmacology (i.e., mood stabilizers) is indicated for treatment (American Psychiatric Association, 2013; Kimmel et al., 2018). Even with unipolar symptomatology, if more severe symptoms are present, the patient may require augmentation with other pharmacotropics, such as mood stabilizers (e.g., lamotrigine and lithium) or atypical antipsychotics with mood stabilizing properties (such as quetiapine, risperidone, or olanzapine).

When medications are implemented during breastfeeding, the risk of untreated symptoms must be considered versus the risk of medication exposure in breastmilk. As described previously, untreated symptoms themselves correlate with significant risk, morbidity, and mortality for the patient and infant. Although no decision is completely risk free, the risk of medication exposure to breastmilk must be weighed against the risk of untreated symptom exposure for the mother and developing baby and against the benefits of breastfeeding (Kimmel et al., 2018). Breastfeeding is recommended by most medical providers due to the numerous benefits for mother and child for the first 6 to 24 months postpartum, depending on the medical organization (American Academy of Pediatrics et al., 2012). There is no universal recommendation; treatment must be individualized and unique for each patient with the goal of balancing overall risk.

As such, as of June 30, 2015, the FDA pregnancy risk categories have been updated to the new Content and Format of Labeling for Human Prescription Drugs and Biological Products; Requirements for Pregnancy and Lactation Labeling (Kimmel et al., 2018). This Pregnancy and Lactation Labeling Rule summarizes medication risks instead of using the former categories modeling. For patients who have been maintained on medication during pregnancy, typically, the placental transfer of medication is going to be greater than the transfer into breastmilk; further, continuation of medication postpartum may help mitigate neonatal adaptation syndrome or withdrawal (Kimmel et al., 2018). When choosing medications during breastfeeding, medications with shorter half-lives, greater levels of protein binding, less lipophilicity, and generally larger molecule size are favorable (Sprague et al., 2020). For premature infants, infants with health conditions, and in general with younger infants, special precaution should be exercised for medications with greater exposure to breastmilk, as the infant will be eliminating medications more slowly and those with less body fat, more immature liver functioning, and less developed blood–brain barrier will have a greater risk for medication toxicity (Sprague et al., 2020).

An excellent resource for clinicians and patients is the National Institute of Health's database, LACTMED, which includes detailed data on medication use during breastfeeding (Health). Tools to gage medication transfer into breastmilk include the milk-to-plasma (M/P) ratio and the relative infant dose (RID). M/P ratios <1, RID <2% (minimal exposure), RID 2–5% (small exposure), and <10%, are considered "safe" exposures. RID >25% is deemed possibly unsafe for the child (2019). Another tool is the infant plasma drug level; however, there are limited data as to whether a plasma drug level in the infant correlates with adverse outcomes for the child (2019). There are no present data to support monitoring blood levels in the infant; however, for some medications (such as lithium), blood levels should be checked as needed for any concerns regarding lethargy, hypotonia, or difficulties feeding in the infant. Furthermore, there are also no data to support "pumping and dumping" for most medications, but this practice might be advised in instances of particular concern for changes in child behavior in the context of exposure to medication with well-established high levels in breastmilk (Kimmel et al., 2018). In general, in all instances of mothers breastfeeding, while taking psychotropic medication, the pediatrician ought to be informed so that all parties can assess and monitor the baby for any changes in sedation, weight gain, milestones, and any possible side effects (Kimmel et al., 2018).

Combination treatment of psychopharmacology with psychotherapy is the gold standard for MDD and similarly for PPD. Treatments will be most efficacious when providers collaborate and work together. Prescribers must be mindful that certain psychotropics can interfere with some modalities of therapy (e.g., an "as needed" dosage of benzodiazepines is contraindicated and interferes with exposure therapy for panic attacks). Additionally, therapists may assist prescribers with certain therapeutic interventions in the instance of some medication side effects, such as insomnia, hypersomnia, or weight gain.

For moderate PPD, repetitive transcranial magnetic stimulation (rTMS) may be a desirable alternative treatment to medication for some patients. rTMS is FDA approved for MDD and also has data demonstrating efficacy and tolerability for PPD (Andriotti et al., 2017; Cox et al., 2020). rTMS utilizes targeted magnetic field pulses applied to the scalp, which generates electrical currents in the brain that stimulate neuroplasticity. It is generally very well tolerated, with scalp pain or headache being the most common side effect. The length of treatment is similar to that for use in MDD outside of the peripartum. Effects are typically more rapid than traditional pharmacotherapy, with results seen within one to two weeks post-treatment. For PPD, this may be particularly desirable if the patient prefers to avoid medication exposure to breastmilk. However, limitations may include the need for daily sessions, five days per week, which can conflict with the need to find childcare.

For more severe PPD, ECT is a viable option. ECT is FDA approved for the treatment of refractory or severe MDD and is also used for bipolar spectrum illness, psychotic disorders, physical decline, severe agitation, and catatonia (Leiknes et al., 2015; Ward et al., 2018). ECT is administered by applying electrodes to the patient's skull that utilize electricity to induce a generalized tonic-clonic seizure that is also thought to stimulate neuroplasticity. Patients undergo anesthesia during treatment. The length of treatment for PPD is similar to that of treatment outside of the peripartum (Leiknes et al., 2015). Benefits of ECT include speed of response and strong efficacy; risks include headache, confusion, myalgias, nausea, vomiting, prolonged seizure, and memory loss. For patients with very severe symptoms of PPD, including treatment-refractory patients, catatonic patients, or patients with psychotic features, ECT should be strongly considered (Bulbul et al., 2013; Bergink et al., 2016).

A novel treatment option for more severe PPD is BRX. BRX is a proprietary formulation of allopregnanolone (a derivative of progesterone) and the first-ever FDA-approved treatment specifically for PPD. BRX is administered intravenously over a course of 60 hours and has demonstrated rapid, effective, and sustained treatment response for PPD. Three randomized, double-blind, placebo-controlled trials were conducted conveying response within an hour of treatment that was sustained through one-month follow-up post-treatment (Meltzer-Brody, Colquhoun, et al., 2018). Patients had onset of depressive symptoms either within the third trimester or within first four weeks following delivery and were no greater than six months postpartum at the time of infusion. Some participants continued to take baseline antidepressant medication, but the dose was stable at least two weeks before infusion through 72 hours post-infusion. BRX was well tolerated, and mild side effects included flushing or hot flashes, dry mouth, sedation, or somnolence, and, in rare instances, brief loss of consciousness; any sedation was remitted within 90 minutes during clinical trials. Data collection investigating safety has been reassuring since clinical trials were completed. However, due to sedation risk, BRX infusion in the United States must be conducted under the Risk Evaluation and Mitigation Strategy (REMS) FDA requirement. REMS specifies particular procedures for healthcare facilities, pharmacies, wholesalers, and the patients themselves to appropriately administer BRX with proper mechanisms and supervision. BRX administration revealed statistically significant reductions in PPD symptoms as compared to placebo, either with or without baseline antidepressant medication; BRX should be considered for either monotherapy or augmentation of baseline antidepressant medication for patients with severe PPD (Meltzer-Brody, Colquhoun, et al., 2018). In the three years that BRX has been commercially available, the drug has continued to be an important clinical treatment tool for patients with severe PPD that is efficacious and well tolerated (Patterson, Krohn, et al., 2022).

Given the progressing, severe symptoms Sarah was experiencing, her psychiatrist referred Sarah for weekly psychotherapy sessions and initiated sertraline while also initiating the process of BRX infusion. Her psychiatrist counseled her on the importance of taking sertraline daily, with the most common potential risks being mild headache and gastrointestinal upset (that should resolve with time if occurs), emphasized that this medication will take four to six weeks to reach a steady state and fully work, and indicated that she may also require steady dose increases to reach full therapeutic effect (which can take more than four to six weeks). Given the severity of her symptoms, Sarah was also felt to be a great candidate for BRX infusion. Her psychiatrist explained the risks of sedation, loss of consciousness, and the need to administer in the hospital setting for the 60-hour infusion. Although Sarah felt that it would be difficult to be away from her baby and spouse for that time interval, she realized that this would be a short-term sacrifice for potential long-term gain and improvement. Notably, Sarah scored positively on EPDS question #10 and was having suicidal thoughts, although her thoughts were passive and not active, making her an appropriate candidate for BRX. As Sarah was still breastfeeding, her psychiatrist advised that her baby's pediatrician should be notified of all medications that she is taking and monitor her baby for any changes or concerns, while noting that both sertraline and BRX have a low transmission into breastmilk.

Sarah began taking sertraline 50 mg daily and was advised to increase to 100 mg daily after one week and within the week was also admitted for the 60-hour BRX infusion. By the end of her infusion, her symptoms had dissipated significantly. At the time of discharge home, her EPDS score had dropped to 12, and she was feeling significantly better. She still had some lingering anxiety and low mood but reported these symptoms were now mild. She began engaging in weekly therapy sessions while continuing sertraline 100 mg daily. Sam also began engaging in his own individual weekly therapy and noted incremental improvement in his symptoms.

Cultural Considerations

It is imperative to also consider differences based on cultural and geographic context. For patients who live in low- and middle-income countries (LMICs), there may be particular disparities and health challenges that exist. Unfortunately, commonly, people in LMICs grapple with more financial disparities, higher rates of food insecurity, greater prevalence of IPV, lower education levels, lower gender status, and, overall, less access to social and health resources than people who do not live in higher-income countries. As a result, perinatal mental health disorders are more frequent in LMICs versus in higher-income countries

(Meltzer-Brody, Howard, et al., 2018). To address these disparities, one must be mindful of low-cost models that will strengthen healthcare systems to incorporate mental healthcare into communities to adequately provide treatment and services for mothers and children. When considering prescriptions for PPD in LMICs, clinicians must be mindful of whether or not certain antidepressants are available for widespread use in that area. Culturally adapted treatment programming in LMICs that utilize peer-based counselors with evidence-based interventions has shown successful outcomes (Meltzer-Brody, Howard, et al., 2018).

Generally speaking, even in higher-income countries, women with lower socioeconomic status and women of color are at heightened risk of experiencing adverse outcomes during pregnancy, delivery, and the newborn stage and are also at increased risk for death during parturition (Beck, Edwards, et al., 2020). Clinicians must first be aware that these disparities exist and are problematic and then work toward education to reduce racism and promote antiracism within our healthcare systems and, finally, allocate resources and programming in a more comprehensive, inclusive, and appropriate manner.

> Sarah and Sam are fortunate to live in a higher-income country, be employed, and have access to healthcare. They were appropriately identified as struggling with mental health concerns at a routine pediatrician's appointment and then quickly seen by a mental health specialist in a timely manner. There was no question or issue with access to basic medication/antidepressants, and, furthermore, Sarah was able to access a novel therapeutic agent, BRX, which she received at a local hospital for a brief inpatient stay. Ensuring that women of all backgrounds and socioeconomic statuses in any geographic location or cultures are able to be appropriately diagnosed and adequately treated is a cornerstone of sufficient medical care that must be addressed across our globe.

Conclusion and Future Directions

The impact of the COVID-19 pandemic on mental health broadly across the globe and in perinatal women specifically has been profound. There has been a marked negative impact on mental health over the course of the pandemic and this has caused an increased prevalence of PPD. The path forward requires innovation in treatment approaches to address the increased prevalence and associated suffering of PPD. This includes a focus on ways to increase access to care and deliver targeted treatment modalities that are specific for the perinatal period and improve response.

Telepsychiatry has been widely deployed since March 2020 and has dramatically increased access to specialty care in perinatal mental health. This has been extremely helpful in light of the fact that most perinatal women do not have local access to specialized mental healthcare. Thus, telepsychiatry can allow for convenient access to treatment and overcome many barriers to care including transportation and child care, which are often most relevant to women living in low-resource settings. Most studies to date have shown good satisfaction and increased access to care with this modality of treatment delivery (Guille, Johnson, et al., 2022; Meltzer-Brody & Kimmel, 2020; Parameswaran, Pentecost, et al., 2022; Singla, Meltzer-Brody, et al., 2022).

Fast-acting antidepressant therapies are an exciting area of investigation that is particularly relevant in PPD. Brexanolone, a neurosteroid, is the first FDA-approved treatment for PPD and is an example of a novel pharmacologic agent with a unique mechanism of action. Because Brexanolone is administered via intravenous injection, the widescale uptake of this modality has not been feasible. Thus, the development of an oral agent with a similar mechanism is of great interest. This includes the study of zuranolone, also a neuroactive steroid, which is a positive allosteric modulator of synaptic and extrasynaptic GABA-A receptors and is currently in phase 3 clinical development as an oral, daily, 14-day treatment course for the treatment of MDD and PPD. There have been multiple, positive, double-blind clinical trials of zuranolone to date that may eventually lead to FDA approval (Deligiannidis, Meltzer-Brody, et al., 2021; Gunduz-Bruce, Takahashi et al., 2022).

Physical activity and yoga show promise as a therapeutic innovation in the treatment of PPD. There are some data showing efficacy in reducing symptoms of PPD, and these may be great modalities for individuals who are more hesitant to pursue traditional therapeutic treatments. However, data are limited, and more studies are needed to fully evaluate exercise and yoga as a treatment for PPD (Eustis et al., 2019).

In sum, there are important innovations that are increasing our ability to effectively treat women with PPD. However, there is much more research needed globally and across diverse cultures and populations to further improve tailored treatment to improve outcomes.

References

American Academy of Pediatrics, Section on Breastfeeding, Johnson, M., Landers, S., Noble, L., Szucs, K., & Viehamm, L. (2012). Breastfeeding and the use of human milk. *Pediatrics, 129*(3), 827–841.

American Psychiatric Association. (2013). *Diagnostic and statistical manual of mental disorders* (5th ed.). American Psychiatric Publishing.

Andriotti, T., Stavale, R., Nafee, T., Fakhry, S., Mohamed, M. M. A., Sofiyeva, N., . . . Boechat-Barros, R. (2017). ASSERT trial – How to assess the safety and efficacy of a high frequency rTMS in postpartum depression? A multicenter, double blinded, randomized, placebo-controlled clinical trial. *Contemporary Clinical Trials Communication, 5*, 86–91.

Ashman, S. G., Dawson, G., Panagiotides, H., Yamada, Y., & Wilkins, C. W. (2002). Stress hormone levels of children of depressed mothers. *Development and Psychopathology, 14*(2), 333–349.

Austin, M.-P., Kildea, S., & Sullivan, E. (2007). Maternal mortality and psychiatric morbidity in the perinatal period: Challenges and opportunities for prevention in the Australian setting. *Medical Journal of Australia, 186*(7), 364–367.

Beck, A. F., Edwards, E. M., Horbar, J. D., Howell, E. A., McCormick, M. C., & Pursley, D. M. (2020). The color of health: How racism, segregation, and inequality affect the health and well-being of preterm infants and their families. *Pediatric Research, 87*, 227–234.

Bergink, V., Rasgon, N., & Wisner, K. L. (2016). Postpartum psychosis: Madness, mania and melancholia in motherhood. *American Journal of Psychiatry, 173*(12), 1179–1188.

Biesmans, K., Franck, E., Ceulemans, C., Jacquemyn, Y., & Van Bogaert, P. (2013). Weight during the postpartum period: What can health care workers do. *Maternal and Child Health Journal, 17*, 996–1004.

Bloch, M., Daly, R. C., & Rubinow, D. R. (2003). Endocrine factors in the etiology of postpartum depression. *Comprehensive Psychiatry, 44*, 234–246.

Bloch, M., Schmidt, P. J., Danaceau, M., Murphy, J., Nieman, L., & Rubinow, D. (2000). Effects of gonadal steroids in women with a history of postpartum depression. *American Journal of Psychiatry, 157*, 924–930.

Bonacquisti, A., Cohen, M., & Schiller, C. (2017). Acceptance and commitment therapy for perinatal mood and anxiety disorders: Development of an inpatient group intervention. *Archives of Women's Mental Health, 20*, 645–654.

Bulbul, F., Alpak, U. C. G., Unal, A., Demir, B., Tastan, M. F., & Savas, H. A. (2013). Electroconvulsive therapy in pregnant patients. *General Hospital Psychiatry, 35*, 636–639.

Cohen, L. S., Viguera, C. A., Bouffard, S. M., et al. (2001). Venlafaxine in the treatment of postpartum depression. *Journal of Clinical Psychiatry, 62*, 592–596.

Cox, E. Q., Frische, S. K. R., McClure, R., Hill, M., Jenson, J., Pearson, B., & Meltzer-Brody, S. E. (2020). Repetitive transcranial magnetic stimulation for the treatment of postpartum depression. *Journal of Affective Disorders, 264*, 193–200.

Cox, E. Q., Sowa, N., Meltzer-Brody, S., & Gaynes, B. (2016). The perinatal depression treatment cascade: Baby steps towards improving outcomes. *Journal of Clinical Psychiatry, 77*(9), 1189–1200.

Cox, J., Holden, J., & Sagovsky, R. (1987). Detection of postnatal depression: Development of the 10-item Edinburgh Postnatal Depression Scale. *British Journal of Psychiatry, 150*, 782–786.

Deligiannidis, K. M., Meltzer-Brody, S., Gunduz-Bruce, H., Doherty, J., Jonas, J., Sankoh, A. J., . . . Lasser, R. (2021). Effect of zuranolone vs placebo in postpartum depression: A randomized clinical trial. *JAMA Psychiatry, 78*(9), 951–959.

Drugs and Lactation Database (LactMed®) [Internet]. Bethesda (MD): National Institute of Child Health and Human Development; 2006–current. Available from: https://www.ncbi.nlm.nih.gov/books/NBK501922/

Earls, M. F., & T. C. o. P. A. o. C. a. F. Health. (2010). Clinical report – Incorporating recognition and management of perinatal and postpartum depression into pediatric practice. *American Academy of Pediatrics.*

Elisei, S., Lucarini, E., Murgia, N., Ferranti, L., & Attademo, L. (2013). Perinatal depression: A study of prevalence and of risk and protective factors. *Psychiatrica Danubina, 25*, S258–262.

Esscher, A., Essén, B., Innala, E., Papdoupoulos, F. C., Skalkidou, A., Sundström, I., & Högberg, U. (2016). Suicides during pregnancy and one year postpartum in Sweden, 1980–2007. *British Journal of Psychiatry, 208*(5), 462–469.

Eustis, E. H., Ernst, S., Sutton, K., & Battle, C. L. (2019). Innovations in the treatment of perinatal depression: The role of yoga and physical activity interventions during pregnancy and the postpartum. *Current Psychiatry Reports, 21*(12), 133.

Frautschi, S., Cerulli, A., & Maine, D. (1994). Suicide during pregnancy and its neglect as a component of maternal mortality. *International Journal of Gynecology & Obstetrics, 47*, 275–284.

Gaynes, B., Gavin, N., & Meltzer-Brody, S. (2005). Perinatal depression: Prevalence, screening accuracy and screening outcomes. *Evidence Report/Technology Assessment, 119*, 1–8.

Gress-Smith, J. L., Luecken, L. J., Lemery-Chalfant, K., & Howe, R. (2012). Postpartum depression prevalence and impact on infant health, weight, and sleep in low-income and ethnic minority women and infants. *Maternal and Child Health, 16*(4), 887–893.

Guille, C., Johnson, E., Douglas, E., Aujla, R., Kruis, R., Beels, R., . . . Sterba, K. (2022). A pilot study examining access to and satisfaction with maternal mental health and substance use disorder treatment via telemedicine. *Telemedicine Reports, 3*(1), 24–29.

Guintivano, J., Sullivan, P. F., Stuebe, A. M., Penders, T., Thorp, J., Rubinow, D. R., & Meltzer-Brody, S. (2018). Adverse life events, psychiatric history, and biological predictors of postpartum depression in an ethnically diverse sample of postpartum women. *Psychological Medicine, 48*(7), 1190–1200.

Gunduz-Bruce, H., Takahashi, K., & Huang M-Y (2022). Development of neuroactive steroids for the treatment of postpartum depression. *Journal of Neuroendocrinology, 34*(2).

Gynecologists, A. C. O. O. A. (2018). ACOG committee opinion no 758: Screening for perinatal depression. *Obstetrics & Gynecology, 132*, 1314–1316.

Herring, S. J., Rich-Edwards, J. W., Oken, E., Rifas-Shiman, S. L., Kleinman, K. P, & Gillman, M. W. (2008). Association of postpartum depression with weight retention 1 year after childbirth. *Obesity, 16*, 1296–1301.

Howard, L. M., Oram, S., Galley, H., Trevillion, K., & Feder, G. (2013). Domestic violence and perinatal mental disorders: A systematic review and meta-analysis. *PLoS Medicine, 10*(5), e10011452.

Kimmel, M. C., Cox, E., Schiller, C., Gettes, E., & Meltzer-Brody, S. (2018). Pharmacologic treatment of perinatal depression. *Obstetrics and Gynecology Clinics of North America, 45*, 419–440.

Lahti, M., Savolainen, K., Tuovinen, S., Pesonen, A.-K., Lahti, J., Heinonen, K., . . . Räikkönen, K. (2017). Maternal depressive symptoms during and after pregnancy and psychiatric problems in children. *Journal of the American Academy of Child and Adolescent Psychiatry, 56*(1), 30–39.

Leiknes, K. A., Cooke, M. J., Jarosch-von Schweder, L., Harboe, I., & Hoie, B. (2015). Electroconvulsive therapy during pregnancy: A systematic review of case studies. *Archives of Women's Mental Health, 18*(1), 1–39.

Levis, B., Negeri, Z., Sun, Y., Benedetti, A., Thombs, B. D., and the Depression Screening Data (DEPRESSED) EPDS Group. (2020). Accuracy of the Edinburgh Postnatal Depression Scale (EPDS) for screening to detect major depression among pregnant and postpartum women: Systematic review and meta-analysis of individual participant data. *British Medical Journal, 371,* m4022.

Lindahl, V., Pearson, J., & Colpe, L. (2005). Prevalence of suicidality during pregnancy and postpartum. *Archives of Women's Mental Health, 8*(2), 77–87.

Luca, D. L., Margiotta, C., Staatz, C., Garlow, E. A., Christensen, A., & Zivin, K. (2020). Financial toll of untreated perinatal mood and anxiety disorders among 2017 births in the United States. *American Journal of Public Health, 110,* 888–896.

Maguire, J., & Mody, I. (2008). GABAAR plasticity during pregnancy: Relevance to postpartum depression. *Neuron, 59*(2), 207–213.

McCabe-Beane, J. E., Segre, L. S., Perkhounkova, Y., Stuart, S., & O'Hara, M. W. (2016). The identification of severity ranges for the Edinburgh Postnatal Depression Scale. *Journal of Reproductive and Infant Psychology, 34,* 293–303.

Meltzer-Brody, S., Bledsoe-Mansori, S. E., Johnson, N., Killian, C., Hamer, R. M., Jackson, C., . . . Thorp, J. (2013). A prospective study of perinatal depression and trauma history in pregnant minority adolescents. *American Journal of Obstetrics and Gynecology, 208*(211), e1–e7.

Meltzer-Brody, S., Colquhoun, H., Riesenberg, R., Epperson, C. N., Deligiannidis, K. M., Rubinow, D. R., . . . Kanes, S. (2018). Brexanolone injection in postpartum depression: Two multicentre, double-blind, randomised, placebo-controlled phase 3 trials. *The Lancet, 392,* 1058–1070.

Meltzer-Brody, S., Howard, L. M., Bergink, V., Vogod, S., Jones, I., Munk-Olsen, T., . . . Milgrom, J. (2018). Postpartum psychiatric disorders. *Nature Review Disease Primers, 4,* 1–18.

Meltzer-Brody, S., & Jones, I. (2015). Optimizing the treatment of mood disorders in the perinatal period. *Dialogues in Clinical Neuroscience, 17*(2), 207–218.

Meltzer-Brody, S., & Kimmel, M. (2020). The promise of telepsychiatry to reduce maternal mortality by increasing access to maternal mental health and addiction services. *Obstetrics & Gynecology, 136*(4), 643–644.

Milgrom, J., Gemmill, A. W., Bilszta, J. L., Hayes, B., Barnett, B., Brooks, J., . . . Buist, A. (2008). Antenatal risk factors for postnatal depression: A large prospective study. *Journal of Affective Disorders, 108,* 147–157.

Nasreen, H.-E., Kabir, Z. N., Forsell, Y., & Edhborg, M. (2013). Impact of maternal depressive symptoms and infant temperament on early infant growth and motor development: Results from a population based study in Bangladesh. *Journal of Affective Disorders, 146*(2), 254–261.

Nonacs R. M., Soares C. N. , Viguera A. C., Pearson K., Poitras J.R., Cohen L.S. Bupropion SR for the treatment of postpartum depression: a pilot study. Int J Neuropsychopharmacol. 2005 Sep;8(3):445-9. doi: 10.1017/S1461145705005079. Epub 2005 Apr 7. PMID: 15817137.

O'Hara, M. W., Stuart, S., Gorman, L. L., & Wenzel, A. (2000). Efficacy of interpersonal psychotherapy for postpartum depression. *Archives of General Psychiatry, 57*(11), 1039–1045.

O'Hara, M. W., & Wisner, K. W. (2014). Perinatal mental illness: Definition, description and aetiology. *Obstetrics & Gynecology, 28*(1), 3–12.

Pahlavan, F., Kazemnejad, A., Razavinia, F., Dayasari, S. R., F., & Najmeh, T. (2020). Biological reflect of Adiponectin hormone in postpartum marital satisfaction and depression scores. *BMC Childbirth, 20,* 525.

Parameswaran, U. D., Pentecost, R., Williams, M., Smid, M., & Latendresse, G. (2022). Experiences with use of technology and telehealth among women with perinatal depression. *BMC Pregnancy and Childbirth, 22*(1), 571.

Patterson, R., Krohn, H., Richardson, E., Kimmel, M., & Meltzer-Brody, S. (2022). A brexanolone treatment program at an academic medical center: Patient selection, 90-day posttreatment outcomes, and lessons learned. *Journal of the Academy of Consultation-Liaison Psychiatry, 63*(1), 14–22.

Putnam, K. T., Wilcox, M., Robertson-Blackmore, E., Sharkey, K., Bergnik, V., Munk-Olsen, T., . . . Meltzer-Brody, S. (2017). Clinical phenotypes of perinatal depression and time of symptom onset: Analysis of data from an international consortium. *Lancet Psychiatry, 4*(6), 477–485.

Rabiee, N. A., Nazari, A. M., Keramat, A., Khosravi, A., & Bolbol-Haghighi, N. (2020). Effect of dialectical behavioral therapy on the postpartum depression, perceived stress, and mental coping strategies in traumatic childbirth: A randomized controlled trial. *International Journal of Health Studies*, 6(2), 41–48.

Rubinow, D., Schmidt, P., & Roca, C. (1998). Estrogen-serotonin interactions: Implications for affective regulation. *Biological Psychiatry*, 44(9), 839–850.

Schiller, C., Dichter, G., Bizzell, J., Johnson, S., Richardson, E., Schmidt, P., . . . Rubinow, D. (2020). Reproductive hormones regulate affect and reward circuit function in women. *Biological Psychiatry*, 87(9), S217.

Shonkoff, J. P., Garner, A. S., Siegel, B. S., Dobbins, M. I., Earls, M. F., McGuinn, L., . . . Wood, D. L. (2011). The lifelong effects of early childhood adversity and toxic stress. *Pediatrics*, 129(1), e232–e246.

Shortis, E., Waarington, D., & Whittaker, P. (2020). The efficacy of cognitive behavioral therapy for the treatment of antenatal depression: A systematic review. *Journal of Affective Disorders*, 272, 485–495.

Singla, D. R., Meltzer-Brody, S., Savel, K., & Silver, R. K. (2022). Scaling up patient-centered psychological treatments for perinatal depression in the wake of a global pandemic. *Frontiers in Psychiatry*, 12.

Slomian, J., Honvo, G., Emonts, P., Reginster, J.-Y., & Bruyère, O. (2019). Consequences of maternal postpartum depression: A systematic review of maternal and infant outcomes. *Women's Health*, 15.

Sprague, J., Wisner, K. L., & Bogen, D. L. (2020). Pharmacotherapy for depression and bipolar disorder during lactation: A framework to aid decision making. *Seminars in Perinatology*, 44(3), 151224.

Stowe, Z., Casarella, J., Landry, J., et al. (1995). Sertraline in the treatment of women with postpartum major depression. *Depression*, 3, 49–55.

Stuebe, A., Grewen, K., Pedersen, C., Popper, C., & Meltzer-Brody, S. (2012). Failed lactation and perinatal depression: Common problems with shared neuroendocrine mechanisms? *Journal of Women's Health*, 21(3), 265–272.

Suri, R., Burt, V. L., & Altshuler, L. L. (2005). Nefazodone for the treatment of postpartum depression. *Archives of Women's Mental Health*, 8, 55–56.

Suri, R., Burt, V. K., Altshuler, L. L., Zuckerbrow-Miller, J., & Fairbanks, L. (2001). Fluvoxamine for postpartum depression. *American Journal of Psychiatry*, 158, 1739–1740.

Vliegen, N., Casalin, S., Luyten, P., Docx, R., Lenaerts, M., Tang, E., & Kempe, S. (2013). Hospitalization-based treatment for postpartum depressed mothers and their babies: Rationale, principles, and preliminary follow-up data. *Psychiatry*, 76(2), 150–168.

Ward, H. B., Fromson, J. A., Cooper, J. J., De Oliveira, G., & Almeida, M. (2018). Recommendations for the use of ECT in pregnancy: Literature review and proposed clinical protocol. *Archives of Women's Mental Health*, 21(6), 715–722.

Warnock, F. K., Craig, K. D., Bakeman, R., Castral, T., & Mirlashan, J. (2016). The relationship of prenatal maternal depression or anxiety to maternal caregiving behavior and infant behavior self-regulation during infant heel lance: An ethological time-based study of behavior. *BMC Pregnancy and Childbirth*, 16, 264.

Winston, R., & Chicot, R. (2016). The importance of early bonding on the long-term mental health and resilience of children. *London Journal of Primary Care*, 8(1), 12–14.

Wisner, K. L., Nahusa, B. H., Perel, J. M., et al. (2006). Postpartum depression: A randomized trial of sertraline versus nortriptyline. *Journal of Clinical Psychopharmacology*, 26, 353–360.

Yonkers, K. A., Lin, H., Howell, H. B., et al. (2008). Pharmacologic treatment of postpartum women with new-onset major depressive disorder: A randomized controlled trial with paroxetine. *Journal of Clinical Psychiatry*, 69, 659–665.

13

POSTPARTUM ANXIETY

Juliana L. Restivo Haney, Gabriella T. Ponzini,
Mira D. H. Snider, Kaley N. Potter, Grace L. Wheeler,
and Shari A. Steinman

Perinatal mental health research has predominantly focused on postpartum depression. Over the past two decades, research has expanded to investigate and highlight other disorders that cause maternal distress, including anxiety disorders. Despite its significant prevalence and the amount of distress it causes many women, many people have never heard of postpartum anxiety (Ponzini et al., 2021). Postpartum anxiety can have adverse effects on both the mother and baby including postpartum depression, disengaged parenting, difficulty bonding, and poor neonatal feeding and nurturing (Araji et al., 2020).

The prevalence of anxiety disorders during the postpartum period is 15% (Dennis et al., 2017). However, the true prevalence of postpartum anxiety is likely underestimated due to the lack of research assessing specific anxiety disorders (e.g., panic, agoraphobia, general anxiety, and social anxiety disorder [SAD]; Fawcett et al., 2019). There is also evidence for the comorbidity of perinatal anxiety and perinatal depression; however, the symptoms do not entirely overlap, and many individuals experience perinatal anxiety without reporting depressive symptoms (Nakić Radoš et al., 2018). This lack of attention in identifying postpartum anxiety risks leaving many mothers undetected and untreated (Dennis et al., 2017).

There is limited evidence for diagnostic accuracy in postpartum anxiety assessment. Some research suggests that postpartum anxiety symptoms are not adequately defined and that a portion of those in the postpartum period experience anxiety symptoms that are not captured by the DSM's anxiety diagnoses (Meades & Ayers, 2011). This is especially concerning because there is no postpartum anxiety diagnosis within the *Diagnostic and Statistical Manual of Mental Disorders* (5th ed.; DSM-5; American Psychiatric Association [APA], 2013). The only diagnostic criteria related to the perinatal period include peripartum onset of brief psychotic disorder, peripartum onset as a specifier for bipolar and related disorders, and peripartum onset as a specifier for depressive disorders.

Anxiety Disorders in the Postpartum Period

Potential causes for new onset of anxiety symptoms during the postpartum period can be triggered by the increase in parenting demands, concerns about the health of the baby, issues with breastfeeding, lack of social support, stress on close relationships, financial

DOI: 10.4324/9781003206903-17

difficulties, personal health issues, lack of self-esteem and self-confidence in parenting skills, body image issues, and the increased pressure to meet the idealized media/social media portrayals of what it means to be the perfect mother (Araji et al., 2020; Kirkpatrick & Lee, 2022; Nakic Radoš et al., 2018; Padoa et al., 2018). During the postpartum period, there is also a significant decrease in both estrogen and progesterone, which has been found to be associated with increased helplessness and anxiety (Schiller et al., 2015). Additionally, changes in oxytocin levels and neuroendocrine responses to lactation can be associated with symptoms of mood and anxiety symptoms (Stuebe et al., 2013).

The features of anxiety disorders are outlined later, along with a brief example of what each disorder may look like in the postpartum period. Note that this chapter does not focus on obsessive-compulsive disorder or posttraumatic stress disorder during the postpartum period—descriptions of those disorders can be found in other chapters in this volume. Unless otherwise noted, for all the following disorders, symptoms must (a) be persistent (e.g., last for at least six months); (b) cause significant distress and/or impairment; (c) not be due to substance use; and (d) not be due to another psychological or medical disorder.

Generalized Anxiety Disorder

Generalized anxiety disorder (GAD) is characterized by excessive and uncontrollable worries about multiple concerns (e.g., family, finances, health of the baby, work). The worries are accompanied by physiological signs of anxiety, such as muscle tension, fatigue, and difficulty concentrating. For example, Gigi is a new mother who excessively worries about her baby's health, her productivity at work following the birth, and financial issues related to caring for a baby.

Social Anxiety Disorder

Social Anxiety Disorder (SAD) is characterized by fear of social situations. Individuals with SAD fear that they may be negatively evaluated or that others will be aware of their anxiety. Consequently, these individuals avoid social situations or endure them with severe distress. For example, Kiana is a new mother who avoids seeing her other "mom friends" because she worries that they will think she is not a good enough mother. She also avoids working in the office (and instead works remotely) so that she will not have to make small talk with her colleagues because she worries that others will think she only talks about the baby.

Specific Phobia

Specific phobia is characterized by an excessive fear of a specific object or situation (e.g., driving in a car, needle injections, and heights). For instance, Joan insists her partner takes her baby to all pediatrician visits and avoids going in for her own postpartum visits because she fears injections and worries that she will faint if she sees blood.

Panic Disorder

A panic attack is a flood of bodily sensations (e.g., sweating, heart palpitations, derealization) that peaks within minutes. An individual with panic disorder experiences recurrent panic attacks that lead to changes in behavior to avoid panic attacks, as well as worry about future panic attacks occurring. Sina had her first panic attack while taking her baby on a brisk walk in the park and her second while following a "mommy and me" exercise routine. Since then, she has avoided going on walks and all other forms of exercise, because she is scared that she will have another panic attack.

Agoraphobia

Agoraphobia involves a fear of situations in which a person may not be able to get help or escape if they experience panic-like (e.g., palpitations, shortness of breath) or embarrassing (e.g., fainting, vomiting) physiological sensations. Commonly feared situations include open places (e.g., a large field), enclosed places (e.g., a theater), public transportation, or being alone outside the home. Maria, for example, is afraid to leave her house with her baby and avoids taking public transportation, because she worries about feeling overheated and throwing up when traveling with the baby.

Separation Anxiety

The defining feature of separation anxiety is a developmentally inappropriate fear of being separated from an important individual (e.g., child, spouse). For example, Kasumi refuses to let anyone watch her young daughter because she worries that something bad will happen to her daughter if they are not always together.

Cognitive Behavioral Model of Postpartum Anxiety

According to cognitive behavioral models of anxiety (Clark & Beck, 2010; Thoma et al., 2015), thoughts, feelings, and behaviors interact to cause and maintain anxiety disorders. Adaptations of this model to perinatal mental health highlight how life stress (e.g., childbirth, lack of partner support, financial instability) increases the likelihood that cognitive vulnerabilities (e.g., dysfunctional beliefs, negative interpretations) are activated, which consequentially lead to unhelpful behavior patterns (avoidance) and anxiety (Wenzel & Kleiman, 2015). Importantly, cognitive vulnerabilities for perinatal anxiety include both general anxiety-relevant beliefs, such as "bad things are likely to happen" and "I will not be able to cope," and specific beliefs related to motherhood, such as "I'm not cut out to be a good enough mother" and "If my baby gets sick it is all my fault."

Cara is a 27-year-old, Caucasian woman who gave birth to her son and first child, Jaime, six months ago. Cara is a high school math teacher and is currently on maternity leave. Cara's husband, Daniel, is also 27 and works full-time as a lawyer. He works long hours in the office every Monday, Wednesday, and Friday and occasionally works from home on Tuesdays and Thursdays. She is nervous about going to an office party with her husband because she is worried that his coworkers will judge her appearance. If she spends too much time getting ready to look nice, they may think that she does not care about the baby; if she does not try to look nice, they will think she let herself go and is not as professional as she was before having a child. She has avoided seeing her friends because she worries that she will bore them if she talks about diapers and the milestones the baby has met so far. She worries that she will not know what else to talk about other than the baby and that they will think she is selfish or not as fun as she used to be.

Her older sister has a daughter who is 3 years old. Jaime is the first grandchild on Daniel's side of the family. Since Jaime's birth, Cara has felt worried that others will judge her parenting skills and her choices. She feels pressure from her sister who always tells her about a better way she could be doing something. She worries that she is being judged by her mother-in-law because she stopped breastfeeding and switched to using formula. Every time the phone rings, she worries that it could be her mother-in-law asking to come over and see the baby. She loves her husband's mother and wants to make sure she has a special relationship with Jaime, but she worries her mother-in-law will think that she is a bad mother and that she does not know how to care for her own son.

Cara is also very concerned about Jaime's health and development. She wonders if he is meeting his milestones. She will time his tummy time and double-check that it matches the recommended time the pediatrician told her. She wakes up multiple times throughout the night to check if he is still breathing. She worries that because she stopped exclusively breastfeeding, he may not be getting all the nutrients that he needs. She also does not want to get together with others, because she wants to keep Jaime from being exposed to any germs (e.g., RSV).

Cara's escalating apprehension about seeing her mother-in-law, meeting up with friends, going to office get-togethers, and seeing her sister and niece is putting a strain on her relationship with her husband. She repeatedly asks him for reassurance that she is making the right decisions and that she is a good mother. Daniel knows she is a good mother, but he becomes frustrated when he must reassure her or when she cancels plans because she is worried about being negatively evaluated by people or that Jaime could become sick.

Prevalence

In the first six months of the postpartum period, the worldwide prevalence of self-reported anxiety symptoms is estimated to be approximately 15% (Dennis et al., 2017) compared to the lifetime prevalence of anxiety in women, which is estimated to be 6% (Hantsoo & Epperson, 2017). In the United States, reports of anxiety symptoms during the early postpartum (i.e., first weeks post-delivery) and late postpartum (i.e., six months post-delivery) periods indicate increased anxiety over time (17.3% to 20.6%, respectively) (Nakić Radoš et al., 2018). These estimates suggest the experience of postpartum anxiety symptoms within the first year after delivery is equal to or greater than the experience of postpartum depression in new mothers (Le Strat et al., 2011). Although there is a lower prevalence for *diagnosed* specific anxiety disorders during the postpartum period (compared with the level of anxiety symptoms in the postpartum period), prevalence estimates are still significant. Specifically, about 9.9% of women worldwide are diagnosed with an anxiety disorder during their postpartum period, with higher rates of anxiety disorders in low- to middle-income countries (Dennis et al., 2017). A meta-analysis examining anxiety disorders in postpartum women reported the prevalence rates for any anxiety disorder during the postpartum period approximating 8.56%, with GAD having the greatest prevalence (3.59%), followed by panic disorder (1.66%), SAD (1.28%), agoraphobia (0.68%), an anxiety disorder not otherwise specified (0.38%), and specific phobias (0.03%) (Goodman et al., 2016). Of note, the prevalence rates from this meta-analysis are likely low, given that many of the studies only assessed women who screened positive for depression. The authors posited that, because of this, women with high anxiety who were not also experiencing depressive symptoms were likely missed (Goodman et al., 2016). These prevalence rates are compared to the general population rates of 3.7% for GAD (Ruscio et al., 2017), 2.4% for panic disorder (Kessler et al., 2012), 1.7% for agoraphobia (Kessler et al., 2012), 7.4% for social anxiety (Kessler et al., 2012), and specific phobias 12.1% (Kessler et al., 2012). These data suggest the widespread experience of postpartum anxiety and the importance of understanding associated risk factors and outcomes to better direct women to effective care.

Correlates and Risk Factors

To date, various risk factors have been identified regarding the development of anxiety disorders in the postpartum period. The strongest predictor of any postpartum anxiety disorder development is prenatal (before birth) anxiety symptoms (e.g., high trait anxiety) and a preexisting diagnosis of an anxiety disorder (Grant et al., 2008; Martini et al., 2015; Reck et al., 2008). That is, women who experience heightened levels of anxiety during their third trimester of pregnancy or women who have been diagnosed with an anxiety disorder prior to or during their pregnancy are especially likely to be diagnosed with an anxiety disorder in the postpartum period. Additionally, women who are younger than 25 years, have experienced one or more pregnancy losses (Giannandrea et al., 2013), have more than one child (Grant et al., 2008), or have low education levels (van der Zee-van den Berg et al., 2021) have a greater incidence of postpartum anxiety. Women who have a lifetime history of depression (van der Zee-van den Berg et al., 2021), experience a depressive disorder during pregnancy (Martini et al., 2015), or have maternity blues at two weeks postpartum (Reck et al., 2009) also have a greater incidence of developing an anxiety disorder postpartum compared to women who do not meet these criteria.

An inverse relation exists between psychosocial factors such as perceived social support (including partner support) (van der Zee-van den Berg et al., 2021), partner satisfaction and self-esteem (Martini et al., 2015), as well as low maternal self-efficacy (van der Zee-van den Berg et al., 2021) with postpartum anxiety disorders. These findings suggest that there are malleable risk factors associated with postpartum anxiety disorder development, which can be targeted in future research. Furthermore, women who experience a higher number of stressful life events during pregnancy (Farr et al., 2014), have a negative life experience during the first week of postpartum, or perceive their infant's crying as excessive (van der Zee-van den Berg et al., 2021) are more likely to develop an anxiety disorder compared to those who have not experienced such events. With regard to health-related risk factors, women who have gestational insomnia (Osnes et al., 2019) or are in poor health (van der Zee-van den Berg et al., 2021) are also at a greater risk of developing postpartum anxiety compared to those who do not have health or sleep issues. Lastly, there is an association between women who recently (i.e., within the last year) experienced interpersonal violence and the development of panic disorder in the postpartum period compared with women who do not report recent interpersonal violence (Cerulli et al., 2011). Understanding risk factors can allow for preventive measures to be considered and implemented across the perinatal period to reduce the risk of anxiety disorders in postpartum women (e.g., education about anxiety disorders and treatment in postpartum, psychotherapy, and/or skills-based training to prevent anxiety development).

Cara acknowledges that her husband Daniel is very supportive, but he often does not share caretaking responsibilities. Even on the days when he works from home, he is busy in his office working. She often feels resentful that he can work while she must take care of their baby. Cara does have additional family support, but she often does not take advantage of this help because she is fearful that something will happen to the baby if she is not the one caring for him. She also believes that it is her responsibility to care for the baby at all times because she is the one on maternity leave. Cara has always held high standards for herself and has been very successful in school and at her job. She places considerable emphasis on how she is perceived by others and whether they view her as successful. She worries that her new role as a mother will interfere with how her coworkers view her at work when she returns. Although she loves her job and is excited to return to work, Cara also worries that her friends who stay home with their children will think she is a bad mother and is choosing her career over her child. She questions whether she will be able to balance family life, the demands of her job, and the needs of her students.

Cara is not characterized by many of the sociodemographic variables mentioned above as risk factors for postpartum anxiety—she is older than 25 years, she has not experienced a previous pregnancy loss, and she and her husband both have graduate degrees in their field. She and her husband both have loans from school but are financially stable. However, throughout areas of her life, she has had a history of perfectionistic tendencies which cause her to over-analyze social interactions, believing that others' approval is conditional on her performance across situations. Additionally, she tries to avoid situations where she does not think she can meet the standards of others. As a new mother, the societal standards of what a good mom should be feel impossible to meet.

Effects on Partner Relationship, Children, and Other Family Members

Entering parenthood is a major life event that will substantially change family dynamics under the best of circumstances. Even when expecting mothers who are in almost perfect health are *not* demonstrating signs or symptoms of a postpartum anxiety disorder, it is expected that they will undergo substantial stressors related to their rapidly changing roles within their own family and community systems. These stressors often arise in response to a major identity shift in which there is conflict between the new parenting role that primarily focuses on the well-being of the new child with the demands from the parents' preexisting social roles. As the challenges of parenting increase, mothers are likely to experience reduced engagement in other meaningful parts of their identity, such as work, hobbies, family relationships, and other friendships (Haga et al., 2012; Seymour-Smith et al., 2017). Thus, the addition of a new child can dramatically change the way that mothers participate in or allocate emotional and physical resources toward their nonparenting relationships. Considering the extent to which changes in social roles are normative for new mothers, it is perhaps unsurprising that these challenges are further exacerbated by clinically significant anxiety symptoms during the perinatal period. As previously described, anxiety disorders during the postpartum period are characterized by excessive worries, fears, and feelings of overwhelm triggered by a multitude of stressors. The distress and impairment from these anxious thoughts, feelings, and behaviors, impact the mothers' relationships and social bonds (Goodman et al., 2016).

The transition from a romantic partnership without children to one in which partners are co-parenting increases the couple's risk for relationship strain and can lower perceptions of relationship quality (Cowan & Cowan, 2000; Glenn & McLanahan, 1982). This may be due to stress caused by increased parenting responsibilities, unequal sharing of parenting responsibilities across gender roles and specific societal pressures placed on new mothers, and declines in new parents' ability to provide and access practical and emotional supports with their partners (Sawers & Wong, 2018; Wardrop & Popadiuk, 2013). Previous research has demonstrated that changes in relationship satisfaction and the mother's individual wellness during the transition to motherhood can be predicted by lower social support from partners (Eller et al., 2022; Haga et al., 2012); and more inconsistency in perceived or observed partner support during this transition has been connected to decreased relationship quality and relationship satisfaction long term for these couples (Eller et al., 2022; Levitt et al., 1993). Conversely, more consistent levels of partner support were related to better relationship quality and mental health (including but not limited to anxiety symptoms) reported by new mothers (Eller et al., 2022).

Predictably, postpartum anxiety has been connected to poorer relationship quality (Goodman et al., 2016). A new mother's perception of social support from their partner and family can be a protective factor against stress and anxiety increases during the perinatal period (Racine et al., 2019). Postpartum mental health concerns, including postpartum anxiety, are often associated with lower perceptions of partner support and relationship satisfaction (Martini et al., 2015; Schmied et al., 2013). Although the relationship strains affiliated with new motherhood can place mothers at risk for postpartum anxiety and other internalizing disorders, the presentation of postpartum anxiety symptoms may also perpetuate or worsen these relationship difficulties. For instance, mothers with postpartum anxiety, compared to mothers who do not experience anxiety, may have greater difficulty regulating strong emotions, be more likely to experience increased conflict with partners because of their attempts to avoid or mitigate anxiety triggers, and become more likely to withdraw from social opportunities as a means of coping, ultimately worsening their presentation in the long term.

Cara is less likely to go to Daniel's work party than she would have been before she had her baby because she is worried about how she might be perceived by others at the party. Daniel may become upset that Cara is not taking the opportunity for a break from parenting responsibilities to spend time with him and his colleagues, or he may feel pressured to leave the work party early to check in on Cara leading to increased conflict about how she is managing her worries.

Another important impact of parenthood on parent relationships concerns changes in sexual and emotional intimacy. Declines in sexual activity, desire, and satisfaction are commonly reported by women during the postpartum period (Acele & Karaçam, 2012; De Judicibus & McCabe, 2002). Reduced perceptions of intimacy after childbirth may be related to changes in attraction after physical body changes, different types of intimacy (emotional vs. sexual), reorganizations around new priorities, and increased pain after childbirth (Stavdal et al., 2019). Women entering new motherhood roles have reported that their intimacy with partners is negatively impacted by increased tiredness, changing lifestyle behaviors, body image concerns, decreased libido, and increased negative emotions such as feelings of guilt or failure in the context of their motherhood role (Ali, 2018; Woolhouse et al., 2012). These concerns can be made worse by anxiety symptoms, in which preoccupations with anxiety triggers and increased distress can reduce desires to engage intimately with partners (Costa et al., 2016).

Importantly, partner relationships are not the only relationships that are impacted by postpartum anxiety; such diagnoses are also associated with significant negative consequences for both the mother and her new baby (Goodman et al., 2016). Compared to women who do not experience anxiety symptoms, women with postpartum anxiety experience decreased mother–infant bonding (Fallon et al., 2021; Field, 2018; Tietz et al., 2014), are more likely to have children who experience excessive infant crying, and have children who are more likely to have poorer motor development at four months postpartum (Petzoldt et al., 2014). Anxious mothers are also more likely than nonanxious mothers to have a reduced duration of breastfeeding and more negative perceptions of infant sleep quality (Davies et al., 2022; Field, 2018). In fact, The American Academy of Pediatrics and others have published data indicating that state anxiety in the postpartum period is associated with reduced duration of breastfeeding (Paul et al., 2013) and increased difficulty maintaining breastfeeding in mothers who wish to breastfeed, impacting an important bonding experience between the mother and the baby (Fallon, Groves, et al., 2016). Moreover, when compared to children born to mothers who do not experience symptoms of anxiety, children of anxious mothers experience greater distress in relation to novel stimuli (Reck et al., 2013). Although the exact mechanisms underlying the relation between postpartum anxiety symptoms, mother–infant bond, and parenting outcomes remain unclear (Ali, 2018), these data illustrate the long-lasting and detrimental impact that postpartum anxiety may have on entire family constellations.

Anxious mothers show the highest level of intrusiveness (e.g., criticism or behavioral corrections) in their interactions with their infants compared to depressed mothers and mothers without such mental health concerns (Feldman et al., 2009). The intrusive parenting style associated with postpartum anxiety may in part be due to the dysfunctional beliefs that women with postpartum anxiety experience. Specifically, women with postpartum anxiety have a heightened experience of maternal responsibility, beliefs of personal inadequacy, and role idealization consistent with high performance (i.e., "perfect") in motherhood (Sockol et al., 2014) compared to mothers who do not experience postpartum anxiety. In fact, perfectionism has been demonstrated as a risk factor for postpartum anxiety development (Arnold & Kalibatseva, 2020). These high-standard beliefs also contribute to experiential avoidance, or the avoidance or suppression of uncomfortable thoughts and feelings (i.e., internal experiences), which consequently affects behaviors and functional outcomes (i.e., external experiences) (Hayes et al., 2006). For example, women who hold increasingly negative beliefs about their maternal responsibility or are concerned with judgment from others may experience heightened anxiety about their maternal performance (Fonseca & Canavarro, 2018), and to suppress such anxiety, these mothers may alter their parent–child interaction styles or may avoid social gatherings with other parents. It is unsurprising, then, that women with any anxiety disorder also scored lower on maternal self-confidence assessments at two weeks postpartum compared to mothers without an anxiety disorder (Reck et al., 2012).

Outcome-related correlates also exist for specific anxiety disorder diagnoses. For example, women with postpartum panic disorder engage in potentially problematic bedtime behaviors, such as greater nighttime feedings, sleeping with their child, and not putting their child to bed while the child is awake (Warren et al., 2006) compared to women who do not have postpartum panic disorder. These intrusive parenting behaviors have been associated with negative infant consequences, including having children with greater salivary cortisol, more disturbed sleep, and less motor activity than children of women without panic disorder (Warren et al., 2006). Likewise, women with SAD demonstrate more anxious behaviors when interacting with strangers, such as less active engagement and less encouragement of infant engagement compared to nonanxious mothers (Murray et al., 2007). Infants of mothers with social anxiety compared to infants of nonanxious mothers demonstrate reduced social responsiveness with strangers (i.e., less positive communication) and increased attention to their anxious mothers. Alternatively, women with GAD have been shown to be less engaged with their infants during face-to-face play time (Murray et al., 2007), compared to those who do not meet the criteria for GAD demonstrating reduced responses to infant vocalizations and less positive emotional tones in their responses when activated by a worry and rumination prime (Stein et al., 2012). Mothers with GAD identify happy infant faces earlier than mothers without GAD, which may suggest that these mothers have an increased difficulty with uncertainty tolerance. Such intolerance of uncertainty likely leads to an increased tendency to focus on environmental stimuli that provide reassurance that negative events will not occur (Arteche et al., 2011). Unfortunately, their heightened awareness and low tolerance for certainty may also impact their self-esteem, as mothers with GAD have also been shown to have greater body image self-consciousness and increased sexual avoidance and fears at ten weeks postpartum (Wenzel et al., 2007) compared to those without GAD. In sum, there are important consequences associated with anxiety disorders in the postpartum period, which render these diagnoses an important focus of perinatal care.

Regarding the social bonds that mothers hold outside of their immediate family system, the research supports that maintaining social connections after having a baby is predictive of better mental health for new mothers (Seymour-Smith et al., 2017). Postpartum anxiety presentations, including excessive preoccupation with worries about the newborn or the maternal role and increased social isolation and avoidance behaviors, may also decrease mothers' ability or capacity to engage meaningfully in friendships and other family roles outside of the home (Seymour-Smith et al., 2017). These fears prevent new mothers with postpartum anxiety from connecting to important social outlets in their communities (e.g., delay going back to work after maternity leave and reduced interaction with religious organizations or hobbies that were important to them before having a child).

Cara is less likely to engage with her friend groups after giving birth due to frequent preoccupations with being seen as a bad mother, or as a mother who is too preoccupied with their newborn. As a result, Cara is less likely to receive much-needed social support from her friend groups that could better help her to cope with these stressors.

Assessment

An accurate and thorough understanding of anxiety symptoms in postpartum populations is needed to effectively treat the symptoms. The use of various general anxiety measures during the postpartum period has been effective in detecting anxiety disorders in postpartum women. Continued validation of general measures of anxiety in postpartum samples is important because normative values and cutoff points may differ within the postpartum period compared to those for the general population and across multiple cultures (Meades & Ayers, 2011). Even so, measures specific to the unique experiences of this life event may have a greater chance of detection of postpartum anxiety than those that are not specific to this life event. There have been multiple anxiety screening assessments developed for the postpartum period. A nonexhaustive list of assessment measures specifically designed for perinatal anxiety as well as general anxiety assessments that have been used during the postpartum period are described later.

Measures Specifically Designed for Perinatal Anxiety

The *Perinatal Anxiety Screening Scale* (PASS) (Somerville et al., 2015) is a 31-item self-report measure designed to assess anxieties unique to prenatal and postpartum women. The PASS was developed for use in a variety of settings, including prenatal clinics, hospitals, and mental health facilities (Somerville et al., 2015). Items are rated on a *Likert Scale* from 0 to 3 with scores ranging from 0 to 93. The prompt for the items is "Over the past month, how often have you experienced the following?" Sample items for the PASS include "Fear that harm will come to the baby" and "A sense of dread that something bad is going to happen." A cutoff score of ≥ 26 has been established for clinical anxiety. The PASS has demonstrated sufficient test–retest reliability (rho = 0.74) (Koukopoulos et al., 2021; Somerville et al., 2015). At the cutoff score of 26, the PASS has a sensitivity of 70% and a specificity of 30% (Koukopoulos et al., 2021; Somerville et al., 2015). The PASS has been validated in Italian, Persian, Turkish, Lebanese, Bangladeshi, Iranian, Sri Lankan, and Saudi Arabian samples (Amiri et al., 2022; Hobeika et al., 2023; Jradi et al., 2020; Koukopoulos et al., 2021; Barzgar-Molan et al., 2020; Priyadarshanie et al., 2020; Somerville et al., 2015).

The *Postpartum Specific Anxiety Scale* (PSAS) (Fallon, Halford, et al., 2016) is a 51-item self-report scale designed to accurately assess anxieties specific to postpartum women. Items are rated on a four-point *Likert Scale*, ranging from 0 = "not at all" to 3 = "almost always." The PSAS has a four-factor structure measuring competence and attachment anxieties, safety and welfare anxieties, practical baby care anxieties, and psychosocial adjustment to motherhood (Fallon, Halford, et al., 2016). The four factors have demonstrated acceptable reliability with Cronbach's alpha values ranging from 0.80 to 0.91 (Fallon, Halford, et al., 2016). Sample items include "I have worried about the way that I feed my baby" and "I have worried that I will not know what to do when my baby cries." The PSAS has a cutoff score of 112 with a sensitivity of 0.75 and a specificity of 0.31, suggesting a detection of clinical levels of anxiety (Fallon, Halford, et al., 2016). A Turkish version of the PSAS has also been validated (Duran, 2020). The PSAS was found to be significantly positively correlated with related measures of anxiety including the *Edinburgh Postpartum Depression Scale-Anxiety* and the *State-Trait Anxiety Inventory* demonstrating convergent validity (Fallon, Halford, et al., 2016).

The *Postpartum Worry Scale-Revised* (PWS-R) (Moran et al., 2014) is a 13-item measure that assesses worry in postpartum women. Compared to the original PWS (Wenzel et al., 2005), the PWS-R added items relating to common concerns about the infant (Moran et al., 201). The PWS-R contains four factors that relate to relationships, the household, time allocations, and health and development which demonstrate adequate reliability.

The *Edinburgh Postpartum Depression Scale* (EPDS) (Cox et al., 1987) is a ten-item self-administered questionnaire that is one of the most widely used screening measures to assess for perinatal distress during pregnancy and postpartum (Lydsdottir et al., 2014). A three-item anxiety subscale (EPDS-3A) has been identified through exploratory factor analysis (Brouwers et al., 2001; Jomeen & Martin, 2007) and has been shown to perform more accurately (Matthey et al., 2013) than the anxiety subscale of other common measures of assessing perinatal anxiety, including the *Hospital Anxiety and Depression Scale* (HADS-A) (Zigmond & Snaith, 1983) and the *Pregnancy Related Anxiety Questionnaire-Revised* (PRAQ-R) (Huizink et al., 2004).

The *Postpartum Distress Measure* (PDM) (Allison et al., 2011) is a ten-item measure that was created to assess postpartum depression and anxiety symptoms. A factor analysis of the PDM yielded a two-factor structure containing a general distress subscale and an obsessive-compulsive subscale. Sample items include "I have recurring thoughts about harm coming to my baby, my family, or myself" and "I am afraid I will never feel better." The PDM total score had a coefficient alpha of 0.84. The PDM has demonstrated evidence of convergent validity with the EPDS (Allison et al., 2011).

Measures for General Anxiety Previously Used in Perinatal Populations

The *Generalized Anxiety Disorder-7* (GAD-7) (Spitzer et al., 2006) is a seven-item scale that was originally developed for primary care physicians to screen for GAD in the general population (Simpson et al., 2014). Items are scored on a Likert-type scale with a total score range of 0 to 21. Respondents are asked to indicate how often they have been bothered by the following problems over the past two weeks. Sample items include "Not being able to stop or control worrying" and "Being so restless that it is hard to sit still." A cutoff score of 13 was found to be the best fit for GAD-7 for use in perinatal populations, instead of the cutoff score of 10 for general populations (Simpson et al., 2014). With the new cutoff score of 13, GAD-7 demonstrated a sensitivity of 61.3% and a specificity of 72.7%, suggesting that it is a reliable initial screening tool.

The *State-Trait Anxiety Inventory* (STAI) (Spielberger et al., 1983) is a 40-item self-report measure containing two subscales to measure state and trait anxiety. The state subscale measures current anxiety, whereas the trait subscale measures average anxiety (Meades & Ayers, 2011). Grant et al. (2008) found that trait anxiety subscale scores of ≥40 correlated with a 600% increase in postpartum anxiety disorders, demonstrating predictive validity (odds ratio = 6.44, 95% confidence interval = 1.28–32–28) (Meades & Ayers, 2011). Grant et al. (2008) found the internal consistency of the STAI to be 0.94 in a postpartum sample. Sample items include "I am tense" and "I feel indecisive" for the state subscale that respondents are instructed to indicate how they are feeling at this moment. For the trait subscale, respondents are instructed to indicate how they generally feel. Trait sample items include "I lack self-confidence" and "I worry too much over something that really doesn't matter." This measure is not specific to the perinatal population but has been validated for use in multiple studies assessing anxiety symptoms in individuals during pregnancy and postpartum (Bayrampour et al., 2014; Grant et al., 2008; Tendais et al., 2014).

The *Depression Anxiety Stress Scales* (DASS) (Lovibond & Lovibond, 1995) contain three subscales measuring depression, anxiety, and stress. The DASS is available for use in a 42-item and a 21-item version. Respondents are asked to indicate how much statement applied to them over the past week. Sample items include "I found it difficult to work up the initiative to do things" and "I tended to over-react to situations." The DASS does not include items related to somatic symptoms that may not be appropriate indicators for those in postpartum, such as quality of sleep, lethargy, and concentration (Meades & Ayers, 2011). The internal consistency for the DASS anxiety subscale is acceptable at 0.77 (Meades & Ayers, 2011; Miller et al., 2006). The DASS correlates positively with the EPDS for detecting clinical levels of anxiety and depression in a postpartum sample indicating convergent validity (Bryson et al., 2021; Miller et al., 2006). Additionally, the DASS was able to identify a subset of mothers who indicated higher clinical distress, as evidenced by symptoms of anxiety and/or stress, on the DASS that were not detected on the EPDS (Miller et al., 2006). This finding demonstrates the importance of identifying depression, anxiety, and stress as distinct emotional states in postpartum mothers.

Challenges to Postpartum Anxiety Assessment

Though there has been a tremendous growth in recognition of the need to assess postpartum anxiety distinctly, there is still a dearth of research on the assessment of perinatal anxiety (Bhat et al., 2022). There is also a lack of current agreement among researchers and clinicians on a specific evidence-based recommendation for a postpartum anxiety screening tool to be used in clinical settings as well as uncertainty about the complexity of differentiating between adaptive anxiety, clinically significant anxiety after childbirth, and whether postpartum anxiety is conceptually distinct from generalized anxiety (Hoberg et al., 2022).

As mentioned earlier, there are distinct symptoms that pertain to the transition to motherhood and the postpartum period experience that are not captured by DSM-5 general anxiety diagnoses (Meades & Ayers, 2011). These symptoms may not be detected by the general self-report measures for anxiety. Alternatively, there are also changes that may happen during this period of transition that are a normal part of pregnancy, postpartum, and lactation that may not indicate mental distress including appetite change, sleep disturbance, tiredness, loss of libido, and concern about the health of the vulnerable newborn. To the authors' knowledge, there are no distinct diagnostic interviews for perinatal anxiety, which could help to further differentiate between the normal and clinical levels of worry and distress for these mothers. Overreliance on self-report can also lead to biased answers from mothers due to societal and specific cultural stigma surrounding negative maternal mental health.

Cara decided to seek treatment for the anxiety she was experiencing. The clinical psychologist she saw assessed her using a few different measures. On the PASS, Cara scored 39, which is above the cutoff score of 26 and indicative of mild–moderate symptoms of anxiety. On the STAI, Cara scored a 50 on the trait anxiety subscale and a 46 on the state anxiety subscale, suggesting clinically significant symptoms of anxiety. On the Generalized Anxiety Disorder-7 measure, Cara scored 15, which is higher than the suggested perinatal cutoff score, 13. Taken together, these scores suggest that Cara is struggling with a significant level of anxiety, and it is appropriate that she continues to seek treatment.

Treatment

Anxiety disorders are one of the most treatable psychological disorders, assuming an individual can find and receive evidence-based treatment. Cognitive behavioral therapy (CBT), or psychotherapies that primarily involve cognitive restructuring and exposures, have been shown to be efficacious in reducing anxiety symptoms across disorders, and results are sustained over time (Abramowitz et al., 2019; Arch & Craske, 2009). Furthermore, medications, such as selective serotonin reuptake inhibitors (SSRIs), have shown strong effects in treating anxiety disorders (Jakubovski et al., 2019). Although anxiety is not eliminated, many find lasting relief through these treatments (Loerinc et al., 2015; Murrough et al., 2015).

Although there is evidence supporting psychosocial treatments and medications for anxiety disorders, there are many fewer studies testing these interventions in postpartum individuals. This is likely due to concerns that medications can transfer to the baby via breastfeeding (Misri & Kendrick, 2007) and barriers faced by mothers to accessing psychosocial treatment (Ponzini et al., 2021). However, there is evidence to suggest that not addressing anxiety disorders with these evidence-based treatments can lead to worse outcomes for the mother, baby, and family in the postpartum period. In the following subsections, we describe interventions that have been successful in reducing and treating postpartum anxiety.

Psychosocial Treatments

The "gold-standard" psychosocial treatment for treating anxiety disorders is CBT (Arch & Craske, 2009). The evidence base for CBT is extensive, with multiple studies demonstrating that CBT is successful at reducing symptoms of GAD (Cuijpers et al., 2014), specific phobias (Choy et al., 2007), SAD (Mayo-Wilson et al., 2014), and panic disorder (Pompoli et al., 2016). Moreover, treatment effects are long lasting, with studies showing maintenance of gains several years post-treatment (Arch & Craske, 2009; Steinman et al., 2016).

A recent meta-analysis suggests that, when compared to controls, CBT administered in an in-person group format (with and without a partner) and an Internet-based format (perinatal individuals alone) both lead to short-term (standardized mean difference = −0.63) and long-term (standardized mean difference = −0.71) effects on anxiety symptoms with 95% confidence (Li et al., 2022). The negative effect size indicates an overall superiority of CBT over the controls (Li et al., 2022). Of note, CBT administered in an in-person individual format (perinatal individuals alone) did not lead to a significant reduction in anxiety symptoms (Li et al., 2022). However, much of the research from randomized controlled trials (RCTs) conducted during the perinatal period utilize CBT interventions designed for perinatal depression (vs. anxiety), and none of the studies emphasize exposure, which is considered a critical component of CBT for anxiety (Arch et al., 2012).

Next, we provide a brief description of CBT and its key components: exposures and cognitive restructuring. We also provide examples of how CBT may be applied to postpartum anxiety. CBT is a time-limited, directive treatment, based on the theory that thoughts, behaviors, and feelings are interconnected, and changing one of these three factors changes the other two factors (Beck, 2021). In CBT for anxiety, patients learn to notice and change their unhelpful thinking patterns (cognitive therapy) and practice approaching feared stimuli (exposure therapy). CBT can also include other components, such as diaphragmatic breathing and mindfulness. However, dismantling studies suggest that exposures are the most impactful and necessary part of CBT (Longmore & Worrell, 2007).

During exposures, individuals gradually approach feared stimuli to learn that their anxiety eventually habituates, or decreases, if they stay in a scary situation (Tolin, 2016). They also learn that their feared outcomes are unlikely to occur (Craske et al., 2022). For instance, a new mother who worries she will get in a car accident with her baby would gradually work her way up to going for drives with her baby in the car. Typically, therapists work with their clients to build an exposure hierarchy, or a list of feared situations ordered from least scary to most scary (Tolin, 2016). Clients then work their way up the hierarchy, eventually completing the scariest tasks on their list. The mother afraid of getting into a car accident would perhaps start by sitting in the car with the baby in the driveway and then as a next step on the hierarchy drive her baby around her neighborhood, and once that became easier, she would move to driving her baby around on main roads and eventually move to driving on the highway with her baby. Exposure therapy often includes over-learning, in which clients practice being in situations that go well beyond normal (Tolin, 2012). For instance, our example mother might practice driving her baby around on the highway during a thunderstorm, while repeatedly telling herself she is going to crash and kill her baby. Once a client can successfully complete exposures such as these, she will find that typical daily driving with her baby is no longer anxiety-provoking. Exposures are not designed to prove to clients that they will always be safe but rather that their feared outcomes are unlikely and that they can tolerate the uncertainty associated with doing these scary actions (Tolin, 2012).

An integral aspect of exposure therapy is to identify and stop safety behaviors, which are overt or covert behaviors designed to reduce anxiety (Salkovskis, 1991). For instance, an overt safety behavior might be only agreeing to drive the baby around if another adult is in the car. A covert safety behavior might be telling oneself "I will be fine" repeatedly while driving. Both behaviors are problematic because they preclude the client from learning that her anxiety will decrease on its own and that her feared outcomes are unlikely to occur. Rather, they teach the mother that her safety and anxiety reduction are conditional on the presence of the safety behavior (e.g., the partner in the car, the internal repetition of affirmations; though see Parrish et al., 2008, suggesting safety behaviors are not always problematic).

Cara has been feeling overwhelmed with responsibilities around the house. She and her therapist came to the realization that she has not been without her son (other than nap time) for the past five months. She knows she could benefit from going to a coffee shop without him to sit and read a book like she used to do before he was born. Cara is worried about all the things that could happen if she leaves him alone with her husband for an hour. Jaime could cry for her and be upset that she left him, her husband could turn his back and the baby could get hurt, or the husband may not know what Jaime wants when he cries. Below, Cara and her therapist are meeting at the local coffee shop for an in-person exposure session.

Therapist: Great job making it to the coffee shop today! On a scale from 0 to 100, how anxious do you feel?

Cara: Really anxious about being away from Jaime. Maybe an 80 out of 100.

Therapist:	I'm proud of you for trying this, even though it is so difficult. What worries are going through your mind as we sit here?
Cara:	I am worried Jaime is going to hurt himself when my husband is not looking at him.
Therapist:	What are some physical sensations you are noticing?
Cara:	My chest feels tight, and my heart is racing. I just want to call and see if everything is ok.
Therapist:	It's good that you are noticing those physical sensations. On that scale from 0 to 100, how anxious do you feel?
Cara:	About a 90. It went up when I started focusing on Jaime getting hurt. Can I call my husband to check if Jaime is ok?
Therapist:	What problems might that cause?
Cara:	It might be reassurance seeking, which is a safety behavior.
Therapist:	Right, so you might find out that Jaime is fine if you call your husband, but . . .
Cara:	This is only a short-term fix for my anxiety, I wouldn't learn to accept that I cannot know everything that is happening to Jaime at all times.
Therapist:	Exactly. How anxious do you feel now?
Cara:	Now I feel about a 75.
Therapist:	It's gone down.
Cara:	Yes, I think just because we've been here for a while and nothing bad has happened yet. I haven't got calls from my husband that something horrible happened or anything.
Therapist:	Good.
Cara:	I also know that my reliance on my husband to reassure me has been straining our relationship.
Therapist:	That makes sense. Our anxiety can put a strain on our relationships. How will stopping the reassurance seeking help your anxiety?
Cara:	Well, it doesn't help my anxiety right now. Not reaching out is making my anxiety very high right now. But if I go home after this and everything is fine my husband may feel that I have more confidence in his parenting. And next time I go out I may not feel as much need to call him.
Therapist:	Right, in the long term not seeking reassurance may help to reduce your anxiety about similar situations.
Cara:	That makes sense.
Therapist:	Ok, I want you to think about the possibility that Jaime is hurt right now at home. Where is your anxiety now?
Cara:	That is a scary thought, it is back to a 90.
Therapist:	I know it can be scary to think about.
Cara:	Yes, but you have explained that thinking about the uncertainty of this happening and feeling this anxiety is important in tackling this fear.
Therapist:	Exactly.
Cara:	My anxiety is closer to 70 now.
Therapist:	Great, it's gone down a bit. Let us sit with this thought for a little longer.

In *cognitive restructuring*, individuals practice identifying, evaluating, and modifying their automatic thoughts that cause anxiety (Arch & Craske, 2009). For instance, a mom fearful of driving with her baby may begin tracking every time she has the thought, "I'm going to get in a car accident," and note how this thought makes her feel (e.g., fearful). Then, the mom will learn to identify *cognitive distortions*, or unhelpful thinking patterns, that underlie their anxious thoughts. Common cognitive distortions in the postpartum period include jumping to conclusions (i.e., overestimating the probability that something bad will happen) and catastrophizing (i.e., overestimating how bad something is or would be if it happened) (Timpano et al., 2011).

Therapist:	What I want to do today is to start noticing some of the thinking errors you have about your worries.
Cara:	Ok.
Therapist:	To do this, we are going to use a tracking form. Every time you have a thought that makes you anxious or upset, I want you to write it down.
Cara:	I'm not really sure what to write on this. I just feel an overwhelming fear that something bad is going to happen to Jaime.
Therapist:	That's ok. Let's take a specific example. When is the last time you felt like that?
Cara:	Last night.
Therapist:	What was going on?
Cara:	I was just watching TV. I put Jaime to bed an hour before, and I couldn't shake the feeling that he wasn't ok.
Therapist:	Good. What was going through your mind last night? While you were watching TV?
Cara:	I was just feeling really anxious.
Therapist:	Ok, that is how you were feeling, not necessarily what you were thinking. But it is still really important. Were there any words or images running through your mind?
Cara:	Just that Jaime might die of Sudden Infant Death Syndrome (SIDS).
Therapist:	Ok, write that down in the thoughts column.
Therapist:	Good. What I want to do next is to think about the list of beliefs we discussed earlier today: jumping to conclusions, catastrophizing, feeling overly responsible, and attributing importance to thoughts . . . does this thought sound like it could be related to any of the beliefs?
Cara:	I guess jumping to conclusions.
Therapist:	Why?
Cara:	Because I know SIDS is really rare, but I keep assuming it will happen to Jaime.
Therapist:	Good. Let's write "jumping to conclusions" in the "beliefs" column. I'm not going to ask you to do anything about the thought or belief right now. I just want you to write it down. We are just focusing on noticing the thoughts and beliefs that underlie them. Just noticing them and recording them can start making a difference.

Next, clients learn to *evaluate the evidence* for and against their anxious thoughts and determine if the original thought is helpful. For example, a mother might consider how she would respond to her friend in a similar situation (i.e., the best friend technique), given that we tend to judge ourselves more critically and are more compassionate and understanding toward others. Finally, clients develop a more balanced, healthier thought (incorporating the evidence from the previous step) and note how the new thought makes them feel. Theoretically, creating healthier, balanced thoughts should result in less anxiety.

Therapist:	Which thought do you want to start with?
Cara:	Jaime is going to roll over and smother himself.
Therapist:	Ok. Can you try to reframe that?
Cara:	Look at past evidence?
Therapist:	Exactly.
Cara:	He hasn't rolled over in his crib yet. [pause.] He hasn't started rolling at all yet. [pause.] I've heard of this happening on the news . . . but I have a lot of friends who have babies, and none of their babies have been smothered. [pause] Melissa's son rolled over a bunch of times. But she said nothing bad happened. She just put him back on his back when she noticed.
Therapist:	Anything else?
Cara:	I've done lots of things to make sure his crib is safe. Like no pillows or blankets.
Therapist:	So how can you put this all together?
Cara:	Although it's possible that Jaime might roll over and suffocate, it's really unlikely.
Therapist:	Good.

In addition to CBT, interpersonal psychotherapy (IPT) is a psychosocial treatment that emphasizes the role that relationships play in psychological distress. IPT, initially developed for the treatment of depression, is time-limited and present-focused psychotherapy with goals of symptom remission, enhanced social support, and improvements to interpersonal functioning (Miniati et al., 2014; Sockol, 2018). When used with perinatal women, IPT tends to focus on role transitions, challenges to interpersonal relationships, low social support, and strain on marital relationships (Sockol, 2018). IPT has been found to be effective in reducing symptoms of perinatal depression symptoms in both prevention and treatment studies of perinatal depression (Sockol, 2018). A systematic review found an overall reduction in perinatal anxiety symptoms across six studies, with a moderate effect size, among participants who were treated for depression using IPT (Bright et al., 2020). Although evidence shows that IPT may be especially appropriate for postpartum women, research has demonstrated that it does not lead to better treatment outcomes than CBT (Wenzel, 2011). IPT can be considered as an alternative to CBT for social anxiety and panic disorder in situations in which childbearing women do not respond to CBT, when their anxiety symptoms or panic attack symptoms are occurring clearly in the context of their transition to the role of a mother, or when there is a clear interpersonal impairment (Wenzel, 2011). Further research should be conducted to investigate the efficacy of IPT for postpartum anxiety specifically.

Medications

Many mothers prefer psychosocial treatment to medication because of the risk that medication can transfer to babies through breastmilk (Misri & Kendrick, 2007). Despite this, there are medications that are effective at reducing anxiety (Jakubovski et al., 2019) that are also considered safe while breastfeeding (Payne, 2019). Antidepressants commonly prescribed to treat postpartum anxiety, including selective SSRIs (e.g., fluoxetine, citalopram) and serotonin and norepinephrine reuptake inhibitors (SNRIs; e.g., venlafaxine), are generally considered safe to use while breastfeeding (Payne, 2019). Studies demonstrate that while these antidepressants are excreted in breastmilk, the amount of medication in breastfeeding infants' blood levels is low or undetectable, and there is a low likelihood of adverse effects on infants (Payne, 2019; Wenzel, 2014). When adverse effects in breastfeeding infants do occur, they tend to be related to mild gastrointestinal or sleep problems. Although the preponderance of research suggests that SSRIs and SNRIs are safe for nursing mothers, it is strongly recommended that mothers and their treating physicians carefully evaluate the risks and benefits of antidepressants prior to use.

Although benzodiazepines can be helpful at reducing maternal anxiety in the short term, they are not recommended for long-term use while breastfeeding. This is because benzodiazepines can lead to infant sedation or potential dependence (Payne, 2019). Moreover, benzodiazepines can serve as a safety behavior (Blakey & Abramowitz, 2016; Westra & Stewart, 1998) which can impair long-term anxiety reduction. Gabapentin is considered moderately safe to use while breastfeeding, although infants should be monitored for sedation, while other antianxiety medications, such as buspirone or pregabalin, have limited data on their effects on breastfeeding infants.

To the authors' knowledge, no studies have evaluated the efficacy of pharmacological therapy for postpartum anxiety specifically (Brown et al., 2021). The efficacy studies of the medications mentioned above may not apply to pregnant and postpartum women as perinatal individuals are generally excluded from these clinical trials (Wenzel, 2011). Future research recommendations include expanding the number of RCTs and increasing the sample sizes of RCTs that evaluate the efficacy and safety of a full range of pharmacological therapies relative to placebo, treatment as usual, and other psychotherapy treatment options for women experiencing postpartum anxiety (Brown et al., 2021).

Cultural Considerations

When considering cultural differences involved in postpartum anxiety, one must first look at the cultural perceptions and norms surrounding motherhood itself. Social, cultural, and political beliefs are intertwined in the transition of motherhood and can be both risk and protective factors for adverse maternal mental health experiences (Sayil et al., 2007). As described earlier in this chapter, there are issues with the validity of measures, diagnostic accuracy, and generalizability for assessing postpartum anxiety. There is an even greater gap in detection tools that are valid for cross-cultural and racially diverse populations. In the United States, in particular, Black, Indigenous, and people of color (BIPOC) are at an increased risk for undetected and therefore untreated perinatal anxiety (Bhat et al., 2022; Kozhimannil et al., 2011; Sidebottom et al., 2021; Weir et al., 2011). At times, cultural perceptions of postpartum depression will be discussed in this section, given the lack of research on postpartum anxiety.

In the United States there are individuals of varying racial and ethnic identities (e.g., BIPOC-identifying individuals) that have been historically excluded from mental health research and have had limited access to mental healthcare. BIPOC individuals in the United States face unique challenges including racism, social and economic inequities, historical trauma, and medical mistrust that can increase their risk of postpartum anxiety, contribute to the lack of detection of anxiety symptoms in these populations, and exacerbate the cultural and societal stigma of negative maternal mental health (Estriplet et al., 2022; Ponting et al., 2022). U.S. immigrant Latinas have also been identified as being at an increased risk for perinatal anxiety, with prevalence rates as high as 19.4% (Lara-Cinisomo et al., 2019). In addition to the pressure of cultural expectations for the role of motherhood for Latina mothers more generally, fear of deportation experienced by immigrant Latinas was found to be significantly correlated with increased rates of postpartum anxiety (Lara-Cinisomo et al., 2019).

Specific societal and cultural expectations for a mother can impact the development and maintenance of postpartum anxiety. For example, a qualitative study by Wardrop and Popadiuk (2013) interviewed women regarding their transition to motherhood. In individualistic Western cultures (e.g., Canada, United States, and Western Europe), nuclear families are expected to care for and raise children without help from extended family or a close community. This structure leads to a lack of social support in the culture, which can then lead to maternal anxiety (Wardrop & Popadiuk, 2013). In these environments, cultural expectations are for mothers to be able to provide fully for their children without outside help. Under such societal norms, if a mother is struggling with raising children, she is failing the culture's expectations.

Wardrop and Popadiuk (2013) also found in their sample of mothers living in a Western culture that women affirmed the notion that there are "taboo" topics in motherhood that are not talked about. Specifically, women noted the avoidance of discussing the difficulty in transitioning into motherhood. Mothers discussed the importance associated with maintaining an image that motherhood is natural and easy. This image also leads to anger, frustration, and anxiety in new mothers who expect a better experience (Wardrop & Popadiuk, 2013). One such example might be having trouble breastfeeding. New mothers may expect this experience to come naturally to them and their child; setbacks, complications, and unplanned circumstances could potentially lead to maternal anxiety.

In some cultures, the transition to motherhood is made easier through assistance from other family members. Korean mothers, for instance, were found not to struggle in their transition to motherhood or the responsibilities of mothering because they received assistance from their mothers and/or mothers-in-law (Lee & Keith, 1999) In this example, a community of support was shown to decrease difficulties in the responsibilities and expectations of the mother. Further research should examine what characteristics or types of social support in different cultures alleviate stress for new mothers most effectively.

However, the emphasis on family in some cultures may lead to difficulty for women with independent careers. One illustration of this is in Malaysia where there is an emphasis on the importance of family and specifically for the women's roles within the family. As such, job autonomy was associated with distress in Malaysian women (Noor, 1999). Similarly, in Italy there is a high cultural importance placed on motherhood, which contributes to the maternal stress of employed Italian mothers who were satisfied with their jobs; in particular, these women had higher maternal stress than stay-at-home mothers (Forgays et al.,

2001). In both communities, such importance on a specific image of what women should do and how motherhood should look could lead to distress and anxiety among women who choose a path outside of the cultural norm.

Whereas some cultures instill expectations for an easy and uncomplicated transition to motherhood, other cultures are more open in discussing potential maternal distress. For instance, in Arabic cultures, postpartum anxiety is conceived as Jinn possession (Hanely & Brown, 2014). Jinn possession has many similarities to postpartum anxiety but is conceptualized as an evil spirit. The Jinn was viewed as being responsible for sadness, anxiety, and emotional distress and could possess new mothers after the birth of their child. Mothers still reported shame in discussing their Jinn possession (Hanely & Brown, 2014). With Jinn possession, postpartum anxiety can be discussed more openly by mothers in the communities; however, feelings of shame and guilt are still associated.

Gender roles and expectations play various roles in different cultures. This carries over into motherhood, as there is an expectation that mothers are the primary caregivers for their children (Wardrop & Popadiuk, 2013) One example of this is in the mother's role of breastfeeding the baby—leading to less time for themselves and less time sleeping during night feeds. The imbalance in responsibility and sometimes lack of support from male partners leads to further maternal distress (Leahy-Warren & McCarthy, 2011). Research has also shown that dissatisfaction with social relations, relationship issues with husbands or mothers-in-law, low social support, and worries about the gender of the baby have all been associated with the development of prenatal and postpartum depression across multiple cultures (Dindar & Erdogan, 2007; Mohammad et al., 2011; Siu et al., 2012).

There are other social norms not related to motherhood that can impact postpartum anxiety. For example, some cultures have very present body image standards and ideals. Western cultures emphasize slim and lean bodies, which can impact a new mother's impression of herself after giving birth. However, other cultures, like Tanzania, do not have such ideals for a thin body and therefore mothers do not categorize body image issues as some of their postpartum worries (Lugina & Sommerfeld, 1994).

Cultural impacts on postpartum anxiety can also affect mothers in different ways and affect the same mother differently at various times during their postpartum period. For instance, in mothers with multiple children, postpartum anxiety decreased over time through the first 24 months (Dipietro et al., 2009). However, for first-time mothers, postpartum anxiety has been shown to increase over time (Wardrop & Popadiuk, 2013). It is possible that cultural expectations may impact first-time mothers more strongly than mothers of multiple children.

As mentioned previously, there are several demographic characteristics that have been linked to postpartum anxiety such as prenatal anxiety, women who are 25 years old or younger, mothers of more than one child, mothers who experience a higher number of stressful life events during pregnancy, and mothers with low education levels (van der Zee-van den Berg et al., 2021). As an example, less education and lower income were both associated with more postpartum anxiety in first-time Nepalese mothers (Shrestha et al., 2014). Particularly, for mothers in low-income households, a primary stressor is completing financial responsibilities; this stress is correlated with poor parent coping skills and lower family cohesion (Dindar & Erdogan, 2007). Taken together with cultural traditions and/or expectations, societal influences of racism and inequity, and norms of social support in different cultures these demographic characteristics may put some mothers at greater risk for postpartum anxiety in some of these cultures compared to others.

Conclusion and Future Directions

Globally, postpartum anxiety is a common and treatable mental health problem, with prevalence rates significantly higher compared to the general adult population (Dennis et al., 2017). Because of this, there is growing recognition of the need to increase awareness, screening, and treatment access for individuals who experience symptoms of postpartum anxiety. Although much has been studied regarding postpartum anxiety over the past two decades, there is still more to learn. This chapter briefly highlighted the current knowledge surrounding the manifestation of symptoms, key risk factors, correlates, impact on relationships, and cultural considerations for postpartum anxiety. We also described the assessment measures and evidence-based treatment options available. Early detection of and intervention for postpartum anxiety symptoms is crucial to reduce distress for the mother, improve family relations, and decrease the risk of adverse child development outcomes.

As research continues to expand in this area, there are a few key aspects where more research is needed. First, further validation of current perinatal-specific assessment measures and their psychometric properties is needed to streamline clinical recommendations for reliable and valid screening measures. Previous research has shown that symptom levels of anxiety are variable during the first year following childbirth, indicating that recommendations for clinical screening should occur at multiple time points. Ideally, screening should be incorporated during pediatrician visits with the newborn, as there are negligible postpartum appointments focused on maternal health. As screening for perinatal anxiety is increased, so must access to effective treatment services including therapists and psychiatrists trained to serve perinatal populations. Additionally, there should be consideration for a specifier of peripartum anxiety in future editions of the DSM because there is no current diagnostic criterion and perinatal mothers do not always fit the diagnosis for other anxiety disorders.

Increasing inclusion of diverse individuals in quantitative and qualitative research studies examining prevalence rates, etiology, validation of measures, and effectiveness of interventions for postpartum anxiety is a necessity in future research. As described, pregnancy, motherhood, family dynamics, and gender roles are intertwined with societal and/or cultural traditions and expectations. Understanding the risk and protective roles that sociocultural factors (e.g., family support, cultural expectations of motherhood, racism, economic status) have in the etiology and maintenance of postpartum anxiety is imperative to adequately assess for clinical levels of distress and implement cross-cultural interventions (Ponting et al., 2022). This recommendation also extends to fathers or parents who are not childbearing individuals and parents who identify as sexual and gender minorities. Inclusion of all parents in postpartum anxiety research, regardless of whether they are the ones giving birth, can help to differentiate between biological (e.g., hormonal) changes that the pregnant individual experiences and the social emotional stress experienced during this transitional period by the other parent (Wenzel, 2011).

Much of the evidence supporting postpartum anxiety interventions comes from studies conducted in nonperinatal samples (i.e., the general population). Studies assessing CBT interventions during the perinatal period for anxiety do not emphasize exposure, which as mentioned is a necessary component of CBT for anxiety. IPT interventions have been shown to reduce anxiety in perinatal samples being treated for postpartum depression, but minimal research has examined IPT interventions for postpartum anxiety specifically (Bright et al., 2020; Miniati et al., 2014). Therefore, there is a critical need for research (specifically RCTs) on interventions designed specifically to treat and prevent postpartum anxiety (vs.

depression). Future researchers should continue to expand testing the efficacy of third-wave behavioral treatments on postpartum anxiety, such as acceptance and commitment therapy, which has been shown to reduce anxiety in nonpregnant samples (Hayes et al., 2006).

In moderation, some degree of worry is practical to protect the vulnerable baby from harm. It is important to validate mothers' fears, worries, stress, and uncertainty that are associated with the transition to parenthood and not over-pathologize their concerns (Wenzel, 2011). As adverse consequences of untreated maternal anxiety are discussed by researchers, clinicians, and the media, it is equally imperative that, on a societal and personal level, we do not increase the guilt mothers experience for these levels of heightened worry, but instead hear her concerns and aid in decreasing her distress. However, excessive levels of anxiety causing clinical levels of impairment and dysfunction in new mothers must not be dismissed and overlooked but addressed using pharmacological means and/or evidence-based psychological therapies such as CBT.

Following 15 sessions of cognitive restructuring and exposure, Cara is doing much better. Her scores on the PASS and the STAI are no longer in the clinically significant ranges. She stopped seeking excessive reassurance from her husband, Daniel, which led to improvements in their relationship. She is more comfortable spending time with others and has enjoyed spending time with friends and colleagues. Additionally, she has stopped checking on Jaime while he sleeps, and she feels more confident spending time out without her son. Although Cara still experiences anxiety and still has worries about Jaime from time to time, the anxiety no longer causes significant distress or impairment. She feels confident applying the skills she learned in therapy to handle her anxiety when it occurs.

Acknowledgments

Preparation of this chapter was supported by the Eunice Kennedy Shriver National Institute of Child Health and Human Development of the National Institutes of Health under Award Number R15HD109689. The content is solely the responsibility of the authors and does not necessarily represent the official views of the National Institutes of Health.

References

Abramowitz, J. S., Deacon, B. J., & Whiteside, S. P. H. (2019). *Exposure therapy for anxiety: Principles and practice* (2nd ed.). Guilford Press. https://psycnet.apa.org/record/2019-19532-000

Acele, E. Ö., & Karaçam, Z. (2012). Sexual problems in women during the first postpartum year and related conditions. *Journal of Clinical Nursing, 21*(7–8), 929–937. https://doi.org/10.1111/J.1365-2702.2011.03882.X

Ali, E. (2018). Women's experiences with postpartum anxiety disorders: A narrative literature review. *International Journal of Women's Health, 10*, 237–249. https://doi.org/10.2147/IJWH.S158621

Allison, K. C., Wenzel, A., Kleiman, K., & Sarwer, D. B. (2011). Development of a brief measure of postpartum distress. *Journal of Women's Health, 20*(4), 617–623. https://doi.org/10.1089/JWH.2010.1989

American Psychiatric Association. (2013). *Diagnostic and statistical manual of mental disorders* (5th ed.). https://doi.org/10.1176/appi.books.9780890425596

Amiri, P., Bahaadinbeigy, K., Asadi, F., Rahmati, S., & Mazhari, S. (2022). Validation of the Persian version of the Perinatal Anxiety Screening Scale (PASS) among antenatal and postnatal women. *BMC Pregnancy and Childbirth*, 22(1). https://doi.org/10.1186/S12884-022-05217-6

Araji, S., Griffin, A., Dixon, L., Spencer, S. K., Peavie, C., & Wallace, K. (2020). An overview of maternal anxiety during pregnancy and the post-partum period. *Journal of Mental Health and Clinical Psychology*, 4(4), 47–56. www.mentalhealthjournal.org

Arch, J. J., & Craske, M. G. (2009). First-line treatment: A critical appraisal of cognitive behavioral therapy developments and alternatives. *Psychiatric Clinics of North America*, 32(3), 525–547. https://doi.org/10.1016/J.PSC.2009.05.001

Arch, J. J., Dimidjian, S., & Chessick, C. (2012). Are exposure-based cognitive behavioral therapies safe during pregnancy? *Archives of Women's Mental Health*, 15(6), 445–457. https://doi.org/10.1007/s00737-012-0308-9

Arnold, M., & Kalibatseva, Z. (2020). Are "superwomen" without social support at risk for post-partum depression and anxiety? *Women & Health*, 61(2), 148–159. https://doi.org/10.1080/03630242.2020.1844360

Arteche, A., Joormann, J., Harvey, A., Craske, M., Gotlib, I. H., Lehtonen, A., . . . Stein, A. (2011). The effects of postnatal maternal depression and anxiety on the processing of infant faces. *Journal of Affective Disorders*, 133(1–2), 197–203. https://doi.org/10.1016/J.JAD.2011.04.015

Barzgar-Molan, S., Farshbaf-Khalili, A., Jafarabadi, M. A., Babapour, J., & Yavarikia, P. (2020). Psychometric properties of the Iranian version of a perinatal anxiety screening scale in Iranian perinatal population: A methodological study. *Crescent Journal of Medical and Biological Sciences*, 7(4), 551–559.

Bayrampour, H., McDonald, S., Fung, T., & Tough, S. (2014). Reliability and validity of three short-ened versions of the state anxiety inventory scale during the perinatal period. *Journal of Psychosomatic Obstetrics & Gynecology*, 35(3), 101–107. https://doi.org/10.3109/0167482X.2014.950218

Beck, J. S. (2021). *Cognitive behavior therapy: Basics and beyond* (3rd ed.). The Guilford Press. https://psycnet.apa.org/record/2020-66930-000

Bhat, A., Nanda, A., Murphy, L., Ball, A. L., Fortney, J., & Katon, J. (2022). A systematic review of screening for perinatal depression and anxiety in community-based settings. *Archives of Women's Mental Health*, 25(1), 33–49. https://doi.org/10.1007/S00737-021-01151-2/METRICS

Blakey, S. M., & Abramowitz, J. S. (2016). The effects of safety behaviors during exposure therapy for anxiety: Critical analysis from an inhibitory learning perspective. *Clinical Psychology Review*, 49, 1–15. https://doi.org/10.1016/J.CPR.2016.07.002

Bright, K. S., Charrois, E. M., Mughal, M. K., Wajid, A., McNeil, D., Stuart, S., . . . Kingston, D. (2020). Interpersonal psychotherapy to reduce psychological distress in perinatal women: A systematic review. *International Journal of Environmental Research and Public Health*, 17(22), 8421. https://doi.org/10.3390/ijerph17228421

Brouwers, E. P. M., van Baar, A. L., & Pop, V. J. M. (2001). Does the Edinburgh Postnatal Depression Scale measure anxiety? *Journal of Psychosomatic Research*, 51(5), 659–663. https://doi.org/10.1016/S0022-3999(01)00245-8

Brown, J. V. E., Wilson, C. A., Ayre, K., Robertson, L., South, E., Molyneaux, E., . . . Khalifeh, H. (2021). Antidepressant treatment for postnatal depression. *The Cochrane Database of Systematic Reviews*, 2(2), CD013560. https://doi.org/10.1002/14651858.CD013560.pub2

Bryson, H., Perlen, S., Price, A., Mensah, F., Gold, L., Dakin, P., & Goldfeld, S. (2021). Patterns of maternal depression, anxiety, and stress symptoms from pregnancy to 5 years postpartum in an Australian cohort experiencing adversity. *Archives of Women's Mental Health*, 24, 987–997. https://doi.org/10.1007/s00737-021-01145-0

Cerulli, C., Talbot, N. L., Tang, W., & Chaudron, L. H. (2011). Co-occurring intimate partner violence and mental health diagnoses in perinatal women. *Journal of Women's Health*, (12), 1797–1803. https://doi.org/10.1089/JWH.2010.2201

Choy, Y., Fyer, A. J., & Lipsitz, J. D. (2007). Treatment of specific phobia in adults. *Clinical Psychology Review*, 27(3), 266–286. https://doi.org/10.1016/J.CPR.2006.10.002

Clark, D. A., & Beck, A. T. (2010). *Cognitive therapy of anxiety disorders: Science and practice*. Guilford Press.

Costa, E. C. V., Castanheira, E., Moreira, L., Correia, P., Ribeiro, D., & Graça Pereira, M. (2016). Predictors of emotional distress in pregnant women: The mediating role of relationship intimacy. *Journal of Mental Health*, 29(2), 152–160. https://doi.org/10.1080/09638237.2017.1417545

Cowan, C. P., & Cowan, P. A. (2000). *When partners become parents: The big life change for couples.* Lawrence Erlbaum Associates Publishers. https://psycnet.apa.org/record/1999-04186-000

Cox, J. L., Holden, J. M., & Sagovsky, R. (1987). Detection of postnatal depression: Development of the 10-item Edinburgh Postnatal Depression Scale. *British Journal of Psychiatry*, *150*(JUNE), 782–786. https://doi.org/10.1192/BJP.150.6.782

Craske, M. G., Treanor, M., Zbozinek, T. D., & Vervliet, B. (2022). Optimizing exposure therapy with an inhibitory retrieval approach and the OptEx nexus. *Behaviour Research and Therapy*, *152*, 104069. https://doi.org/10.1016/J.BRAT.2022.104069

Cuijpers, P., Sijbrandij, M., Koole, S., Huibers, M., Berking, M., & Andersson, G. (2014). Psychological treatment of generalized anxiety disorder: A meta-analysis. *Clinical Psychology Review*, *34*(2), 130–140. https://doi.org/10.1016/j.cpr.2014.01.002

Davies, S. M., Todd-Leonida, B. F., Fallon, V. M., & Silverio, S. A. (2022). Exclusive breastfeeding duration and perceptions of infant sleep: The mediating role of postpartum anxiety. *International Journal of Environmental Research and Public Health*, *19*, 4494. https://doi.org/10.3390/IJERPH19084494

De Judicibus, M., & McCabe, M. (2002). Psychological factors and the sexuality of pregnant and postpartum women. *Journal of Sex Research*, *39*(2), 94–103. www.jstor.org/stable/3813191

Dennis, C. L., Falah-Hassani, K., & Shiri, R. (2017). Prevalence of antenatal and postnatal anxiety: Systematic review and meta-analysis. *British Journal of Psychiatry*, *210*(5), 315–323. https://doi.org/10.1192/BJP.BP.116.187179

Dindar, I., & Erdogan, S. (2007). Screening of Turkish women for postpartum depression within the first postpartum year: The risk profile of a community sample. *Public Health Nursing*, *24*(2), 176–183. https://doi.org/10.1111/J.1525-1446.2007.00622.X

Dipietro, J. A., Costigan, K. A., & Sipsma, H. L. (2009). Continuity in self-report measures of maternal anxiety, stress, and depressive symptoms from pregnancy through two years postpartum. *Journal of Psychosomatic Obstetrics and Gynecology*, *29*(2), 115–124. https://doi.org/10.1080/01674820701701546

Duran, S. (2020). Postpartum Specific Anxiety Scale (PSAS): Reliability and validity of the Turkish version. *Perspectives in Psychiatric Care*, *56*(1), 95–101. https://doi.org/10.1111/PPC.12385

Eller, J., Girme, Y. U., Don, B. P., Rholes, W. S., Mickelson, K. D., & Simpson, J. A. (2022). Here one time, gone the next: Fluctuations in support received and provided predict changes in relationship satisfaction across the transition to parenthood. *Journal of Personality and Social Psychology.* https://doi.org/10.1037/PSPI0000408

Estriplet, T., Morgan, I., Davis, K., Crear Perry, J., & Matthews, K. (2022). Black perinatal mental health: Prioritizing maternal mental health to optimize infant health and wellness. *Frontiers in Psychiatry*, *13*. https://doi.org/10.3389/FPSYT.2022.807235

Fallon, V., Groves, R., Halford, J. C. G., Bennett, K. M., & Harrold, J. A. (2016). Postpartum anxiety and infant-feeding outcomes. *Journal of Human Lactation*, *32*(4), 740–758. https://doi.org/10.1177/0890334416662241

Fallon, V., Halford, J. C. G., Mary Bennett, K., & Allison Harrold, J. (2016). The postpartum specific anxiety scale: Development and preliminary validation. *Archives of Women's Mental Health*, *19*, 1079–1090. https://doi.org/10.1007/s00737-016-0658-9

Fallon, V., Silverio, S. A., Halford, J. C. G., Bennett, K. M., & Harrold, J. A. (2021). Postpartum-specific anxiety and maternal bonding: Further evidence to support the use of childbearing specific mood tools. *Journal of Reproductive and Infant Psychology*, *39*(2), 114–124. https://doi.org/10.1080/02646838.2019.1680960

Farr, S. L., Dietz, P. M., O'Hara, M. W., Burley, K., & Ko, J. Y. (2014). Postpartum anxiety and comorbid depression in a population-based sample of women. *Journal of Women's Health*, *23*(2), 120–128. https://doi.org/10.1089/JWH.2013.4438

Fawcett, E. J., Fairbrother, N., Cox, M. L., White, I. R., & Fawcett, J. M. (2019). The prevalence of anxiety disorders during pregnancy and the postpartum period: A multivariate Bayesian meta-analysis. *Journal of Clinical Psychiatry*, *80*(4), Article 18r12527. https://doi.org/10.4088/JCP.18R12527

Feldman, R., Granat, A., Pariente, C., Kanety, H., Kuint, J., & Gilboa-Schechtman, E. (2009). Maternal depression and anxiety across the postpartum year and infant social engagement, fear regulation, and stress reactivity. *Journal of the American Academy of Child and Adolescent Psychiatry*, *48*(9), 919–927. https://doi.org/10.1097/CHI.0b013e3181b21651

Field, T. (2018). Postnatal anxiety prevalence, predictors and effects on development: A narrative review. *Infant Behavior & Development*, *51*, 24–32. https://doi.org/10.1016/J.INFBEH.2018.02.005

Fonseca, A., & Canavarro, M. C. (2018). Exploring the paths between dysfunctional attitudes towards motherhood and postpartum depressive symptoms: The moderating role of self-compassion. *Clinical Psychology & Psychotherapy, 25*(1), e96–e106. https://doi.org/10.1002/CPP.2145

Forgays, D. K., Ottaway, S. A., Guarino, A., & D'Alessio, M. (2001). Parenting stress in employed and at-home mothers in Italy. *Journal of Family and Economic Issues, 22*(4), 327–351. https://doi.org/10.1023/A:1012703227992/METRICS

Giannandrea, S. A. M., Cerulli, C., Anson, E., & Chaudron, L. H. (2013). Increased risk for postpartum psychiatric disorders among women with past pregnancy loss. *Journal of Women's Health, 22*(9). https://doi.org/10.1089/jwh.2012.4011

Glenn, N. D., & McLanahan, S. (1982). Children and marital happiness: A further specification of the relationship. *Journal of Marriage and the Family, 44*(1), 63–72. https://doi.org/10.2307/351263

Goodman, J. H., Watson, G. R., & Stubbs, B. (2016). Anxiety disorders in postpartum women: A systematic review and meta-analysis. *Journal of Affective Disorders, 203*, 292–331. https://doi.org/10.1016/J.JAD.2016.05.033

Grant, K. A., McMahon, C., & Austin, M. P. (2008). Maternal anxiety during the transition to parenthood: A prospective study. *Journal of Affective Disorders, 108*(1–2), 101–111. https://doi.org/10.1016/J.JAD.2007.10.002

Haga, S. M., Lynne, A., Slinning, K., & Kraft, P. (2012). A qualitative study of depressive symptoms and well-being among first-time mothers. *Scandinavian Journal of Caring Sciences, 26*(3), 458–466. https://doi.org/10.1111/J.1471-6712.2011.00950.X

Hantsoo, L., & Epperson, C. N. (2017). Anxiety disorders among women: A female lifespan approach. *Focus (American Psychiatric Publishing), 15*(2), 162–172. https://doi.org/10.1176/APPI.FOCUS.20160042

Hanely, J., & Brown, A. (2014). Cultural variations in interpretation of postnatal illness: Jinn possession amongst Muslim communities. *Community Mental Health Journal, 50*(3), 348–353. https://doi.org/10.1007/S10597-013-9640-4/TABLES/1

Hayes, S. C., Luoma, J. B., Bond, F. W., Masuda, A., & Lillis, J. (2006). Acceptance and commitment therapy: Model, processes, and outcomes. *Behaviour Research and Therapy, 44*(1), 1–25. https://doi.org/10.1016/J.BRAT.2005.06.006

Hobeika, E., Malaeb, D., Obeid, S., Salameh, P., Hobeika, E., Outayek, M., . . . Hallit, S. (2023). Postpartum depression and anxiety among Lebanese women: Correlates and scales psychometric properties. *Healthcare (Basel, Switzerland), 11*(2), Article 201. https://doi.org/10.3390/HEALTHCARE11020201

Hoberg, M., Demirci, J. R., Sereika, S. M., Levine, M. D., & Devito Dabbs, A. (2022). Descriptive exploratory study to understand postpartum anxiety using multiple measures. *Journal of Obstetric, Gynecologic, and Neonatal Nursing, 52*(1), 50–61. https://doi.org/10.1016/j.jogn.2022.09.003

Huizink, A. C., Mulder, E. J. H., Robles De Medina, P. G., Visser, G. H. A., & Buitelaar, J. K. (2004). Is pregnancy anxiety a distinctive syndrome? *Early Human Development, 79*(2), 81–91. https://doi.org/10.1016/J.EARLHUMDEV.2004.04.014

Jakubovski, E., Johnson, J. A., Nasir, M., Müller-Vahl, K., & Bloch, M. H. (2019). Systematic review and meta-analysis: Dose–response curve of SSRIs and SNRIs in anxiety disorders. *Depression and Anxiety, 36*(3), 198–212. https://doi.org/10.1002/DA.22854

Jomeen, J., & Martin, C. R. (2007). Confirmation of an occluded anxiety component within the Edinburgh Postnatal Depression Scale (EPDS) during early pregnancy. *BMC Psychology, 23*(2), 143–154. https://doi.org/10.1080/02646830500129297

Jradi, H., Alfarhan, T., & Alsuraimi, A. (2020). Validation of the Arabic version of the Perinatal Anxiety Screening Scale (PASS) among antenatal and postnatal women. *BMC Pregnancy and Childbirth, 20*(1), Article 758. https://doi.org/10.1186/S12884-020-03451-4

Kessler, R. C., Petukhova, M., Sampson, N. A., Zaslavsky, A. M., & Wittchen, H. U. (2012). Twelve-month and lifetime prevalence and lifetime morbid risk of anxiety and mood disorders in the United States. *International Journal of Methods in Psychiatric Research, 21*, 169–184.

Kirkpatrick, C. E., & Lee, S. (2022). Comparisons to picture-perfect motherhood: How Instagram's idealized portrayals of motherhood affect new mothers' well-being. *Computers in Human Behavior, 137*, 107417. https://doi.org/10.1016/J.CHB.2022.107417

Koukopoulos, A., Mazza, C., De Chiara, L., Sani, G., Simonetti, A., Kotzalidis, G. D., . . . Angeletti, G. (2021). Psychometric properties of the perinatal anxiety screening scale administered to Italian women in the perinatal period. *Frontiers in Psychiatry, 12*, Article 684579. https://doi.org/10.3389/FPSYT.2021.684579

Kozhimannil, K. B., Trinacty, C. M., Busch, A. B., Huskamp, H. A., & Adams, A. S. (2011). Racial and ethnic disparities in postpartum depression care among low-income women. *Psychiatric Services*, 62(6), 619–625. https://pubmed.ncbi.nlm.nih.gov/21632730/

Lara-Cinisomo, S., Fujimoto, E. M., Oksas, C., Jian, Y., & Gharheeb, A. (2019). Pilot study exploring migration experiences and perinatal depressive and anxiety symptoms in immigrant Latinas. *Maternal and Child Health Journal*, 23, 1627–1647. https://doi.org/10.1007/s10995-019-02800-w

Leahy-Warren, P., & McCarthy, G. (2011). Maternal parental self-efficacy in the postpartum period. *Midwifery*, 27(6), 802–810. https://doi.org/10.1016/J.MIDW.2010.07.008

Lee, S. C., & Keith, P. M. (1999). The transition to motherhood of Korean women. *Journal of Comparative Family Studies*, 30(3), 453–470. www.jstor.org/stable/41603645

Le Strat, Y., Dubertret, C., & Le Foll, B. (2011). Prevalence and correlates of major depressive episode in pregnant and postpartum women in the United States. *Journal of Affective Disorders*, 135(1–3), 128–138. https://doi.org/10.1016/J.JAD.2011.07.004

Levitt, M. J., Coffman, S., Guacci-Franco, N., & Loveless, S. (1993). Social support and relationship change after childbirth: An expectancy model. *Health Care for Women International*, 14(6), 503–512. https://doi.org/10.1080/07399339309516080

Li, X., Laplante, D. P., Paquin, V., Lafortune, S., Elgbeili, G., & King, S. (2022). Effectiveness of cognitive behavioral therapy for perinatal maternal depression, anxiety and stress: A systematic review and meta-analysis of randomized controlled trials. *Clinical Psychology Review*, 92, 102129. https://doi.org/10.1016/J.CPR.2022.102129

Loerinc, A. G., Meuret, A. E., Twohig, M. P., Rosenfield, D., Bluett, E. J., & Craske, M. G. (2015). Response rates for CBT for anxiety disorders: Need for standardized criteria. *Clinical Psychology Review*, 42, 72–82. https://doi.org/10.1016/J.CPR.2015.08.004

Longmore, R. J., & Worrell, M. (2007). Do we need to challenge thoughts in cognitive behavior therapy? *Clinical Psychology Review*, 27(2), 173–187. https://doi.org/10.1016/J.CPR.2006.08.001

Lovibond, P. F., & Lovibond, S. H. (1995). The structure of negative emotional states: Comparison of the Depression Anxiety Stress Scales (DASS) with the beck depression and anxiety inventories. *Behaviour Research and Therapy*, 33(3), 335–343. https://doi.org/10.1016/0005-7967(94)00075-U

Lugina, H. I., & Sommerfeld, D. M. P. (1994). Postpartum concerns: A study of Tanzanian mothers. *Health Care for Women International*, 15(3), 225–233. https://doi.org/10.1080/07399339409516114

Lydsdottir, L. B., Howard, L. M., Olafsdottir, H., Thome, M., Tyrfingsson, P., Psych, C., & Sigurdsson, J. F. (2014). The mental health characteristics of pregnant women with depressive symptoms identified by the Edinburgh Postnatal Depression Scale. *Journal of Clinical Psychiatry*, 75(4), 11633. https://doi.org/10.4088/JCP.13M08646

Martini, J., Petzoldt, J., Einsle, F., Beesdo-Baum, K., Höfler, M., & Wittchen, H. U. (2015). Risk factors and course patterns of anxiety and depressive disorders during pregnancy and after delivery: A prospective-longitudinal study. *Journal of Affective Disorders*, 175, 385–395. https://doi.org/10.1016/J.JAD.2015.01.012

Matthey, S., Valenti, B., Souter, K., & Ross-Hamid, C. (2013). Comparison of four self-report measures and a generic mood question to screen for anxiety during pregnancy in English-speaking women. *Journal of Affective Disorders*, 148(2–3), 347–351. https://doi.org/10.1016/J.JAD.2012.12.022

Mayo-Wilson, E., Dias, S., Mavranezouli, I., Kew, K., Clark, D. M., Ades, A. E., & Pilling, S. (2014). Psychological and pharmacological interventions for social anxiety disorder in adults: A systematic review and network meta-analysis. *The Lancet Psychiatry*, 1(5), 368–376. https://doi.org/10.1016/S2215-0366(14)70329-3

Meades, R., & Ayers, S. (2011). Anxiety measures validated in perinatal populations: A systematic review. *Journal of Affective Disorders*, 133(1–2), 1–15. https://doi.org/10.1016/J.JAD.2010.10.009

Miller, R. L., Pallant, J. F., & Negri, L. M. (2006). Anxiety and stress in the postpartum: Is there more to postnatal distress than depression? *BMC Psychiatry*, 6(1), 1–11. https://doi.org/10.1186/1471-244X-6-12/TABLES/1

Miniati, M., Callari, A., Calugi, S., Rucci, P., Savino, M., Mauri, M., & Dell'Osso, L. (2014). Interpersonal psychotherapy for postpartum depression: A systematic review. *Archives of Women's Mental Health*, 17(4), 257–268. https://doi.org/10.1007/s00737-014-0442-7

Misri, S., & Kendrick, K. (2007). Treatment of perinatal mood and anxiety disorders: A review. *Canadian Journal of Psychiatry*, 52(8), 489–498. https://doi.org/10.1177/070674370705200803

Mohammad, K. I., Gamble, J., & Creedy, D. K. (2011). Prevalence and factors associated with the development of antenatal and postnatal depression among Jordanian women. *Midwifery*, 27(6), e238–e245. https://doi.org/10.1016/J.MIDW.2010.10.008

Moran, T. E., Polanin, J. R., & Wenzel, A. (2014). The Postpartum Worry Scale–Revised: An initial validation of a measure of postpartum worry. *Archives of Women's Mental Health*, 17(1), 41–48. https://doi.org/10.1007/S00737-013-0380-9

Murray, L., Cooper, P., Creswell, C., Schofield, E., & Sack, C. (2007). The effects of maternal social phobia on mother-infant interactions and infant social responsiveness. *Journal of Child Psychology and Psychiatry, and Allied Disciplines*, 48(1), 45–52. https://doi.org/10.1111/J.1469-7610.2006.01657.X

Murrough, J. W., Yaqubi, S., Sayed, S., & Charney, D. S. (2015). Emerging drugs for the treatment of anxiety. *Expert Opinion on Emerging Drugs*, 20(3), 393–406. https://doi.org/10.1517/14728214.2015.1049996

Nakic Radoš, S., Tadinac, M., & Herman, R. (2018). Anxiety during pregnancy and postpartum: Course, predictors and comorbidity with postpartum depression. *Acta Clinica Croatica*, 57(1), 39–51. https://doi.org/10.20471/acc.2018.57.01.05

Noor, N. M. (1999). Roles and women's well-being: Some preliminary findings from Malaysia. *Sex Roles*, 41(3–4), 123–145. https://doi.org/10.1023/A:1018846010541/METRICS

Osnes, R. S., Roaldset, J. O., Follestad, T., & Eberhard-Gran, M. (2019). Insomnia late in pregnancy is associated with perinatal anxiety: A longitudinal cohort study. *Journal of Affective Disorders*, 248, 155–165. https://doi.org/10.1016/J.JAD.2019.01.027

Padoa, T., Berle, D., & Roberts, L. (2018). Comparative social media use and the mental health of mothers with high levels of perfectionism. *Journal of Social and Clinical Psychology*, 37(7), 514–535. https://doi.org/10.1521/JSCP.2018.37.7.514

Parrish, C. L., Radomsky, A. S., & Dugas, M. J. (2008). Anxiety-control strategies: Is there room for neutralization in successful exposure treatment? *Clinical Psychology Review*, 28(8), 1400–1412. https://doi.org/10.1016/J.CPR.2008.07.007

Paul, I. M., Downs, D. S., Schaefer, E. W., Beiler, J. S., & Weisman, C. S. (2013). Postpartum anxiety and maternal-infant health outcomes. *Pediatrics*, 131(4), e1218–e1224. https://doi.org/10.1542/PEDS.2012-2147

Payne, J. L. (2019). Psychopharmacology in pregnancy and breastfeeding. *Medical Clinics of North America*, 103(4), 629–650. https://doi.org/10.1016/J.MCNA.2019.02.009

Petzoldt, J., Wittchen, H. U., Wittich, J., Einsle, F., Höfler, M., & Martini, J. (2014). Maternal anxiety disorders predict excessive infant crying: A prospective longitudinal study. *Archives of Disease in Childhood*, 99(9), 800–806. https://doi.org/10.1136/ARCHDISCHILD-2013-305562

Pompoli, A., Furukawa, T. A., Imai, H., Tajika, A., Efthimiou, O., & Salanti, G. (2016). Psychological therapies for panic disorder with or without agoraphobia in adults: A network meta-analysis. *Cochrane Database of Systematic Reviews*, 2016(4). https://doi.org/10.1002/14651858

Ponting, C., Urizar, G. G., & Dunkel Schetter, C. (2022). Psychological interventions for prenatal anxiety in Latinas and Black women: A Scoping review and recommendations. *Frontiers in Psychiatry*, 13. https://doi.org/10.3389/FPSYT.2022.820343

Ponzini, G. T., Snider, M. D. H., Evey, K. J., & Steinman, S. A. (2021). Women's knowledge of postpartum anxiety disorders, depression, and cognitive behavioral therapy. *Journal of Nervous and Mental Disease*, 209(6), 426–433. https://doi.org/10.1097/NMD.0000000000001315

Priyadarshanie, M. N., Waas, M. D. I. A., Goonewardena, C. S. E., Balasuriya, A., Senaratna, B. C. V., & Fernando, D. M. S. (2020). Sinhala translation of the perinatal anxiety screening scale: A valid and reliable tool to detect anxiety disorders among antenatal women. *BMC Psychiatry*, 20(1). https://doi.org/10.1186/S12888-020-02757-Z

Racine, N., Plamondon, A., Hentges, R., Tough, S., & Madigan, S. (2019). Dynamic and bidirectional associations between maternal stress, anxiety, and social support: The critical role of partner and family support. *Journal of Affective Disorders*, 252, 19–24. https://doi.org/10.1016/J.JAD.2019.03.083

Reck, C., Müller, M., Tietz, A., & Möhler, E. (2013). Infant distress to novelty is associated with maternal anxiety disorder and especially with maternal avoidance behavior. *Journal of Anxiety Disorders*, 27(4), 404–412. https://doi.org/10.1016/J.JANXDIS.2013.03.009

Reck, C., Noe, D., Gerstenlauer, J., & Stehle, E. (2012). Effects of postpartum anxiety disorders and depression on maternal self-confidence. *Infant Behavior and Development*, 35(2), 264–272. https://doi.org/10.1016/J.INFBEH.2011.12.005

Reck, C., Stehle, E., Reinig, K., & Mundt, C. (2009). Maternity blues as a predictor of DSM-IV depression and anxiety disorders in the first three months postpartum. *Journal of Affective Disorders, 113*(1–2), 77–87. https://doi.org/10.1016/J.JAD.2008.05.003

Reck, C., Struben, K., Backenstrass, M., Stefenelli, U., Reinig, K., Fuchs, T., . . . Mundt, C. (2008). Prevalence, onset and comorbidity of postpartum anxiety and depressive disorders. *Acta Psychiatrica Scandinavica, 118*(6), 459–468. https://doi.org/10.1111/J.1600-0447.2008.01264.X

Ruscio, A. M., Hallion, L. S., Lim, C. C. W., Aguilar-Gaxiola, S., Al-Hamzawi, A., Alonso, J., . . . Scott, K. M. (2017). Cross- sectional comparison of the epidemiology of DSM- 5 generalized anxiety disorder across the globe. *JAMA Psychiatry, 74*, 465–475.

Salkovskis, P. M. (1991). The importance of behaviour in the maintenance of anxiety and panic: A cognitive account. *Behavioural and Cognitive Psychotherapy, 19*(1), 6–19. https://doi.org/10.1017/S0141347300011472

Sawers, M., & Wong, G. (2018). Pregnancy and childbirth: Postpartum Anxiety (PPA) and support for new mothers. *Journal of the Motherhood Initiative for Research and Community Involvement, 9*(2), 45–59. https://jarm.journals.yorku.ca/index.php/jarm/article/view/40507

Sayil, M., Güre, A., & Uçanok, Z. (2007). First time mothers' anxiety and depressive symptoms across the transition to motherhood: Associations with maternal and environmental characteristics. *Women and Health, 44*(3), 61–77. https://doi.org/10.1300/J013V44N03_04

Schiller, C. E., Meltzer-Brody, S., & Rubinow, D. R. (2015). The role of reproductive hormones in postpartum depression. *CNS Spectrums, 20*(1), 48–59. https://doi.org/10.1017/S1092852914000480

Schmied, V., Johnson, M., Naidoo, N., Austin, M. P., Matthey, S., Kemp, L., Mills, A., Meade, T., & Yeo, A. (2013). Maternal mental health in Australia and New Zealand: A review of longitudinal studies. *Women and Birth: Journal of the Australian College of Midwives, 26*(3), 167–178. https://doi.org/10.1016/J.WOMBI.2013.02.006

Seymour-Smith, M., Cruwys, T., Haslam, S. A., & Brodribb, W. (2017). Loss of group memberships predicts depression in postpartum mothers. *Social Psychiatry and Psychiatric Epidemiology, 52*(2), 201–210. https://doi.org/10.1007/S00127-016-1315-3

Shrestha, S., Adachi, K., Petrini, M. A., & Shrestha, S. (2014). Factors associated with post-natal anxiety among primiparous mothers in Nepal. *International Nursing Review, 61*(3), 427–434. https://doi.org/10.1111/INR.12118

Sidebottom, A., Vacquier, M., Larusso, E., Erickson, D., & Hardeman, R. (2021). Perinatal depression screening practices in a large health system: Identifying current state and assessing opportunities to provide more equitable care. *Archives of Women's Mental Health, 24*, 133–144. https://doi.org/10.1007/s00737-020-01035-x

Simpson, W., Glazer, M., Michalski, N., Steiner, M., & Frey, B. N. (2014). Comparative efficacy of the Generalized Anxiety Disorder 7-Item Scale and the Edinburgh Postnatal Depression Scale as screening tools for generalized anxiety disorder in pregnancy and the postpartum period. *Canadian Journal of Psychiatry, 59*(8), 434–440. https://doi.org/10.1177/070674371405900806

Siu, B. W. M., Leung, S. S. L., Ip, P., Hung, S. F., & O'Hara, M. W. (2012). Antenatal risk factors for postnatal depression: A prospective study of Chinese women at maternal and child health centres. *BMC Psychiatry, 12*, Article 22. https://doi.org/10.1186/1471-244X-12-22

Sockol, L. E. (2018). A systematic review and meta-analysis of interpersonal psychotherapy for perinatal women. *Journal of Affective Disorders, 232*, 316–328. https://doi.org/10.1016/j.jad.2018.01.018

Sockol, L. E., Epperson, C. N., & Barber, J. P. (2014). The relationship between maternal attitudes and symptoms of depression and anxiety among pregnant and postpartum first-time mothers. *Archives of Women's Mental Health, 17*(3), 199–212. https://doi.org/10.1007/S00737-014-0424-9

Somerville, S., Byrne, S. L., Dedman, K., Hagan, R., Coo, S., Oxnam, E., . . . Page, A. C. (2015). Detecting the severity of perinatal anxiety with the Perinatal Anxiety Screening Scale (PASS). *Journal of Affective Disorders, 186*, 18–25. https://doi.org/10.1016/J.JAD.2015.07.012

Spielberger, C. D., Gorsuch, R. L., Lushene, R., Vagg, P. R., & Jacobs, G. A. (1983). *Manual for the state-trait anxiety inventory.* Consulting Psychologists Press.

Spitzer, R. L., Kroenke, K., Williams, J. B. W., & Löwe, B. (2006). A brief measure for assessing generalized anxiety disorder: The GAD-7. *Archives of Internal Medicine, 166*(10), 1092–1097. https://doi.org/10.1001/archinte.166.10.1092

Stavdal, M. N., Skjævestad, M. L. L., & Dahl, B. (2019). First-time parents' experiences of proximity and intimacy after childbirth – A qualitative study. *Sexual & Reproductive Healthcare, 20*, 66–71. https://doi.org/10.1016/J.SRHC.2019.03.003

Stein, A., Craske, M. G., Lehtonen, A., Harvey, A., Savage-McGlynn, E., Davies, B., . . . Counsell, N. (2012). Maternal cognitions and mother – Infant interaction in postnatal depression and generalized anxiety disorder. *Journal of Abnormal Psychology, 121*(4), 795. https://doi.org/10.1037/A0026847

Steinman, S. A., Wootton, B. M., & Tolin, D. F. (2016). Exposure therapy for anxiety disorders. In H. Friedman (Ed.), *Encyclopedia of mental health* (2nd ed., pp. 186–191). Academic Press. https://doi.org/10.1016/B978-0-12-397045-9.00266-4

Stuebe, A. M., Grewen, K., & Meltzer-Brody, S. (2013). Association between maternal mood and oxytocin response to breastfeeding. *Journal of Women's Health (2002), 22*(4), 352–361. https://doi.org/10.1089/JWH.2012.3768

Tendais, I., Costa, R., Conde, A., & Figueiredo, B. (2014). Screening for depression and anxiety disorders from pregnancy to postpartum with the EPDS and STAI. *Spanish Journal of Psychology, 17*, Article E7. https://doi.org/10.1017/SJP.2014.7

Thoma, N., Pilecki, B., & McKay, D. (2015). Contemporary cognitive behavior therapy: A review of theory, history, and evidence. *Psychodynamic Psychiatry, 43*(3), 423–462. https://doi.org/10.1521/PDPS.2015.43.3.423

Tietz, A., Zietlow, A. L., & Reck, C. (2014). Maternal bonding in mothers with postpartum anxiety disorder: The crucial role of subclinical depressive symptoms and maternal avoidance behaviour. *Archives of Women's Mental Health, 17*(5), 433–442. https://doi.org/10.1007/S00737-014-0423-X

Timpano, K. R., Abramowitz, J. S., Mahaffey, B. L., Mitchell, M. A., & Schmidt, N. B. (2011). Efficacy of a prevention program for postpartum obsessive – Compulsive symptoms. *Journal of Psychiatric Research, 45*(11), 1511–1517. https://doi.org/10.1016/J.JPSYCHIRES.2011.06.015

Tolin, D. F. (2012). *Face your fears: A proven plan to beat anxiety, panic, phobias, and obsessions.* John Wiley & Sons.

Tolin, D. F. (2016). *Doing CBT: A comprehensive guide to working with behaviors, thoughts, and emotions.* Guilford Press.

van der Zee-van den Berg, A. I., Boere-Boonekamp, M. M., Groothuis-Oudshoorn, C. G. M., & Reijneveld, S. A. (2021). Postpartum depression and anxiety: A community-based study on risk factors before, during and after pregnancy. *Journal of Affective Disorders, 286*, 158–165. https://doi.org/10.1016/J.JAD.2021.02.062

Wardrop, A. A., & Popadiuk, N. E. (2013). Women's experiences with postpartum anxiety: Expectations, relationships, and sociocultural influences. *Qualitative Report, 18*(6), 1–24. www.nova.edu/ssss/QR/QR18/wardrop6.pdf

Warren, S. L., Racu, C., Gregg, V., & Simmens, S. J. (2006). Maternal panic disorder: Infant prematurity and low birth weight. *Journal of Anxiety Disorders, 20*(3), 342–352. https://doi.org/10.1016/J.JANXDIS.2005.02.007

Weir, S., Posner, H. E., Zhang, J., Willis, G., Baxter, J. D., & Clark, R. E. (2011). Predictors of prenatal and postpartum care adequacy in a Medicaid managed care population. *Women's Health Issues, 21*(4), 277–285. https://doi.org/10.1016/j.whi.2011.03.001

Wenzel, A. (2011). *Anxiety in childbearing women: Diagnosis and treatment.* American Psychological Association.

Wenzel, A. (Ed.). (2014). *The Oxford handbook of perinatal psychology.* Oxford University Press. https://doi.org/10.1093/OXFORDHB/9780199778072.001.0001

Wenzel, A., Haugen, E. N., & Goyette, M. (2007). Sexual adjustment in postpartum women with generalized anxiety disorder. *Journal of Reproductive and Infant Psychology, 23*(4), 365–366. https://doi.org/10.1080/02646830500273723

Wenzel, A., Haugen, E. N., Jackson, L. C., & Brendle, J. R. (2005). Anxiety symptoms and disorders at eight weeks postpartum. *Journal of Anxiety Disorders, 19*(3), 295–311. https://doi.org/10.1016/j.janxdis.2004.04.001

Wenzel, A., & Kleiman, K. R. (2015). *Cognitive behavioral therapy for perinatal distress.* Routledge.

Westra, H. A., & Stewart, S. H. (1998). Cognitive behavioural therapy and pharmacotherapy: Complementary or contradictory approaches to the treatment of anxiety? *Clinical Psychology Review, 18*(3), 307–340. https://doi.org/10.1016/S0272-7358(97)00084-6

Woolhouse, H., McDonald, E., & Brown, S. (2012). Women's experiences of sex and intimacy after childbirth: Making the adjustment to motherhood. *Journal of Psychosomatic Obstetrics and Gynaecology, 33*(4), 185–190. https://doi.org/10.3109/0167482X.2012.720314

Zigmond, A. S., & Snaith, R. P. (1983). The hospital anxiety and depression scale. *Acta Psychiatrica Scandinavica, 67*(6), 361–370. https://doi.org/10.1111/J.1600-0447.1983.TB09716.X

14

POSTPARTUM OBSESSIVE-COMPULSIVE DISORDER

Linda Jüris

In the postpartum period, there is a heightened risk of onset or exacerbation of obsessive-compulsive disorder (OCD) (Russell et al., 2013). It is common for persons with pre-existing symptoms to experience a worsening of symptoms, sometimes resulting in full-blown OCD (Guglielmi et al., 2014). The prevalence of OCD symptoms has been reported at 6.2% in pregnant women (Miller et al., 2022) and between 2.2% and 16.9% in postpartum women (Fairbrother et al., 2016, 2021; Fawcett et al., 2020; Miller et al., 2022; Osnes et al., 2019; Russell et al., 2013). If untreated, OCD may result in serious consequences for the patient, her family, and the newborn (Brandes et al., 2004).

Naturally, many parents worry about the safety or well-being of their children, but in some cases this normal worry develops into OCD. According to the *Diagnostic and Statistical Manual of Mental Disorders* (DSM-5), OCD is defined as the presence of obsessions, compulsions, or both. *Obsessions* are defined as recurrent and persistent thoughts, urges, or images that are experienced, at some time during the disturbance, as intrusive and unwanted, and that cause marked anxiety or distress. Often, the obsessions do not correspond with the person's values and are, therefore, perceived as frightening or aversive. The individual attempts to ignore, suppress, or otherwise counteract such thoughts, urges, images, or the disastrous core fear they represent. Nevertheless, intrusive thoughts are a normal part of human psychology, even thoughts with aggressive content. Avoidance, and the performance of certain behaviors (i.e., compulsions) may reinforce the notion common intrusive thought as threatening, a clinical presentation that can develop into OCD.

Compulsions are defined as willful behaviors that the individual performs to obtain relief from the anxiety and/or discomfort, and/or to prevent the core fearful event from happening. Compulsions may be overt behaviors (e.g., excessive hand washing or repeatedly turning lights on and off) or covert acts (e.g., praying or repeating words or sentences backward silently) that the person feels obliged to perform in response to an obsession, or according to specific rules that must be applied rigidly. However, these behaviors or mental acts either are not connected in a realistic way to what they are meant to prevent or are clearly excessive. In most cases, the patient has good insight into the process in that they know their behavior is unnecessary or excessive but that they cannot stop due to the discomfort.

DOI: 10.4324/9781003206903-18

To meet the criteria as a disorder, the obsessions and/or compulsions must be time consuming (e.g., take more than one hour per day) or cause clinically significant distress or impairment in social, occupational, or other important areas of functioning. OCD can be a very disabling disorder associated with significant interference in social functioning, in the workplace, and at home (Ruscio et al., 2010).

Usually, the OCD patient suffers from multiple obsessions and compulsions (Ruscio et al., 2010). At least ten factor analyses have delineated more or less clinically meaningful OCD symptom dimensions (Mataix-Cols et al., 2005). While fairly similar in content, the number of factors reported ranges from three to six. Often, the dimensions constitute similar overt behaviors, such as checking. An alternative scheme to categorize OCD subtypes is based on the *function* of the compulsive behavior—what the patient is trying to flee by performing them. A widely used base for subtyping in functional themes is established by Abramowitz et al. (2003), in four categories:

1. *Contamination*—the patient is afraid for their own life and health, the fear is *often* manifesting in avoidance of germs and viruses, and cleaning behaviors
2. *Responsibility for harm and mistakes*—the patient is afraid to accidentally harm others, *often* showing in checking and asking for reassurance
3. *Symmetry/ordering*—the patient fears the so-called *not just right experience*, as this either might indicate an upcoming catastrophe or just feels awful, and it is *often* showing in repeating behaviors
4. *Unacceptable thoughts*—the patient is afraid of being an awful person, such as a murderer, a pedophile, or a blasphemer. Often these persons avoid situations where they might prove themselves to be a person as mentioned earlier

A recent analysis of OCD themes using The Dimensional YBOCS (DY-BOCS) (Rosario-Campos et al., 2006) resulted in a slightly different set of themes (Cervin et al., 2021). Eight dimensions emerged through factor analysis, including disturbing thoughts, incompleteness, contamination, hoarding, transformation, body focus, superstition, and loss/separation.

Clinically, knowledge of the common subtypes can make it easier for the clinician to recognize OCD and differentiate it from other disorders. Also, the templates that constitute subtypes or dimensions that are based on the function of the compulsive behavior, rather than the behavior itself, make a logical basis for exposure therapy and simplify the analysis, goal setting, and creation of exposure hierarchies. For instance, a patient who washes her hands excessively may suffer from many different fears, perhaps fear of either catching a disease herself, or infecting others, or perhaps fear of infidelity by spreading her genital fluids; three different dimensions that would result in three completely different exposure strategies. The patients might also find it useful to know about different types of OCD, if themselves, or someone they know develops OCD or relapses.

Clara is a 30-year-old preschool teacher, who gave birth to her first child 18 months ago. Since then, she has developed a debilitating OCD. Clara recognizes having some mild obsessions in childhood, mostly concerning "not just right" experiences when walking outdoors, resulting mainly in avoidance of cracks in the pavement when walking to school. She also experienced anxiety in test situations in school but nothing of a psychiatric nature that required attention from a healthcare provider.

Clara's pregnancy progressed without physical complications for both her and her baby. She looked after herself when pregnant, tried to get enough sleep and exercise, and studied diet recommendations closely. To ensure that she would not harm her fetus, she stayed away from any food or drink that could contain alcohol, caffeine, or bacteria, such as listeria or salmonella. Clara avoided consuming fish and cheese, and she stayed clear of the pets belonging to family and friends. She also avoided gardening and stayed out of parks. To be completely sure to keep safe, she got rid of all the plants in her home. When her partner asked about her behavior, she explained she knew she behaved a little strangely, but this would surely end as soon as she entered the third trimester, as she had been informed that most risks would be much lower after that point in time. When the time did arrive, though, she found it best to continue these routines for the rest of the pregnancy, and again "to be completely safe," also change her diet to vegan.

After this period, baby Alba was born, a delivery without complications. A couple of days after the family arrived home with their new family member, there was a discussion on TV about the consequences for children after the COVID-19 pandemic, specifically their heightened sensitivity to infections. This made Clara worry about different germs and viruses that could potentially harm her child. She naturally felt a high level of responsibility as a parent to make sure this did not happen. The following days she went through the home to find possible dangerous or dirty areas and made sure to clean them properly. She discussed her worries with her partner, and they decided on several measures to ensure Alba's safety, including an elaborate cleaning schedule, the agreement to use hand sanitizer much more often, and also, as an extra precaution, the decision to look into the possible chemical dangers of the fabric of the baby's clothing and diapers. They decided to keep the baby away from situations that they perceived as potentially harmful, mainly contact with other individuals, especially other children.

In a matter of weeks, the cleaning and avoidance behaviors had grown to affect the family's preferred routines in many ways. The cleaning had become time-consuming and included their home, their belongings, and themselves. The washing machine was always running. In addition, the family avoided an increasing number of outside-the-home environments, such as grocery stores and the homes of relatives and friends. Clara had planned to breastfeed for at least six months, if possible. She stopped after three weeks due to "the impossibility of knowing the exact contents of the breastmilk."

Today, Clara spends all her time inside the house with her child. Her partner continues to go to work and runs the necessary errands, however, when he returns home, he is required to complete a complicated cleaning ritual before entering the house. The child has no contact with persons apart from her parents, to her grandparents' great sorrow. Clara and her partner have managed to take their child to almost all doctors' appointments but are now dreading an upcoming important vaccination appointment.

Clara's partner wants their child to be healthy and for Clara to be relieved of her anxiety, so he reassures Clara thoroughly if she asks him to do so, or even if he only vaguely perceives that her anxiety is rising. He performs many compulsions to help her. His perspective on OCD is clearer than Clara's, he notices her lack of insight in many situations and has, therefore, with strong support from all grandparents, urged her to seek psychiatric evaluation.

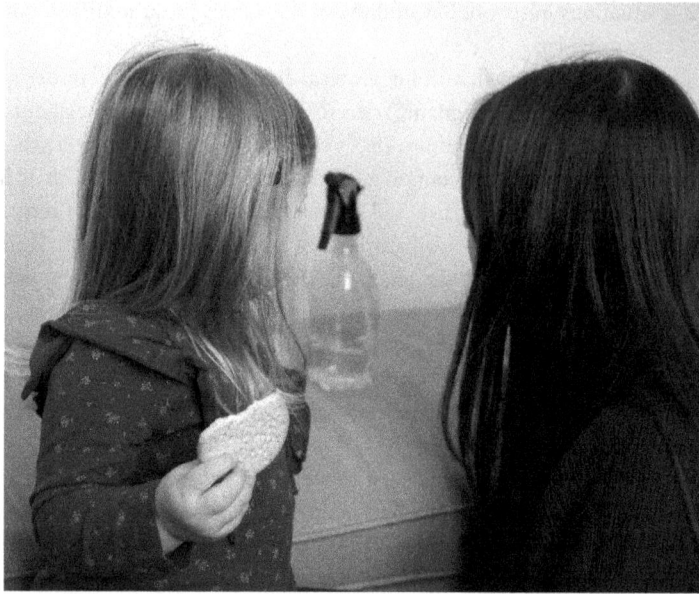

Figure 14.1   Clara with Alba

Development of OCD

Intrusive thoughts, or mental images that disturb the normal line of thought, occur among most people (Rachman & De Silva, 1978). If the intrusive thought is disturbing enough, many persons try actively not to think about it. Unfortunately, research on thought suppression shows that this type of behavior leads to the opposite effect—even more unwanted thoughts emerge (Wegner, 1994). According to the behavioral model of OCD, with roots in the work of Orval Hobart Mowrer (1947), an intrusive thought at some point has occurred simultaneously as a person is experiencing anxiety or other discomfort, connecting the two via classical conditioning. Furthermore, the person starts avoiding the stimuli that relate to discomfort to reduce the risk of named discomfort or other catastrophe. The intrusive thought is viewed as being of great importance and develops into an obsession when the individual chooses to change their behavior to relieve themselves associated with the anxiety associated with the obsession. The compulsion reduces the anxiety or discomfort in the short run, encouraging the individual to continue to perform the behavior, such that the behavior is negatively reinforced. Avoidance and the performance of compulsive behaviors lead to greater focus on the obsessions, in turn leading to more time and effort devoted to compulsions, more avoidance, and so on, establishing OCD at a clinical level. When a person suffers from OCD, their concurrent anxiety and discomfort increase over time (Najmi et al., 2009).

OCD has also been understood from a cognitive perspective. According to the cognitive model, OCD develops when a person catastrophically misinterprets the significance of normal, distressing intrusive thoughts (Salkovskis, 1985). The compulsions that follow are problematic because they prevent the disconfirmation of the obsessional fear (Salkovskis, 1996). Some patients' obsessions may have developed from dysfunctional core beliefs and life rules that are viewed as absolute truths and are not at all questioned by the patient. Consensus ratings from a group of experienced OCD clinicians and researchers indicated that three belief domains are likely to be important in OCD: (a) overestimation of threat and inflated responsibility; (b) importance of and need to control thoughts; and (c) perfectionism and intolerance of uncertainty (OCCWG, 1997, 2001, 2003, 2005). Research on cognitive differences between persons with and without OCD demonstrates that these belief domains appear relevant (Hezel & McNally, 2016).

The main difference between postpartum OCD and OCD with onset at other times in life is, not surprisingly, that the content of the obsessions often relates to the baby (Fairbrother et al., 2016; Russell et al., 2013; Speisman et al., 2011). Apart from the very common stressors of sleep deprivation, physical problems from giving birth, and relational problems due to new priorities in life, most new parents report intrusive thoughts concerning harm toward their children. Half of all new mothers report intrusive thoughts of *intentionally* harming their infant (Abramowitz et al., 2006, 2007; Fairbrother & Woody; 2008; Collardeau et al., 2019). Both mothers and fathers report a higher frequency of this type of thoughts when the baby is crying, relative to adults who are not parents (Fairbrother et al., 2019). The most common type of intrusive thought among new mothers is fear of having an unhealthy baby at birth, contamination, the baby being taken away, and infant death. The most common behavioral responses are repeating rituals, asking for reassurance, checking, and cleaning (Lord et al., 2011).

A well-established explanation for the increase in the incidence of OCD is that new parents are naturally focused on the safety of their child and experience a great responsibility for their newborn (Fairbrother & Abramowitz, 2007). Intrusive thoughts containing accidentally or willfully harming their child, or sexual behavior toward their child are, therefore, very disturbing. For a person prone to developing OCD, these normal intrusive thoughts may be misinterpreted as significant threats to the baby's safety and evoke avoidance and compulsive behaviors.

Clinical manifestations of postpartum OCD differ from those of pregnant women with OCD and from women with OCD who are in other periods of their lives (Starcevic et al., 2020). Postpartum women report a significantly higher incidence of aggressive obsessions and lesser incidence of washing/cleaning compulsion compared to pregnant women and women not in the perinatal period. Usually, OCD-related behaviors are more avoidant and less compulsive (Fairbrother & Abramowitz, 2007; House et al., 2016). Checking compulsions, self-reassurance, and seeking reassurance from others are, nevertheless, relatively common in this group. Interestingly, frequencies of various obsessions and compulsions do not differ between pregnant women with OCD and women not in the perinatal period (Starcevic et al., 2020).

In one study, it was shown that behavioral responses to postpartum harm thoughts predicted the frequency and total duration of accidental harm thoughts, and interference in parenting by intentional harm thoughts. These findings provide support for cognitive behavioral conceptualizations of postpartum OCD (Fairbrother et al., 2018).

A complication factor in the development of OCD is that perinatal and postpartum OCD often are missed by healthcare professionals (Brand & Brennan, 2009). Many medical and mental health providers are not adequately trained to recognize and accurately diagnose anxiety disorders in the postpartum period and might, thereby, regard the obsessions as true beliefs and intentions of the new parent (Challacombe & Wroe, 2013). Subsequently, persons suffering from postpartum OCD are often hesitant to seek help, as they are afraid authorities might see them as unfit parents. Whereas maternal unwanted and intrusive thoughts of infant-related harm are known to be associated with OCD and depression, there is evidence that they are not associated with an increased risk of harm to infants. The prevalence of child abuse is actually lower than reported in other groups (Fairbrother et al., 2022). Reassuringly, the children of mothers with OCD do not differ from controls when it comes to suffering from insecure attachment (Challacombe et al., 2017).

Correlates and Risk Factors

Understanding biological factors in perinatal OCD can help destigmatize mental illness during this vulnerable time in a woman's life. In the literature, different neurochemical, neuroanatomical, and genetic factors are of interest in general OCD and in explaining why OCD and anxiety symptoms seem to intensify in women when they're pregnant. First, the neurotransmitter serotonin has often been discussed as a possible factor in OCD, as selective serotonin reuptake inhibitors (SSRIs) and also clomipramine, a tricyclic antidepressant (TCA), have proved to have an effect on treating OCD. Nevertheless, persons with OCD often suffer from other psychiatric disorders, and sometimes it can be difficult to know which disorder was actually targeted by the change in serotonin reuptake.

Second, there are many theories about structural and functional abnormalities in the brain, (e.g., abnormalities of the cortico-striato-thalamic circuits) causing OCD (Pauls et al., 2014), but no hard evidence. Thirdly, there are a few genetic studies on OCD, but no clear proof of specific genes that may explain the onset of OCD (Mattheisen et al., 2015; Noh et al., 2017; IOCDF-GC & OCGAS, 2018). Much more research is needed even though there is some evidence for an overlap in the origins of postpartum depression and perinatal OCD symptoms. Two biomarkers, TTC9B and HP1BP3, were found to predict the development of postpartum depression and may also be used to forecast the exacerbation of OCD symptoms during pregnancy. In one study, those gene biomarkers predicted the exacerbation of OCD with about 75% accuracy (Kaminsky et al., 2020).

A range of perinatal risk factors are associated with a higher risk of developing OCD *in the child* such as maternal smoking during pregnancy, cesarean section, preterm birth, low birth weight, and Apgar distress scores (Brander et al., 2016). Maternal OCD has been associated with many increased risks for the mother as well, for instance gestational diabetes, both elective and emergency cesarean delivery, and preeclampsia (Fernández de la Cruz et al., 2023). Women with OCD taking SSRIs during pregnancy have shown an overall increased risk of these outcomes, compared with those not taking SSRIs. However, women with OCD not taking SSRIs had increased risks compared with women without OCD (Fernández de la Cruz et al., 2023).

For the mothers, predictors for peripartum anxiety and depressive disorders are anxiety and depressive disorders prior to pregnancy, but psychosocial, individual, and interpersonal factors are also important, such as level of education and social support (Martini et al., 2015). In another study, it was concluded that two risk factors for mothers in developing OCD later in life were edema during pregnancy and prolonged labor (Vasconcelos et al., 2007).

With regard to cognitive biases, postpartum women reported significantly higher scores of responsibility interpretations regarding baby-related intrusions, compared to both non-baby-related intrusions and women without children, even though the groups were not significantly different regarding general responsibility ratings. These responsibility interpretations were shown to predict obsessive-compulsive symptomatology (Barret et al., 2016).

From a clinical perspective, aspects of the patient's environment, mainly the accommodating behavior repertoire of others, can constitute a risk factor. Accommodating behaviors to manage OCD logically leads to a more restricted life for all involved and might also lead to conflict, as avoidance and compulsive behavior exacerbate symptoms. Some relatives also support the sufferer financially or with different everyday chores that the sufferer does not have time to do, also exacerbating symptoms and likely preventing or postponing the suffering person from seeking professional care. When it comes to parents with children suffering from OCD, it has been shown that accommodation mediates the relation between OCD symptom severity and functional impairment (Caporino et al., 2012; Storch et al., 2007). Accommodation has also been shown to be positively associated with parental distress in pediatric OCD (Storch et al., 2007) and with anxiety and depression in relatives of adults with OCD (Amir et al., 2000).

When studying accommodation in romantic couples, Boeding et al. (2013) concluded that "Unless couples learn how to change their interaction patterns that include accommodation, the long-term effectiveness of exposure-based cognitive behavioral therapy (CBT) for OCD patients is likely to be limited" (p. 321). The group of researchers investigated accommodation behaviors in 20 romantic couples before and after treatment and noticed accommodation to be associated with the patient's OCD symptoms at pre-treatment and negatively associated with the partners', but not the patients', self-reported relationship satisfaction. Accommodation was shown to be associated with poorer individual functioning, as well as with poorer relationship functioning. Post-treatment, partner accommodation was also associated with poorer response to treatment. A complex problem is a stressful situation where the relationship stress in itself affects and exacerbates OCD symptoms, causing the partner to accommodate and, in turn, feel less satisfied with the relationship. OCD clearly can have a strong negative impact on the affected person's close romantic relationships (Boeding et al., 2013). Furthermore, criticism and hostility from family members are associated with greater symptom severity and worse treatment outcomes (Chambless & Steketee, 1999; Renshaw et al., 2003; Van Noppen & Steketee, 2009).

There are not many known risk factors in Clara's history, apart from her mother being a heavy smoker and being unable to refrain from smoking during her pregnancy. Clara's partner David, as part of Clara's interpersonal environment, has a learning history that could be affecting the maintenance of OCD. David grew up with a highly anxious mother and has had a couple of romantic partners with untreated anxiety disorders. David perceived them all to be in great need of his accommodating of behaviors, which he offered as much as he could. David sees himself as a good listener and problem-solver, and both he and Clara view his ability to manage other people's anxiety to be one of his greatest skills.

Comorbidity

The most common comorbid diagnosis along with OCD in general is major depressive disorder, followed by generalized anxiety disorder, panic disorder, and social anxiety disorder (Crino & Andrews, 1996). Around 12% of women in the perinatal period fulfill the criteria for clinical depression (Woody et al., 2017), but not much has been researched in this group when it comes to comorbidity between OCD and depression, or comorbidity with other disorders. Comorbidity between depression and any anxiety disorder, OCD included, has been reported at 4.2% in a smaller sample at some point in either pregnancy or the first three months postpartum (Fairbrother et al., 2016).

> In addition to OCD, Clara fulfills the clinical diagnosis for depression. After some time with OCD, life inevitably changes. What were once the most valued activities in Clara's life have turned into terrible situations where she, in her mind, experiences her worst fears. Clara, like most people with OCD, avoids a great number of situations. This loss leads to sadness, of course, but also to general inactivity. This inactivity can include increasing difficulties in getting started with most activities in life, both those that are necessary, and can carry a feeling of being productive, and those that are mainly pleasurable.

Effects on the Partner Relationship, Children, and Other Family Members

Families, friends, and other persons close to someone suffering from OCD are often involved in and affected by the disorder. Unfortunately, they often unwillingly contribute to the worsening of symptoms. Almost 90% of caregivers of adult OCD patients report accommodating to some extent (Calvocoressi et al., 1995, 1999). Most disabled patients are sometimes totally dependent on their relatives. A common clinical observation is that family members and other persons around the OCD sufferer try to accommodate by helping to avoid triggers, answer questions repeatedly, or perform certain compulsive behaviors with or instead of the patient. Usually, the relative has no intention to harm the person suffering from OCD, but, of course, the accommodating behaviors lead to a worsening of OCD symptoms in the long run, in both treated and untreated patients (Thompson-Hollands et al., 2015; Van Noppen & Steketee, 2009).

> Clara's case shows the range and complexity of how OCD can play in a relation context. Clara's partner, David, has an extensive history of helping out with family members' and romantic partners' problems with anxiety. He has since long been the primary caretaker for baby Alba, including assuming full responsibility for taking her to all doctor's appointments. He has concluded it is best for the family, as the visits seem to be too anxiety-provoking for Clara, and also too anxiety-provoking for himself, as he finds it difficult to endure Clara's emotional distress. If there is something he can do about her suffering, he very much wants

to help. David also suspects that the baby probably reacts to the heightened levels of anxiety in the family as well. Moreover, Clara's excursions outside of the home have become quite time consuming with all the rituals that must be performed when leaving and re-entering their home, the extra laundry, and the extra checking of the baby the following days. Besides, David reasons that the baby obviously needs to go to the doctor, and believes that it is better that he takes Alba there on his own.

David and Clara perform many excessive compulsive cleaning behaviors together. David also changes his work clothes in the garage to take a shower before entering the home in his "home clothes." David gives Clara all the answers that he may give her if she asks for reassurance about germs and viruses and whether her behavior in protecting the baby is adequate. He also helps her investigate different bacteria and such on the Internet. Another time-consuming task is cooking for the family, as it has to be performed according to complicated rules and rituals with only a few specific foods and high temperatures.

Assessment

Mulcahy et al. (2023) have delineated specific clinical practice recommendations for OCD in the perinatal period by Delphi survey methodology (Jorm, 2015), compiling views of expert professionals with persons with experience of perinatal OCD. In sum, most of the items on psychoeducation, screening, assessment, differential diagnosis, case care considerations, treatment, partners and families, and cultural and diversity considerations do not differ from general recommendations of OCD treatment. Nevertheless, the researchers emphasize to specifically include perinatal OCD in general information provided to expectant and new parents and to normalize the experience of intrusive thoughts in the general population as well as the increase or onset of intrusive thoughts in the perinatal period.

Mulcahy et al. urged practitioners to recognize that many parents may decline OCD assessment or withhold OCD symptoms due to fearfulness of the consequences for the child. Practitioners are recommended to directly ask about, while also normalizing, the presence of taboo/aggressive/sexual intrusions and corresponding compulsions. The researchers also stressed the level of education of the healthcare professionals. Specifically, there is a need to improve the recognition and treatment of postpartum OCD in medical staff, requiring, better training (Brakoulias et al., 2020), and careful assessment and reporting can help in this regard.

An important aspect of specific measures is the opportunity for both clinicians and patients to openly normalize and discuss intrusions. There are many assessment tools and measures for OCD in general but not much research on the specific assessment of perinatal OCD. Clinicians can use their preferred diagnostic tool to investigate whether their patient fulfills diagnostic criteria for OCD and its specific nature and severity.

The Yale-Brown Obsessive-Compulsive Scale

The YBOCS (Goodman et al., 1989a, 1989b) is regarded as the "gold standard" in the measurement of OCD symptom severity and treatment response (Woody et al., 1995; Moritz et al., 2002). It is a semistructured interview that consists of ten core items, the first five of them measuring time, interference, distress, resistance, and control of obsessions, and another five identical items measuring compulsions. The items are rated from 0 (no symptoms) to 4 (severe symptoms) and result in a global severity score (range 0–40). YBOCS scores of 0–13 correspond to *mild* symptoms, 14–25 to *moderate* symptoms, 26–34 to *moderate-severe* symptoms, and 35–40 to *severe* symptoms (Storch et al., 2015). The scale also exists in a self-report version, the YBOCS-SR, with strong internal consistency, test–retest reliability, and construct validity (Storch et al., 2011). The measure has been used in the study of postpartum women (House et al., 2016).

The Dimensional Obsessive-Compulsive Scale

The *Dimensional Obsessive-Compulsive Scale* (DOCS) (Abramowitz et al., 2010) is a 20-item self-report questionnaire that assesses the severity of the four most consistently replicated OCD symptom dimensions, corresponding to the measure's four subscales: (a) contamination, (b) responsibility for harm and mistakes, (c) symmetry/ordering, and (d) unacceptable thoughts. In a study, the *Edinburgh Postnatal Depression Scale* (EPDS, Cox et al., 1996) was compared to the screening accuracy of the DOCS. The EPDS is a commonly used scale but does not include questions related to obsessions or intrusive thoughts. The DOCS total score demonstrated a higher level of accuracy in the identification of OCD than the EPDS (Fairbrother et al., 2023).

The Perinatal Obsessive-Compulsive Scale

The *Perinatal Obsessive-Compulsive Scale* (POCS) (Lord et al., 2011) is a self-report scale of perinatal obsessions and compulsions developed to help professionals detect perinatal OCD. The POCS has good construct validity, high internal consistency, good concurrent validity, and discriminative capacity according to the researchers, although the measure has rarely been used in studies.

The Parental Thoughts and Behaviors Checklist

The *Postpartum Thoughts and Behaviors Checklist*, later changed to *Parental Thoughts and Behaviors Checklist* (PTBC) (Abramowitz et al., 2006), is a semistructured interview that assesses clinically relevant thoughts (e.g., obsessions about puncturing the baby's fontanel or "soft spot") and behaviors (e.g., compulsive praying) in the perinatal period. This scale has also been converted into a self-report measure (Thiséus et al., 2019).

The Postpartum Distress Measure

Another very brief screening measure, including a six-item general distress scale and a four-item postpartum-specific OCD symptoms scale, is the *Postpartum Distress Measure* (Allison et al., 2011). The OCD subscale includes items assessing postpartum checking behaviors, fear of harm, illness anxiety, and intrusive thoughts.

Assessment of Themes or Subtypes

OCD often presents with a variety of obsessions and compulsions. Sometimes these are logically connected, but, in many cases, they are difficult to understand for both the person suffering from them and the people around them. Also, it might be hard for professionals to distinguish OCD from other mental disorders, such as depression, delusions, and health anxiety. Even though obsessions and compulsions can vary widely, the main principle is that the obsessions cause discomfort, and the purpose of the willful performance of the compulsion is to relieve the discomfort. The patient may suffer from a particular type, or theme, of OCD, or several others. The combination of themes often complicates the analysis of the disorder, in the planning and implementation of CBT. The DOCS, mentioned earlier, measures the specific themes established by Abramowitz et al. (2003): contamination, responsibility for harm and mistakes, symmetry/ordering, and unacceptable thoughts.

Clara completed the scales above plus a depression index that indicated a moderate level of depression. Her YBOCS total score was 32, which is in the moderate-severe range. The most informative item for the clinician was that Clara stated the amount of time she was occupied by obsessive thoughts was nearly constant. She stated her level of distress as extreme, and her level of insight to be fair. On the DOCS, Clara scored the maximum number of points on the second scale, that of concerns about being responsible for harm. The third and fourth scales showed nothing of clinical interest, but the first scale, contamination, also yielded a high score. Furthermore, Clara answered "yes" on the PTBC items about fear of the child falling ill by contamination (items 24 and 25), worry about chemicals in the household, insects, animals, and contamination associated with diseases (items 26–28). Also, Clara answered affirmatively on the item about fear of damaging the baby's fontanel or "soft spot" (item 10). Her total scores of the time, anxiety, and disability items were very high.

The clinical impression of Clara is that she is primarily afraid to harm her baby and that being responsible for contaminating her with bacteria and germs is only one of the presentations. The treatment should accordingly focus on exposure tasks in which Clara takes risks to harm the baby, at times including exposure to bacteria and viruses. Results of the assessment suggested that the response prevention component should focus on cleaning and checking behaviors, as well as reassurance seeking.

Treatment

Pharmacological Treatment

Antidepressants are commonly used in the treatment of OCD and have been shown to be effective, with a mean effect size of 0.91, and a median of 0.73 reported (Eddy et al., 2004), although the treatment effect does not always last after discontinuation of medication. *Clomipramine*, a tricyclic antidepressant (TCA), is a common choice in OCD due to studies showing its advantages over other SSRIs (Eddy et al., 2004, Greist et al., 1995) but has been associated with adverse birth outcomes when prescribed to pregnant women (Källén, 2007; ter Horst et al., 2012). The SSRIs, sertraline and paroxetine, and TCAs, nortriptyline and imipramine, are the most evidence-based medications for use during breastfeeding (Lanza di Scalea & Wisner, 2009), but more research is required to assess the role of SSRIs in the postpartum period (Brakoulias et al., 2020). Benzodiazepines are often prescribed for OCD but generally not recommended due to their addictive properties and also due to an increased risk of spontaneous abortion (Sheehy et al., 2019). Benzodiazepine use in the third trimester has been associated with preterm birth (Shyken et al., 2019). In one study, postpartum women stated that restarting medication postpartum was the reason they did not continue breastfeeding (Challacombe et al., 2016).

Psychotherapy

CBT is the psychotherapy of choice for OCD, with meta-analyses yielding large effect sizes. For example, one meta-analysis found effect sizes of 1.31 when CBT was compared to waitlist control conditions and 1.33 when CBT was compared to placebo conditions (Öst et al., 2015). Other researchers have calculated similar results (van Balkom et al., 1994; American Psychiatric Association, NICE, Ferrando & Selai, 2021). There are CBT protocols that have a primarily behavioral focus and those that have a primarily cognitive focus. The major difference is the framework, such that the behavioral models focus on the extinction of fear responses, acceptance of emotions, and seeing thoughts as uncontrollable, whereas the cognitive model focuses on changing the interpretation of the feared stimuli. Exposure with response prevention (ERP) is a behaviorally focused CBT that has been studied most often (Abramowitz & Jacoby, 2015; van Noppen et al., 2021) and is concluded to be more effective than other psychotherapies and placebo in reducing symptoms (Ferrando & Selai, 2021). *Exposure* is defined as gradually and systematically exposing the patient to what they fear in a preplanned and controlled fashion (e.g., to a specific situation, an emotion, an urge, or a thought). Before, during, and after exposure, the patient shall not perform any compulsive behaviors, but instead take part in so-called *response prevention*, which allows the patient a new experience with their anxiety or that the anxiety is bearable (i.e., that it disappears even without the compulsion being performed). Intensive CBT treatment, in some cases performed in the patients' homes, has also been studied (Challacombe & Salkovskis, 2011; Challacombe et al., 2017).

Individuals experiencing postpartum OCD should be offered CBT that includes ERP as a core component as a first-line treatment option. This treatment is to be given by specially trained professionals who are also receiving qualified clinical supervision. Healthcare professionals should specifically focus on encouraging bonding between the parent and the infant by reducing avoidance behavior and involving the baby in the exposure when necessary (Mulcahy et al., 2023). CBT for pregnant and postpartum women has been studied to at least some extent. There is a debate on whether exposure is safe for the baby when treating pregnant women, and an often-seen clinical choice is to postpone exposure treatment until after delivery. Unfortunately, this delay may result in a worsening of symptoms. There may also be practical difficulties in attending treatment together with a baby. An important consideration when deciding on the type of treatment is that women often state they prefer anxiety-related treatment that includes psychotherapy (Pearlstein et al., 2006). Preference for psychotherapy alone is even stronger among pregnant women relative to women in general (Arch, 2014).

To initiate the exposure component of CBT, the clinician completes a functional analysis, or an explanation of the problem's emergence and how it is maintained, as well as a treatment plan as the basis for clinical interventions to come. There are many different templates in the literature in which OCD clinicians and/or researchers have described themes and subtypes. Incidentally, McGuinness et al. (2011) reviewed the literature in 2011 and concluded that there was not enough evidence for postpartum OCD to be considered a distinct subtype in itself, suggesting the utility of a general approach to the delivery of exposure (Hudepohl et al., 2022).

Exposure may be conducted both as *in vivo* exposure and as *imaginal* exposure (Foa et al., 2012). *Exposure in vivo* refers to performing the exposure in real life, such as if Clara were to take her baby out in the garden for two minutes, letting her touch a plant for a moment. *Imaginal exposure* includes the clinician's guidance of the patient to mentally experience the feared context, such as if Clara were to *imagine* she took the baby out in the garden. Another possibility for imaginal exposure in this setting would be to imagine the feared consequences of touching the plant. The clinician guides the patient through exposure in the patient's mind. The patient sits comfortably, often with eyes closed, and tries to experience the situation as described by the clinician. Imaginal exposure may be performed in those cases when the feared situation is impossible to treat with exposure in vivo, or as a step on the way when the goal is to reach in vivo exposure. Another reason to use imaginal exposure is if the patient refuses in vivo exposure.

To facilitate exposure, the clinician and the patient, together, construct a list of difficult situations together, from simpler situations to the most difficult the patient can imagine in the service of reaching the agreed-upon treatment goals. Hierarchies, or ordered sequences of exposure exercises, are constructed for every specific fear, which means, in OCD, for every specific OCD theme. For example, if the patient suffers from debilitating OCD in two different dimensions, then two hierarchies need to be constructed. Exposure starts on an intermediate level of difficulty and escalates to more and more difficult situations. Exposure is carried out in sessions with the therapist and in between sessions as homework, often with a co-therapist, such as the patient's partner. Traditionally, it has been recommended that the exposure trial continue until the experienced anxiety had dropped in half, but more recent research has shown this is not crucial for the treatment effect and that treatment may be optimized by varying the contexts to a higher extent and performing exposure to several fears in parallel (Craske et al., 2014).

When all items on the hierarchies have been addressed, and most of the treatment goals are met, it is important to focus on the patient returning to their normal life. Some patients will easily take up their old habits when it comes to work, education, and social activities. For others, the loss of an often long and important time in life leads to sadness and sometimes depression. Strategies associated with behavioral activation (Jacobson et al., 2001), a well-established treatment program for depression, are often used to help patients reduce the impacts of negative mood and return to pre-OCD behavior. Usually, a relapse prevention program is established at the end of treatment, and it is also common to arrange booster sessions.

An interesting prevention program designed to target postpartum obsessive-compulsive symptoms has been developed and studied by Timpano et al. (2011). Pregnant women and their partners were randomly assigned to either the prevention program plus childbirth education or a control condition with traditional childbirth education only. The OCD material added to the prevention program consisted of psychoeducation about anxiety and anxiety disorders, psychoeducation about postpartum anxiety and obsessive-compulsive symptoms, psychoeducation about the cognitive model, and training in the cognitive restructuring of dysfunctional "obsessive" beliefs and instruction in using behavioral experiments and exposure techniques as a way of testing and modifying faulty beliefs. The material focused on the beliefs about the importance of, and the need to control, intrusive thoughts about the child. Results indicated that participants in the prevention group were not as distressed by naturally occurring obsessions as were those in the control group, and at one, three, and six months postpartum, participants in the prevention program had significantly lower levels of obsessions and compulsions.

Family members and/or other important persons can assist in both assessment and treatment of OCD. The key issue to teach the significant other is how to provide supportive but nonaccommodating responses, as described in a treatment manual by Jonathan Abramowitz et al. (2013). The manual includes a description of the information gathering and psychoeducation, followed by the rationale and procedures for exposure and response prevention techniques, including specific OCD-related beliefs of the patient, and accommodation-related beliefs and behaviors of the partner. The partner is instructed on how to assist with exposure, and the couple is assigned exposure exercises to conduct between sessions in combination with the reduction of accommodation behaviors. An important factor is to help the couple find alternative support strategies that do not involve avoidance, providing reassurance, or helping with rituals. The last phase of treatment focuses on how OCD has impacted the couple's relationship, what shifts they have seen with symptom reduction, and how to handle general communication issues within the relationship (Abramowitz et al., 2013).

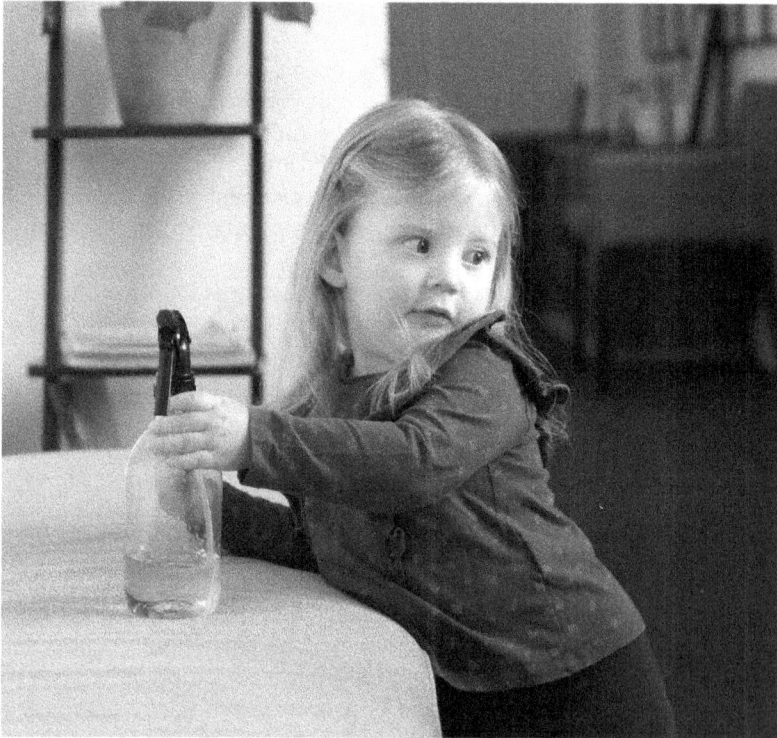

Figure 14.2 Exposure with Alba

When Clara began psychotherapy, her partner was also invited to the assessment sessions to include his input and to provide him with information so that he could play a helpful role. He was also present at some of the treatment sessions and assisted with homework. The clinician started by normalizing the occurrence of intrusive thoughts, such as by communicating that such thoughts naturally revolve around the now most important thing in Clara's life, Alba.

Clara's obsessions belong in the subtype or dimension of harming. Many of Clara's behaviors could easily be mistaken for contamination OCD, but viewing the function of the cleaning behaviors as protecting her child and making sure she is not responsible for harming her, makes the hierarchy of exposure more logical in light of the manifestation of CBT at this time in Clara's life. The clinician made sure to assess for the other subtypes to be able to exclude them and to prepare Clara for possibly recurring problems in the future.

In the psychoeducation phase of treatment, the clinician explained the criteria for the diagnosis of OCD, its prevalence, and how common the onset is during the perinatal period. Then, the CBT model of onset was taught, including the role of avoidance and compulsive behaviors as crucial in the exacerbation of symptoms. After this, the clinician outlined the treatment plan, explaining the principles of exposure and response prevention in a gradual manner, making sure that Clara understood that she would have full control over the speed of progress. Goal setting for treatment was done simultaneously with the construction of exposure hierarchies. Some of Clara's goals for treatment were to (a) independently take the baby to 50% of her doctor's appointments; (b) meet with her parents at least twice a month, with the baby present; and (c) wash hands according to recommendations only d) shower for no more than ten minutes, every other day.

Hierarchies in exposure contain graduated anxiety-arousing stimuli focusing on a specific theme. As Clara's main OCD theme was harming, there was only one hierarchy to set up for her. The hierarchy included situations such as "letting grandma hold the baby for five minutes," "bringing the baby with me to the psychiatric clinic," "letting the clinician enter my home," and so on. A corresponding list of response prevention tasks included gradual weekly changes in the compulsive behaviors of washing her hands and showering by, for example, establishing time limits and amounts of soap and shampoo that could be used.

The course of exposure started at the lower end of the hierarchy, such that Clara was instructed to perform the behavior stated without doing anything to lower her anxiety, meaning no compulsions such as washing or asking for reassurance. The first exposure session took place in Clara's home where the clinician gradually entered the home, via the kitchen and living room to the baby's room, getting as close as one meter away from the baby during the course of the 100-minute session. Clara's partner was in the room at all times, watching the procedure, but not interfering. After the session, he made sure to praise Clara's courage and progress without giving reassurance.

Clara and the clinician agreed on homework between sessions. The first week, her homework was to invite her mother to her home several times, gradually getting closer and closer to her grandchild. After some time in treatment, a spray bottle was introduced (see picture 2).

Clara and her partner learned to contaminate the water in the spray with different particles, such as fruit and so, of which Clara was fearful. They then sprayed the areas in their home to expose Clara to the perceived heightened risk of harming her child. The use of spray bottles can be a simple way to expose a person to a feared substance. After spraying, the possibility of performing compulsive behavior is usually more difficult as well, as the substance has spread in an uncontrollable way.

After five sessions in the family's home and another 15 sessions at the clinic and in different public areas, treatment was considered completed, as Clara had reached her goals and her scores on YBOCS, the primary measure for treatment effect, had dropped significantly.

Cultural Considerations

Scholars have suggested that investigating the patient's educational background, access to health services, food, religion, religiosity, and the genetic structure of populations may increase our understanding of the importance of culture in OCD and its treatment (Nicolini et al., 2017). However, there are very few studies comparing the different manifestations of OCD across cultures, and it appears there are none when it comes to cultural aspects of perinatal OCD. For OCD in general, it has been shown that the disorder appears similar in the different cultures studied but that the content of the obsessions may differ (Fontenelle et al., 2004). In one study, the rates of incidence of OCD for the different countries Canada, Puerto Rico, Germany, Korea, Hong Kong, Taiwan, and New Zealand, were similar with the exception of Taiwan, where incidence rates were lower. The clinical presentations of OCD were also studied with the result that the United States, Canada, Puerto Rico, and New Zealand demonstrated larger proportions of individuals with only obsessions, and in Korea, the proportion of people presenting only with compulsions was higher (Horwath & Weissman, 2000).

People probably also differ in their view of how meaningful intrusive thoughts are and the degree of so-called thought-action fusion. The cognitive behavioral view of intrusive thoughts is that thoughts are uncontrollable and that any thought may enter any person's mind without specific reason. It is easy to imagine the possible complications if a pregnant woman's aggressive intrusive thoughts about her child are seen as sent from God or sent from the devil or demons and followed by her experiencing more anxiety, naturally leading to avoidance of the thoughts in different ways. Higher religiosity/spirituality and magical ideation scores have been associated with increased obsessive-compulsive traits (Koenig et al., 1993).

Other possible areas of interest can be values in societies and gender roles. In many cultures, one of the parents, usually the mother, is considered to have a greater responsibility for the upbringing of children. The mother more often stays at home. For a person suffering from OCD, staying at home with a child may, on the one hand, lead to more opportunities for exposure, resulting in fewer problems with OCD but, on the other, to more stress, exacerbating the OCD.

Other important areas to consider are quality of available healthcare, especially when it comes to maternal and psychiatric healthcare. How society sees mental illness in the perinatal period might play a great role in this. Cultural explanations of psychiatric disorders differ and could possibly affect the onset, course, assessment, and treatment, of OCD in perinatal women.

Clara lives in one of the Nordic European countries, where expectations are for both parents to take equal interest and responsibility in bringing their children up but also for both parents to remain connected to their workplace and most certainly go back to work after a limited amount of time. Normally, parental leave is paid for by the state for the first 15 months of the child's life. Clara and David had earlier decided that Clara was to stay at home for the first eight months of Alba's life and then David for five months before Alba was to go to nursery during the workdays. Unfortunately, when OCD struck, the plans changed. Instead, both Clara and David stayed at home for six months together, Clara on sick leave, and David taking care of both her and the baby. After that time, David has worked part time. Clara has now quit her job as she deems herself unfit to look after other people's children as she cannot take care of her own.

Clara's parents had reared Clara to be a self-sufficient person who values her education and profession. The parents and most of Clara's other relatives and friends pressure her to go back to work. Clara's doctor and other healthcare professionals that she has met during the first year and a half of Alba's life often bring up the fact that Clara chose not to breastfeed after three weeks despite their message that breastfeeding is the best option for children in general, and for some reason they seem to think, for Alba in particular. Before Clara entered treatment, she felt more and more stressed and sad when she thought about her failure as a mother, but also as a professional, leading to more anxiety, less sleep, and most certainly more obsessions and compulsions. Thus, the interplay between the tone of Clara's family culture and her experience of societal expectations for work and child care presents an ongoing challenge.

Conclusion and Future Directions

Postpartum OCD is OCD that develops after the delivery of the baby. It is very common for intrusive thoughts to arise in new mothers and often also in fathers, involving the infliction of harm on the baby. If avoidance behavior and compulsive behaviors arise, there is a risk that the new parent develops OCD, which is a highly debilitating disorder for the patient and highly impacting on those around them. Fortunately, there is effective psychosocial treatment in ERP, as long as the problems are correctly diagnosed and there are qualified professionals available.

Many areas of perinatal OCD are understudied. There is for instance a scarcity of studies about cultural differences in perinatal OCD. In Western countries, there is evidence for OCD that includes worry about harming the child particularly in women during the perinatal period and also in new fathers. The knowledge of whether this is true in other cultural contexts could improve psychoeducation for pregnant women and their partners.

In many countries around the world, there is a shortage of CBT clinicians. Furthermore, not all CBT clinicians specialize in OCD. The diagnosis of OCD can be complex when it comes to conducting functional analyses of obsessions and compulsions, especially when several dimensions/subtypes are present. ERP is sometimes difficult to conduct practically, as many of the problematic situations are outside the clinic, and there might be rules preventing the clinician from conducting therapy outside their workplace or other difficulties such as lack of time to travel between the office and the patient's home. Sometimes, quite a few sessions are needed for good results, and relatives have to attend and also take an active part in treatment, or at least discontinue their accommodating behavior. Therefore, it might be difficult to find evidence-based psychotherapy for OCD.

One way to partly solve the scarcity of effective treatment is prevention. Further investigating how psychoeducation in and by itself can affect the prevalence of perinatal OCD would be highly interesting. Psychoeducation in CBT often includes knowledge of intrusive thoughts, their escalation during the perinatal period, and the CBT model of OCD. This could be delivered by many different professions, giving more patients the opportunity to see a clinician and hopefully preventing the development of OCD. It has also been reasoned that if perinatal care providers and policy makers, as well as new parents, are presented with evidence-based information to respond appropriately to these types of thoughts, it could be less frightening for parents to seek treatment (Collardeau et al., 2019; Fairbrother et al., 2022).

Another remedy to the lack of available clinicians is to condense treatment, and there are many interesting intensive programs available around the globe, some of them residential. For instance, Norwegian professor Gerd Kvale and her team have condensed ERP treatment into a four-day intensive model (Hansen et al., 2018). Family-based intensive treatments could be an interesting area of future research, where the family plus other significant persons in the patient's life attend (Abramowitz et al., 2013).

More research is necessary on what happens *after* successful treatment of perinatal OCD. In the clinic, we see many success stories when it comes to reducing anxiety, compulsions, and fear of the obsessions in which patients return to their life pre-OCD without too much difficulty. But, for some, relief from OCD does not make their quality of life much better. They might have lost several years otherwise spent on educating themselves, starting relationships, spending time with their children, taking part in different activities, and even if, in theory, they have the possibility to do so after treatment, some do not. Many feel sad or depressed they lost all that time, or they feel shame that they are so inexperienced in areas relative to their age or guilt toward their children. The development of some type of post-ERP-back-to-life intervention, over a longer period of time, could be a possible solution.

Finally, the consequences of the pandemic on the prevalence and presentation of OCD and other anxiety disorders will soon be seen in clinical practice. Mixed results have already been published as some studies report an elevation of anxiety and depression symptoms in pregnant women during the pandemic compared to before (Lebel et al., 2020; Pereira et al., 2022) and some do not (Uguz et al., 2022). More studies are on their way and will prepare patients, families, and clinicians for similar events in the future.

References

Abramowitz, J. S., Baucom, D. H., Wheaton, M. G., Boeding, S., Fabricant, L. E., Paprocki, C., & Fisher, M. S. (2013). Enhancing exposure and response prevention for OCD: A couple-based approach. *Behaviour Modification*, 37, 189–210.

Abramowitz, J. S., Deacon, B. J., Olatunji, B. O., Wheaton, M. G., Berman, N. C., Losardo, D., . . . Hale, L. R. (2010). Assessment of obsessive-compulsive symptom dimensions: Development and evaluation of the dimensional obsessive-compulsive scale. *Psychological Assessment*, 22(1), 180–198.

Abramowitz, J. S., Franklin, M. E., Schwartz, S. A., & Furr, J. M. (2003). Symptom presentation and outcome of cognitive-behavioural therapy for obsessive-compulsive disorder. *Journal of Consulting and Clinical Psychology*, 71(6), 1049–1057.

Abramowitz, J. S., & Jacoby, R. J. (2015). *Obsessive-compulsive disorder in adults: Advances in psychotherapy – Evidence-based practice*. Hogrefe Publishing.

Abramowitz, J. S., Khandker, M., Nelson, C. A., Deacon, B. J., & Rygwall, R. (2006). The role of cognitive factors in the pathogenesis of obsessive-compulsive symptoms: A prospective study. *Behaviour Research and Therapy, 44*(9), 1361–1374.

Abramowitz, J. S., Nelson, C. A., Rygwall, R., & Khandker, M. (2007). The cognitive mediation of obsessive-compulsive symptoms: A longitudinal study. *Journal of Anxiety Disorders, 21*(1), 91–104.

Allison, K. C., Wenzel, A., Kleiman, K., & Sarwer, D. B. (2011). Development of a brief measure of postpartum distress. *Journal of Women's Health, 20*(4), 617–623.

Amir, N., Freshman, M., & Foa, E. B. (2000). Family distress and involvement in relatives of obsessive-compulsive disorder patients. *Journal of Anxiety Disorders, 14*(3), 209–217.

Arch, J. J. (2014). Cognitive behavioural therapy and pharmacotherapy for anxiety: Treatment preferences and credibility among pregnant and non-pregnant women. *Behaviour Research and Therapy, 52*(1), 53–60.

Barret, R., Wroe, A. L., & Challacombe, F. L. (2016). Context is everything: An investigation of responsibility beliefs and interpretations and the relationship with obsessive-compulsive symptomatology across the perinatal period. *Behavioural and Cognitive Psychotherapy, 44*(3), 318–330.

Boeding, S. E., Paprocki, C. M., Baucom, D. H., Abramowitz, J. S., Wheaton, M. G., Fabricant, L. E., & Fischer, M. S. (2013). Let me check that for you: Symptom accommodation in romantic partners of adults with obsessive compulsive disorder. *Behaviour Research and Therapy, 51*(6), 316–322.

Brakoulias, V., Viswasam, K., Dwyer, A., Raine, K. H., & Starcevic, V. (2020). Advances in the pharmacological management of obsessive-compulsive disorder in the postpartum period. *Expert Opinion on Pharmacotherapy, 21*(2), 163–165.

Brand, S. R., & Brennan, P. A. (2009). Impact of antenatal and postpartum maternal mental illness: How are the children? *Clinical Obstetrics and Gynaecology, 52*(3), 441–455.

Brander, G., Rydell, M., Kuja-Halkola, R., Fernández de la Cruz, L., Lichtenstein, P., Serlachius, E., . . . Mataix-Cols, D. (2016). Association of perinatal risk factors with obsessive-compulsive disorder: A population-based birth cohort, sibling control study. *JAMA Psychiatry, 73*(11), 1135–1144.

Brandes, M., Soares, C. N., & Cohen, L. S. (2004). Postpartum onset obsessive-compulsive disorder: Diagnosis and management. *Archives of Women's Mental Health, 7*(2), 99–110.

Calvocoressi, L., Lewis, B., Harris, M., Trufan, S. J., Goodman, W. K., McDougle, C. J., & Price, L. H. (1995). Family accommodation in obsessive-compulsive disorder. *The American Journal of Psychiatry, 152*(3), 441–443.

Calvocoressi, L., Mazure, C., Kasl, S. V., Skolnick, J., Fisk, D., Vegso, S. J., . . . Price, L. H. (1999). Family accommodation of obsessive-compulsive symptoms: Instrument development and assessment of family behaviour. *Journal of Nervous and Mental Disease, 187*, 636–642.

Caporino, N. E., Morgan, J., Beckstead, J., Phares, V., Murphy, T. K., & Storch, E. A. (2012). A structural equation analysis of family accommodation in pediatric obsessive-compulsive disorder. *Journal of Abnormal Child Psychology, 40*(1), 133–143.

Cervin, M., Miguel, E. C., Güler, A. S., Ferrão, Y. A., Erdoğdu, A. B., Lazaro, L., . . . Mataix-Cols, D. (2021). Towards a definitive symptom structure of obsessive-compulsive disorder: A factor and network analysis of 87 distinct symptoms in 1366 individuals. *Psychological Medicine, 52*(14), 3267–3279.

Challacombe, F. L., & Salkovskis, P. M. (2011). Intensive cognitive-behavioural treatment for women with postnatal obsessive-compulsive disorder: A consecutive case series. *Behaviour Research and Therapy, 49*, 422–426.

Challacombe, F. L., Salkovskis, P. M., Woolgar, M., Wilkinson, E. L., Read, J., & Acheson, R. (2016). Parenting and mother-infant interactions in the context of maternal postpartum obsessive-compulsive disorder: Effects of obsessional symptoms and mood. *Infant Behavior and Development, 44*, 11–20.

Challacombe, F. L., Salkovskis, P. M., Woolgar, M., Wilkinson, E. L., Read, J., & Acheson, R. (2017). A pilot randomized controlled trial of time-intensive cognitive – Behaviour therapy for postpartum obsessive – Compulsive disorder: Effects on maternal symptoms, mother-infant interactions and attachment. *Psychological Medicine, 47*(8), 1478–1488.

Challacombe, F. L., & Wroe, A. L. (2013). A hidden problem: Consequences of the misdiagnosis of perinatal obsessive-compulsive disorder. *British Journal of General Practice, 63*(610), 275–276.

Chambless, D. L., & Steketee, G. (1999). Expressed emotion and behavior therapy outcome: A prospective study with obsessive-compulsive and agoraphobic outpatients. *Journal of Consulting and Clinical Psychology, 67*(5), 658–665.

Collardeau, F., Corbyn, B., Abramowitz, J. S., Janssen, P. A., Woody, S., & Fairbrother, N. (2019). Maternal unwanted and intrusive thoughts of infant-related harm, obsessive-compulsive disorder and depression in the perinatal period: Study protocol. *BMC Psychiatry, 21, 19*(1), 94.

Cox, J. L., Chapman, G., Murray, D., & Jones, P. (1996). Validation of the Edinburgh Postnatal Depression Scale (EPDS) in non-postnatal women. *Journal of Affective Disorders, 39*(3), 185–189.

Craske, M., Treanor, M., Conway, C., Zbozinek, T., & Vervliet, B. (2014). Optimizing inhibitory learning during exposure therapy. *Behaviour Research and Therapy, 46*(1), 5–27.

Crino, R. D., & Andrews, G. (1996). Obsessive-compulsive disorder and axis I comorbidity. *Journal of Anxiety Disorders, 10*(1), 37–46.

Eddy, K. T., Dutra. L., Bradley, R., & Westen, D. (2004). A multidimensional meta-analysis of psychotherapy and pharmacotherapy for obsessive-compulsive disorder. *Clinical Psychology Review, 24*, 1011–1030.

Fairbrother, N., & Abramowitz, J. (2007). New parenthood as a risk factor for the development of obsessional problems. *Behaviour Research and Therapy, 45*(9), 2155–2163.

Fairbrother, N., Albert, A., Keeney, C., Tchir, D., & Cameron, R. B. (2023). Screening for perinatal OCD: A comparison of the DOCS and the EPDS. *Assessment, 30*(4), 1028–1039.

Fairbrother, N., Barr, R. G., Chen, M., Riar, S., Miller, E., Brant, R., & Ma, A. (2019). Prepartum and postpartum mothers' and fathers' unwanted, intrusive thoughts in response to infant crying. *Behavioural and Cognitive Psychotherapy, 47*(2), 129–147.

Fairbrother, N., Collardeau, F., Albert, A., Challacombe, F. L., Thordarson, D. S., Woody, S. R., & Janssen, P. A. (2021). High prevalence and incidence of obsessive-compulsive disorder among women across pregnancy and the postpartum. *Journal of Clinical Psychiatry, 82*(2).

Fairbrother, N., Collardeau, F., Woody, S. R., Wolfe, D. A., & Fawcett, J. M. (2022). Postpartum thoughts of infant-related harm and obsessive-compulsive disorder: Relation to maternal physical aggression toward the infant. *The Journal of Clinical Psychiatry, 83*(2).

Fairbrother, N., Janssen, P., Antony, M. M., Tucker, E., & Young, A. H. (2016). Perinatal anxiety disorder prevalence and incidence. *Journal of Affective Disorders, 200*, 148–155.

Fairbrother, N., Thordarson, D. S., Challacombe, F. L., & Sakaluk, J. K. (2018). Correlates and predictors of new mothers' responses to postpartum thoughts of accidental and intentional harm and obsessive compulsive symptoms. *Behavioural and Cognitive Psychotherapy, 46*(4), 437–453.

Fairbrother, N., & Woody, S. R. (2008). New mothers' thoughts of harm related to the newborn. *Archives of Women's Mental Health, 11*(3), 221–229.

Fawcett, E. J., Power, H., & Fawcett, J. M. (2020). Women are at greater risk of OCD than men: A meta-analytic review of OCD prevalence worldwide. *Journal of Clinical Psychiatry, 81*(4).

Fernández de la Cruz, L., Joseph, K. S., Wen, Q., Stephansson, O., Mataix-Cols, D., & Razaz, N. (2023). Pregnancy, delivery, and neonatal outcomes associated with maternal obsessive-compulsive disorder: Two cohort studies in Sweden and British Columbia, Canada. *JAMA Network Open, 6*(6).

Ferrando, C., & Selai, C. (2021). A systematic review and meta-analysis on the effectiveness of exposure and response prevention therapy in the treatment of obsessive-compulsive disorder. *Journal of Obsessive-Compulsive and Related Disorders, 83*(2).

Foa, E., Yadin, E., & Lichner, T. K. (2012). *Exposure and response (ritual) prevention for obsessive compulsive disorder.* Oxford University Press.

Fontenelle, L. F., Mendlowicz, M. V., Marques, C., & Versiani, M. (2004). Trans-cultural aspects of obsessive-compulsive disorder: A description of a Brazilian sample and a systematic review of international clinical studies. *Journal of Psychiatric Research, 8*(4), 403–411.

Goodman, W. K., Price, L. H., Rasmussen, S. A., Mazure, C., Delgado, P., Heninger, G. R., & Charney, D. S. (1989b). The Yale-Brown Obsessive Compulsive Scale: II validity. *Archives of General Psychiatry, 46*, 1012–1016.

Goodman, W. K., Price, L. H., Rasmussen, S. A., Mazure, C., Fleischmann, R., Hill, C. L., . . . Charney, D. S. (1989a). The Yale-Brown Obsessive-Compulsive Scale I: Development, use, and reliability. *Archives of General Psychiatry, 46*, 1006–1011.

Greist, J. H., Jefferson, J. W., Kobak, K. A., Katzelnick, D. J., & Serlin, R. C. (1995). Efficacy and tolerability of serotonin transport inhibitors in obsessive-compulsive disorder: A meta-analysis. *Archives of General Psychiatry, 52*(1), 53–60.

Guglielmi, V., Vulink, N. C. C., Denys, D., Wang, Y., Samuels, J. F., & Nestadt, G. (2014). Obsessive-compulsive disorder and female reproductive cycle events: Results from the OCD and reproduction collaborative study. *Depression and Anxiety, 31*(12), 979–987.

Hansen, B., Kvale, G., Hagen, K., Havnen, A., & Öst, L. G. (2018). The Bergen 4-day treatment for OCD: Four years follow-up of concentrated ERP in a clinical mental health setting. *Cognitive Behaviour Therapy*, 48(2), 89–105.

Hezel, A. M., & McNally, R. J. (2016). A Theoretical review of cognitive biases and deficits in obsessive-compulsive disorder. *Biological Psychology*, 121(Pt B), 221–232.

Horwath, E., & Weissman, M. M. (2000). The epidemiology and cross-national presentation of obsessive-compulsive disorder. *Psychiatric Clinics of North America*, 23, 493–507.

House, S. J., Tripathi, S. P., Knight, B. J., Morris, N., Newport., D. J., & Stowe, Z. N. (2016). Obsessive-compulsive disorder in pregnancy and the postpartum period: Course of illness and obstetrical outcome. *Archives of Women's Mental Health*, 19(1), 3–10.

Hudepohl, N., MacLean, J. V., & Osborne, L. M. (2022). Perinatal obsessive-compulsive disorder: Epidemiology, phenomenology, etiology, and treatment. *Current Psychiatry Reports*, 24(4), 229–237.

International Obsessive Compulsive Disorder Foundation Genetics Collaborative (IOCDF-GC), & OCD Collaborative Genetics Association Studies (OCGAS). (2018). Revealing the complex genetic architecture of obsessive-compulsive disorder using meta-analysis. *Molecular Psychiatry*, 23, 1181–1188.

Jacobson, N. S., Martell, C. R., & Dimidjian, S. (2001). Behavioral activation treatment for depression: Returning to contextual roots. *Clinical Psychology: Science and Practice*, 8, 255–270.

Jorm, A. F. (2015). Using the Delphi expert consensus method in mental health research. *Australian and New Zealand Journal of Psychiatry*, 49(10), 887–897.

Kaminsky, Z. A., Osborne, L. M., Guglielmi, V., Jones, I., Grenier, W., Clark, K., . . . Nestadt, G. (2020). Postpartum depression biomarkers predict exacerbation of OCD symptoms during pregnancy. *Psychiatry Research*, 293, 113332.

Koenig, H. G., Ford, S. M., George, L. K., Blazer, D. G., & Meador, K. G. (1993). Religion and anxiety disorder: An examination and comparison of associations in young, middle-aged, and elderly adults. *Journal of Anxiety Disorders*, 7, 321–342.

Källén, B. (2007). The safety of antidepressant drugs during pregnancy. *Expert Opinion on Drug Safety*, 6(4), 357–370.

Lanza di Scalea, T., & Wisner, K. L. (2009). Antidepressant medication use during breastfeeding. *Clinical Obstetrics and Gynaecology*, 52(3), 483–497.

Lebel, C., MacKinnon, A., Bagshawe, M., Tomfohr-Madsen, L., & Giesbrecht, G. (2020). Elevated depression and anxiety symptoms among pregnant individuals during the COVID-19 pandemic. *Journal of Affective Disorders*, 277, 5–13.

Lord, C., Rieder, A., Hall, G. B., Soares, C. N., & Steiner, M. (2011). Piloting the Perinatal Obsessive-Compulsive Scale (POCS): Development and validation. *Journal of Anxiety Disorders*, 25(8), 1079–1084.

Martini, J., Petzoldt, J., Einsle, F., Beesdo-Baum, K., Höfler, M., & Wittchen, H. U. (2015). Risk factors and course patterns of anxiety and depressive disorders during pregnancy and after delivery: A prospective-longitudinal study. *Journal of Affective Disorders*, 175, 385–395.

Mataix-Cols, D., Rosario-Campos, M. C., & Leckman, J. F. (2005). A multidimensional model of obsessive-compulsive disorder. *American Journal of Psychiatry*, 162, 228–238.

Mattheisen, M., Samuels, J. F., Wang, Y., Greenberg, B. D., Fyer, A. J., McCracken, J. T, . . . Nestadt, G. (2015). Genome-wide association study in obsessive-compulsive disorder: Results from the OCGAS. *Molecular Psychiatry*, 20(3), 337–344.

McGuinness, M., Blissett, J., & Jones, C. (2011). OCD in the perinatal period: Is postpartum OCD (ppOCD) a distinct subtype? A review of the literature. *Behavioural and Cognitive Psychotherapy*, 5(39), 3.

Miller, M. L., Roche, A. I., Lemon, E., & O'Hara, M. W. (2022). Obsessive-compulsive and related disorder symptoms in the perinatal period: Prevalence and associations with postpartum functioning. *Archives of Women's Mental Health*, 25(4), 771–780.

Moritz, S., Meier, B., Kloss, M., Jacobsen, D., Wein, C., Fricke, S., & Hand, I. (2002). Dimensional structure of the Yale-Brown Obsessive-Compulsive Scale (Y-BOCS). *Psychiatry Research*, 109(2), 193–199.

Mowrer, O. H. (1947). On the dual nature of learning – A reinterpretation of "conditioning" and "problem-solving". *Harvard Education Review*, 17, 102–148.

Mulcahy, M., Long, C., Morrow, T., Galbally, M., Rees, C., & Anderson, R. (2023). Consensus recommendations for the assessment and treatment of perinatal Obsessive-Compulsive Disorder (OCD): A Delphi study. *Archives of Women's Mental Health*, 26(3), 389–399.

Najmi, S., Riemann, B., & Wegner, D. (2009). Managing unwanted intrusive thoughts in obsessive-compulsive disorder: Relative effectiveness of suppression, focused distraction and acceptance. *Behaviour Research and Therapy, 47*(6), 494–503.

Nicolini, H., Salin-Pascual, R., Cabrera, B., & Lanzagorta, N. (2017). Influence of culture in obsessive-compulsive disorder and its treatment. *Current Psychiatry Reviews, 13*(4), 285–292.

Noh, H. J., Tang, R., Flannick, J., O'Dushlaine, C., Swofford, R., Howrigan, D., . . . Lindblad-Toh, K. (2017). Integrating evolutionary and regulatory information with a multispecies approach implicates genes and pathways in obsessive-compulsive disorder. *Nature Communications, 8*(1), 774.

OCCWG, Obsessive Compulsive Cognitive Work Group. (1997). Cognitive assessment of obsessive-compulsive disorder. *Behaviour Research and Therapy, 35*(7), 667–681.

OCCWG, Obsessive Compulsive Cognitive Work Group. (2001). Development and initial validation of the obsessive beliefs' questionnaire and the interpretation of intrusions inventory. *Behaviour Research and Therapy, 39*, 987–1006.

OCCWG, Obsessive Compulsive Cognitive Work Group. (2003). Psychometric validation of the obsessive beliefs questionnaire and the interpretation of intrusions inventory: Part 1. *Behaviour Research and Therapy, 41*, 863–878.

OCCWG, Obsessive Compulsive Cognitive Work Group. (2005). Psychometric validation of the obsessive belief questionnaire and interpretation of intrusions inventory: Part 2: Factor analyses and testing of a brief version. *Behaviour Research and Therapy, 43*, 1527–1542.

Osnes, R. S., Roaldset, J. O., Follestad, T., & Eberhard-Gran, M. (2019). Insomnia late in pregnancy is associated with perinatal anxiety: A longitudinal cohort study. *Journal of Affective Disorders, 248*, 155–165.

Öst, L.-G., Havnen, A., Hansen, B., & Kvale, G. (2015). Cognitive behavioural treatments of obsessive – Compulsive disorder: A systematic review and meta-analysis of studies published 1993–2014. *Clinical Psychology Review, 40*, 156–169.

Pauls, D. L., Abramovitch, A., Rauch, S. L., & Geller, D. A. (2014). Obsessive-compulsive disorder: An integrative genetic and neurobiological perspective. *Nature Reviews Neuroscience, 15*(6), 410–424.

Pearlstein, T., Zlotnick, C., Battle, C., Stuart, S., O'Hara, M. W., Price, A. B., Grause, M. A., & Howard, M. (2006). Patient choice of treatment for postpartum depression: A pilot study. *Archives of Women's Mental Health, 9*, 303–308.

Pereira, D., Wildenberg, B., Gaspar, A., Cabaços, C., Madeira, N., Macedo, A., & Pereira, A. T. (2022). The impact of COVID-19 on anxious and depressive symptomatology in the postpartum period. *International Journal of Environmental Research and Public Health, 19*(13), 7833.

Rachman, S., & De Silva, P. (1978). Abnormal and normal obsessions. *Behaviour Research and Therapy, 16*(4), 233–248.

Renshaw, K. D., Chambless, D. L., & Steketee, G. (2003). Perceived criticism predicts severity of anxiety symptoms after behavioral treatment in patients with obsessive-compulsive disorder and panic disorder with agoraphobia. *Journal of Clinical Psychology, 59*(4), 411–421.

Rosario-Campos, M. C., Miguel, E. C., Quatrano, S., Chacon, P., Ferrao, Y., Findley, D., . . . Leckman, J. F. (2006). The Dimensional Yale-Brown Obsessive-Compulsive Scale (DY-BOCS): An instrument for assessing obsessive-compulsive symptom dimensions. *Molecular Psychiatry, 11*(5), 495–504.

Ruscio, A. M., Stein, D. J., Chiu, W. T., & Kessler, R. C. (2010). The epidemiology of obsessive-compulsive disorder in the national comorbidity survey replication. *Molecular Psychiatry, 15*, 53–63.

Russell, E. J., Fawcett, J. M., & Mazmanian, D. (2013). Risk of obsessive-compulsive disorder in pregnant and postpartum women: A meta-analysis. *Journal of Clinical Psychiatry, 74*(4), 377–385.

Salkovskis, P. M. (1985). Obsessional-compulsive problems: A cognitive-behavioural analysis. *Behaviour Research and Therapy, 23*, 571–583.

Salkovskis, P. M. (1996). The cognitive approach to anxiety: Threat beliefs, safety seeking behaviour, and the special case of health anxiety and obsessions. In P. M. Salkovskis (Ed.), *Frontiers of cognitive therapy* (pp. 48–74). Guilford.

Sheehy, O., Zhao, J., & Bérard, A. (2019). Association between incident exposure to benzodiazepines in early pregnancy and risk of spontaneous abortion. *JAMA Psychiatry, 76*(9), 948–957.

Shyken, J. M., Babbar, S., Babbar, S., & Forinash, A. (2019). Benzodiazepines in pregnancy. *Clinical Obstetrics and Gynecology, 62*(1), 156–167.

Speisman, B. B., Storch, E. A., & Abramowitz, J. S. (2011). Postpartum obsessive-compulsive disorder. *Journal of Obstetric, Gynecologic and Neonatal Nursing, 40*(6), 680–690.

Starcevic, V., Eslick, G. D., Viswasam, K., & Berle, D. (2020). Symptoms of obsessive-compulsive disorder during pregnancy and the postpartum period: A systematic review and meta-analysis. *Psychiatric Quarterly, 91*, 965–981.

Storch, E. A., Benito, K., & Goodman, W. (2011). Assessment scales for obsessive-compulsive disorder. *Neuropsychiatry, 1*(3), 243–250.

Storch, E. A., De Nadai, A. S., do Rosário, M. C., Shavitt, R. G., Torres, A. R., Ferrão, Y. A., . . . Fontenelle, L. F. (2015). Defining clinical severity in adults with obsessive-compulsive disorder. *Comprehensive Psychiatry, 63*, 30–35.

Storch, E. A., Geffken, G. R., Merlo, L. J., Jacob, M. L., Murphy, T. K., & Goodman, W. K. (2007). Family accommodation in pediatric obsessive-compulsive disorder. *Journal of Clinical Child and Adolescent Psychology, 36*(2), 207–216.

Ter Horst, P. G. J., van der Linde, S., Smit, J. P., den Boon, J., van Lingen, R. A., Jansman, F. G. A., . . . Wilffert, B. (2012). Clomipramine concentration and withdrawal symptoms in 10 neonates. *British Journal of Clinical Pharmacology, 73*, 295–302.

Thiséus, C. J., Perrin, S., & Cervin, M. (2019). Intrusive thoughts and compulsive behaviours in postpartum women: Psychometric properties of the parental thoughts and behaviours checklist. *Psychiatry Research, 278*, 194–198.

Thompson-Hollands, J., Abramovitch, A., Tompson, M. C., & Barlow, D. H. (2015). A randomized clinical trial of a brief family intervention to reduce accommodation in obsessive-compulsive disorder: A preliminary study. *Behavior Therapy, 46*(2), 218–229.

Timpano, K. R., Abramowitz, J. S., Mahaffey, B. L., Mitchell, M. A., & Schmidt, N. B. (2011). Efficacy of a prevention program for postpartum obsessive – Compulsive symptoms. *Journal of Psychiatric Research, 45*(11), 1511–1517.

Uguz, F., Kirkas, A., Yalvac, T., Gundogan, K. M., & Gezginc, K. (2022). Is there a higher prevalence of mood and anxiety disorders among pregnant women during the COVID-19 pandemic? A comparative study. *Journal of Psychosomatic Research, 155*.

Van Balkom, A., van Oppen, P., Vermeulen, A., van Dyck, R., Nauta, M., & Vorst, H. (1994). A meta-analysis on the treatment of obsessive compulsive disorder: A comparison of antidepressants, behaviour, and cognitive therapy. *Clinical Psychology Review, 14*(5), 359–381.

Van Noppen, B., Sassano-Higgins, S., Appasani, R., & Sapp, F. (2021). Cognitive-behavioral therapy for obsessive-compulsive disorder: 2021 update. *Focus (American Psychiatry Publishings), 19*(4), 430–443.

Van Noppen, B., & Steketee, G. (2009). Testing a conceptual model of patient and family predictors of Obsessive Compulsive Disorder (OCD) symptoms. *Behaviour Research and Therapy, 47*(1), 18–25.

Vasconcelos, M. S., Sampaio, A. S., Hounie, A. G., Akkerman, F., Curi, M., Lopes, A. C., & Miguel, E. C. (2007). Prenatal, perinatal, and postnatal risk factors in obsessive-compulsive disorder. *Biological Psychiatry, 61*(3), 301–307.

Wegner, D. M. (1994). *White bears and other unwanted thoughts: Suppression, obsession and the psychology of mental control.* Guilford Press.

Woody, C. A., Ferrari, A. J., Siskind, D. J., Whiteford, H. A., & Harris, M. G. (2017). A systematic review and meta-regression of the prevalence and incidence of perinatal depression. *Journal of Affective Disorders, 219*, 86–92.

Woody, S. R., Steketee, G., & Chambless, D. L. (1995). Reliability and validity of the Yale-Brown Obsessive-Compulsive Scale. *Behaviour Research and Therapy, 33*(5), 597–605.

15

CHILDBIRTH-RELATED POST-TRAUMATIC STRESS DISORDER

Sharon Dekel, Sabrina J. Chan, and Kathleen M. Jagodnik

Over the course of their lifetime, each person will experience, on average, at least one significant traumatic event (Watkins et al., 2018). Post-traumatic stress disorder (PTSD) is the common psychopathology associated with exposure to such an event. According to the American Psychiatric Association's *Diagnostic and Statistical Manual of Mental Disorders*, 5th edition (DSM-5) (2013), this event could entail a personal experience of actual or threatened death, serious injury, or sexual violence, or could involve witnessing such an event. Four clusters of symptoms characterize PTSD: trauma-specific intrusive psychological or physiological phenomena, such as recurrent involuntary memories or distressing dreams of the trauma, and pronounced physiological reactions to cues related to the event; habitual avoidance of reminders of the trauma; negative alterations in cognition and mood, such as negative beliefs about oneself and the world, and feelings of detachment, guilt, and shame; and alterations in arousal and reactivity such as hypervigilance and sleep disturbances. For diagnosis, symptoms are required to endure for more than one month and cause significant distress or impaired functioning. In the general community, the lifetime incidence of PTSD is estimated to be 8.3% (Watkins et al., 2018).

Each year, about 140 million women give birth worldwide. Although childbirth is often regarded as a positive experience, about one-third of these women have a highly stressful birth experience (Dekel et al., 2017). Among them, a significant subset will proceed to develop a form of PTSD resulting from a childbirth-related traumatic experience; this is termed childbirth-related PTSD (CB-PTSD) (Dekel et al., 2017). This disorder can occur in at-term deliveries with healthy infants, and it is not limited to pregnancy loss or prematurity (Chan et al., 2020). Although evidence supports the validity of a PTSD condition triggered by childbirth (Dekel et al., 2017; Horesh et al., 2021; Lai et al., 2022), there is no formal recognition of PTSD with postpartum onset in the DSM-5. The traumatic elements of childbirth commonly pertain to objective aspects, namely, medical complications/interventions, in which there is danger to the woman's life or her newborn. However, beyond physical morbidity, other nonmedical elements can contribute to a woman's traumatic appraisal of childbirth. These factors will be described in the section on risk factors and correlates of CB-PTSD.

CB-PTSD is highly comorbid with postpartum depression (PPD) symptoms (Dekel et al., 2020). Co-occurrence of symptoms is generally manifested in increased functional

DOI: 10.4324/9781003206903-19

impairment, symptom burden, and medical costs, compared with each condition experienced separately. Although CB-PTSD includes dysphoric symptoms such as diminished interest in pleasurable activities, its core symptoms are trauma-specific. The strong comorbidity of CB-PTSD and PPD may result in underdiagnosis or misdiagnosis of CB-PTSD. Another common comorbidity of CB-PTSD is mother-to-infant bonding impairment (Chan et al., 2020; Mayopoulos et al., 2021), with such bonding impairment being a common feature of CB-PTSD, beyond the DSM-5 symptoms of general PTSD (Dekel, Thiel, et al., 2019). This impaired bonding is described in detail in the section on the effects of CB-PTSD on family relationships.

CB-PTSD is characterized by both physiological and psychological manifestations (Chan et al., 2020, 2022; Thiel & Dekel, 2020; Thiel et al., 2018). In a task involving mental imagery of their traumatic childbirth experiences, women with CB-PTSD demonstrated higher response in heart rate and skin conductance than women without this disorder (Chan et al., 2022). The heightened physiological responsivity in CB-PTSD is similar to abnormalities observed in combat veterans in response to war imagery. These findings offer strong validation for CB-PTSD as a condition triggered by traumatic childbirth. Pilot evidence also shows neural alterations in fear processing involving amygdalar hyper-responsivity in women with CB-PTSD (Berman et al., 2020). This again underscores that concrete biological abnormalities characterize CB-PTSD.

CB-PTSD can become an enduring maternal mental health disorder in the first postpartum month (Dikmen-Yildiz et al., 2018). Sleep deprivation and insomnia, in part related to infant care, are documented as important factors that contribute to the persistence of CB-PTSD symptoms. Limited social support and prior trauma are additional factors that can maintain this disorder (Garthus-Niegel et al., 2015). It is also hypothesized that frequent contact with the infant, involving re-exposure to a cue representing the traumatic event, may trigger maternal distress and maintain CB-PTSD symptoms.

The patient, a White-Hispanic 41-year-old woman at the time of the first interview, endorsed symptoms of CB-PTSD after delivering her first child, a male, five years previously. At the time of delivery, the patient had been living in the United States for approximately two years, having immigrated from another country. She was married and working at a prestigious university as a postdoctoral fellow in physics. Despite some concerns regarding her career path and difficulties involving living in a new country, her pregnancy was planned and described by the patient as "very good." There were no obstetric complications. She had no concerns about the forthcoming delivery, and she reported that her mood was good; she was physically active; and she had a strong social support system during her pregnancy. The patient and her husband attended weekly group meetings with a doula in preparation for childbirth. She developed a written birth plan that she provided to medical staff at the hospital, detailing her wish for a birth as natural as possible.

The stressful peripartum experience began at the end of her pregnancy. During her weekly routine perinatal visit at week 37, medical staff repeatedly pressured her to undergo an induced delivery, as they had concerns about the growth of her fetus. She was instructed to visit the Labor and Delivery (L&D) Unit "just to see the room," and upon arrival, it was suggested that she undergo induction immediately. She eventually refused, and she was asked to sign a consent form, in which she documented that she understood the risk of choosing to go home. Her decision was based on her significant research about the risks involved in induction.

At the end of her weekly doctor's visit at 39 weeks' gestation, after two weeks of negotiation, she recalls having no energy remaining to argue against staff and "gave in" to having an induced delivery. Her birth plan was completely disregarded; that plan included a natural-as-possible delivery with no medication or interventions. Now admitted to L&D, she received the induction and then experienced contractions for several hours. The medical staff subsequently recommended an epidural, which again disregarded her birth plan. During this period, a nurse entered her room to check the heart rate of the fetus. The nurse could not locate the heartbeat, and their concern was clear to the patient; at least six medical staff subsequently rushed into her room. The patient was fitted with an oxygen mask while medical staff continued to search for the heartbeat, and she recalls feeling extremely stressed and thinking "the baby's gone." Following this crisis situation, her contractions suddenly stopped completely, which the doctor attributed to the high-stress situation that had just occurred. With labor stopped for several hours, the medical team returned and recommended a Cesarean delivery. She felt as if she had no option but to agree: they informed her that she could not stay in the hospital room since she was not in labor, but she could not return home since her baby's life would be endangered. Heading into the operating room while significantly deprived of sleep, the patient felt sad, defeated, and fearful.

Prevalence

In the general population of women who recently underwent childbirth, ~3% to 6% are estimated to suffer from full CB-PTSD in the first postpartum months (Dekel et al., 2017). This translates to a conservative rate of approximately 4.2 million affected women per year globally. This number may not reflect the relatively high rates of CB-PTSD occurrence in certain childbirth-related situations. These data are derived from mean values of women who may or may not have had a traumatic childbirth; consequently, averaged statistics that do not stratify women into categories should be interpreted with caution. Systematic reviews show that ~15% to 18+% of high-risk women, such as those with medically complicated delivery, will develop CB-PTSD (Dekel et al., 2017). Among women who undergo unplanned Cesarean section, ~20% are likely to suffer from CB-PTSD. Additionally, most research on CB-PTSD is conducted on samples of women giving birth in the Western world; limited knowledge exists about the prevalence of CB-PTSD in other regions.

An important distinction involves differentiating women who have PTSD from another trauma unrelated to childbirth from women who develop CB-PTSD as the result of a traumatic childbirth (Dekel et al., 2017). Pre-existing PTSD has been associated with severe postpartum maternal morbidity (Duval et al., 2022). Because this involves trauma unrelated to childbirth, it should be considered a general PTSD condition that may impact how the mother copes in the postpartum period. Of women with CB-PTSD, ~20% had PTSD due to prior trauma, but ~80% did not (Dekel et al., 2020). Therefore, in the majority of cases, CB-PTSD represents a new-onset trauma-related psychopathology triggered by childbirth.

Beyond fully diagnosed cases of CB-PTSD, subclinical cases that involve symptoms not meeting the threshold for formal diagnosis, yet causing significant impairment, should be considered. Around 25% of women who delivered a healthy baby at term will show clinically significant levels of CB-PTSD symptoms without meeting diagnostic criteria (Dekel et al., 2017). These cases are usually not captured in reports of the disorder's prevalence, but they represent a population of women significantly impaired by their distress levels.

As is often the case for maternal mental health conditions, women tend to underreport their symptoms. A common barrier to diagnosis and treatment of postpartum mental illness is women's reluctance to disclose their feelings and symptoms (Dennis & Chung-Lee, 2006). This may be due to stigma and shame (Vigod & Dennis, 2020), or fear of being separated from their infant. Women tend not to seek medical help (Dennis & Chung-Lee, 2006), suggesting that many cases are simply not identified. For these reasons, perinatal mental health disorders are often underdiagnosed or undiagnosed, and undertreated or untreated (Vigod & Dennis, 2020). Although no study has specifically examined rates of disclosure of CB-PTSD, survivors of trauma with PTSD tend to keep their experiences private (Bedard-Gilligan et al., 2012), and in the context of societal expectation of childbirth being a happy event, this may further hinder patient reporting of CB-PTSD.

Current knowledge of CB-PTSD prevalence is heavily based on the patient's self-report of their symptoms using questionnaires; this may limit capturing the full magnitude of the rates of this disorder. Research using formal clinical diagnosis assessment is limited, and objective biomarkers to inform accurate identification of patients remain to be discovered. This raises the challenge that reporting may not be standardized and can vary by the individual respondent, depending on their education level and cultural background, as well as their willingness to disclose their symptoms. Furthermore, prevalence rates are heavily based on the first postpartum month. Data involving longer timeframes will be required to understand how CB-PTSD develops and persists over time, subsequently guiding the timing for assessment and intervention.

Risk Factors and Correlates

Understanding risk factors for the development of CB-PTSD can guide the early identification of women at risk and may serve as the first step in implementing treatment before the condition fully develops. Existing research reveals a range of factors associated with CB-PTSD development, as well as its reinforcement and maintenance. To date, however, models to inform the early stratification of at-risk women based on risk factors remain lacking, as does the classification of necessary and sufficient causal factors. Information about risk factors is often derived from retrospective assessments. This section classifies the factors associated with the development of CB-PTSD to include prenatal, peripartum, and postpartum factors.

Prenatal Factors

Distal factors related to demographics, previous trauma, and mental health status may contribute to CB-PTSD development. Demographic risk factors include young age and low income (Chan et al., 2020). As in general PTSD, trauma history is strongly associated with CB-PTSD (O'Donovan et al., 2014). Trauma in relation to prior pregnancy and/or childbirth, including stillbirth, prematurity, and postpartum hemorrhage (Sentilhes et al., 2017), as well as exposure to lifetime traumatic events, mainly sexual assault, may increase CB-PTSD risk (Chan et al., 2020; Dekel et al., 2017). Endorsement of mental disorders prior to childbirth (Khsim et al., 2022), and in particular PTSD involving another trauma, can make the mother more susceptible to developing CB-PTSD compared with women without a history of mental health disorders, including PTSD (Dekel et al., 2017). An important factor is the role of race and ethnicity, as is described later in the chapter.

Proximal risk factors have also been identified in understanding CB-PTSD. Prenatal stress due to significant fear of forthcoming childbirth is strongly associated with subsequent CB-PTSD (O'Donovan et al., 2014). Other nonspecific risk factors related to adverse postpartum mental outcomes include depression in pregnancy and limited social support (Khsim et al., 2022). Evidence also suggests having an unplanned pregnancy is a risk factor (Andersen et al., 2012).

Peripartum Factors

Peripartum factors pertain to the time period shortly before, during, and immediately after giving birth. These factors mainly entail the elements that may make childbirth a traumatic experience, and therefore, some may serve as causal risk factors (Dekel et al., 2017). In the following subsections, we review the objective, subjective, and environmental factors involving childbirth that increase the risk for CB-PTSD. In general PTSD, it is arguable that factors during and immediately after trauma exposure have a stronger effect than pre-trauma factors (Brewin et al., 2000).

Objective Factors

Severe maternal morbidity (SMM), which involves an actual threat to the woman's life, places a delivering woman at heightened risk for CB-PTSD (Duval et al., 2022). In the most severe cases, obstetric complications, including hemorrhaging and puerperal sepsis, as well as maternal hypertension, may result in maternal near-miss (MNM), which involves nearly escaping death.

Obstetric interventions during labor may further increase the traumatic nature of childbirth; this pertains primarily to the method of delivery (Khsim et al., 2022). Unplanned/emergency Cesarean delivery, which is performed to prevent maternal morbidity and mortality, is associated with a threefold increase in probable CB-PTSD, controlling for obstetric and infant medical complications (Dekel, Ein-Dor et al., 2019). With rates of Cesarean procedures exceeding the World Health Organization's (WHO's) recommended rate of 10% to 15% (World Health Organization, 2023) in numerous global regions (Boerma et al., 2018), many delivering women may be at risk for psychiatric morbidity. The use of medication for labor induction, as well as prolonged birth and sleep deprivation before giving birth, have also been associated with CB-PTSD (Chan et al., 2020).

Medical complications in infant health are an important factor that can strongly contribute to the overall traumatic experience of childbirth and increase the risk for CB-PTSD in the context of a complicated delivery (Grekin & O'Hara, 2014). Women with newborns who had medical complications, often resulting in neonatal intensive care unit (NICU) admission, are nearly twice as likely to report probable CB-PTSD than women with infants who did not have medical complications (Chan et al., 2020).

Beyond infant medical complications, CB-PTSD has been associated with a lack of skin-to-skin and rooming-in contact (Chan et al., 2020; Mayopoulos et al., 2021). Reduced maternal bonding behaviors may also indicate early signs of CB-PTSD in which the woman is avoiding cues of the trauma. Whether these bonding behaviors should be promoted following traumatic childbirth to support infant and mother health is unclear.

Subjective Factors

The negative appraisal and immediate negative emotional response to childbirth strongly reflect the subjective impact of trauma on the individual. For many women undergoing birth trauma, there is a critical discrepancy between their birth plan and expectations, and their actual experience (Khsim et al., 2022). Unsurprisingly, the subjective elements of traumatic childbirth, rather than objective factors, appear as a more salient predictor of CB-PTSD (Chan et al., 2020; Dekel et al., 2017). Subjective emotional distress at a clinical level in L&D has been repeatedly linked with subsequent CB-PTSD (Andersen et al., 2012; Mayopoulos et al., 2021). A sense of helplessness and lack of control, dissociative response to childbirth, and high levels of perceived pain during L&D are also reported as risk factors (Chan et al., 2020; Dekel et al., 2017).

Environmental Factors

Environmental factors represent aspects of the childbirth experience that do not relate to obstetrical factors or related psychological distress. For example, women's interactions with medical staff can influence their perceptions of the childbirth event (Grekin & O'Hara, 2014). Perceived low support from medical staff during childbirth and perceived poor quality of medical care are associated with CB-PTSD (Stramrood & Slade, 2017). During the COVID-19 pandemic, hospitals implemented visitation restrictions, which resulted in lack of a support person in childbirth and potentially increased the traumatic experience of childbirth and CB-PTSD (Mayopoulos et al., 2021).

Postpartum Factors

Postpartum factors influence not only the development of CB-PTSD but also its severity and persistence. Psychological factors that may contribute to the development of CB-PTSD include intrusive and negative birth memories (James, 2015), as well as negative post-traumatic cognitions (e.g., persistent negative emotional state involving feelings of guilt, shame, anger, or fear; exaggerated negative beliefs about oneself, others, or the world) (Dekel et al., 2017). How trauma is remembered is a factor that can maintain CB-PTSD: women endorsing CB-PTSD symptoms tend to provide childbirth narratives characterized by less coherent childbirth memories and use more sensory and emotional details than narratives provided by women without CB-PTSD (Thiel et al., 2021). These narratives are characterized by fewer positive emotions and more cognitive descriptions (characterized by using words such as "know," "cause," and "ought"). Negative cognitive coping styles including self-blame and rumination have been associated with CB-PTSD, as was a perception that social resources (e.g., support by family and friends) had been lost (Tomsis et al., 2018).

A central factor contributing to CB-PTSD persistence and severity involves the newborn's health. NICU admission has been consistently shown to increase the mother's risk for CB-PTSD (Chan et al., 2020). Another infant-related factor associated with CB-PTSD concerns breastfeeding: lack of exclusive breastfeeding not explained by infant medical complications (Chan et al., 2020) is common in mothers with CB-PTSD (Mayopoulos et al., 2021). Similar to reduced immediate bonding behaviors, this may represent early signs of the disorder and its complications. Additionally, because a mother experiencing CB-PTSD may re-experience the trauma via repeated exposure to stimuli that remind her of the traumatic childbirth experience, such as interactions with her infant, these environmental factors may complicate her recovery process. Furthermore, the demands of infant care that may cause sleep deprivation and insomnia are important factors contributing to the persistence of CB-PTSD symptoms.

There remains a critical gap in knowledge of physiological risk and other biological factors associated with CB-PTSD and its development. Excessive blood loss may increase CB-PTSD risk in women following vaginal delivery (Sentilhes et al., 2017). Heightened physiological reactivity to the childbirth memory may serve not only as a manifestation of CB-PTSD, but an early sign of the disorder before the full syndrome develops (Chan et al., 2022). It remains to be examined whether alterations in hypothalamic–pituitary–adrenal axis reactivity (Pitman et al., 2012) in general PTSD and the oxytocinergic system (Rashidi et al., 2022), as well as inflammatory processes, and other systems and processes, may play a critical role in CB-PTSD development.

Protective Factors

Research on the protective factors against CB-PTSD is lacking. Social support in the perinatal period is often associated with positive postpartum outcomes in general, particularly with respect to the mother having a reliable social alliance (Milgrom et al., 2019). Being psychologically prepared for birth, having a birth plan, and use of a midwifery team, may contribute to more positive childbirth experiences (Hernández-Martínez et al., 2020). Experiences of traumatic childbirth that eventually result in the endorsement of *post-traumatic psychological growth*, in which a woman develops a stronger appreciation of her life and a sense of strength and connections with others, are also associated with psychological benefits and may protect against CB-PTSD development (Babu et al., 2022; Berman et al., 2021). Additionally, accumulating studies in nonpostpartum samples show that physical exercise can improve mood and reduce stress (Hearing et al., 2016), and may therefore support postpartum adjustment.

As a Hispanic woman who immigrated to the United States, the patient's demographic factors may have contributed to psychological vulnerability, despite having a strong social support system and high educational level. Her physiological risk factors included a significant lack of sleep: before her Cesarean, the patient had around an hour of sleep the previous night. Although she reports no prior mental health problems or family history of mental health disorders, she reports an uncomfortable sexual experience in the past. She also experienced a prior abortion. Despite an otherwise healthy pregnancy, the patient was considered medically high-risk due to her age of 36 years.

At the patient's 37-week routine obstetrical appointment, induction was recommended based on the ultrasound's measurement of the fetus's size. She did not think this was the right decision, as her pregnancy had been going well, and she and her husband decided to wait.

Nevertheless, she was sent to the delivery floor to obtain more information, where she was admitted into a room for the induction. The patient describes that this possible miscommunication "felt like a trap." She returned home against medical advice.

The following week, the ultrasound measurement was deemed normal, but induction was still recommended due to a problem with the amniotic fluid. The patient reports that the medical staff emphasized that her baby was at risk and that "the baby could die tonight" because she was refusing the induction. After two more weeks of feeling pressured by the staff, she agreed to be induced for labor.

Her planned vaginal delivery with no medication was substituted with an unplanned Cesarean section with local anesthesia, to which she warily agreed. Although her baby boy was born at term and healthy, his glucose levels had dropped. The patient reports that the medical staff were paying attention to her, but less to the baby, and he may have simply become cold. Her baby had to have multiple blood draws, which was difficult for her to watch. While the baby stayed in the room with the patient and her husband, she felt exhausted and was briefly taken to the sensitive care unit.

Contributing to the development of her CB-PTSD symptoms may have included the loss of control she felt as her birth plan was repeatedly disregarded; her elevated emotional distress; the objectively stressful event of undergoing an unplanned Cesarean surgery, in the context of her body being prepared for a vaginal delivery (via induction); significant sleep deprivation; and the alarming concern related to her infant's health.

The patient experienced ongoing challenges in the postpartum period. Ten days postpartum, she experienced chest pain and difficulty breathing. The doctor in the urgent care center immediately suspected pulmonary embolism, a complication from the Cesarean section, and she was sent immediately in an ambulance to the hospital. She stayed one night with her baby and was treated with medication before being discharged and subsequently monitored daily by a nurse at home. During the interview, the patient recalls feeling extremely exhausted during the postpartum period, and she was chronically deprived of sleep from waking up each night to breastfeed her baby.

Effects of CB-PTSD on Family Relationships

Maternal CB-PTSD develops in temporal proximity to childbirth and during a critical time for the formation of mother–infant attachment and the child's growth. It may also affect the mother's other children and her intimate partner. This section reviews the literature on the effects of CB-PTSD on familial relationships.

Effects on the Infant

Daily positive interactions between mother and infant are instrumental for healthy child social emotional development (Shorey et al., 2021). Among the core behavioral symptoms of CB-PTSD are avoidance and hypervigilance, which may interfere with the mother's ability to engage in healthy interactions during a period when the welfare of the child is highly dependent on the caregiver. This suggests that CB-PTSD can impair the mother–infant dyad (Ionio & Di Blasio, 2014; Van Sieleghem et al., 2022).

Knowledge about the impact of CB-PTSD on the developing infant remains limited. A body of research does show that CB-PTSD can adversely influence the formation of mother–infant bonding (Dekel, Thiel, et al., 2019; Ionio & Di Blasio, 2014; Mayopoulos et al., 2021), and these impairments may remain enduring across the first postpartum year (Kjerulff et al., 2021). Early signs of bonding impairment are also often manifested in reduced immediate postpartum bonding behaviors known to support healthy child outcomes, such as skin-to-skin contact and exclusive breastfeeding (Chan et al., 2020). Furthermore, some evidence supports adverse effects of CB-PTSD on the child's temperament, behavior, and sleep habits. Because optimal child development is a salient predictor of adult offspring's mental health, more research that provides insight into CB-PTSD and child development, especially focusing on the underlying mechanisms of maternal psychopathology transmission, is warranted.

Effects on Other Children

Maternal psychopathology not specific to CB-PTSD during the postpartum period can adversely impact the cognitive, psychological, and behavioral development of other children raised by an affected mother (Ribaudo et al., 2022; Vänskä et al., 2011). For example, maternal major depressive disorder is associated with infant withdrawal behaviors at six months postpartum (Burtchen et al., 2022). Additionally, longitudinal data show that mothers who developed PTSD due to interpersonal violence and had an elevated *Clinician-Administered PTSD Scale* (CAPS) (Blake et al., 1995) score when their child was toddler age had school-age children with increased risk of attention-deficit/hyperactivity disorder and PTSD (Glaus et al., 2021). Research in nonpostpartum samples indicates that PTSD resulting from non-childbirth trauma can result in cross-generational effects via both biological and behavioral mechanisms (Bowers & Yehuda, 2016). Children of mothers with PTSD are more likely to suffer from mental illness as adults than those with mothers without PTSD (Bowers & Yehuda, 2016). The unique adverse effects that CB-PTSD may have on other children in the family are unknown.

Effects on Intimate Partner Relationships

CB-PTSD may negatively affect the woman's relationship with her intimate partner (McKenzie-McHarg et al., 2015). Women with this disorder are likely to avoid sexual intimacy and may suffer from sexual dysfunction. They show reduced communication with their partner, increased negative emotions, and disagreement during interactions. Another significant potential complication is a fear of becoming pregnant again (Stramrood & Slade, 2017). Because of the strong association between CB-PTSD and symptoms of postpartum depression (Dekel et al., 2020), symptoms of depression may significantly account for the adversity of CB-PTSD in the couple's relationship (Garthus-Niegel et al., 2018).

In accordance with the DSM-5, PTSD can develop not only in those directly experiencing the traumatic event but also in individuals witnessing the trauma. Some data support the adverse effect of a traumatic childbirth experience on the father's mental health. Fathers, like mothers, may endorse symptoms of an acute stress reaction in response to childbirth (McKenzie-McHarg et al., 2015) and further develop enduring traumatic stress symptoms, although rates are relatively lower (Kress et al., 2021). Also, similarly to maternal CB-PTSD, paternal CB-PTSD is associated with complicated deliveries and negative birth experiences, as well as mental health problems before childbirth (Kress et al., 2021). Additional risk factors include low education, high job burden, and being a first-time father. Because of the important role of social support in successful postpartum adaptation, future research is warranted to examine how paternal CB-PTSD may adversely influence maternal CB-PTSD as well as child development (McKenzie-McHarg et al., 2015).

Although the patient engaged in skin-to-skin contact with her baby immediately after delivery, she reports difficulties bonding with her child in the subsequent weeks at home, partially due to feeling physically exhausted. She reports: "It took a while to feel connected." Her husband assumed many of the parenting activities. She recalls her husband's anxiety about their baby, to the point where she deemed his behavior concerning. This was surprising to her, as her husband had wanted to have a child. She recalls that since the time of childbirth, he became angry and verbally aggressive. The two never discussed what had happened during the birth, and the patient's husband most likely never knew the impact of the stressful birth experience on his wife. She recalls that the childbirth experience and parenting clearly exacerbated the existing stress and discord in their relationship, and the couple divorced four years later. The patient and her now ex-husband share joint custody of the child, although their relationship remains tense.

Assessment

Over the past years, screening for postpartum mental health has been integrated into routine perinatal care in the United States and other Western countries. This screening assesses symptoms of peripartum depression and is typically performed using the *Edinburgh Postnatal Depression Scale* (Cox & Holden, 2003). Although recommendations exist for a full psychological well-being assessment during postpartum visits (American College of Obstetricians and Gynecologists (ACOG), 2018), no screening for CB-PTSD is performed in routine care, and no standard recommended screening protocol exists. Currently, no biomarkers for CB-PTSD exist that could be developed into screening tools. This section reviews potential measures to guide CB-PTSD screening in the clinic.

Instruments for CB-PTSD Measurement

To date, various instruments have been used in research to assess CB-PTSD (Dekel et al., 2017; O'Carroll et al., 2024), with no single instrument considered as the recommended tool to be translated into the clinic. Although the gold-standard strategy to confirm CB-PTSD, similarly to general PTSD, is a clinician diagnostic interview, patient self-report instruments can serve as a first step in initial screening and offer feasible, low-cost protocols with low patient burden. Typically, the measures used for CB-PTSD assessment are PTSD symptom instruments validated in adult populations exposed to other, non-childbirth trauma. For CB-PTSD assessment, these measures are modified such that patients are asked to report their PTSD symptoms in relation to their childbirth. More recently, a questionnaire has been developed for the assessment of childbirth trauma, and its reliability has been confirmed in the postpartum population (Ayers et al., 2018).

The following is a selection of commonly used instruments to assess CB-PTSD. Refer to recent review papers (Dekel et al., 2017; O'Carroll et al., 2024; Williams, Strobino & Holliday, 2022) for a more comprehensive list of instruments for patient self-report. The following measures assess PTSD; these have been adopted for postpartum samples.

The *PTSD Checklist* (PCL) (Weathers et al., 1993) is the standard self-report measure for the assessment of provisional PTSD recommended by the U.S. Department of Veterans Affairs (VA). Its most current version is the PCL-5 (Blevins et al., 2015), which lists the 20 DSM-5 PTSD symptoms and assesses their frequency over the past month. The PCL strongly corresponds with diagnostic measures. A review recommends that the PCL be used in postpartum populations (Cirino & Knapp, 2019). Recent studies show that the PCL-5 adapted to childbirth has high reliability (Dekel et al., 2020), and importantly, when assessing symptoms of CB-PTSD, this tool has strong predictive validity when compared with the gold-standard clinician diagnostic assessment for PTSD (*Clinician-Administered PTSD Scale for DSM-5* [CAPS-5]) (Arora et al., 2024) for informing accurate diagnosis of CB-PTSD following birth trauma.

The *Posttraumatic Diagnostic Scale* (PDS) (Foa, 1995), in its current version, the PDS-5 (Foa et al., 2016), is a 24-item self-report questionnaire based on the DSM-5 PTSD symptom criteria. It assesses symptoms severity and level of functioning over the past month. The PDS-5 showed good internal consistency, test-retest reliability, and convergent validity with other PTSD assessments in the general population (Foa et al., 2016), and has been used in partpartum samples (Roberts et al., 2022; Tasuji et al., 2020).

The *Impact of Event Scale* (IES) (Horowitz et al., 1979) is a 20-item self-report questionnaire assessing the intensity and frequency of PTSD symptoms over the past week. The updated version, the *Impact of Event Scale—Revised* (IES-R) (Weiss & Marmar, 1997), is a 22-item self-report questionnaire corresponding to the DSM-IV criteria. Both versions of this questionnaire have been used in postpartum samples (Ayers, 2001; Abdollahpour et al., 2016; De Schepper et al., 2016; Froeliger et al., 2022).

The *Posttraumatic Stress Disorder Questionnaire* (PTSD-Q) (Cross & McCanne, 2001) is another self-report measure used to assess CB-PTSD. It includes 17 items that accord with the PTSD Interview (PTSD-I) (Watson et al., 1991). This questionnaire has been used in numerous postpartum samples (Andersen et al., 2012; Williams, Strobino & Holliday, 2022).

Peripartum PTSD Measures

The *City Birth Trauma Scale* (City BiTS) was designed to assess symptoms of CB-PTSD over the past week (Ayers et al., 2018). Its 29 items cover the DSM-5 symptoms, as well as two items from the DSM-IV (criterion A2) measuring the subjective emotional reaction to childbirth (i.e., emotional numbing and feelings of intense fear, helplessness, or horror) through self-reporting. The instrument has strong reliability (Nakic Rados et al., 2020).

The *Perinatal Posttraumatic Stress Disorder Questionnaire* (PPQ) (Hynan, 1998) is a 14-item self-report instrument developed to identify PTSD symptoms over the past month in mothers with high-risk babies based on the DSM-III-R criteria. The current version, the PPQ-II (Callahan et al., 2006), accords with the DSM-IV-TR PTSD symptom criteria and assesses symptom severity. The reliability and validity of both of these questionnaires have been confirmed, compared against other questionnaires (Callahan & Hynan, 2002; Komurcu Akik & Durak Batigun, 2020; Zhang et al., 2018).

The *IES—German* (IES-G) (Stadlmayr et al., 2009) is adapted from the IES, and it specifically assesses childbirth-related PTSD symptoms six weeks postpartum. This 15-question instrument assesses CB-PTSD symptoms over the past week. Reliability of this scale has been confirmed (Sommerlad et al., 2021).

Additionally, a childbirth-specific version of the *Peritraumatic Distress Inventory* (PDI) questionnaire, which assesses acute distress response following trauma, can accurately detect women likely to develop CB-PTSD (Jagodnik et al., 2024).

Most recently, Bartal et al. (2023, 2024) used machine learning (ML) methods, which involve the use of statistical models to draw inferences from data, to analyze brief narratives generated by mothers, describing the most traumatic aspects of their childbirth experience. Their ML models, which employed Natural Language Processing, achieved good accuracy in identifying women with CB-PTSD using only the childbirth narratives as the data source. The advantage of using these narratives as a data source is that they can be efficiently and inexpensively collected during the early postpartum period, while the new mother remains under medical supervision.

Diagnostic Assessment

The CAPS (Blake et al., 1995) is the gold standard in PTSD (nonpostpartum) assessment. It is a clinician rating scale used to confirm both current and lifetime PTSD diagnosis. Its most current version, adapted to the DSM-5 criteria, is the CAPS-5 (Weathers et al., 2018). It assesses symptom severity and frequency in regard to a specific trauma, levels of overall distress, and impaired functioning, as well as PTSD with specifiers (e.g., dissociative symptoms and delayed reaction). The CAPS-5 has strong psychometric properties (Weathers et al., 2018), and symptoms severity correlates strongly with scores on the PCL-5. The CAPS and CAPS-5 have been used in postpartum samples to assess CB-PTSD (Burtchen et al., 2022; van Steijn et al., 2021), although due to their resource-intensive nature, their use is rare in research studies (Vesel & Nickasch, 2015; Zaat et al., 2018).

Physiological Assessment

To date, no biomarkers for CB-PTSD have been identified that have been implemented in clinical settings. A pioneering study reports heightened heart rate and skin conductance in women with CB-PTSD in response to childbirth recollection (Chan et al., 2022). Neuroimaging research on CB-PTSD is currently being conducted using functional magnetic resonance imaging (fMRI) to characterize the impact of traumatic childbirth on the maternal brain, and possibly reveal unique abnormalities of CB-PTSD differentiating it from postpartum depression or other forms of PTSD (Berman et al., 2020). Once better characterized, these physiological characteristics will assist in improving the accuracy of CB-PTSD diagnosis in the future.

Timeframes of CB-PTSD Assessment

Early symptoms of CB-PTSD can appear in the days and weeks following childbirth. This suggests that early screening for CB-PTSD symptoms is recommended to identify women at risk of developing CB-PTSD before the condition fully develops. Assessing symptoms of emotional distress in the acute period following childbirth-related trauma via the PDI tool is an accurate strategy for identifying women likely to develop CB-PTSD (Jagodnik et al., 2024). Based on the DSM-5, the duration of the disturbance is required to be more than one month to confirm diagnosis. Additionally, screening women who are likely to endorse chronic CB-PTSD would aid in allocating resources to this risk group. Some evidence suggests that symptoms of CB-PTSD remain enduring (Dikmen-Yildiz et al., 2018), and a better characterization of the CB-PTSD symptom trajectory may inform the timing for screening.

Challenges of Postpartum Assessment

Numerous challenges exist when conducting postpartum mental health screening. Many women do not attend follow-up postpartum doctor visits (ACOG, 2018), making it difficult to identify women who may benefit from treatment. A significant portion of affected postpartum women avoid seeking treatment or underreport their symptoms; in general, <40% of women with perinatal mental health challenges seek professional medical help (Daehn et al., 2022). Perinatal women have cited knowledge-related, structural, and attitudinal barriers to seeking help (Daehn et al., 2022); women with CB-PTSD often feel shame and guilt, and avoid talking about their traumatic childbirth. *Knowledge-related barriers* involve a lack of knowledge required to identify relevant symptoms of perinatal mental health problems. Educational campaigns to inform perinatal women, clinicians, and the public are needed to overcome these challenges. *Structural barriers* include the cost of treatments and the inability to attend appointments due to challenges including transportation, childcare, time constraints, and unavailability of medical providers. *Attitudinal barriers* include the fact that some women want to avoid a label of mental illness; affected women often report not seeking help due to feelings of shame or embarrassment. Others may fear being separated from their infant if they report a mental health problem. More broadly, societal stigma has been suggested as a factor preventing women from seeking mental health-related treatment (Daehn et al., 2022).

Upon returning to work after three months away, the patient recalls simply trying "to survive [each] day," not even considering the idea that the events she experienced could possibly be traumatic. This belief, as well as lack of awareness, are barriers to the diagnosis and treatment of CB-PTSD.

At approximately five years postpartum, the patient's CB-PTSD symptoms based on PCL-5 assessment were associated with a score of 50, suggesting symptoms at a clinical level warranting further assessment. She reported "extremely" for the following symptoms: having strong negative beliefs about yourself, other people, or the world; having strong negative feelings such as fear, horror, anger, guilt, or shame; loss of interest in activities that you used to enjoy; feeling distant or cut off from other people; irritable behavior, angry outbursts, or acting aggressively; feeling jumpy or easily startled; having difficulty concentrating; and trouble falling asleep. A positive PTSD screen was confirmed in the assessment six months later, using the CAPS-5.

Like many other women, the patient was reluctant to report her symptoms, seek treatment, or discuss her experience. For many years, the patient avoided talking with friends and family about the events that had unfolded, trying her best to avoid the memories despite their constant presence in her mind. During routine pediatric and postpartum visits, her mental health issues were never discussed. These medical visits provided only general recommendations about the importance of taking care of oneself, but no assessment of psychological distress.

Treatment

This section reviews the available treatment options for CB-PTSD, including psychotherapies, pharmacotherapies, and other interventions. It also includes research studies on early interventions to potentially prevent CB-PTSD. Although maternal psychopathologies are the most common complication of childbirth, the majority of postpartum women do not receive the necessary treatment to achieve recovery (Vigod & Dennis, 2020). Due to the numerous challenges described in the previous sections, including the lack of routine screening for CB-PTSD and women's hesitance to seek medical help, CB-PTSD remains an underdiagnosed and undertreated psychiatric morbidity. Society-wide changes will be needed to address these problems, including recognition of birth-related traumatic stress, as well as continuing efforts to destigmatize mental health problems and encourage those affected to seek treatment.

Based on guidelines from the U.S. Department of Veterans Affairs (VA) (2017), trauma-focused psychotherapy (TFPT) should be considered as the first-line treatment for PTSD before pharmacotherapies. In general, psychotherapies are more time-intensive than drugs, but they avoid the side effects common in psychiatric medications (Bryant, 2019). Nursing mothers may be concerned about medication transmission to the infant via breastmilk. For this and other reasons, postpartum women often prefer psychological interventions over medications (Battle et al., 2013).

Psychotherapies

Trauma-focused psychotherapy (TFPT) is the most frequently recommended treatment for PTSD (Bryant, 2019; Watkins et al., 2018). This class of interventions involves reprocessing of and exposure to the traumatic memory. Among them, first-line trauma-focused cognitive behavioral therapies (CBTs) include a series of structured interventions involving Prolonged Exposure (PE) or Cognitive Processing Therapy (CPT). These therapies have been shown to ease symptoms of non-postpartum PTSD (Bisson & Olff, 2021). PE involves *in vivo* and imaginal exposure to the trauma and emotional processing to extinguish the fear response. CPT mainly targets maladaptive trauma-related thoughts to establish a new understanding of the trauma. Evidence also exists for the benefit of using another TFPT, Eye Movement Desensitization and Reprocessing (EMDR). This is also a structured intervention involving multiple sessions in which the trauma memory is processed during bilateral stimulation of the eyes, similar to REM sleep, and is thought to decrease the physiological and psychological intensity of the memory. Additionally, Expressive Writing (EW) is a strategy that may be useful in treating CB-PTSD, although evidence remains very preliminary (Slade et al., 2021).

Knowledge remains limited about the efficacy of psychotherapeutic treatments for PTSD in postpartum women, as applied to CB-PTSD (Furuta et al., 2018). A small number of randomized clinical trials (RCTs) (to date, 26 RCTs) are available (reviewed in Dekel et al., 2024; Furuta et al., 2018; Shorey et al., 2021; Slade et al., 2021; Taylor Miller et al., 2021). Early studies focused on individual counseling therapies and debriefing, showing mixed results. More recent work includes TFPT interventions (Furuta et al., 2018), as described earlier. Although TFPT treatments, as noted regarding non-postpartum samples, appear promising and acceptable for treating CB-PTSD by reducing CB-PTSD symptoms, more studies are needed to fully determine the utility of these interventions. Beyond treating the mother, herself, four RCTs to date have tested interventions involving mother–infant interactions, with some trials showing benefits, and others showing no effects (Dekel et al., 2024).

Future work should ensure the use of statistically meaningful sample sizes, assess long-term outcomes, include mechanistic biomarkers to complement the standard patient self-report questionnaires commonly used, and identify the key time window following childbirth that would optimize treatment (Dekel et al., 2024). Systematic reviews of treatment studies are available in the literature (Furuta et al., 2018; Shorey et al., 2021; Slade et al., 2021; Taylor Miller et al., 2021).

Pharmacotherapies

Pharmacotherapies are often used as a second-line treatment for general PTSD for those who have not benefited from psychotherapy, to whom psychotherapy is not available, or for those who prefer not to engage in psychotherapy (Cirino & Knapp, 2019). Pharmacological treatments offer the advantage of requiring far less time and effort by the patient, compared with psychotherapy. However, medications typically have smaller effect sizes than psychotherapeutic interventions and are often associated with adverse effects, and relapse upon discontinuing the medication is a concern (Bryant, 2019). Antidepressant selective serotonin reuptake inhibitors (SSRIs) are the most commonly prescribed medications to treat PTSD and are supported by moderate-certainty evidence (Williams, Phillips et al., 2022). Only two drugs, both SSRIs, have been approved by the U.S. Food and Drug Administration to treat PTSD: sertraline and paroxetine. As mentioned earlier, concerns about medications being transmitted from mother to infant via breastmilk is a significant concern to many women (Battle et al., 2013), and often results in women opting for non-pharmacological treatments. To date, the benefit of pharmacological interventions for CB-PTSD remains unknown (Cirino & Knapp, 2019; Dekel et al., 2024).

Secondary (Preventive) Interventions for CB-PTSD

Because of the biological underpinnings of PTSD, early intervention following trauma exposure may avert the trajectory of PTSD (Taylor Miller et al., 2021). The early postpartum window offers a unique opportunity for preventing CB-PTSD if a traumatic childbirth experience has occurred. In the case of other forms of trauma, it is often not possible to identify individuals at risk, due to the unpredictable nature of most forms of trauma. In contrast, when considering early interventions for CB-PTSD, women could be identified and offered treatment during their maternity hospitalization stay. This window of time to intervene is critical, because many women do not attend their postpartum appointments (ACOG, 2018).

Currently, there is no recommended protocol for secondary preventive interventions (i.e., intervention delivered after traumatic exposure) for CB-PTSD (de Graaff et al., 2018; Taylor Miller et al., 2021), and existing research on secondary preventive intervention for CB-PTSD that uses RCTs is limited. Nevertheless, existing studies support the acceptability of interventions delivered by a midwife or clinician at the time around L&D, in the first days following childbirth during maternity hospitalization stay, or in the first postpartum weeks. As described next, these interventions include trauma-focused CBT, individual counseling, and EMDR (Taylor Miller et al., 2021). Evidence suggests that these interventions are more helpful than standard clinical care. The interventions appear more promising when delivered to at-risk women, defined as those reporting early symptoms of acute stress and/or in the context of complicated deliveries, than as a universal approach. Brief trauma-focused psychotherapies (CBT and EMDR) as well as EW about traumatic childbirth have been associated with symptom reduction. Published research about secondary prevention strategies also supports at a preliminary level individual counseling, and interventions to promote mother–infant bonding. At present, insufficient empirical data exist to strongly recommend a first-line treatment of choice, and whether the effects of these therapies endure for the long term remains to be studied (Furuta et al., 2018; Taylor Miller et al., 2021). Psychological debriefing involves an unstructured intervention to normalize acute psychological responses; it does not appear to be helpful in reducing acute postpartum stress responses (Bastos et al., 2015). Psychoeducation provided to women following birth trauma is insufficient as a standalone approach, but it could be considered in addition to the interventions listed earlier.

Women in labor who receive continuous, one-on-one support from another person throughout the peripartum period have significantly more positive experiences, and have clinically meaningful benefits for themselves and their infants, compared with women who did not receive this type of support (Hodnett et al., 2011). Additionally, with the goal of preventing traumatic childbirth experiences, interventions that can modify various aspects of commonly cited risk factors for developing CB-PTSD, such as pain during labor and negative interactions with medical staff, should be further researched and implemented.

The patient endorsed enduring symptoms of CB-PTSD but did not seek treatment for her condition. Her recognition of the impact of her traumatic childbirth on her mental health became more apparent in the context of psychological therapy that she sought during the process of divorce five years after giving birth. The patient engaged in weekly insight-oriented eclectic individual psychotherapy for three years and reports benefiting from it. Through revisiting her birth experience, and thoughts and perceptions regarding her self-esteem, she was able to acknowledge the various traumatic aspects of her experience, her sense of helplessness stemming from needing to "give in" and follow the recommendation of the medical staff, as well as her sense of strength and enhanced sense of meaning related to motherhood. This reflects manifestations of post-traumatic growth. It also became important to her to share her story with others and educate people. She shared her birth trauma experience in an educational event open to the public. Overall, her symptoms were not impairing her functioning; she maintained a steady professional job and an active social life, and she was strongly attached to her son and showed many signs of maternal sensitivity in her ability to parent him. At the same time, however, she continued to endorse short-lived emotional and physiological stress when reminded of her childbirth experience. She presented intermittently with dysphoric mood, problems with sleep, and a tendency toward withdrawal, which in part may reflect her emotional struggle following traumatic childbirth.

Cultural Considerations for CB-PTSD

Trauma-related psychological disorders are recognized and medically treated differently across cultures globally. The same applies to maternal psychiatric illness with respect to symptoms disclosure, seeking therapy, and type of therapy. To date, knowledge of cultural differences in CB-PTSD rates and symptoms manifestation is largely lacking. Research on low-resource regions of the world with high rates of maternal mortality is underway and may address a critical gap in our knowledge about CB-PTSD in developing countries.

Societal and Cultural Characteristics

Collectivist cultures tend to be characterized by tighter and more supportive social networks than individualistic cultures (Triandis et al., 1988), and cultures with high levels of social support may provide a buffer against post-traumatic stress symptoms (Zalta et al., 2021). In general, collectivist cultures are associated with increased well-being and less distress (Scott et al., 2004); at the same time, collectivist societies have also been associated with higher levels of stigma, compared with Western countries (Krendl & Pescosolido, 2020).

Societies also differ in their regard for and treatment of women, with some cultures holding women in a subordinate position. This could influence whether women are likely to report postpartum mental health challenges; whether these women's concerns are taken seriously by healthcare providers; and which forms of treatment are available. As mentioned previously, women may be dissuaded from seeking treatment due to the common societal stigma involving maternal mental illness (Vigod & Dennis, 2020). Furthermore, a woman's religious culture and beliefs can shape her attitudes toward maternal mental illness and her willingness to seek treatment.

Medical Aspects of Culture

As described previously, MNM occurs when a woman experiences life-threatening complications during or following pregnancy and childbirth. MNM, which entails severe maternal (physical) morbidity (SMM), is strongly linked to the development of CB-PTSD. Hemorrhage and hypertensive disorders are among the leading causes of SMM globally. Consistent with rates of maternal mortality, the rates of SMM are significantly higher in low- and middle-income countries than in high-income countries (Geller et al., 2018). Strategies to prevent SMM are expected not only to reduce cases of maternal death but also to improve the mental health of mothers and the well-being of their infants.

The unplanned Cesarean section procedure increases threefold the risk of developing CB-PTSD, even when obstetric and infant medical complications are controlled for (Dekel, Ein-Dor et al., 2019). Although this procedure is performed to support optimal birth outcomes, the rates in different regions sometimes critically exceed the proposed acceptable rates of 10% to 15% advised by the WHO (World Health Organization, 2023). More research is needed to examine across cultures the extent to which medical obstetrical interventions are performed, and their role in CB-PTSD development.

Minorities

In the United States, marginalized racial and ethnic minority women are almost three times more likely to endorse acute childbirth-related stress and are therefore at increased risk for CB-PTSD (Iyengar et al., 2022). The prevalence of maternal traumatic stress, as well as postpartum depression, is disproportionally higher in Black women when compared with White women, and is not explained by background factors, prior trauma history, or prior mental health. Of the ~4 million women who give birth in the United States annually, ~15% are Black, and these women experience maternal mortality and severe morbidity with at least double the rates of White women (Creanga et al., 2014).

A variety of factors may contribute to the increased risk of postpartum mental health disorders among marginalized minority women. The role of racial discrimination has been suggested to explain racial disparities in traumatic experiences of childbirth (Iyengar et al., 2022). Access to appropriate healthcare resources is often reduced for minority women. Additionally, the cultural stigma against mental illness and lack of mental health literacy may increase the susceptibility to remaining untreated when experiencing mental health challenges (Beck, 2022).

Summary: Cultural Considerations for CB-PTSD

When the screening, diagnosis, and treatment of CB-PTSD are considered, cultural factors should be taken into account, as these may significantly impact a woman's risk of developing this disorder, as well as her likelihood of reporting her symptoms and receiving treatment. As symptom manifestations of general PTSD in Western culture may differ from those in non-Western cultures (Marsella, 2010), it is likely that these symptom expressions may extend to CB-PTSD; more research is needed to provide insight into these potential differences in CB-PTSD symptoms manifestation across cultures.

The patient is Hispanic and had immigrated to the United States two years prior to giving birth. She reports that if she were to have another child, she would choose not to deliver in the United States due to cultural differences, especially the American focus on medication and induced labor. According to the patient, the medical team's case for the urgent need for induction and the Cesarean section was not based on clear-cut evidence and followed a protocol and timeline based on the hospital's priorities rather than the patient's desires or needs. To the patient, the risks of the Cesarean section were minimized by the hospital staff, and the risks of waiting for labor to occur again were exaggerated because the medical staff were focused on the time-saving aspects of their proposed medical care instead of "letting [her] body have its natural time for things to go." She may have experienced inequities in her perinatal care due to her ethnic background, language barriers, and immigration status. Her sense of helplessness and tension with the treating team may have, in part, reflected her unfamiliarity with American culture.

Conclusion and Future Directions

This section summarizes key points from this chapter and provides suggestions for future research directions. Childbirth-related PTSD (CB-PTSD) is a psychiatric disorder triggered by experiencing a traumatic childbirth and/or associated proximal highly stressful events. It is a debilitating condition because symptoms develop in proximity to the birth of the child—during a time of pressing parenting demands—and the child may become a constant traumatic cue. These two factors may hinder recovery, affect maternal and infant welfare, and result in a condition of heavy societal costs.

Although over the past decade recognition of the broader spectrum of postpartum mental health conditions has increased, much work remains to inform the accurate identification of women at risk for CB-PTSD and the development of effective treatments and preventive strategies. The following section describes current gaps in knowledge about CB-PTSD and future directions for research to address these gaps.

Biological Mechanisms of CB-PTSD

Much remains to be understood about the biological basis of CB-PTSD. Presently, no biomarkers for this disorder are available. Current research is characterizing the physiological and neural mechanisms underlying this disorder, with the goal of revealing such markers to be implemented in the clinic. Biomarkers may inform screening, treatment choice, and even treatment response. Understanding the biological basis of CB-PTSD will aid in further distinguishing it from other postpartum psychopathologies (including postpartum depression) and also clarify the extent to which CB-PTSD resembles general PTSD or entails a distinct form of psychopathology. Because CB-PTSD may result in problems with maternal responsiveness to the infant, it is critical to understand the biological mechanisms of impairment in maternal attachment behavior; these are presently unknown.

Prediction of CB-PTSD

Although many distal and proximal factors have been identified as associated with CB-PTSD and may be considered risk factors, this has not yet yielded a highly accurate model for use in the clinic to detect CB-PTSD. The ability to forecast this disorder before it develops remains elusive. Because CB-PTSD entails multiple risk factors that interact, using advanced computational models that can efficiently identify trends in large datasets is a natural next step in research. Some efforts have entailed using existing information in patients' medical records to develop ML models for CB-PTSD diagnosis (Zafari et al., 2021). Alternatively, the use of rich information in patient reports of their childbirth experience may aid in the early identification of CB-PTSD. As described previously, ML methods including Natural Language Processing have been used to analyze brief maternal childbirth narratives describing the most traumatic aspects of their childbirth experience (Bartal et al., 2023, 2024).

To further improve the accuracy of ML models to assess risk for developing CB-PTSD, future work should integrate both electronic medical record data and other data sources, such as childbirth narratives, into these predictions. Once reliable ML models have been developed using data types accessible in clinical settings, these models could be expanded into commercial-grade software that can be made available to healthcare providers. This will facilitate a more consistent, standardized strategy for screening for CB-PTSD to complement subsequent clinician-based assessments.

Diagnosis of CB-PTSD

The formal definition of PTSD based on the DSM-5 does not include PTSD with a specifier of postpartum onset (Dekel, 2024). The common recognition of postpartum psychopathology pertains to mood and anxiety disorders, omitting the traumatic stress domain. More research is needed to determine whether CB-PTSD has distinctive features from general PTSD. The inclusion of CB-PTSD in the DSM would improve the diagnosis and treatment of CB-PTSD, and increase awareness about this condition for both patients and healthcare providers (Dekel, 2024).

Treatment of CB-PTSD

Beyond trauma-focused psychotherapies and the use of antidepressants, alternative treatment strategies are being tested for general PTSD and remain to be studied for postpartum women endorsing CB-PTSD. "Mind–body" or "person-centered" strategies include mindfulness, metacognitive therapy, and yoga. Mindfulness therapy involves focusing attention on the present moment in a nonjudgmental way (Lang, 2017). Metacognitive therapies target worry, rumination, and threat-monitoring cognitive processes, rather than focusing on the traumatic memory (Brown et al., 2022). Some of these mind-body therapies have demonstrated moderate to large effect sizes for reducing general PTSD symptoms (Niles et al., 2018). Other treatment strategies that appear promising for non-postpartum individuals include transcranial magnetic stimulation, neurofeedback, and acupuncture (Bisson et al., 2020). Additionally, physical exercise is documented as a helpful adjunct treatment for PTSD (Björkman & Ekblom, 2022). Studies are needed to determine the utility and safety of novel nonpharmacological therapies for treating CB-PTSD.

A range of novel pharmacological therapies to treat PTSD in the general population continues to be studied; however, their efficacy, safety, and feasibility in the maternal postpartum population remains to be determined. This includes the consideration of whether the drug may be transmitted to the infant via breastmilk. The psychedelic drug MDMA has outperformed standard pharmacotherapies in early trials (Bisson & Olff, 2021). Cannabis and synthetic cannabinoids may be promising for improving PTSD symptoms, including reducing anxiety, improving sleep, and modulating memory processes. Novel pharmacotherapies that target cannabinoid, cholinergic, neuropeptide, glutamate, GABA, and monoamine systems are currently being developed and tested in the general population. Promising pharmacological agents to treat PTSD include cannabidiol, ketamine, pregnenolone and allopregnanolone, dronabinol, and brexanolone, as well as the psychedelic, psilocybin (Singewald et al., 2023).

Because CB-PTSD involves the mother–infant unit, future directions in treatment entail developing interventions to facilitate and support maternal sensitivity; to date, nonpharmacological interventions exist. The neuromodulator, oxytocin, influences social attachment and other aspects of social behavior and reduces fear memories (Rashidi et al., 2022). Intranasally administered oxytocin may have the potential to promote healthy mother–infant bonding after childbirth. More research is needed to understand the underlying biology of CB-PTSD to inform the development of pharmacological agents.

Secondary Interventions: Prevention of CB-PTSD

CB-PTSD is an excellent candidate for prevention because its symptoms develop following a specific event (childbirth) and during a period when women are treated as part of routine obstetric care. Research is ongoing to investigate a variety of secondary interventions to be administered in the hours and days following childbirth trauma to mitigate or prevent CB-PTSD development. Similar to general PTSD, interventions that are trauma-focused and work through exposure to and reprocessing of the traumatic memory appear potentially promising in reducing early symptoms of traumatic stress following childbirth; these include primarily CBT and EMDR. Other work supports the benefits of EW. Novel research has been conducted on interventions delivered during or even before childbirth. These include visual biofeedback and a visuospatial Tetris task (Dekel et al., 2024); the latter focuses on preventing traumatic memory consolidation. Nevertheless, RCTs to inform treatment recommendations remain limited in number. Future research is warranted to evaluate the long-term benefits of these and other interventions and to use biological assessments to inform the mechanisms of action.

When considering potential pharmacological prophylactic agents, moderate-certainty evidence supports a range of compounds, including hydrocortisone, propranolol, gabapentin, paroxetine, dexamethasone, 5-hydroxytryptophan, and omega-3 fatty acids (Bertolini et al., 2022) to prevent PTSD development. Prophylactic glucocorticoid-based therapies are supported by moderate-certainty evidence (Florido et al., 2023). The appropriateness of these treatments for the postpartum population remains to be studied.

In summary, most studies of therapies for general PTSD to date have not included postpartum women. Based on our survey of the published literature (Dekel et al., 2024), studies examining CB-PTSD interventions have largely involved psychological interventions, and none have involved pharmacological therapies. Developing effective interventions that could be administered around the time of childbirth to prevent CB-PTSD development is an important future research direction.

Internet-Based Assessment and Treatment of CB-PTSD

The Internet is a promising tool for CB-PTSD diagnosis and treatment. Bartal et al. (2023, 2024) collected brief narratives about women's childbirth experiences via web data collection, and they reported that the birth stories analyzed via Natural Language Processing may inform the provisional diagnosis of CB-PTSD. Additionally, a preliminary study has suggested that telehealth interventions entailing psychologically based, structured, individualized treatments delivered via the Internet may be effective in treating CB-PTSD (Nieminen et al., 2016). A remote intervention could represent an exciting strategy for making treatments more accessible to a broader range of postpartum women, particularly those for whom in-person medical visits are a barrier to treatment. The evidence for the value of Internet-based psychotherapies, based on non-postpartum samples, remains preliminary. More research is needed to understand the benefits and limitations of Internet-based therapies in the treatment of CB-PTSD relative to in-person interventions.

Additional Topics for Future Research

Societal attitudes toward pregnancy and childbirth influence women's experiences in the peripartum and postpartum periods. Further research is needed to characterize how different societies conceptualize and handle childbirth-related traumatic events, and how these attitudes influence women's childbirth experiences and their subsequent management of trauma-related sequelae, including CB-PTSD development. The long-term and potentially intergenerational effects of CB-PTSD on an affected woman, her infant, and other children in the family, remain to be studied in more depth. Understanding secondary traumatization is also important. This entails studying paternal CB-PTSD, as well as the impact of birth trauma on the treating staff on the delivery floor.

Whereas PTSD in the general population is recognized as a significant public health problem that is associated with high costs, particularly when this disorder remains untreated, the public health costs of untreated maternal CB-PTSD are unknown. When this condition remains untreated, maternal work time is lost due to mental illness, and other potential medical expenses are associated with untreated CB-PTSD and the probable effects of this disorder on the infant. Acquiring critical knowledge about the adversity associated with CB-PTSD is likely to guide modifications in healthcare policies and improve the perinatal care of women globally.

Acknowledgments

Dr. Sharon Dekel was supported by grants from the Eunice Kennedy Shriver National Institute of Child Health and Human Development (R01HD108619, R21HD100817, R21HD109546, and R03HD101724) and the Mass General Executive Committee on Research (ECOR) (ISF award).

References

Abdollahpour, S., Khosravi, A., & Bolbolhaghighi, N. (2016). The effect of the magical hour on post-traumatic stress disorder (PTSD) in traumatic childbirth: A clinical trial. *Journal of Reproductive and Infant Psychology, 34*(4), 403–412. https://doi.org/10.1080/02646838.2016.1185773

American College of Obstetricians and Gynecologists. (2018). Optimizing postpartum care. ACOG committee opinion No. 736. *Obstetrics & Gynecology, 131*(5), e140–e150. https://doi.org/10.1097/AOG.0000000000002633

American Psychiatric Association. (2013). *Diagnostic and Statistical Manual of Mental Disorders* (5th ed.). https://doi.org/10.1176/appi.books.9780890425787

Andersen, L. B., Melvaer, L. B., Videbech, P., Lamont, R. F., & Joergensen, J. S. (2012). Risk factors for developing post-traumatic stress disorder following childbirth: A systematic review. *Acta Obstetricia et Gynecologica Scandinavica, 91*(11), 1261–1272. https://doi.org/10.1111/j.1600-0412.2012.01476.x

Arora, I. H., Woscoboinik, G. G., Mokhtar, S., Quagliarini, B., Bartal, A., Jagodnik, K. M., . . . Dekel, S. (2024). Establishing the validity of a diagnostic questionnaire for childbirth-related posttraumatic stress disorder. *American Journal of Obstetrics and Gynecology.* Advance online publication. https://doi.org/10.1016/j.ajog.2023.11.1229

Ayers, S. (2001). Assessing psychopathology in pregnancy and postpartum. *Journal of Psychosomatic Obstetrics & Gynecology, 22*(2), 91–102. https://doi.org/10.3109/01674820109049959

Ayers, S., Wright, D. B., & Thornton, A. (2018). Development of a measure of postpartum PTSD: The City Birth Trauma Scale. *Frontiers in Psychiatry, 9*, 409. https://doi.org/10.3389/fpsyt.2018.00409

Babu, M. S., Chan, S. J., Ein-Dor, T., & Dekel, S. (2022). Traumatic childbirth during COVID-19 triggers maternal psychological growth and in turn better mother-infant bonding. *Journal of Affective Disorders, 313*, 163–166. https://doi.org/10.1016/j.jad.2022.06.076

Bartal, A., Jagodnik, K. M., Chan, S. J., Babu, M. S., & Dekel, S. (2023). Identifying women with post-delivery posttraumatic stress disorder using natural language processing of personal childbirth narratives. *American Journal of Obstetrics & Gynecology MFM, 5*(3), 100834. https://doi.org/10.1101/2022.08.30.22279394

Bartal, A., Jagodnik, K.M., Chan, S.J., & Dekel, S. (2024). AI and narrative embeddings detect PTSD following childbirth via birth stories. *Scientific Reports, 14*(1), 8336. https://doi.org/10.1038/s41598-024-54242-2

Bastos, M. H., Furuta, M., Small, R., McKenzie-McHarg, K., & Bick, D. (2015). Debriefing interventions for the prevention of psychological trauma in women following childbirth. *The Cochrane Database of Systematic Reviews,* (4), CD007194. https://doi.org/10.1002/14651858.CD007194.pub2

Battle, C. L., Salisbury, A. L., Schofield, C. A., & Ortiz-Hernandez, S. (2013). Perinatal antidepressant use: Understanding women's preferences and concerns. *Journal of Psychiatric Practice, 19*(6), 443–453. https://doi.org/10.1097/01.pra.0000438183.74359.46

Beck, C.T., 2023. Experiences of postpartum depression in women of color. *MCN: The American Journal of Maternal/Child Nursing, 48*(2), 88–95. https://doi.org/10.1097/NMC.0000000000000889

Bedard-Gilligan, M., Jaeger, J., Echiverri-Cohen, A., & Zoellner, L. A. (2012). Individual differences in trauma disclosure. *Journal of Behavior Therapy and Experimental Psychiatry, 43*(2), 716–723. https://doi.org/10.1016/j.jbtep.2011.10.005

Berman, Z., Kaim, A., Reed, T., Felicione, J., Hinojosa, C., Oliver, K., . . . Dekel, S. (2020). Amygdala response to traumatic childbirth recall is associated with impaired bonding behaviors in mothers with childbirth-related PTSD symptoms: Preliminary findings. *Biological Psychiatry, 87*(9), S142. https://doi.org/10.1016/j.biopsych.2020.02.378

Berman, Z., Thiel, F., Dishy, G. A., Chan, S. J., & Dekel, S. (2021). Maternal psychological growth following childbirth. *Archives of Women's Mental Health, 24*, 313–320. https://doi.org/10.1007/s00737-020-01053-9

Bertolini, F., Robertson, L., Bisson, J. I., Meader, N., Churchill, R., Ostuzzi, G., . . . Barbui, C. (2022). Early pharmacological interventions for universal prevention of post-traumatic stress disorder (PTSD). *Cochrane Database of Systematic Reviews*, (2), CD013443. https://doi.org/10.1002/14651858.CD013443.pub2

Bisson, J. I., & Olff, M. (2021). Prevention and treatment of PTSD: The current evidence base. *European Journal of Psychotraumatology*, *12*(1), 1824381. https://doi.org/10.1080/20008198.2020.1824381

Bisson, J. I., van Gelderen, M., Roberts, N. P., & Lewis, C. (2020). Non-pharmacological and non-psychological approaches to the treatment of PTSD: Results of a systematic review and meta-analyses. *European Journal of Psychotraumatology*, *11*(1), 1795361. https://doi.org/10.1080/20008198.2020.1795361

Björkman, F., & Ekblom, Ö. (2022). Physical exercise as treatment for PTSD: A systematic review and meta-analysis. *Military Medicine*, *187*(9–10), e1103–e1113. https://doi.org/10.1093/milmed/usab497

Blake, D. D., Weathers, F. W., Nagy, L. M., Kaloupek, D. G., Gusman, F. D., Charney, D. S., & Keane, T. M. (1995). The development of a Clinician-Administered PTSD Scale. *Journal of Traumatic Stress*, *8*(1), 75–90. https://doi.org/10.1002/jts.2490080106

Blevins, C. A., Weathers, F. W., Davis, M. T., Witte, T. K., & Domino, J. L. (2015). The Posttraumatic Stress Disorder Checklist for DSM-5 (PCL-5): Development and initial psychometric evaluation. *Journal of Traumatic Stress*, *28*(6), 489–498. https://doi.org/10.1002/jts.22059

Boerma, T., Ronsmans, C., Melesse, D. Y., Barros, A. J., Barros, F. C., Juan, L., . . . Neto, D. D. L. R. (2018). Global epidemiology of use of and disparities in caesarean sections. *The Lancet*, *392*(10155), 1341–1348. https://doi.org/10.1016/S0140-6736(18)31928-7

Bowers, M. E., & Yehuda, R. (2016). Intergenerational transmission of stress in humans. *Neuropsychopharmacology*, *41*(1), 232–244. https://doi.org/10.1038/npp.2015.247

Brewin, C. R., Andrews, B., & Valentine, J. D. (2000). Meta-analysis of risk factors for posttraumatic stress disorder in trauma-exposed adults. *Journal of Consulting and Clinical Psychology*, *68*(5), 748–766. https://doi.org/10.1037//0022-006x.68.5.748

Brown, R. L., Wood, A., Carter, J. D., & Kannis-Dymand, L. (2022). The metacognitive model of post-traumatic stress disorder and metacognitive therapy for post-traumatic stress disorder: A systematic review. *Clinical Psychology & Psychotherapy*, *29*(1), 131–146. https://doi.org/10.1002/cpp.2633

Bryant, R. A. (2019). Post-traumatic stress disorder: A state-of-the-art review of evidence and challenges. *World Psychiatry*, *18*(3), 259–269. https://doi.org/10.1002/wps.20656

Burtchen, N., Alvarez-Segura, M., Urben, S., Giovanelli, C., Mendelsohn, A. L., Guedeney, A., & Schechter, D. S. (2022). Effects of maternal trauma and associated psychopathology on atypical maternal behavior and infant social withdrawal six months postpartum. *Attachment & Human Development*, *24*(6), 750–776. https://doi.org/10.1080/14616734.2022.2142894

Callahan, J. L., Borja, S. E., & Hynan, M. T. (2006). Modification of the perinatal PTSD questionnaire to enhance clinical utility. *Journal of Perinatology*, *26*(9), 533–539. https://doi.org/10.1038/sj.jp.7211562

Callahan, J. L., & Hynan, M. T. (2002). Identifying mothers at risk for postnatal emotional distress: Further evidence for the validity of the Perinatal Posttraumatic Stress Disorder Questionnaire. *Journal of Perinatology*, *22*(6), 448–454. https://doi.org/10.1038/sj.jp.7210783

Chan, S. J., Ein-Dor, T., Mayopoulos, P. A., Mesa, M. M., Sunda, R. M., McCarthy, B. F., . . . Dekel, S. (2020). Risk factors for developing posttraumatic stress disorder following childbirth. *Psychiatry Research*, *290*, 113090. https://doi.org/10.1016/j.psychres.2020.113090

Chan, S. J., Thiel, F., Kaimal, A. J., Pitman, R. K., Orr, S. P., & Dekel, S. (2022). Validation of childbirth-related posttraumatic stress disorder using psychophysiological assessment. *American Journal of Obstetrics and Gynecology*, *227*(4), 656–659. https://doi.org/10.1016/j.ajog.2022.05.051

Cirino, N. H., & Knapp, J. M. (2019). Perinatal posttraumatic stress disorder: A review of risk factors, diagnosis, and treatment. *Obstetrical & Gynecological Survey*, *74*(6), 369–376. https://doi.org/10.1097/OGX.0000000000000680

Cox, J., & Holden, J. (2003). *Perinatal Mental Health: A Guide to the Edinburgh Postnatal Depression Scale (EPDS)*. Royal College of Psychiatrists.

Creanga, A. A., Bateman, B. T., Kuklina, E. V., & Callaghan, W. M. (2014). Racial and ethnic disparities in severe maternal morbidity: A multistate analysis, 2008–2010. *American Journal of Obstetrics and Gynecology*, *210*(5), 435, e1–435, e4358. https://doi.org/10.1016/j.ajog.2013.11.039

Cross, M. R., & McCanne, T. R. (2001). Validation of a self-report measure of posttraumatic stress disorder in a sample of college-age women. *Journal of Traumatic Stress*, *14*(1), 135–147. https://doi.org/10.1023/A:1007843800664

Daehn, D., Rudolf, S., Pawils, S., & Renneberg, B. (2022). Perinatal mental health literacy: Knowledge, attitudes, and help-seeking among perinatal women and the public – A systematic review. *BMC Pregnancy and Childbirth*, 22(1), 574. https://doi.org/10.1186/s12884-022-04865-y

de Graaff, L. F., Honig, A., van Pampus, M. G., & Stramrood, C. A. I. (2018). Preventing post-traumatic stress disorder following childbirth and traumatic birth experiences: A systematic review. *Acta Obstetricia et Gynecologica Scandinavica*, 97(6), 648–656. https://doi.org/10.1111/aogs.13291

Dekel, S. (2024). A call for a formal diagnosis for childbirth-related PTSD. *Nature Mental Health*, 1–2. 2, 259–260. https://doi.org/10.1038/s44220-024-00213-5

Dekel, S., Ein-Dor, T., Berman, Z., Barsoumian, I. S., Agarwal, S., & Pitman, R. K. (2019). Delivery mode is associated with maternal mental health following childbirth. *Archives of Women's Mental Health*, 22(6), 817–824. https://doi.org/10.1007/s00737-019-00968-2

Dekel, S., Ein-Dor, T., Dishy, G. A., & Mayopoulos, P. A. (2020). Beyond postpartum depression: Posttraumatic stress-depressive response following childbirth. *Archives of Women's Mental Health*, 23(4), 557–564. https://doi.org/10.1007/s00737-019-01006-x

Dekel, S., Papadakis, J. E., Quagliarini, B., Pham, C. T., Pacheco-Barrios, K., Hughes, F., . . . Nandru, R. (2024). Preventing posttraumatic stress disorder following childbirth: A systematic review and meta-analysis. *American Journal of Obstetrics and Gynecology*. Advance online publication. https://doi.org/10.1016/j.ajog.2023.12.013

Dekel, S., Stuebe, C., & Dishy, G. (2017). Childbirth induced posttraumatic stress syndrome: A systematic review of prevalence and risk factors. *Frontiers in Psychology*, 8, 560. https://doi.org/10.3389/fpsyg.2017.00560

Dekel, S., Thiel, F., Dishy, G., & Ashenfarb, A. L. (2019). Is childbirth-induced PTSD associated with low maternal attachment? *Archives of Women's Mental Health*, 22(1), 119–122. https://doi.org/10.1007/s00737-018-0853-y

Dennis, C. L., & Chung-Lee, L. (2006). Postpartum depression help-seeking barriers and maternal treatment preferences: A qualitative systematic review. *Birth*, 33(4), 323–331. https://doi.org/10.1111/j.1523-536X.2006.00130.x

De Schepper, S., Vercauteren, T., Tersago, J., Jacquemyn, Y., Raes, F., & Franck, E. (2016). Posttraumatic stress disorder after childbirth and the influence of maternity team care during labour and birth: A cohort study. *Midwifery*, 32, 87–92. https://doi.org/10.1016/j.midw.2015.08.010

Dikmen-Yildiz, P., Ayers, S., & Phillips, L. (2018). Longitudinal trajectories of post-traumatic stress disorder (PTSD) after birth and associated risk factors. *Journal of Affective Disorders*, 229, 377–385. https://doi.org/10.1016/j.jad.2017.12.074

Duval, C. J., Youssefzadeh, A. C., Sweeney, H. E., McGough, A. M., Mandelbaum, R. S., Ouzounian, J. G., & Matsuo, K. (2022). Association of severe maternal morbidity and post-traumatic stress disorder. *AJOG Global Reports*, 2(4), 100111. https://doi.org/10.1016/j.xagr.2022.100111

Florido, A., Velasco, E. R., Monari, S., Cano, M., Cardoner, N., Sandi, C., . . . Perez-Caballero, L. (2023). Glucocorticoid-based pharmacotherapies preventing PTSD. *Neuropharmacology*, 109344. https://doi.org/10.1016/j.neuropharm.2022.109344

Foa, E. B. (1995). *Post-traumatic Diagnostic Scale Manual*. National Computer Systems.

Foa, E. B., McLean, C. P., Zang, Y., Zhong, J., Powers, M. B., Kauffman, B. Y., . . . Knowles, K. (2016). Psychometric properties of the Posttraumatic Diagnostic Scale for DSM – 5 (PDS – 5). *Psychological Assessment*, 28(10), 1166–1171. https://doi.org/10.1037/pas0000258

Froeliger, A., Deneux-Tharaux, C., Seco, A., & Sentilhes, L. (2022). Posttraumatic stress disorder symptoms 2 months after vaginal delivery. *Obstetrics & Gynecology*, 139(1), 63–72. https://doi.org/10.1097/AOG.0000000000004611

Furuta, M., Horsch, A., Ng, E. S. W., Bick, D., Spain, D., & Sin, J. (2018). Effectiveness of trauma-focused psychological therapies for treating post-traumatic stress disorder symptoms in women following childbirth: A systematic review and meta-analysis. *Frontiers in Psychiatry*, 9, 591. https://doi.org/10.3389/fpsyt.2018.00591

Garthus-Niegel, S., Ayers, S., von Soest, T., Torgersen, L., & Eberhard-Gran, M. (2015). Maintaining factors of posttraumatic stress symptoms following childbirth: A population-based, two-year follow-up study. *Journal of Affective Disorders*, 172, 146–152. https://doi.org/10.1016/j.jad.2014.10.003

Garthus-Niegel, S., Horsch, A., Handtke, E., von Soest, T., Ayers, S., Weidner, K., & Eberhard-Gran, M. (2018). The impact of postpartum posttraumatic stress and depression symptoms on couples' relationship satisfaction: A population-based prospective study. *Frontiers in Psychology*, 9, 1728. https://doi.org/10.3389/fpsyg.2018.01728

Geller, S. E., Koch, A. R., Garland, C. E., MacDonald, E. J., Storey, F., & Lawton, B. (2018). A global view of severe maternal morbidity: Moving beyond maternal mortality. *Reproductive Health*, *15*(1), 31–43. https://doi.org/10.1186/s12978-018-0527-2

Glaus, J., Pointet Perizzolo, V., Moser, D. A., Vital, M., Rusconi Serpa, S., Urben, S., . . . Schechter, D. S. (2021). Associations between maternal post-traumatic stress disorder and traumatic events with child psychopathology: Results from a prospective longitudinal study. *Frontiers in Psychiatry*, *12*, 718108. https://doi.org/10.3389/fpsyt.2021.718108

Grekin, R., & O'Hara, M. W. (2014). Prevalence and risk factors of postpartum posttraumatic stress disorder: A meta-analysis. *Clinical Psychology Review*, *34*(5), 389–401. https://doi.org/10.1016/j.cpr.2014.05.003

Hearing, C. M., Chang, W. C., Szuhany, K. L., Deckersbach, T., Nierenberg, A. A., & Sylvia, L. G. (2016). Physical exercise for treatment of mood disorders: A critical review. *Current Behavioral Neuroscience Reports*, *3*, 350–359. https://doi.org/10.1007/s40473-016-0089-y

Hernández-Martínez, A., Rodríguez-Almagro, J., Molina-Alarcón, M., Infante-Torres, N., Rubio-Álvarez, A., & Martínez-Galiano, J. M. (2020). Perinatal factors related to post-traumatic stress disorder symptoms 1–5 years following birth. *Women and Birth: Journal of the Australian College of Midwives*, *33*(2), e129–e135. https://doi.org/10.1016/j.wombi.2019.03.008

Hodnett, E. D., Gates, S., Hofmeyr, G. J., Sakala, C., & Weston, J. (2011). Continuous support for women during childbirth. *The Cochrane Database of Systematic Reviews*, (2), CD003766. https://doi.org/10.1002/14651858.CD003766.pub3

Horesh, D., Garthus-Niegel, S., & Horsch, A. (2021). Childbirth-related PTSD: Is it a unique post-traumatic disorder? *Journal of Reproductive and Infant Psychology*, *39*(3), 221–224.

Horowitz, M., Wilner, N., & Alvarez, W. (1979). Impact of Event Scale: A measure of subjective stress. *Psychosomatic Medicine*, *41*(3), 209–218.

Hynan, M. (1998). The Perinatal Posttraumatic Stress Disorder (PTSD) Questionnaire (PPQ). In C. Zalaquett & R. Wood (Eds.), *Evaluating Stress: A Book of Resources* (199–200). Scarecrow Press.

Ionio, C., & Di Blasio, P. (2014). Post-traumatic stress symptoms after childbirth and early mother-child interactions: An exploratory study. *Journal of Reproductive and Infant Psychology*, *32*(2), 163–181. https://doi.org/10.1080/02646838.2013.841880

Iyengar, A. S., Ein-Dor, T., Zhang, E. X., Chan, S. J., Kaimal, A. J., & Dekel, S. (2022). Increased traumatic childbirth and postpartum depression and lack of exclusive breastfeeding in Black and Latinx individuals. *International Journal of Gynaecology and Obstetrics*, *158*(3), 759–761. https://doi.org/10.1002/ijgo.14280

Jagodnik, K. M., Ein-Dor, T., Chan, S. J., Titelman Ashkenazy, A., Bartal, A., Barry, R. L., & Dekel, S. (2024). Screening for post-traumatic stress disorder following childbirth using the Peritraumatic Distress Inventory. *Journal of Affective Disorders*, *348*, 17–25. https://doi.org/10.1016/j.jad.2023.12.010

James, S. (2015). Women's experiences of symptoms of posttraumatic stress disorder (PTSD) after traumatic childbirth: A review and critical appraisal. *Archives of Women's Mental Health*, *18*(6), 761–771. https://doi.org/10.1007/s00737-015-0560-x

Khsim, I. E. F., Rodríguez, M. M., Riquelme Gallego, B., Caparros-Gonzalez, R. A., & Amezcua-Prieto, C. (2022). Risk factors for post-traumatic stress disorder after childbirth: A systematic review. *Diagnostics (Basel, Switzerland)*, *12*(11), 2598. https://doi.org/10.3390/diagnostics12112598

Kjerulff, K. H., Attanasio, L. B., Sznajder, K. K., & Brubaker, L. H. (2021). A prospective cohort study of post-traumatic stress disorder and maternal-infant bonding after first childbirth. *Journal of Psychosomatic Research*, *144*, 110424. https://doi.org/10.1016/j.jpsychores.2021.110424

Kömürcü Akik, B., & Durak Batigun, A. (2020). Perinatal Post Traumatic Stress Disorder Questionnaire-II (PPQ-II): Adaptation, validity, and reliability study. *Dusunen-Adam-Journal of Psychiatry and Neurological Sciences*, *33*(4). https://doi.org/10.14744/DAJPNS.2020.00102

Krendl, A. C., & Pescosolido, B. A. (2020). Countries and cultural differences in the stigma of mental illness: The East – West divide. *Journal of Cross-Cultural Psychology*, *51*(2), 149–167. https://doi.org/10.1177/0022022119901297

Kress, V., von Soest, T., Kopp, M., Wimberger, P., & Garthus-Niegel, S. (2021). Differential predictors of birth-related posttraumatic stress disorder symptoms in mothers and fathers – A longitudinal cohort study. *Journal of Affective Disorders*, *292*, 121–130. https://doi.org/10.1016/j.jad.2021.05.058

Lai, X., Chen, J., Li, H., Zhou, L., Huang, Q., Liao, Y., . . . Xie, R.-H. (2022). The incidence of post-traumatic stress disorder following traumatic childbirth: A systematic review and meta-analysis. *International Journal of Gynecology & Obstetrics.* https://doi.org/10.1002/ijgo.14643

Lang, A. J. (2017). Mindfulness in PTSD treatment. *Current Opinion in Psychology, 14,* 40–43. https://doi.org/10.1016/j.copsyc.2016.10.005

Marsella, A. J. (2010). Ethnocultural aspects of PTSD: An overview of concepts, issues, and treatments. *Traumatology, 16*(4), 17–26. https://doi.org/10.1177/1534765610388062

Mayopoulos, G. A., Ein-Dor, T., Dishy, G. A., Nandru, R., Chan, S. J., Hanley, L. E., . . . Dekel, S. (2021). COVID-19 is associated with traumatic childbirth and subsequent mother-infant bonding problems. *Journal of Affective Disorders, 282,* 122–125. https://doi.org/10.1016/j.jad.2020.12.101

McKenzie-McHarg, K., Ayers, S., Ford, E., Horsch, A., Jomeen, J., Sawyer, A., . . . Slade, P. (2015). Post-traumatic stress disorder following childbirth: An update of current issues and recommendations for future research. *Journal of Reproductive and Infant Psychology, 33*(3), 219–237. https://doi.org/10.1080/02646838.2015.1031646

Milgrom, J., Hirshler, Y., Reece, J., Holt, C., & Gemmill, A. W. (2019). Social support – A protective factor for depressed perinatal women? *International Journal of Environmental Research and Public Health, 16*(8), 1426. https://doi.org/10.3390/ijerph16081426

Nakić Radoš, S., Matijaš, M., Kuhar, L., Anđelinović, M., & Ayers, S. (2020). Measuring and conceptualizing PTSD following childbirth: Validation of the City Birth Trauma Scale. *Psychological Trauma: Theory, Research, Practice, and Policy, 12*(2), 147–155. https://psycnet.apa.org/doi/10.1037/tra0000501

Nieminen, K., Berg, I., Frankenstein, K., Viita, L., Larsson, K., Persson, U., . . . Wijma, K. (2016). Internet-provided cognitive behaviour therapy of posttraumatic stress symptoms following childbirth – A randomized controlled trial. *Cognitive Behaviour Therapy, 45*(4), 287–306. https://doi.org/10.1080/16506073.2016.1169626

Niles, B. L., Mori, D. L., Polizzi, C., Pless Kaiser, A., Weinstein, E. S., Gershkovich, M., & Wang, C. (2018). A systematic review of randomized trials of mind-body interventions for PTSD. *Journal of Clinical Psychology, 74*(9), 1485–1508. https://doi.org/10.1002/jclp.22634

O'Carroll, J., Blake, H., Ando, K., Beaven, A., Patrick, A., Ke, J., . . . Sultan, P. (2024). A systematic review of patient-reported outcome measures in maternal postpartum post-traumatic stress disorder. Manuscript in Preparation.

O'Donovan, A., Alcorn, K. L., Patrick, J. C., Creedy, D. K., Dawe, S., & Devilly, G. J. (2014). Predicting posttraumatic stress disorder after childbirth. *Midwifery, 30*(8), 935–941. https://doi.org/10.1016/j.midw.2014.03.011

Pitman, R. K., Rasmusson, A. M., Koenen, K. C., Shin, L. M., Orr, S. P., Gilbertson, M. W., . . . Liberzon, I. (2012). Biological studies of post-traumatic stress disorder. *Nature Reviews Neuroscience, 13*(11), 769–787. https://doi.org/10.1038/nrn3339

Rashidi, M., Maier, E., Dekel, S., Sütterlin, M., Wolf, R. C., Ditzen, B., . . . Herpertz, S. C. (2022). Peripartum effects of synthetic oxytocin: The good, the bad, and the unknown. *Neuroscience and Biobehavioral Reviews, 141,* 104859. https://doi.org/10.1016/j.neubiorev.2022.104859

Ribaudo, J., Lawler, J. M., Jester, J. M., Riggs, J., Erickson, N. L., Stacks, A. M., . . . Rosenblum, K. L. (2022). Maternal history of adverse experiences and posttraumatic stress disorder symptoms impact toddlers' early socioemotional wellbeing: The benefits of infant mental health-home visiting. *Frontiers in Psychology, 12,* 792989. https://doi.org/10.3389/fpsyg.2021.792989

Roberts, L., Henry, A., Harvey, S.B., Homer, C.S., & Davis, G.K. (2022). Depression, anxiety and posttraumatic stress disorder six months following preeclampsia and normotensive pregnancy: A P4 study. *BMC Pregnancy and Childbirth, 22*(1), 108. https://doi.org/10.1186/s12884-022-04439-y

Scott, G., Ciarrochi, J., & Deane, F. P. (2004). Disadvantages of being an individualist in an individualistic culture: Idiocentrism, emotional competence, stress, and mental health. *Australian Psychologist, 39*(2), 143–154. https://doi.org/10.1080/00050060410001701861

Sentilhes, L., Maillard, F., Brun, S., Madar, H., Merlot, B., Goffinet, F., & Deneux-Tharaux, C. (2017). Risk factors for chronic post-traumatic stress disorder development one year after vaginal delivery: A prospective, observational study. *Scientific Reports, 7*(1), 1–9. https://doi.org/10.1038/s41598-017-09314-x

Shorey, S., Downe, S., Chua, J. Y. X., Byrne, S. O., Fobelets, M., & Lalor, J. G. (2021). Effectiveness of psychological interventions to improve the mental well-being of parents who have experienced traumatic childbirth: A systematic review and meta-analysis. *Trauma, Violence, & Abuse,* 15248380211060808. https://doi.org/10.1177/15248380211060808

Singewald, N., Sartori, S. B., Reif, A., & Holmes, A. (2023). Alleviating anxiety and taming trauma: Novel pharmacotherapeutics for anxiety disorders and posttraumatic stress disorder. *Neuropharmacology, 226*, 109418. https://doi.org/10.1016/j.neuropharm.2023.109418

Slade, P., Molyneux, R., & Watt, A. (2021). A systematic review of clinical effectiveness of psychological interventions to reduce post traumatic stress symptoms following childbirth and a meta-synthesis of facilitators and barriers to uptake of psychological care. *Journal of Affective Disorders, 281*, 678–694. https://doi.org/10.1016/j.jad.2020.11.092

Sommerlad, S., Schermelleh-Engel, K., La Rosa, V. L., Louwen, F., & Oddo-Sommerfeld, S. (2021). Trait anxiety and unplanned delivery mode enhance the risk for childbirth-related post-traumatic stress disorder symptoms in women with and without risk of preterm birth: A multi sample path analysis. *PLOS ONE, 16*(8), e0256681. https://doi.org/10.1371/journal.pone.0256681

Stadlmayr, W., Cignacco, E., Surbek, D., & Büchi, S. (2009). Screening-Instrumente zur Erfassung von Befindlichkeitsstörungen nach der Geburt. *Hebamme, 22*(1), 13–19. https://doi.org/10.1055/s-0029-1213450

Stramrood, C., & Slade, P. (2017). A woman afraid of becoming pregnant again: Posttraumatic stress disorder following childbirth. In K. Paarlberg & H. van de Wiel (Eds.), *Bio-Psycho-Social Obstetrics and Gynecology* (pp. 33–49). Springer. https://doi.org/10.1007/978-3-319-40404-2_2

Tasuji, T., Reese, E., van Mulukom, V., & Whitehouse, H., (2020). Band of mothers: Childbirth as a female bonding experience. *PLOS ONE, 15*(10), e0240175. https://doi.org/10.1371/journal.pone.0240175

Taylor Miller, P. G., Sinclair, M., Gillen, P., McCullough, J. E. M., Miller, P. W., Farrell, D. P., . . . Klaus, P. (2021). Early psychological interventions for prevention and treatment of post-traumatic stress disorder (PTSD) and post-traumatic stress symptoms in post-partum women: A systematic review and meta-analysis. *PLOS ONE, 16*(11), e0258170. https://doi.org/10.1371/journal.pone.0258170

Thiel, F., Berman, Z., Dishy, G. A., Chan, S. J., Seth, H., Tokala, M., . . . Dekel, S. (2021). Traumatic memories of childbirth relate to maternal postpartum posttraumatic stress disorder. *Journal of Anxiety Disorders, 77*, 102342. https://doi.org/10.1016/j.janxdis.2020.102342

Thiel, F., & Dekel, S. (2020). Peritraumatic dissociation in childbirth-evoked posttraumatic stress and postpartum mental health. *Archives of Women's Mental Health, 23*, 189–197. https://doi.org/10.1007/s00737-019-00978-0

Thiel, F., Ein-Dor, T., Dishy, G., King, A., & Dekel, S. (2018). Examining symptom clusters of childbirth-related posttraumatic stress disorder. *The Primary Care Companion for CNS Disorders, 20*(5), 18m02322. https://doi.org/10.4088/PCC.18m02322

Tomsis, Y., Gelkopf, M., Yerushalmi, H., & Zipori, Y. (2018). Different coping strategies influence the development of PTSD among first-time mothers. *Journal of Maternal-Fetal & Neonatal Medicine, 31*(10), 1304–1310. https://doi.org/10.1080/14767058.2017.1315658

Triandis, H. C., Bontempo, R., Villareal, M. J., Asai, M., & Lucca, N. (1988). Individualism and collectivism: Cross-cultural perspectives on self-ingroup relationships. *Journal of Personality and Social Psychology, 54*(2), 323–338. https://doi.org/10.1037/0022-3514.54.2.323

United States Department of Veterans Affairs. (2017). VA/DOD clinical practice guideline for the management of posttraumatic stress disorder and acute stress disorder. *Department of Veterans Affairs Department of Defense.* Retrieved November 27, 2022, from www.tricare.mil

Van Sieleghem, S., Danckaerts, M., Rieken, R., Okkerse, J. M., de Jonge, E., Bramer, W. M., & Lambregtse-van den Berg, M. P. (2022). Childbirth related PTSD and its association with infant outcome: A systematic review. *Early Human Development, 174*, 105667. https://doi.org/10.1016/j.earlhumdev.2022.105667

Vänskä, M., Punamäki, R.-L., Tolvanen, A., Lindblom, J., Flykt, M., Unkila-Kallio, L., . . . Tulppala, M. (2011). Maternal pre- and postnatal mental health trajectories and child mental health and development: Prospective study in a normative and formerly infertile sample. *International Journal of Behavioral Development, 35*(6), 517–531. https://doi.org/10.1177/0165025411417505

van Steijn, M. E., Scheepstra, K. W. F., Zaat, T. R., van Rooijen, D. E., Stramrood, C. A., Dijksman, L. M., . . . van Pampus, M. G. (2021). Severe postpartum hemorrhage increases risk of posttraumatic stress disorder: A prospective cohort study. *Journal of Psychosomatic Obstetrics & Gynecology, 42*(4), 335–345. https://doi.org/10.1080/0167482X.2020.1735343

Vesel, J., & Nickasch, B. (2015). An evidence review and model for prevention and treatment of postpartum posttraumatic stress disorder. *Nursing for Women's Health*, *19*(6), 504–525. https://doi.org/10.1111/1751-486X.12234

Vigod, S. N., & Dennis, C. L. (2020). Advances in virtual care for perinatal mental disorders. *World Psychiatry*, *19*(3), 328–329. https://doi.org/10.1002/wps.20775

Watkins, L. E., Sprang, K. R., & Rothbaum, B. O. (2018). Treating PTSD: A review of evidence-based psychotherapy interventions. *Frontiers in Behavioral Neuroscience*, *12*, 258. https://doi.org/10.3389/fnbeh.2018.00258

Watson, C. G., Juba, M. P., Manifold, V., Kucala, T., & Anderson, P. E. (1991). The PTSD interview: Rationale, description, reliability, and concurrent validity of a DSM-III-based technique. *Journal of Clinical Psychology*, *47*(2), 179–188. https://doi.org/10.1002/1097-4679(199103)47:2<179::aid-jclp2270470202>3.0.co;2-p

Weathers, F. W., Bovin, M. J., Lee, D. J., Sloan, D. M., Schnurr, P. P., Kaloupek, D. G., . . . Marx, B. P. (2018). The Clinician-Administered PTSD Scale for DSM-5 (CAPS-5): Development and initial psychometric evaluation in military veterans. *Psychological Assessment*, *30*(3), 383–395. https://doi.org/10.1037/pas0000486

Weathers, F. W., Litz, B., Herman, D., Huska, J., & Keane, T. (1993, October). *The PTSD Checklist (PCL): Reliability, validity, and diagnostic utility*. Paper presented at the Annual Convention of the International Society for Traumatic Stress Studies (Vol. 462).

Weiss, D. S., & Marmar, C. R. (1997). The Impact of Event Scale: Revised. In J. P. Wilson & T. M. Keane (Eds.), *The Impact of Event Scale–Revised: Assessing Psychological Trauma and PTSD*. Guilford Press.

Williams, M. E., Strobino, D. M., & Holliday, C. N. (2022). Measuring post-traumatic stress after childbirth: A review and critical appraisal of instruments. *Journal of Reproductive and Infant Psychology*, 1–15. https://doi.org/10.1080/02646838.2022.2030052

Williams, T., Phillips, N. J., Stein, D. J., & Ipser, J. C. (2022). Pharmacotherapy for post traumatic stress disorder (PTSD). *The Cochrane Database of Systematic Reviews*, *3*(3), CD002795. https://doi.org/10.1002/14651858.CD002795.pub3

World Health Organization. *WHO statement on caesarean section rates*. Retrieved January 31, 2023, from www.who.int/publications/i/item/WHO-RHR-15.02

Zaat, T. R., van Steijn, M. E., de Haan-Jebbink, J. M., Olff, M., Stramrood, C. A., & van Pampus, M. G. (2018). Posttraumatic stress disorder related to postpartum haemorrhage: A systematic review. *European Journal of Obstetrics & Gynecology and Reproductive Biology*, *225*, 214–220. https://doi.org/10.1016/j.ejogrb.2018.04.012

Zafari, H., Kosowan, L., Zulkernine, F., & Signer, A. (2021). Diagnosing post-traumatic stress disorder using electronic medical record data. *Health Informatics Journal*, *27*(4), 14604582211053259. https://doi.org/10.1177/14604582211053259

Zalta, A. K., Tirone, V., Orlowska, D., Blais, R. K., Lofgreen, A., Klassen, B., . . . Dent, A. L. (2021). Examining moderators of the relationship between social support and self-reported PTSD symptoms: A meta-analysis. *Psychological Bulletin*, *147*(1), 33–54. https://doi.org/10.1037/bul0000316

Zhang, D., Zhang, J., Gan, Q., Wang, Q., Fan, N., Zhang, R., & Song, Y. (2018). Validating the psychometric characteristics of the Perinatal Posttraumatic Stress Disorder Questionnaire (PPQ) in a Chinese context. *Archives of Psychiatric Nursing*, *32*(1), 57–61. https://doi.org/10.1016/j.apnu.2017.09.016

16

POSTPARTUM EATING DISORDERS AND BODY IMAGE DISTURBANCE

Alyssa M. Minnick, Nathaniel Holmes,
Molly Moore, and Kelly C. Allison

The postpartum period is a major life transition across multiple domains, including physical health, psychological, and social experiences. Changes to the body and eating behavior are natural aspects of every pregnancy; however, body image disturbances and eating pathology that persist from pregnancy can impact outcomes for both mother and baby. Therefore, it is important to understand and address body image and eating factors during the postpartum period.

Description and Salient Features

Body Image Disturbances During the Postpartum Period

Body image is a multifaceted construct that includes perceptions, thoughts, feelings, and attitudes toward the body (Grogan, 2021). Body image disturbances developed during pregnancy can continue during the postpartum period. Even for new mothers without an eating disorder (ED) history, dietary restraint, body shape concerns, and/or weight concerns significantly increase from the early-mid pregnancy period to the early postpartum period (Baskin, Meyer, et al., 2021). There are distinct features of body image concerns following pregnancy to consider.

Similar to prenatal body image appraisals, there is diversity among women in their feelings toward their bodies postpartum. Some women report being amazed by their bodies' ability to create life, which leads to feeling strong and appreciative of their bodies, whereas other women express shame, sadness, and loss of self after pregnancy (Raspovic et al., 2020). These sentiments were reflected in a qualitative study (Clark et al., 2009), in which only three out of ten postpartum women reported positive attitudes toward their bodies following pregnancy. The other seven women reported dramatic changes to their bodies postpartum and described the sense of having a "new" body after delivery. They indicated more difficulties with adapting to their postpartum bodies than with body changes during pregnancy. In part, women reported that they no longer felt they had an "excuse" to have a larger body because they were no longer carrying their babies. These experiences were distressing particularly because they felt it was not apparent to others that their body shapes

DOI: 10.4324/9781003206903-20

and sizes were due to recently having a baby; this experience differed from pregnancy in which their baby belly was easily visible to others.

Women also no longer spoke of their bodily changes as functional to support their babies, as they had felt during pregnancy. There was the sense that they should now be in full control over their body weight, shape, and size again. Women indicated that they often received messages that the postpartum body is a sort of "project" that should be focused on to return to pre-pregnancy weight and shape; some women even perceived more body image pressure postpartum compared to prior to pregnancy (Hodgkinson et al., 2014).

Women also reported unrealistic expectations about their bodies' abilities to quickly return to pre-pregnancy weights and shapes and expressed surprise that they needed to continue wearing maternity clothes postpartum (Clark et al., 2009). New Danish mothers indicated, in qualitative interviews, that losing weight was a measure of successful recovery and rehabilitation from pregnancy; they described the pressure of "not looking like a mother." The process and challenges of losing weight were often discussed in postpartum mothers' groups (Prinds et al., 2020). They identified other sources of information on beauty and appearance postpartum, including magazines, social media, books, blogs, and their social environment (e.g., family, friends, colleagues, mothers' groups, and acquaintances; Prinds et al., 2020). Some women reported that these unrealistic expectations about their body postpartum had a negative impact on their mood; however, most women indicated that body image became less of a priority postpartum because they were more focused on motherhood and caring for their child(ren) (Clark et al., 2009). Danish women also reported that they did not judge other new mothers' bodies, whereas they were judgmental of themselves regarding weight loss postpartum (Prinds et al., 2020).

Postpartum Eating Disorders

Women may be at heightened risk for disordered eating due to the pressures to lose weight postpartum and adhere to these body ideals, whether or not they have a history of ED (Astrachan-Fletcher et al., 2008). The body ideal pressures and body image disturbances could contribute to disordered eating, in that restrictive eating patterns and/or compensatory behaviors may be used to achieve weight loss (Burns & Gavey, 2004; Reba-Harrelson et al., 2009). Binge eating may also be used as a strategy for managing stress or negative emotions (Schaefer et al., 2020), which are common during the postpartum period (Ayers et al., 2019; Miller et al., 2006).

A detailed description of ED behaviors and diagnoses is found in the prenatal chapter for body image disturbances and EDs. The ED diagnostic categories do not change as applied to the postpartum period and include anorexia nervosa (AN), bulimia nervosa (BN), binge eating disorder (BED), and otherwise specified feeding and eating disorders (OS-FED), previously known as eating disorder, not otherwise specified (ED-NOS), including purging disorder (PD) and night eating syndrome (NES). The feeding disorders in the DSM-5 pertinent to postpartum include pica. Pre-pregnancy EDs may also persist into the postpartum period. For women with an ED, relapse in postpartum was driven by being less concerned that their behaviors will have a direct negative impact on their baby, in addition to irregular eating and sleep patterns and additional stress related to caring for a newborn (Astrachan-Fletcher et al., 2008).

Introduction to the Case

Victoria is a 30-year-old White woman from the United States. She developed anorexia nervosa (AN) during her first year of college. She felt overwhelmed by the setting, living away from her family for the first time, and the load of her coursework. She focused on trying to control her eating as a means of coping and to avoid the "freshman 15" (i.e., a common experience of gaining weight during the first year of college due to constant availability of food, alcohol consumption, and changes in physical activity routine). She received outpatient eating disorder treatment intermittently in college and maintained a body mass index (BMI) of 19 kg/m² (i.e., within the normal range) in her 20s; however, she continued to have an entrenched body image and fear of weight gain concerns.

Victoria met her partner just after college. They exercised together and focused on healthy eating as a shared value. They are both image sensitive and prided themselves on their appearance and being in shape. Victoria wanted a family but was concerned that she would gain weight with pregnancy and her body would not be the same afterward. She worried that her partner would find her less desirable and that she would lose her identity. After pregnancy, she suffered from postpartum depression, which impacted her bonding with her baby initially and her ability to breast feed within the first month after giving birth.

Prevalence

A large-scale, population-based study of over 77,000 participants in the Norwegian Mothers and Child Cohort study (MoBa; Knoph et al., 2013) tracked the course of EDs from pre-pregnancy through 36 months postpartum. The most common ED reported prior to pregnancy was BED (3.5%), which was also true for EDs with onset during pregnancy and at 18 months and 36 months postpartum. The second-most common ED at these timepoints was BN, at less than 1% of the sample.

This large-scale study also found that for women who reported an ED prior to pregnancy or who developed an ED during pregnancy, 39% (for BN) to 50% (for AN) of them no longer met the criteria for an ED at 18 months postpartum, indicating remittance of these EDs; remission rates for BED and EDNOS-purging type fell between this range (Knoph et al., 2013). These remission rates ranged from 30% to 59% at 36 months postpartum and followed a similar pattern as at 18 months postpartum. The other women in this sample whose symptoms did not remit continued to either meet full ED criteria, meet subthreshold symptomology, or cross over into meeting criteria for a different ED. The study found that, specifically for women who developed BED during pregnancy, 66% and 57% of them were in remission at 18 months and 36 months postpartum, respectively.

The pattern observed across most studies for the prevalence of EDs in the peripartum period is a decrease in full threshold EDs and ED symptoms during pregnancy, followed by a resurgence in the postpartum period, albeit to a lesser extent than the pregravid period (Nunes et al., 2014; Chan et al., 2019; Pettersson et al., 2016). Pettersson et al. (2016) surveyed Swedish women longitudinally and found that 7.2% screened positive for any ED in the postpartum period, an increase from 3% during pregnancy. Chan et al. (2019) also found this resurgence among 1,470 women from Hong Kong, reporting disordered eating (defined as being above the cut score on the *Eating Attitudes Test*) of 2.5% at six weeks postpartum but then falling to 1.2% at six months postpartum, which was similar to levels reported during pregnancy. Pregravid disordered eating history was associated with disordered eating at each subsequent peripartum time. One note of caution is that there was significant attrition of the sample in the postpartum period.

Nunes et al. (2014) used a brief version of the *Eating Disorders Examination-Questionnaire* (EDE-Q) to assess ED symptoms among a disadvantaged population of 712 women in Brazil. They found that risk scores for global ED symptoms in the pregravid (retrospectively assessed), pregnancy, and postpartum periods, respectively, were 0%, 0.2%, and 2.3%; restraint and eating concerns showed similar prevalence at all three timepoints: 0%, 0.2%, and 1.4%; shape concerns showed a higher prevalence: 11.5%, 4.2%, and 19%; followed by weight concerns: 1.3%, 4.6%, and 16.9%. Endorsement of objective binge episodes (OBEs) was common across this period, respectively: 27.6, 19.2, and 17.1%; and to a lesser extent, so were inappropriate compensatory behaviors, with vomiting at 6.8%, 1.4%, and 2.6%; laxative use at 6.3%, 0%, and 1.9%; diuretic misuse at 3.3%, 0%, and 0.7%, and excessive exercise at 0%, 1.6%, and 2.1%. They stated that ED symptoms seemed to reappear around five months postpartum (Nunes et al., 2014). These levels are higher than in European and U.S. populations and should be assessed further in South American populations.

A prospective study of women in the United States diagnosed with EDs included 42 women who became pregnant during the study's four-year observation period (Crow et al., 2008). Using the EDE interview every six months, Crow et al. (2008) found that EDE restraint, weight concerns, and shape concerns fell during pregnancy and rebounded to similar levels as those reported pregravid. However, OBEs and compensatory behaviors fell during pregnancy and remained lower following pregnancy, particularly in those with BN. Unfortunately, those with AN showed no significant difference in binge eating or restrictive eating from the pre- to postpartum periods.

In another sample of women who had a diagnosed ED prior to pregnancy but had been in remission, 50% (*n* = 12) experienced a relapse of their ED after birth. Furthermore, 50% of those who relapsed had postpartum depression, 33% (*n* = 4) of whom had low birth weight babies (none of the other 50% had low birth weight babies; Makino et al., 2020). The authors cautioned that it is difficult to predict who might relapse, and that this indicates a need for monitoring these patients through the postpartum period when they might experience compounded clinical issues.

There is limited research on pica during the postpartum period, as well as specific forms of OSFED (formerly EDNOS). Thus, we are not able to report on the prevalence of these disorders in the postpartum period. However, it is likely that for pica, nutritional deficits that might have influenced its onset during pregnancy resolve in the postpartum period, suggesting that symptoms may abate.

Correlates and Risk Factors

Depression and Anxiety

Depression and anxiety can be prevalent during the postpartum period. Specifically, postpartum depression (PPD) is a common disorder characterized by the onset of a mood disorder within four weeks after birth (Wisner et al., 2010). According to a recent meta-analysis, the global rate of postpartum depression is 17.2% (Wang et al., 2021), whereas generalized anxiety disorder in the postpartum period can reach rates between 4.4% and 8.2% (Ross & McLean, 2006).

Past and current depression and/or anxiety symptoms are associated with EDs in the postpartum period. In one study, participants were classified into four groups based on their ED symptomology: "lower disorder eating," "increasing risk," "sub-clinical," and "clinical" (Baskin, Galligan et al., 2021). Results indicated that both depression and anxiety in the postpartum period were associated with an increased risk of falling into the three ED groups. Specifically, falling into the "clinical" ED group was more than four times as likely if women had depression (odds ratio (OR) = 4.48) and more than three times as likely if women had anxiety (OR= 3.17; Baskin, Galligan et al., 2021). This is supported by other research in a Chinese sample, in which depressive symptoms and disordered eating were related in the postpartum period (Lai et al., 2006).

Furthermore, due to the bidirectional association between these disorders, EDs can be a risk factor for the development of depression and anxiety in the postpartum period. Depressive symptomology during the postpartum period is found among individuals with a history of all subtypes of EDs in comparison to those in a no-ED diagnosis control group (Mazzeo et al., 2006). For example, individuals with prior BN or BED were three times more vulnerable to developing postpartum depression compared to individuals with no history of these two EDs; this risk remained after controlling for a history of major depressive disorder (Mazzeo et al., 2006). They also discovered that concern over mistakes, one facet of perfectionism, might be a contributing factor to the severity of an individual's postpartum depression symptomology (Mazzeo et al., 2006). Concern over mistakes, and more broadly perfectionism, are also common features of EDs. Women who strive for perfection might be less likely to disclose that they are struggling with their doctor and may also be less likely to ask for help with PPD than women who do not struggle with perfectionism (Mazzeo et al., 2006).

Individuals with a history of ED or ED symptoms in pregnancy and prior depression have approximately four to six times the risk of depression in the postpartum period (Micali et al., 2011). History of depression, history of an ED, and current ED are all predictors of high anxiety in the postpartum period (Micali et al., 2011). Interestingly, one study found that the *Eating Attitudes Test* (EAT; used to assess eating attitudes, disturbances, and behavior, such as poor body image, having binge episodes, or vomiting after eating) in pregnancy was not significantly related to anxiety and depressive symptoms in the prenatal period or four months postpartum (Carter et al., 2000). However, eating attitudes were related to anxiety and depression 14 months into the postpartum period (Carter et al., 2000). The authors speculated that negative eating attitudes are not as prevalent during pregnancy and early postpartum because the weight fluctuations that women have during these times are more socially accepted, and, therefore, are less likely to be related to anxiety and depression (Carter et al., 2000). However, at 14 months, a woman's weight fluctuation is less socially accepted and instead criticized. This may lead to changes in eating attitudes, and anxiety and depression may result. Overall, a history of or current depression, anxiety, and EDs may all interact throughout an individual's lifetime, particularly during the perinatal period, increasing the risk of experiencing multiple psychopathologies.

Infant Feeding

A large body of research has focused on infant feeding (i.e., bottle feeding, formula feeding, and breastfeeding), EDs, and body image, with mostly mixed findings. There is no consensus on the association between maternal EDs and the initiation of breastfeeding (Kaß et al., 2021). Some research has found no differences between mothers with and without EDs at the initial start of breastfeeding (Torgersen et al., 2010), whereas other work indicates differences between these groups of women (Micali et al., 2009; Nguyen et al., 2017). Clinically significant levels of ED symptoms may also put individuals at risk for early discontinuation of breastfeeding and lower breastfeeding self-efficacy (Kapa et al., 2022). Cessation of breastfeeding at six months was higher among mothers with AN or EDNOS in one study (Torgersen et al., 2010), but remained high for at least partial breastfeeding at six months at 64% in another study (Martini et al., 2019). Authors of a review article found that the literature on this topic is varied (Kaß et al., 2021). Articles finding that EDs were significantly related to the short duration of breastfeeding generally had a larger sample size, whereas those that found no differences between mothers with EDs and mothers with no EDs had smaller sample sizes (Kaß et al., 2021).

Research on breastfeeding and postpartum weight retention and weight loss is not clearly established. A common belief is that breastfeeding is related to postpartum weight loss. Some studies have supported this claim (da Silva et al., 2015; Neville et al., 2014); however, several studies have found no association between breastfeeding and postpartum weight loss (Neville et al., 2014). The full picture surrounding breastfeeding and weight loss is complicated, considering that women are advised to eat more to produce milk. The National Institutes of Health recommend taking an extra 450 to 500 calories per day to support the production of breastmilk (2017), which may be distressing for mothers who are overly concerned about losing their pregnancy weight. More rigorous research is needed to clarify the relationship between breastfeeding and weight loss.

The decision to breastfeed or bottle feed is often nuanced and complex. In individuals with EDs, it may be an especially complicated decision to make considering the added concern surrounding weight and body image. A qualitative study examined mothers with EDs and found that some women wanted to use formula so that they could revert back to their ED tendencies and lose their pregnancy weight (Stapleton et al., 2008). Other mothers wanted to breastfeed because it made them feel like a good mother, they felt they could eat more, and some believed that breastfeeding could help them lose weight (Stapleton et al., 2008). These dilemmas are especially important for women with EDs to understand because physical breastfeeding issues that may influence a decision to breastfeed or bottle feed (e.g., sore nipples or low milk supply) are common experiences for women (Kaß et al., 2021). Therefore, the emotional and cognitive problems that are specifically related to EDs may better explain the added degree of difficulty that mothers with EDs experience regarding breastfeeding (Kaß et al., 2021).

Maternal eating behaviors can also impact whether mothers decide to breast or bottle feed. Individuals with restrained eating or external eating behaviors (i.e., eating in response to the food environment) had an increased likelihood of using formula from birth and had a decreased likelihood of continuing to breastfeed if they had started (Brown, 2014). Furthermore, both restrained and external eating were related to having a "mother-led routine" (vs. a "baby-led routine") when feeding their baby (Brown, 2014). A mother-led routine is indicative of wanting control over their infant's feeding behaviors and formula feeding can allow for this to happen (Brown, 2014). Although recommendations support the benefits of breastfeeding, particularly for the first six months of life (Meek & Noble, 2022), it is also important to assist women in developing self-efficacy in whatever method they choose to feed their babies, whether by breast or bottle.

Maternal EDs have also been linked to general feeding difficulties. Specifically, an ED during pregnancy was found to be a predictor for difficulty with feeding (i.e., slow feeding, no routine, refusing solids) at one month postpartum (Micali et al., 2009). A lifetime history of EDs predicted difficulties with feeding at both one month and six months after birth (Micali et al., 2009). Maternal distress (i.e., anxiety and depressed mood) can, in part, explain the connection between an ED and feeding difficulties (Micali, Simonoff, Stahl, et al., 2011). Specifically, there was a direct association between an ED and feeding difficulties, and this association was partially mediated by anxiety and maternal distress (Micali, Simonoff, Stahl, et al., 2011).

Furthermore, the feeding behavior of infants is affected by the status of EDs in mothers. Individuals with EDs tend to feed their offspring irregularly, and female infants have faster suckling behaviors and a difficult time weaning off of a bottle compared to the infants of mothers without an ED (Agras et al., 1999). Between the ages of two and five, mothers with EDs become significantly more concerned about their daughter's weight than mothers without an ED; however, there is no difference in the daughters' body mass index (BMI) between these groups. Interestingly, mothers with an ED did not demonstrate significant concern regarding their male infants' weight and shape. These results demonstrate that female infants may be at a greater risk for developing an ED based on their own early behaviors (i.e., tendency to have feeding issues) and their mother's concerns (i.e., weight concerns; Agras et al., 1999).

There is also noteworthy research that has investigated breastfeeding in relation to body image. Breastfeeding self-efficacy (i.e., breastfeeding confidence) and positive breastfeeding experiences (i.e., enjoyment, infant growth, and satisfaction) are both related to body image satisfaction (Kapa et al., 2022). The authors speculated that women who view their body in terms of its physical ability to feed their infant have better experiences with breastfeeding compared to women who are more focused on their outward appearance (Kapa et al., 2022). Breastfeeding self-efficacy can also predict breastfeeding duration (De Jager et al., 2015). Furthermore, body image is related to breastfeeding duration, as women with various body image issues across the perinatal period had an increased likelihood of discontinuing breastfeeding early (Brown et al., 2015; De Jager et al., 2015; Swanson et al., 2017).

Body Image Concerns

Issues surrounding body image are addressed throughout the chapter; however, it is important to note how these issues relate specifically to EDs and disordered eating. A recent Australian study found that postpartum body dissatisfaction can put women at risk for developing disordered eating (especially binge eating) via an increase in negative affect (O'Loghlen & Galligan, 2022). Binge eating can act as a way to regulate negative affect and distress surrounding body image (O'Loghlen & Galligan, 2022). In a qualitative study conducted in the United Kingdom, three groups of postpartum mothers (individuals with an ED, individuals at risk for an ED, and a nonclinical comparison group) were interviewed about their body image and eating habits (Patel et al., 2005). Regardless of group, women expressed concern about their postpartum appearance and pregnancy-related weight gain (Patel et al., 2005). Many women were distressed about the changes that occurred to their bodies, and those women in the ED group seemed to express the most distress (Patel et al., 2005).

In the postpartum period, mothers can feel pressure to lose their pregnancy weight and return to their pre-pregnancy body. Sociocultural influences from social media play a part in this pressure. Specifically, social media usage in the German population was related to body image dissatisfaction in the postpartum period. This relation was mediated by the internalization of the thin ideal and appearance-related social comparisons. Moreover, social media usage was also associated with ED symptoms in postpartum (Nagl et al., 2021).

Weight, Diet, and Exercise

EDs and body image issues have also been linked to BMI throughout the perinatal period. Specifically, high BMI during pregnancy (greater than 25.0 kg/m²) was associated with disordered eating in a Chinese sample during the postpartum period (Lai et al., 2006). High BMI before and after pregnancy are also predictors of the continuation of BED in the late postpartum period (Knoph et al., 2013). In a Polish sample of women, the majority (68.8%) were dissatisfied with their body weight and shape in the postpartum period (Grajek et al., 2022). However, individuals with a higher BMI had more body shape dissatisfaction than those with a lower BMI (below 25 kg/m²) (Grajek et al., 2022).

An individual's diet may influence EDs in the postpartum period. In Australian mothers, those who practiced intuitive eating (i.e., bringing awareness to and accepting one's body's hunger and satiety cues, not restricting or feeling guilty about food, having compassion for oneself) had higher body image satisfaction and healthier eating attitudes (Lee et al., 2020). Intuitive eating was also linked to lower levels of EDs (Lee et al., 2020). Importantly, this study included individuals with kids from a wide age range, between six months and four years old. Given that this study stretches well beyond the postpartum period, it demonstrates that these influences can have lasting consequences.

Exercise is also an important factor in relation to body image, and mothers may engage in physical activity in the postpartum period to lose the weight gained during pregnancy. One study divided women into three body image profiles: "average profile," (i.e., average scores on both body dissatisfaction and body appreciation; 55.73% of the sample) "dissatisfied profile," (i.e., higher body dissatisfaction and lower body appreciation; 21.37%) and "appreciative profile" (e.g., higher body appreciation and lower body dissatisfaction; 22.90%). Women with the dissatisfied profile engaged in significantly less exercise than those with the appreciative body image profile (Raspovic et al., 2022). Perhaps women who were appreciative of their bodies and thus had a positive body image engaged in physical activity in an attempt to take care of their bodies. Alternatively, a negative body image may result in shame and reluctance to engage in physical activity, particularly around other people. The interaction between EDs and exercise is complex (Brunet et al., 2021), and much of the research surrounding exercise in postpartum women involves weight management (Nascimento et al., 2014) and its impact on postpartum depression (Marconcin et al., 2021). Surprisingly, little research has been done specifically investigating EDs and exercise in the postpartum period. More research needs to be done to explore these associations.

Infant Health

In the postpartum period, a mother's ED can impact the baby, its development, and its health. In an observational study from the United Kingdom, the one-year-old babies of mothers with EDs weighed significantly less than the babies of mothers in the non-ED control group (Stein et al., 1994). More specifically, this study investigated behaviors during meal times and found that increased conflict during mealtime was associated with lower weight of the infant (Stein et al., 1994). The authors hypothesized that infants may eat less food because they engage in conflict with their mothers. Furthermore, mothers with EDs were unable to successfully mediate these conflicts due to their own difficulties surrounding food (Stein et al., 1994).

Mothers with EDs may also influence their infants' diets, but the evidence is mixed. Research demonstrated that when introducing food to their children, differences can occur between mothers with EDs and those without. One study showed that women with BN were less likely than women without an ED to feed their infant homemade food in comparison to jarred baby food (Torgersen et al., 2015). This is in contrast to another article (Hoffman et al., 2014) that found no differences in the diet composition between mothers with and without a history of an ED. Furthermore, restrictive feeding style scores were actually lower in individuals with a history of ED compared to those in the control group. However, mothers with a history of EDs also anecdotally reported more restricting and controlling of the food quality than the control group, often feeding their infants organic rather than processed foods. Furthermore, the authors noted that the small sample size of this study could limit the ability to find effects (Hoffman et al., 2014). The research is varied, and more work is needed to determine the exact consequences that the infant diet has on current and long-term health (Torgersen et al., 2015). Future research should also focus on parent-infant feeding behaviors to determine if they lead to healthy eating behaviors or lead to restrictive behaviors in children as they grow older (Hoffman et al., 2014).

Sleep

Sleep is also an important factor to consider during this time, particularly given that caregivers need to wake up throughout the night for several months to attend to their babies. Night eating in mothers can start during this time and can continue even after the children sleep through the night (Allison et al., 2004). Short sleep has also been linked with excessive caloric intake (Dashti et al., 2015). Individuals with BED during pregnancy were more dissatisfied with their sleep than those without an ED, even at 18 months postpartum (Ulman et al., 2012). BE episodes commonly occur at night (Raymond et al., 2003). As the evening approaches, the body adapts to anticipate the stress of the binge-eating event, even if an individual does not actually have a binge-eating episode. This may lead to increased cortisol levels, which make it difficult to sleep (Ulman et al., 2012). Alternatively, eating a large amount of food prior to lying down to sleep can be uncomfortable and interrupt sleep. Finally, hunger signals related to daytime eating restriction, which can occur in any of the EDs, may also impair sleep duration and quality (Allison et al., 2016). This is an understudied area that deserves more attention in the postpartum period.

Effects on Relationships

Body image disturbance and EDs may influence the relationships in the mother's life, and relationships in her life may impact eating behaviors and perceptions about the body. Of note, some research in this area focuses on the perinatal period, which encompasses approximately 20 weeks' gestation through four weeks postpartum and does not necessarily separate findings for the postpartum period specifically. However, this research still provides essential insights into ED and body image concerns following birth.

Social Support and Partner Relationships

Relationship satisfaction and spousal support can influence postpartum EDs in mothers. Baskin et al. (2021) investigated EDs across pregnancy and postpartum in four different groups of individuals ("lower disordered eating," "increasing risk," "sub-clinical," and "clinical") across three time points. In the postpartum period, they found that relationship satisfaction along with self-compassion were both associated with a lower chance of being in the sub-clinical ED group (Baskin, Galligan et al., 2021). No other significant associations were found between the other ED risk groups and relationship satisfaction in the postpartum period (Baskin, Galligan et al., 2021). Other research supports this finding, as one study established that high levels of relationship satisfaction were correlated with BED remission in the postpartum period (Knoph et al., 2013). High relationship satisfaction in early pregnancy also predicted a decrease in a woman's concern about body shape during postpartum (Baskin, Meyer et al., 2021). Low partner support during pregnancy was related to disordered eating six months into the postpartum period (Lai et al., 2006). Clearly, the quality of the relationship between the mother and her partner during the pregnancy period can have important repercussions even into postpartum.

A qualitative study identified three groups of mothers (individuals with an ED, individuals at risk for an ED, and a nonclinical comparison group) and interviewed them about their body image and eating habits during the postpartum period (Patel et al., 2005). Individuals across all of the groups mentioned feeling "helpless," "frustrated," and "inadequate" when discussing their family and partner relationships (Patel et al., 2005). However, individuals with an ED during the postpartum period viewed their partner's support in a negative manner. They interpreted comments from their partners as critical (i.e., reinforcing the women's ideas of the importance of a thin body for their relationship) even if the partner did not have that intention. Contrary to this, women in the nonclinical comparison group were more likely to view their family and partners as helpful in confronting any diet attempts or unusual eating patterns (Patel et al., 2005).

In a study investigating body dissatisfaction in postpartum individuals, internalization of the thin ideal and appearance comparison mediated the association between sociocultural pressure (i.e., pressure from the media, the partner, and peers to lose weight or be thin) and eating and body image concerns (Lovering et al., 2018). The authors speculated that positive feedback from partners about individuals' postpartum bodies can be a crucial way they can provide support for women during the postpartum period. This study also established that family influence had a direct relation with body dissatisfaction and was not mediated by the thin ideal and appearance comparison (Lovering et al., 2018). Therefore, messages from family can influence body dissatisfaction. The authors speculated that in families where weight is often discussed and a drive for thinness is idealized, postpartum women may have increased levels of body dissatisfaction (Lovering et al., 2018).

Relationship With the Baby

Poor maternal-fetal attachment during pregnancy and a poor mother–infant relationship postpartum are both related to disordered eating during the postpartum period (Lai et al., 2006). Women with high maternal-fetal attachment are more likely to choose breastfeeding than bottle feeding (Huang et al., 2004). However, breastfeeding can prove to be a difficult adjustment for mothers with EDs, as now they have to pay more attention to their bodies and food intake during this time as compared to times when they are not sustaining their babies' nutrition (Carwell & Spatz, 2011). Individuals with EDs may be uncomfortable with the idea that the baby is relying on them for nutrients via breastfeeding, and some individuals with EDs may think about breastfeeding in terms of their own weight loss (Patel et al., 2005). Breastfeeding, however, can provide an important bonding time for mothers and their infants, and focusing on breastfeeding could help mothers overcome their EDs by casting their ability to feed their babies as a positive purpose for their bodies.

Furthermore, the relationship between the mother and her infant can be influenced by a maternal ED even beyond the breastfeeding period. In one observational study of mothers and their 12-month-old children, mothers with EDs had increased intrusiveness during meals and playtimes and increased negative affect during mealtimes than mothers without an ED (Stein et al., 1994). The infants with maternal EDs also were not as "cheerful" when compared to the infants of the non-ED control group (Stein et al., 1994). Thus, important parent–child interactions can be disrupted if the mother suffers from an ED, which can influence their relationship.

Therapist: What has it been like to adjust to motherhood?

Victoria: It has been really tough. I was honestly excited to have the baby and start to get rid of this baby weight and not worry that my urges to restrict eating would impact my baby, but it's still there, but in a different way.

T: Can you explain that more? That there's a worry but in a different way.

V: Yeah. When I was pregnant, I forced myself to eat more because I knew that the baby needed nutrition to grow. It was uncomfortable seeing and feeling my body getting bigger, but I tried to remind myself that it was all for my baby. Now, she is here, and I'm trying to lose the baby weight, but I'm also told that I still need to eat to make milk for breastfeeding. So, I'm still feeling a battle between the urge to restrict to lose weight but also feed my baby.

T: That's a lot to manage while also taking care of your baby.

V: Yes, it's hard because I still feel the postpartum depression; not as bad as it was right after she was born, but it's still there.

T: Tell me more about the postpartum depression and how it's affecting your eating.

V: I just don't really have an appetite to eat, and in a way, I'm not too bothered by it because I want to lose the baby weight. But, I also know that I need to eat to produce milk. I'm already having issues with milk production, I think because I'm not eating enough, so it makes me feel like a bad mother, which makes the depression worse, too.

T: It does sound like a tough situation and like a cycle between the depression and eating.

V: It is a cycle, and I don't know how to get out of it. The part that makes me feel the worst is that I feel like I lost out on bonding with my baby after she was first born. Between the postpartum depression, not making enough milk for her, and having trouble getting her to latch, I felt distant from her. The stress of all of that plus not sleeping at night, just with normal nighttime feedings, was making the urge to restrict even more intense because I wanted some sort of control over my life.

Assessment

Although individuals in the postpartum period may be returning toward some normalcy, or perhaps a new normal, their bodies are still changing and their energy needs and drive to eat may fluctuate depending on factors such as whether they are breastfeeding, how much sleep debt they are accumulating, and whether they are experiencing postpartum distress. Despite these differences, most studies have used established eating disorder assessment tools to measure disordered eating in the postpartum period.

Some studies have used interview or survey items that map onto the DSM-IV or DSM-5, depending on when the studies were conducted. For example, the Norwegian Mother and Child Cohort study (MoBa) used this approach in its large, population-based study of EDs in pregnancy and the postpartum periods (Knoph et al., 2013). Some have used such items as a follow-up to survey questions to confirm a diagnosis (Makino et al., 2020).

The *Eating Attitudes Test*-26 (EAT-26; Garner & Garfinkel, 1979) has been used more frequently than DSM-based items. This self-report measure assesses broad eating pathology with a standardized, clinical cut score of 20 indicating the likely presence of an ED. Several studies have used the EAT-26 in the postpartum period to assess ED symptoms, including U.S. (Thompson & Bardone-Cone, 2021), Chinese (Chan et al., 2019), and Japanese samples (Makino et al., 2020). These researchers used versions of the EAT-26 that were validated for use with their native populations and/or translations but did not show much validation data for these postpartum samples. Thompson and Bardone-Cone (2021) indicated a coefficient alpha of 0.88 suggesting high internal consistency, but no such measures were indicated in the other two papers.

The *Eating Disorder Examination-Questionnaire* (EDE-Q; Fairburn et al., 2008) has been used most frequently in research of EDs in the postpartum period. The EDE-Q is based on the original interview version of the EDE and measures four factors related to disordered eating attitudes, as well as specific ED behaviors over the past 28 days. The four subscales validated in general samples include dietary restraint, eating concerns, shape concerns, and weight concerns, as well as a global score. These subscales have shown strong internal consistency (αs = 0.78 to 0.93; Luce & Crowther, 1999) and concurrent validity (rs = 0.68 to 0.84; Mond et al., 2004) in past studies. Several studies have used the original EDE-Q, including U.S. (Vanderkruik et al., 2022) and Brazilian samples (Nunes et al., 2014), with Vanderkruik et al. reporting Cronbach's alpha of 0.94, presumably for the global score, and no validation data reported from Nunes et al. (2014).

The only adaptation found in the literature for the EDE-Q, or any other ED measure, for the postpartum period, was published by Pettersson et al. (2016). These researchers administered the EDE-Q at several postpartum clinics in Stockholm, with data from 335 women between six and eight weeks postpartum. They performed an exploratory factor analysis that yielded a three-factor model, instead of the four-factor model found in general samples and named them: (a) dissatisfaction with shape and weight, (b) eating concern, and (c) avoidance of eating. Pettersson et al. removed low-loading items, leaving 14 items of the ED-related attitudes questions, and the six items assessing ED behaviors (e.g., binge-eating and compensatory behaviors). They removed items referring to a desire for a flat stomach, fear of weight gain, reaction to prescribed weighing, importance of weight, preoccupation with food, eating in secret, desire for an empty stomach, and restraint over eating. The "optimized version" estimated a higher percent of new mothers as scoring above the clinical cut score for ED attitudes, at 12.8%, compared to 7.2% using the original version. However, there were low levels of ED behaviors overall, with 1.2 days of objective overeating, 0.1 episodes of loss of control eating, 0.1 objective binge episodes, 0 vomiting or laxative use episodes, and 0.2 days of excessive exercise over the past 28. This suggests that the ED behaviors may be low during this time, but that disordered eating attitudes are fairly common.

Given this version of the EDE-Q is six items shorter than the original, it may be easier to use as a screening questionnaire in clinical practice, although a 20-item survey is still considered long for a screener. As referenced in the previous chapter in this volume on EDs during pregnancy, the SCOFF, a five-item questionnaire designed to screen for AN and BN (Morgan et al., 1999), may be the best brief measure to use by practitioners during the postpartum period in a clinical setting. The SCOFF is an abbreviation for the symptoms assessed in each item: 1. Do you make yourself *Sick* (vomit) because you feel uncomfortably full? 2. Do you worry that you have lost *Control* over how much you eat? 3. Have you lost more than *One* stone (15 lb) in a three-month period? 4. Do you believe yourself to be *Fat* when others say you are too thin? and 5. Would you say that *Food* dominates your life? It is evident that more work is needed in this area to determine if the currently used assessment tools are valid in this population, and new screeners for clinical practice are especially needed.

OB/GYN:	It's nice to see you for your six-week postpartum visit. How is everything going?
Victoria:	It's going okay. I still have some trouble with breastfeeding but we are supplementing with formula when needed to make sure the baby gets enough.
O:	That's good. You have to do what works best for you and your family. The most important part if that she is fed. You completed a screening questionnaire for me in the waiting room. Can you talk about that?
V:	Yes, sure.
O:	It looks like you are having some concerns about your body and your eating.
V:	Yes, I have never been this big before and I thought the baby weight would be easier to lose after she was born. I'm finding myself counting calories again and sort of restricting things that I eat.
O:	You are not alone in these types of feelings, and I also want to make sure you are getting support to deal with them.
V:	Yes, I know. I am still meeting with my therapist weekly, and we are talking about these things. I appreciate that you checked in on them, though.

Treatment

It is recommended that treatment for EDs during the postpartum period involve a multidisciplinary team approach (Astrachan-Fletcher et al., 2008), similar to recommendations for prenatal treatment. A combination of psychological (individual, group, and/or family therapy), pharmacotherapy, medical treatment, and nutritional counseling should be considered. Level of care is dependent upon multiple factors, including medical status (e.g., weight status, cardiac functioning, vital signs, and/or bloodwork/laboratory abnormalities), severity of disordered eating behaviors, comorbid psychopathology, motivation for recovery, insuf-ficient or excessive weight gain during pregnancy, high preoccupation with weight during and/or after pregnancy, and environmental stress (Astrachan-Fletcher et al., 2008; Bye et al., 2021). Similar to the prenatal period, there are limited treatment protocols for the treatment of EDs in the postpartum period; however, treatments for EDs in general may be applied.

Multiple forms of psychotherapy can be considered and have been reviewed with addi-tional considerations for the postpartum period (Astrachan-Fletcher et al., 2008). Cogni-tive behavioral therapy (CBT) is relatively short term (16 to 20 sessions) and focuses on the thoughts and behaviors of the ED. It aims to normalize eating patterns (i.e., establish a regular pattern of eating throughout the day), reduce body shape/weight/eating concerns and dysfunctional beliefs, and develop coping strategies to manage triggers for restricting, binge-eating, and/or compensatory behaviors. Interpersonal therapy (IPT), on the other hand, focuses on interpersonal difficulties, including role transitions (e.g., becoming a par-ent), that can impact the re-emergence of EDs following the birth of a child. Dialectical behavior therapy (DBT) focuses on developing coping strategies, including mindfulness and emotion regulation, in addition to skills in interpersonal effectiveness and distress toler-ance. Authors of this review and recommendations for treatment of EDs with postpartum women also suggest that special attention be given to simultaneously treating postpartum depression during psychotherapy, if indicated, due to high comorbidity. Treatment should also address mother–infant interactions, particularly during feeding and mealtimes, to improve the mother's ability to respond to their child's cues, and mealtime conflicts, and increase infant/child autonomy (Astrachan-Fletcher et al., 2008). Pharmacotherapy may also be used in combination with psychotherapy to treat disordered eating behaviors (e.g., reduce binge eating or loss of control eating) and treat comorbid depression and/or anxiety (Astrachan-Fletcher et al., 2008); however, it is important to include a psychiatrist or other informed medical provider when including psychotropic medication in a treatment plan.

Family, partners, and/or other important support persons/people should be included in the care plan to improve support in the home environment (Bye et al., 2021). There are a few couples-based interventions that have been developed for adults with EDs, which could be used with those who are transitioning into parenthood. The Uniting Couples in the treatment of Anorexia Nervosa (UCAN; Bulik et al., 2011) and the UNIting Couples in the Treatment of Eating disorders (UNITE; Kirby et al., 2015) focus on AN and binge-eating type disorders, respectively. These treatments integrate CBT for couples therapy, CBT for EDs, and DBT principles to assist couples in making joint decisions about the treatment process, adapting to their role transition as new parents (if they just had a baby), and managing environmental stressors. These interventions include three treatment targets: (a) reduce ED symptoms and stress by improving communication between partners about the symptoms; (b) enhance interpersonal, problem-solving, and behavior change skills; and (c) develop emotion regulation strategies, in part to manage triggers, mealtimes, stressors, and ED urges and behaviors. These treatments also aim to increase partner support and intimacy, trust, communication, and relapse prevention to facilitate the treatment goals, which can improve parenting.

There is an extreme paucity of literature examining these treatments, although it seems that a randomized trial to test UNITE versus CBT for eating disorders (CBT-E) was recently completed, with final results not yet published (Bulik & Baucom, 2019, clinicaltrials.gov NCT03784820). In a case study of UCAN, both partners reported high satisfaction with the treatment (Kirby et al., 2016). These partners were parents, but it did not appear they were new parents. The woman partner (with AN) had a significant reduction in dietary restraint but not eating, shape, or weight concerns subscales of the EDE semi-structured clinical interview assessment. There was also a significant improvement in relationship satisfaction and communication between partners. Furthermore, in an open pilot trial for UNITE for BED, 11 couples completed 22 weekly sessions of treatment (Runfola et al., 2018). An impressive 81.8% of participants reported abstinence from OBEs by the end of treatment, with a significant reduction in total OBEs in the past 28 days from pre- to post-treatment (pre-treatment: $M = 11.4$, $SD = 11.02$ vs. post-treatment: $M = .9$, $SD = 2.51$, $p = .009$). There were also significant reductions in depression symptoms ($d = .89$ for the patient and $d = .11$ for the partner) and improvements in emotion regulation for the partner with an ED ($d = .97$ for the patient and $d = -.20$ for the partner; Sadeh-Sharvit et al., 2016).

The Parent-Based Prevention (PBP) of Eating Disorders similarly focuses on parents with EDs and their children aged 5 years and younger (Sadeh-Sharvit et al., 2020). It targets three risk mechanisms: (a) feeding behaviors influenced by the mother's (with history or current ED) concerns rather than by the child's own hunger/satiety cues; (b) any comorbid psychopathology (with the ED) that may further impact parental functioning; and (c) issues in parental communication regarding the child's feeding behaviors and/or daily routines. The protocol includes group therapy for the parent with an ED (current or lifetime), family sessions, and spousal sessions. A pilot study of 16 families (with a 25% attrition rate) indicated significant post-treatment reductions in the mother's (with EDs) concerns about their child's eating ($d = 1.15$) and weight ($d = .62$), monitoring of the child's eating ($d = .11$), pressures of the child to eat ($d = .61$), and maternal symptomology ($d = 3.56$ for eating symptoms and $d = .68$ for comorbid symptoms). The mothers did not perceive differences from pre- to post-treatment in their child's eating-related symptoms, whereas their spouse did perceive a significant reduction in these symptoms at the end of treatment ($d = .48$). This pilot study provides promising results for these prevention efforts, although additional research is needed.

The chapter in this volume on prenatal body image disturbances and EDs discusses other body image-focused interventions that can be considered for use during the postpartum period as well. These include a cognitive dissonance-based intervention called The Body Project, that targets thin ideal internalization. It helps people identify the consequences of internalizing the thin ideal and uses exercises to think and act counter to these negative body-focused beliefs (Becker & Stice, 2017). Vanderkruik et al. (2022) conducted a qualitative study to identify important body- and eating-related concerns for perinatal women and indicated that the themes could be easily incorporated into The Body Project. Another study tested a self-compassion meditation program, among a combined group of prenatal and postpartum women, that focused on reducing body shame and body dissatisfaction, while increasing body appreciation and self-compassion (Papini et al., 2022). Findings indicated that, after controlling for covariates and baseline scores, the treatment group (compared to the control group) predicted lower body shame ($R^2 = .71$) and body dissatisfaction ($R^2 = .70$), as well as body appreciation ($R^2 = .75$) and higher self-compassion ($R^2 = .61$).

As stated previously, women with EDs may be at a higher risk for postpartum depression than women without EDs. Psychoeducation should be provided during the prenatal period to the patient and their partner, when appropriate (Harris, 2010). It is suggested that women with EDs should be scheduled for visits at one and two weeks postpartum to assess for postpartum depression, ED symptoms, and adjustment to motherhood. These early visits can include education about the normal feelings and emotions experienced postpartum, as well as developing and/or reinforcing coping strategies to manage the adjustment to motherhood. Providers may also discuss the risk of unplanned pregnancy during the postpartum period given that some women with EDs have an irregular menstrual cycle and may believe they cannot get pregnant again.

Therapist:	You said previously that your urge to restrict increases when a situation feels out of control. Is that the primary way that you cope with or manage stressors?
Victoria:	Yes, I guess so.
T:	What are typical triggers for these urges to restrict?
V:	I don't know, it can be anything that's unexpected or stressful.
T:	That often describes parenthood.
V:	Yes! I didn't realize or expect that I couldn't plan for or anticipate things that happen with kids. It is like being in a constant state of unknown.
T:	That can be uncomfortable.
V:	I'm very uncomfortable in those feelings, so controlling my calories kind of calms me and gives me something to focus on that I can fully plan and control.
T:	Does your partner know this? The stress you are experiencing as a new mother and how it affects the eating disorder?
V:	Yes, kind of. I'm not sure if we've ever talked about it specifically.
T:	Do you think it could be a helpful conversation?
V:	Sure, to give my perspective on why it's been especially hard for me since the baby was born.
T:	If restriction was used to cope with stress, we don't want to leave you without other strategies or skills. What are other ways you can cope in these situations?
V:	. . . I don't really know. This has been my go-to. Perhaps going for a walk? I can do that with the baby in the stroller, and we can do it as a family since my partner and I would work out together before the baby was born.
T:	That sounds like a great idea. Perhaps a family walk could also be a time for you and your partner to talk about the week and plan for events, whether it's childcare duties, mealtimes, or other activities?
V:	That could be a good time to make sure we're talking about things, not just about the baby, and also planning for how to divide up the daily household duties. Then maybe it wouldn't be as hectic in the moment.
T:	We can continue to discuss your plans for how often you plan to go on these family walks and how to talk to your partner about this idea, as well as other strategies to use if a walk isn't feasible at a particular time.

Cultural Considerations

Research concerned with investigating the association between postpartum individuals' culturally relevant identities and disordered eating and body image is sparse. This section aims to highlight the existing research on postpartum individuals' racial/ethnic background and socioeconomic status (SES) in relation to their pathology to demonstrate the importance of these factors.

Racial and Ethnic Backgrounds

Research suggests differences in postpartum body image satisfaction between racial and/or ethnic groups. Two studies found that postpartum Black women experienced significantly higher levels of body satisfaction when compared to women who identified as White, Hispanic, or another racial/ethnic identity (Gjerdingen et al., 2009; Walker et al., 2002). Providing similar results, another study utilized the *Stunkard Figure Rating Scale* (FRS) to measure women's perceived current and ideal body sizes. The Stunkard FRS has participants select 1 of 9 body figures (1 having the smallest body size and 9 having the largest body size) that resemble their current, as well as ideal, body, (Stunkard et al., 1983). Black women in this study had lower discrepancies between their perceived current body size and ideal body size ($M = 1.7, SD = 0.1$), indicating lower body dissatisfaction when compared to White women ($M = 2.3, SD = 2.3, p <$ .001; Carter-Edwards et al., 2010). It is important to highlight, however, that Black women still experience body image disturbances in the postpartum period. For instance, a study of 105 low-income, postpartum Black women utilized the *Reese Scale*, which is a culturally sensitive, validated figure rating scale (Boyington et al., 2007). The average body satisfaction score—defined as an individual's preferred (also termed "ideal") size score subtracted from their current size score—was reported as –0.92 ($SD = 1.81, p < .001$). This, coupled with the study finding that over 50% of participants desired to lose weight, and nearly 75% were not satisfied with the size of their bodies (Boyington et al., 2007), indicates body dissatisfaction. Future research is warranted to elucidate this issue, but it is clear that racial and ethnic background can influence body image postpartum. Studies should also address differences in eating disorder symptoms and presentations appropriately to inform assessment and treatment.

Socioeconomic Status

Although limited, research suggests that SES may impact body image and eating disorders postpartum. Authors of one study reported that women of high SES had greater confidence in achieving their postpartum weight loss goals and retained less weight when compared to women of medium and lower SES (Shrewsbury et al., 2008). When compared to women of high SES, women with a lower SES had greater differences between their pre-pregnancy weight and their ideal weight in the future (Shrewsbury et al., 2008). The authors also found that there was no difference in body dissatisfaction or the desire to lose weight. Other researchers observed disordered eating and body image in a sample of Brazilian women with high rates of unemployment in addition to low levels of schooling and family income (Nunes et al., 2014). These women reported higher levels of body image dissatisfaction during the postpartum period—with the highest level of dissatisfaction occurring at six months postpartum—when compared to their prepregnant and pregnant self-perceptions. Weight retention during the postpartum period was associated with eating disorder symptomatology. Reports indicate that although postpartum women exhibited high levels of ED-related cognitions (e.g., over-concern about weight), they did not exhibit inappropriate compensatory behaviors (e.g., self-induced vomiting and laxative abuse; Nunes et al., 2014).

Food insecurity also may be related to disordered eating, and it exists in low-, middle-, and high-income countries, primarily affecting marginalized communities (Hazzard et al., 2020). Individuals with marginally insecure or food insecure households had higher levels of disordered eating behaviors in the postpartum period (Laraia et al., 2015). Further research is encouraged to expand upon the impact of SES on postpartum experiences. It is imperative that disparities are illuminated in an effort to provide equitable care.

Therapist:	Are there any early childhood experiences that you think influenced your eating?
Victoria:	You know, now that I think about it, maybe some of my restrictions started as a kid when my family didn't have enough food for all of us.
T:	Tell me more about that.
V:	We didn't have a lot of money growing up, so we had to make our meals stretch throughout the month, especially at the end of the month when our benefits would run out. I would purposely not eat as much to make sure my younger siblings had enough to eat; and maybe it was also to have some sort of control over the situation since I couldn't do anything to help my parents. I guess I got used to it, in a way, and now it shades how I think about what is "enough" for me to eat instead of "what does my body need right now?
T:	How do you think replacing the thought, "What is enough?" with "What does my body need?" might impact what and how much you eat?
V:	I could try to ask myself that each time I eat to help me think about food as something that I need instead of something bad or something I'm not worthy enough to have.

Conclusion and Future Directions

It is evident that body image issues and eating disorders are important to address during postpartum. These pathologies significantly impact the mother, child, and her relationships. For some women, the postpartum period is particularly difficult as ED symptoms re-emerge that may have reduced or remitted during pregnancy. Multidisciplinary treatment teams are needed to provide proper care, and further research must validate assessment methods and treatment options that are effective across postpartum patients' identities.

Future researchers are encouraged to examine the multitude of factors surrounding disordered eating and/or body image during the postpartum period. Of importance, assessment and screening tools should be prioritized to improve the prediction of relapse of ED symptoms postpartum. Interventions for postpartum people and their support system, including the Uniting Couples in the treatment of Anorexia Nervosa (UCAN), the UNIting Couples in the Treatment of Eating disorders (UNITE), and the Parent-Based Prevention (PBP) of Eating Disorders should continue to be validated. Postpartum providers should prioritize staying abreast of the research as our knowledge of this population continues to develop.

Psychoeducation provided to the mother on factors surrounding breastfeeding, her attachment style, and the link between these constructs may prove fruitful in developing a healthy relationship with her child. Providing education to the mother's partner, family, and peers is essential as this may help mitigate potential issues by informing others on how to properly support the mother throughout the postpartum period, including understanding that those with EDs may interpret their support through the lens of their ED and not as their support person intended. Future research should investigate methods to increase the effectiveness of and streamline the education of the mother, partners, family members, peers, and medical providers.

Finally, it is vital for future researchers to study and develop an understanding of cultural factors affecting individuals in the postpartum period suffering from EDs and disordered body image. Once cultural factors are identified, their application to modern care practice is crucial to providing proper care. These factors do not exist in a vacuum; medical providers must take a patient-centered approach by accounting for their patients' multi-faceted backgrounds to deliver care that is genuine and effective.

References

Agras, S., Hammer, L., & McNicholas, F. (1999). A prospective study of the influence of eating-disordered mothers on their children. *International Journal of Eating Disorders, 25*(3), 253–262. https://doi.org/10.1002/(SICI)1098-108X(199904)25:3<253::AID-EAT2>3.0.CO;2-Z

Allison, K. C., Spaeth, A., & Hopkins, C. M. (2016). Sleep and eating disorders. *Current Psychiatry Reports, 18*(10), 92. https://doi.org/10.1007/s11920-016-0728-8

Allison, K. C., Stunkard, A. J., & Thier, S. L. (2004). *Overcoming night eating syndrome: A step-by-step guide to breaking the cycle.* New Harbinger Publications.

Astrachan-Fletcher, E., Veldhuis, C., Lively, N., Fowler, C., & Marcks, B. (2008). The reciprocal effects of eating disorders and the postpartum period: A review of the literature and recommendations for clinical care. *Journal of Women's Health, 17*(2), 227–239. https://doi.org/10.1089/jwh.2007.0550

Ayers, S., Crawley, R., Webb, R., Button, S., & Thornton, A. (2019). What are women stressed about after birth? *Birth, 46*(4), 678–685. https://doi.org/10.1111/birt.12455

Baskin, R., Galligan, R., & Meyer, D. (2021). Disordered eating from pregnancy to the postpartum period: The role of psychosocial and mental health factors. *Appetite, 156*, 104862. https://doi.org/10.1016/j.appet.2020.104862

Baskin, R., Meyer, D., & Galligan, R. (2021). Predicting the change in perinatal disordered eating symptoms: An examination of psychosocial factors. *Body Image, 37*, 162–171. https://doi.org/10.1016/j.bodyim.2021.02.002

Becker, C. B., & Stice, E. (2017). From efficacy to effectiveness to broad implementation: Evolution of the body project. *Journal of Consulting and Clinical Psychology, 85*(8), 767–782. https://doi.org/10.1037/ccp0000204

Boyington, J., Johnson, A., & Carter-Edwards, L. (2007). Dissatisfaction with body size among low-income, postpartum Black women. *Journal of Obstetric, Gynecologic & Neonatal Nursing, 36*(2), 144–151. https://doi.org/10.1111/j.1552-6909.2007.00127.x

Brown, A. (2014). Maternal restraint and external eating behaviour are associated with formula use or shorter breastfeeding duration. *Appetite, 76*, 30–35. https://doi.org/10.1016/j.appet.2013.12.022

Brown, A., Rance, J., & Warren, L. (2015). Body image concerns during pregnancy are associated with a shorter breast feeding duration. *Midwifery, 31*(1), 80–89. https://doi.org/10.1016/j.midw.2014.06.003

Brunet, J., Del Duchetto, F., & Wurz, A. (2021). Physical activity behaviors and attitudes among women with an eating disorder: A qualitative study. *Journal of Eating Disorders, 9*(1). https://doi.org/10.1186/s40337-021-00377-w

Bulik, C. M., & Baucom, D. H. (2019). Uniting couples in the treatment of binge eating disorder (UNITE). *ClinicalTrials.gov identifier: NCT03784820.* Updated April 11, 2023. Retrieved October 6, 2023, from https://clinicaltrials.gov/study/NCT03784820

Bulik, C. M., Baucom, D. H., Kirby, J. S., & Pisetsky, E. (2011). Uniting Couples (in the treatment of) Anorexia Nervosa (UCAN). *International Journal of Eating Disorders, 44*(1), 1928. https://doi.org/10.1002/eat.20790

Burns, M., & Gavey, N. (2004). "Healthy weight" at what cost? "Bulimia" and a discourse of weight control. *Journal of Health Psychology, 9*(4), 549–565. https://doi.org/10.1177/1359105304044039

Bye, A., Martini, M. G., & Micali, N. (2021). Eating disorders, pregnancy and the postnatal period: A review of the recent literature. *Current Opinion in Psychiatry, 34*(6), 563–568. https://doi.org/10.1097/YCO.0000000000000748

Carter, A. S., Baker, C. W., & Brownell, K. D. (2000). Body mass index, eating attitudes, and symptoms of depression and anxiety in pregnancy and the postpartum period. *Psychosomatic Medicine, 62*(2), 264–270.

Carter-Edwards, L., Bastian, L. A., Revels, J., Durham, H., Lokhnygina, Y., Amamoo, M. A., & Ostbye, T. (2010). Body image and body satisfaction differ by race in overweight postpartum mothers. *Journal of Women's Health, 19*(2), 305–311. https://doi.org/10.1089/jwh.2008.1238

Carwell, M. L., & Spatz, D. L. (2011). Eating disorders and breastfeeding. *MCN: The American Journal of Maternal/Child Nursing, 36*(2), 112–117. https://doi.org/10.1097/NMC.0b013e318205775c

Chan, C. Y., Lee, A. M., Koh, Y. W., Lam, S. K., Lee, C. P., Leung, K. Y., & Tang, C. S. K. (2019). Course, risk factors, and adverse outcomes of disordered eating in pregnancy. *International Journal of Eating Disorders, 52*(6), 652–658. https://doi.org/10.1002/eat.23065

Clark, A., Skouteris, H., Wertheim, E. H., Paxton, S. J., & Milgrom, J. (2009). My baby body: A qualitative insight into women's body-related experiences and mood during pregnancy and the postpartum. *Journal of Reproductive and Infant Psychology, 27*(4), 330–345. https://doi.org/10.1080/02646830903190904

Crow, S. J., Agras, W. S., Crosby, R., Halmi, K., & Mitchell, J. E. (2008). Eating disorder symptoms in pregnancy: A prospective study. *International Journal of Eating Disorders, 41*(3), 277–279. https://doi.org/10.1002/eat.20496

Dashti, H. S., Scheer, F. A., Jacques, P. F., Lamon-Fava, S., & Ordovás, J. M. (2015). Short sleep duration and dietary intake: Epidemiologic evidence, mechanisms, and health implications. *Advances in Nutrition, 6*(6), 648–659.

da Silva, M. D. C. M., Oliveira Assis, A. M., Pinheiro, S. M. C., de Oliveira, L. P. M., & da Cruz, T. R. P. (2015). Breastfeeding and maternal weight changes during 24 months post-partum: A cohort study. *Maternal & Child Nutrition, 11*(4), 780–791. https://doi.org/10.1111/mcn.12071

De Jager, E., Broadbent, J., Fuller-Tyszkiewicz, M., Nagle, C., McPhie, S., & Skouteris, H. (2015). A longitudinal study of the effect of psychosocial factors on exclusive breastfeeding duration. *Midwifery, 31*(1), 103–111. https://doi.org/10.1016/j.midw.2014.06.009

Fairburn, C. G., Cooper, Z., & O'Connor, M. (2008). Eating disorder examination (Edition 16.0 D). In C. Fairburn (Ed.), *Cognitive behavior therapy and eating disorders* (pp. 265–308). Guilford Press.

Garner, D. M., & Garfinkel, P. E. (1979). The eating attitudes test: An index of the symptoms of anorexia nervosa. *Psychological Medicine, 9*(2), 273–279. https://doi.org/10.1017/s0033291700030762

Gjerdingen, D., Fontaine, P., Crow, S., McGovern, P., Center, B., & Miner, M. (2009). Predictors of mothers' postpartum body dissatisfaction. *Women & Health, 49*(6–7), 491–504. https://doi.org/10.1080/03630240903423998

Grajek, M., Krupa-Kotara, K., Grot, M., Kujawińska, M., Helisz, P., Gwioździk, W., . . . Kobza, J. (2022). Perception of the body image in women after childbirth and the specific determinants of their eating behavior: Cross-sectional study (Silesia, Poland). *International Journal of Environmental Research and Public Health, 19*(16), 10137. https://doi.org/10.3390/ijerph191610137

Grogan, S. (2021). *Understanding body dissatisfaction in men, women and children* (4th ed.). Routledge. https://doi.org/10.4324/9781003100041

Harris, A. A. (2010). Practical advice for caring for women with eating disorders during the perinatal period. *Journal of Midwifery & Women's Health, 55*(6), 579–586. https://doi.org/10.1016/j.jmwh.2010.07.008

Hazzard, V. M., Loth, K. A., Hooper, L., & Becker, C. B. (2020). Food insecurity and eating disorders: A review of emerging evidence. *Current Psychiatry Reports, 22*(12), 74. https://doi.org/10.1007/s11920-020-01200-0

Hodgkinson, E. L., Smith, D. M., & Wittkowski, A. (2014). Women's experiences of their pregnancy and postpartum body image: A systematic review and meta-synthesis. *BMC Pregnancy and Childbirth, 14*, 330. https://doi.org/10.1186/1471-2393-14-330

Hoffman, E. R., Bentley, M. E., Hamer, R. M., Hodges, E. A., Ward, D. S., & Bulik, C. M. (2014). A comparison of infant and toddler feeding practices of mothers with and without histories of eating disorders. *Maternal & Child Nutrition, 10*(3), 360–372. https://doi.org/10.1111/j.1740-8709.2012.00429.x

Huang, H.-C., Wang, S.-Y., & Chen, C.-H. (2004). Body image, maternal-fetal attachment, and choice of infant feeding method: A study in Taiwan. *Birth, 31*(3), 183–188. https://doi.org/10.1111/j.0730-7659.2004.00303.x

Kapa, H. M., Litteral, J. L., Keim, S. A., Jackson, J. L., Schofield, K. A., & Crerand, C. E. (2022). Body image dissatisfaction, breastfeeding experiences, and self-efficacy in postpartum women with and without eating disorder symptoms. *Journal of Human Lactation, 38*(4), 633–643. https://doi.org/10.1177/08903344221076529

Kaß, A., Dörsam, A. F., Weiß, M., Zipfel, S., & Giel, K. E. (2021). The impact of maternal eating disorders on breastfeeding practices: A systematic review. *Archives of Women's Mental Health, 24*(5), 693–708. https://doi.org/10.1007/s00737-021-01103-w

Kirby, J. S., Fischer, M. S., Raney, T. J., Baucom, D. H., & Bulik, C. M. (2016). Couple-based interventions in the treatment of adult anorexia nervosa: A brief case example of UCAN. *Psychotherapy*, *53*(2), 241–250. https://doi.org/10.1037/pst0000053

Kirby, J. S., Runfola, C. D., Fischer, M. S., Baucom, D. H., & Bulik, C. M. (2015). Couple-based interventions for adults with eating disorders. *Eating Disorders*, *23*(4), 356–365. https://doi.org/1 0.1080/10640266.2015.1044349

Knoph, C., Von Holle, A., Zerwas, S., Torgersen, L., Tambs, K., Stoltenberg, C., . . . Reichborn-Kjennerud, T. (2013). Course and predictors of maternal eating disorders in the postpartum period. *International Journal of Eating Disorders*, *46*(4), 355–368. https://doi.org/10.1002/eat.22088

Lai, B. P., Tang, C. S., & Tse, W. K. (2006). A longitudinal study investigating disordered eating during the transition to motherhood among Chinese women in Hong Kong. *International Journal of Eating Disorders*, *39*(4), 303–311. https://doi.org/10.1002/eat.20266

Laraia, B., Vinikoor-Imler, L. C., & Siega-Riz, A. M. (2015). Food insecurity during pregnancy leads to stress, disordered eating, and greater postpartum weight among overweight women. *Obesity*, *23*(6), 1303–1311. https://doi.org/10.1002/oby.21075

Lee, M. F., Williams, S. L., & Burke, K. J. (2020). Striving for the thin ideal post-pregnancy: A cross-sectional study of intuitive eating in postpartum women. *Journal of Reproductive and Infant Psychology*, *38*(2), 127–138. https://doi.org/10.1080/02646838.2019.1607968

Lovering, M. E., Rodgers, R. F., George, J. E., & Franko, D. L. (2018). Exploring the tripartite influence model of body dissatisfaction in postpartum women. *Body Image*, *24*, 44–54. https://doi.org/10.1016/j.bodyim.2017.12.001

Luce, K. H., & Crowther, J. H. (1999). The reliability of the Eating Disorder Examination-Self-Report Questionnaire version (EDE-Q). *International Journal of Eating Disorders*, *25*(3), 349–351. https://doi.org/10.1002/(sici)1098-108x(199904)25:3<349::aid-eat15>3.0.co;2-m

Makino, M., Yasushi, M., & Tsutsui, S. (2020). The risk of eating disorder relapse during pregnancy and after delivery and postpartum depression among women recovered from eating disorders. *BMC Pregnancy and Childbirth*, *20*(1), 323. https://doi.org/10.1186/s12884-020-03006-7

Marconcin, P., Peralta, M., Gouveia, É. R., Ferrari, G., Carraça, E., Ihle, A., & Marques, A. (2021). Effects of exercise during pregnancy on postpartum depression: A systematic review of meta-analyses. *Biology*, *10*(12), 1331. https://doi.org/10.3390/biology10121331

Martini, M. G., Taborelli, E., Schmidt, U., Treasure, J., & Micali, N. (2019). Infant feeding behaviours and attitudes to feeding amongst mothers with eating disorders: A longitudinal study. *European Eating Disorders Review: The Journal of the Eating Disorders Association*, *27*(2), 137–146. https://doi.org/10.1002/erv.2626

Mazzeo, S. E., Slof-Op't Landt, M. C. T., Jones, I., Mitchell, K., Kendler, K. S., Neale, M. C., . . . Bulik, C. M. (2006). Associations among postpartum depression, eating disorders, and perfectionism in a population-based sample of adult women. *International Journal of Eating Disorders*, *39*(3), 202–211. https://doi.org/10.1002/eat.20243

Meek, J. Y., & Noble, L. (2022). Policy statement: Breastfeeding and the use of human milk. *Pediatrics*, *150*(1), e2022057988. https://doi.org/10.1542/peds.2022-057988

Micali, N., Simonoff, E., Stahl, D., & Treasure, J. (2011). Maternal eating disorders and infant feeding difficulties: Maternal and child mediators in a longitudinal general population study. *Journal of Child Psychology and Psychiatry*, *52*(7), 800–807. https://doi.org/10.1111/j.1469-7610.2010.02341.x

Micali, N., Simonoff, E., & Treasure, J. (2009). Infant feeding and weight in the first year of life in babies of women with eating disorders. *Journal of Pediatrics*, *154*(1), 55–60, e1. https://doi.org/10.1016/j.jpeds.2008.07.003

Micali, N., Simonoff, E., & Treasure, J. (2011). Pregnancy and post-partum depression and anxiety in a longitudinal general population cohort: The effect of eating disorders and past depression. *Journal of Affective Disorders*, *131*(1), 150–157. https://doi.org/10.1016/j.jad.2010.09.034

Miller, R. L., Pallant, J. F., & Negri, L. M. (2006). Anxiety and stress in the postpartum: Is there more to postnatal distress than depression? *BMC Psychiatry*, *6*(1), 12. https://doi.org/10.1186/1471-244X-6-12

Mond, J. M., Hay, P. J., Rodgers, B., Owen, C., & Beumont, P. J. V. (2004). Validity of the Eating Disorder Examination Questionnaire (EDE-Q) in screening for eating disorders in community samples. *Behaviour Research and Therapy*, *42*(5), 551–567. https://doi.org/10.1016/S0005-7967(03)00161-X

Morgan, J. F., Reid, F., & Lacey, J. H. (1999). The SCOFF questionnaire: Assessment of a new screening tool for eating disorders. *British Medical Journal, 319*(7223), 1467–1468.

Nagl, M., Jepsen, L., Linde, K., & Kersting, A. (2021). Social media use and postpartum body image dissatisfaction: The role of appearance-related social comparisons and thin-ideal internalization. *Midwifery, 100*, 103038. https://doi.org/10.1016/j.midw.2021.103038

Nascimento, S. L., Pudwell, J., Surita, F. G., Adamo, K. B., & Smith, G. N. (2014). The effect of physical exercise strategies on weight loss in postpartum women: A systematic review and meta-analysis. *International Journal of Obesity, 38*, 626–635. https://doi.org/10.1038/ijo.2013.183

National Institutes of Health, Eunice Kennedy Shriver National Institute of Child Health and Human Development. (2017, January 31). *When breastfeeding, how many calories should moms and babies consume?* www.nichd.nih.gov/health/topics/breastfeeding/conditioninfo/calories#:~:text=The%20 increased%20caloric%20need%20for,to%20500%20calories%20per%20day

Neville, C. E., McKinley, M. C., Holmes, V. A., Spence, D., & Woodside, J. V. (2014). The relationship between breastfeeding and postpartum weight change – A systematic review and critical evaluation. *International Journal of Obesity, 38*(4), 577–590. https://doi.org/10.1038/ijo.2013.132

Nguyen, A. N., de Barse, L. M., Tiemeier, H., Jaddoe, V. W. V., Franco, O. H., Jansen, P. W., & Voortman, T. (2017). Maternal history of eating disorders: Diet quality during pregnancy and infant feeding. *Appetite, 109*, 108–114. https://doi.org/10.1016/j.appet.2016.11.030

Nunes, M. A., Pinheiro, A. P., Hoffmann, J. F., & Schmidt, M. I. (2014). Eating disorders symptoms in pregnancy and postpartum: A prospective study in a disadvantaged population in Brazil. *International Journal of Eating Disorders, 47*(4), 426–430.

O'Loghlen, E., & Galligan, R. (2022). Disordered eating in the postpartum period: Role of psychological distress, body dissatisfaction, dysfunctional maternal beliefs and self-compassion. *Journal of Health Psychology, 27*(5), 1084–1098. https://doi.org/10.1177/1359105321995940

Papini, N. M., Mason, T. B., Herrmann, S. D., & Lopez, N. V. (2022). Self-compassion and body image in pregnancy and postpartum: A randomized pilot trial of a brief self-compassion meditation intervention. *Body Image, 43*, 264–274. https://doi.org/10.1016/j.bodyim.2022.09.010

Patel, P., Lee, J., Wheatcroft, R., Barnes, J., & Stein, A. (2005). Concerns about body shape and weight in the postpartum period and their relation to women's self-identification. *Journal of Reproductive and Infant Psychology, 23*(4), 347–364. https://doi.org/10.1080/02646830500273657

Pettersson, C. B., Zandian, M., & Clinton, D. (2016). Eating disorder symptoms pre-and postpartum. *Archives of Women's Mental Health, 19*(4), 675–680. https://doi.org/10.1007/s00737-016-0619-3

Prinds, C., Nikolajsen, H., & Folmann, B. (2020). Yummy mummy – The ideal of not looking like a mother. *Women and Birth, 33*(3), e266–e273. https://doi.org/10.1016/j.wombi.2019.05.009

Raspovic, A. M., Hart, L. M., Zali, Y., & Prichard, I. (2022). Body image profiles and exercise behaviours in early motherhood: A latent profile analysis. *Journal of Health Psychology, 27*(9), 2056–2067. https://doi.org/10.1177/13591053211019114

Raspovic, A. M., Prichard, I., Yager, Z., & Hart, L. M. (2020). Mothers' experiences of the relationship between body image and exercise, 0–5 years postpartum: A qualitative study. *Body Image, 35*, 41–52. https://doi.org/10.1016/j.bodyim.2020.08.003

Raymond, N. C., Neumeyer, B., Warren, C. S., Lee, S. S., & Peterson, C. B. (2003). Energy intake patterns in obese women with binge eating disorder. *Obesity Research, 11*(7), 869–879. https://doi.org/10.1038/oby.2003.120

Reba-Harrelson, L., Holle, A. V., Hamer, R. M., Swann, R., Reyes, M. L., & Bulik, C. M. (2009). Patterns and prevalence of disordered eating and weight control behaviors in women ages 25–45. *Eating and Weight Disorders, 14*(4), e190–e198. https://doi.org/10.1007/BF03325116

Ross, L. E., & McLean, L. M. (2006). Anxiety disorders during pregnancy and the postpartum period: A systematic review. *Journal of Clinical Psychiatry, 67*(8), 1285–1298. https://doi.org/10.4088/jcp.v67n0818

Runfola, C. D., Kirby, J. S., Baucom, D. H., Fischer, M. S., Baucom, B. R. W., Matherne, C. E., . . . Bulik, C. M. (2018). A pilot open trial of UNITE-BED: A couple-based intervention for binge-eating disorder. *International Journal of Eating Disorders, 51*(9), 1107–1112. https://doi.org/10.1002/eat.22919

Sadeh-Sharvit, S., Sacks, M. R., Runfola, C. D., Bulik, C. M., & Lock, J. D. (2020). Interventions to empower adults with eating disorders and their partners around the transition to parenthood. *Family Process, 59*(4), 1407–1422. https://doi.org/10.1111/famp.12510

Sadeh-Sharvit, S., Zubery, E., Mankovski, E., Steiner, E., & Lock, J. D. (2016). Parent-based prevention program for the children of mothers with eating disorders: Feasibility and preliminary outcomes. *Eating Disorders*, 24(4), 312–325. https://doi.org/10.1080/10640266.2016.1153400

Schaefer, L. M., Smith, K. E., Anderson, L. M., Cao, L., Crosby, R. D., Engel, S. G., . . . Wonderlich, S. A. (2020). The role of affect in the maintenance of binge-eating disorder: Evidence from an ecological momentary assessment study. *Journal of Abnormal Psychology*, 129(4), 387. https://doi.org/10.1037/abn0000517

Shrewsbury, V. A., Robb, K. A., Power, C., & Wardle, J. (2008). Socioeconomic differences in weight retention, weight-related attitudes and practices in postpartum women. *Maternal and Child Health Journal*, 13(2), 231–240. https://doi.org/10.1007/s10995-008-0342-4

Stapleton, H., Fielder, A., & Kirkham, M. (2008). Breast or bottle? Eating disordered childbearing women and infant-feeding decisions. *Maternal & Child Nutrition*, 4(2), 106–120. https://doi.org/10.1111/j.1740-8709.2007.00121.x

Stein, A., Woolley, H., Cooper, S. D., & Fairburn, C. G. (1994). An observational study of mothers with eating disorders and their infants. *Journal of Child Psychology and Psychiatry*, 35(4), 733–748. https://doi.org/10.1111/j.1469-7610.1994.tb01218.x

Stunkard, A. J., Sørensen, T., & Schulsinger, F. (1983). Use of the Danish Adoption Register for the study of obesity and thinness. *Research Publications – Association for Research in Nervous and Mental Disease*, 60, 115–120.

Swanson, V., Keely, A., & Denison, F. C. (2017). Does body image influence the relationship between body weight and breastfeeding maintenance in new mothers? *British Journal of Health Psychology*, 22(3), 557–576. https://doi.org/10.1111/bjhp.12246

Thompson, K. A., & Bardone-Cone, A. M. (2021). 2019-nCOV distress and depressive, anxiety and OCD-type, and eating disorder symptoms among postpartum and control women. *Archives of Women's Mental Health*, 24(4), 671–680. https://doi.org/10.1007/s00737-021-01120-9

Torgersen, L., Ystrom, E., Haugen, M., Meltzer, H. M., Von Holle, A., Berg, C. K., . . . Bulik, C. M. (2010). Breastfeeding practice in mothers with eating disorders. *Maternal & Child Nutrition*, 6(3), 243–252. https://doi.org/10.1111/j.1740-8709.2009.00208.x

Torgersen, L., Ystrom, E., Siega-Riz, A. M., Knoph Berg, C., Zerwas, S., Reichborn-Kjennerud, T., & Bulik, C. M. (2015). Maternal eating disorder and infant diet: A latent class analysis based on the Norwegian Mother and Child Cohort Study (MoBa). *Appetite*, 84, 291–298.

Ulman, T. F., Von Holle, A., Torgersen, L., Stoltenberg, C., Reichborn-Kjennerud, T., & Bulik, C. M. (2012). Sleep disturbances and binge eating disorder symptoms during and after pregnancy. *Sleep*, 35(10), 1403–1411. https://doi.org/10.5665/sleep.2124

Vanderkruik, R., Ellison, K., Kanamori, M., Freeman, M. P., Cohen, L. S., & Stice, E. (2022). Body dissatisfaction and disordered eating in the perinatal period: An underrecognized high-risk timeframe and the opportunity to intervene. *Archives of Women's Mental Health*, 25(4), 739–751. https://doi.org/10.1007/s00737-022-01236-6

Walker, L., Timmerman, G. M., Kim, M., & Sterling, B. (2002). Relationships between body image and depressive symptoms during postpartum in ethnically diverse, low income women. *Women & Health*, 36(3), 101–121. https://doi.org/10.1300/J013v36n03_07

Wang, Z., Liu, J., Shuai, H., Cai, Z., Fu, X., Liu, Y., . . . Yang, B. X. (2021). Mapping global prevalence of depression among postpartum women. *Translational Psychiatry*, 11(1), 543. https://doi.org/10.1038/s41398-021-01663-6

Wisner, K. L., Moses-Kolko, E. L., & Sit, D. K. Y. (2010). Postpartum depression: A disorder in search of a definition. *Archives of Women's Mental Health*, 13(1), 37–40. https://doi.org/10.1007/s00737-009-0119-9

17

POSTPARTUM ALCOHOL AND DRUG MISUSE

Tracy Moran Vozar, Stephanie Pinch, Amy Van Arsdale, Kelly Elliott, and Dakota Staren

"Emily" was an experienced mom and healthcare professional feeling lucky to be expecting her fourth child. Her job was stressful and caring for four young children would be challenging, but she felt well supported by her large network of family and friends. She felt ready. She had friends who experienced high-risk pregnancies and she worked with countless women who had experienced difficulties during their pregnancies and deliveries including infant loss. Her C-section delivery was planned, and she prepared to bring the baby home with her husband after a few days' recovery time in the hospital, as she had with her prior deliveries. Delivery and recovery went smoothly, but not without pain. To manage the pain, she began taking physician-prescribed opioids during her C-section recovery. After a few days, over-the-counter pain relief was sufficient, and she forgot about that prescription bottle in her medicine cabinet. A few months later, her stress and anxiety level increased. Things were tough at work, tough at home, and she was not sleeping. She went days without a good night's sleep before remembering the prescription pain medicine in her cabinet had also helped her relax and fall asleep. She told herself she would just take one for just one full night's rest. Emily was not sure how many pills were left in the bottle, but over the next few weeks, she went through all that remained. Desperate to continue sleeping through the night, she remembered where the same medication was stored at her work. She thought she could sneak a few pills from that supply and not get caught. In her mind, no one needed to know; however, she was discovered, forced to resign, and enter treatment. Suddenly, she needed to disclose to her friends and family and seek care for her addiction while juggling being an unemployed mom of four young children.

Prevalence of Use, Abuse, and Disorder

Emily is just one of thousands of mothers struggling with a substance use disorder (SUD). However, accurately understanding just how prevalent substances are used and abused during the postpartum period is extremely challenging from available epidemiologic survey data for a variety of reasons. Prevalence rates for postpartum (i.e., throughout this chapter

DOI: 10.4324/9781003206903-21

meaning loss/termination/labor/delivery through at least one year postpartum) substance use, misuse, and disorders are difficult to accurately determine and vary widely across cultures and types of substance being assessed. Some prevalence studies do not distinguish among types of substances used when reporting results. Moreover, many epidemiological surveys lump pregnant and postpartum women together in one group, making it difficult to ascertain substance use rates among postpartum women, specifically. Furthermore, definitions of use, abuse, and disorder are often blurred, complicating the meaning of the prevalence data. Throughout this chapter, we differentiate among substance use, abuse, and disorder in the postpartum period, as each may have different implications for the woman, child, and family.

The authors wish to draw attention to the use of outdated and cisgender terminology (e.g., mothers, women) throughout this chapter, as is largely consistent with the overall literature in the perinatal mental health field. Although the literature reviewed within this chapter was conducted without an emphasis on inclusion of LGBTQIA+ families, future research needs to be more inclusive of sexual and gender minorities. The use of the term, "birthing persons", throughout would be a notable step towards inclusivity and an affirming stance.

A review of international studies of postpartum substance use suggests the need for more international research on this topic. We can extrapolate some from international studies of substance use with broader samples. Historically, men have had higher rates of substance use, abuse, and SUDs than women across cultures, but this gender gap is narrowing worldwide (Steingrimsson et al., 2012), likely reflecting differential access to substances as well as cultural shifts away from traditional gender roles (McHugh et al., 2018). A Brazilian study of postpartum women found that 10% reported substance use; of those, half reported they had tried to stop using but could not (Lamus et al., 2021). A 2019 study of 308 Australian women, recruited from hospitals and clinics, found 65% reported drinking alcohol and 6% tobacco at eight weeks postpartum (Rossen et al., 2019). Prevatt et al. (2016) studied lifespan substance use in a community-based sample of Canadian women who were three months or less postpartum and found that 43% of participants reported behaviors indicative of lifetime substance abuse, and 25% experienced substance dependence at some point in their lifetime. Considering the interaction of substance abuse and other mental health issues, they found that substance use, particularly drug use, was strongly associated with postpartum mood disorders and posttraumatic stress disorder (PTSD). These authors encouraged researchers to consider asking about lifetime use, as opposed to current use, to capture women's mental health and comorbid substance use more fully.

Understandably, many women underreport postpartum substance use due to fear of stigma from family or friends, as well as concerns about interventions from the criminal justice system. Policies, laws, and cultural norms around substance use vary greatly both across countries and within countries, impacting reporting, screening, and treatment. Additionally, many laws and policies relating to substance abuse during pregnancy are developed based on historical stigmas rooted in discrimination toward historically marginalized populations. Similarly, individual and societal attitudes toward substance use vary widely. For example, one author (A.V.) who is an American observed while living in France that some French mothers smoked cigarettes at the local playground. This behavior is not commonly observed in this author's home state of Colorado and is culturally frowned upon; meanwhile in Colorado, cannabis is legal and used among some postpartum mothers—behavior that would be taboo in many cultures.

Given the difficulties described in estimating the prevalence of postpartum substance use, abuse, and dependence, we focus on research on specific substances when summarizing epidemiological research.

Alcohol Use

The National Epidemiologic Study of Alcohol and Related Conditions (NESARC) is a large, independent, nationally representative survey of Americans aged 18 years and older. This survey asks female participants whether they have been pregnant in the past 12 months and, thus, categorizes women into a single group—"pregnant and postpartum." Analyzing these data, Tebeka et al. (2020) found in 2001–2002, more than half (57.8%) of pregnant and postpartum women reported alcohol use in the past year, but ten years later, more than two-thirds (66.2%) reported prior year alcohol use, corresponding to an increased risk of 35%. Heavy episodic drinking among pregnant and postpartum women significantly increased (17.9% in 2001–2002 and 28.2% in 2012–2013, corresponding to a 70% increase). Ninety-six percent of women who drink heavily reported stopping during pregnancy, yet 51% of women relapsed three months postpartum (Forray & Foster, 2015; Forray et al., 2015). In a review of survey data in the United States and New Zealand, Chapman and Wu (2013) found that postpartum alcohol (prevalence range 30.1% to 49%) and drug use (4.5% to 8.5%) were higher than use among pregnant women (5.4% to 11.6%, 3.7% to 4.3%, respectively). Postpartum alcohol use increased compared to alcohol use during pregnancy. Board et al. (2022) found that 51.5% of 1,790 postpartum women reported consuming alcohol, and 15.6% of postpartum respondents endorsed binge drinking. A South Korean study found that Korean mothers' alcohol use during the six years postpartum fell into four categories: stable low use (49.9%), increasing use (25.0%), chronic modest use (18.3%), and chronic high use (6.8%), with about half of Korean mothers increasing their alcohol use (Kim, 2020). Additional research is needed to better understand global postpartum alcohol consumption.

Alcohol consumed by a breastfeeding mother can pass to the infant via breastfeeding in a reduced capacity. As a result, the World Health Organization (WHO) recommends avoiding alcohol while breastfeeding (WHO, 2018). After an alcoholic drink is consumed, alcohol can be detected in breastmilk within 30 to 60 minutes and can be present as long as two to three hours per consumed drink (CDC, 2022).

Another drug in the depressant class, benzodiazepines, is researched less than alcohol in prevalence studies of postpartum women. For reference, one study in the United States examined prevalence rates of benzodiazepine dispensing during the post-labor/delivery period and found a significant decrease from 2.4% to 2.1% ($p = 0.02$) between the years 2007 and 2015 (Qato & Gandhi, 2015).

Nicotine Use

The percentage of postpartum women who use nicotine varies across the world, yet some trends emerge. Global nicotine and tobacco use have shifted with increases in prevalence of use among younger women as well as increasing use of additional tobacco products such as waterpipes and e-cigarettes (WHO, 2013; Samet & Yoon, 2011). About one-third to one-half of American women report quitting smoking either just before or around the time of finding out they are pregnant (Orton et al., 2014, Rodriguez & Smith, 2019); however, up to 60% relapse in the postpartum period (Cooper et al., 2017). Jones et al. (2016), in the United Kingdom, found that 43% of postpartum women who had previously received a smoking cessation intervention relapsed. Rodriguez and Smith (2019) found that 16% of women who stopped smoking during pregnancy resumed after delivery. Similarly, a study in Spain found that 17.6% of women who abstained from smoking during pregnancy relapsed two months postpartum (Míguez & Pereira, 2021). Nordhagen et al. (2019) found that 5.6% of Swedish and Norwegian women endorsed using nicotine products, with 95.1% of postpartum women not reporting any nicotine use.

Postpartum women exposed to secondhand smoke who previously smoked were found to be more likely to relapse (Ashford et al., 2009). Secondhand smoke can also have detrimental effects on children. Children exposed to secondhand smoke may be associated with lower growth outcomes of children (e.g., height and head circumference), attention-deficit hyperactivity disorder (ADHD), behavior disorders, and conduct disorders (Huang et al., 2021; Kabir et al., 2011; Nadhiroh et al., 2020).

Cannabis Use

Cannabis is the most widely used illicit substance among both the general and postpartum population in many places (Bayrampour et al., 2019). Rates of cannabis use among postpartum women vary widely across, and within, countries. Whereas use rates in the United States vary between states, cannabis use has been increasing across the country as more states legalize its medicinal and recreational use for adults (Chang, 2020), increasing the general perception it is more acceptable and less harmful (Conner et al., 2016). A population-based study in these authors' home state of Colorado—where cannabis has been legal since 2012—found that 5% of postpartum women reported using cannabis (Crume et al., 2018). In a 2015 survey, lactation support providers estimated that 15% of their patients used cannabis postpartum (Bergeria & Heil, 2015). Forray and colleagues found that 41% of women who had abstained during pregnancy relapsed during the postpartum period (Forray et al., 2015).

Stimulant Use

The class of drugs known as stimulants, including prescriptions, cocaine, methamphetamines, ecstasy, and others, are the second-most commonly used/abused class of medications during pregnancy and are related to a host of negative postpartum outcomes (Smid et al., 2019). Little research examines postpartum stimulant use, specifically. Prevalence rates are rarely reported in the postpartum period, with most estimates reported during pregnancy or at labor/delivery via urine toxicology. Across studies, approximately 15% of women report using some form of stimulant medication, such as Adderall (i.e., dextroamphetamine-amphetamine) or Ritalin (i.e., methylphenidate HCl), during the postpartum period. Specifics of the prevalence of nonprescription stimulant medication are less well known in the postpartum (England et al., 2020).

Opioid Use

Opioid use, prescribed and nonprescribed, among women of childbearing age has significantly increased over the past decade in the United States. Women of childbearing age (i.e., 15 to 44) who reported past-month heroin use increased by 31% from 2011 to 2014 (SAMHSA, 2015) and reported past-month misuse of prescription pain relievers such as oxycodone increased by 5% in the same period (SAMHSA, 2015). Similar to stimulant use data, there are fewer specific studies of postpartum opioid prevalence.

As illustrated in Emily's case, many women who develop opioid use disorder begin their substance use postpartum through a prescription. Opioids are often prescribed after delivery for pain reduction. In the United States from 2012 to 2014, over 50% of women who gave birth with either Medicaid or private insurance had an opioid prescription filled within seven days of delivery (Ali et al., 2020). Notably, this sample was without a history of opioid use prior to or during pregnancy. Ali et al. (2020) found that women with Medicaid insurance who had cesarean deliveries had an increased likelihood of a postpartum opioid prescription filled (93%) compared with vaginal delivery (65%). Women with private insurance had similar correlations, with a higher rate of 82% of prescription opioids filled with a cesarean delivery compared to 44% with a vaginal delivery (Ali et al., 2020). Despite prescription opioids being filled by new mothers, less than 5% of these women developed an opioid use disorder within 18 months of the first prescription fill (Ali et al., 2020).

Polysubstance Use

Adding to the complications of estimating prevalence rates of various substances used in the postpartum period is the understanding that polysubstance use is likely in those who use a single substance. Research into rates of polysubstance use in the postpartum period is rare and difficult to conduct given likely reduced rates of reporting out of stigma, child abuse reporting, and other concerns. However, in the general population, co-use of opioids and benzodiazepines is rampant, suggesting a need to further understand polysubstance use postnatally (Qato & Gandhi, 2021).

Risk Factors and Correlates

Reviewing the literature on risk factors and correlates associated with substance use during the postpartum period feels a bit like untangling a web. It is a messy, "sticky" literature with few clear connections. To somewhat clarify the findings, next, we distinguish risk factors and correlates by type of substance and note the nationalities of the participants. Much of the literature on postpartum use focuses on concentrations of the substance in breastmilk and infant outcomes. Fewer studies examine the impact of use on the postpartum mother and/or the dyadic relationship. Research on breastmilk concentrations of various substances and related safety and risk information quickly evolves with new methodologies and is outside the scope of the current chapter. For more information on breastfeeding guidelines for women using substances please reference up-to-date review articles and toolkits, such as Gray's (2018) report from the Canadian Agency for Drugs and Technologies in Health.

A small body of research examines the effects of postpartum substance use, specifically, on parenting, with broader studies included in the larger child abuse and neglect literature. In a review of 13 studies, Canfield et al. (2017) examined factors associated with mothers who use substances losing custody of their children. Those factors included some related to postpartum substance use, such as specific patterns of use (e.g., prenatal cocaine use, injection drug use), lack of treatment for substance use, and fewer prenatal care visits. Hatters

Friedman et al. (2009) studied the custody status of mothers who did not receive prenatal care. Mothers with substance use without prenatal care were 30 times more likely to lose custody of their child than mothers who did not use substances without prenatal care (Hatters Friedman et al., 2009).

In line with research available on prenatal substance use, research on postpartum substance use is limited, mostly focusing on American samples (Chapman & Wu, 2013). Important differences in risk factors for African women can include the influence of traditional African value systems, customs, and prenatal exposure to societal stress (Wittkowski et al., 2013). As another example, a Brazilian study found that drug use was connected to conditions of social vulnerability such as poverty, teenage pregnancy, a lack of education, or not practicing a religion (Pereira et al., 2018). More research within and across international samples is needed to understand the social contextual factors related to postpartum substance use.

Depressive disorders and substance use in the postpartum period are risk factors for one another (Swendsen & Merikangas, 2000). In one study including Black mothers in an inner-city hospital program in the United States, symptoms of depression, stress, and need for social support were related to alcohol use (Barnet et al., 1995). Stress and the need for social support were also related to illicit drug use. Both smoking cigarettes and experiencing depressive symptoms were related to greater use of alcohol and illicit drug use (Barnet et al., 1995). Furthermore, receiving alcohol intervention treatment was related to less depression (Wilton et al., 2009), which highlights the need for effective treatments for comorbid mental health and substance use as well as more research to distinguish causal pathways between substance use and depression for the postpartum period.

Alcohol

Although research supports the notion that pregnant and postpartum women use alcohol at lower rates than nonpregnant women, alcohol use is more prevalent in the postpartum period compared to the prenatal period (Chapman & Wu, 2013). The complexities and challenges associated with identifying risk factors and correlates of substance use during the prenatal period discussed in the previous chapter (Jacobs et al., this volume) are also present in the postpartum period as well as risk factors and correlates unique to the postpartum period. Research has also established several prenatal factors associated with postpartum use (Homish et al., 2004; Salisbury et al., 2007; Wilton et al., 2009). Above and beyond race, employment, marital status, social support, cigarette use, depressive symptoms, and binge drinking, postpartum alcohol use is related to depressive symptoms, cigarette use, and binge drinking across pregnancy. Being unmarried during the second trimester and experiencing anxiety in the third trimester is related to postpartum alcohol use (Homish et al., 2004). These findings highlight the importance of prenatal substance use and mental health screening.

Correlates of postpartum problem drinking—defined as binge drinking or more than seven drinks per week—were being unemployed, unmarried, and a cigarette smoker. Collectively, in the United States problem drinkers were characterized by being predominately White and low-income (Chapman & Wu, 2013). Single marital status, never marrying, lower income, unemployment, history of smoking, being multiparous, being White, partners engaging in risky alcohol use, women not breastfeeding, depression, tobacco use, post high school, and college education were all factors associated with postpartum alcohol use

(Chapman & Wu, 2013). Depression may also play a role in postpartum alcohol binge use, with around 15% of depressed postpartum women reporting binge drinking, a higher rate than for women who are not postpartum and for those who are postpartum but not depressed (England et al., 2020).

Stimulants

The use of prescription and nonprescription stimulant use in the postpartum is of growing concern, in part due to deleterious effects on maternal and infant health and parenting. In one study, prenatal cocaine use and experiencing depression were associated with postpartum cocaine use more so than cocaine use without experiencing depression (Salisbury et al., 2007). Generally, a review of the literature suggests a lack of clear guidelines and recommendations for healthcare providers on the use of prescribed stimulants during this period for infant and maternal-infant relationship development.

Nicotine

In a Dutch study of nearly 2,000 mothers of young children, researchers found that the partner's smoking status during pregnancy and postpartum was the strongest predictor of the mother's smoking (Scheffers-van Schayck et al., 2019). Women who had quit smoking during pregnancy and relapsed postpartum more often had a partner who continued smoking postpartum or a partner who did not smoke at all compared to women who did not relapse postpartum.

Cannabis

Several studies have found that pregnancy and parenting are important predictors of cannabis cessation in women. Compared to tobacco and alcohol use, individuals are more likely to "age out" of cannabis use (Nelson et al., 2015). Desistance often occurs at the same time many women first give birth. In life course theory, the birth of a child represents an important "turning point" in the life span that may shape patterns of substance use (Teruya & Hser, 2010). Longitudinal research has found that younger mothers are more likely than older mothers to use cannabis during the postpartum period (DeGenna et al., 2015), and younger mothers have been found to be more likely to use cannabis at ten years postpartum (DeGenna et al., 2015).

Opioid Prescriptions

Among people aged 12 or older in 2020 who misused prescription pain relievers in the past year, the most common main reason given for their last misuse was to relieve physical pain (64.6%). This is a significant finding for the perinatal population, given that physical pain is an aspect of childbirth, and many women experience ongoing pain-related issues postpartum. In a nationwide survey of women undergoing cesarean delivery, 85% received an opioid prescription upon discharge (Bateman et al., 2017). The Centers for Disease Control and Prevention (CDC) estimates that one-third of reproductive-age women enrolled in Medicaid and more than one-quarter of those with private insurance filled a prescription for an opioid pain medication each year between 2008 and 2012 (Ailes et al., 2015).

Women who developed opioid use disorder were more likely to have higher average days of opioids prescribed (eight days for Medicaid insurers and nine days for private insurers) and have more prescriptions filled (seven for both Medicaid and private insurance; Ali et al., 2020).

Polysubstance Use

Relative to the use of any one substance, polysubstance use may be most highly correlated with depression and anxiety in the postpartum period (Pentecost et al., 2021) and with overall risk for comorbid mental health concerns, broadly defined. Pentecost et al. (2021) noted the lack of research on comorbid postpartum mental health concerns and substance use, suggesting that more research on the impact of and efficacious treatments for comorbid postpartum substance use and mental health concerns is needed.

Emily's friends and family were shocked by her substance misuse. They had considered her to be strong and a superhero who had "it all together." In treatment, her partner took on more of the parenting of their four children and he reached out to the family to ask for help. He did not understand how this could have happened without him knowing. He knew Emily was having trouble sleeping but thought she had gotten that under control on her own. He had no idea she was using substances to sleep, which was frightening to him. The older children did not understand why mom had to leave her job in medicine and why she was now a patient. She did not seem sick, so why did she need to see the doctor daily? Emily and her partner attempted explanations that their children could understand, but they realized the kids were stressed because of all the changes for mom and in the household. Emily also struggled with feelings of guilt and shame related to being away from the baby for so long. She had been looking forward to this time in her infant's life—milestones were happening fast, but Emily missed many due to full-time treatment. With Emily out of work and the increased need for childcare, the household suffered financially. Her partner was stressed, wondering how they would get back to making ends meet. Emily was lucky—through her prior medical connections, she identified treatment providers with whom she could work. But she also felt very different from the others in her group treatment sessions. Few in her Medication-Assisted Treatment (MAT) program were parents and even fewer were newly postpartum. She struggled to feel supported in treatment and struggled more to feel understood by family members. It was a lonely and isolating time of "recovery" for Emily.

Ripple Effects of Postpartum Substance Use

"Having a partner who drinks too much or uses drugs is very much like throwing a stone into a still pond: the effects ripple out and influence all that is near" (Fals-Stewart, n.d.). Although evidence indicates substance use in the perinatal period adversely impacts child development, parenting, and the parent–child relationship, only a small percentage of women in the perinatal period are receiving substance use services, and even fewer are receiving concurrent parenting supports. Infants and children of substance-abusing caregivers are more likely to experience harm, enter the foster care system, and have associated negative outcomes related to child protection than infants and children of non-substance-abusing caregivers (Wallman et al., 2011). Substance abuse is linked to both child abuse and neglect in families involved with the child welfare system (McGlade et al., 2009). Early identification through patient self-report screening conducted in a more relational, empathic, and nonjudgmental manner can be preventive and protective for children's safety and well-being.

Substance use can contribute to difficulties within the partner relationship, including financial strain and discord, contributing to the likelihood of intimate partner violence, arguments regarding the distribution of household responsibilities, and isolation from social supports including family members, among other concerns. The partner's role in families affected by postpartum substance use is seldom examined. More attention to partners in the household is essential, as they can be supportive or damaging toward mothers in recovery. Furthermore, parenting partners can provide essential care to infants and children in the household, acting as a protective factor for child development (Twomey, 2007).

The World Health Organization (WHO) projects that tobacco use will be responsible for eight million deaths per year by 2030. There are numerous health risks of nicotine use and secondhand smoke exposure for both mother and child. For example, the risk for sudden infant death syndrome (SIDS) is increased among the offspring of women who smoked during or after pregnancy (WHO, 2013). Furthermore, the WHO notes that money spent on tobacco can have a very high opportunity cost; for the poor, money spent on tobacco is money not spent on necessities, such as food, transportation, housing, and healthcare, thus increasing the risk of adverse health outcomes for pregnant and postpartum women and their families.

Screening and Assessment

Potential screening tools for perinatal substance use are described in the prenatal substance use chapter in this volume (Jacobs et al., this volume) and any could be used with a postpartum population depending on the intended purpose. Screening and assessing substance use in the postpartum period, a seemingly straightforward task of asking women whether and how much they use various substances, is unfortunately complicated by societal and cultural factors. In the United States and other countries, mothers' concerns regarding the implications of endorsing substance use during the postpartum period result in underreporting. Concerns may stem from state or national policies regarding parental substance use endorsement, historical trauma, and related stories of children being removed from the parents' care because of endorsing substances, and more. In the United States, reporting requirements vary by state. At the time of writing, 24 states and the District of Columbia report substance use during pregnancy to be child abuse, 25 states and the District of Columbia require healthcare practitioners to report suspected prenatal drug use, 19 states have created or funded drug treatment programs for pregnant individuals, and 10 states prohibit publicly funded drug treatment programs from discriminating against pregnant people (Guttmacher Institute, 2024).

Universal screening for substance use using patient report screening tools is identified as a best practice by numerous oversight organizations, including the World Health Organization (WHO), the American College of Obstetricians and Gynecologists (ACOG), the Centers for Disease Control and Prevention (CDC), and the American Academy of Pediatrics

(AAP; see Chasnoff et al., 2007; Coleman-Cowger et al., 2019, for reviews). However, practices regarding screening via patient reports, toxicology testing, and reporting requirements for postpartum care, generally, and substance use during the postpartum period, specifically, vary widely across clinics, hospitals, states, and countries. Urine toxicology testing should not be used in place of patient report screening, as urine drug testing can discourage postpartum women from seeking care (ACOG, 2018). Women identified as using substances at any point during the pregnancy should be offered coordinated multidisciplinary care through the postpartum period (Gopman, 2014), as relapse or increase in use following labor and delivery is possible. The postpartum period is an ideal time to screen patients again, ideally within the context of a trusting patient–provider relationship (Jones et al., 2014).

When substance misuse is identified, providers can feel understandably uncertain about how best to proceed to support patients and their infants. Hospitals and clinics have differing protocols for positive screens depending on local recommendations and requirements. Providers feeling knowledgeable and supported in making referrals that patients can confidently follow is essential to the effectiveness of screening efforts. If providers feel uncertain about what to do following a positive screen or wonder about referral availability for substance-using women with infants, screening is likely to fall short of needed efficacy. The next steps following a positive screen may include a referral for substance use treatment, mental health counseling, a care coordination evaluation for needed resources, and/or screening and toxicology tests of mother and child urine or newborn meconium in the case of a positive screen while in a labor and delivery unit. Based on these findings, in the United States, a referral to Child Protective Services or a similar resource within the jurisdiction may also occur and providers need to be knowledgeable of potential outcomes of postpartum substance use disclosure within their area.

Treatment

Treatment programs for postpartum women with substance misuse or SUD are imperative for the well-being of the mother and the infant and can vary from behavioral approaches, teaching parent skills, dyadic relational work between the mother and infant, decreasing barriers to receiving treatment, and group therapy. Treatment within this population is essential to mitigate the deleterious effects substance use can have on the mother–infant dyad and the future psychological and physical health of the child. Timeliness of treatment is also vital, as perinatal women who use opioids, cocaine, and amphetamines are at an increased risk of being readmitted for drug use within six weeks of delivery (Salemi et al., 2020). Chapman and Wu (2013) noted that the initial decrease in substance use during pregnancy followed by an increase in use postpartum to pre-pregnancy rates suggests that women who seemingly *stop* substance use during pregnancy more accurately *pause* use and that this is a missed prevention opportunity. Additionally, infants can have an increased risk of exposure to drugs in utero and, thus, can experience the physiological and neurobehavioral signs of withdrawal and develop neonatal abstinence syndrome (NAS; Patrick et al., 2015). The total number of infants diagnosed with NAS has increased by five times from 2004 to 2013 (Tolia et al., 2015).

A handful of studies show efficacious interventions for substance-using parents (Barnard & McKeganey, 2004; Preis et al., 2020). Cognitive behavioral therapy (CBT) approaches are commonly used to treat postpartum mood and anxiety disorders (see Li et al., 2022, for a review) as well as substance use throughout the lifespan (see Carroll & Kiluk, 2017, for a review). However, the authors struggled to find studies of CBT for postpartum substance use, specifically. When examining previously evaluated interventions for substance use reduction and improved family management, Barnard and McKeganey (2004) noted that existing interventions often do not directly focus on parenting or children and that this is especially lacking with the perinatal and postpartum populations. Many parents consider parenting an essential role important to their self-concept (Troutman et al., 2012), suggesting substance use interventions that focus on enhancing parenting self-efficacy as well as centering the child's development and relationship development as treatment goals could be effective in diminishing maladaptive substance use.

Successful interventions include behavioral approaches with an emphasis on parenting, the dyadic relationship between the mother and infant, reflective functioning, environmental stressors, and mindfulness (Preis et al., 2020; Barnard & McKeganey, 2004; Catalano et al., 1999; Black et al., 1994; Ernst et al., 1999; Grant et al., 1999; Camp & Finkelstein, 1997; Horton & Murray, 2015; Gannon et al., 2017; Suchman et al., 2011, 2017; Suchman, 2016). Emphasis on the mother–child dyadic relationship can be important for the mother's recovery from substance use because substance-using mothers often have histories of parenting difficulties (Luthar & Walsh, 1995). Stress from parenting can increase the likelihood that a mother experiences a relapse (Sinha, 2001; Rutherford & Mayes, 2019). Mothers with chronic substance misuse can experience a change in their neural circuitry compared to mothers who do not use substances (Potenza & Mayes, 2011). This change can affect the mothers' neural reward system which makes caring for their children less rewarding and thus the mothers are less reactive to their child's emotions (Landi et al., 2011).

In a study by Gannon et al. (2017), mothers with opioid use disorder participated in a mindfulness-based parenting curriculum for two hours a week for 12 weeks. The program included mother–child dyad education, knowledge of the impact of trauma on parenting, and mindfulness practices. Mothers in this study found a clinically significant increase in measured quality of parenting on the *Keys to Interactive Parenting Scale* (KIPS) from low-to-moderate quality parenting after the 12-week trauma-informed mindfulness-based parenting program. The higher mindful parenting scores led to an increase in the quality of parenting behaviors, which can have a positive impact on mothers' relationships with their children (for more information see Gannon et al., 2017).

Suchman and colleagues (Suchman et al., 2011, 2017; Suchman, 2016) created an evidence-based treatment, Mothering from the Inside Out (MIO). MIO provides an individual, manualized, psychotherapeutic 12-week intervention for mothers who are in treatment for drug use and have children under the age of five. MIO focuses on increasing the mother's reflective functioning, such as the ability to make sense of behaviors in oneself as well as understand the behaviors, thoughts, emotions, and intentions of others (Lowell et al., 2021). In a randomized clinical trial comparing mothers in the MIO group to a control group of a 12-week, manualized, psychoeducation parenting group, both groups of mothers were evaluated on reflective functioning, representations of caregiving, mother–child interaction quality, and child attachment, measuring at baseline, posttreatment, three-month follow-up, and 12-month follow-up (Suchman et al., 2017). Compared to the control group, MIO mothers showed greater reflective functioning, and the mother–child dyad showed greater reciprocity while the children showed greater involvement. The study also found that these protective factors for mothers in MIO were consistent when controlling for addiction severity. Mothers with reflective functioning can be better equipped to recognize and manage their emotional stress related to parenting, as evaluated in a randomized study with mothers with children from zero to three (Suchman et al., 2011). This program's findings included: (a) attachment-based interventions can be done in a substance use treatment center; (b) abstinence alone does not improve caregiving; (c) emotional exploration of the self and mother–child relationship does not interfere with prolonged abstinence; and (d) reflective functioning can improve well-being (Suchman et al., 2011). The MIO intervention suggests reflective functioning can be a protective factor for mothers to mitigate the effects of stress from parenting.

Another attachment-based intervention, Circle of Security-Parenting (COS-P; Powell et al., 2009), can be conducted in individual or group formats and includes a DVD and/or manual-based format. Although training for COS is widespread, treatment efficacy and effectiveness studies are fewer in number. An exploratory effectiveness study conducted with a small sample (i.e., n = 15) in a group therapy setting with mothers living in residential substance abuse treatment settings showed improvements on three variables when mothers attended the majority of the nine sessions: the *Emotion Regulation Questionnaire*; the *Parenting Scale*; and the *Parent Attrition Test* (Horton & Murray, 2015) calculated using the Reliable Change Index, of which scores above ±1.96 are clinically significant at the $p < .05$ level (RCI; Jacobson & Truax, 1991).

In a larger multisite study of treatment efficacy for COS-P (Maxwell et al., 2021), a sample of 256 parents of young children ages birth to 6 was recruited across four child and family health organizations. Note that this study was not specific to substance-affected families. COS-P showed significant improvements compared to controls on several outcomes including (a) improvements in self-efficacy and mentalizing toward the child, (b) reductions in hostility toward the child and caregiving-related helplessness, and (c) reductions in caregiver depressive symptoms. No significant difference was found in the perception of child difficulty across groups. Another review of effectiveness and efficacy studies of COS-P in Norway (Gerdts-Andresen, 2021) found seven studies examining the interventions used with "multi-problem families" (i.e., families in which at least two risk factors were endorsed). The review found improvements in COS-P participants on parental stress reduction, increased self-efficacy, improved parenting skills, and enhanced understanding of child behavior. The review did not find evidence of improvement in attachment security based on COS-P treatment involvement. Overall, the author suggested that more studies on the efficacy of COS-P are needed, especially with special populations (e.g., high-risk families, substance-using families, and families involved in child protection services).

Describing all treatment programs for postpartum substance use is outside of the scope of this chapter, however, we wanted to highlight several additional promising programs and their effectiveness here. Some additional successful treatments for parents with SUDs include the following researched programs.

Focus on Families, an experimental intervention, provided 33 small group sessions of family training delivered twice a week plus nine months of home-based case management to parents recruited from methadone clinics (Catalano et al., 1999). Compared to the control group, this program resulted in a reduction of cocaine and heroin use, adoption of family rules, and less domestic conflict, especially in families with younger children. Black et al. (1994) studied a randomized treatment program for 60 prenatal women with drug problems that provided support and advocacy, parenting and child development coaching, and linked mothers with community support through 18 months postpartum. Mothers were provided twice-weekly, hour-long home visits. This study found a modest impact on the intervention mothers compared to the control group, with slightly decreased drug use, slightly greater primary healthcare participation, and a slightly better home environment.

The Seattle Birth-to-Three Program (Ernst et al., 1999; Grant et al., 1999) provided home visits by well-trained, motivated, and well-supported paraprofessionals to work with high-risk substance-using mothers of children from birth to age three. The program provided six weekly visits and thereafter twice weekly or more as needed to provide motivation and assistance, facilitate community resources, and offer guidance. Seattle Birth-to-Three found participating mothers benefitted from lower or absent drug use, a higher likelihood of retaining custody of children, and a higher likelihood of children living in appropriate home situations. In a residential drug environment, Camp and Finkelstein (1997) studied a program that provided weekly 2.5-hour long parent training over 23 weeks from staff who received three days of intensive training on healthy parenting. Only one-third of the mothers finished the program, and the researchers noted substantial methodological inconsistencies in the uniform delivery of the treatment, but the results did show significant improvements in self-esteem, parenting knowledge and attitudes, empathy, role reversal, and improved average levels of parenting from seriously deficient to average.

The *Mothers and Toddlers Program* provides a 12-session, attachment-based individual therapy for substance-using mothers to improve maternal capacity for reflective functioning and to adjust distorted mental representations of parenting (Suchman et al., 2011). It found improvement along these metrics, along with notable decreased substance use, less depression, better communication to and from children, and increased scores on Total and Contingent Caregiving Behavior evaluation.

The *Children and Recovering Mothers (CHARM) Collaborative*, a multidisciplinary group founded in Vermont serving opioid-affected families during the postpartum period, supports around 150 to 200 families in that state each year. CHARM has since been replicated in other states and studied by the Substance Abuse and Mental Health Services Administration (SAMHSA, 2014). CHARM aims to enroll opioid-using women as soon as possible, ideally during pregnancy, reduce cravings using medication for opioid use disorder (MOUD) treatment, initiate substance use counseling services, and promote social support and social determinants of health for the woman and family.

Treatment Barriers and Motivators

As described in this chapter, there are many promising interventions for postpartum alcohol and drug misuse. From reading as well as our own experiences in clinical practice, we also realize numerous barriers can prevent women from receiving such treatment or from continuing with treatment services, including not wanting to leave children or a partner at home, fear of punitive measures or loss of parental custody, lack of childcare, lack of transportation, and limited availability in program treatment openings (Frazer et al., 2019; Kuo et al., 2013). The shame or guilt women experience surrounding the disclosure of their substance use to providers correlates with self-critical thoughts and a belief they will be judged by others around them, which can prevent women from undergoing essential substance use treatment (Paris et al., 2020). The perceived stigma of receiving treatment has been found to be a stronger barrier for women compared to men (Stringer & Baker, 2018).

The postpartum period can also be a time of high motivation for women to seek treatment and services for the well-being of their infant and themselves (Kuo et al., 2013). Chou et al. (2020) found improvement in client care when transportation was provided, children remained with their mothers, and consistency was maintained among clinical team members. Furthermore, many postpartum women question their substance use in consideration of breastfeeding their infants and may seek services to have their questions answered. Providing support and resources around breastfeeding that include substance use considerations is beneficial from a harm reduction perspective to the mother and infant and from a holistic treatment perspective. Additionally, peer support can positively impact women's postpartum substance use treatment (Gruss et al., 2021). The opportunity for women to build peer relationships that can hold them accountable, as well as create a community around motherhood and shared experiences, supports mothers in their recovery (Gruss et al., 2021). As an example, one treatment program used a conceptual framework for understanding population health and included women's personal and medical history, their currently available mental, social, and physical resources, and their cultural and biomedical needs (Preis et al., 2020). Evaluators of this program found that when women's needs and vulnerabilities are addressed and acknowledged, women feel better equipped to overcome treatment barriers (Preis et al., 2020).

Since the COVID-19 pandemic, telehealth has been used as an effective means of decreasing barriers by eliminating the need for transportation and childcare and allowing patients to participate from their homes or other convenient locations (Sadicario et al., 2021). However, downsides of telehealth include that some patients are less likely to disclose information relative to the inside of the clinic, attendance can decrease, and there is a decrease in "warm handoffs: between providers, decreasing patients' participation in treatment programs (Sadicario et al., 2021).

Cultural Considerations

Cultural humility and curiosity are increasingly understood to be essential components of effective treatments. In a recent review of empirical studies on cultural humility, psychotherapy, and supervision, Zhang et al. (2022) discovered a myriad of treatment benefits related to therapist cultural humility (e.g., positive working alliances, therapy continuance, effectiveness, outcomes, therapist competence ratings by clients). For treatment effectiveness and efficacy as well as social justice, equity, and inclusion considerations, it is imperative to respect women's cultural backgrounds when considering treatment for postpartum women who are substance using. The impact of substance use on postpartum women across cultures has been examined by a few researchers, though there is a need for additional research on this topic.

Postpartum women who use and abuse substances exist across all cultures, though there are certain characteristics that help define or identify this population. Internationally and across cultures, research has found that the recognized postpartum period across cultures on average is around 40 days (about one and a half months), with many cultures having specific rituals and customs associated with this period (Eberhard-Gran et al., 2010). Within the United States, postpartum women who did receive SUD treatment are more likely to be older, White, and live in a large metropolitan city compared with mothers of infants with neonatal abstinence syndrome or prenatal substance exposure who did not receive postpartum SUD treatment (Faherty et al., 2021). Screening and treatment for mothers with SUD are impacted by racial disparities. For example, parents of Black and Hispanic children are more likely than parents of White children to be asked about household smokers, household drug use, or household alcohol use (Kogan et al., 2004). Socioeconomic factors are relevant as well, as mothers with publicly funded health insurance whose infant had in utero substance exposure received postpartum substance use treatment only 15% of the time (Faherty et al., 2021).

Internationally, one study compared the prevalence and characteristics of patients at risk for substance use disorders in Tijuana and East Los Angeles. Researchers found a need for interventions to be tailored toward pregnant drug users (Gelberg et al., 2017). Wittkowski et al. (2013) found that women in sub-Saharan Africa experience postpartum depression at similar rates as women in developed countries. Another study examining American Indians and Alaska Natives found that culturally competent care is essential to treatment programs (Croff et al., 2014). Culturally competent care in this study included training for clinical staff about tribal traditions and customs, awareness of historical and intergenerational trauma, the relations between Native individuals and the U.S. government as well as tailoring of evidence-based treatments for American Indian and Alaskan Native populations (Croff et al., 2014). These studies focused on different cultural groups, yet all elucidated how culturally competent care tailored to postpartum women can be impactful.

There is a need for more research into culturally competent treatments for substance use, abuse, and disorders with postpartum women to provide practitioners with a robust understanding of how to support those from different cultural backgrounds.

In Emily's case, Emily's demographics, professional connections, and level of education positively influenced the likelihood she would receive SUD treatment. Although she struggled during recovery, Emily was lucky. She received treatment quickly due to her connections in the medical field. She had the financial means and social support to access and remain in her MAT program. She has since changed careers to a profession she finds less stressful and is able to enjoy her time as a partner, mother, friend, and individual. Emily's example is notable for all of its strengths during a time of adversity. It is also notable as anyone can find themselves abusing substances and in need of treatment.

Conclusion and Future Directions

Access to addictive substances through legal and illegal means is rampant. Affordable, culturally attuned, effective care for substance use should be equally or more so accessible. Care for postpartum women using or abusing substances needs to acknowledge: (a) childcare considerations for the infant and any siblings; (b) the impact of maternal substance use on the partner, child(ren), and family system; (c) comorbid mental health concerns prevalent during the postpartum period; and (d) associated guilt, shame, and other considerations mothers using substances can experience during the postpartum period. Furthermore, a provider stance of transparency around what patients can expect regarding substance use screening, toxicology testing, treatment, policies, and regulations is needed to promote patient discussion of use.

There are knowledge and treatment gaps contributing to the lack of effective and accessible comorbid mental health and substance use treatments. First, we need improved access to data on the prevalence of use of substances in the postpartum period. Accurate data are hard to find for many reasons detailed earlier in this chapter, but de-identified sources of prevalence data, such as the National Survey on Drug Use and Health (SAMHSA, 2021), could be used to gather large samples of pregnant and postpartum participants while protecting confidentiality. Specific recruitment efforts for pregnant and postpartum populations would be beneficial to the larger body of work on perinatal substance use screening, assessment, and treatment. Second, few mental health professionals receive training in substance use care provision, and few substance use counselors receive training in comorbid psychopathology—particularly in perinatal, infant, and early childhood (i.e., Perinatal through age 5 of P-5) mental health. Training substance use and mental health providers across P-5 mental health and substance use screening, assessment, and treatment is needed to address the shortage of services.

Interdisciplinary training for introductory through advanced levels addressing multidisciplinary professionals is needed to address this gap. The authors of this chapter were part of one example of a comprehensive mental health and substance use training initiative designed for psychology graduate trainees, the Colorado Opioid Use Disorder (OUD) SUD Training (COST) program at the University of Denver. A team of faculty across two departments in Clinical and Counseling Psychology developed the Health Resources and Services Administration (HRSA) funded COST program to train students in screening, assessment, and treatment of comorbid substance use. Trainees in the COST program receive didactic and experiential training in working with comorbid OUD/SUD symptoms, provision of services via telehealth to increase access to care, working with medical colleagues on interdisciplinary care teams, and provision of culturally competent services. Rather than training in a particular model of treatment, trainees receive exposure to the incorporation of substance use informed screening, assessment, and treatment approaches across all of their work. Students enrolled in the COST program select an area of specialty for their training, including one option to focus on P-5 mental health. Trainees apply for the two-year commitment and enroll in related coursework, field placement practica, supervision, and additional training and workshops. Training partners include local hospitals, clinics, and community locations that benefit immediately from trainees with additional experience working with comorbid OUD/SUD, including a within-department P-5 mental health training clinic, the Caring for You and Baby (CUB) Clinic. The long-term goal of the COST program is a strengthened clinical workforce with enhanced preparedness to meet clients' needs in the comorbid mental health and OUD/SUD space.

In addition to training programs for mental health providers, specifically, interdisciplinary, integrated substance use screening, treatment, and referral training for multidisciplinary providers who serve perinatal individuals is needed to address service gaps. One example is an introductory training developed for Colorado in collaboration with several statewide initiatives: Postpartum Support International Colorado Chapter (CO-PSI), Colorado Department of Public Health and Environment (CDPHE), Colorado's Maternal Mortality Review Committee, The COST program, Tough as a Mother, Colorado Hospital Substance Exposed Newborns Collaborative (CHoSEN), and 20/20 Mom as well as numerous content experts (Jacobs et al., 2023). The Connecting the Dots: Maternal Mental Health and Substance Use During Pregnancy and Early Parenthood training is offered in-person and asynchronously online and provides introductory information on treating comorbid substance use within the context of mental health treatment. Future training is in development for more advanced content, as there is a need for ongoing, more in-depth, and specialized training following participation in this introductory coursework.

Professionals considering developing and disseminating training on perinatal substance use within their communities will benefit from developing similar multidisciplinary partnerships for support, guidance, and feedback as well as assistance with dissemination. In our experience, content expert partners provided an invaluable lens related to their specific areas of focus. They each were able to review our training from a unique outlook, founded on years of specific training and experience. Their knowledge, constructive feedback, and guidance provided credibility and quality assurance.

One barrier to finding or referring for treatment is the unfortunate turnover in services. Keeping referral networks and resources regularly updated and accessible online is essential. One resource in the United States is a SAMSHA site (i.e., Home-FindTreatment.gov). The resource promotes treatment accessibility by developing an updated provider database, thereby promoting efficiency in referral making. Chapters of perinatal mental health organizations can assist referral connections by providing a similar list of regularly updated comorbid substance use and mental health treatment providers within their directories. For example, Colorado's Postpartum Support International website has an online directory that is searchable by specialty, and searching "substance use" results in a provider list of perinatal mental health and substance use trained clinicians.

The Alliance for Innovation on Maternal Health (AIM) created a quality improvement project, which provides free online and print materials for professionals on numerous topics, including, Care for Pregnant and Postpartum People with Substance Use Disorder | AIM (saferbirth.org). They take a harm reduction stance by promoting early universal screening, brief, on-the-spot conversations including psychoeducation, and referrals to substance use treatment are efficacious in improving maternal and infant outcomes. AIM recommends a multidisciplinary approach without fear of criminal repercussions, judgment, or stigma is best for improving outcomes for families. Video and print materials describe how to implement a coordinated care plan for substance use during pregnancy and the first year postpartum. The goals of the substance use disorder bundle include providing guidance on the creation of multidisciplinary care teams, screening and recognition of SUDs, and supports and services that reduce risks and improve outcomes for mothers and infants, in an equitable manner.

Beyond training and accessing treatment, additional upstream changes are needed to address postpartum substance use, abuse, and disorders. Following training, treatment and screening recommendations need to be well implemented in mental health, physical health, and substance use clinics. Remaining provider biases or uncertainties in providing treatment for comorbid substance use and mental health concerns need to be explored and addressed, perhaps in supervision and via program-level interventions, as well as broader policy changes.

U.S. Policies Impacting Substance-Using Postpartum Caregivers

The literature reviewed in the prenatal alcohol and drug misuse chapter on U.S. state and federal policies regarding prenatal substance use largely applies to the postpartum period. Here, we highlight policy findings and recommendations specific to the postpartum population.

Many U.S. policies pertaining to postpartum substance use do not align with promoting patient disclosure of use, treatment seeking, or evidence-based practices of reducing substance use. Postpartum caregivers experience stigma and fear of legal and caregiving repercussions when seeking care. Weber and colleagues (2021) found that parents with substance use disorders reported 49% greater odds of experiencing stigma compared to nonparenting individuals with the same disorder. Evidence strongly suggests that punitive policies are not effective in reducing the incidence of postpartum substance use. Instead, policies such as decriminalization and legalization of all substances, universal drug testing, and availability of safe consumption sites have all shown promise in reducing substance use (Weber et al., 2021). Unfortunately, stigma limits policy changes that would improve substance use treatment for postpartum individuals. Reduction of stigma through provider education and public campaigns is critical to improving policymaker perceptions of postpartum substance use and resulting policy change.

Policy experts also note the need for increased investments in community-based organizations and rural hospitals that provide treatment to vulnerable populations. Progress has been made at the federal level, and it will be critical to review how the increased funding impacts access to care, the prevalence of neonatal abstinence syndrome, and resources available for those in need of substance use treatment.

Future Directions

As mentioned throughout the chapter, there are several directions the literature on postpartum alcohol and drug misuse could lean toward to benefit our knowledge and practices. More research on dyadic and family-focused interventions for postpartum SUD is needed. Research on prevalence, risk factors, screening, assessment, and treatment for postpartum SUD within and across cultures, and especially internationally, is needed. Additionally, research on LGBTQIA+ families and birthing persons, is lacking in perinatal mental health, broadly, and in the perinatal substance use literature, specifically. Research conducted in a more inclusive manner is needed. Furthermore, research that examines polysubstance use with the postpartum population is lacking. Substance use researchers would do well to partner with perinatal mental health professionals in developing, recruiting, and disseminating such work.

As a final note, the authors of this chapter overlap some and collaborate with the authors of the prior prenatal substance use chapter. We found it particularly challenging to summarize the literature on postpartum use in isolation from prenatal use, as these literatures are strongly overlapping and populations included in this work are not always clearly defined (e.g., perinatal, prenatal, postpartum). Future literature could more proactively examine the trajectory and patterns of use prior to pregnancy, through pregnancy, and into the postpartum period and could describe use trajectories in a more clear and detailed manner.

References

Ailes, E. C., Dawson, A. L., Lind, J. N., Gilboa, S. M., Frey, M. T., Broussard, C. S., . . . Centers for Disease Control and Prevention (CDC). (2015). Opioid prescription claims among women of reproductive age – United States, 2008–2012. *Morbidity and Mortality Weekly Report, 64*(2), 37–41.

Ali, M. M, West, K., & Nye, E., & HHS Office of the Assistant Secretary for Planning and Evaluation. (2020, December). *Postpartum opioid prescription fills, opioid use disorder and utilization of medication-assisted treatment among women with Medicaid and private health insurance coverage (4).* https://aspe.hhs.gov/sites/default/files/migrated_legacy_files//197941/PostpartOUDIB.pdf

American College of Obstetrics and Gynecologists (ACOG). (2018). *Opposition to criminalization of individuals during pregnancy and the postpartum period.* www.acog.org/clinical-information/policy-and-position-statements/statements-of-policy/2020/opposition-criminalization-of-individuals-pregnancy-and-postpartum-period

Ashford, K. B., Hahn, E., Hall, L., Rayens, M. K., & Noland, M. (2009). Postpartum smoking relapse and secondhand smoke. *Public Health Reports, 124*(4), 515–526. https://doi.org/10.1177.003335490912400408

Barnard, A., & McKeganey, N. (2004). The impact of parental problem drug use on children: What is the problem and what can be done to help? *Addiction, 99*(5), 552–559. https://doi.org/10.1111/j.1360-0443.2003.00664.x

Barnet, Duggan, A. K., Wilson, M. D., & Joffe, A. (1995). Association between postpartum substance use and depressive symptoms, stress, and social support in adolescent mothers. *Pediatrics*, *96*(4), 659–666. https://doi.org/10.1542/peds.96.4.659

Bateman, B. T., Cole, N. M., Maeda, A., Burns, S. M., Houle, T. T., Huybrechts, K. F., . . . Leffert, L. R. (2017). Patterns of opioid prescription and use after cesarean delivery. *Obstetrics & Gynecology*, *130*(1), 29–35.

Bayrampour, H., Zahradnik, M., Lisonkova, S., & Janssen, P. (2019). Women's perspectives about cannabis use during pregnancy and the postpartum period: An integrative review. *Preventive Medicine*, *119*, 17–23. https://doi.org/10.1016/j.ypmed.2018.12.002

Bergeria, C. L., & Heil, S. H. (2015). Surveying lactation professionals regarding marijuana use and breastfeeding. *Breastfeeding Medicine*, *10*(7), 377–380. https://doi.org/10.1089/bfm.2015.0051

Black, M., Nair, P., Kight, C., Wachtel, R., Roby, P., & Schuler, M. (1994). Parenting and early development among children of drug-misusing women: Effects of a home intervention. *American Journal of Pediatrics*, *94*, 440–448.

Board, A., Park, Y., Denny, C. H., Salvesonvon Essen, B., Miele, K., & D'Angelo, D. (2022). Prevalence of alcohol use, screening and counseling among postpartum persons: Six U.S. states, 2019. *Obstetrics & Gynecology*, *139*. https://doi.org.10.1097/01.AOG.0000825720.19010.94

Camp, J. M., & Finkelstein, N. (1997). Parenting training for women in residential substance abuse treatment: Results of a demonstration project. *Journal of Substance Abuse Treatment*, *15*, 411–422. https://doi.org/10.1016/s0740-5472(97)00004-4

Canfield, M., Radcliffe, P., Marlow, S., Boreham, M., & Gilchrist G. (2017, August). Maternal substance use and child protection: a rapid evidence assessment of factors associated with loss of child care. *Child Abuse Negl*. 70:11–27. doi: 10.1016/j.chiabu.2017.05.005. Epub 2017 May 25. PMID: 28551458.

Carroll, K. M., & Kiluk, B. D. (2017). Cognitive behavioral interventions for alcohol and drug use disorders: Through the stage model and back again. *Psychology of Addictive Behaviors*, *31*(8), 847–861. https://doi.org/10.1037/adb0000311

Catalano, R. F., Gainey, R. R., Fleming, C. B., Haggerty, K. P., & Johnson, N. O. (1999). An experimental intervention with families of substance abusers: One year follow-up of the focus on families project. *Addiction*, *94*, 241–254. https://doi.org/10.1046/j.1360-0443.1999.9422418.x

Centers for Disease Control and Prevention (CDC). (2022, October 4). Alcohol. *Centers for Disease Control and Prevention*. Retrieved March 4, 2023, from www.cdc.gov/breastfeeding/breast-feeding-special-circumstances/vaccinations-medicationsdrugs/alcohol.html#:~:text=Alcohol%20levels%20are%20usually%20highest,more%20alcohol%20a%20mother%20consumes.

Chang, G. (2020). Maternal substance use: Consequences, identification, and interventions. *Alcohol Research: Current Review*, *40*(2), 1–10. https://doi.org/10.35946/arcr.v40.2.06

Chapman, S. L., & Wu, L. T. (2013). Postpartum substance use and depressive symptoms: A review. *Women & Health*, *53*(5), 479–503. https://doi.org/10.1080/03630242.2013.804025

Chasnoff, I. J., Wells, A. M., McGourty, R. F., & Bailey, L. K. (2007). Validation of the 4P's plus screen for substance use in pregnancy validation of the 4P's plus. *Journal of Perinatology*, *27*(12), 744–748. https://doi.org/10.1038/sj.jp.7211823

Chou, J. L., Muruthi, B. A., Ibrahim, M., Janes, E., Pennington, L. B., Seiler, R., . . . Herbert, D. (2020). A process evaluation of a substance use program for pregnant women: Lessons learned from the field. *International Journal of Mental Health and Addiction*. https://doi.org/10.1007/s11469-020-00374-1

Coleman-Cowger, V. H., Oga, E. A., Peteers, E. N., Trocin, K. E., Koszowski, B., & Mark, K. (2019). Accuracy of three screening tools for prenatal substance use. *Obstetrics & Gynecology*, *133*(5), 952–961. https://doi.org/10.1097/AOG0000000000003230

Conner, S. N., Bedell, V., Lipsey, K., Macones, G. A., Cahill, A. G., & Tuuli, M. G. (2016). Maternal marijuana use and adverse neonatal outcomes. *Obstetrics & Gynecology*, *128*(4), 713–723. http://doi.org/10.1097/AOG.0000000000001649

Cooper, S., Orton, S., Leonardi-Bee, J., Brotherton, E., Vanderbloemen, L., Bowker, K., . . . Coleman, T. (2017). Smoking and quit attempts during pregnancy and postpartum: A longitudinal UK cohort. *BMJ Open*, *7*(11). https://doi.org/10.1136/bmjopen-2017-018746

Croff, R. L., Rieckmann, T. R., & Spence, J. D. (2014). Provider and state perspectives on implementing cultural-based models of care for American Indian and Alaska native patients with substance use disorders. *Journal of Behavioral Health Services & Research*, *41*(1), 64–79. https://doi.org/10.1007/s11414-01309322-6

Crume, T. L., Juhl, A. L., Brooks-Russell, A., Hall, K. E., Wymore, E., & Borgelt, L. M. (2018). Cannabis use during the perinatal period in a state with legalized recreational and medical marijuana: The association between maternal characteristics, breastfeeding patterns, and neonatal outcomes. *Journal of Pediatrics, 197*, 90–96. https://doi.org/10.1016/j.jpeds.2018.02.005

DeGenna, N. M., Cornelius, M. D., Goldschmidt, L., & Day, N. L. (2015). Maternal age and trajectories of cannabis use. *Drug and Alcohol Dependence, 156*, 199–206. https://doi.org.du.idm.oclc.org/10.1016/j.drugalcdep.2015.09.014

Eberhard-Gran, M., Garthus-Niegel, S., Garthus-Niegel, K., & Eskild, A. (2010). Postnatal care: A cross-cultural and historical perspective. *Archives Women's Mental Health, 13*, 459–466. https://doi.org/10.1007/s00737-010-0175-1

England, L. J., Bennett, C., Denny, C. H., Honein, M. A., Gilboa, S. M., Kim, S. Y., . . . Boyle, C. A. (2020). Alcohol use and co-use of other substances among pregnant females aged 12–44 years – United States, 2015–2018. *Morbidity and Mortality Weekly Report, 69*(31), 1009–1014. https://doi.org/10.15585/mmwr.mm6931a1

Ernst, C. C., Grant, T. M., Streissguth, A. P., & Sampson, P. D. (1999). Interventions with high risk alcohol and drug abusing mothers: Three year findings for the Seattle model of paraprofessional advocacy. *Journal of Community Psychology, 27*(1), 19–38. https://doi.org/10.1002/(SICI)1520-6629(199901)27:1<19::AID-JCOP2>3.0.CO;2-K

Fals-Stewart, W. (n.d.). Substance abuse and intimate relationships. Advanced Solutions International. Retrieved June 30, 2022, from www.aamft.org/Consumer_Updates/Substance_Abuse_and_Intimate_Relationships.aspx#:~:text=Having%20a%20partner%20who%20drinks,friends%2C%20and%20co%2Dworkers

Faherty, L. J., Heins, S., Kranz, A. M., & Stein, B. D. (2021). Postpartum treatment for substance use disorder among mothers of infants with neonatal abstinence syndrome and prenatal substance exposure. *Women's Health Reports, 2*(1), 163–172. https://doi.org/10.1089/whr.2020.0128

Forray, A., & Foster, D. (2015). Substance use in the perinatal period. *Current Psychiatry Reports, 17*(91). https://doi.org/10.1007/s11920-015-0626-5

Forray, A., Merry, B., Lin, H., Prah Ruger, J., & Yonkers, K. A. (2015). Perinatal substance use: A prospective evaluation of abstinence and relapse. *Drug and Alcohol Dependence, 150*, 147–155. https://doi.org/10.1016/j.drugalcdep.2015.02.027

Frazer, Z., McConnell, K., & Jansson, L. M. (2019). Treatment for substance use disorders in pregnant women: Motivators and barriers. *Drug and Alcohol Dependence, 205*. https://doi.org/10.1016/j.drugalcdep.2019.107652

Gannon, M., Mackenzie, M., Kaltenback, K., & Abatemarco, D. (2017). Impact of mindfulness-based parenting on women in treatment for opioid use disorder. *Journal of Addictive Medicine, 11*(5), 368–376. https://doi.org/10.1097/ADM.0000000000000336

Gelberg, L., Natera Rey, G., Andersen, R. M., Arroyo, M., Bojorquez-Chapela, I., Rico, M. W., . . . Serota, M. (2017). Prevalence of substance use among patients of community health centers in east Los Angeles and Tijuana. *Substance Use and Misuse, 52*(3), 359–372. https://dx.doi.org/10/1080/10826084.2016.12227848

Gerdts-Andresen, T. (2021). Circle of security-parenting: A systematic review on effectiveness of use of the parent training program within multi-problem families. *Nordic Journal of Social Research, 12*, 1–26. https://doi.org.10.7577/njsr.3482

Gopman, S. (2014). Prenatal and postpartum care of women with substance use disorders. *Obstetrics and Gynecology Clinics of North America, 41*(2), 213–228. https://dx.doi.org/10.1016/j.ogc.2014.02.004

Grant, T. M., Ernst, C. C., & Streissguth, A. P. (1999). Interventions with high risk alcohol and drug abusing mothers 1: Administrative strategies of the Seattle model of paraprofessional advocacy. *Journal of Community Psychology, 27*, 1–18. https://doi.org/10.1002/(SICI)1520-6629(199901)27:1<1::AID-JCOP1>3.0.CO;2-3

Gray, C. (2018, September 13). *Substance use in breastfeeding parents: A review of safety and guidelines.* National Center for Biotechnology Information. https://www.ncbi.nlm.nih.gov/books/NBK538536/

Gruss, I., Firemark, A., & Davidson, A. (2021). Motherhood, substance use and peer support: Benefits of an integrated group program for pregnant and postpartum women. *Journal of Substance Abuse Treatment, 131*, 108450. https://doi.org/10.1016/j.jsat.2021.108450

Guttmacher Institute. (2024, March 15). *Substance use during pregnancy.* Guttmacher Institute. www.guttmacher.org/state-policy/explore/substance-use-during-pregnancy

Hatters Friedman, S., Heneghan, A., & Rosenthal, M. (2009). Disposition and health outcomes among infants born to mothers with no prenatal care. *Child Abuse & Neglect, 33,* 116–122. https://doi.org/10.1016/j.chiabu.2008.05.009

Homish, G. G., Cornelius, J. R., Richardson, G. A., & Day, N. L. (2004). Antenatal risk factors associated with postpartum comorbid alcohol use and depressive symptomatology. *Alcoholism: Clinical and Experimental Research, 28*(8), 1242–1248. https://doi.org/10.1097/01.alc.0000134217.43967.97

Horton, E., & Murray, C. (2015). A quantitative exploratory evaluation of the circle of security-parenting program with mothers in residential substance-abuse treatment. *Infant Mental Health Journal, 36*(3), 320–336. https://doi.org/10.1002/imhj.21514

Huang, A., Wu, K., Cai, Z., Lin, Y., Zhang, X., & Huang, Y. (2021). Association between postnatal second – Hand smoke exposure and ADHD in children: A systematic review and meta – Analysis. *Environmental Science and Pollution Research, 28,* 1370–1380. https://doi.org/10.1007/s11356-020-11269-y

Jacobs, J., Moran Vozar, T. E., Thornton, K., Lavin Elliott, K., & Holmberg, J. (2023). What to expect when you're expecting . . . and in recovery. *General Hospital Psychiatry, 83,* 172–178.

Jacobson, N. S., & Truax, P. (1991). Clinical significance: A statistical approach to defining meaningful change in psychotherapy research. *Journal of Consulting and Clinical Psychology, 59*(1), 12–19. https://doi.org/10.1037/0022-006X.59.1.12

Jones, H. E., Deppen, K., Hudak, M. L., Leffert, L., McClellan, C., Sahin, L., . . . Creanga, A. A. (2014). Clinical care for opioid-using pregnant and postpartum women: The role of obstetric providers. *American Journal of Obstetrics & Gynecology, 210*(4), 302–310. https://10.1016/j.ajog.2013.10.010

Jones, M., Lewis, S., Parrott, S., Wormall, S., & Coleman, T. (2016). Re-starting smoking in the postpartum period after receiving a smoking cessation intervention: A systematic review. *Addiction, 111,* 981–990. https://doi.org/10.1111/add.13309

Kabir, Z., Connolly, G. N., & Alpert, H. R. (2011). Secondhand smoke exposure and neurobehavioral disorders among children in the United States. *Pediatrics, 128*(2), 263–270. https://doi.org/10.1542/peds.2011-0023

Kim, Y. H. (2020). Korean mothers' alcohol consumption trajectories form childbirth to 6 years postpartum and children's executive function difficulties at first grade. *Social Psychiatry and Psychiatric Epidemiology, 55,* 497–506. https://doi.org/10.1007/s00127-019-01804-9

Kogan, M. D., Schuster, M. A., Yu, S. M., Park, C. H., Olson, L. M., Inkelas, M., . . . Halfon. (2004). Routine assessment of family and community health risks: Parent views and what they receive. *Pediatrics, 113,* 1934–1943. https://doi.org/10.1542/peds.113.6.S1.1934

Kuo, C., Chatav Schonbrun, Y., Zlotnick, C., Bates, N., Todorova, R., Chien-Wen Kao, J., & Johnson, J. (2013). A qualitative study of treatment needs among pregnant and postpartum women with substance use and depression. *Substance Use and Misuse, 48,* 1498–1508. https://doi.org/10.3109/10826084.2013.800116

Li, X., Laplante, D. P., Paquin, V., Lafortune, S., Elgbeili, G., & King, S. (2022). Effectiveness of cognitive behavioral therapy for perinatal maternal depression, anxiety and stress: A systematic review and meta-analysis of randomized controlled trials. *Clinical Psychology Review, 92,* 102129. https://doi.org/10.1016/j.cpr.2022.102129

Lamus, M. N., Pabon, S., MPoca, C., Guida, J. P., Parpinelli, M. A., Cecatti, J. G., . . . Costa, M. L. (2021). Giving women WOICE postpartum: Prevalence of maternal morbidity in high-risk pregnancies using the WHO-WOICE instrument. *BMC Pregnancy and Childbirth, 21*(1), 357. https://doi.org/10.1186/s12884-021-03727-3

Landi, N., Montoya, J., Kober, H., Rutherford, H. J. V., Mencl, W. E., Worhunsky, P. D., . . . Mayes, L. C. (2011). Maternal neural responses to infant cries and faces: Relationships with substance use. *Frontiers in Psychiatry, 2*(32), 1–13. https://doi.org/10.3389/fpsyt.2022.00032

Lowell, A. F., Peacock-Chambers, E., Zayde, A., DeCoste, C. L., McMahon, T. J., & Suchman, N. E. (2021). Mothering from the inside out: Addressing the intersection of addiction, adversity, and attachment with evidence-based parenting intervention. *Current Addiction Reports, 8,* 605–615. https://doi.org/10.1007/s40429-021-00389-1

Luthar, S. S., & Walsh, K. G. (1995). Treatment needs of drug-addicted mothers: Integrated parenting psychotherapy interventions. *Journal of Substance Abuse Treatment, 12*(5), 341–348. https://doi.org/10.1016/0740-5472(95)02010-1

Pentecost, R., Latendresse, G., & Smid, M. (2021). Scoping review of the associations between peri-natal substance use and perinatal depression and anxiety. *Journal of Obstetric, Gynecologic & Neonatal Nursing, 50*(4), 382–391. https://doi.org/10.1016/j.jogn.2021.02.008

Potenza, M. N., & Mayes, L. C. (2011). Maternal neural responses to infant cries and faces: Relation-ships with substance use. *Frontiers in Psychiatry, 2*(32). https://doi.org/10.3389.fpsyt.2011.00032

Powell, B., Cooper, G., Hoffman, K., & Marvin, R. S. (2009). The circle of security. In C. H. Zeanah, Jr. (Ed.), *Handbook of infant mental health* (pp. 450–467). Guilford Press.

Maxwell, A. M., McMahan, C., Huber, A., Reay, R. E., Hawkins, E., & Barnett, B. (2021). Examining the effectiveness of Circle of Security Parenting (COS-P): A multi-site noon-randomized study with waitlist control. *Journal of Child and Family Studies, 30*, 1123–1140. https://doi.org/10.1007/s10826-021-01932-4

McGlade, A., Ware, R., & Crawford, M. (2009). Child protection outcomes for infants of substance-using mothers: A matched-cohort study. *Pediatrics, 124*, 285–293. https://doi.org/10.1542/peds.2008–0576

McHugh, R. K., Votaw, V. R., Sugarman, D. E., & Greenfield, S. F. (2018). Sex and gender differ-ences in substance use disorders. *Clinical Psychology Review, 66*, 12–23. https://doi.org/10.1016/j.cpr.2017.10.012

Míguez, M. C., & Pereira, B. (2021). Factors associated with smoking relapse in the early postpar-tum period: A prospective longitudinal study in Spain. *Maternal and Child Health Journal, 25*, 998–1006. https://doi.org/10.1007/s10995-020-03019-w

Nadhiroh, S. R., Djokosujono, K., & Utari, D. M. (2020). The association between secondhand smoke exposure and growth outcomes of children: A systematic literature review. *Tobacco Induced Diseases, 18*(12). https://doi.org/10.18332/tid/117958

Nelson, S. E., Van Ryzin, M. J., & Dishion, T. J. (2015). Alcohol, marijuana, and tobacco use trajectories from age 12 to 24 years: Demographic correlates and young adult substance use problems. *Devel-opment and Psychopathology, 27*(1), 253–277. https://doi.org/10.1017/S0954579414000650

Nordhagen, L. S., Kreyberg, I., Bains, K. E. S., Carlsen, K. H., Glavin, K., Skjerven, H. O., . . . Lodrup Carlsen, K. C. (2019). Maternal use of nicotine products and breastfeeding 3 months postpartum. *Acta Paediatricia, 109*, 2594–2603. https://doi.org/10.1111/apa.15299

Orton, S., Bowker, K., Cooper, S., Naughton, F., Ussher, M., Pickett, K. E., . . . Coleman, T. (2014). Longitudinal cohort survey of women's smoking behaviour and attitudes in pregnancy: Study methods and baseline data. *BMJ Open, 4*(5). https//doi.org/10.1136/bmjopen-2014-004915

Paris, R., Herriott, A. L., Maru, M., Hacking, S. E., & Sommer, A. R. (2020). Secrecy versus disclo-sure: Women with substance use disorders share experiences in help seeking during pregnancy. *Maternal and Child Health Journal, 24*, 1396–1403. https://doi.org/10.1007/s10995-020-03006-1

Patrick, S. W., Dudley, J., Martin, P. R., Harrell, F. E., Warren, M. D., Hartmann, K. E., . . . Cooper, W. O. (2015). Prescription opioid epidemic and infant outcomes. *Pediatrics, 135*(5), 842–850. https://doi.org/10.1542/peds.2014-3299

Pereira, C. M., Pacagnella, R. C., Parpinelli, M. A., Andreucci, C. B., Zanardi, D. M., Souza, R. T., . . . Cecatti, J. G. (2018). Postpartum psychoactive substance abuse after severe maternal morbidity. *International Federation of Gynecology and Obstetrics, 147*, 368–374. https://10.1002/ijgo.12967

Preis, H., Garry, D. J., Herrera, K., Garretto, D. J., & Lobel, M. (2020). Improving assessment, treat-ment, and understanding of pregnant women with opioid use disorder: The importance of life context. *Women's Reproductive Health, 7*(3), 153–163. https://doi.org/10.1080/23293691.2020.1780395

Prevatt, Desmarais, S. L., & Janssen, P. A. (2016). Lifetime substance use as a predictor of postpar-tum mental health. *Archives of Women's Mental Health, 20*(1), 189–199. https://doi.org/10.1007/s00737-016-0694-5

Qato, D. M., & Gandhi, A. B. (2021). Opioid and benzodiazepine dispensing and co – Dispensing patterns among commercially insured pregnant women in the United States, 2007–2015. *BMC Pregnancy & Childbirth, 62*(1), 168–184. https:doi.org/10.1097/GRF.000000000000418

Rodriguez, J. J., & Smith, V. C. (2019). Epidemiology of perinatal substance use: Exploring trends in maternal substance use. *Seminars in Fetal and Neonatal Medicine, 24*, 86–89. https://doi.org/10.1016/j.siny.2019.01.006

Rossen, L., Mattick, R. P., Wilson, J., Clare, P. J., Burns, L., Allsop, S., . . . Hutchinson, D. (2019). Mother – Infant bonding and emotional availability at 12 months of age: The role of early post-natal bonding, maternal substance use and mental health. *Maternal and Child Health Journal, 23*(12), 1686–1698. https://doi.org/10.1007/s10995-019-02809-1

Rutherford, J. V., & Mayes, L. C. (2019). Parenting stress: A novel mechanism of addiction vulnerability. *Neurobiology of Stress, 11*. https://doi.org/10.1016/j.ynstr.2019.100172

Sadicario, J. S., Parlier-Ahmad, A. B., Brechbiel, J. K., Islam, L. Z., & Martin, C. E. (2021). Caring for women with substance use disorders through pregnancy and postpartum during the COVID-19 pandemic: Lessons learned from psychology trainees in an integrated OBGYN/substance use disorder outpatient treatment program. *Journal of Substance Abuse Treatment, 122*. https://doi.org/10.1016/j.jsat.2020.108200

Salemi, J. L., Raza, S. A., Modal, S., Fields-Gilmore, J. A. R., Mejia de Grubb, M. C., & Zoorob, R. J. (2020). The association between use of opioids, cocaine, and amphetamines during pregnancy and maternal postpartum readmission in the United States: A retrospective analysis of the nationwide readmissions database. *Drug and Alcohol Dependence, 210*. https://doi.org/10.1016/j.drugalcdep.2020.107963

Salisbury, A. L., Lester, B. M., Seifer, R., Lagasse, L., Bauer, C. R., Shankaran, S., . . . Poole, K. (2007). Prenatal cocaine use and maternal depression: Effects on infant neurobehavior. *Neurotoxicology and Teratology, 29*(3), 331–340. https://doi.org/10.1016/j.ntt.2006.12.001

Samet, J. M., & Yoon, S. Y. (2011). *Women and the tobacco epidemic: Challenges for the 21st century*. WHO, Institute for Global Tobacco Control, Johns Hopkins School of Public Health.

Scheffers-van Schayck, T., Tuithof, M., Otten, R., Engels, R., & Kleinjan, M. (2019). Smoking behavior of women before, during, and after pregnancy: Indicators of smoking, quitting, and relapse. *European Addiction Research, 25*(3), 132–144. https://doi.org/10.1159/000498988

Smid, M. C., Metz, T. D., & Gordon, A. J. (2019). Stimulant use in pregnancy: An under – Recognized epidemic among pregnant women. *Clinical Obstetrics and Gynecology, 62*(1), 168–184. Https://doi.org/10.1097/GRF.0000000000000418

Sinha, R. (2001). How does stress increase risk of drug abuse and relapse? *Psychopharmacology, 158*, 343–359. https://doi.org/10.1007/s002130100917

Steingrimsson, S., Carlsen, H. K., Sigfusson, S., & Magnusson, A. (2012). The changing gender gap in substance use disorder: A total population-based study of psychiatric in-patients. *Addiction, 107*(11), 1957–1962. https://dx.doi.org/10.1111/j.1360-0443. 2012.03954.x

Stringer, K. L., & Baker, E. H. (2018). Stigma as a barrier to substance abuse treatment among those with unmet need: An analysis of parenthood and marital status. *Journal of Family Issues, 39*(1), 3–27. https://doi.org/10.1177/0192513X15581659

Substance Abuse and Mental Health Services Administration (SAMHSA). (2014). *SAMHSA's concept of trauma and guidance for a trauma-informed approach*. HHS Publication No. (SMA) 14-4884. Substance Abuse and Mental Health Services Administration.

Substance Abuse and Mental Health Services Administration. (2015). *The center for behavioral health statistics and quality report*. SAMHSA.

Substance Abuse and Mental Health Services Administration (SAMHSA). (2021, March 15). *National survey on drug use and health (NSDUH). Releases (samhsa.gov)*. SAMHSA. www.samhsa.gov/data/release/2021-national-survey-drug-use-and-health-nsduh-releases#annual-national-report

Suchman, N. E. (2016). Mothering from the inside out: A mentalization-based therapy for mothers in treatment for drug addiction. *International Journal of Birth and Parent Education, 3*(4), 19–24. https://doi.org/10.1017/S0954579417000220

Suchman, N. E., Decoste, C., McMahon, T. J., Dalton, R., Mayes, L., & Borelli, J. (2017). Mothering from the inside out: Results of a second randomized clinical trial testing a mentalization-based intervention for mothers in addiction treatment. *Developmental and Psychopathology, 29*, 617–636. https://doi.org/10.1017/S0954579417000220

Suchman, N. E., Decoste, C., McMahon, T. J., Rounsaville, B., & Mayes, L. (2011). The mothers and toddlers program, an attachment-based parenting intervention for substance-using women: Results at 6-week follow-up in a randomized clinical pilot. *Infant Mental Health Journal, 32*(4), 427–449. https://doi.org/10.1002/imhj.20303

Swendsen, J. D., & Merikangas, K. R. (2000). The comorbidity of depression and substance use disorders. *Clinical Psychology Review, 20*(2), 173–189. https://doi.org/10.1016/s0272-7358(99)00026-4

Tebeka, S., De Premorel Higgons, A., Dubertret, C., & Le Strat, Y. (2020). Changes in alcohol use and heavy episodic drinking in U.S. Women of childbearing-age and peripartum between 2001–2002 and 2012–2013. *Addictive Behaviors, 107*, 1–7. https://doi.org/10.1016/j.addbeh.2020.106389

Teruya, C., & Hser, Y. (2010). Turning points in the life course: Current findings and future directions in drug use research. *Current Drug Abuse Review*, 3, 189–195. https://doi. org/10.2174/1874473711003030189

Tolia, V. N., Patrick, S. W., Bennett, M. M., Murthy, K, Sousa, J., Smith, P. B., . . . Spitzer, A. R. (2015). Increasing incidence of the neonatal abstinence syndrome in U.S. neonatal ICUs. *New England Journal of Medicine*, 372, 2118–2126. https://doi.org/10.1056/NEJMsa1500439

Troutman, B., Moran, T. E., Arndt, S., Johnson, R. F., & Chmielewski, M. (2012). Development of parenting self-efficacy in mothers of infants with high negative emotionality. *Infant Mental Health Journal*, 33(1), 45–50. https://doi.org/10.1002/imhj.20332.

Twomey, J. E. (2007). Partners of perinatal substance users: Forgotten, failing or fit to father? *American Journal of Orthopsychiatry*, 77(4), 563–572. https://doi.org/10/1037/0002-9432.77.4.563

Wallman, C. M., Bohling Smith, P., & Moore, K. (2011). Implementing a perinatal substance abuse screening tool. *Advanced Neonatal Care*, 11(4), 255–267. https://doi.org/10.1097/ANC.0b013e318225a20b

Weber, A., Miskle, B., Lynch, A., Arndt, S., & Acion, L. (2021). Substance use in pregnancy: Identifying stigma and improving care. *Substance Abuse and Rehabilitation*, 12, 105–121. https://doi. org/10.2147/SAR.S319180

Wilton, G., Moberg, D. P., & Fleming, M. F. (2009). The effect of brief alcohol intervention on postpartum depression. *MCN: The American Journal of Maternal Child Nursing*, 34(5), 297–302. https://doi.org/10.1097/01.NMC.0000360422.06486.c4

Wittkowski, A., Gardner, P. L., Bunton, P., & Edge, D. (2013). Culturally determined risk factors for postnatal depression in Sub-Saharan Africa: A mixed method systematic review. *Journal of Affective Disorders*, 163, 115–124. https://dx.doi.org/10.1016/j.jad.2013.12.028

World Health Organization (WHO). (2013). WHO *recommendations for the prevention and management of tobacco use and second-hand smoke exposure in pregnancy*. WHO.

World Health Organization (WHO). (2018). *Global status report on alcohol and health*. WHO.

Zhang, H., Watkins, C. E., Hook, J. N., Hodge, A. S., Davis, C. W., Norton, J., . . . Owen, J. (2022). Cultural humility in psychotherapy and clinical supervision: A research review. *Counselling and Psychotherapy Research*, 22, 548–557. https://doi.org/10.1002/capr.12481

18

POSTPARTUM PSYCHOSIS

Anja Wittkowski

Postpartum psychosis, which is sometimes referred to as puerperal psychosis, postpartum psychosis, or psychosis after childbirth, is considered to be the most severe form of postpartum mood disorders, despite being relatively rare (e.g., Robertson et al., 2005; Bergink et al., 2015; Robertson Blackmore et al., 2016; NICE, 2014/2020). For example, one to two women in 1,000 deliveries develop symptoms of postpartum psychosis (e.g., Kendell et al., 1987; Munk-Olsen et al., 2006; Sit et al., 2006). VanderKruik et al. (2017) identified an incidence rate of 0.80 to 2.6 per 1,000 births and a prevalence of 5 in 1,000 women. The incidence rate of first-onset postpartum psychosis is thought to range from 0.24 to 0.6 women per 1,000 births (Munk-Olsen et al., 2006; Valdimarsdóttir et al., 2009; Brockington, 2014). However, in terms of epidemiology, some caution is required due to the variety of how postpartum psychosis has been defined (Robertson Blackmore et al., 2016). Nowadays, postpartum psychosis, thought to be distinct from non-postpartum psychosis in many ways (Friedman et al., 2023), is used as an umbrella term for mania, psychosis, and depression with psychotic features in the postpartum period (Kapfhammer et al., 2014; Bergink et al., 2015, 2016).

Although postpartum psychosis is considered to be rare compared to other postpartum mental health presentations, the impact of postpartum psychosis on women and their family members is often severe, especially in the acute phase, as highlighted by various campaign groups raising awareness of this disorder through their websites (see *Action on Postpartum Psychosis* [2023a] and *Postpartum Support International* [2023]) and via increased media coverage targeting the public and healthcare professionals, especially in the United Kingdom (see U.K. documentaries like *Louis Theroux: Mothers on the Edge* [Casebow et al., 2019] or *My Baby, My Psychosis and Me* [Burrell et al., 2019]). Roberts et al. (2018) examined the effects of increased public awareness on women who had experienced postpartum psychosis, following a storyline about postpartum psychosis in 2016 in *Eastenders*, a popular British television soap opera. Website visits to the charity *Action on Postpartum Psychosis* had doubled, with a fourfold increase in people registering for email peer support. Interviews revealed that women felt it was easier to disclose their experiences of postpartum psychosis after the storyline was shown on television.

DOI: 10.4324/9781003206903-22

The impact of postpartum psychosis on women and their families is likely related to its rapid onset, the acuity and kaleidoscopic nature of symptoms, and the fact that women often lack insight into what is happening to them. Family members may not be aware of the symptoms of postpartum psychosis at all and, hence, cannot look out for them (Friedman et al., 2023). In addition, most women who have given birth are often discharged from their maternity hospital within one to two days, when postpartum psychosis typically develops on day 3.

This combination of factors can lead to devastating consequences and situations in which the safety and well-being of the mother and her baby are threatened (Wisner et al., 1994; Sit et al., 2006). For this reason, guidance from the National Institute of Clinical Excellence (NICE) in the U.K. classified postpartum psychosis as a medical emergency and women should be assessed by a mental health team within four hours (NICE, 2014/2020). The initial evaluation of a woman presenting with suspected postpartum psychosis requires a thorough assessment, which may often take part in an emergency setting given the rapid onset of symptoms, to exclude an organic cause for acute psychosis. A differential diagnosis may include ruling out infection, thyroid disease, blood loss, tumor, autoimmune disease, or anoxia (e.g., Sit et al., 2006; Friedman et al., 2023).

In the U.K., the National Health Service (NHS, 2023) website on postpartum psychosis (www.nhs.uk/mental-health/conditions/post-partum-psychosis/) urges to contact whoever is already involved in this woman's care including her general physician (GP) or midwife or a healthcare professional from a mental health team that the woman is already involved with, requesting an assessment on the same day. If necessary, this should be escalated to ringing the emergency services or presenting at the hospital, especially if the woman or baby is believed to be in danger. Crucially, the NHS website also states the following: "Be aware that if you have postpartum psychosis, you may not realise you're ill. Your partner, family or friends may spot the signs and have to take action."

Once a diagnosis is made, the woman usually requires admission to a psychiatric inpatient unit, ideally to a Mother and Baby Unit (MBU), so that the mother can be jointly admitted with her baby for assessment and treatment (Jones & Craddock, 2007; Doucet et al., 2011; Gillham & Wittkowski, 2015; NICE, 2014/2020; NHS, 2023; Wittkowski, 2021).

Symptoms and Clinical Features

Brockington (1996, cited in Sit et al., 2006, p. 353) described a mother with postpartum psychosis as presenting with *"an odd affect, withdrawn, distracted by auditory hallucinations, incompetent, confused, catatonic; or alternatively, elated, labile, rambling in speech, agitated or excessively active."* This description highlights a complex picture of symptoms. Symptoms can range from paranoid, grandiose, or bizarre delusions and hallucinations to mood swings, confused thinking, and disorganized behavior (e.g., Wisner et al., 1994; Sit et al., 2006; Robertson Blackmore et al., 2016; Perry et al., 2021). The most common psychotic symptoms appear to be persecutory delusions and delusions of reference (Kamperman et al., 2017), with grandiose delusions being rarer (Ganjekar et al., 2013).

Ye it was a big, ye unexpected, no previous unwellness, no, no fore warning because it's so sudden, and just, ye, it, umm the unravelling meant a complete loss of functioning really.

(Woman 9, cited in Forde et al., 2019, p. 418)

Postpartum psychosis is seen as presenting a "kaleidoscopic" clinical picture (NICE, 2014/2020; Perry et al., 2021) because its presentation may range from symptoms of mania (e.g., elation, excess energy, racing thoughts and restlessness) to symptoms more typical of depression (e.g., beliefs and feelings of helplessness, hopelessness and worthlessness; see Berrisford et al., 2015) alongside brief periods of lucidity (Klompenhouwer et al., 1995). Drawing on Brockington et al. (1981), Brockington (1996), and Robertson Blackmore et al. (2016) pointed out that the majority of episodes may be more affective than psychotic in presentation because manic symptoms (e.g., elation, rambling speech, flight of ideas, lability of mood, distractability, euphoria, excessive activity) tend to be more frequent and severe, especially in the first two weeks after childbirth. However, it is also estimated that in more than 70% of women, psychotic symptoms are present, sometimes co-occurring with other symptoms (Kamperman et al., 2017). Furthermore, perplexity and visual hallucinations are more frequently reported by women with postpartum psychosis compared to women presenting with episodes of mania or psychosis unrelated to childbirth (Ganjekar et al., 2013; Gordon-Smith et al., 2020). According to Gordon-Smith et al. (2020), women with postpartum psychosis showed more depressive symptoms, more complexity and self-reproach, and fewer classic manic symptoms (e.g., pressured speech and sociability), compared to women with postpartum mania.

In terms of clinical presentation, it is also very important to pay attention to disturbances in consciousness and behavior, characterized by cognitive disorganization, confusion, bewilderment, or perplexity and unusual, disorganized behavior that is markedly different from the woman's usual functioning (e.g., Wisner et al., 1994; Bergink et al., 2016). It is possible that these disturbances explain why women often do not realize that they are in the grip of a severe mental illness. As a consequence, it is often family members who first notice the acute signs and seek help from healthcare professionals.

Onset of Postpartum Psychosis

It is now widely accepted that the immediate postpartum period places mothers at increased risk for presenting with a mental health problem. Compared to any other period in a woman's life, the risk of the first onset of a postpartum disorder (not just postpartum psychosis) was found to be 23 times higher in the four weeks after childbirth (Munk-Olsen et al., 2006). Using a U.K. population sample, Kendell et al. (1987) also noted that the risk of psychiatric admission for a psychotic or mood disorder was 22 greater in the first month after childbirth, with psychiatric admissions being 35 times more likely if a woman had given birth to her first baby. Thus, the postpartum period is a time of increased risk for women's mental health to deteriorate.

Postpartum psychosis onset is considered to be rapid because acute symptoms typically emerge within the first two weeks after childbirth (Brockington et al., 1981; NICE, 2014/2020), with 90% of episodes beginning in this timeframe (Heron et al., 2007). Typical onset is by day 3 after childbirth (Sit et al., 2006; Heron et al., 2008; NICE, 2014/2020). The risk of an onset decreases over time; for example, after the first three months of their baby's life, mothers were found to be less at risk of developing postpartum psychosis (Valdimarsdóttir et al., 2009).

Infanticide and Filicide in the Context of Postpartum Psychosis

Postpartum psychosis is often considered an emergency because of the increased risk of infanticide, child harm, and suicide (Friedman et al., 2023). Delusional beliefs with a focus

407

on childbirth or obsessive and/or delusional thoughts about their baby are common (Brockington, 1996; Chandra et al., 2006; Bergink et al., 2016). For example, women may believe that her baby has changed (e.g., into an evil spirit or the devil) and/or she feels persecuted by her baby (Brockington, 1996; Ramsauer & Achtergarde, 2018). She may also believe her baby to be in danger of being stolen or hurt (Ramsauer & Achtergarde, 2018), as illustrated by this quote:

> You know they would never say to a woman that had been attacked "well that's no big deal" but people will separate psychosis, because to them it's not real, to them it never happened, but it did happen to me, something was coming up my hill, it was going to kill my kid and if I didn't kill myself he was going to die. You know it's as simple as that, I really believed my baby was going to die and be killed.
>
> *(Woman 7 cited in Forde et al., 2019, p. 418)*

Depending on their exact nature, these beliefs may elicit protective or more harmful (or neglectful) responses in the mother (Brockington, 2017). Although this may sound alarming, infanticide is rare (Brockington, 2017). Robertson Blackmore et al. (2016) suggested that infanticide occurred in 1 to 3 in 50,000 births. Citing Kumar et al.'s survey (1995), Sit et al. (2006) reported that 28% to 35% of women hospitalized for postpartum psychosis expressed delusions about their infant, but only 9% had thoughts of harming their infant. Furthermore, only 8% of 130 women admitted to a Mother and Baby Unit experienced infanticidal thoughts in Kamperman et al.'s study (2017).

However, having thoughts of harming one's child does not mean that the mother will go on to harm her infant or child intentionally. In his review, Brockington (2017) reported that less than 1% of mothers killed their child and that some of these mothers had no intention of harming their child. However, he also noted that the filicide rate appeared to be higher (4.5%) in mothers presenting with depressive psychoses. Thus, he warned that severely depressed mothers present with the risk of melancholic filicide, especially if these mothers also show suicidal actions. Interestingly, filicides are not common during the acute postpartum episode (Brockington, 2017). One could argue that the rapid onset of symptoms translates into help-seeking and the implementation of treatment, clinical observation, and relevant safeguarding.

Another important aspect to consider is the fact that women experiencing postpartum psychosis can fluctuate between lucid and delusional states. The Postpartum Psychosis International website addresses perinatal psychosis related tragedies by advising the following: "Perinatal psychosis is a temporary illness that needs to be looked at differently than chronic psychiatric disorders. This difference must be understood as individuals are assessed, defended and evaluated for alleged crimes committed during a temporary and treatable delusional state. Legal insanity definitions can be misleading, because the individual experiencing postpartum can at moments be able to differentiate right from wrong, yet in the delusional state be influenced by extreme compelling delusional beliefs, hallucinations, or commands which might instruct them to harm their baby" (www.postpartum.net/learn-more/postpartum-psychosis/).

However, as women can present with a wide range of symptoms, including mood disturbances and confusion, they are more at risk of accidentally harming their infant through neglect or unsafe childcaring practices (e.g., Sit et al., 2006; Robertson Blackmore et al., 2016). As healthcare professionals have child safeguarding duties, they should sensitively ask mothers about the nature of their delusions and inquire about her childcaring behaviors by liaising with family members as well. With depressive psychosis being a potential risk factor, the presence of depressive symptoms should also be established to implement a more tailored treatment approach.

Suicide and Suicide Risk in the Context of Postpartum Psychosis

Maternal suicide remains the leading cause of direct deaths occurring within a year after the end of pregnancy in a number of high-income countries (e.g., Knight et al., 2020; Reid et al., 2022). In their meta-analysis of 14 studies, Rao et al. (2021) identified that the worldwide prevalence of suicide attempts during pregnancy was 680 per 100,000, and during the postpartum period, it was 210 per 100,000 births. In their comprehensive systematic review of 59 studies, Reid et al. (2022) investigated 32 different risk factors they deemed to be modifiable in mothers during the perinatal period. They noted that the link between recent and historic abuse and maternal suicide ideation, attempted suicide, and death was consistently evidenced in the reviewed studies. Perception of social support also played a role, but more so for women with suicide attempts. However, Reid et al. (2022) did not examine diagnosis-specific risk factors.

In terms of postpartum psychosis, women have been found to be at greater risk of suicide when compared to mothers with psychiatric disorders with an onset at other times (Johannsen et al., 2016). It is more common for women with postpartum psychosis to present with thoughts of self-harm and suicide (Kamperman et al., 2017). Using a broad definition of postpartum psychosis and drawing on older Confidential Enquiries into Maternal Death (CEMD, 2001, 2004), Robertson Blackmore et al. (2016) noted that the majority of women who had died by suicide had experienced a severe psychotic illness with an abrupt onset within days of childbirth. However, this finding is somewhat in contrast to Brockington's (2017) interpretation of the literature (rather than data on maternal deaths), which led him to state that suicide is rare during an acute episode of postpartum psychosis, but that the risk is raised after recovery or later in a mother's life as well as in mothers with first degree relatives who died by suicide. Furthermore, compared to rates in age-matched women without children, the rates of completed suicides in postpartum women are lower (Lysell et al., 2018). In their Danish registry study (with a mean follow-up of 26.26 years), Johannsen et al. (2016) noted that 29 of 2,699 women who had inpatient or outpatient contact with psychiatry within three months of giving birth had died by suicide (i.e., 0.01%). This study collected data from 1970 to 2011, but women's episodes could have been less severe if outpatient contact was sufficient. In contrast, in their Danish register study with data from 1973 to 1993, Appleby et al. (1998) noted a suicide rate of 3.3%. Furthermore, Gilden et al. (2020a) identified that three of the six studies in their review reported high suicide rates (4% to 11%) in women with first-onset postpartum psychosis (e.g., Kapfhammer et al., 2014; Videbech & Gouliaev, 1995; Schöpf & Rust, 1994). These rates underscore the need to view the emergence of symptoms as a psychiatric emergency, especially for women with a first-onset postpartum psychosis. The risk seems increased during untreated acute episodes, following hospital discharge and also when depressive symptoms are present (Kessler et al., 1999; Qin & Nordentoft, 2005).

Postpartum Psychosis and the Link to Bipolar Disorder

For approximately 40% to 50% of women postpartum psychosis is the first severe psychiatric disorder they experienced (e.g., Martin et al., 2016; Perry et al., 2021). The other 60% appear to present with a recurrence of an existing psychiatric disorder (Munk-Olsen et al.,

2006; Martin et al., 2016). The evidence points to a particular link with bipolar disorder, which has been outlined well in various reviews (e.g., Sit et al., 2006; Robertson Blackmore et al., 2016; Meltzer-Brody et al., 2018; Perry et al., 2021; Sharma et al., 2022). For example, Jones and Craddock (2001) identified that in women with a history of bipolar disorder and in women with a history of bipolar disorder alongside a family history of postpartum psychosis, the base rate for postpartum psychosis increased from 1 to 260 and 570 in 1,000 deliveries, respectively. In addition, Robertson Blackmore et al. (2016) highlighted the link between postpartum psychosis and bipolar disorder by pointing out the possibility of a lifetime diagnosis of bipolar disorder or schizoaffective bipolar disorder (see also Brockington et al., 1981; Videbech & Gouliaev, 1995; Robling et al., 2000). Women with a diagnosis of bipolar disorder may also go on to develop postpartum psychosis; a meta-analysis by Wesseloo et al. (2016) reported this prevalence to be 17%.

The development of better predictive risk models of postpartum psychosis has been advocated in the literature (Perry et al., 2021), and technology including machine learning approaches using electronic health data of pregnant women or childbirth data is an area of growing interest (Friedman et al., 2023).

Classification of Postpartum Psychosis

One of the difficulties in presenting an accurate picture of the prevalence of postpartum psychosis and its clinical features relates to its definition and how this has changed and been applied. The nosology of postpartum psychosis remains controversial (Perry et al., 2021; Sharma et al., 2022). For example, postpartum psychosis has been considered to be a disorder or condition in its own right as well as linked to bipolar disorder, as mentioned previously (e.g., Bergink et al., 2016; Kendell et al., 1987; Sit et al., 2006; Sharma et al., 2022). Robertson Blackmore et al. (2016) highlighted that postpartum psychosis was included in ICD-8 and in DSM-II, albeit with qualifiers to only use this diagnosis when other diagnoses could not be used or could not be excluded. In subsequent versions of the ICD and DSM classification systems, postpartum psychosis is no longer seen as a separate diagnostic category and nosological entity (Robertson Blackmore et al., 2016; Sharma et al., 2022). According to Bergink et al. (2015), postpartum psychosis is considered an atypical presentation of a mood disorder and not primarily a disorder of psychosis. The authors also explained that the term psychosis was used because this disorder was grouped with affective psychoses, which included "endogeneous depression" and "manic depressive psychosis," but that the term was no longer used in DSM-III. Despite having no official nosological status in DSM-IV, DSM-V, or ICD-10, the term postpartum psychosis continues to be widely used by clinicians and researchers (Bergink et al., 2015).

Spinelli (2021) argued that postpartum psychosis should be made a separate diagnostic entity, whereas Di Florio et al. (2021) promoted the idea that first-onset postpartum psychosis should be a separate entity within the bipolar disorder spectrum (see Sharma et al., 2022). In 2015, Bergink, Boyce and Munk-Olsen had welcomed this debate by terming postpartum psychosis "a valuable misnomer" (p. 102), arguing that the term should be used regardless, because it emphasizes that episodes are uniquely related to childbirth and childbearing. According to Bergink et al. (2015), a classification of postpartum psychosis, if it is the first episode, as a distinct gender-specific diagnostic entity would be advantageous for women and for research purposes. Hopefully, the inclusion of postpartum psychosis in future editions of the DSM can be justified and implemented (Spinelli, 2021).

Etiology of Postpartum Psychosis and the Role of Contributing Factors

In terms of the etiology of postpartum psychosis, various underlying or contributing factors have already been presented and discussed in the literature and, consequently, these will only be detailed briefly here (e.g., please see Sit et al., 2006; Robertson Blackmore et al., 2016; Meltzer-Brody et al., 2018; Perry et al., 2021; Sharma et al., 2022). Although the mechanisms remain poorly understood (Sharma et al., 2022), it is now thought that a complex interaction of biological, psychological, and social factors contribute to the etiology of postpartum psychosis (e.g., Perry et al., 2021; Davies, 2017; Aas et al., 2020).

Perry et al. (2021) reviewed the possible contribution of a) obstetric factors, b) psychological and social stressors, c) sensitivity to hormone changes in relation to labor, d) sleep and circadian rhythm disruptions, e) immunological factors, and f) genetic factors. Primiparity appears to be the most reliable obstetric factor associated with the onset of postpartum psychosis (Kendell et al., 1981; Munk-Olsen et al., 2014; Di Florio et al., 2014), with the nature of this association possibly explained by significant biological and/or psychosocial changes associated with pregnancy and childbirth. Interestingly, no consistent associations were noted between postpartum psychosis and psychological/social factors (e.g., adverse life events in pregnancy or the year prior to delivery, nor those occurring during childhood). Perry et al. (2021) noticed more compelling evidence for the role of hormonal factors, including estrogen and progesterone, but they also raised the possibility that there are interactions with other reproductive hormones and neurotransmitters (see Perry et al., 2021, for more details). As few studies have investigated sleep loss and the onset of postpartum psychosis, with the findings so far appearing rather inconclusive. Evidence for the role of immunological factors is more promising, with Perry et al. (2021) drawing in part on circumstantial evidence. A strong link has been found between genetic factors and postpartum psychosis, with about 40% to 50% of women who experienced postpartum psychosis also reporting to have a family history of mood disorders in first- and second-degree relatives (e.g., Robertson et al, 2005; Da Silva & Johnstone, 1981; Schöpf & Rust, 1994), which is higher when compared to the general population. Although Perry et al. (2021) concluded that more research is required with much larger sample sizes to determine the link between postpartum psychosis and contributing factors, perhaps the better line of investigation would be an exploration of risk factors that are modifiable through pharmacological and/or psychological treatment with a view to preventing the onset or to reduce the severity of the episode. However, although researchers strive to investigate associations, it is important to remember that many women struggle to identify any specific factors that could have predisposed them to develop postpartum psychosis.

> Cos you think, well I must have done something to make, you know, make myself ill, 'cos why would I get ill and not somebody else, sort of thing, obviously you start thinking it's your own fault for being ill, or that you've done something, not done something, erm, that kind of thing, and I think it takes a while to realise well actually it's just, that's, it's just something that happened, that it's just unfortunate that it happened, but it's very difficult to get your head round that.
>
> *(Woman 13, cited in Forde et al., 2019, p. 417)*

Treatment and the Clinical Management of Postpartum Psychosis

As a medical and psychiatric emergency with fluctuating symptoms, women suspected to experience postpartum psychosis should be assessed by a mental health team as soon as possible, ideally within four hours (NICE, 2014/2020). Given the kaleidoscopic presentation and the potential risk to the mother and the infant, in most cases outpatient treatment is not considered to be safe (Meltzer-Brody et al., 2018). According to the U.K. NICE guidelines (2014/2020), these mothers should receive specialist assessment and treatment through a joint admission with their baby to a Mother and Baby Unit (MBU), with its multidisciplinary team of psychiatrists, psychiatric nursing staff, nursery nurses and clinical psychologists. Apart from pharmacological and psychiatric treatment (e.g., NICE, 2014/2020), MBUs typically offer a range of interventions, including psychosocial and psychological ones, targeting the mother only, the baby only, the dyad or even whole family, at least in England (e.g., Gillham & Wittkowski, 2015; Garrett et al., 2018; Wittkowski & Santos, 2017). In a review of outcomes, Gillham and Wittkowski (2015) found that admission to a MBU led to improvements in the mother's mental health, in the mother–infant relationship and in the child's development.

In the U.K., women have improved access to a MBU admission, with more MBUs being planned under the current NHS plan (2019). Although a joint admission of the mother with her baby to a psychiatric facility has widely been advocated because of its benefits (e.g., Jones & Craddock, 2007; Doucet et al., 2011; Gillham & Wittkowski, 2015; NICE, 2014/2020; NHS, 2019; Wittkowski, 2021), MBUs are not available in every country (e.g., Gillham & Wittkowski, 2015; Meltzer-Brody et al., 2018). As a consequence, other types of admissions as well as intensive home treatment options may need to be considered (Meltzer-Brody et al., 2018).

Medication also plays a major role in the treatment of women with postpartum psychosis (e.g., Doucet et al., 2011; NICE, 2014/2020), including antipsychotics, mood stabilizers, and benzodiazepines (Robertson Blackmore et al., 2016). Antipsychotics are typically the first medication prescribed to women with postpartum psychosis to address any manic and psychotic symptoms, including delusions and hallucinations. Mood stabilizers (which may include lithium) are offered to stabilize any fluctuating moods and emotions, whereas antidepressants are offered specifically to address significant symptoms of depression. Benzodiazepines may also be considered, especially if lack of sleep has been a problem. For example, Bergink et al. (2015) noted that a stepwise sequence of short-term benzodiazepines, antipsychotics, and lithium was effective in their sample of 68 patients, with a remission rate of 98.4% in the acute phase. Electroconvulsive therapy (ECT) may also be considered for women presenting with catatonic or depressed psychotic features or if they express a preference for this intervention (Bergink et al., 2016; Friedman et al., 2023).

However, the clinical management and treatment of a woman with postpartum psychosis will, in part, be dependent on her past psychiatric history, the severity of her symptoms, and her symptom profile (e.g., Sit et al., 2006; Meltzer-Brody et al., 2018). Meltzer-Brody et al. (2018) pointed out that the aim of any clinical management should be the limitation of the current episode and ideally the prevention of bipolar disorder with multiple episodes.

One aspect that needs to be carefully considered and discussed with the mother is her desire to continue breastfeeding (Sit et al., 2006; Doucet et al., 2011). Robertson Blackmore et al. (2016) noted that breastfeeding may become impossible for many mothers due to the severity of the illness, Although the potential benefits of breastfeeding should be considered alongside any possible risks to the infant, especially given the fact that all antipsychotic medications pass into breastmilk.

In their systematic review of interventions for the prevention and treatment of postpartum psychosis, Doucet et al. (2011) examined 26 studies but concluded that evidence-based recommendations could not yet be made due to the methodological limitations of the included studies and that multicenter prospective studies are required. Doucet et al.'s review focused on pharmacological treatments only, potentially because psychological treatments for perinatal mental health conditions tend to focus on postpartum depression and anxiety (Howard & Khalifeh, 2020). To date there does not appear to be a specific psychological intervention for the treatment of postpartum psychosis. Although NICE guidelines (2014/2020) refer to psychological interventions recommended for psychosis and/or bipolar disorder, without considering the perinatal context and the needs of the baby and the mother-baby attachment. If the mother has been admitted to a MBU with her baby, various psychological and psychosocial interventions might be offered, at least in England (e.g., Garrett et al., 2018; Wittkowski & Santos, 2017), but these are not necessarily specific to addressing postpartum psychosis only.

It may also be important to consider that psychological support remains in place after the mother and her baby are discharged from the MBU, partly because psychological difficulties may remain after the acute symptoms have resolved. Qualitative studies have highlighted the nonlinear nature of recovery from postpartum psychosis (e.g., see McGrath et al., 2013; Forde et al., 2019; Forde et al., 2020). Helpful interventions may include support to enhance the mother-baby relationship and their interaction and access to information as well as access to support groups (e.g., Heron et al., 2012; Plunkett et al., 2017; NHS, 2023). The NHS website on postpartum psychosis advises that talking to others can be helpful and recommends the charity Action on Postpartum Psychosis (APP). This charity in the U.K. has produced several guides covering topics such as recovery, supporting partners, planning pregnancy and parenting after postpartum psychosis. APP also offers a forum which allows women and family members to connect with other people whose lives were impacted by postpartum psychosis. Talking to other women about experiences can help normalize feelings and help with recovery as illustrated in the following quote.

> I think it's helped me not to feel like I'm alone because . . . reading things from umm, Action on Postpartum Psychosis [APP] and talking to the other women on the ward where I was, we all had different things, some people had had psychosis, and knowing I wasn't on my own umm and that I wasn't going mad and it was a real thing and . . . umm, that we would get better, definitely, definitely helped
> *(Woman 8, cited in Forde et al., 2019, p. 419).*

As postpartum psychosis can significantly impact the woman's partner, her family and friends, they may also require psychological support (e.g., COPE, 2023; NHS, 2023).

Prognosis

Despite the necessity for urgent treatment and when available an inpatient admission to a specialist psychiatric unit, with prompt treatment and intervention, the prognosis of recovery has been found to be good. Irrespective of diagnosis, an average MBU admission in the United Kingdom can last up to seven weeks (Wittkowski & Santos, 2017), but women generally recover from an acute episode of postpartum psychosis within a few weeks (Jones & Smith, 2009). Thus, the short-term prognosis is generally excellent. Burgerhout et al. (2017) noted that most women, who had been admitted to an inpatient unit, reported to have made a full recovery by nine months post-birth. For example, 88% had resumed their work and home responsibilities by that point.

However, women who experience postpartum psychosis are at an increased risk of subsequent postpartum and non-postpartum mental health episodes, including depression and anxiety (Robertson et al., 2005; Nager et al., 2013). In their review of the long-term outcomes, Gilden et al. (2020a) noted that 36% of 645 women with a first-onset postpartum psychosis had no further episodes and remained well during their longitudinal follow-up (with a mean of 16 years). Although 6.1% had a recurrence, this episode occurred after a subsequent pregnancy. Thus, 43.5% of women had an isolated postpartum psychosis, limited to the postpartum period only. The remaining women had at least one subsequent experience of mental illness. Gilden et al. (2020a) also noted that in their review, only 35% of women reported a subsequent pregnancy and of those 27% had a severe postpartum recurrence. This percentage is comparable to the 29% reported by Wesseloo et al. (2016). Although Gilden et al.'s review and meta-analysis identified only six relevant studies for inclusion, their findings were similar to other reported rates in the literature. For example, in a prospective longitudinal study, Rommel et al. (2021) examined the long-term outcomes of 106 women with postpartum psychosis over a four-year period. Seventy-two women (67.9%) did not experience a recurrence, whereas 34 women (32.1%) had at least one episode outside of the postpartum period. Of those 34 women, 14 experienced an episode of (hypo) mania, 11 had an episode of depression/anxiety, and nine had a psychotic episode with or without an affective component. Rommel et al. (2021) noted the difference in recurrence rate in their study, when compared to Gilden et al.'s (2020a) review (i.e., 32.1% and 56.5%, respectively). They wondered if this difference was attributable to the different lengths in follow-ups and the possibility of recurrence rates increasing over time. However, they also wondered if the lower relapse rates were linked to specialist healthcare including follow-ups and continued medication use in the study setting. Interestingly, in their large prospective study, Rommel et al. (2021) did not observe length of the episode or the woman's age to be linked to higher risk of developing a more severe disorder with non-postpartum episode, unlike previous retrospective studies had (Sit et al., 2006; Terp et al., 1999; Blackmore et al., 2013).

Overall, it seems to be important to consider that there are some women for whom postpartum psychosis signals the probability of a long-term course of mental ill health, usually within the bipolar spectrum, whereas there are also some women whose postpartum psychosis was a one-off episode and strictly limited to the postpartum period (e.g., Bergink et al., 2016; Wesseloo et al., 2016; Gilden et al., 2020a, 2020b).

Postpartum Psychosis and Future Pregnancies

Although the prognosis is good for their return to their usual, often termed high, functioning within a few months, healthcare professionals are likely to advise that women should remain on their psychotropic medication for at least a year and that they should allow themselves time to recover by avoiding becoming pregnant in this timeframe. In the U.K., after an MBU admission, women would be referred to their local NHS perinatal community mental health team (NICE, 2014/2020; NHS, 2019) and advised to continue on medication, with regular contact with their care coordinator for symptom monitoring.

If women are contemplating having another child, they are advised to seek preconception counseling so that they can base their decision on all the information available to them (NICE, 2014/2020). Despite the risk of recurrence with a subsequent pregnancy as indicated earlier, healthcare professionals should include a carefully discussed cost-benefit analysis as part of their preconception counseling, if possible. For example, the NHS website on postpartum psychosis (www.nhs.uk/mental-health/conditions/post-partum-psychosis/) states the following:

> Many people who've had postpartum psychosis go on to have more children. Although there is about a 1 in 2 chance you will have another episode after a future pregnancy, you should be able to get help quickly with the right care and the risks can be reduced with appropriate interventions.

Impact of Postpartum Psychosis on Mother and Baby Bonding

Given the fact that most women recover quickly from the acute phase of postpartum psychosis with appropriate treatment and care, it stands to reason that their ability to care for their babies can be resumed relatively quickly. However, the association between postpartum psychosis and mothers' bonding with their babies has received little research attention so far (Gilden et al., 2020b). Depending on the woman's specific clinical presentation and illness severity, family members may be required to help look after the baby initially. If the woman has been admitted to a MBU, as part of her treatment plan she would be supported by MBU staff to care more and more for her baby when she begins to recover. Staff would ensure that the mother has time to strengthen the bond with her baby and to build up her confidence in caring for her baby, as illustrated in this quote:

> I think that being in the Mother and Baby Unit was a key factor because they kept us together and they encourage you, they help you with things like baby massage, they encourage you to do as much as you can for them when you're well enough, erm, yeah, I don't really know how we would have been affected if we hadn't been together.
> *(Participant 6, cited in Plunkett et al., 2016, p. 1104)*

In a prospective cohort study, Gilden et al. (2020b) compared bonding in women with postpartum psychosis ($n = 91$) with bonding in women with severe postpartum depression ($n = 64$) during their admission to a MBU in the Netherlands, in which both groups received the same types of interventions. Using the self-report *Postpartum Bonding Questionnaire* (PBQ, Brockington et al., 2001), which is a well validated and researched questionnaire (Wittkowski et al., 2020), 17.6% of women with postpartum psychosis and 57.1% of women with postpartum depression scored above the PBQ cut off score of 26 (indicative of medium to severe impaired bonding) at admission. These percentages reduced to 5.9% and 18.2%, respectively, at discharge. When the cut off score of 40 was used, 5.7% of women with postpartum psychosis and 37.5% of women with postpartum depression were thought to present with severely impaired bonding at admission, with these percentages decreasing to 1.2% and 5.5%, respectively, at discharge. Citing studies on impaired bonding in the general population, Gilden et al. (2020b) concluded that at discharge the prevalence rate of impaired bonding in women with a diagnosis of postpartum psychosis was equal to that in women from the general population.

Impairments in bonding had previously been noted in 29.4% of women with postpartum psychosis in contrast to 61.1% of women with postpartum depression (Hornstein et al., 2006). However, these differences are seen as expressions of the underlying mental health presentations. For example, depressed mothers typically express negative beliefs, feelings of inadequacy and self-doubt which are likely to influence how she evaluates her bond with her baby in a self-report questionnaire. In contrast, mothers with postpartum psychosis are likely to lack insight into their difficulties and/or experience symptoms of mania (Gilden et al., 2020b), evaluating their bond with their baby more favorably.

Encouragingly, these relatively positive findings in relation to bonding were reinforced by Hill et al.'s study (2019) of 25 mothers admitted with their babies to an Australian MBU: all mothers were discharged with their infants in their care. Furthermore, 64% of those mothers agreed to be admitted voluntarily and although all were treated with antipsychotic medication, 36% were able to continue breastfeeding. Importantly, observations indicated that all of their babies developed normally during the admission.

Despite these positive findings, further research should be conducted comparing bonding in MBU as well as outpatient settings including the use of longer follow-up studies using self-report and observer-rated measures and ideally measures of the child's psychosocial development. Ideally, these future studies should not just be restricted to mothers with postpartum psychosis either but include other perinatal mental health conditions.

The Psychological Recovery From Postpartum Psychosis—A Closer Look

As outlined earlier, the short-term prognosis of recovery from postpartum psychosis is excellent for most women, with many resuming their usual functioning within a year. Although historically research has focused on the biomedical and psychiatric management of postpartum psychosis, there has been a growing body of psychological literature exploring postpartum psychosis from an experiential perspective. Studies revealed that mothers with postpartum psychosis felt ashamed and guilty about not being able to care for or respond appropriately to their babies (Engqvist et al., 2011; Engqvist & Nilsson, 2013) and that family members struggled to understand this illness, which then impeded the woman's recovery (Glover et al., 2014).

> So, my family, have found it VERY hard to understand my illness, and, er, and, (sigh) and the impact, so for the, the sort of, er, ripple effect, if you like, that goes on after your illness and during your illness is really strong.
>
> *(Woman 10, cited in Forde et al., 2019, p. 418)*

These insights into women's lived experiences of postpartum psychosis and their recoveries allow us to understand their experiences better and hopefully this knowledge can then also inform the development of novel psychosocial and/or psychological intervention approaches and the refinement of existing ones. Existing psychological interventions for psychosis or bipolar disorder can help to inform the psychological support offered to women presenting with postpartum psychosis during an inpatient admission or even whilst being treated by a community mental health team (NICE, 2014/2020). However, they were developed and tested with adults in general and not tailored to the needs of mothers with young babies. The NHS website on postpartum psychosis (2023) recommends cognitive behavioral therapy, without providing further details as to what clinical features should be addressed specifically.

Psychological recovery is often not straightforward. By psychological recovery we mean a process that does not just focus on symptom reduction but strengthens resilience and control over problems and challenges (Jacob, 2015). In three separate, consecutive studies (McGrath et al., 2013; Plunkett et al., 2017; Forde et al., 2019), my colleagues and I explored the lived experiences of women and family members to capture this recovery process. In our first inter-view-based study, 12 women described their recovery as a complex, ongoing psychological process. Understanding their experience was an important strategy that helped them recover (McGrath et al., 2013). Our method of data analysis (i.e., constructivist grounded theory, Charmaz, 2006) deemed this sample size to be appropriate and we actively sought women with diverse onsets to explore a broad range of experiences of postpartum psychosis (inter-views took place at four months to 23 years post-birth). We developed four overarching or main themes from the interview data covering the process of recovery, their need to develop an understanding of their lived experience of postpartum psychosis to use certain strategies for recovery, with these aspects occurring within their sociocultural context.

Women's initial understanding of postpartum psychosis was rather limited, but this evolved over time. In the early and acute stages, women acknowledged that they relied on support (termed crisis management) from healthcare professions but could not yet use psychological strategies to help their own recovery. However, noticing changes in their mental health and being told about improvements by professionals or family members allowed women to feel hopeful about getting better. Their recovery process, however, included the need to accept losses (e.g., women reported feeling sad, angry and guilty about not being able to care for or bond with their baby in the early weeks) and negotiate stigma they felt and/or experienced in relation to their diagnosis. Although women often talked of quite traumatic experiences, they resolutely focused on finding something positive in their experiences, valuing qualities like empathy and patience more. They also spoke of positive changes in relationships and of their desire to help other women through similar experiences. Although initially it seemed as if the experience of postpartum psychosis was incongruent with the way that they saw themselves as women and mothers, they described that this focus on positive outcomes helped them to accept the experience and develop a narrative they were happy to share with others.

The narratives revealed that recovery was nonlinear and often ongoing: women did remain preoccupied with worry about the recurrence of postpartum psychosis and were actively trying to maintain their well-being through the use of a range of recovery strategies. Importantly, we noted that our group of women were "active agents rather than passive recipients of 'treatment'" (McGrath et al., 2013, p. 7) whose understanding of their experi-ences and recovery evolved. Women reflected on the changes, positive and negative, in their sense of selves. Using their experience positively, finding a sense of purpose, was an impor-tant part in their recovery and supported the integration of these experiences into their own narrative about what had happened to them. The existence of different recovery styles should be acknowledged here, with the use of "integration" appearing to be more adaptive and helpful compared to "sealing over" the experience (i.e., the significance of symptoms and the experience of a mental health condition is minimized) (McGlashan et al., 1977).

Although women emphasized that the support from family and friends was one of the most important factors in their recovery, they did not specifically talk about their babies (McGrath et al., 2013). This is why we conducted another study. Using thematic analysis this time (Braun & Clark, 2006, 2013), we interviewed another group of mothers (*n* = 12), whose postpartum psychosis onset ranged from six weeks to 26 years, about the specific role their baby had in their recovery (see Plunkett et al., 2017, for full details). Women's responses revealed that their baby, although central to recovery, was experienced as simul-taneously helpful *and* unhelpful. The baby could be a barrier to recovery because he or she did increase the mother's emotional distress and hindered her from accessing help and looking after herself but the baby interacting with her also reduced her emotional distress and increased her confidence as a parent.

> I thought if she goes, I'll get better. But I didn't realise actually, she needs to stay and I need to be her mum to get better, it was actually the opposite thing that ended up making it better, which comes a bit later down the line but actually being her mum and growing to love her and feeling competent and all those things that were absolutely central to me getting better.
>
> *(Participant 10, cited in Plunkett et al., 2017, p. 1102)*

In our efforts to understand the psychological aspects involved in recovering from postpartum psychosis even further, we interviewed another group of mothers ($n = 13$) but also included the experiences of partners/family members ($n = 8$) in an attempt to synthesize findings from different perspectives (see Forde et al., 2019, for full details). The qualitative data were again analyzed using thematic analysis (Braun & Clark, 2006). The nuances of our findings are illustrated in Figure 18.1. Essentially, recovery appeared to be happening in three interlinked phases

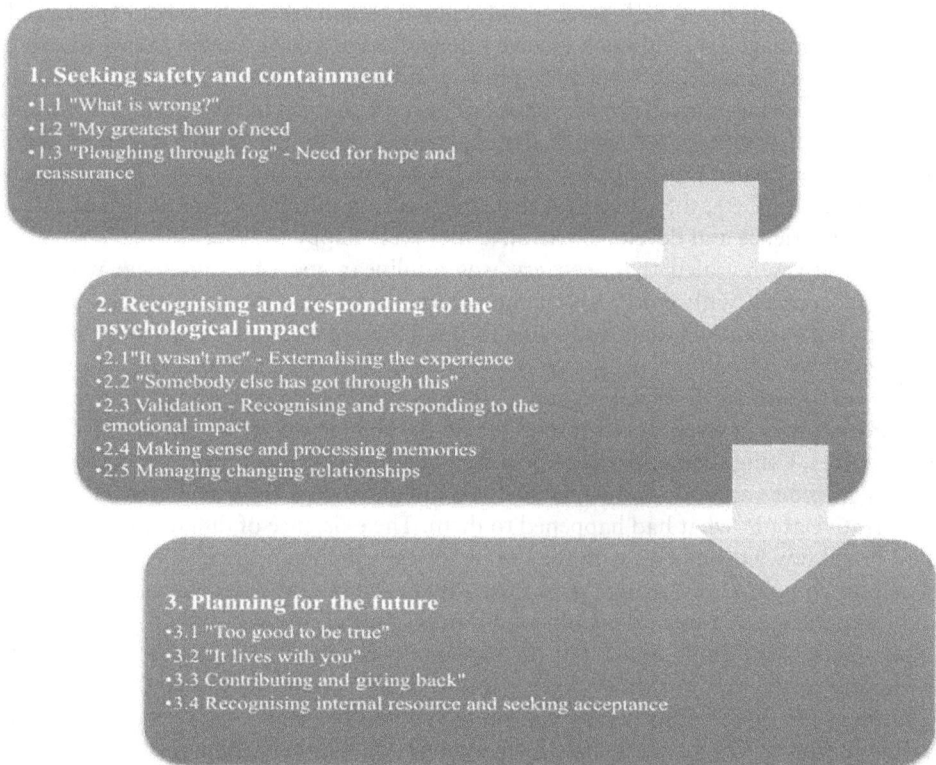

1. Seeking safety and containment
- 1.1 "What is wrong?"
- 1.2 "My greatest hour of need
- 1.3 "Ploughing through fog" - Need for hope and reassurance

2. Recognising and responding to the psychological impact
- 2.1 "It wasn't me" - Externalising the experience
- 2.2 "Somebody else has got through this"
- 2.3 Validation - Recognising and responding to the emotional impact
- 2.4 Making sense and processing memories
- 2.5 Managing changing relationships

3. Planning for the future
- 3.1 "Too good to be true"
- 3.2 "It lives with you"
- 3.3 Contributing and giving back"
- 3.4 Recognising internal resource and seeking acceptance

Figure 18.1 Recovery from postpartum psychosis from the perspective of women and family members

Source: From "Psychological interventions for managing postpartum psychosis: a qualitative analysis of women's and family members' experiences and preferences," by R. Forde, S. Peters & A. Wittkowski, 2019, *BMC Psychiatry*, 19(411), p. 7. CC BY-NC-ND.

represented as three main themes that follow a temporal order in which symptoms of postpartum psychosis reduce over time from acute and severe to mild or minimal.

The first theme or phase represents confusion (*What's wrong?* and *Ploughing through the fog*) and the need for seeking safety and containment to manage distress (*My greatest hour of need*) in order for women and family members to feel a sense of hope that recovery was possible (Forde et al., 2019).

> She was a bit like the frog climbing out of the well, she'd, you know, would climb up a bit, then slip back into the well, a bit like that, but she didn't see that, she didn't perceive that she was getting better for a long time.
>
> *(Family member 14, cited in Forde et al., 2019, p. 416)*

Once women and family members developed an understanding of what postpartum psychosis was, they could recognize and respond to its psychological impact.

> At the time, it felt that those things were really happening, that I felt that I really did experience the death of all of my family members and err . . . I wouldn't have been able to speak like this about that, you know maybe even a year ago, I don't know. Umm, err, it was hugely traumatic.
>
> *(Woman 9, cited in Forde et al., 2019, p. 419)*

This second phase is characterized by making sense of the experience and processing, sometimes emotionally painful, memories of the initial phase. During this time the women and their family are reassessing their relationships and how to interact with each other.

> Even over a long period of time that's [memory] never come back but hmm obviously from my ex describing it and from the doctors as well, because you learn about these things through other people when you're not quite with it yourself, but it was like I wasn't even there. I was kind of, it wasn't me at all. I could have killed everybody you know, in the whole town and I wouldn't have been aware of it . . . you know.
>
> *(Woman 5, cited in Forde et al., 2019, p. 418)*

The second phase seemed necessary for women and family members to engage with the process of planning for the future (i.e., the final theme). Comparable to the findings outlined by McGrath et al. (2013), there were initial worries about recovery not lasting but this was followed by acceptance and the recognition of their own personal strength. It is also possible that the lack of insight during the acute phase when women might have been quite confused adds to this concern of not recognizing a potential relapse as illustrated well by the following quote.

> One of the things that was really bothering me, was when [partner] would say things like "are you feeling ok?" if I was saying something, or you know, just look at me, really concerned, sort of, yeah just, it just made me feel, like it would always, like really shook me, because I'd be like "oh gosh, am I not ok?" because I had no, no, umm self-awareness before anyway, it made me just think "OH MY GOD, maybe something's wrong with me again" and I just can't even tell.
>
> *(Woman 11, cited in Forde et al., 2019, p. 421)*

Another finding noted previously by McGrath et al. (2013) was also emerging in the narratives analyzed by Forde et al. (2019): The desire to share their experiencing and to help others was also part of the final phase of planning for the future.

> Ye, ye, ye, and more recently I can think about it much more positively, you know, because I used to think things like, "why on earth did that happen to me?" sort of thing and now, I think of some of the. you know, it's made me very strong I think and it's also helped me to, maybe help other people going through it so I think of it, you know much more positively now.
>
> *(Woman 12, as quoted in Forde et al., 2019, p. 419)*

Although we interviewed 37 women and eight family members in total about their experiences of postpartum psychosis which happened as recently as three months ago and as long ago as 26 years across all three studies, it is important to acknowledge that qualitative research is always context-specific and findings may be less transferrable to other groups of women and their family members and to other countries and healthcare settings. However, these experiences were not restricted to these particular mothers and family members but they were universal as captured by two reviews of the qualitative literature on postpartum psychosis (see Wicks et al., 2019; Forde et al., 2020).

As part of the more recent systematic review, Forde et al. (2020) identified and reviewed 15 qualitative studies published in Sweden, the United States, Canada and the United Kingdom. We set out to include studies not published in English, but our search did not identify any for inclusion. The included 15 studies represented the voices of 103 women and 42 family members (of which 32 were partners) who drew on experiences from 3 months to 32 years ago (for details, see Forde et al., 2020). Figure 18.2 provides an overview of the review findings.

The findings from this review reflect aspects noted in the aforementioned qualitative studies, namely the initial shock and confusion characterized by the acute phase, the realization of the impact that this experience had and the process of integrating the experience of postpartum psychosis and its impact into one's existing self which could be indicative of acceptance. This systematic review summarized women's and family members' experiences in terms of experiencing "the unspeakable" (Forde et al., 2020, p. 603), highlighting loss, disruption and stigma. The process of learning to come to terms with the experience and accepting it to gain new strengths was clear in the narratives of these included studies, as was the temporal aspect to their recovery even if recovery was not experienced as linear. In addition, women reflected on the crucial role of other people in allowing them to undergo this process, including the support offered by healthcare staff and family members, even the baby, during treatment. However, the narratives synthesized in this review also highlighted a lack of awareness shown by healthcare professionals as well as friends and family.

Forde et al. (2020) considered what psychological needs there were for the women with postpartum psychosis, their family members but also for healthcare professionals who are trying to support these families. Their recommendations are outlined in Table 18.1.

A conceptual model of the psychological recovery from postpartum psychosis was developed based on the findings from these qualitative studies (McGrath et al., 2013; Plunkett et al., 2017; Forde et al., 2019) alongside related reviews of the literature (e.g., McGrath et al., 2013; Plunkett et al., 2016; Plunkett et al., 2017; Forde et al., 2019; Wicks et al., 2019). Figure 18.3 shows that the woman's wider psychosocial context, including her relationships

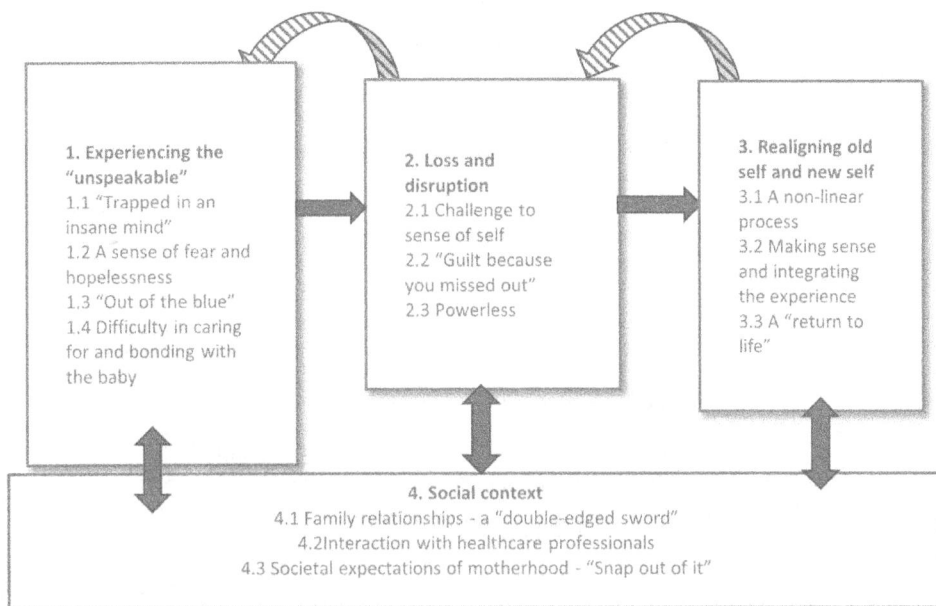

Figure 18.2 A conceptual model of recovery from postpartum psychosis drawing on women's and family members' views

Source: From "Recovery from postpartum psychosis: a systematic review and metasynthesis of women's and families' experiences," by R. Forde, S. Peters & A. Wittkowski, 2020, *Archives of Women's Mental Health, 23,* p. 603. CC BY-NC-ND.

Table 18.1 Suggested Clinical Implications and Recommendations

Target group	Recommendations
Women	• Accurate information should be provided, alongside access to peer support to help normalize women's experiences
	• Women should be offered psychological and psychosocial input during the latter stages of recovery
	• Longer-term psychological needs should also be addressed, which incorporate the reported feelings of guilt, loss, and difficulties transitioning to their new perceived role
	• Practical considerations are required to enable access to psychological support; this should be flexible and consider childcare provision
	• Women/partners should be offered more proactive support when reaching decisions about future pregnancies
Partners and family	• The needs of the family should be considered and incorporated into any assessment and intervention plan
	• Family members' well-being should be monitored, and they should be signposted to appropriate support and peer networks as required
	• Family members should be informed of reputable sources to obtain accurate information
	• Families may benefit from a therapeutic space in which they can openly explore and seek to resolve any difficulties within their relationships

(Continued)

Table 18.1 (Continued)

Target group	Recommendations
Healthcare professionals	• Specialist training and support is required to develop healthcare professionals' confidence and competence meeting the needs of women experiencing PP and their family • It is important that professionals maintain a compassionate and nonjudgmental stance; to develop a therapeutic relationship which promotes optimism and hope for the future • Healthcare professionals should pay particular attention to women who do not have supportive family structures in place • Help-seeking behavior should be targeted; through provision of accurate information (e.g., during prenatal classes) and by improving public awareness of PP

Source: From "Recovery from postpartum psychosis: a systematic review and metasynthesis of women's and families' experiences," by R. Forde, S. Peters & A. Wittkowski, 2020, *Archives of Women's Mental Health*, 23, p. 603. CC BY-NC-ND)

with her partner, family members and her baby, need to be considered. Women generally recover successfully over time, as they navigate four main phases: Once women can understand that they experienced an acute episode of postpartum psychosis, characterized by confusion and possibly unawareness that they were ill (Phase 1), they can begin to accept that they have been extremely unwell, but that this experience was beyond their control (Phase 2). Recognition and acceptance allow women, and their family members, to seek and accept personal and professional support, which also helps them to recognize that they are recovering and bonding with their babies (Phase 3). Women then realize that recovery is a process, but one they can master with less reliance on others (Phase 4).

Figure 18.3 summarizes how women move on from a sense of shock toward help-seeking and coping to regain a sense of self and their self-confidence, while their symptoms reduce in severity. The need for support by healthcare professionals decreases over time, whilst partner and family support and self-management increases. In addition, the bond with their baby is strengthened over time. This proposed model may assist family members and healthcare professionals alike on how and when to support these women and women, in turn, may retain a sense of hope that recovery remains obtainable.

Thankfully, Action on Postpartum Psychosis produced a very useful guide for mothers on recovery (APP, 2023b), which largely addresses the findings outlined earlier. The guide consists of three main sections covering (a) the first couple of months after diagnosis, (b) rebuilding confidence in the first six months to a year, and (c) living life to the full after postpartum psychosis. Both the NHS postpartum psychosis website (www.nhs.uk/mental-health/conditions/post-partum-psychosis/) and the Postpartum Psychosis International website (www.postpartum.net/learn-more/postpartum-psychosis/) recommend this guide for further information alongside a range of other resources.

As the importance of particularly male partners in supporting their partner's recovery from perinatal mental health problems and their baby's development is increasingly recognized, their experiences have also received more prominence in the literature (e.g., Ruffell et al., 2019; Holford et al., 2018) and even led to a good clinical practice guide for involving and supporting partners and other family members in specialist perinatal mental health

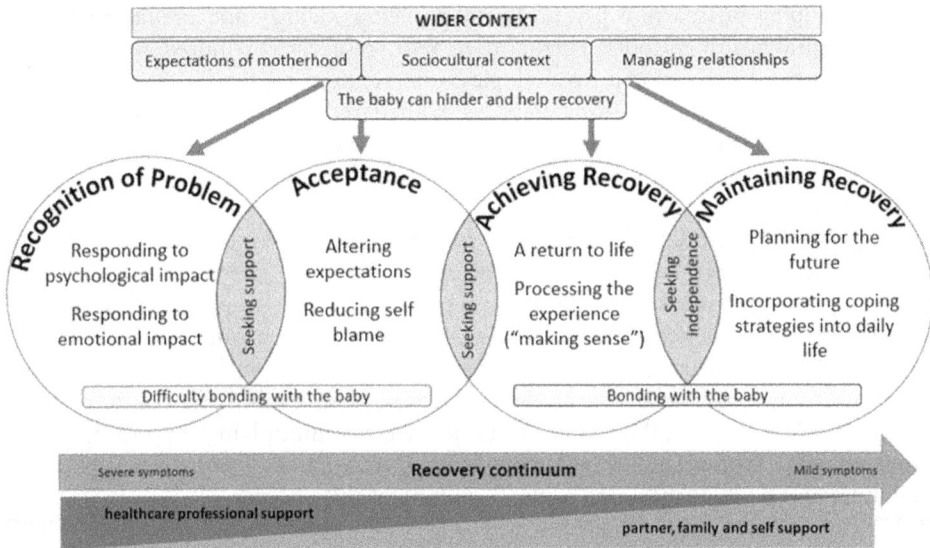

Figure 18.3   The conceptual model of the psychological process of recovery from postpartum psychosis

services in England (Darwin et al., 2021). However, a review of clinical psychological guidance for perinatal mental health by O'Brien et al. (2023) noted that the needs of partners, families and carers were only address in two recommendations outlined in five of the seven included guidelines.

In terms of postpartum psychosis specific support for partners, the insider guide for partners by Action on Postpartum Psychosis (2023c) offers information on postpartum psychosis and its treatment as well as advising what the partner's role during admission and recovery entails. Planning for the future is also considered. Importantly, this guide also advises partners to look after their own mental health and well-being.

Overall, there are resources and information guides readily available for women, family members and healthcare professionals alike. Online and peer support are also offered by APP as well as by Postpartum Psychosis International. By raising awareness of the seriousness of postpartum psychosis and its psychological impact on the mother, her baby and her family the stigma surrounding this mental health condition can be reduced and symptoms, when emerging, can be recognized, assessed and treated quickly.

Conclusions and Future Directions

Postpartum psychosis is a rare but severe mental health condition in the context of childbirth and the postpartum period. As a medical emergency it requires prompt assessment and treatment, ideally in a specialist Mother and Baby Unit setting. Its kaleidoscopic nature and the debate about its nosology contribute to the confusing picture of what postpartum psychosis is and how it should be classified. However, accurate diagnosis and assessment are important for suicide risk assessments and treatment planning and to minimize the impact on family members as well. More research studies are required using different types of methodologies including prospective studies to better identify pregnant women at high risk of developing postpartum psychosis and to better identify and predict their risks of recurrent mental health episodes. Furthermore, more research is required in terms of developing more refined and tailored psychological interventions to, firstly, assist those women with isolated postpartum psychosis episodes in their recovery by allowing them to truly integrate (and not seal over) their sometimes traumatic experiences and regain their sense of self and to, secondly, support those women who go on to have another mental health episode or who are on the bipolar spectrum by allowing them to cope better with recurrent mental health episodes. The important roles that the baby and other family members, including their partners, play in their recovery will have to be acknowledged, with any intervention seeking to make them an integral part, whilst also supporting their well-being. Furthermore, the influence of depressive symptoms in postpartum psychosis on illness course and recovery processes warrants more research attention because depression has been identified as a particular risk factor for mothers posing more of a risk to their infant and to themselves. Finally, the advances in this area, the multiplying support options, and positive recovery stories should be acknowledged. Awareness of postpartum psychosis is raised more and more as indicated in the beginning of this chapter.

References

Aas, M., Vecchio, C., Pauls, A., Mehta, M., Williams, S., Hazelgrove, K., . . . Dazzan, P. (2020). Biological stress response in women at risk of postpartum psychosis: The role of life events and inflammation. *Psychoneuroendocrinology, 113*, 104558. https://doi.org/10.1016/j.psyneuen.2019.104558

Action on Postpartum Psychosis (APP). (2023a). *The charity for mums and families affected by postpartum psychosis.* Retrieved October, 2023, from www.app-network.org/

Action on Postpartum Psychosis (APP). (2023b). *Insider guide: Recovery after postpartum psychosis.* Retrieved October, 2023, from www.app-network.org/wp-content/uploads/2013/07/APP-Insider-Guide-Recovery.pdf

Action on Postpartum Psychosis (APP). (2023c). *Insider guide: Postpartum psychosis: A guide for partners.* Retrieved October, 2023, from www.app-network.org/wp-content/uploads/2013/12/Postpartum-Psychosis-a-Guide-for-Partners.pdf

Appleby, L., Mortensen, P. B., & Faragher, E. B. (1998). Suicide and other causes of mortality after post-partum psychiatric admission. *The British Journal of Psychiatry, 173*, 209–211. https://doi.org/10.1192/bjp.173.3.209

Beraud, V., Burgerhout, K. M., Koorengevel, K. M., Kamperman, A. M., Hoogendijk, W. J., Lambregtse-van den Berg, M. P., & Kushner, S. A. (2015). Treatment of psychosis and mania in the postpartum period. *American Journal of Psychiatry, 172*(2), 115–123. https://doi.org/10.1176/appi.ajp.2014.13121652

Berginkeck, V., Rasgon, N., & Wisner, K. L. (2016). Postpartum psychosis: Madness, mania, and melancholia in motherhood. *American Journal of Psychiatry, 173*(12), 1179–1188. https://doi.org/10.1176/appi.ajp.2016.16040454

Berrisford, G., Lambert, A., & Heron, J. (2015). Understanding postpartum psychosis. *Community Practitioner, 88*(5), 22–24.

Blackmore, E. R., Rubinow, D. R., O'Connor, T. G., Liu, X., Tang, W., Craddock, N., & Jones, I. (2013). Reproductive outcomes and risk of subsequent illness in women diagnosed with postpartum psychosis. *Bipolar Disorders, 15*(4), 394–404. https://doi.org/10.1111/bdi.12071

Braun, V., & Clarke, V. (2006). Using thematic analysis in psychology. *Qualitative Research in Psychology, 3*(2), 77–101. https://doi.org/10.1191/1478088706qp063oa

Braun, V., & Clarke, V. (2013). *Successful qualitative research: A practical guide for beginners.* Sage.

Brockington, I. F. (1996). *Puerperal psychosis: Motherhood and mental health.* Oxford University Press.

Brockington, I. F. (2014). *What is worth knowing about "puerperal psychosis".* Eyry Press.

Brockington, I. F. (2017). Suicide and filicide in postpartum psychosis. *Archives of Women's Mental Health, 20*, 63–69. https://doi.org/10.1007/s00737-016-0675-8

Brockington, I. F., Cernik, K. F., Schofield, E. M., Downing, A. R., Francis, A. F., & Keelan, C. (1981). Puerperal psychosis: Phenomena and diagnosis. *Archives of General Psychiatry, 38*(7), 829–833. https://doi.org/10.1001/archpsyc.1981.01780320109013

Brockington, I. F., Oates, J., George, S., Turner, D., Vostanis, P., Sullivan, M., . . . Murdoch, C. (2001). A screening questionnaire for mother-infant bonding disorders. *Archives of Women's Mental Health, 3*, 133–140. https://doi.org/10.1007/s007370170010

Burgerhout, K. M., Kamperman, A. M., Roza, S. J., Lambregtse-Van den Berg, M. P., Koorengevel, K. M., Hoogendijk, W. J., . . . Bergink, V. (2017). Functional recovery after postpartum psychosis: A prospective longitudinal study. *The Journal of Clinical Psychiatry, 78*(1), 7510. https://doi.org/10.4088/jcp.15m10204

Burrell, R. (Director), Burrell, R., Carter, G., Gourlay, B., Merkin, J., & Wilson, R. (Producers). (2019, May 23). *My baby, psychosis and me* [TV Documentary]. United Kingdom, Matchlight & Sprout Pictures.

Casebow, M. (Director), Barrow, F., Dale, P., Fellows, A., Loach, E., Podmore, S., . . . Theroux, L. (Producers). (2019 May 12). *Mothers on the edge* (Louis Theroux Specials) [TV Documentary]. United Kingdom, BBC Studios.

Centre of Perinatal Excellence (COPE). (2023). *Effective mental health care in the perinatal period: Australian clinical practice guideline.* www.cope.org.au/health-professionals/health-professionals-3/review-of-new-perinatal-mental-health-guidelines/

Chandra, P. S., Bhargavaraman, R. P., Raghunandan, V. N. G. P., & Shaligram, D. (2006). Delusions related to infant and their association with mother – Infant interactions in postpartum psychotic disorders. *Archives of Women's Mental Health, 9*, 285–288. https://doi.org/10.1007/s00737-006-0147-7

Charmaz, K. (2006). *Constructing grounded theory: A practical guide through qualitative analysis.* Sage publications.

Confidential Enquiries into Maternal Deaths [CEMD]. (2001). *Why mothers die 1997–1999.* Royal College of Obstetricians and Gynaecologists.

Confidential Enquiries into Maternal Deaths [CEMD]. (2004). *Why mothers die 2000–2002: The sixth report on the confidential enquiries into maternal deaths in the United Kingdom.* Royal College of Obstetricians and Gynaecologists Press.

Darwin, Z., Domoney, J., Iles, J., Bristow, F., McLeish, J., & Sethna, V. (2021). Involving and supporting partners and other family members in specialist perinatal mental health services. *Good Practice Guide.* Retrieved October, 2023, from www.england.nhs.uk/publication/involving-and-supporting-partners-and-other-family-members-in-specialist-perinatal-mental-health-services-good-practice-guide/

Da Silva, L., & Johnstone, E. C. (1981). A follow-up study of severe puerperal psychiatric illness. *The British Journal of Psychiatry, 139*(4), 346–354. https://doi.org/10.1192/bjp.139.4.346

Davies, W. (2017). Understanding the pathophysiology of postpartum psychosis: Challenges and new approaches. *World Journal of Psychiatry, 7*(2), 77. https://doi.org/10.5498%2Fwjp.v7.i2.77

Di Florio, A., Jones, L., Forty, L., Gordon-Smith, K., Blackmore, E. R., Heron, J., . . . Jones, I. (2014). Mood disorders and parity – A clue to the aetiology of the postpartum trigger. *Journal of Affective Disorders, 152*, 334–339. https://doi.org/10.1016/j.jad.2013.09.034

Di Florio, A., Yang, J. M. K., Crawford, K., Leonenko, G., Pardiñas, A. F., . . . Jones, I. (2021). Post-partum psychosis and its association with bipolar disorder in the UK: A case-control study using polygenic risk scores. *The Lancet Psychiatry, 8*(12), 1045–1052. https://doi.org/10.1016/S2215-0366(21)00253-4

Doucet, S., Jones, I., Letourneau, N., Dennis, C. L., & Blackmore, E. R. (2011). Interventions for the prevention and treatment of postpartum psychosis: A systematic review. *Archives of Women's Mental Health, 14*, 89–98. https://doi.org/10.1007/s00737-010-0199-6

Engqvist, I., Ferszt, G., Åhlin, A., & Nilsson, K. (2011). Women's experience of postpartum psychotic episodes – Analyses of narratives from the Internet. *Archives of Psychiatric Nursing, 25*(5), 376–387. https://doi.org/10.1016/j.apnu.2010.12.003

Engqvist, I., & Nilsson, K. (2013). Experiences of the first days of postpartum psychosis: An interview study with women and next of kin in Sweden. *Issues in Mental Health Nursing, 34*(2), 82–89. https://doi.org/10.3109/01612840.2012.723301

Forde, R., Peters, S., & Wittkowski, A. (2019). Psychological interventions for managing postpartum psychosis: A qualitative analysis of women's and family members' experiences and preferences. *BMC Psychiatry, 19*, 1–17. https://doi.org/10.1186/s12888-019-2378-y

Forde, R., Peters, S., & Wittkowski, A. (2020). Recovery from postpartum psychosis: A systematic review and metasynthesis of women's and families' experiences. *Archives of Women's Mental Health, 23*, 597–612. https://doi.org/10.1007/s00737-020-01025-z

Friedman, S. H., Reed, E., & Ross, N. E. (2023). Postpartum psychosis. *Current Psychiatry Reports, 25*(2), 65–72. https://doi.org/10.1007/s11920-022-01406-4

Ganjekar, S., Desai, G., & Chandra, P. S. (2013). A comparative study of psychopathology, symptom severity, and short-term outcome of postpartum and nonpostpartum mania. *Bipolar Disorders, 15*(6), 713–718. https://doi.org/10.1111/bdi.12076

Garrett, C., Turner, B., & Wittkowski, A. (2018). Psychological and psychosocial interventions for improving the mental health of women admitted to mother and baby units in the United Kingdom. *Women's Health Research, 2*(1), Women-s. https://doi.org/10.1057/whr0000009

Gilden, J., Kamperman, A. M., Munk-Olsen, T., Hoogendijk, W. J., Kushner, S. A., & Berink, V. (2020a). Long-term outcomes of postpartum psychosis: A systematic review and meta-analysis. *The Journal of Clinical Psychiatry, 81*(2), 10750. https://doi.org/10.4088/JCP.19r12906

Gilden, J., Molenaar, N. M., Smit, A. K., Rommel, A.-S., Kamperman, A. M., & Berink, V. (2020b). Mother-to-infant bonding in women with postpartum psychosis and severe postpartum depression: A clinical cohort study. *Journal of Clinical Medicine, 19*, 9(7), 291. https://doi.org/10.3390/jcm9072291

Gillham, R., & Wittkowski, A. (2015). Outcomes for women admitted to a mother and baby unit: A systematic review. *International Journal of Women's Health*, 459–476. https://doi.org/10.2147/IJWH.S69472

Glover, L., Jomeen, J., Urquhart, T., & Martin, C. R. (2014). Puerperal psychosis – A qualitative study of women's experiences. *Journal of Reproductive and Infant Psychology, 32*(3), 254–269. https://doi.org/10.1080/02646838.2014.883597

Gordon-Smith, K., Perry, A., Di Florio, A., Forty, L., Fraser, C., Dias, M. C., . . . Jones, I. (2020). Symptom profile of postpartum and non-postpartum manic episodes in bipolar I disorder: A within-subjects study. *Psychiatry Research, 284*, 112748. https://doi.org/10.1016/j.psychres.2020.112748

Heron, J., Gilbert, N., Dolman, C., Shah, S., Beare, I., Dearden, S., . . . Ives, J. (2012). Information and support needs during recovery from postpartum psychosis. *Archives of Women's Mental Health, 15*, 155–165. https://doi.org/10.1007/s00737-012-0267-1

Heron, J., McGuinness, M., Blackmore, E. R., Craddock, N., & Jones, I. (2008). Early postpartum symptoms in puerperal psychosis. *BJOG: An International Journal of Obstetrics & Gynaecology, 115*(3), 348–353. https://doi.org/10.1111/j.1471-0528.2007.01563.x

Heron, J., Robertson Blackmore, E., McGuinness, M., Craddock, N., & Jones, I. (2007). No "latent period" in the onset of bipolar affective puerperal psychosis. *Archives of Women's Mental Health, 10*, 79–81. https://doi.org/10.1007/s00737-007-0174-z

Hill, R., Law, D., Yelland, C., & Sved Williams, A. (2019). Treatment of postpartum psychosis in a mother-baby unit: Do both mother and baby benefit? *Australasian Psychiatry, 27*(2), 121–124. https://doi.org/10.1177/1039856218822

Holford, N., Channon, S., Heron, J., & Jones, I. (2018). The impact of postpartum psychosis on partners. *BMC Pregnancy and Childbirth, 18*(1), 1–10. https://doi.org/10.1186/s12884-018-2055-z

Hornstein, C., Trautmann-Villalba, P., Hohm, E., Rave, E., Wortmann-Fleischer, S., & Schwarz, M. (2006). Maternal bond and mother – Child interaction in severe postpartum psychiatric disorders: Is there a link? *Archives of Women's Mental Health, 9*, 279–284. https://doi.org/10.1007/s00737-006-0148-6

Howard, L. M., & Khalifeh, H. (2020). Perinatal mental health: A review of progress and challenges. *World Psychiatry, 19*(3), 313–327. https://doi.org/10.1002/wps.20769

Jacob, K. S. (2015). Recovery model of mental illness: A complementary approach to psychiatric care. *Indian Journal of Psychological Medicine, 37*(2), 117–119. https://doi.org/10.4103/0253-7176.155605

Johannsen, B. M. W., Larsen, J. T., Laursen, T. M., Berink, V., Meltzer-Brody, S., & Munk-Olsen, T. (2016). All-cause mortality in women with severe postpartum psychiatric disorders. *American Journal of Psychiatry, 173*(6), 635–642. https://doi.org/10.1176/appi.ajp.2015.14121510

Jones, I., & Craddock, N. (2001). Familiality of the puerperal trigger in bipolar disorder: Results of a family study. *American Journal of Psychiatry, 158*(6), 913–917. https://doi.org/10.1176/appi.ajp.158.6.913

Jones, I., & Craddock, N. (2007). Searching for the puerperal trigger: Molecular genetic studies of bipolar affective puerperal psychosis. *Psychopharmacology Bulletin, 40*(2), 115.

Jones, I., & Smith, S. (2009). Puerperal psychosis: Identifying and caring for women at risk. *Advances in Psychiatric Treatment, 15*(6), 411–418. https://doi.org/10.1192/apt.bp.107.004333

Kamperman, A. M., Veldman-Hoek, M. J., Wesseloo, R., Robertson Blackmore, E., & Bergink, V. (2017). Phenotypical characteristics of postpartum psychosis: A clinical cohort study. *Bipolar Disorders*, *19*(6), 450–457. https://doi.org/10.1111/bdi.12523

Kapfhammer, H. P., & Lange, P. (2012). Suicidal and infanticidal risks in puerperal psychosis of an early onset. *Neuropsychiatrie*, *26*, 129–138. https://doi.org/10.1007/s40211-012-0023-9

Kapfhammer, H. P., Reininghaus, E. Z., Fitz, W., & Lange, P. (2014). Clinical course of illness in women with early onset puerperal psychosis: A 12-year follow-up study. *The Journal of Clinical Psychiatry*, *75*(10), 2725. https://doi.org/10.4088/jcp.13m08769

Kendell, R. E., Chalmers, J. C., & Platz, C. (1987). Epidemiology of puerperal psychoses. *The British Journal of Psychiatry*, *150*(5), 662–673. https://doi.org/10.1192/bjp.150.5.662

Kendell, R. E., Rennie, D., Clarke, J. A., & Dean, C. (1981). The social and obstetric correlates of psychiatric admission in the puerperium. *Psychological Medicine*, *11*(2), 341–350. https://doi.org/10.1017/s0033291700052156

Kessler, R. C., Borges, G., & Walters, E. E. (1999). Prevalence of and risk factors for lifetime suicide attempts in the national comorbidity survey. *Archives of General Psychiatry*, *56*(7), 617–626. https://doi.org/10.1001/archpsyc.56.7.617

Klompenhouwer, J. L., Van Hulst, A. M., Tulen, J. H. M., Jacobs, M. L., Jacobs, B. C., & Segers, F. (1995). The clinical features of postpartum psychoses. *European Psychiatry*, *10*(7), 355–367. https://doi.org/10.1016/0924-9338(96)80337-3

Knight, M. B. K., Tuffnell, D., Shakespeare, J., Kotnis, R., Kenyon, S., Kurinczuk, J. J., & MBRRACE-UK. (2020). *Saving lives, improving mothers' care. Lessons learned to inform maternity care from the UK and Ireland confidential enquiries into maternal deaths and morbidity 2016–18*. https://www.npeu.ox.ac.uk/assets/downloads/mbrrace-uk/reports/maternal-report-2020/MBRRACE-UK_Maternal_Report_Dec_2020_v10_ONLINE_VERSION_1404.pdf

Kumar, R., Marks, M., Platz, C., & Yoshida, K. (1995). Clinical survey of a psychiatric mother and baby unit: Characteristics of 100 consecutive admissions. *Journal of Affective Disorders*, *33*(1), 11–22. https://doi.org/10.1016/0165-0327(94)00067-j

Lysell, H., Dahlin, M., Viktorin, A., Ljungberg, E., D'Onofrio, B. M., Dickman, P., & Runeson, B. (2018). Maternal suicide – Register based study of all suicides occurring after delivery in Sweden 1974–2009. *PLoS One*, *13*(1), e0190133. https://doi.org/10.1371/journal.pone.0190133

Martin, J. L., McLean, G., Cantwell, R., & Smith, D. J. (2016). Admission to psychiatric hospital in the early and late postpartum periods: Scottish national linkage study. *BMJ Open*, *6*(1), e008758. http://dx.doi.org/10.1136/bmjopen-2015-008758

McGlashan, T. H., Wadeson, H. S., Carpenter, W. T., & Levy, S. T. (1977). Art and recovery style from psychosis. *The Journal of Nervous and Mental Disease*, *164*(3), 182–190. https://doi.org/10.1097/00005053-197703000-00004

McGrath, L., Peters, S., Wieck, A., & Wittkowski, A. (2013). The process of recovery in women who experienced psychosis following childbirth. *BMC Psychiatry*, *13*, 1–10. https://doi.org/10.1186/1471-244X-13-341

Meltzer-Brody, S., Howard, L. M., Bergink, V., Vigod, S., Jones, I., Munk-Olsen, T., . . . Milgrom, J. (2018). Postpartum psychiatric disorders. *Nature Reviews Disease Primers*, *4*(1), 1–18. https://doi.org/10.1038/nrdp.2018.22

Munk-Olsen, T., Jones, I., & Laursen, T. M. (2014). Birth order and postpartum psychiatric disorders. *Bipolar Disorders*, *16*(3), 300–307. https://doi.org/10.1111/bdi.12145

Munk-Olsen, T., Laursen, T. M., Pedersen, C. B., Mors, O., & Mortensen, P. B. (2006). New parents and mental disorders: A population-based register study. *JAMA*, *296*(21), 2582–2589. https://doi.org/10.1001/jama.296.21.2582

Nager, A., Szulkin, R., Johansson, S. E., Johansson, L. M., & Sundquist, K. (2013). High lifelong relapse rate of psychiatric disorders among women with postpartum psychosis. *Nordic Journal of Psychiatry*, *67*(1), 53–58. https://doi.org/10.3109/08039488.2012.675590

National Health Service (NHS). (2019). *Mental Health Implementation Plan 2019/20–2023/24*. Retrieved December 8, 2020, from www.longtermplan.nhs.uk/wp-content/uploads/2019/07/nhs-mental-health-implementation-plan-2019-20-2023-24.pdf

National Health Service (NHS). (2023). *Postpartum psychosis*. Retrieved October, 2023, from www.nhs.uk/mental-health/conditions/post-partum-psychosis/

National Institute for Health and Care Excellence (NICE). (2014, updated in 2020). Antenatal and Postnatal Mental Health: The NICE guideline on clinical management and service guidance updated edition. [online] *National Collaborating Centre for Mental Health (NCCMH)*. www.nice.org.uk/guidance/cg192/evidence/full-guideline-pdf-4840896925

O'Brien, J., Gregg, L., & Wittkowski, A. (2023). A systematic review of clinical psychological guidance for perinatal mental health. *BMC Psychiatry*, 23, 790. https://doi.org/10.1186/s12888-023-05173-1

Perry, A., Gordon-Smith, K., Jones, L., & Jones, I. (2021). Phenomenology, epidemiology and aetiology of postpartum psychosis: A review. *Brain Sciences*, 11(1), 47. https://doi.org/10.3390/brainsci11010047

Plunkett, C., Peters, S., Wieck, A., & Wittkowski, A. (2017). A qualitative investigation in the role of the baby in recovery from postpartum psychosis. *Clinical Psychology & Psychotherapy*, 24(5), 1099–1108. https://doi.org/10.1002/cpp.2074

Plunkett, C., Peters, S., & Wittkowski, A. (2016). Mothers' experiences of recovery from postnatal mental illness: A systematic review of the qualitative literature and metasynthesis. *JSM Anxiety and Depression*, 1(4). www.jscimedcentral.com/Anxiety/anxiety-1-1019.pdf

Postpartum Support International. (2023). *Postpartum Psychosis*. Retrieved October, 2023, from www.postpartum.net/learn-more/postpartum-psychosis/

Qin, P., & Nordentoft, M. (2005). Suicide risk in relation to psychiatric hospitalization: Evidence based on longitudinal registers. *Archives of General Psychiatry*, 62(4), 427–432. https://doi.org/10.1001/archpsyc.62.4.427

Ramsauer, B., & Achtergarde, S. (2018). Mothers with acute and chronic postpartum psychoses and impact on the mother-infant interaction. *Schizophrenia Research*, 197, 45–58. https://doi.org/10.1016/j.schres.2018.02.032

Rao, W. W., Yang, Y., Ma, T. J., Zhang, Q., Ungvari, G. S., Hall, B. J., & Xiang, Y. T. (2021). Worldwide prevalence of suicide attempt in pregnant and postpartum women: A meta-analysis of observational studies. *Social Psychiatry and Psychiatric Epidemiology*, 56, 711–720. https://doi.org/10.1007/s00127-020-01975-w

Reid, H. E., Pratt, D., Edge, D., & Wittkowski, A. (2022). Maternal suicide ideation and behaviour during pregnancy and the first postpartum year: A systematic review of psychological and psychosocial risk factors. *Frontiers in Psychiatry*, 13, 349. https://doi.org/10.3389%2Ffpsyt.2022.765118

Roberts, L., Berrisford, G., Heron, J., Jones, L., Jones, I., Dolman, C., & Lane, D. A. (2018). Qualitative exploration of the effect of a television soap opera storyline on women with experience of postpartum psychosis. *British Journal of Psychiatry Open*, 4(2), 75–82.

Robertson Blackmore, E. R., Heron, J., & Jones, I. (2016). Severe psychopathology during pregnancy and the postpartum period In A. Wenzel (Ed.), *The Oxford handbook of perinatal psychology*. Oxford Library of Psychology. https://doi.org/10.1093/oxfordhb/9780199778072.013.15

Robertson, E., Jones, I., Haque, S., Holder, R., & Craddock, N. (2005). Risk of puerperal and non-puerperal recurrence of illness following bipolar affective puerperal (post-partum) psychosis. *The British Journal of Psychiatry*, 186(3), 258–259. https://doi.org/10.1192/bjp.186.3.258

Robling, S. A., Paykel, E. S., Dunn, V. J., Abbott, R., & Katona, C. (2000). Long-term outcome of severe puerperal psychiatric illness: A 23-year follow-up study. *Psychological Medicine*, 30(6), 1263–1271. https://doi.org/10.1017/S0033291799003025

Rommel, A. S., Molenaar, N. M., Gilden, J., Kushner, S. A., Westerbeek, N. J., Kamperman, A. M., & Bergink, V. (2021). Long-term outcome of postpartum psychosis: A prospective clinical cohort study in 106 women. *International Journal of Bipolar Disorders*, 9(1), 31. https://doi.org/10.1186/s40345-021-00236-2

Ruffell, B., Smith, D. M., & Wittkowski, A. (2019). The experiences of male partners of women with postnatal mental health problems: A systematic review and thematic synthesis. *Journal of Child and Family Studies*, 28, 2772–2790. https://doi.org/10.1007/s10826-019-01496-4

Schöpf, J., & Rust, B. (1994). Follow-up and family study of postpartum psychoses: Part IV: Schizophreniform psychoses and brief reactive psychoses: Lack of nosological relation to schizophrenia. *European Archives of Psychiatry and Clinical Neuroscience*, 244, 141–144. https://doi.org/10.1007/BF02191889

Sharma, V., Mazmanian, D., Palagini, L., & Bramante, A. (2022). Postpartum psychosis: Revisiting the phenomenology, nosology, and treatment. *Journal of Affective Disorders Reports*, 100378. https://doi.org/10.1016/j.jadr.2022.100378

Sit, D., Rothschild, A. J., & Wisner, K. L. (2006). A review of postpartum psychosis. *Journal of Women's Health, 15*(4), 352–368. https://doi.org/10.1089/jwh.2006.15.352

Spinelli, M. (2021). Postpartum psychosis: A diagnosis for the DSMV. *Archives of Women's Mental Health*, 1–6. https://doi.org/10.1007/s00737-021-01175-8

Terp, I. M., Engholm, G., Meller, H., & Mortensed, P. B. (1999). A follow-up study of postpartum psychoses: Prognosis and risk factors for readmission. *Acta Psychiatrica Scandinavica, 100*(1), 40–46. https://doi.org/10.1111/j.1600-0447.1999.tb10912.x

Valdimarsdóttir, U., Hultman, C. M., Harlow, B., Cnattingius, S., & Sparén, P. (2009). Psychotic illness in first-time mothers with no previous psychiatric hospitalizations: A population-based study. *PLoS Medicine, 6*(2), e1000013. https://doi.org/10.1371/journal.pmed.1000013

VanderKruik, R., Barreix, M., Chou, D., Allen, T., Say, L., & Cohen, L. S. (2017). The global prevalence of postpartum psychosis: A systematic review. *BMC Psychiatry, 17*, 1–9. https://doi.org/10.1186/s12888-017-1427-7

Videbech, P., & Gouliaev, G. (1995). First admission with puerperal psychosis: 7–14 years of follow-up. *Acta Psychiatrica Scandinavica, 91*(3), 167–173. https://doi.org/10.1111/j.1600-0447.1995.tb09761.x

Wesseloo, R., Kamperman, A. M., Munk-Olsen, T., Pop, V. J., Kushner, S. A., & Bergink, V. (2016). Risk of postpartum relapse in bipolar disorder and postpartum psychosis: A systematic review and meta-analysis. *American Journal of Psychiatry, 173*(2), 117–127. https://doi.org/10.1176/appi.ajp.2015.15010124

Wicks, S., Tickle, A., & Dale-Hewitt, V. (2019). A meta-synthesis exploring the experience of postpartum psychosis. *Journal of Prenatal & Perinatal Psychology & Health, 34*(1), 3–35

Wisner, K. L., Peindl, K., & Hanusa, B. H. (1994). Symptomatology of affective and psychotic illnesses related to childbearing. *Journal of Affective Disorders, 30*(2), 77–87. https://doi.org/10.1016/0165-0327(94)90034-5

Wittkowski, A. (2021). "What is postpartum psychosis?" In P. Tomasi & J. Charlebois (Eds.), *You are not alone: An anthology of perinatal mental health stories from conception to postpartum.* Wintertickle Press.

Wittkowski, A., & Santos, N. (2017). Psychological and psychosocial interventions promoting the mother-infant interaction on mother and baby units in the United Kingdom. *JSM Anxiety and Depression, 2*(1). www.jscimedcentral.com/Anxiety/anxiety-2-1022.pdf

Wittkowski, A., Vatter, S., Muhinyi, A., Garrett, C., & Henderson, M. (2020). Measuring bonding or attachment in the parent-infant-relationship: A systematic review of parent-report assessment measures, their psychometric properties and clinical utility. *Clinical Psychology Review, 82*, 101906. https://doi.org/10.1016/j.cpr.2020.101906

PART IV

Intervention

19

SCREENING AND ASSESSMENT OF PERINATAL MENTAL HEALTH DISORDERS

Gracia Fellmeth, Siân Harrison, and Fiona Alderdice

Mental health disorders including depression, anxiety, and posttraumatic stress disorder (PTSD) are common during the perinatal period and contribute significantly to the global disease burden (Howard & Khalifeh, 2020). Left untreated, perinatal mental health disorders are associated with significant maternal morbidity and mortality including adverse pregnancy outcomes and death from suicide (Howard & Khalifeh, 2020). In addition, perinatal mental health disorders are associated with adverse infant and child outcomes: perinatal depression, in particular, has been associated with poor physical, cognitive, and emotional outcomes among infants as well as poorer mental health in later childhood (Stein et al., 2014). More severe disorders such as bipolar disorder, affective psychosis, and schizophrenia, although less common, are also associated with serious negative outcomes: without treatment, severe mental disorders can result in disruption of the bond between mothers and their infants and have long-term implications on the well-being of the woman and her baby (Jones et al., 2014). Identifying women with perinatal mental health disorders is paramount to ensuring that effective and appropriate treatment and support is offered as early as possible. Initiating treatment in a timely manner can help to prevent progression of the disorder and ensure that adverse outcomes for women and their infants are minimized.

Unlike many physical health conditions, which can be diagnosed through visible or measurable symptoms or clinical signs, the identification of mental health disorders is more challenging (Harrison & Alderdice, 2020). Ambiguities in definitions and diagnostic criteria can make it difficult to determine the point at which symptoms such as low mood and anxiety—which in their mildest form constitute part of the spectrum of "normal" mood—become sufficiently severe or persistent to be considered a disorder (Harrison & Alderdice, 2020; O'Hara & Wisner, 2014). Diagnostic classification systems list criteria based on the frequency, severity, and impact of symptoms, which can help to establish when a mental health disorder is present. However, in practice, boundaries between wellness and ill health are not always easily defined and conceptual challenges remain. During pregnancy and the postpartum period in particular, worries and fears about the pregnancy and birth, feelings of irritability as well as physical symptoms of fatigue, and a change in appetite are all common. It can be difficult to disentangle which of these symptoms are normal manifestations of the perinatal period and which might be indicative of mental ill health (Alderdice, 2020).

DOI: 10.4324/9781003206903-24

Additional challenges around the identification of mental health disorders relate to the disclosure and recognition of symptoms. Women may not recognize symptoms of mental health disorders as being significant, considering them to be a normal part of the adjustment to pregnancy and motherhood. High levels of persisting stigma around mental illness across many societies and cultures make it more difficult to disclose symptoms. Women experiencing poor mental health may feel uncomfortable or reluctant to talk about their symptoms, and this may negatively affect their willingness to seek help (Daehn et al., 2022; Fonseca et al., 2018). In studies of perinatal women with mental health disorders in the United Kingdom, participants have reported being afraid to mention their symptoms to healthcare professionals for fear of being perceived as inadequate and worry that their baby could be taken away from them into care (Button et al., 2017; Sambrook Smith et al., 2019). Underdetection may also be driven by a lack of expertise around mental health disorders among healthcare staff, often as a result of inadequate training in mental health. As well as leading to symptoms of mental health disorders going unrecognized or being misattributed to other causes, a lack of training can affect healthcare professionals' confidence in enquiring about symptoms as they would not know what support to offer or what steps to take if a mental health disorder were identified (Sambrook Smith et al., 2019).

Screening for Perinatal Mental Health Disorders

One way of overcoming these challenges in identifying women with perinatal mental health disorders is to routinely ask perinatal women whether they have experienced symptoms that may be indicative of a mental health disorder—a process commonly referred to as screening. Though definitions vary, *screening* generally refers to a test or clinical examination offered to healthy or asymptomatic individuals with the aim of detecting a risk factor for or precursor to the condition of interest (Speechley et al., 2017). The underlying assumption of screening is that early detection can be followed by an intervention, which will lead to an improved health outcome for the individual and reduce the harm caused by a disorder or its complications (Lewis et al., 2014; Speechley et al., 2017). In the context of perinatal mental health, screening involves systematically administering a set of questions to women attending routine prenatal or postpartum appointments. Screening can be universally applied to all perinatal women attending care or targeted to those considered to be at high risk of mental health disorders.

The types of tests that are used to assess an individual's mental health status fall broadly into two categories: diagnostic clinical interviews and standardized self-report measures. *Diagnostic clinical interviews* are the "gold standard" test for mental health disorders. They are conducted by a trained health professional who assesses for the presence or absence of a condition (Trevethan, 2017). Diagnostic clinical interviews follow a structured or semi-structured format and provide in-depth information which, combined with the health professional's clinical judgment, allows a diagnosis to be reached. Commonly used diagnostic clinical interviews include the *Structured Clinical Interview for the Diagnosis of DSM-5 Disorders* (SCID) (First et al., 2016), the *Mini International Neuropsychiatric Interview* (MINI) (Sheehan et al., 1998) and the *World Mental Health Composite International Diagnostic Interview* (WMH-CIDI) (World Health Organization (WHO), 1994). These clinical interviews rely on diagnostic criteria, such as the *Diagnostic and Statistical Manual of Mental Disorders* (DSM), currently in its fifth edition, or the *International Classification of Diseases* (ICD), currently in its eleventh edition (American Psychiatric Association, 2013; World Health Organization (WHO), 2019).

The advantage of using diagnostic interviews is that they combine professional clinical judgment with established diagnostic criteria to derive a specific diagnosis. However, a significant drawback is the high level of expertise, training, and skills required to conduct clinical interviews, which renders them a resource-intensive means of assessing for the presence of a mental health disorder. Clinical interviews are also time-consuming to administer: typically, a comprehensive assessment takes an hour or more to complete. These extensive time and resource commitments represent important limitations with regard to screening, as they cannot easily be administered on a large scale.

The second type of test used to assess mental health status are standardized self-report measures. *Standardized self-report measures* are questionnaires, which consist of a set of questions that can be completed by respondents or administered verbally by healthcare workers. The questions relate to symptoms that are indicative or typical for a particular mental health disorder and assess the frequency with which these symptoms are experienced by the respondent. Importantly, standardized measures do not provide a diagnosis; instead, they indicate the presence or absence of symptoms which *may* be indicative of a disorder (Lewis et al., 2014). Responses to the questions are scored using pre-defined criteria, and those who score above an agreed threshold or cutoff are considered to be at elevated risk of the disorder. Further assessment, usually in the form of a diagnostic clinical interview, is required for individuals who score above the cutoff to confirm the presence or absence of the disorder.

Standardized self-report measures have a number of advantages over diagnostic interviews. They are significantly less time-consuming: many of the more commonly used self-report measures can be completed in around ten minutes. Minimal or no training is required for their use, and they can be administered by non-healthcare professionals in non-healthcare settings. Overall, they offer an efficient means of identifying women at risk of mental health disorders. However, self-report measures also have drawbacks. Although they are a useful aid, assessment using self-report measures lacks clinical judgment, and important factors such as the course and duration of symptoms are often not considered (Harrison & Alderdice, 2020). Because they do not provide a definitive diagnosis, further confirmatory assessment is required for those who score above the cutoff and mechanisms need to be in place for this follow-up to occur. If sensitivity and specificity of a given self-report measure are poor, individuals who do not have the condition of interest may be incorrectly identified as being at risk (i.e., false positives) and individuals who have the condition of interest may be incorrectly identified as not being at risk (i.e., false negatives) (Trevethan, 2017).

Besides diagnostic clinical interviews and standardized self-report measures, there is some evidence to suggest that asking women a single, direct question about their mental health may be helpful in identifying the presence of mental health disorders. A direct question might be phrased as, "During your pregnancy, have you experienced anxiety?" or "Do you feel depressed?" (Fellmeth et al., 2022; Williams et al., 1999). Direct comparisons of postpartum women's scores on standardized self-report measures and their responses to direct questions on depression and anxiety in the United Kingdom found that despite some overlap, these two different ways of assessing for symptoms identified different groups of women (Fellmeth, Harrison, et al., 2022; Fellmeth et al., 2019). An advantage of a direct question is that it opens the possibility of a wider and more nuanced discussion around a woman's mental health status that can go beyond the more specific questions included on standardized measures. However, this more direct approach may not suit all women: for example, findings from the United Kingdom found that women from ethnic minority backgrounds were less likely to report depression and anxiety in response to the direct question compared with reporting symptoms on a standardized measure (Fellmeth, Harrison, et al., 2022; Fellmeth et al., 2019). The direct question approach also relies on women having sufficient understanding and insight to know what it means to experience anxiety or depression.

Guidance and Recommendations on Screening for Perinatal Mental Health Disorders

A number of national and professional organizations have developed guidance around screening for perinatal mental health disorders (O'Hara & Wisner, 2014). In the United Kingdom, for example, the National Institute for Health and Care Excellence (NICE) recommends asking all perinatal women two questions about symptoms of depression and two questions about symptoms of anxiety (the *Whooley* questions for depression and the two-item *Generalized Anxiety Disorder Scale*, respectively) during their first prenatal appointment and in the early postpartum period (National Institute for Health and Care Excellence (NICE), 2014; Whooley et al., 1997). Those women with positive responses require further, more detailed assessment. In the United States, the American College of Obstetricians and Gynecologists recommends that women are screened at least once during the perinatal period for depression and anxiety symptoms using a standardized, validated tool, with follow-up for diagnosis and treatment for those women who screen positive (American College of Obstetricians and Gynecologists, 2018). In Australia, the National Health and Medical Research Council recommends screening for depression and anxiety as early as possible during pregnancy and again in later pregnancy using the *Edinburgh Postnatal Depression Scale* (EPDS) (Australian Government: Department of Health and Aged Care, 2018; Cox et al., 1987). However, in most settings, these are recommendations for practice rather than requirements, and there may be inconsistencies across settings and across healthcare providers in the extent to which screening is administered. Notably, to date, such national-level guidance exists largely in high-income countries and examples from low- and middle-income countries remain lacking.

Validation of Standardized Self-Report Measures

Psychometric Validity

Before a standardized self-report measure is used in a given context, it should undergo psychometric evaluation and validation within the local setting and target population. This is required to determine whether the measure can correctly detect symptoms of the mental health disorder of interest. Psychometric validation consists of testing the self-report measure against a "gold standard"—ideally in the form of a diagnostic clinical interview—so that the sensitivity, specificity, positive predictive value (PPV), negative predictive value (NPV), accuracy and optimal cutoff scores of the self-report measure can be calculated. Figure 19.1 and Table 19.1 summarize the key psychometric terminology and properties that should be assessed and how they are derived.

Results of the 'gold standard' diagnostic test

Results of the screening test		Condition is present	Condition is absent
	Positive	True positive (a)	False positive (b)
	Negative	False negative (c)	True negative (d)

Figure 19.1 True positives, false positives, true negatives and false negatives in screening

Table 19.1 Key Terms in Psychometric Assessment of Self-Report Measures

Term	Definition	Calculation
Sensitivity	The proportion of people with a condition who are correctly identified by a screening test as indeed having that condition	$[a/(a+c)] \times 100$
Specificity	The proportion of people without a condition who are correctly identified by a screening test as indeed not having the condition	$[d/(b+d)] \times 100$
Positive predictive value (PPV)	The probability that people with a positive screening test result indeed do have the condition of interest	$[a/(a+b)] \times 100$
Negative predictive value (NPV)	The probability that people with a negative screening test result indeed do not have the condition of interest	$[d/(c+d)] \times 100$
Accuracy	The ability of a test to correctly identify individuals with and without the condition of interest. It is the true positives and true negatives, expressed as a proportion of all individuals tested	$[a+d]/[a+b+c+d] \times 100$

The psychometric properties of a screening tool provide an important indication of how confident we can be in the information they provide (Harrison & Alderdice, 2020). A tool with high sensitivity suggests that we can be fairly confident that an individual who screens positive has clinically significant symptoms of the condition. A tool with high specificity suggests that we can be fairly confident that an individual who screens negative does not have clinically significant symptoms of the condition. Screening tools with low specificity are poor at ruling out those without the condition and are thus overly inclusive, which risks inflating prevalence estimates and overwhelming health services through a large number of unnecessary referrals for further assessment. Conversely, screening tools with low sensitivity risk missing individuals with clinically significant symptoms, thus failing to identify those in need of support (Harrison & Alderdice, 2020). In practice, a balance between sensitivity and specificity is sought, and a cutoff point is usually selected based on the point at which sensitivity and specificity are maximized (Trevethan, 2017).

Cultural and Linguistic Validity

As well as ensuring the psychometric validity of the selected measure, it is also important to assess whether it is linguistically and culturally acceptable and appropriate. The World Health Organization (WHO) has developed guidance for the translation and adaptation of instruments which outline a number of steps (WHO, 2013). First, a forward translation of the measure from the original language into the target language is conducted. This initial translation should be carried out by a health professional familiar with the subject-specific terminology and fluent in the target language. Emphasis should be on conceptual rather than literal translation and language should be simple and acceptable for a broad audience. During the second step, an expert panel of bilingual experts in the field identifies and resolves any inadequate terminology or expressions. Any disagreements are resolved through discussion and a complete translated version of the measure is agreed upon. The third step is a back-translation of the measure from the target language into the original language. This should be done by an independent translator fluent in the original language who has not seen the original version of the standardized measure. As with the forward translation, back translation should focus on conceptual and cultural equivalence rather than linguistic equivalence. Step four is the pre-testing of the measure within the target population group. The measure is administered to a group of individuals who are representative of the target population. This group will be asked to explain in their own words what they feel each of the questions is asking them. This systematic debriefing, item by item, is known as cognitive interviewing and helps to highlight any terms or expressions that are unclear or are perceived as inappropriate or not acceptable within the local context. In step five, a final version of the translated measure is established drawing upon any feedback from cognitive interviews (WHO, 2013).

The rigorous translation and culturally sensitive adaptation of self-report measures is essential not only due to linguistic differences but also because of cultural differences in the manifestations of mental health disorders and nuances in the terminology that might be used to describe symptoms of mental ill health. Without rigorous evaluation of the cultural validity of a measure in a given setting, the measure may not be assessing relevant symptoms or eliciting the most relevant information. The validity of the *Edinburgh Postnatal Depression Scale* (EPDS), for example, has been found to vary significantly according to the language of administration, the geographical and cultural setting as well as respondents' educational backgrounds and levels of literacy (Gibson et al., 2009; Ing et al., 2017). A systematic review of validation studies of the EPDS reported that applying the standard threshold of ≥13, sensitivity ranged from 34% to 100% and specificity ranged from 49% to 100% across different settings globally (Gibson et al., 2009). Differences can exist even within a single country: a systematic review of measures to identify perinatal mental disorders in India found that the sensitivity and specificity of the EPDS varied from 64.7% to 100% and 84.8% to 100%, respectively, across different regions of India (Fellmeth et al., 2021).

Self-Report Measures for Perinatal Mental Health Disorders

Multiple standardized self-report measures have been developed to facilitate the identification of mental health disorders. An umbrella review of screening tools for common mental disorders identified 72 self-report measures that have been validated in perinatal women (Sambrook Smith et al., 2022). Measures can be specific to the perinatal period or designed for the general population. Most existing self-report measures for mental health disorders were originally developed for use in the general population and have subsequently been validated in perinatal groups. Administering measures that were designed for the general population to perinatal women can be problematic because of the overlap between normal somatic manifestations of pregnancy and the postpartum period—such as a change in appetite, weight gain, fatigue or sleeplessness—and symptoms of depression (Harrison & Alderdice, 2020). Without rigorous validation of these general population measures in a perinatal sample, there is a risk of self-report measures misattributing normal symptoms of pregnancy to a mental health disorder and over-estimating the presence of a disorder (Sambrook Smith et al., 2022). More broadly, the distribution of symptoms across different population groups will also differ, as will the most appropriate cutoffs and, therefore, care needs to be taken to ensure that a general population measure remains meaningful in perinatal groups (Meades & Ayers, 2011). To address some of these challenges, a number of self-report measures have been developed specifically for use among perinatal populations. These measures tend to place more emphasis on psychological and cognitive rather than physical symptoms of mental health disorders and some include questions directly addressing concerns around the pregnancy or the infant.

In addition to some measures being developed for specific populations, some measures are developed for specific mental health disorders, such as depression or anxiety, whereas others assess more broadly for symptoms of general psychopathology. Women can experience a range of mental health disorders during the perinatal period, and symptoms can vary. Comorbidity of perinatal mental health disorders is also high: up to 50% of women with mood disorders are thought to have comorbid depression and anxiety (Meades & Ayers, 2011). More generalized measures that assess for a broader range of symptoms have the advantage of casting a wider net: they are designed to identify women with symptoms of any mental health disorder, the details of which can be explored in more depth at a subsequent diagnostic interview for anyone who screens positive. On the other hand, if measures for single conditions are used, several measures might be required to ensure that symptoms of different disorders are captured (Coates et al., 2020). However, given that depression and anxiety are the most common mental health disorders, these conditions might be prioritized meaning that only two condition-specific measures are required. Some might argue that two measures specific to depression and anxiety may be more helpful and less burdensome than longer generalized measures.

In the following section, self-report measures for mental health disorders that have been validated in perinatal populations are listed and described. This is not intended to be an exhaustive list; rather, the most commonly used measures are highlighted.

Measures of General Psychopathology and Multiple Conditions

The *Kessler Psychological Distress Scale* (K10) is a self-report measure of general psychological distress originally developed for use in population surveys in the United States (Kessler et al., 2002). It includes ten questions on symptoms of anxiety and depression experienced during the past four weeks, each scored from 1 (minimal distress) to 5 (maximal distress) with scores of ≥30 indicative of likely severe mental disorder in the general population (Andrews & Slade, 2001; Kessler et al., 2002). The K10 has been validated as a measure of anxiety disorders among perinatal women: in a study of women in early pregnancy, sensitivity and specificity ranges of the K10 were 50% to 100% and 75% to 98%, respectively (Spies et al., 2009).

The *General Health Questionnaire* (GHQ) is a measure of general psychopathology designed for use in general populations (Goldberg, 1972; Goldberg et al., 1970). The complete version consists of 60 items, each scored on a four-point scale from 0 to 3, with higher scores indicating greater likelihood of a mental disorder (Goldberg, 1972; Goldberg et al., 1970). Several shortened versions of the GHQ exist, including 12-, 28- and 30-item versions (Goldberg & Hillier, 1979). The validity of the GHQ-12, GHQ-28, and GHQ-30 has been assessed in perinatal populations, with some evidence suggesting that the GHQ-12 and modified GHQ-30 offer the best sensitivity and specificity (Meades & Ayers, 2011). However, other studies have reported poor validity of the GHQ among postpartum groups suggesting it may not be a helpful measure of mental well-being in this group (Webb et al., 2018).

The *Clinical Outcomes in Routine Evaluation* (CORE-10) is a ten-item self-report tool covering symptoms of anxiety, depression, trauma, physical problems, functioning and risk to self (Barkham et al., 2013). It is designed to support monitoring of change and outcomes to psychological therapies. It includes two items on anxiety and depression, an item each on sleep, trauma, and risk to self and three items on functioning, each scored from 0 (not at all) to 4 (most or all of the time). A validation study of the CORE-10 among pregnant women found that with a cutoff of ≥10, sensitivity and specificity were 75.2% and 67.6%, respectively (Coates et al., 2020).

The *Hospital Anxiety and Depression Scale* (HADS) consists of an *Anxiety Subscale* (HADS-A) and a *Depression Subscale* (HADS-D) and was designed for use in hospital settings (Zigmond & Snaith, 1983). Each subscale consists of seven items, each scored on a four-point scale ranging from 0 to 3. Total scores of 8 to 10 are considered suggestive of a mood disorder, and scores of ≥11 are considered to indicate a probable mood disorder (Snaith, 2003). The validity of the HADS-A as a stand-alone measure of anxiety has been assessed in perinatal samples, and a cutoff of ≥8 has been recommended to indicate possible anxiety disorder (Meades & Ayers, 2011). However, another study found that the HADS did not reliably identify anxiety and depression in early pregnancy (Jomeen & Martin, 2004). Overall, the evidence base is limited, and it is, therefore, difficult to draw conclusions about the use of this measure in pregnant and postpartum samples.

Depression

Two measures developed specifically for perinatal populations are the *Edinburgh Postnatal Depression Scale* (EPDS) (Cox et al., 1987) and the *Postpartum Depression Screening Scale* (PDSS) (Beck & Gable, 2000). The EPDS is the most commonly used self-report measure for perinatal depression globally (Sambrook Smith et al., 2022). It consists of ten items which assess the presence of cognitive and affective symptoms of depression during the past seven days (Cox et al., 1987). Each item is scored from 0 (absent) to 3 (always) to a maximum score of 30; scores of 10 or higher and 13 or higher are indicative of "possible" and "probable" depression, respectively. A cutoff of ≥13 yielded sensitivity of 86% and specificity of 78% in the original validation study of postpartum women (Cox et al., 1987). Although the most appropriate cutoffs vary depending on context, the original threshold of

≥13 remains the most commonly applied across diverse global settings (Park & Kim, 2023). The EPDS has been widely translated and is available in over 30 languages and dialects (Gibson et al., 2009; Sambrook Smith et al., 2022).

The PDSS is aimed at perinatal groups (Beck & Gable, 2000). The PDSS consists of 35 items covering feelings of anxiety and insecurity, emotional lability, guilt and shame, cognitive impairment, thoughts of self-harm, disturbances in eating and sleeping and a sense of loss of self. Women initially complete the first seven items; those scoring ≥14 on these items complete the additional 28 items to further explore symptoms and severity. Women with scores of ≥60 on the full PDSS are considered to be at risk of minor or major postpartum depression, whereas those with scores of ≥80 are considered to have current major depression. A cutoff of ≥80 yields a sensitivity of 94% and a specificity of 98% (Beck & Gable, 2000).

Other depression measures were designed for use in the general population but have been validated within perinatal groups. The *Patient Health Questionnaire* (PHQ-9) is a nine-item measure designed for use among general populations in primary care settings (Kroenke et al., 2001). Each item is scored 0 (not at all) to 3 (nearly every day), and scores of ≥10 are indicative of depressive disorder with a specificity of 88% and a sensitivity of 88% (Kroenke et al., 2001). The PHQ-9 has been validated in perinatal populations and is a commonly used measure. A two-item version of the PHQ (PHQ-2) has also been validated in general and obstetric samples and found to have similar sensitivity (83%) and specificity (92%) at a cutoff of ≥3, compared with using the full PHQ-9 (Kroenke et al., 2003). The two-item version can be used as a brief screen, with those scoring above the cutoff being asked to complete the remaining seven items. Since the original validation study, the PHQ has shown good psychometric properties across diverse global settings (Sambrook Smith et al., 2022).

The *Centre for Epidemiologic Studies Depression Scale* (CES-D) is a 20-item measure designed for the general population which asks about symptoms of restlessness, poor sleep, loss of appetite and feelings of loneliness over the past week (Radloff, 1977). Each item is scored 0 (rarely or none of the time) to 3 (most or almost all of the time) with scores ≥16 considered to indicate a higher risk of clinical depression. The CES-D has been validated in prenatal and postpartum populations (Sambrook Smith et al., 2022).

Anxiety Disorders

Two measures designed to assess for anxiety disorders specifically within perinatal populations are the *Perinatal Anxiety Screening Scale* (PASS) (Somerville et al., 2014) and the *Postpartum-Specific Anxiety Scale* (PSAS) (Fallon et al., 2016). The PASS is a 31-item self-report measure which assesses symptoms including worry, specific fears, perfectionism, trauma and social anxiety. Items are scored between 0 (not at all) and 3 (almost always) (Somerville et al., 2014). In the original validation study conducted in pregnant and postpartum women, a cutoff of ≥26 yielded the optimal sensitivity and specificity of 70% and 30%, respectively (Somerville et al., 2014). Severity scores have also been developed for the PASS: scores of 21–41 are considered to be indicative of mild to moderate anxiety, whereas scores of 42–93 are considered indicative of severe anxiety (Somerville et al., 2015).

The PSAS is a 51-item measure of postpartum anxiety which assesses the frequency of maternal and infant focused anxieties experienced by women over the last week (Fallon et al., 2016). Items relate to maternal competence, infant safety and welfare anxieties, practical infant care anxieties and psychological adjustment to motherhood. Each item is scored between 1 and 4, with higher scores indicating higher levels of anxiety. In the original validation study conducted with postpartum women, a cutoff of ≥112 yielded a sensitivity and specificity of 75% and 31%, respectively (Fallon et al., 2016). The PASS and the PSAS were developed and validated in Australia and the United Kingdom, respectively, and there are little data on the validity of these measures across other global settings (Silverwood et al., 2022).

Although the EPDS is primarily a self-report measure of depression, it includes three items that assess for symptoms of anxiety. These three items have been validated independently of the full EPDS for use as an *Anxiety Subscale* (EPDS-3A), and evidence suggests that the subscale can distinguish depression from anxiety (Jomeen & Martin, 2005; Matthey, 2008; Swalm et al., 2010). The three anxiety items are scored 0 to 3. A threshold of ≥6 has been suggested to indicate possible anxiety with a sensitivity of 66.7% and specificity of 88.2% (Matthey, 2008), though other analyses have suggested a threshold of ≥4 may be preferable (Matthey et al., 2013).

The *Generalized Anxiety Disorder Scale* (GAD-7) is designed to identify symptoms of generalized anxiety in general populations (Spitzer et al., 2006). Respondents are asked to rate the frequency with which they have experienced symptoms of anxiety over the previous two weeks. Each item is scored on a four-point *Likert Scale* from 0 (not at all) to 3 (nearly every day), with the total score ranging from 0 to 21. Scores of ≥8 are indicative of possible anxiety disorder in the general population, with sensitivity and specificity of 86% and 83%, respectively (Kroenke et al., 2007). The first two items of the GAD-7 can be administered as a two-item version (GAD-2); a cutoff of ≥3 on the two-item version is suggested to constitute a positive screen and requires further assessment using the remaining five items of the GAD-7 (Kroenke et al., 2007). There is limited evidence on the validity of the GAD-7 and GAD-2 in perinatal populations (Sambrook Smith et al., 2022). One study assessing the validity of the GAD-2 in pregnant women reported a sensitivity of 69% and a specificity of 91%, suggesting that the GAD-2 may not be helpful as a screening tool in maternity services due to the high number of false positives it generates (Nath et al., 2018). Despite this lack of evidence the GAD-2 is recommended in the United Kingdom for routine screening during the perinatal period (National Institute for Health and Care Excellence (NICE), 2014).

The *State-Trait Anxiety Inventory* (STAI) is a measure of anxiety consisting of two subscales, each with 20 items (Spielberger et al., 1970). The state subscale assesses anxiety related to a specific situation or time period, whereas the trait subscale assesses the more stable individual attribute or tendency to experience anxiety. Although it was not originally intended to be used as a screening measure, a cutoff of ≥40 is often applied to indicate clinically significant anxiety (Julian, 2011). The STAI was developed for use in general populations but has shown good validity among pregnant women, for example yielding a sensitivity of 81% and specificity of 80% at a cutoff of ≥40 in one study (Grant et al., 2008).

Posttraumatic Stress Disorder

PTSD in the perinatal period may result from birth-related trauma or other trauma. Studies on perinatal PTSD often do not differentiate between these two forms of trauma, but evidence suggests that for many women with perinatal PTSD, trauma is unrelated to childbirth (Harrison et al., 2021). Self-report measures which assess for any type of trauma, rather than those that are limited to birth-related trauma, may therefore be helpful in identifying a broader group of women with symptoms of PTSD.

There are several PTSD measures that were designed specifically for perinatal populations. One of the most commonly used is the *City Birth Trauma Scale* (Ayers et al., 2018). The measures consists of 29 items which assess birth-related PTSD according to the DSM-5 criteria which cover the stressor, symptoms of re-experiencing, avoidance, negative cognitions and mood and hyper-arousal as well as the duration of symptoms and levels of distress and impairment caused. The frequency of symptoms over the past week are scored on a scale ranging from 0 (not at all) to 3 (5 or more times), and higher scores indicate greater severity of PTSD symptoms (Ayers et al., 2018). The *City Birth Trauma Scale* has been validated across many geographical settings but to date its psychometric properties have been assessed only in Brazil (Osório et al., 2022).

There are also several self-report measures for PTSD developed for general populations that have been used in perinatal women. The *Posttraumatic Diagnostic Scale* (PDS-5) is a 24-item measure which assesses PTSD symptom severity and diagnosis using DSM-5 criteria (Foa et al., 2016). The PDS-5 includes an item on the index trauma, followed by questions about symptoms, their onset and duration and the distress caused by symptoms. Items are scored from 0 (not at all) to 4 (6 or more times a week/severe). A score of ≥28 is suggestive of a probable diagnosis of PTSD with sensitivity and specificity of 79% and 78%, respectively (Foa et al., 2016). If respondents do not report an index trauma, they are not required to complete the remaining items of the PDS. This is potentially problematic in the perinatal context, as women may not think of a difficult pregnancy or birth-related traumas as comparable to the events such as earthquakes and sexual violence which are listed as examples. Women who report no index trauma would not continue with the remainder of the PDS, and any symptoms of PTSD related to birth trauma could potentially be missed (Ayers, 2004).

Measures of Suicidality

To date, no measure exists that assesses specifically for symptoms of suicidality in perinatal groups (Dudeney et al., 2023). Instead, suicidality is usually assessed as part of a depression measure, many of which include an item or a subscale on symptoms of self-harm or suicidal thoughts. The EPDS includes an item assessing thoughts of self-harm, with response options of "never" (0), "hardly ever" (1), "sometimes" (2) and "quite often" (3) (Cox et al., 1987). Scores of either ≥1 or ≥2 have been suggested as indicative of a significant risk of suicidality, with sensitivity ranging between 37% and 77% and specificity ranging between 82% and 92% across different validation studies (Dudeney et al., 2023; Rochat et al., 2013; van Heyningen et al., 2019).

The final item of the PHQ-9 asks about suicidal ideation and thoughts of self-harm, with response options of "not at all" (0), "several days" (1), "more than half the days" (2) and "nearly every day" (3) (Kroenke et al., 2001). A score of ≥1 on this single item is considered to represent an elevated risk of suicidality, with a wide range of sensitivity from 28% to 100% and specificity from 72% to 81% reported across validation studies of perinatal populations (Dudeney et al., 2023; van Heyningen et al., 2019).

The PDSS includes a five-item suicidal thoughts subscale which assesses for symptoms of suicidal ideation and self-harm (Beck & Gable, 2000). Response options range from "strongly disagree" (1) to "strongly agree" (5) and a score of ≥1 on any of the five items is considered a positive screen. The PDSS subscale has been validated among perinatal groups with results indicating good correlations with other measures of depression; however, evidence assessing how well the subscale performs against gold standard measures of suicidality remains lacking (Dudeney et al., 2023).

None of the earlier measures are ideal for identifying women at risk of self-harm or suicide. Suicide is a significant cause of maternal mortality globally (Fuhr et al., 2014). Although depression and suicidal ideation are overlapping and often co-morbid, suicidality can occur independently and in the absence of depression; using depression measures as a proxy for suicidality therefore is likely to under-detect women at risk (Dudeney et al., 2023; Fellmeth, Nosten, et al., 2022; Garman et al., 2019). Furthermore, an analysis of maternal deaths in the United Kingdom between 2017 and 2019 found that over half of women who died by suicide in the postpartum period had not been in contact with social services (Knight et al., 2021). These findings highlight the urgent need to improve detection through appropriate screening mechanisms.

Severe Mental Disorders

Despite their importance during the perinatal period, guidance around the management of severe mental disorders in pregnancy and the postpartum period remains lacking (Jones et al., 2014). Severe mental disorders including bipolar disorder, affective psychosis, and schizophrenia often present acutely, and, therefore, their identification often relies on clinical diagnosis rather than screening. Because they occur more rarely than disorders such as depression, anxiety and PTSD, there has been less emphasis on routine screening for severe mental disorders in the perinatal period. Because bipolar disorder may present with depression symptoms, it may be picked up by self-report measures for depression and there is a risk of it being misdiagnosed as depressive disorder. Some guidelines suggest that individuals with a positive screening result for depression who exhibit signs of manic or hypomanic behavior should have a follow-up screen for bipolar disorder or undergo a diagnostic interview to differentiate between depression and bipolar disorders (Demers et al., 2023).

Several self-report measures exist for bipolar disorder and a number of these have been validated and used in perinatal populations (Chessick & Dimidjian, 2010). However, *The Highs* is the only measure developed specifically for perinatal populations (Glover et al., 1994). This measure consists of seven items which cover feelings of elation, increased activity, racing thoughts, grandiosity, distractibility, and lack of sleep. Each item is scored between 0 (no change) and 2 (a lot more than normal), and a cutoff of 8 is used to indicate the presence of possible bipolar disorder requiring further assessment (Glover et al., 1994).

Effectiveness of Screening Programs

Screening programs should be evaluated to assess their effectiveness and ensure that they are beneficial to the perinatal population. Evidence around the extent to which screening improves the detection and treatment of mental health disorders remains debated (The Lancet, 2016; Tomlinson & Rotheram-Borus, 2022). However, a recent and comprehensive meta-analysis suggests a number of indicators of effectiveness. Waqas et al. (2022) found that screening for perinatal depression and anxiety was associated with a reduction in rates of perinatal depression (odds ratio 0.55; 95% confidence interval [CI] = 0.45 to 0.66, $n = 9,009$), an improvement in anxiety symptoms (standardized mean difference –0.18;

95% CI = –0.25 to –0.12), improvements in parenting stress scores and higher levels of marital satisfaction (Waqas et al., 2022). Furthermore, screening was associated with small improvements in social emotional development among children and improved parent–child interactions, but no improvements in children's physical development (Waqas et al., 2022). Few studies have assessed adverse effects of screening programs but the small number that did reported none.

The cost-effectiveness of screening for perinatal depression and anxiety has been assessed in two studies: the first found screening to be cost-effective at an incremental cost-effectiveness ratio or US$13,000 per QALY gained, whereas the second found that the probability of cost-effectiveness was over 70% among women who underwent CBT after being identified through screening to have depression or anxiety (Morrell et al., 2009; Wilkinson et al., 2017). Importantly, this evidence stems exclusively from high-income countries and does not reflect the effectiveness or cost-effectiveness of screening programs in low- and middle-income countries. One approach that has been used effectively in low-income settings is task-sharing, whereby nonspecialists including community health workers and other health-care providers are trained to deliver screening and psychosocial interventions. This model has been successful in non-perinatal mental health treatment programs and shows promise for use in perinatal settings (Manolova et al., 2023). Studies assessing the effectiveness and efficiency of perinatal mental health screening programs in low- and middle-income settings are an urgent research priority.

Sociocultural Considerations

There are a number of other considerations besides the effectiveness and clinical outcomes of screening programs. These relate to sociocultural contextual factors, which can introduce challenges to the implementation of screening. In resource-constrained settings, where mental health services may already be over-stretched, screening diverts time and resources away from other health activities (Waqas et al., 2022). The choice of measure becomes a crucial consideration, as measures with low specificity can result in a large number of individuals who have screened positive but do not have the mental health disorder being unnecessarily referred for further evaluation, which may overwhelm health systems that are already stretched (Tomlinson & Rotheram-Borus, 2022). Additional uncertainties exist regarding the optimal timing and frequency of screening to maximize the detection of women needing support (Milgrom & Gemmill, 2014; Sambrook Smith et al., 2019). Partly as a result of these remaining uncertainties, routine screening for perinatal mental health disorders is not yet universally implemented in most parts of the world (Sambrook Smith et al., 2022).

Characteristics of the population must also be taken into consideration. Women who are at particularly high risk of experiencing mental health disorders may benefit from more regular or more frequent screening. This might include women with a pre-existing mental health disorder, women who have experienced interpersonal violence, women from migrant and refugee backgrounds, women who have had negative or traumatic birth experiences and those whose infant requires admission to neonatal intensive care (Gong et al., 2023; Stevenson et al., 2023). In addition, it is increasingly recognized that partners may experience perinatal mental disorders, and there is some evidence around screening both parents: notably, the EPDS, CES-D and *Beck Depression Inventory* have been validated to identify paternal depression in the first year postpartum (Berg et al., 2022).

Challenges in Detection

There may be additional barriers to identifying symptoms of perinatal mental disorder among certain groups. Linguistic and literacy barriers may be important for women who are not proficient in the language of country in which they are living. This might include migrant and refugee groups who have relocated to other countries, for whom it may be challenging to find the words to describe their feelings and symptoms in a language that is not their own (Ing et al., 2017). Questions from self-report measures may be difficult to understand for women who are not fluent in that language. The availability of rigorously translated measures as well as professional interpreters can help to facilitate these conversations and ensure that women are given the opportunity to express themselves in a language with which they feel comfortable. It is important to be mindful that reliance on family members or other nonprofessionals to interpret questions may create a barrier for women who do not feel comfortable or safe disclosing such personal information. Low levels of literacy can also pose a challenge, with evidence suggesting that poor mental health literacy in particular represents a major barrier to help-seeking for mental health disorders (Daehn et al., 2022). In addition to the ability to read and write in itself, cultures with a strong oral tradition may find the use of numerical response scales unfamiliar and the emphasis on quantifying frequency of symptoms (e.g., questions about how many times per week a certain symptom occurs) rather than the more qualitative impact of symptoms (e.g., how symptoms might be experienced and how they impact functioning and daily life) may be challenging. In certain contexts, it may be more appropriate to use visual scales or for self-report measures to be administered verbally to women (Downe et al., 2007; Fellmeth et al., 2018). In some cultures, open-ended questions as offered by diagnostic tests may be easier to administer than standardized measures and, paradoxically, be more efficient to use (Fellmeth et al., 2018; Ing et al., 2017).

Women's social, cultural, and ethnic backgrounds can influence the ways in which mental health disorders manifest, the ways in which symptoms are interpreted and expressed, and the ways in which women might disclose their symptoms and seek help (Sorsa et al., 2021). As discussed previously, women from certain backgrounds may prefer completing self-report measures, whereas others may prefer the option of being asked a direct question (Fellmeth, Harrison, et al., 2022). Stigmatization of mental health disorders remains prevalent across many societies and may hinder the disclosure of symptoms within certain groups more than others (Watson et al., 2019). Social desirability may also be important: within cultures where a hierarchical status is given to healthcare professionals or where there is a perceived power imbalance between the respondent and the assessor, it may be common for women to give answers which they perceive as being more acceptable. Among some groups there may be lower awareness of what constitutes a mental health disorder, leading to under-disclosure of symptoms. Self-report measures which have not undergone culturally sensitive adaptation and translation may fail to identify culturally diverse manifestations of mental health disorders (Bhat et al., 2022). Evidence suggests that in settings where screening is universally recommended, women from certain backgrounds are less likely to be asked (Harrison et al., 2023; Redshaw & Henderson, 2016). Given that women from minority groups are at greater risk of experiencing perinatal mental health disorders, it is particularly important to ensure that screening systems in place can account for cultural differences (Fellmeth et al., 2018; Gennaro et al., 2020; Nielsen-Scott et al., 2022).

Referral and Treatment Pathways

Alongside any screening programs implemented within perinatal settings, referral pathways must be in place so that women who are identified as having symptoms of a mental health disorder can be offered the appropriate follow-up. This follow-up will include establishing a definitive diagnosis, usually through a diagnostic clinical interview administered by a qualified mental health professional, as well as referral for treatment and care if the diagnosis is confirmed. Introducing perinatal mental health screening can significantly impact the burden on mental health services, which will need to conduct confirmatory assessments on all those who screen positive. Careful planning and mapping of existing services must be carried out to ensure that there is capacity to safely manage any increase in referrals and cases identified by a screening program. This is especially relevant in resource-constrained settings, where any existing mental health services may already be over-stretched. Without robust referral systems in place, screening may lead to women being identified as having symptoms of mental health disorders who can then not be offered any support or treatment. This becomes especially problematic for women who are identified as being at risk of harming themselves or others. If a women discloses active suicidal ideation or symptoms of acute psychosis or mania, it is imperative that these women can be immediately supported, effectively treated and kept safe (Waqas et al., 2022).

Women who are identified as having a mental health disorder should have access to information about what this means and their options for follow-up and treatment. Healthcare professionals involved in administering and scoring the self-report measures require training in communicating sensitively as well as in the process of the screening program, including the processes required to refer for further follow-up and any standard operating procedures for anyone found to be at immediate risk to themselves or others. Training for healthcare professional should be continuous to ensure knowledge remains up-to-date. There should also be support structures in place for staff, as well as regular opportunities for discussion and debrief. It can be emotionally taxing to hear about difficult experiences and emotional challenges women face, and it is important that staff are able to speak to supportive colleagues when needed.

Conclusion and Future Directions

Screening for perinatal mental health disorders is paramount to ensuring that effective and appropriate support and treatment is offered as early as possible to those women who need it. Diagnostic clinical interviews are the gold standard test for identifying women with perinatal mental health disorders, but these are often unfeasible for universal use in busy, resource-limited settings. Standardized self-report measures offer an alternative and efficient way of screening. Careful consideration is needed when introducing a measure to clinical practice as low sensitivity and specificity can lead to under-detection or overburdening of health services. Despite the availability of many standardized self-report measures, few have been developed specifically for or validated among perinatal populations, and even fewer are available in multiple languages. Future work should focus on the cultural validation and adaptation of self-report measures within target populations to ensure that they are acceptable to and effective within the given context. In terms of implementation of screening, efforts must be made to integrate screening programs into maternal and child health services, whilst ensuring that existing resources and health systems are not over-burdened. Alongside clear referral pathways and robust treatment systems, screening for symptoms of perinatal mental health disorders has the potential to significantly improve outcomes for women.

References

Alderdice, F. (2020). Supporting psychological well-being around the time of birth: What can we learn from maternity care? *World Psychiatry*, *19*(3), 332–333. https://doi.org/10.1002/wps.20778

American College of Obstetricians and Gynecologists. (2018). ACOG committee opinion no. 757: Screening for perinatal depression. *Obstetrics and Gynecology*, *132*(5), e208–e212. https://doi.org/10.1097/aog.0000000000002927

American Psychiatric Association. (2013). *Diagnostic and statistical manual of mental disorders* (5th ed.). American Psychiatric Association.

Andrews, G., & Slade, T. (2001). Interpreting scores on the Kessler Psychological Distress Scale (K10). *Australian and New Zealand Journal of Public Health*, *25*(6), 494–497. https://doi.org/10.1111/j.1467-842x.2001.tb00310.x

Australian Government: Department of Health and Aged Care. (2018). *Pregnancy care guidelines: Screening for depressive and anxiety disorders*. www.health.gov.au/resources/pregnancy-care-guidelines/part-e-social-and-emotional-screening/screening-for-depressive-and-anxiety-disorders#274-practice-summary-depression-and-anxiety

Ayers, S. (2004). Delivery as a traumatic event: Prevalence, risk factors, and treatment for postnatal posttraumatic stress disorder. *Clinical Obstetrics and Gynecology*, *47*(3), 552–567. https://doi.org/10.1097/01.grf.0000129919.00756.9c

Ayers, S., Wright, D. B., & Thornton, A. (2018). Development of a measure of postpartum PTSD: The City Birth Trauma Scale. *Frontiers in Psychiatry*, *9*, 409. https://doi.org/10.3389/fpsyt.2018.00409

Barkham, M., Bewick, B., Mullin, T., Gilbody, S., Connell, J., Cahill, J., . . . Evans, C. (2013). The CORE-10: A short measure of psychological distress for routine use in the psychological therapies. *Counselling and Psychotherapy Research*, *13*(1), 3–13. https://doi.org/10.1080/14733145.2012.729069

Beck, C. T., & Gable, R. K. (2000). Postpartum depression screening scale: Development and psychometric testing. *Nursing Research*, *49*(5), 272–282. https://doi.org/10.1097/00006199-200009000-00006

Berg, R. C., Solberg, B. L., Glavin, K., & Olsvold, N. (2022). Instruments to identify symptoms of paternal depression during pregnancy and the first postpartum year: A systematic scoping review. *American Journal of Men's Health*, *16*(5). https://doi.org/10.1177/15579883221114984

Bhat, A., Nanda, A., Murphy, L., Ball, A. L., Fortney, J., & Katon, J. (2022). A systematic review of screening for perinatal depression and anxiety in community-based settings. *Archives of Women's Mental Health*, *25*(1), 33–49. https://doi.org/10.1007/s00737-021-01151-2

Button, S., Thornton, A., Lee, S., Shakespeare, J., & Ayers, S. (2017). Seeking help for perinatal psychological distress: A meta-synthesis of women's experiences. *British Journal of General Practice*, *67*(663), e692–e699. https://doi.org/10.3399/bjgp17X692549

Chessick, C. A., & Dimidjian, S. (2010). Screening for bipolar disorder during pregnancy and the postpartum period. *Archives of Women's Mental Health*, *13*(3), 233–248. https://doi.org/10.1007/s00737-010-0151-9

Coates, R., Ayers, S., de Visser, R., & Thornton, A. (2020). Evaluation of the CORE-10 to assess psychological distress in pregnancy. *Journal of Reproductive and Infant Psychology*, *38*(3), 311–323. https://doi.org/10.1080/02646838.2019.1702631

Cox, J. L., Holden, J. M., & Sagovsky, R. (1987). Detection of postnatal depression: Development of the 10-item Edinburgh Postnatal Depression Scale. *British Journal of Psychiatry*, *150*, 782–786. https://doi.org/10.1192/bjp.150.6.782

Daehn, D., Rudolf, S., Pawils, S., & Renneberg, B. (2022). Perinatal mental health literacy: Knowledge, attitudes, and help-seeking among perinatal women and the public – a systematic review. *BMC Pregnancy Childbirth*, *22*(1), 574. https://doi.org/10.1186/s12884-022-04865-y

Demers, C. J., Walker, R., Rossi, N. M., & Bradford, H. M. (2023). Management of bipolar disorder during the perinatal period. *Nursing for Women's Health*, *27*(1), 42–52. https://doi.org/10.1016/j.nwh.2022.11.001

Downe, S. M., Butler, E., & Hinder, S. (2007). Screening tools for depressed mood after childbirth in UK-based South Asian women: A systematic review. *Journal of Advanced Nursing*, *57*(6), 565–583. https://doi.org/10.1111/j.1365-2648.2006.04028.x

Dudeney, E., Coates, R., Ayers, S., & McCabe, R. (2023). Measures of suicidality in perinatal women: A systematic review. *Journal of Affective Disorders*, *324*, 210–231. https://doi.org/10.1016/j.jad.2022.12.091

Fallon, V., Halford, J. C. G., Bennett, K. M., & Harrold, J. A. (2016). The postpartum specific anxiety scale: Development and preliminary validation. *Archives of Women's Mental Health*, *19*(6), 1079–1090. https://doi.org/10.1007/s00737-016-0658-9

Fellmeth, G., Harrison, S., Opondo, C., Nair, M., Kurinczuk, J. J., & Alderdice, F. (2021). Validated screening tools to identify common mental disorders in perinatal and postpartum women in India: A systematic review and meta-analysis. *BMC Psychiatry*, *21*(1), 200. https://doi.org/10.1186/s12888-021-03190-6

Fellmeth, G., Harrison, S., Quigley, M. A., & Alderdice, F. (2022). A comparison of three measures to identify postnatal anxiety: Analysis of the 2020 national maternity survey in England. *International Journal of Environmental Research and Public Health*, *19*(11). https://doi.org/10.3390/ijerph19116578

Fellmeth, G., Nosten, S., Khirikoekkong, N., Oo, M. M., Gilder, M. E., Plugge, E., . . . McGready, R. (2022). Suicidal ideation in the perinatal period: Findings from the Thailand-Myanmar border. *Journal of Public Health (Oxf)*, *44*(4), e514–e518. https://doi.org/10.1093/pubmed/fdab297

Fellmeth, G., Opondo, C., Henderson, J., Redshaw, M., McNeill, J., Lynn, F., & Alderdice, F. (2019). Identifying postnatal depression: Comparison of a self-reported depression item with Edinburgh Postnatal Depression Scale scores at three months postpartum. *Journal of Affective Disorders*, *251*, 8–14. https://doi.org/10.1016/j.jad.2019.03.002

Fellmeth, G., Plugge, E., Fazel, M., Charunwattana, P., Nosten, F., Fitzpatrick, R., . . . McGready, R. (2018). Validation of the refugee health screener-15 for the assessment of perinatal depression among Karen and Burmese women on the Thai-Myanmar border. *PLoS One*, *13*(5), e0197403. https://doi.org/10.1371/journal.pone.0197403

First, M. B., Williams, J. B. W., Karg, R. S., & Spitzer, R. L. (2016). *User's guide for the SCID-5-CV structured clinical interview for DSM-5® disorders: Clinical version*. American Psychiatric Association.

Foa, E. B., McLean, C. P., Zang, Y., Zhong, J., Powers, M. B., Kauffman, B. Y., . . . Knowles, K. (2016). Psychometric properties of the Posttraumatic Diagnostic Scale for DSM-5 (PDS-5). *Psychological Assessment*, *28*(10), 1166–1171. https://doi.org/10.1037/pas0000258

Fonseca, A., Moura-Ramos, M., & Canavarro, M. C. (2018). Attachment and mental help-seeking in the perinatal period: The role of stigma. *Community Mental Health Journal*, *54*(1), 92–101. https://doi.org/10.1007/s10597-017-0138-3

Fuhr, D. C., Calvert, C., Ronsmans, C., Chandra, P. S., Sikander, S., De Silva, M. J., & Patel, V. (2014). Contribution of suicide and injuries to pregnancy-related mortality in low-income and middle-income countries: A systematic review and meta-analysis. *The Lancet Psychiatry*, *1*(3), 213–225. https://doi.org/10.1016/s2215-0366(14)70282-2

Garman, E. C., Cois, A., Schneider, M., & Lund, C. (2019). Association between perinatal depressive symptoms and suicidal risk among low-income South African women: A longitudinal study. *Social Psychiatry and Psychiatric Epidemiology*, *54*(10), 1219–1230. https://doi.org/10.1007/s00127-019-01730-w

Gennaro, S., O'Connor, C., McKay, E. A., Gibeau, A., Aviles, M., Hoying, J., & Melnyk, B. M. (2020). Perinatal anxiety and depression in minority women. *MCN American Journal of Maternal and Child Nursing*, *45*(3), 138–144. https://doi.org/10.1097/nmc.0000000000000611

Gibson, J., McKenzie-McHarg, K., Shakespeare, J., Price, J., & Gray, R. (2009). A systematic review of studies validating the Edinburgh Postnatal Depression Scale in antepartum and postpartum women. *Acta Psychiatrica Scandinavia*, *119*(5), 350–364. https://doi.org/10.1111/j.1600-0447.2009.01363.x

Glover, V., Liddle, P., Taylor, A., Adams, D., & Sandler, M. (1994). Mild hypomania (the highs) can be a feature of the first postpartum week: Association with later depression. *British Journal of Psychiatry*, *164*(4), 517–521. https://doi.org/10.1192/bjp.164.4.517

Goldberg, D. P. (1972). *The detection of psychiatric illness by questionnaire*. Oxford University Press.

Goldberg, D. P., Cooper, B., Eastwood, M. R., Kedward, H. B., & Shepherd, M. (1970). A standardized psychiatric interview for use in community surveys. *British Journal of Preventive and Social Medicine*, *24*(1), 18–23. https://doi.org/10.1136/jech.24.1.18

Goldberg, D. P., & Hillier, V. F. (1979). A scaled version of the general health questionnaire. *Psychological Medicine*, *9*(1), 139–145. https://doi.org/10.1017/s0033291700021644

Gong, J., Fellmeth, G., Quigley, M. A., Gale, C., Stein, A., Alderdice, F., & Harrison, S. (2023). Prevalence and risk factors for postnatal mental health problems in mothers of infants admitted to neonatal care: Analysis of two population-based surveys in England. *BMC Pregnancy Childbirth*, *23*(1), 370. https://doi.org/10.1186/s12884-023-05684-5

Grant, K. A., McMahon, C., & Austin, M. P. (2008). Maternal anxiety during the transition to parenthood: A prospective study. *Journal of Affective Disorders*, *108*(1–2), 101–111. https://doi.org/10.1016/j.jad.2007.10.002

Harrison, S., & Alderdice, F. (2020). Challenges of defining and measuring perinatal anxiety. *Journal of Reproductive and Infant Psychology*, *38*(1), 1–2. https://doi.org/10.1080/02646838.2020.1703526

Harrison, S., Ayers, S., Quigley, M. A., Stein, A., & Alderdice, F. (2021). Prevalence and factors associated with postpartum posttraumatic stress in a population-based maternity survey in England. *Journal of Affective Disorders*, *279*, 749–756. https://doi.org/10.1016/j.jad.2020.11.102

Harrison, S., Pilkington, V., Li, Y., Quigley, M. A., & Alderdice, F. (2023). Disparities in who is asked about their perinatal mental health: An analysis of cross-sectional data from consecutive national maternity surveys. *BMC Pregnancy Childbirth*, *23*(1), 263. https://doi.org/10.1186/s12884-023-05518-4

Howard, L. M., & Khalifeh, H. (2020). Perinatal mental health: A review of progress and challenges. *World Psychiatry*, *19*(3), 313–327. https://doi.org/10.1002/wps.20769

Ing, H., Fellmeth, G., White, J., Stein, A., Simpson, J. A., & McGready, R. (2017). Validation of the Edinburgh Postnatal Depression Scale (EPDS) on the Thai-Myanmar border. *Tropical Doctor*, *47*(4), 339–347. https://doi.org/10.1177/0049475517717635

Jomeen, J., & Martin, C. R. (2004). Is the hospital anxiety and depression scale (HADS) a reliable screening tool in early pregnancy? *Psychology & Health*, *19*(6), 787–800. https://doi.org/10.1080/0887044042000272895

Jomeen, J., & Martin, C. R. (2005). Confirmation of an occluded anxiety component within the Edinburgh Postnatal Depression Scale (EPDS) during early pregnancy. *Journal of Reproductive and Infant Psychology*, *23*(2), 143–154. https://doi.org/10.1080/02646830500129297

Jones, I., Chandra, P. S., Dazzan, P., & Howard, L. M. (2014). Bipolar disorder, affective psychosis, and schizophrenia in pregnancy and the post-partum period. *The Lancet*, *384*(9956), 1789–1799. https://doi.org/10.1016/s0140-6736(14)61278-2

Julian, L. J. (2011). Measures of anxiety: State-Trait Anxiety Inventory (STAI), Beck Anxiety Inventory (BAI), and Hospital Anxiety and Depression Scale-Anxiety (HADS-A). *Arthritis Care Research (Hoboken)*, *63*(Suppl 11, 11), S467–S472. https://doi.org/10.1002/acr.20561

Kessler, R. C., Andrews, G., Colpe, L. J., Hiripi, E., Mroczek, D. K., Normand, S. L., . . . Zaslavsky, A. M. (2002). Short screening scales to monitor population prevalences and trends in non-specific psychological distress. *Psychological Medicine*, *32*(6), 959–976. https://doi.org/10.1017/s0033291702006074

Knight, M., Bunch, K., Tuffnell, D., Patel, R., Shakespeare, J., Kotnis, R., . . . on behalf of MBRRACE-UK. (2021). *Saving lives, improving mothers' care – Lessons learned to inform maternity care from the UK and Ireland confidential enquiries into maternal deaths and morbidity 2017–19*. National Perinatal Epidemiology Unit, University of Oxford. https://www.npeu.ox.ac.uk/assets/downloads/mbrrace-uk/reports/maternal-report-2021/MBRRACE-UK_Maternal_Report_2021_-_FINAL_-_WEB_VERSION.pdf

Kroenke, K., Spitzer, R. L., & Williams, J. B. (2001). The PHQ-9: Validity of a brief depression severity measure. *Journal of General Internal Medicine*, *16*(9), 606–613. https://doi.org/10.1046/j.1525-1497.2001.016009606.x

Kroenke, K., Spitzer, R. L., & Williams, J. B. (2003). The patient health questionnaire-2: Validity of a two-item depression screener. *Medical Care*, *41*(11), 1284–1292. https://doi.org/10.1097/01.Mlr.0000093487.78664.3c

Kroenke, K., Spitzer, R. L., Williams, J. B., Monahan, P. O., & Löwe, B. (2007). Anxiety disorders in primary care: Prevalence, impairment, comorbidity, and detection. *Annals of Internal Medicine*, *146*(5), 317–325. https://doi.org/10.7326/0003-4819-146-5-200703060-00004

The Lancet. (2016). Screening for perinatal depression: A missed opportunity. *The Lancet*, *387*(10018), 505. https://doi.org/10.1016/s0140-6736(16)00265-8

Lewis, G., Sheringham, J., Lopez Bernal, J., & Crawford, T. (2014). *Mastering public health: A postgraduate guide to examinations and revalidation* (2nd ed.). CRC Press.

Manolova, G., Waqas, A., Chowdhary, N., Salisbury, T. T., & Dua, T. (2023). Integrating perinatal mental healthcare into maternal and perinatal services in low and middle income countries. *British Medicine Journal, 381*, e073343. https://doi.org/10.1136/bmj-2022-073343

Matthey, S. (2008). Using the Edinburgh Postnatal Depression Scale to screen for anxiety disorders. *Depression and Anxiety, 25*(11), 926–931. https://doi.org/10.1002/da.20415

Matthey, S., Fisher, J., & Rowe, H. (2013). Using the Edinburgh Postnatal Depression Scale to screen for anxiety disorders: Conceptual and methodological considerations. *Journal of Affective Disorders, 146*(2), 224–230. https://doi.org/10.1016/j.jad.2012.09.009

Meades, R., & Ayers, S. (2011). Anxiety measures validated in perinatal populations: A systematic review. *Journal of Affective Disorders, 133*(1–2), 1–15. https://doi.org/10.1016/j.jad.2010.10.009

Milgrom, J., & Gemmill, A. (2014). Screening for perinatal depression. *Best Practice & Research Clinical Obstetrics & Gynaecology, 28*(1), 13–23.

Morrell, C. J., Warner, R., Slade, P., Dixon, S., Walters, S., Paley, G., & Brugha, T. (2009). Psychological interventions for postnatal depression: Cluster randomised trial and economic evaluation: The PoNDER trial. *Health Technology Assessment, 13*(30), iii–iv, xi–xiii, 1–153. https://doi.org/10.3310/hta13300

Nath, S., Ryan, E. G., Trevillion, K., Bick, D., Demilew, J., Milgrom, J., . . . Howard, L. M. (2018). Prevalence and identification of anxiety disorders in pregnancy: The diagnostic accuracy of the two-item Generalised Anxiety Disorder scale (GAD-2). *BMJ Open, 8*(9), e023766. https://doi.org/10.1136/bmjopen-2018-023766

National Institute for Health and Care Excellence (NICE). (2014). *Antenatal and postnatal mental health: Clinical management and service guidance (CG192)*. NICE.

Nielsen-Scott, M., Fellmeth, G., Opondo, C., & Alderdice, F. (2022). Prevalence of perinatal anxiety in low- and middle-income countries: A systematic review and meta-analysis. *Journal of Affective Disorders, 306*, 71–79. https://doi.org/10.1016/j.jad.2022.03.032

O'Hara, M. W., & Wisner, K. L. (2014). Perinatal mental illness: Definition, description and aetiology. *Best Practice and Research in Clinical Obstetrics and Gynaecology, 28*(1), 3–12. https://doi.org/10.1016/j.bpobgyn.2013.09.002

Osório, F. L., Rossini Darwin, A. C., Bombonetti, E. A., & Ayers, S. (2022). Posttraumatic stress following childbirth: Psychometric properties of the Brazilian version of the City Birth Trauma Scale. *Journal of Psychosomatic Obstetrics and Gynaecology, 43*(3), 374–383. https://doi.org/10.1080/0167482x.2021.1977278

Park, S. H., & Kim, J. I. (2023). Predictive validity of the Edinburgh Postnatal Depression Scale and other tools for screening depression in pregnant and postpartum women: A systematic review and meta-analysis. *Archives of Gynecology and Obstetrics, 307*(5), 1331–1345. https://doi.org/10.1007/s00404-022-06525-0

Radloff, L. S. (1977). The CES-D scale: A self-report depression scale for research in the general population. *Applied Psychological Measurement, 1*(3), 385–401. https://doi.org/10.1177/014662167700100306

Redshaw, M., & Henderson, J. (2016). Who is actually asked about their mental health in pregnancy and the postnatal period? Findings from a national survey. *BMC Psychiatry, 16*(1), 322. https://doi.org/10.1186/s12888-016-1029-9

Rochat, J., Bland, R. M., Tomlinson, M., & Stein, A. (2013). Suicide ideation, depression and HIV among pregnant women in rural South Africa. *Health, 5*(3A), 650–661.

Sambrook Smith, M., Cairns, L., Pullen, L. S. W., Opondo, C., Fellmeth, G., & Alderdice, F. (2022). Validated tools to identify common mental disorders in the perinatal period: A systematic review of systematic reviews. *Journal of Affective Disorders, 298*(Pt A), 634–643. https://doi.org/10.1016/j.jad.2021.11.011

Sambrook Smith, M., Lawrence, V., Sadler, E., & Easter, A. (2019). Barriers to accessing mental health services for women with perinatal mental illness: Systematic review and meta-synthesis of qualitative studies in the UK. *BMJ Open, 9*(1), e024803. https://doi.org/10.1136/bmjopen-2018-024803

Sheehan, D. V., Lecrubier, Y., Sheehan, K. H., Amorim, P., Janavs, J., Weiller, E., . . . Dunbar, G. C. (1998). The Mini-International Neuropsychiatric Interview (M.I.N.I.): The development and validation of a structured diagnostic psychiatric interview for DSM-IV and ICD-10. *Journal of Clinical Psychiatry, 59*(Suppl 20), 22–33; quiz 34–57.

Silverwood, V. A., Bullock, L., Turner, K., Chew-Graham, C. A., & Kingstone, T. (2022). The approach to managing perinatal anxiety: A mini-review. *Frontiers in Psychiatry, 13*, 1022459. https://doi.org/10.3389/fpsyt.2022.1022459

Snaith, R. P. (2003). The hospital anxiety and depression scale. *Health and Quality of Life Outcomes, 1*, 29. https://doi.org/10.1186/1477-7525-1-29

Somerville, S., Byrne, S. L., Dedman, K., Hagan, R., Coo, S., Oxnam, E., . . . Page, A. C. (2015). Detecting the severity of perinatal anxiety with the Perinatal Anxiety Screening Scale (PASS). *Journal of Affective Disorders, 186*, 18–25. https://doi.org/10.1016/j.jad.2015.07.012

Somerville, S., Dedman, K., Hagan, R., Oxnam, E., Wettinger, M., Byrne, S., . . . Page, A. C. (2014). The perinatal anxiety screening scale: Development and preliminary validation. *Archives of Women's Mental Health, 17*(5), 443–454. https://doi.org/10.1007/s00737-014-0425-8

Sorsa, M. A., Kylmä, J., & Bondas, T. E. (2021). Contemplating help-seeking in perinatal psychological distress-a meta-ethnography. *International Journal of Environmental Research and Public Health, 18*(10). https://doi.org/10.3390/ijerph18105226

Speechley, M., Kunnilathu, A., Aluckal, E., Balakrishna, M. S., Mathew, B., & George, E. K. (2017). Screening in public health and clinical care: Similarities and differences in definitions, types, and aims – A systematic review. *Journal of Clinical and Diagnostic Research, 11*(3), Le01–Le04. https://doi.org/10.7860/jcdr/2017/24811.9419

Spielberger, C. D., Gorsuch, R. L., & Lushene, R. E. (1970). *Manual for the State-Trait Anxiety Inventory (STAI)*. Consulting Psychologists Press.

Spies, G., Stein, D. J., Roos, A., Faure, S. C., Mostert, J., Seedat, S., & Vythilingum, B. (2009). Validity of the Kessler 10 (K-10) in detecting DSM-IV defined mood and anxiety disorders among pregnant women. *Archives of Women's Mental Health, 12*(2), 69–74. https://doi.org/10.1007/s00737-009-0050-0

Spitzer, R. L., Kroenke, K., Williams, J. B., & Löwe, B. (2006). A brief measure for assessing generalized anxiety disorder: The GAD-7. *Archives of Internal Medicine, 166*(10), 1092–1097. https://doi.org/10.1001/archinte.166.10.1092

Stein, A., Pearson, R. M., Goodman, S. H., Rapa, E., Rahman, A., McCallum, M., . . . Pariante, C. M. (2014). Effects of perinatal mental disorders on the fetus and child. *The Lancet, 384*(9956), 1800–1819. https://doi.org/10.1016/s0140-6736(14)61277-0

Stevenson, K., Fellmeth, G., Edwards, S., Calvert, C., Bennett, P., Campbell, O. M. R., & Fuhr, D. C. (2023). The global burden of perinatal common mental health disorders and substance use among migrant women: A systematic review and meta-analysis. *Lancet Public Health, 8*(3), e203–e216. https://doi.org/10.1016/s2468-2667(22)00342-5

Swalm, D., Brooks, J., Doherty, D., Nathan, E., & Jacques, A. (2010). Using the Edinburgh Postnatal Depression Scale to screen for perinatal anxiety. *Archives of Women's Mental Health, 13*(6), 515–522. https://doi.org/10.1007/s00737-010-0170-6

Tomlinson, M., & Rotheram-Borus, M. J. (2022). When less is more: The way forward for mental health interventions during the perinatal period. *PLoS Med, 19*(12), e1004138. https://doi.org/10.1371/journal.pmed.1004138

Trevethan, R. (2017). Sensitivity, specificity, and predictive values: Foundations, pliabilities, and pitfalls in research and practice. *Frontiers in Public Health, 5*, 307. https://doi.org/10.3389/fpubh.2017.00307

van Heyningen, T., Myer, L., Tomlinson, M., Field, S., & Honikman, S. (2019). The development of an ultra-short, maternal mental health screening tool in South Africa. *Global Mental Health, 6*, e24. https://doi.org/10.1017/gmh.2019.21

Waqas, A., Koukab, A., Meraj, H., Dua, T., Chowdhary, N., Fatima, B., & Rahman, A. (2022). Screening programs for common maternal mental health disorders among perinatal women: Report of the systematic review of evidence. *BMC Psychiatry, 22*(1), 54. https://doi.org/10.1186/s12888-022-03694-9

Watson, H., Harrop, D., Walton, E., Young, A., & Soltani, H. (2019). A systematic review of ethnic minority women's experiences of perinatal mental health conditions and services in Europe. *PLoS One, 14*(1), e0210587. https://doi.org/10.1371/journal.pone.0210587

Webb, R., Ayers, S., & Rosan, C. (2018). A systematic review of measures of mental health and emotional wellbeing in parents of children aged 0–5. *Journal of Affective Disorders, 225*, 608–617. https://doi.org/10.1016/j.jad.2017.08.063

Whooley, M. A., Avins, A. L., Miranda, J., & Browner, W. S. (1997). Case-finding instruments for depression. *Journal of General Internal Medicine, 12*(7), 439–445.

Wilkinson, A., Anderson, S., & Wheeler, S. B. (2017). Screening for and treating postpartum depression and psychosis: A cost-effectiveness analysis. *Maternal and Child Health Journal, 21*(4), 903–914. https://doi.org/10.1007/s10995-016-2192-9

Williams, J. W., Jr., Mulrow, C. D., Kroenke, K., Dhanda, R., Badgett, R. G., Omori, D., & Lee, S. (1999). Case-finding for depression in primary care: A randomized trial. *American Journal of Medicine, 106*(1), 36–43. https://doi.org/10.1016/s0002-9343(98)00371-4

World Health Organization (WHO). (1994). *Composite International Diagnostic Interview (CIDI) researcher's manual. Version 1.1.* World Health Organization.

World Health Organization (WHO). (2013). *Guidelines on translation and adaptation of instruments.* www.mhinnovation.net/sites/default/files/files/WHO%20Guidelines%20on%20Translation%20and%20Adaptation%20of%20Instruments.docx#:~:text=Process%20of%20translation%20and%20adaptation%20of%20instruments&text=That%20is%2C%20the%20instrument%20should,than%20on%20linguistic%2Fliteral%20equivalence

World Health Organization (WHO). (2019). *International statistical classification of diseases and related health problems* (11th ed.). https://icd.who.int/

Zigmond, A. S., & Snaith, R. P. (1983). The hospital anxiety and depression scale. *Acta Psychiatrica Scandinavia, 67*(6), 361–370. https://doi.org/10.1111/j.1600-0447.1983.tb09716.x

20

PRENATAL PHARMACOTHERAPY

Jessica Pineda MD and Millicent Fugate MD

In this chapter, we review the currently known risks of medication in pregnancy to better help clinicians discuss the risks and benefits of continued medication in pregnancy as well as to inform decisions surrounding choice of new medications in the perinatal period. It is important to combine the information that follows with information of the risks of untreated mental illness in both pregnancy and the postpartum period. The discussion of these risks is out of the scope of this chapter, but it should be noted that untreated mental illness has been associated with numerous complications in pregnancy that pose a risk to both mother and infant. Adverse outcomes associated with major depressive disorder (MDD) in pregnancy include preeclampsia premature birth, low birth weight, and future behavioral disturbances in offspring (Davis et al., 2005; Li et al., 2009). One of the most important and repeatedly validated findings of untreated depression in pregnancy is worsening depression in the postpartum period (Bonari et al., 2004). Untreated maternal psychiatric symptoms have been shown to impact a child's development, attachment, behavior, and long-term academic achievement (Bonari et al., 2004; Grace et al., 2003; Weissman et al., 2006). It is important to remember that suicide is one of the leading causes of death in the perinatal period (Lindahl et al., 2005), and, therefore, depression and other mood disorders should be treated as potentially life-threatening illnesses.

The best way to prevent acute decompensation in the postpartum period is for mothers to receive treatment for any mood symptoms present in pregnancy and to maintain this euthymia throughout pregnancy (Suri et al., 2017). A clinician's understanding of these risks is critical to provide an accurate risk-benefit discussion with patients regarding psychiatric treatment in the perinatal period. Often, patients and clinicians focus on the known and unknown risks of medication, with this becoming the totality of risks discussed with patients. The risks of untreated mental illness are often not reviewed and, therefore, not included in the calculation of treatment decisions, including psychopharmacology. This pattern leads to a bias of risk to medications and an inaccurate decision-making process in the treatment of mental illness in the perinatal period.

A patient's individual risks regarding psychiatric decompensation should be included in discussions of initiating or continuing psychotropics in the perinatal period. Such historical features could include suicide attempts, inpatient psychiatric admissions, chronicity of illness,

DOI: 10.4324/9781003206903-25

time since last relapse and any current symptoms. These risks alter potential for decompensation, severity of decompensation, risks of suicide, and harm to infant. For example, someone with a remote history of depression that did not require multiple inpatient psychiatric admissions and current remission of symptoms greater than six months may not benefit from prophylactic antidepressant treatment (Yonkers et al., 2011); however, a currently asymptomatic patient with a suicide attempt in the past six months with repeated inpatient psychiatric admissions would likely require more aggressive medication management and could greatly benefit from continued psychotropics in pregnancy (Cohen et al., 2006).

When prescribing psychotropic medications in pregnancy, there are several clinical practices (Table 20.1) that can help guide treatment decisions to help minimize overall exposure risk—either to maternal mental health concerns or to medications themselves. For instance, it is recommended that clinicians use the lowest effective dose of medication to obtain mood stabilization. It is important to clarify the recommendation of lowest effective dose, as the dose that achieves euthymia, rather than a dose that provides nominal symptom improvement or maintenance of basic functionality. Euthymia should be identified as a goal of treatment to minimize exposure and potential complications from suboptimal treatment of perinatal mental health disturbances. Dosages of medication should be maximized to avoid multiple medication trials and polypharmacy, which would further increase fetal exposure risks. We recommend that medication be chosen that can be used both during pregnancy and during the breastfeeding period, as switching medication in the immediate postpartum period potentiates risk of an acute decompensation during a very vulnerable time for women. Importantly, stopping medication at the time of delivery puts patients at high risk for decompensation in the postpartum period, which is one of the very goals for treatment in pregnancy. The choice of pharmacotherapy should be individualized to each patient's needs, rather than attempting to follow a one-size-fits-all algorithm for prescription of medication in pregnancy. Decisions surrounding choice of medication should include the patient's own treatment history with efficacious and nonefficacious medication trials, known risks of medication in pregnancy, and breastfeeding, evidence for use of medication for presenting illness, as well as patient's values, and preferences.

In addition to these prescribing guidelines, it is important to consider the changing pharmacokinetics of psychotropic medication during pregnancy. These physiologic changes (Table 20.2) can accelerate the metabolism of psychotropics, thereby lowering serum concentration

Table 20.1 General Prescribing Guidelines

• Use monotherapy when able
• Treat symptoms to remission
• Limit use of polypharmacy
• Minimize medication changes
• Do not stop effective medication prior to delivery
• Prioritize medications that have worked in the past

Table 20.2 Physiologic Changes in Pregnancy

• Renal blood flow and glomerular filtration rate increase 50% to 80%
• Increased estrogen levels lead to accelerated drug glucuronidation
• Reduced serum albumin affect protein binding and total plasma clearance
• Increased plasma volume/increased total body water

levels resulting in decreased efficacy. It is not uncommon for pregnant individuals to require higher doses of medication to maintain efficacy (Reimers & Brodtkorb, 2012).

In the pages that follow, we attempt to elucidate the available safety data regarding exposure of psychotropic medications during pregnancy. The gold standard for evaluating cause and effect of medication treatment is the use of randomized, placebo controlled double blind studies. However, pregnant women are not eligible for these studies; therefore, the ability to minimize bias and establish cause and effect of an intervention during pregnancy is compromised. When evaluating findings with psychotropic exposure, it is nearly impossible to separate the impact of medication versus the impact of illness (including severity of illness and behaviors associated with illness) on adverse outcomes. Studies have little information regarding adherence to medication, dosage, duration of treatment, and timing of fetal exposure. Other variables, including severity of psychiatric symptoms, socioeconomic status, age, previous pregnancy loss, polypharmacy, substance use and comorbid medical illnesses, are not always addressed in the methodology of available studies (Chaudron, 2013). These limitations, combined with inherent stigma related to mental illness and hesitancy to treat women during pregnancy, can often leave physicians feeling hesitant to employ pharmacologic interventions. It is our hope that by detailing the available data, we can help minimize this hesitancy and provide a framework for the treatment of perinatal mood and anxiety disorders during pregnancy and the postpartum period.

It had been the previous practice by clinicians to determine safety of a medication by reviewing pregnancy risk categories. This simplified process included Categories A, B, C, D, and X, as described in Table 20.3. Although these guidelines were meant to be simplified for busy clinicians, simply using these categories did not allow for clinicians to have a nuanced discussion and shared decision-making with patients. For instance, based on these criteria, an "older" medication may be considered Category D due to a small relative risk of increasing congenital defects; however, a novel medication may be considered Category B due to an absence of risk in animal studies despite lack of adequate human trials. We would argue that a medication with an abundance of human data provides greater reassurance and the opportunity for a more thorough informed consent discussion

Table 20.3 Former FDA Pregnancy Categories

Category	
A	Controlled studies show no risk: Adequate, well controlled studies in pregnant women have failed to demonstrate risk to women.
B	No evidence of risk in humans: Either animal studies show no risk, but human findings do not, or, if no adequate human studies have been done animal findings are negative.
C	Risk cannot be ruled out: Human studies are lacking, and animal studies are either positive for fetal risk or lacking as well. However, potential benefits may justify potential risk.
D	Positive evidence of risk: Investigational or postmarketing data show risk to the fetus. Nevertheless, potential benefits may outweigh the risks.
X	Contraindicated in pregnancy: Studies in animals or humans, or investigational or postmarketing reports, have shown fetal risks that clearly outweighs any possible benefit to the patient.

as compared to a medication in which only animal data are available. Simplifying risk to a graded category system, while convenient, can asperse medications that are otherwise compatible with pregnancy, while simultaneously providing a false sense of security regarding medications lacking in human data.

Currently, the Federal Drug Administration (FDA) is using a narrative summary of medications including three sections: pregnancy, lactation, and reproductive potential. Each of these sections includes a detailed risk summary, clinical considerations, and a data section. The FDA announced this shift upon publication of the *Content and Format of Labeling for Human Prescription Drug and Biological Products; Requirements for Pregnancy and Lactation Labeling* (The Pregnancy and Lactation Rule) on December 4, 2014. In the Pregnancy and Lactation Rule, the FDA noted that including more detailed information on the risk of and benefits of medication in pregnancy would support "healthcare providers' understanding of drug product risks and benefits" and facilitate "informed prescribing decisions and patient counseling." The Pregnancy and Lactation Rule also specified that the pregnancy categories A, B, C, D, and X be removed from all drug labeling. The FDA found that the "pregnancy categories were confusing and did not accurately and consistently communicate differences in degree of fetal risk" and were "heavily relied upon by clinicians but were often misinterpreted and misused." This shift from pregnancy categories to narrative summary has allowed clinicians and patients to discuss in more detail the risks and benefits of medication during pregnancy and better tailor treatment interventions to a patient's needs, rather than feeling stifled by the limitation inherent in a category system.

Antidepressants

Case A: Patient A is a 27-year-old gravida 0 parity 0 (no previous pregnancies) with a past psychiatric history of recurrent major depressive disorder, first diagnosed at 15 years of age. Patient A's history is notable for three prior inpatient hospitalizations for suicidal ideation and one previous suicide attempt via acetaminophen overdose, which required medication admission and stabilization for acute liver failure. She has been trialed on numerous medications, including fluoxetine, sertraline, escitalopram, and citalopram. Per the patient, these medications provide some symptomatic relief; however, remission of symptoms were not achieved even on maximum doses of the aforementioned medications. Patient A is planning a pregnancy and has recently been restarted on sertraline by her obstetrician due to persistent depressive symptoms impacting her ability to function socially and professionally. Prominent symptoms include low mood, anhedonia, hopelessness, hypersomnia, and increased appetite. Patient A also endorses prominent anxious ruminations regarding the potential viability of any future pregnancies and her ability to meet the needs of future offsprings. On exam, she appears depressed with constricted affect, downcast gaze, and psychomotor slowing. Patient Health Questionnaire (PHQ9) score was elevated at 17 without current suicidal ideation.

Case A Discussion: Patient A is currently experiencing significant depressive symptoms that are impairing her ability to function, and, therefore, we agree with the obstetrician's decision to initiate pharmacotherapy for ongoing mood symptoms. Given her previous history of a serious suicide attempt as well as recurrent severe depressive symptoms, she would likely benefit from medication management in pregnancy, even if symptoms remit, to prevent relapse during pregnancy or the postpartum period. Although sertraline is often the preferred agent of many obstetricians, lack of response to multiple selective serotonin reuptake inhibitor (SSRI) trials suggests that sertraline may not adequately achieve euthymia for this patient. An astute clinician may consider a trial of another medication to potentially achieve a more robust response. As Patient A is not currently pregnant, this is an excellent opportunity to provide preconception consultation regarding treatment options during and after pregnancy, including a thorough discussion of risk/benefits of medication and untreated illness, including risks of miscarriage, teratogenicity, delivery complications and long-term complications of infant development. This also provides time to try alternative treatment options, such as switching to another medication class, which is often discouraged in pregnancy to minimize potential exposures.

Selective serotonin reuptake inhibitors (SSRIs) are one of the most studied medication classes in pregnancy, with sertraline—the most commonly prescribed antidepressant during the perinatal period—having the largest amount of safety data. As a class, SSRIs have not been associated with early pregnancy loss when compared to pregnancies in which perinatal mood and anxiety disorders are prominent (Kjaersgaard et al., 2013). Historically, these data have been misinterpreted, as individuals with symptoms of depression and anxiety during pregnancy appear to have higher rates of pregnancy loss; however, there are no data to suggest that SSRI exposure in the early perinatal period alters this risk in any significant way. This can be reassuring information for women with recurrent or persistent mood disorders who require continued treatment with SSRIs for mood stabilization when trying to conceive or during their early stages of pregnancy.

SSRIs are not teratogens and have not been associated with teratogenicity. There have been reports of atrial septal and ventricular septal defects seen with sertraline and other SSRIs (Louik et al., 2014; Pedersen et al., 2009); however, upon larger review of data, there does not appear to be an association between sertraline and cardiac malformations (Huybrechts et al., 2014). Initial data likely reflected evidence of confounders including gestational diabetes and obesity. Previous data suggested that another SSRI, paroxetine, was associated with cardiac outflow tract obstructions (Alwan et al., 2007; Louik et al., 2014; Wurst et al., 2010), although subsequent evaluations, including a 2014 paper published in the *New England Journal of Medicine*, demonstrated insufficient evidence to support this association (Huybrechts et al., 2014). Understandably, remnants of this historical concern linger, making paroxetine one of the lesser prescribed SSRIs during the perinatal period. Prominent anticholinergic properties of paroxetine, including sedation, and weight gain; its short half-life and propensity for discontinuation syndrome if dosing is delayed or missed; and the high prevalence of sexual dysfunction (Stahl & Grady, 2011) often make it a less desirable medication for the majority of the population.

A phenomenon reported as *post neonatal adaptation syndrome* (PNAS) has been described with serotonergic medications and has been most studied with SSRIs (Kieviet et al., 2013). It should be noted that this phenomenon lacks distinct diagnostic criteria, but rather has, historically, been reported at the time of delivery. Literature suggests that 30% or less of infants exposed to serotonergic medications in utero may develop abnormal behavioral and autonomic symptoms within the first few days of life (Kieviet et al., 2013). Prominent symptoms associated with PNAS include tremor, irritability, poor feeding, respiratory challenges, low muscle tone, and high muscle tone (Kieviet et al., 2013). These symptoms are self-limited, often resolving within 48 hours to seven days of life (Sie et al., 2012; Oberlander et al., 2004; Ferreira et al., 2007) and do not appear to be related to long-term complications (Oberlander et al., 2004). It is also important to note that there are a number of limitations in the literature regarding the study of this phenomenon. For instance, PNAS lacks a specific definition as well as diagnostic criteria, which limits the ability to evaluate for the presence or absence of the syndrome at birth, as evidenced by the lack of a validated screening tool. Additionally, the literature lacks a blinded rating of this phenomenon and studies regarding possible treatment or prevention (Payne & Meltzer-Brody, 2009).

It is plausible that the symptoms observed at the time of delivery are consistent with an absence of exposure to serotonin (Kieviet et al., 2013), as argued by symptom profile and improvement in symptom severity when mothers breastfeed (Kieviet et al., 2013). However, this possibility does not appear to be substantiated when reviewing data regarding transmission of sertraline in breastfeeding. Sertraline is transmitted in relatively low amounts via breastmilk, with negligible amounts seen in infants' serum. It seems likely that the sucking motion, inherent in breastfeeding, is likely more of a support than any delivery of medication. Additionally, studies of individuals who stopped their serotonergic medications weeks prior to delivery did not demonstrate a statistically significant difference in the rates of PNAS when compared to individuals who continued serotonergic medications through parturition (Sie et al., 2012). This suggests that PNAS symptoms may reflect an interaction between serotonin and the developing fetus earlier in gestation and cannot simply be described as a discontinuation or withdrawal-like syndrome. It is likely that higher dosages and multiple medications, including adjunct therapy with benzodiazepines, elevate the risk of PNAS (Oberlander et al., 2004).

When discussing PNAS with patients, it is important to balance the need to provide comprehensive risk stratification, without being overly sensational regarding the severity of the risk. It can be helpful to identify that PNAS is a potentially common phenomenon, and therefore, one that should be included in any informed consent discussion. Nonetheless, PNAS is not considered a dangerous or life-threatening condition, but rather is benign and self-limiting. PNAS rarely requires intervention and has not been associated with any long-term complications in the infant (Moses-Kolko et al., 2005).

There have been reports of respiratory complications in infants when mothers take SSRIs during pregnancy. This phenomenon, referred to as *persistent pulmonary hypertension of the newborn* (PPHN), is a heterogeneous phenomenon with several etiologies and a wide range of severity. In essence, PPHN is a failure of the pulmonary vasculature to decrease resistance at birth (Payne & Meltzer-Brody, 2009). It is a rare condition affecting 1–2/1,000 births (Hageman et al., 1984) and can be related to a variety of etiologies, the most common of which being cesarean section, meconium aspiration, and preterm delivery (Hernández-Díaz et al., 2007). Most cases result in full recovery of the infant; however, severe and life-threatening etiologies of PPHN can occur. Several studies attempted to evaluate the association of serotonergic medication and PPHN, although confounding variables, including maternal smoking, maternal obesity, and preterm delivery, were often not controlled for in the studies' methodology. Although the literature does suggest a slightly increased relative risk for PPHN with exposure to SSRIs in pregnancy, the absolute risk remains low (Grigoriadis et al., 2014). Understandably, the potential for respiratory complications in the offspring can be an upsetting possibility for many parents. We have found that when discussing this risk with patients it can be important to provide reassurance regarding the lack of associated morbidity and mortality, but also provide statistical data to help patients better conceptualize this risk. Whereas physicians and other medical professionals can understand the statistical implications of an elevated relative risk but low absolute risk, patients often prefer to have this information presented in a franker manner. For instance, by reporting that PPHN occurs in approximately 1–2/1,000 live births in the general populations, with an increase to 2–3/1,000 live births with SSRI exposure (Grigoriadis et al., 2014).

One of the major concerns for many patients regarding psychotropic medications during pregnancy is the potential impact on neurobehavioral complications, particularly the risk for autism spectrum disorder (ASD). The risk of SSRI exposure on the development of ASD is not well understood and may be better represented by the risk of underlying illness. SSRI exposure during pregnancy is a marker for increased risk of ASD in the offspring; however, the risk is reduced, and is likely no longer statistically significant, when adjusting for maternal psychiatric illness (Andrade, 2017).

Serotonin–norepinephrine reuptake inhibitors (SNRIs) are also considered for the treatment of depression and/or anxiety during pregnancy. We would not typically recommend starting an SNRI as a first-line treatment approach during pregnancy, given the larger quantity of data for SSRIs in pregnancy as compared to SNRIs. Nevertheless, it is likely that one could encounter a scenario in which prescription of an SNRI would be preferred, such as current euthymia achieved with SNRI, failed trials of at least two SSRIs, and comorbid pain syndromes such as fibromyalgia. In general, if a patient is responding well to an SNRI, careful consideration should be taken prior to altering the patient's treatment regimen. In general, SNRIs carry many of the same risks of SSRIs including PNAS and PPHN; however, SNRIs also confer additional risks, which should be discussed and reviewed with patients.

A Danish registry suggested that duloxetine use might be associated with an increased risk of spontaneous abortion; however, there are several limitations to this finding (Kjaersgaard et al., 2013). Primarily, the sample size of women prescribed duloxetine was smaller than that of women prescribed SSRIs in this analysis, which suggests that the study may not have sufficient power to accurately represent the risk associated with duloxetine. Additionally, data were not collected regarding the severity of maternal mental illness, which represents a limitation because the women prescribed an SNRI during pregnancy may have more severe or treatment-resistant symptoms.

Data vary regarding the potential for physical malformations with exposure to SNRIs during pregnancy. Duloxetine exposure in utero does not seem to confer a statistically significant increased risk of congenital malformations over that of the general population (Hoog et al., 2013; Lassen et al., 2016). Venlafaxine, however, has been associated with an elevated risk of birth defects, particularly cardiac defects, when compared to other antidepressants (Anderson et al., 2020). Once again, the generalizability of these data is questionable given limitations in sample size and failure to account for the severity of underlying conditions that are often comorbid with use of SNRIs.

SNRIs act on both serotonin and norepinephrine; therefore, concerns have arisen regarding the impact of elevated norepinephrine during pregnancy, particularly regarding the potential to elevate blood pressure and theoretically contribute to decreased fetal growth or preterm birth. Women with psychiatric disorders are at an elevated risk for hypertensive disorders of pregnancy (Hu et al., 2015; Rusner et al., 2016; Thombre et al., 2015; Vigod et al., 2014), with some data suggesting a three-fold elevated risk on women taking SNRI throughout pregnancy (Frayne et al., 2021). The literature does demonstrate a small, yet statistically significant, increased risk of postpartum hemorrhage associated with SNRIs; however, given the inconsistency of the findings, small overall risk, and the potential for decompensation if psychotropic medications are held prior to delivery, there is not compelling evidence to suggest that SNRIs should be held during delivery to mitigate the risk of postpartum hemorrhage (Huybrechts et al., 2020).

Tricyclic antidepressants (TCAs) are effective medications in the management of depression, anxiety, and obsessive-compulsive symptoms and have potential additional benefits in the treatment of migraines, pain, and insomnia. However, due to their unfavorable side effect profile, including sedation, weight gain, dry mouth, and constipation, as well as dangerous cardiac arrhythmias with overdose (Stahl & Grady, 2011), their use has decreased with availability of SSRIs. Despite the longer tenure of TCAs for the treatment of psychiatric disorders when compared to SSRIs and SNRIs, less overall data are available regarding the risks and outcomes in pregnancy and breastfeeding. This lack of data likely reflects the relatively low percentage of individuals of childbearing age being prescribed TCAs as the primary pharmacological intervention. Current data do not demonstrate an association between in utero TCA exposure and increased risk of congenital malformations (Altshuler et al., 1996). Data do, however, suggest that there may be an elevated risk for preeclampsia, and blood pressure should be monitored closely for individuals continued on TCAs during pregnancy (Gentile, 2014). Similar to SSRIs and SNRIs, descriptions of PNAS have been described, most commonly with clomipramine (Gentile, 2014). No developmental or long-term behavioral complications have been reported (Nulman et al., 1997; Wisner et al., 1999). In light of this evidence, TCAs can be considered for the treatment of anxiety and depressive disorders during pregnancy when an individual has completed two failed trials of SSRIs and may be excellent options for women with OCD or comorbid migraines, insomnia, or pain syndromes.

Bupropion is an aminoketone antidepressant that affects both the dopaminergic and noradrenergic systems and is classified as a norepinephrine-dopamine reuptake inhibitor (NDRI) (Stahl & Grady, 2011). It is prescribed not only for MDD but also for attention-deficit/hyperactivity disorder (ADHD), and smoking cessation (Stahl & Grady, 2011). Given the wide range of indications for this medication, careful consideration must be taken when reviewing the literature to accurately assess the risk of underlying illness to pregnancy outcomes. Bupropion may be a preferable monotherapy for numerous patients, including those with prominent neurovegetative symptoms, or comorbid ADHD, or nicotine use disorder. It is often found to exacerbate anxiety symptoms and should be avoided in those with epilepsy or active eating disorders as it can lower the seizure threshold.

Overall, data are favorable regarding the risk of spontaneous abortion following prenatal bupropion exposure. In fact, studies in which the incidence of miscarriage is elevated over that of control groups, the rate of miscarriage is still within the realm of population norms (Chun-Fai-Chan et al., 2005). At this time, there are no data to suggest that bupropion increases the risk of pregnancy loss or that bupropion should be avoided in the first trimester to prevent or minimize the likelihood of spontaneous abortions.

Bupropion is not considered a teratogenic medication. Data from the Bupropion Pregnancy Registry demonstrates that the rate of birth defects with first trimester bupropion exposure is 3.6%, which is consistent with the rate of birth defects in the general population. One retrospective study demonstrated an elevated risk of cardiac malformations (i.e., left ventricular outflow tract defects); however, the number of exposed offspring with this condition was relatively small and likely contributed to an overestimation of risk (Alwan et al., 2010). Subsequent studies demonstrated consistent concerns regarding the potential for cardiac malformations although the absolute risk of such conditions remains relatively low (Louik et al., 2014; Turner et al., 2019). A study of long-term effects of prenatal exposure to bupropion found an elevated risk of ADHD diagnosis, even when controlling for underlying maternal illness (Ornoy, 2018).

Mirtazapine is a tetracyclic antidepressant with serotonergic, noradrenergic, and antihistamine properties (Stahl & Grady, 2011). Although mirtazapine is primarily prescribed for treatment of depressive symptomatology, in pregnancy and the postpartum period it can often be prescribed in an effort to take advantage of its side effect profile, namely sedation and appetite stimulation. Additionally, mirtazapine has antiemetic properties through antagonism of the 5-HT3 receptor (Stahl & Grady, 2011), which can be especially useful for patients struggling with morning sickness, or hyperemesis gravidarum. Current data do not suggest that mirtazapine is associated with spontaneous abortion, intrauterine fetal demise, or neonatal death, nor is it associated with elevated risk of congenital malformations (Ostenfeld et al., 2022). Although the appetite stimulating properties of mirtazapine can be beneficial for patients who are not gaining weight appropriately for gestational age, critics have expressed concern regarding the potential for elevating risk of gestational diabetes mellitus (GDM). Data from the Norwegian Mother, Father, and Child Cohort Study suggest that antidepressant medications with a high affinity for the histamine H1 receptor, such as mirtazapine, may confer an elevated risk for GDM (Lupattelli et al., 2022; Salvi et al., 2016). It is important to note that a relative risk could not be calculated in this study due to the small sample size of pregnancies exposed to high H1 affinity medications. At this time, further studies are warranted to better understand the clinical implications of these data, although it would be fair to consider alternative medications in women at high risk of GDM. Reports of perinatal adaptations syndrome, symptoms at the time of delivery, or neurodevelopmental outcomes are not currently available for mirtazapine.

Trazodone is an antidepressant belonging to the class of medications called serotonin receptor antagonists and reuptake inhibitors (SARIs) (Stahl & Grady, 2011). Trazodone is rarely used as monotherapy for treatment of MDD, but is rather used as adjunct treatment, specifically for associated insomnia. Therefore, the risk/benefit discussion for the prescription of trazodone should be structured around the risk of insomnia, sedation, and polypharmacy. There are limited data available regarding the impact of trazodone in pregnancy, which is likely related to the hesitancy of providers to prescribe psychotropic medications in pregnancy, especially those which are considered adjunct therapies. Current data do not suggest an increased risk of major congenital malformations with trazodone exposure in the first trimester (Einarson et al., 2003, 2009).

Case A: After a thorough discussion of risks and benefits of SSRIs, SNRIs, TCAs, bupropion, and mirtazapine, Patient A decided to continue sertraline. Patient A felt that the larger amount of safety data, including in early pregnancy, were more reassuring than the data available for other medications. Patient A also felt more comfortable continuing with this medication, as their obstetrician had recommended and endorsed its safety in pregnancy.

Case A Discussion: Continuing sertraline and titrating dose to address residual depressive symptoms is an appropriate option for this patient. Importantly, this decision aligns with the patient's preferences (i.e., to use medications with the most data), which should always be a crucial component of any informed consent discussion. Several of the other options would be suboptimal choices for this patient: TCAs should often be avoided in patients at an elevated risk of suicide or overdose (as evidenced in Patient A's history of serious suicide attempt), bupropion could worsen anxiety symptoms, and mirtazapine could exacerbate hypersomnia and elevated appetite. SNRIs could be a viable option for Patient A, given her history of failed trials with multiple SSRIs, although her individual risks for hypertension and hemorrhage should be taken into consideration.

Although sertraline is a viable option, concerns remain that Patient A may once again have inadequate response to medication treatment, resulting in fetal exposure to both sertraline as well as complications of maternal illness. Preconception counseling offers the opportunity to discuss trials of new medications to potentially achieve euthymia. Trialing new medications in the preconception period is preferred to trialing new medications in pregnancy to minimize the risks of fetal exposure to multiple medications as well as exposure to ongoing maternal illness. Ideally, a new medication may result in complete remission of symptoms prior to pregnancy and exposure could be limited to one medication.

Anxiolytics

Case A: Patient A titrated sertraline dose to 200mg with improvement of depressive symptoms. At 20 weeks' gestation, Patient A noticed worsening anxiety symptoms with development of panic attacks approximately two to three times/week. She described these events as terrifying and reported that worrying about having another attack has resulted in several absences from work and an overall decrease in work performance. During one panic attack, Patient A presented to the emergency room and was given a prescription for lorazepam 1 mg three times/day as needed. She has been hesitant to use lorazepam in pregnancy as she read it was considered Pregnancy Category D and, thus, has only used lorazepam one time since this emergency room visit. Patient A reports good response to lorazepam and some improvement of overall anxiety due to availability of lorazepam in case of panic attack.

Case A Discussion: Benzodiazepines are controlled substances, meaning they have potential for misuse and physiologic dependence, and should always be prescribed with caution and are not recommended as the primary agent for daily persistent anxiety. Rather, can be used for the treatment of acute intermittent anxiety or as an adjunct for anxiety while medications such as SSRIs take effect. Patient A has tolerated lorazepam use well and has been able to limit its use with good overall response. At this stage in pregnancy, our concern for malformations would be relatively low. Additionally, at current frequency and dosage, risks of infant intoxication, withdrawal, or other complications at the time of delivery would likely be minimal. We would suggest that if intermittent use of lorazepam for panic is helpful and maintains adequate mood stabilization, it can be continued. Continuation of low-dose lorazepam as needed for panic is likely preferable to switching sertraline to another agent or adding a second daily medication as an augmentation strategy.

Benzodiazepines are effective medications for the treatment of acute anxiety and panic and can be used as an adjunctive treatment for mania, psychosis, premenstrual dysphoric disorder, and other psychiatric conditions. Benzodiazepines, as a class, confer an increased risk of tolerance and dependence, and, therefore, it is recommended to prescribe these medications only for short courses or on an intermittent basis. Challenges arise in reviewing the safety data of these medications in pregnancy due to the broad variations in use patterns. For instance, some patients may take a low-dose benzodiazepine once every one to two weeks, whereas other patients may be prescribed a high dose scheduled numerous times throughout the day. Further complicating the discussion is the potential for misuse or abuse of benzodiazepines.

There are data to support increased risk of spontaneous abortion when benzodiazepines are used during the early perinatal period (Sheehy et al., 2019). Increased risk of facial clefts has been described (McElhatton, 1994). In a study examining 278 children with cleft lip and/or palate, diazepam ingestion was found to be four times more common during pregnancy (Safra & Oakley, 1975). In a study evaluating mothers who used anxiolytics during the first trimester where the most commonly prescribed medication was diazepam, infants were found to have a threefold relative risk for cleft lip with or without cleft palate (Saxén, 1975). Many of the women included in these studies had multiple comorbidities, including epilepsy, diabetes, and psychiatric illnesses that carry their own risks for pregnancy and neonatal outcomes. Additionally, medical, obstetric, and family histories of malformations were not always evaluated; thus, understanding the risk associated with benzodiazepines is difficult. In most studies involving first trimester use of benzodiazepines, the majority of infants were normal at birth (McElhatton, 1994).

Diazepam and its metabolites have been detected in infants for up to eight days after delivery (Cree et al., 1973). Abnormal infant behavior at the time of delivery has been reported and includes floppy baby syndrome, low Apgar scores, apenic spells, hypotonia, reluctance to feed and impaired metabolic responses to cold stress (Cree et al., 1973). Risks of infant benzodiazepine withdrawal have been reported and should be monitored, especially when maternal dosages are significant and have been used chronically. Symptoms of neonatal infant benzodiazepine withdrawal have included tremor, irritability, diarrhea, vomiting, vigorous sucking and hypertonicity (Briggs et al., 2021).

Long-term neurobehavioral complications have been reported with maternal benzodiazepine use, including motor and developmental delays, although, typically, children will catch up and exhibit normal development by four years of age (McElhatton, 1994). Reports of persistent developmental delay associated with maternal benzodiazepine use is challenging to prove a cause-effect association. It is possible that additional or alternative factors contribute to developmental delays including social and economic stressors.

Buspirone is an anxiolytic medication classified as an azapirone (Stahl & Grady, 2011). The FDA currently approves buspirone for treatment of generalized anxiety disorder, although buspirone is typically used as an adjunct treatment rather than monotherapy. Minimal data are available regarding the risks and outcomes of buspirone in pregnancy, which likely reflects a tendency toward optimizing monotherapy in pregnancy and discontinuing adjunctive medications. In a recent study looking at 68 women prescribed buspirone during the first trimester, no malformations in offspring were observed (Freeman et al., 2022).

Case A: Patient A continued sertraline 200 mg throughout the remainder of her pregnancy and required lorazepam less than one time per week. She had a spontaneous vaginal delivery at 38 weeks' gestation. Infant did not require any intervention, nor did Patient A observe any abnormal behavior following parturition. She is currently exclusively breastfeeding and has not noticed any abnormal behavior or signs in offspring. Patient A's anxiety has stabilized and she has not required lorazepam in the postpartum period.

Mood Stabilizers

Case B: Patient B is a 32-year-old gravida 0 parity 0 (no prior pregnancies) with a past psychiatric history of bipolar I disorder presenting for preconception consultation. She was diagnosed with bipolar disorder during a manic episode necessitating inpatient hospitalization at age 23 and has tried numerous agents in the past, including lithium, valproic acid, olanzapine, risperidone, and quetiapine. The majority of agents are typically effective for addressing mood symptoms, although lithium, valproic acid, and olanzapine were discontinued secondary to intolerable weight gain. History is significant for four prior inpatient hospitalizations, the most recent of which was nine months ago for mania. Patient B is currently managed on lamotrigine 250 mg daily, which she finds effective and tolerable. In the past, Patient B has required monotherapy with lamotrigine and a second-generation antipsychotic for acute mania; however, antipsychotic agents are typically titrated and discontinued after a few months. She reports absence of mood symptoms for the past five months, with the most recent episode being depressive in nature. Patient B reports that she and her partner are considering trying to conceive within the next year, but she is concerned about taking medications during pregnancy.

Case B Discussion: Patient B has been diagnosed with bipolar I disorder, which confers an elevated risk of mood decompensation in pregnancy and postpartum, with some data suggesting a greater than 80% risk of mood episodes in unmedicated pregnancies. One of the most significant risks associated with bipolar disorder in pregnancy is the risk of postpartum psychosis. Postpartum psychosis is considered a psychiatric emergency requiring inpatient hospitalization given elevated risk of infanticide. Patient B's history is significant for several inpatient hospitalizations and two known mood episodes during the last year. While Patient B endorses euthymia at present, substantial risk of decompensation with medication discontinuation should be weighed against risks of potential medication options.

Lamotrigine is an FDA-approved medication for maintenance treatment of bipolar I disorder. Additionally, lamotrigine has data supporting its use in bipolar depression and as an adjunct therapy for both bipolar mania and unipolar depression. A significant amount of safety data exists for the use of lamotrigine in pregnancy as it is often first-line for management of epilepsy in reproductive-age women. For this reason, lamotrigine is often considered for treatment of bipolar spectrum illnesses during the perinatal period, although, it should be noted that the data are somewhat skewed, given that the studies are focused on a different patient cohort with unique underlying illnesses and risk profiles.

According to the North America Antiepileptic Drug (AED) Pregnancy Registry, an increased risk of oral cleft has been associated with lamotrigine use in pregnancy. These findings are not consistent throughout the literature, although lamotrigine doses less than 300 mg/day do not seem to be associated with malformations (Reimers & Brodtkorb, 2012). These data are reassuring, as lamotrigine doses for mood stabilization do not typically exceed 300 mg/day. Long-term studies do not demonstrate IQ or behavioral differences in offspring exposed to lamotrigine in utero (Meador et al., 2009; Cummings et al., 2011). Unique considerations exist when prescribing lamotrigine in pregnancy secondary to increased drug glucuronidation and increased overall clearance of medication. Some data suggest that serum lamotrigine levels can decrease by up to 30% during pregnancy (Tran et al., 2002). Therefore, it is often necessary to increase lamotrigine doses throughout pregnancy to maintain euthymia. One potential tool to help guide lamotrigine dosing in pregnancy is to obtain serum lamotrigine levels. The use of lamotrigine levels is often not part of routine clinical care or guidelines in the treatment of bipolar illness, given the lack of formal reference ranges for euthymia. However, for women on lamotrigine maintenance, obtaining a pre-pregnancy lamotrigine level consistent with euthymia can provide a baseline value to help guide dosing throughout pregnancy. A repeat lamotrigine level during pregnancy that is lower than the pre-pregnancy baseline can help guide clinicians when deciding between increasing the lamotrigine dose or adding an augmentation agent in the setting of emergence of symptoms.

Lithium has been used for the treatment of bipolar illness as well as depression augmentation. Its data in the treatment and prevention of postpartum psychosis have shown greater efficacy than other mood stabilizers and antipsychotics, and, therefore, may be an important tool for a select group of women. Lithium does demonstrate complete placental passage, with an infant: mother ratio of 1.05 (Newport, 2005). This medication has often been avoided or stopped in pregnancy due to the known risk of Ebstein's Anomaly—a cardiac malformation in which there is a downward displacement of the tricuspid valve into the right ventricle, leading to variable degrees of right ventricular hypoplasia. Although risk for this anomaly does exist when there is exposure in the first trimester, the absolute risk is relatively low—1/1,000 of exposed infants (Altshuler et al., 1996). For some women, the efficacy of this medication for management of mood disorder outweighs the small but elevated risk of cardiac malformations. However, some women may choose alternative strategies for mood stabilization during pregnancy, or specifically for the first trimester.

During pregnancy, there is increased renal excretion of lithium that may require increased dosages of this medication. In order to minimize fetal exposure, we recommend increasing dosages based on an emergence of mood symptoms rather than to maintain a specific lithium level.

Neonatal symptoms at the time of delivery include *floppy baby syndrome*, which can include respiratory distress, cardiac arrhythmias, hypotonia, lethargy as well as neonatal hypothyroidism. How to manage lithium dosing at the time of delivery has been debated, as higher levels of lithium at delivery increase the risk of neonatal symptoms. It has been suggested to hold lithium surrounding time of delivery (between 24 and 48 hours), maintain adequate hydration, and return to preconception lithium dose immediately postpartum in anticipation of decreased renal clearance after gestation (Newport, 2005). Additional studies have suggested that with maternal lithium levels < 0.6 at the time of delivery, minimal, if any, adverse outcomes are seen with infants and there have been no reports of maternal toxicity (Newport, 2005) and, therefore, changes to dosages of lithium at the time of delivery may not be necessary in these cases. Careful balance of adequate psychotropic support postpartum to prevent severe decompensation, which can include depression, mania, or psychosis, should be balanced with any risk of toxicity or adverse drug event. No long-term developmental delay has been associated with perinatal lithium use.

Valproic acid is a known teratogen that has been associated with neural tube defects, atrial septal defects, cleft palate, hypospadias, polydactyly and craniostenosis (Jentink et al., 2010). Additionally, in utero exposure is a risk factor for cognitive impairment in children, which appears to be dose dependent (Meador et al., 2013). It is recommended that valproic acid be completely avoided in pregnancy due to high risk of teratogenicity and cognitive impairments. It is worth noting that nearly half of all pregnancies are unplanned, contraceptives can fail, and opportunities to change medication prior to conception may be limited, elevating risk of teratogenic effects of valproic acid before knowledge of pregnancy. We would, therefore, discourage the use of valproic acid to any woman of reproductive age.

Case B: After thorough discussion of the risks associated with untreated bipolar disorder during pregnancy and postpartum and the safety data associated with lamotrigine, Patient B elected to continue lamotrigine during pregnancy. Patient B felt reassured by the vast amount of safety data available for lamotrigine in pregnancy and expressed concern for recurrence of mood episodes during pregnancy or after parturition. She was amenable to having lamotrigine levels ordered to help guide dosing during pregnancy. Lamotrigine level associated with euthymia pre-pregnancy was 6 µg/mL.

Case B Discussion: Lamotrigine is an excellent choice for a mood stabilizing agent during pregnancy, especially considering that Patient B has, historically, responded well to this agent. Bipolar disorder is associated with a high risk of mood episode recurrence in pregnancy and postpartum, and, thus, we would be hesitant to discontinue an effective medication for which there are an abundance of safety data. Obtaining a lamotrigine level can be an effective strategy to help guide dosing during pregnancy, given increased glucuronidation and clearance; however, this is not considered a standard of care. It is our experience that having a pre-pregnancy lamotrigine level associated with euthymia can be an effective strategy when discussing dose increases in symptomatic patients who are reluctant to take or increase medications during pregnancy.

Antipsychotics

Case B: Patient B is continued on lamotrigine 250 mg daily and quickly conceives after removal of her IUD. Pregnancy is uncomplicated medically with the exception of mild anemia. Patient B denies obstetric concerns for gestational diabetes mellitus or pre-eclampsia. Routine ultrasound was unremarkable, with no evidence of craniofacial anomalies. Mood is fairly stable through the first and second trimesters; however, at 28 weeks' gestation Patient B begins to experience worsening mood symptoms consistent with a depressive episode. Lamotrigine level at the time of mood decompensation is 4 µg/mL.

Lamotrigine dose is steadily increased to 350 mg daily (lamotrigine level 6 µg/mL) without full amelioration of symptoms. Patient B reports ongoing feelings of sadness, anhedonia, insomnia, low appetite, and difficulty attending to activities of daily living. Quetiapine was started as an adjunct treatment and steadily increased to 200 mg at bedtime. Patient B reports gradual improvement and remission of depressive symptoms as well as improved sleep and appetite.

Case B Discussion: Addition of quetiapine was an effective strategy for addressing Patient B's depressive symptoms. Although starting quetiapine represents an additional fetal exposure, it was likely a necessary choice given failure to achieve euthymia by increasing lamotrigine dose. Quetiapine is FDA-approved for bipolar depression, which suggests that it would likely be more effective than attempting to advance lamotrigine dose. Quetiapine has been associated with increased risk of gestational diabetes and should therefore be used with caution in patients with history of or risks factors for gestational diabetes. Thankfully, Patient B does not appear to be at elevated risk of gestational diabetes, although this risk should be discussed with her obstetrician prior to starting quetiapine.

Atypical/second-generation antipsychotics are frequently used for the management of bipolar disorder, primary psychotic disorders such as schizophrenia, as well as depression augmentation. Increasing off-label use for these medications has included treatment of anxiety disorders and insomnia. There have not been data to confirm any consistent pattern of malformation or teratogenicity for second-generation antipsychotics (McCauley-Elsom et al., 2010; Yaeger et al., 2006). Due to their metabolic profile, dietary counseling should be offered to women who require medication in pregnancy. Consequences of weight gain in pregnancy can include gestational diabetes, hypertension, preeclampsia and neural tube defects. Data suggest that both quetiapine and olanzapine are associated with development of gestational diabetes in pregnancy (Park et al., 2018). Known consequences of gestational diabetes include infant hypoglycemia, large-for-gestational-age, and birth trauma for both infant and mother, including infant shoulder dystocia, fractures, and nerve palsies (Kc et al., 2015). Normal development has been documented for children up to five years of age (McCauley-Elsom et al., 2010).

Typical/first-generation antipsychotics are primarily used for the management of psychotic disorders, such as schizophrenia, and have not been associated with malformations (Einarson et al., 2009). Due to elevations of prolactin as result of D2 antagonism in the tubularinfidibular pathway, there is a risk for infertility in women taking these medications prior to pregnancy (Robinson, 2012). At the time of delivery, there have been symptoms reported in newborns including respiratory distress, difficulty feeding, floppy baby syndrome, hypertonicity, sluggish primitive reflexes, extrapyramidal symptoms, tremor, abnormal movements, irritability, and agitation (Kohen, 2004). Although most symptoms when reported have resolved within days (Kohen, 2004), there have been reports in which extrapyramidal signs lasted for weeks to months prior to resolution (Solt et al., 2002). There have been reports of decreased motor skills at six months (Johnson et al., 2012), but normal IQ at age 4 (Slone et al., 1977) and reports of normal behavior, socialization and cognition at ages 9 and 10 (Kris, 1965; Stika et al., 1990).

Conclusion and Future Directions

For years the plight of perinatal mental health disorders has been under-diagnosed, under-treated, and under-discussed. Current data suggest that one in five childbearing patients will develop a perinatal mood and anxiety disorder, with maternal suicide representing one of the leading causes of peripartum mortality, accounting for up to 20% of all postpartum deaths (Lindahl et al., 2005). Ongoing symptoms of maternal psychiatric illness during pregnancy can confer negative ramifications to mother, fetus, and pregnancy, including poor compliance with prenatal care, increased risk of spontaneous abortion, elevated rates of pre-eclampsia, neonatal growth retardation, higher rate of operative deliveries, pre-term delivery, low birth weight, and higher rates of NICU admissions (Bonari et al., 2004; Henry et al., 2004). Additionally, symptomatic disturbances during pregnancy place patients at elevated risk of postpartum decompensation, which is associated with decreased rate of initiation and continuation of breastfeeding, decreased compliance with pediatric care, and poor maternal-infant bonding (Minkovitz et al., 2005; Olson et al., 2002). Aberrations in maternal-infant bonding have been associated with offspring developing long-term difficulties in peer relationships, lower scores on cognitive testing, and higher rates of depression, anxiety, ADHD, behavioral outbursts, and substance dependence (Davis et al., 2005). Suffice to say, prenatal mental health disorders are not benign conditions, irrespective of the suffering of the patient, which we would argue is sufficient rationale for treatment in and of itself.

It is paramount that all clinicians understand the risk of untreated perinatal mental health disorders and have the knowledge and ability to counsel women during preconception, pregnancy, and the postpartum period. Over half of pregnancies in the United States are believed to be unplanned, and most women will not present for in-depth preconception counseling with an expert in reproductive psychiatry. Rather, many women will reach out to their primary psychiatric provider, primary care provider, or obstetrician upon confirmation of conception. As it is often the first point of contact and first counseling session for patients, it is important that all providers have a general understanding of the treatment of perinatal mental health disorders to provide patients with accurate and unbiased information. At minimum, clinicians should be aware that psychiatric symptoms confer an elevated risk to mother, fetus, and pregnancy, and that there are several medication options that are compatible with pregnancy and breastfeeding, and be able to refer patients if needed.

It is our hope that as the field of reproductive psychiatry continues to grow, this knowledge will become more commonplace in the educational training of mental health providers so that every clinician would have the basic information necessary to achieve the aforementioned goals. Grander than this hope, however, is the aspiration to enhance our understanding of the complexities of psychotropic medication exposure during pregnancy. Whereas there is an abundance of data available for commonly used psychotropic medications—SSRIs, SNRIs, lithium, lamotrigine, and second-generation antipsychotics—the same cannot be said for all medications that fall under the purview of a mental health specialist. For example, although benzodiazepines are a commonly prescribed medication class, the available data are often inconsistent and difficult to interpret based on the variable patterns of use. Further study to explore the impact and differentiation of common prescribing patterns (i.e., as needed administration, scheduled dosage one to three times a day) could help provide a better framework for navigating the informed consent discussion regarding benzodiazepines in pregnancy. Additionally, little is known about newer psychotropic medications that are often a necessary component of treatment for patients with treatment-resistant disorders, or those who experienced intolerable side effects from other treatment options. The impact of exposure to newer antidepressants (e.g., vortioxetine, vilazodone) or antipsychotics (e.g., lurasidone, iloperidone, brexpiprazole) will likely become more apparent as data are collected the longer the medications are on the market. Similarly, information regarding the impact of novel or interventional treatment options, such as ketamine or transcranial magnetic stimulation (TMS) will become important as these treatments become more widely available.

References

Altshuler, L. L., Cohen, L., Szuba, M. P., Burt, V. K., Gitlin, M., & Mintz, J. (1996). Pharmacologic management of psychiatric illness during pregnancy: Dilemmas and guidelines. *American Journal of Psychiatry, 153*(5), 592–606. https://doi.org/10.1176/ajp.153.5.592

Alwan, S., Reefhuis, J., Botto, L. D., Rasmussen, S. A., Correa, A., Friedman, J. M., & National Birth Defects Prevention Study. (2010). Maternal use of bupropion and risk for congenital heart defects. *American Journal of Obstetrics and Gynecology, 203*(1), 52.e1–52.e56. https://doi.org/10.1016/j.ajog.2010.02.015

Alwan, S., Reefhuis, J., Rasmussen, S. A., Olney, R. S., Friedman, J. M., & National Birth Defects Prevention Study. (2007). Use of selective serotonin-reuptake inhibitors in pregnancy and the risk of birth defects. *New England Journal of Medicine, 356*(26), 2684–2692. https://doi.org/10.1056/NEJMoa066584

Anderson, K. N., Lind, J. N., Simeone, R. M., Bobo, W. V., Mitchell, A. A., Riehle-Colarusso, T., Polen, K. N., & Reefhuis, J. (2020). Maternal use of specific antidepressant medications during early pregnancy and the risk of selected birth defects. *JAMA Psychiatry, 77*(12):1246–1255. https://doi.org/10.1001/jamapsychiatry.2020.2453

Andrade, C. (2017). Antidepressant exposure during pregnancy and risk of autism in the offspring, 1: Meta review of meta-analyses. *Journal of Clinical Psychiatry, 78*(8), e1047–e1051. https://doi.org/10.4088/jcp.18f11903

Bonari, L., Pinto, N., Ahn, E., Einarson, A., Steiner, M., & Koren, G. (2004). Perinatal risks of untreated depression during pregnancy. *Canadian Journal of Psychiatry. Revue Canadienne de Psychiatrie, 49*(11), 726–735. https://doi.org/10.1177/070674370404901103

Briggs, G. G., Freeman, R. K., Towers, C. V., & Forinash, A. B. (2021). *Drugs in pregnancy and lactation* (12th ed.). Lippincott Williams & Wilkins.

Chaudron, L. H. (2013). Complex challenges in treating depression during pregnancy. *American Journal of Psychiatry, 170*(1), 12–20. https://doi.org/10.1176/appi.ajp.2012.12040440

Chun-Fai-Chan, B., Koren, G., Fayez, I., Kalra, S., Voyer-Lavigne, S., Boshier, A., Sakir, S., & Einarson, A. (2005). Pregnancy outcome of women exposed to bupropion during pregnancy: A prospective comparative study. *American Journal of Obstetrics and Gynecology, 192*(3), 932–936. https://doi.org/10.1016/j.ajog.2004.09.027

Cohen, L. S., Altshuler, L. L., Harlow, B. L., Nonacs, R., Newport, D. J., Viguera, A. C., Suri, R, Burt, V. K., Hendrick, V., Reminick, A. M., Loughead, A., Vitonis, A. F., & Stowe, Z. N. (2006). Relapse of major depression during pregnancy in women who maintain or discontinue antidepressant treatment. *JAMA, 295*(5), 499–507. https://doi.org/10.1001/jama.295.499

Cree, J. E., Meyer, J., & Hailey, D. M. (1973). Diazepam in labour: Its metabolism and effect on the clinical condition and thermogenesis of the newborn. *British Medical Journal, 4*(5887), 251–255. https://doi.org/10.1136/bmj.4.5887.251

Cummings, C., Stewart, M., Stevenson, M., Morrow, J., & Nelson, J. (2011). Neurodevelopment of children exposed in utero to lamotrigine, sodium valproate and carbamazepine. *Archives of disease in childhood, 96*(7), 643–647. https://doi.org/10.1136/adc.2009.176990

Davis, E. P., Glynn, L. M., Dunkel Schetter, C., Hobel, C., Chicz-Demet, A., Sandman, C. A. (2005). Corticotropin-releasing hormone during pregnancy is associated with infant temperament. *Developmental Neuroscience, 27*(5), 299–305. https://doi.org/10.1159/000086709

Einarson, A., Bonari, L., Voyer-Lavigne, S., Addis, A., Matsui, D., Johnson, Y., & Koren, G. (2003). A multicentre prospective controlled study to determine the safety of trazodone and nefazodone use during pregnancy. *Canadian Journal of Psychiatry. Revue Canadienne de psychiatrie, 48*(2), 106–110. https://doi.org/10.1177/070674370304800207

Einarson, A., Choi, J., Einarson, T. R., & Koren, G. (2009). Incidence of major malformations in infants following antidepressant exposure in pregnancy: Results of a large prospective cohort study. *Canadian Journal of Psychiatry. Revue Canadienne de Psychiatrie, 54*(4), 242–246. https://doi.org/10.1177/070674370905400405

Ferreira, E., Carceller, A. M., Agogué, C., Martin, B. Z., St-André, M., Francoeur, D., & Bérard, A. (2007). Effects of selective serotonin reuptake inhibitors and venlafaxine during pregnancy in term and preterm neonates. *Pediatrics, 119*(1), 52–59. https://doi.org/10.1542/peds.2006-2133

Frayne, J., Watson, S., Snellen, M., Nguyen, T., & Galbally, M. (2021). The association between mental illness, psychotropic medication use and hypertensive disorders in pregnancy: A multicentre study. *Pregnancy Hypertension, 24*, 22–26. https://doi.org/10.1016/j.preghy.2021.02.002

Freeman, M. P., Szpunar, M. J., Kobylski, L. A., Harmon, H., Viguera, A. C., & Cohen, L. S. (2022). Pregnancy outcomes after first trimester exposure to buspirone: Prospective longitudinal outcomes from the MGH National Pregnancy Registry for Psychiatric Medications. *Archives of Women's Mental Health, 10*, 1007/s00737-022-1250-8. Advance online publication https://doi.org/10.1007/s007/s00737-022-01250-8.

Gentile, S. (2014). Tricyclic antidepressants in pregnancy and puerperium. *Expert Opinion on Drug Safety, 13*(2), 207–225. https://doi.org/10.1517/14740338.2014.869582

Grace, S. L., Evindar, A., & Stewart, D. E. (2003). The effect of postpartum depression on child cognitive development and behavior: A review and critical analysis of the literature. *Archives of Women's Mental Health, 6*(4), 263–274. https://doi.org/10.1007/s99737-003-0024-6

Grigoriadis, S., Vonderporten, E. H., Mamisashvili, L., Tomlinson, G., Dennis, C. L., Koren, G., Steiner, M., Mousmanis, P., Cheung, A., & Ross, L. E. (2014). Prenatal exposure to antidepressants and persistent pulmonary hypertension of the newborn: Systematic review and meta-analysis. *British Medical Journal (Clinical Research Ed.), 348*, f6932. https://doi.org/10.1136/bmj.f6932

Hageman, J. R., Adams, M. A., & Gardner, T. H. (1984). Persistent pulmonary hypertension of the newborn: Trends in incidence, diagnosis, and management. *American Journal of Diseases of Children (1960), 138*(6), 592–595. https://doi.org/10.1001/archpedi.1984.02140440076021

Henry, A. L., Beach, A. J., Stowe, Z. N., & Newport, D. J. (2004). The fetus and maternal depression: Implications for antenatal treatment guidelines. *Clinical Obstetrics and Gynecology, 47*(3), 535–546. https://doi.org/10.1097/01.grf.0000135341.48747.f9

Hernández-Díaz, S., Van Marter, L. J., Werler, M. M., Louik, C., & Mitchell, A, A. (2007). Risk factors for persistent pulmonary hypertension of the newborn. *Pediatrics, 120*(2), e272–e282. https://doi.org/10.1542/peds.2006-3037

Hoog, S. L., Cheng, Y., Elpers, J., & Dowsett, S. A. (2013). Duloxetine and pregnancy outcomes: Safety surveillance findings. *International Journal of Medical Sciences, 10*(4), 413–419. https://doi.org/10.7150/ijms.5213

Hu, R., Li, Y., Zhang, Z., & Yan, W. (2015). Antenatal depressive symptoms and the risk of preeclampsia or operative deliveries: A meta-analysis. *PLoS One, 10*(3), e0119018. https://doi.org/10.1371/journal.pone.0119018

Huybrechts, K. F., Bateman, B. T., Pawar, A., Bessett, L. G., Mogun, H., Levin, R., Li, H., Motsko, S., Scantamburlo Fernandes, M. F., Upadhyaya, H. P., & Hernandez-Diaz, S. (2020). Maternal and fetal outcomes following exposure to duloxetine in pregnancy: Cohort study. *British Medical Journal (Clinical Research Ed.), 368*, m237. https://doi.org/10.1136/bmj.m237

Huybrechts, K. F., Palmsten, K., Avorn, J., Cohen, L. S., Holmes, L. B., Franklin, J. M., Mogun, H., Levin, R., Kowal, M., Setoguchi, S., & Hernández-Díaz, S. (2014). Antidepressant use in pregnancy and the risk of cardiac defects. *New England Journal of Medicine, 370*(25), 2397–2407. https://doi.org/10.1056/NEJMoa1312828

Jentink, J., Loane, M. A., Dolk, H., Barisic, I., Garne, E., Morris, J. K., de Jong-van den Berg, L. T., & EUROCAT Antiepileptic Study Working Group. (2010). Valproic acid monotherapy in pregnancy and major congenital malformations. *New England Journal of Medicine, 362*(23), 2185–2193. https://doi.org/10.1056/NEJMoa0907328

Johnson, K. C., LaPrairie, J. L., Brennan, P. A., Stowe, Z. N., & Newport, D. J. (2012). Prenatal antipsychotic exposure and neuromotor performance during infancy. *Archives of General Psychiatry, 69*(8), 787–794. https://doi.org/10.1001/archgenpsychiatry.2012.160

Kc, K., Shakya, S., & Zhang, H. (2015). Gestational diabetes mellitus and macrosomia: A literature review. *Annals of Nutrition & Metabolism, 66*(Suppl. 2), 14–20.

Kieviet, N., Doman, K. M., & Honig, A. (2013). The use of psychotropic medication during pregnancy: How about the newborn? *Neuropsychiatric Disease and Treatment, 9*, 1257–1266. https://doi.org/10.2147/NDT.S36394

Kjaersgaard, M. I., Parner, E. T., Vestergaard, M., Sørensen, M. J., Olsen, J., Christensen, J., Bech, B. H., & Pedersen, L. H. (2013). Prenatal antidepressant exposure and risk of spontaneous abortion: A population-based study. *PLoS One, 8*, e72095. https://doi.org/10.1371/journal.pone.0072095

Kohen, D. (2004). Psychotropic medication in pregnancy. *Advances in Psychiatric Treatment, 10*(1), 59–66. https://doi.org/10.1192/apt.10.1.59

Kris, E. B. (1965). Children of mothers maintained on pharmacotherapy during pregnancy and postpartum. *Current Therapeutic Research, Clinical and Experimental, 7*(12), 785–789.

Lassen, D., Ennis, Z. N., & Damkier, P. (2016). First-trimester pregnancy exposure to venlafaxine or duloxetine and risk of major congenital malformations: A systematic review. *Basic & Clinical Pharmacology & Toxicology, 118*(1), 32–36. https://doi.org/19.1111/bcpt.12497

Li, D., Liu, L., & Odouli, R. (2009). Presence of depressive symptoms during early pregnancy and the risk of preterm delivery: A prospective cohort study. *Human Reproduction (Oxford, England), 24*(1), 146–153. https://doi.org/10.1093/humrep/den342

Lindahl, V., Pearson, J. L., & Colpe, L. (2005). Prevalence of suicidality during pregnancy and the postpartum. *Archives of Women's Mental Health, 8*(2), 77–87. https://doi.org/10.1007/s00737-005-0080-1

Louik, C., Kerr, S., & Mitchell, A. A. (2014). First-trimester exposure to bupropion and risk of cardiac malformations. *Pharmacoepidemiology and Drug Safety, 23*(10), 1066–1075. https://doi.org/10.1002/pds.3661

Lupattelli, A., Barone-Adesi, F., & Nordeng, H. (2022). Association between antidepressant use in pregnancy and gestational diabetes mellitus: Results from the Norwegian Mother, Father and Child Cohort study. *Pharmacoepidemiology and Drug Safety, 31*(2), 247–256. https://doi.org/10.1002/pds.5388

McCauley-Elsom, K., Gurvich, C., Elsom, S. J., & Kulkarni, J. (2010). Antipsychotics in pregnancy. *Journal of Psychiatric and Mental Health Nursing, 17*(2), 97–104. https://doi.org/10.1111/j.1365-2850.2009.01481.x

McElhatton, P. R. (1994). The effects of benzodiazepine use during pregnancy and lactation. *Reproductive Toxicology (Elmsford, N.Y.), 8*(6), 461–475. https://doi.org/10.1016/0890-6238(94)90029-9

Meador, K. J., Baker, G. A., Browning, N., Clayton-Smith, J., Combs-Cantrell, D. T., Cohen, M., Kalayjian, L. A., Kanner, A., Liporace, J. D., Pennell, P. B., Privitera, M., Loring, D. W., & NEAD Study Group. (2009). Cognitive function at 3 years of age after fetal exposure to antiepileptic drugs. *The New England Journal of Medicine, 360*(16), 1597–1605. https://doi.org/10.1056/NEJMoa0803531

Meador, K. J., Baker, G. A., Browning, N., Cohen, M. J., Bromley, R. L., Clayton-Smith, J., Kalayjian, L. A., Kanner, A., Liporace, J. D., Pennell, P. B., Privitera, M., Loring, D. W., & NEAD Study Group. (2013). Fetal antiepileptic drug exposure and cognitive outcomes at age 6 years (NEAD study): A prospective observational study. *The Lancet. Neurology, 12*(3), 244–252. https://doi.org/10.1016/S1474-4422(12)70323-X

Minkovitz, C. S., Strobino, D., Scharfstein, D., Hous, W., Miller, T., Mistry, K. B., & Swartz, K. (2005). Maternal depressive symptoms and children's receipt of health care in the first 3 years of life. *Pediatrics, 115*(2), 306–314. https://doi.org/10.1542/peds.2004-0341

Moses-Kolko, E. L., Bogen, D., Perel, J., Bregar, A., Uhl, K., Levin, B., & Wisner, K. L. (2005). Neonatal signs after late in utero exposure to serotonin reuptake inhibitors: Literature review and implications for clinical applications. *JAMA, 293*(19), 2372–2383. https://doi.org/10.1001/jama.293.19.2372

Newport. (2005). Lithium placental passage and obstetrical outcome: Implications for clinical management during late pregnancy. *American Journal of Psychiatry, 162*(11), 2162–2170. https://doi.org/10.1176/appi.ajp.162.11.2162

Nulman, I., Rovet, J., Stewart, D. E., Wolpin, J., Gardner, H. A., Theis, J. G., Kulin, N., & Koren, G. Neurodevelopment of children exposed in utero to antidepressant drugs. *New England Journal of Medicine, 336*(4), 258–262. https://doi.org/10.1056/NEJM199701233360404

Oberlander, T. F., Misri, S., Fitzgerald, C. E., Kostaras, X., Rurak, D., & Riggs, W. (2004). Pharmacologic factors associated with transient neonatal symptoms following prenatal psychotropic medication exposure. *Journal of Clinical Psychiatry, 65*(2), 230–237. https://doi.org/10.4088/jcp.v65n0214

Olson, A. L., Kemper, K. J., Kelleher, K. J., Hammond, C. S., Zuckerman, B. S., & Dietrich, A. J. (2002). Primary care pediatricians' roles and perceived responsibilities in the identification and management of maternal depression. *Pediatrics*, *110*(6), 1169–1176. https://doi.org/10.1542/peds.110.6.1169

Ornoy, A. (2018). Pharmacological treatment of attention deficit hyperactivity disorder during pregnancy and lactation. *Pharmaceutical Research*, *35*(3), 46. https://doi.org/10.1007/s11095-017-2323-z

Ostenfeld, A., Petersen, T. S., Pedersen, L. H., Westergaard, H. B., Løkkegaard, E., & Andersen, J. T. (2022). Mirtazapine exposure in pregnancy and fetal safety: A nationwide cohort study. *Acta Psychiatrica Scandinavica*, *145*(6), 557–567. https://doi.org/10.1111/acps.13431

Park, Y., Hernandez-Diaz, S., Bateman, B. T., Cohen, J. M., Desai, R. J., Patorno, E., Glynn, R. J., Cohen, L. S., Mogun, H., & Huybrechts, K. F. (2018). Continuation of atypical antipsychotic medication during early pregnancy and the risk of gestational diabetes. *American Journal of Psychiatry*, *175*(6), 564–574. https://doi.org/10.1176/appi.ajp.2018.17040393

Payne, J. L., & Meltzer-Brody, S. (2009). Antidepressant use during pregnancy: Current controversies and treatment strategies. *Clinical Obstetrics Gynecology*, *52*(3), 469–482. https://doi.org/10.1097/GRF.Ob013e3181b52e20

Pedersen, L. H., Henriksen, T. B., Vestergaard, M., Olsen, J., & Bech, B. H. (2009). Selective serotonin reuptake inhibitors in pregnancy and congenital malformations: Population based cohort study. *British Medical Journal (Clinical Research Ed.)*, *339*, b3569. https://doi.org/10.1136/bmj.b3569

Reimers, A., & Brodtkorb, E. (2012). Second-generation antiepileptic drugs and pregnancy: A guide for clinicians. *Expert Review of Neurotherapeutics*, *12*(6), 707–717. https://doi.org/10.1586/ern.12.32

Robinson, G. E. (2012). Treatment of schizophrenia in pregnancy and postpartum. *Journal of Population Therapeutics and Clinical Pharmacology = Journal de la Therapeutique des Populations et de la Pharmacologie Clinique*, *19*(3), e380–e386.

Rusner, M., Berg, M., & Begley, C. (2016). Bipolar disorder in pregnancy and childbirth: A systematic review of outcomes. *BMC Pregnancy Childbirth*, *16*(1), 331. https://doi.org/10.1186/s12884-016-1127-1

Safra, M. J., & Oakley, G. P., Jr. (1975). Association between cleft lip with or without cleft palate and prenatal exposure to diazepam. *The Lancet (London, England)*, *2*(7933), 478–480. https://doi.org/10.1016/s0140-6736(75)90548-6

Salvi, V., Barone-Adesi, F., D'Ambrosio, V., Albert, U., & Maina, G. (2016). High H1-affinity antidepressants and risk of metabolic syndrome in bipolar disorder. *Psychopharmacology*, *233*(1), 49–56. https://doi.org/10.1007/s00213-015-4085-9

Saxén, I. (1975). Associations between oral clefts and drugs taken during pregnancy. *International Journal of Epidemiology*, *4*(1), 37–44. https://doi.org/10.1093/ije/4.1.37

Sheehy, O., Zhao, J. P., & Bérard, A. (2019). Association between incident exposure to benzodiazepines in early pregnancy and risk of spontaneous abortion. *JAMA Psychiatry*, *76*(9), 948–957. https://doi.org/10.1001/jamapsychiatry.2019.0963

Sie, S. D., Wennink, J. M., van Driel, J. J., te Winkel, A. G., Boer, K., Casteelen, G., & van Weissenbruch, M. M. (2012). Maternal use of SSRIs, SNRIs and SaSSAs: Practical recommendations during pregnancy and lactation. *Archives of Disease in Childhood Fetal and Neonatal Edition*, *97*(6), F472–F476. https://doi.org/10.1136/archdischild-2011-214239

Slone, D., Siskind, V., Heinonen, O. P., Monson, R. R., Kaufman, D. W., & Shapiro, S. (1977). Antenatal exposure to the phenothiazines in relation to congenital malformations, perinatal mortality rate, birth weight, and intelligence quotient score. *American Journal of Obstetrics and Gynecology*, *128*(5), 486–488. https://doi.org/10.1016/0002-9378(77)90029-1

Solt, I., Ganadry, S., & Weiner, Z. (2002). The effect of meperidine and promethazine on fetal heart rate indices during the active phase of labor. *The Israel Medical Association Journal: IMAJ*, *4*(3), 178–180.

Stahl, S. M., & Grady, M. M. (2011). *Stahl's essential psychopharmacology: The prescriber's guide* (4th ed.). Cambridge University Press.

Stika, L., Elisová, K., Honzáková, L., Hrochová, H., Plechatová, H., Strnadová, J., Skop, B., Svihovec, J., Váchova, M., & Vinar, O. (1990). Effects of drug administration in pregnancy on children's school behavior. *Pharmaceutisch weekblad. Scientific Edition*, *12*(6), 252–255. https://doi.org/10.1007/BF01967827

Suri, R., Stowe, Z. N., Cohen, L. S., Newport, D. J., Burt, V. K., Aquino-Elias, A. R., Knight, B. T., Mintz, J., & Altshuler, L. L. (2017). Prospective longitudinal study of predictors of postpartum-onset depression in women with a history of major depressive disorder. *Journal of Clinical Psychiatry, 78*(8), 1110–1116. https://doi.org/10.4088/JCP.15m10427

Thombre, M. K., Talge, N. M., & Holzman, C. (2015). Association between pre-pregnancy depression/anxiety symptoms and hypertensive disorders of pregnancy. *Journal of Women's Health (2002), 24*(3), 228–236. https://doi.org/10.1089/jwh.2014.4902

Tran, T. A., Leppik, I. E., Blesi, K., Sathanandan, S. T., & Remmel, R. (2002). Lamotrigine clearance during pregnancy. *Neurology, 59*(2), 251–255. https://doi.org/10.1212/wnl.59.2.251

Turner, E., Jones, M., Vaz, L. R., & Coleman, T. (2019). Systematic review and meta-analysis to assess the safety of bupropion and varenicline in pregnancy. *Nicotine & Tobacco Research, 21*(8), 1001–1010. https://doi.org/10.1093/ntr/nty055

Vigod, S. N., Kurdyak, P. A., Dennis, C. L., Gruneir, A., Newman, A., Seeman, M. V., Rochon, P. A, Anderson, G. M., Grigoriadis, S., & Ray, J. G. (2014). Maternal and newborn outcomes among women with schizophrenia: A retrospective population-based cohort study. *British Journal of Obstetrics and Gynaecology, 121*(5), 566–574. https://doi.org/10.1111/1471-0528.12567

Weissman, M. M., Wickramaratne, P., Nomura, Y., Warner, V., Pilowsky, D., & Verdeli, H. (2006). Offspring of depressed parents: 20 years later. *American Journal of Psychiatry, 163*(6), 1001–1008. https://doi.org/10.1176/ajp.2006.163.6.1001

Wisner, K. L., Gelenberg, A. J., Leonard, H., Zarin, D., & Frank, E. (1999). Pharmacologic treatment of depression during pregnancy. *JAMA, 282*(13), 1264–1269. https://doi.org/10.1001/jama.282.13.1264

Wurst, K. E., Poole, C., Ephross, S. A., & Olshan, A. F. (2010). First trimester paroxetine use and the prevalence of congenital, specifically cardiac, defects: A meta-analysis of epidemiological studies. *Birth Defects Research. Part A, Clinical and Molecular Teratology, 88*(3), 159–170. https://doi.org/10.1002/bdra.20627

Yaeger, D., Smith, H. G., & Altshuler, L. L. (2006). Atypical antipsychotics in the treatment of schizophrenia during pregnancy and the postpartum. *American Journal of Psychiatry, 163*(12), 2064–2070. https://doi.org/10.1176/ajp.2006.163.12.2064

Yonkers, K. A., Gotman, N., Smith, M. V., Foray, A., Belanger, K., Brunetto, W. L., Lin, H., Burkman, R. T., Zelop, C. M., & Lockwood, C. J. (2011). Does antidepressant use attenuate the risk of major depressive episode in pregnancy? *Epidemiology (Cambridge, Mass), 22*(6), 848–854. https://doi.org/10.1097/EDE.0b013e3182306847

21

POSTPARTUM PHARMACOTHERAPY

Sophie Grigoriadis, Morgan Sterling, and Gail Erlick Robinson

Postpartum depression (PPD) is a depressive episode that occurs during the postpartum period. For the purposes of this chapter, we define postpartum as referring to the first year following childbirth. The *Diagnostic and Statistical Manual of Mental Disorders* (American Psychiatric Association, 2022) refers to the first month after birth to describe this condition, whereas the International Classification of Diseases-11 refers to it as the first six weeks (World Health Organization, 2019). Some women may experience their first depressive episode during the postpartum, whereas others experience a recurrence if they have previously suffered from depression. Women with bipolar disorder can also experience a new or recurrent depressive episode. New mothers face pressures and challenges especially during the early postpartum period, which can have an impact on their desire to seek, select, and then adhere to treatment (Mammen et al., 1997).

One of the greatest worries for new mothers in the treatment of such episodes is the potential for psychiatric medication to pass through to the infant through lactation (Pearlstein et al., 2009). One way to alleviate some of this worry is through education about the risks and benefits of taking these medications during the postpartum period. Empowering mothers through providing them with knowledge is also helpful in promoting compliance to treatment. This chapter reviews the various psychopharmacological interventions available for PPD and related conditions, with a consideration for lactation. Antidepressants, benzodiazepines, and non-benzodiazepine hypnotics, antipsychotics, and mood stabilizers are reviewed. Although stimulation treatments are not drug interventions, they are included in this chapter because they are somatic treatments and are often used when pharmacotherapy fails.

Pharmacological Interventions

Antidepressants

Antidepressants are indicated for moderate to severe depression during the postpartum, and *selective serotonin reuptake inhibitor (SSRI)* antidepressants are currently favored by most guidelines (ACOG, 2008; Austin et al., 2017; MacQueen et al., 2016; Yonkers et al., 2009). They pass through into breastmilk at different levels (Schoretsanitis et al., 2019).

DOI: 10.4324/9781003206903-26

Typically, it is recommended that the level of antidepressant found in breastmilk should be less than 10% of the mother's own level (relative infant dose, RID) to be compatible with breastfeeding. However, it has not been established that even if a drug is not detectable in breastmilk, it is indeed "safe" (Eberhard-Gran et al., 2006; Sachs & the Committee on Drugs, 2013; Stowe, 2007). Conversely, it is also not clear if measurable amounts are cause for concern (Lanza di Scalea & Wisner, 2009). Levels vary in milk according to several factors, including milk pH and lipid amounts. Milk tends to be more acidic than blood and, thus, medications that are weak bases can accumulate as opposed to more acidic ones. In general, *hind milk* (i.e., milk during second phase of feeding) is fattier and may contain more medication than the *foremilk*. Drugs that reach peak plasma concentration quickly (i.e., less than three hours, generally immediate release), if taken right after the feed, would be at low levels after a few hours (Kronenfeld et al., 2017).

SSRI antidepressants, such as sertraline, have been shown to be present in very low or undetectable amounts in the serum of the child and not thought to pose risk to the well-being of the child (Berle & Spigset, 2011; Schoretsanitis et al., 2019). Research suggests that the low levels within the child's serum do not significantly increase the reuptake of serotonin within the brain, which is the main mechanism of action for SSRIs (Lanza di Scalea & Wisner, 2009). Although case reports of babies experiencing untoward effects such as colic, irritability, and feeding problems, have been reported with exposure to SSRIs, they are confounded by indication and are nonspecific and, thus, may be due to other causes. For example, colic is also a risk when a mother is experiencing depression; longitudinal studies have found PPD associated with infant cholic (Akman et al., 2006; Bang et al., 2020). Factors such as prematurity or kidney/liver impairment can affect the levels found in the infant (Kim et al., 2014). Data on long-term neurodevelopment for the infant exposed to medication via lactation are limited, but to our knowledge, there is no evidence of significance (Orsolini, 2015). The prenatal literature is also reassuring, as exposure in pregnancy (where the concentrations are much higher than through lactation) has not been associated with consistent neurocognitive issues (Rommel et al., 2020).

Although there are preferred antidepressants as "first-line" (e.g., sertraline, escitalopram, citalopram) (MacQueen et al., 2016), it is not recommended a mother switch an antidepressant from pregnancy to postpartum if she is responding to the medication. This is because the infant will receive less during lactation than in pregnancy (about five to ten times) (Kim et al., 2014) and there are no data showing significant risk within the SSRI class or one drug being safer than another (Howard et al., 2014; Ray & Stowe, 2014; Schoretsanitis et al., 2019). Switching also increases the risk for recurrence or relapse in the mother, and the infant will have two medication exposures (Howard et al., 2014). However, the child should always be monitored for changes in behavior, such as sedation or agitation, irritability, excessive crying, or poor weight gain. A breastmilk serum analysis can be requested specifically if there are concerns, as this is not routinely done regardless of SSRI used. In general, it is not recommended a women pump out her breastmilk at the time of expected peak concentration, as there are no data to support this practice, and it creates an extra burden on the mother (Berle & Spigset, 2011; McAllister-Williams et al., 2017).

The *serotonin and norepinephrine reuptake inhibitors* (SNRIs), such as venlafaxine, desvenlafaxine or duloxetine, are not first-line, as less is known about them during lactation. The limited observational studies have not reported adverse events in the exposed infants, but the levels in breastmilk of venlafaxine/desvenlafaxine have been found to be higher than the SSRIs, although undetectable levels have also been found (Anderson, 2021; Briggs et al.,

2009; Collin-Lévesque et al., 2018; Ilett et al., 2002; Newport et al., 2009; Schoretsanitis et al., 2019). Other antidepressants like bupropion and mirtazapine have also not been well studied, but data suggest levels in milk are low (Davis et al., 2009; Kristensen et al., 2007). There have been two case reports of seizure in infants exposed to bupropion (Chaudron & Schoenecker, 2004; Neuman et al., 2014). Too little information is known about vortioxetine, vilazodone, and trazodone to recommend it for lactating mothers. The older *tricyclic antidepressants* (TCAs) are not used as often as SSRIs, but nortriptyline has been found to be present in low levels in breastmilk. Other TCAs like imipramine, amitriptyline, clomipramine and desipramine are found in low levels (Burt et al., 2001; Fortinguerra et al., 2009; Misri & Sivertz, 1991; Yoshida et al., 1997), but these drugs have more side effects than the SSRIs, including sedation, orthostatic hypotension, and constipation and can be lethal in overdose and generally are not used. Doxepin is also not used because its active metabolite has a long half-life and can accumulate (Gentile, 2014; Lanza di Scalea & Wisner, 2009). *Monoamine oxidase inhibitors* (MAOIs) are also not recommended while a mother is breastfeeding her baby, again because there is not enough information on them, and there is a danger of sudden increase in blood pressure (Calvi et al., 2021; Eberhard-Gran et al., 2006; Payne & Meltzer-Brody, 2009).

Recently, a GABA-A modulator class has been introduced in the United States. In 2019, the FDA-approved *brexanolone* for the treatment of moderate to severe PPD. This drug is an exogenous analog of allopregnanolone, a progesterone metabolite derivative. Its mechanism of action is not totally understood, but it is thought to involve $GABA_A$ receptors (Leader et al., 2019). GABA is a neurotransmitter that affects the central nervous system. The drug may reestablish the effects of $GABA_A$ receptors, re-establish $GABA_A$ transmembrane channels that are not functioning properly, and act like a progesterone metabolite (Edinoff et al., 2021). It must be administered as an intravenous infusion and delivered over 60 hours. Thus, it can only be administered in specialized centers. Initially 30 µg/kg/hour is given from hour 0 to 4, then 60 µg/kg/hour infused from hour 4 to 24, and lastly 90 µg/kg/hour infused for the past 24 to 52 hours. The dosage is reduced from hours 52 to 56 to 60 µg/kg/hour, 30 µg/kg/hour for hours 56–60 hours, and then stopped at the 60-hour mark. The most common side effects are sedation or somnolence, dry mouth, loss of consciousness, and flushing. The mother cannot breastfeed during treatment, as this was not done in the studies with the drug. The available evidence, however, showed the medication rapidly disappeared from breastmilk (Dyer, 2019; Food and Drug Administration, 2021). The advantage of this new medication is that it has a rapid onset of action, within 60 hours, but it is only available through a restricted program to those who can afford it. To our knowledge, it is not available worldwide.

Benzodiazepines and Non-Benzodiazepine Hypnotics

Benzodiazepines are often prescribed as an adjunct to an antidepressant at treatment initiation for PPD or for occasional use when anxiety is overwhelming. There is not a large amount of research on the topic of benzodiazepine use during the postpartum, and the data generally suggest that there is passage into the breastmilk in low amounts. Infants under six weeks have difficulty metabolizing benzodiazepines, so they should be used very cautiously. To reduce infant exposure, mothers can avoid breastfeeding when the levels would be highest in breastmilk after ingestion. It is recommended to use the medication only occasionally, if possible, as opposed to regularly. When starting a benzodiazepine with an antidepressant for very anxious mothers, perinatal psychiatrists recommend keeping daily use to about two weeks (Stewart & Vigod, 2019). Generally, intermediate acting benzodiazepines with known lower levels in breastmilk, such as lorazepam, are preferred (ACOG, 2008; Kelly et al., 2012). Shorter acting ones (i.e., alprazolam) run the risk of rebound anxiety in the mother. There have been reports of infants experiencing sedation and respiratory distress likely due to benzodiazepine accumulation but the risk of these, and other adverse effects, occurring is extremely low. As a precaution, mothers may want to assess their infant for any signs of central nervous system depression, irritability, or issues with feeding and weight gain. Mothers with infants who have medical issues with known risk to poorly metabolize drugs should be especially cautious.

Hypnotics, which are generally known as the "z" drugs, can be used for insomnia during the postpartum. Paying attention to half-life is recommended. Zolpidem and zopiclone have shorter half-lives than that of benzodiazepines, which makes them the preferred choice (Fortinguerra et al., 2009). Regardless however, they do pass into the breastmilk, albeit at low levels, and the infant should be monitored for sedation (Pons et al., 1989). Alternate options that can be used for sleep, off label, in a lactating woman include sedating antihistamines, such as doxylamine (doxylamine combined with pyridoxine is used as an antinausea agent in pregnant women); diphenhydramine and hydroxyzine are also options and although less studied, are found in low levels in breastmilk (So et al., 2010). Antidepressants with sedating side effects are also options such as trazodone, mirtazapine, and amitriptyline (McLafferty et al., 2018). Low-dose (10–20 mg) amitriptyline is as an effective nonaddictive sleep agent and preferred because of known low levels in breastmilk.

Antipsychotics

There are at least two indications for using an antipsychotic in treating PPD. Severe depressive episodes can present with psychotic symptoms (i.e., hallucinations, delusions and/ or thought disorder), and these symptoms would require specific treatment. Women with known bipolar disorder can also develop depression during this time and antipsychotics can be used as mood stabilizers. Depression with psychotic features generally requires admission to a hospital and is likely a psychiatric emergency (Nager et al., 2008). A psychotic depression has predominantly depressive symptoms and requires antidepressant treatment; the antipsychotic would target the psychotic symptoms and would not be used for as long as the antidepressant. Depression in women with bipolar disorder is generally similar to a unipolar depressive episode in terms of presentation but differs in treatment. The use of antipsychotics in bipolar depression is for their mood stabilization as recommended by several guidelines (Royal Australian and New Zealand College of Psychiatrists Clinical Practice Guidelines Team for Bipolar Disorder, 2004; Yatham et al., 2018).

Nursing at such a difficult time may pose further risks, but there is some information on the safety of older antipsychotics, although limited, and less so for the newer atypical antipsychotics. Drugs that have been available for many years, such as haloperidol alongside the atypical antipsychotics' quetiapine, and olanzapine pass in low quantities into breastmilk (Pacchiarotti et al., 2016). Chlorpromazine has also been available for decades, and we have data that it can be associated with developmental delay in children who are exposed to high quantities in terms of percentage in breastmilk (Klinger et al., 2013) but this may have been a function of polytherapy. Clozapine, which is used in cases of refractory treatment should only be used when explicitly necessary and should be paired with ongoing monitoring of white blood cell count in the child as is done in adults who take the drug (Cohen & Monden, 2013). Ziprasidone and aripiprazole are drugs with limited data and thus not first choice when the mother is lactating (Gentile, 2004).

Mood Stabilizers

Mood stabilizers are indicated for treatment of bipolar disorder. Women with this condition are vulnerable to experience a depressive episode, as the sleep deprivation of this life stage can be a trigger (Gold & Sylvia, 2016). As with the nature of the illness, a depressive episode may be followed by a manic episode, which may include unpredictable behavior, and other risks for harm (Sharma et al., 2020). As a result, the decision to breastfeed must take into account how to manage the nights to minimize sleep disruption. Mood stabilizers carry the most potential for adverse effects on the child exposure during lactation, among the currently used psychotropics.

Lithium is commonly used to treat bipolar disorder in the general population. Unfortunately, it is excreted at relatively high levels in breastmilk (as high as 50% of mother's level) (Moretti et al., 2003). In the past, it was contraindicated in breastfeeding, but now is a relative contraindication. It can be used safely at appropriate doses but requires infant monitoring. For example, it can lead to gastric issues for the child, such as vomiting and diarrhea, which in turn increases the risk for dehydration (Newmark et al., 2019). At very high doses, a child may experience cyanosis, hypotonia, and hypothermia which would indicate toxicity (Fortinguerra et al., 2009). Therefore, child's blood lithium, thyroid, and kidney function should be monitored on a two- to three-month continuing schedule (Khan et al., 2016). This vigilance however, may pose further stress on a postpartum mother, which can also increase her risk for destabilization.

Lamotrigine, the mood stabilizer of choice for use in pregnancy, has the potential to be present in quantities of up to 50% of the mother's serum concentration (which spikes postdelivery) in breastmilk (Blume, 2003). Despite this, however, there have been no significant effects on the infant reported (Blume, 2003; Uguz & Sharma, 2016). Lamotrigine has the very rare but extremely dangerous side effect of Steven-Johnson syndrome, which occurs in 1 in 1,000 people who use it. Theoretically, this risk also occurs through exposure during lactation, but to date, it has not been reported in breastfeeding infants (Biederman et al., 2010; Newport et al., 2008). Valproic acid and carbamazepine, although thought to be compatible with breastfeeding, have been associated with liver abnormalities in adults and, therefore, recommended that the child is monitored for hepatic dysfunction, drug levels, and general liver functioning (Perucca, 2002) if used at all. It is important to mention that valproic acid is associated with serious side effects in women, such as poly cystic ovarian disease and generally should be avoided (Okanović, 2016).

Brain Stimulation

Repetitive Transcranial Magnetic Stimulation

Repetitive transcranial magnetic stimulation (rTMS) is a noninvasive method for treating depression and is particularly appealing for nursing mothers. A magnetic coil is held against the patient's skull, and an electric current is sent through the coil and into the brain to change the rate of neuronal activity in that particular area. It is well tolerated, with few side effects, and if they occur, they are typically mild and temporary, such as headaches and temporary dizziness. Severe adverse effects are exceedingly rare (Hebel et al., 2020), but an epileptic seizure is possible and mitigated with safety guidelines (Rossi et al., 2021). It also has an advantage over electroconvulsive therapy (ECT), as it does not require anesthesia, nor does it induce significant downtime. The one not insignificant barrier to treatment especially for postpartum mothers is the time commitment. As the "repetitive" name suggests, women can be expected to attend clinic for treatment five days a week for up to eight weeks. There are studies looking at at-home options for more convenience, but there are little data for this population currently. This commitment for postpartum women to attend daily appointments may be overwhelming.

Electroconvulsive Therapy

Electroconvulsive therapy (ECT) is an effective treatment reserved for severe PPD. It is also an option when other treatments have failed and has an advantage when a rapid response is necessary. When offering this therapy to mothers, it is particularly important to dispel myths associated with the treatment that stem from how it is portrayed in media and common culture. Current procedures involve a lower level of electric stimulation, which lowers the chances and severity of any side effects (Sackeim, 2017). ECT is performed under general anesthesia with a muscle relaxant to avoid discomfort during the process. Following sedation, minor electric current is applied to the brain, which, in turn, triggers an intentional mild seizure. This seizure is thought to dramatically alter brain chemistry and aid in symptom regression (Bolwig, 2011).

After the procedure, some may experience confusion that may last a few hours up to a few days. There is the potential for some minor retrograde amnesia, but this usually resolves a few weeks after treatment ends (Brodaty et al., 2001). Some people may experience some jaw pain, headaches, or nausea the day of treatment, but these too subside quickly in general. This procedure also carries the general risks of anesthesia; these drugs do transfer into breastmilk but at very low levels, posing low risk for the child (Dalal et al., 2014). Recommending ECT in lactating women is consistent with treatment guidelines around the world, and feeds can be resumed when the mother recovers from the anesthesia (MacQueen et al., 2016; McAllister-Williams et al., 2017; National Institute for Health and Care Excellence., 2014).

ECT can be done in both outpatient and inpatient settings. ECT requires a series of treatments repeated two to three times per week for three to four weeks, so the time commitment may also be a barrier for some new mothers. It requires follow-up, which may include the addition of medication, psychotherapy, or continued treatment with ECT periodically. ECT should not be used in patients who have heart conditions or recent brain bleeds.

Efficacy and Effectiveness

Antidepressants

There is a paucity of studies on the effectiveness of antidepressants in the treatment of depression during the postpartum, but the results generally compare to the effectiveness of non-postpartum populations (National Institute for Health and Care Excellence, 2014). There are about ten randomized control trials (RCTs) that examine antidepressants for PPD. One of the first studied with fluoxetine compared it to placebo (both had adjunct counseling) (Appleby et al., 1997). The only study to compare an SSRI to a TCA found that sertraline was not superior to nortriptyline (Wisner et al., 2006). Most existing studies have examined SSRIs (i.e., sertraline, paroxetine, citalopram) either to placebo (Hantsoo et al., 2014; Yonkers et al., 2008) another drug or psychotherapy (Bloch et al., 2012;

Milgrom et al., 2015; Misri et al., 2004; O'Hara et al., 2019); One study compared a variety of antidepressants mostly SSRIs (Sharp et al., 2010). In a four-week trial, 254 mothers with PPD taking a number of antidepressants (mostly SSRIs) or with usual care found women on medication showed greater improvement (45% compared to 20%). Over 40% of the women in the trial were breastfeeding. The RCT examining a TCA was amitriptyline compared to a group problem-solving therapy (Chibanda et al., 2014; Misri et al., 2006); Uncontrolled studies exist for venlafaxine (Cohen et al., 2001), bupropion (Nonacs et al., 2005), as well as sertraline (Stowe et al., 1995). Most of the existing evidence is based on small sample sizes, some have high dropout rates (i.e., with nortriptyline), and all have only short-term follow-up.

A recent Cochrane review found 11 RCTs including 1,016 women who were treated with antidepressants, mostly SSRIs, for 4 to 12 weeks (Brown et al., 2021); The women were primarily from English-speaking high-income countries, with only two from middle income. Meta-analysis of the effect sizes found SSRIs were superior to placebo in women for both response (55% compared to 43%; pooled risk ratio [RR] = 1.27, 95% confidence interview [CI] = 0.97 to 1.66) and especially remission (42% compared to 27%; RR = 1.54, 95% CI = 0.99 to 2.41). Interestingly, although it was not possible to summarize data for adverse effects, there were no differences in acceptability of SSRIs and placebo. Although effects on breastfed infants were limited, no adverse effects were reported. High rates of attrition were noted, as well as possible bias, and this affected the certainty of the evidence. It was not possible to summarize data on SSRIs compared to other classes of antidepressants nor to other kinds of treatments. The authors concluded the evidence remains limited.

The efficacy for brexanolone is supported by an open label study and three RCTs (Kanes et al., 2017; Kanes et al., 2017; Meltzer-Brody et al., 2018). Women received the drug intravenously over a 60-hour duration and then followed up within a week and one month. A statistically significant reduction in depression scores was demonstrated over placebo in all three RCTs. Regardless of illness severity, drug was superior to placebo at hour 60, and this was maintained at day 30. Interestingly women's depression scores improved by hour 24. Response and remission were 50% versus 25% and 75% versus 55% (brexanolone vs. placebo) at 60 hours. The side effects, however, included sedation and loss of consciousness; this led to the drug being available only through a special program for women who can afford it.

Other Drugs

The efficacy of mood stabilizers, antipsychotics, and benzodiazepines during the postpartum is extrapolated from the general adult literature. In small studies in which these drugs were used during the postpartum, safety during lactation is typically examined, but the literature is not extensive.

Brain Stimulation

There have been several studies evaluating the use of rTMS for treating PPD in which rTMS was found to be beneficial, safe, and well tolerated with high remission rates (Brock et al., 2016; Cox et al., 2020; Garcia et al., 2010; Myczkowski et al., 2012). A recent meta-analysis of five studies found the effect size of rTMS peripartum depression was significant at 1.40 (95% CI = 0.94 to 1.84). The treatment was found to be tolerable without significant side effects (Lee et al., 2021). Observational studies have shown that ECT is helpful for PPD and safe in lactation (Anderson & Reti, 2009; McAllister-Williams et al., 2017; Robakis & Williams, 2013). A review of 87 postpartum women demonstrated that ECT was efficacious and well tolerated (Gressier et al., 2015). Another study that was also a retrospective review that used a registry locating 99 postpartum depressed patients showed that 81% responded (Rundgren et al., 2018). However, given that the data are only based on case reports, further investigation is necessary. With regard to rTMS, multicenter RCTs have yet to be done; thus, we need more information to know who would be the best candidate for this intervention.

Cultural Considerations

Postpartum mental health disorders are experienced by women around the world. Antidepressants are generally available across the globe, albeit more readily available in some countries. Moreover, medications are typically more available across the world than structured psychotherapies. It is known that postpartum rituals can have an impact on the disorder (Bina, 2008; Grigoriadis et al., 2009). What is less well understood is the impact of culture on treatment availability and selection by the mother. In European countries and Australia, there are many mother-baby units available where mother and baby are admitted together. There, pharmacotherapy would be readily available as needed. In the United Kingdom, the public health system provides home monitoring often through general practitioners or midwives. In Sweden, almost all perinatal women come in contact with services (in pregnancy and then postpartum). In Australia, the government has set up specific initiatives for the best provision of postpartum care. In the United States and Canada, programs for the identification of women at risk for depression during the perinatal period also exist (Evagorou et al., 2016). It is not a leap to assume, then, that in those countries, women who could benefit from pharmacotherapy may be more readily identified. In countries where the illness is not recognized as a serious one, such as in some South American counties, Africa, the Middle East, or Asian countries, access to pharmacotherapy may be limited. These countries leave the care of the postpartum woman to the family where many have postpartum rituals aimed at providing the mother with support and rest and a smoother transition (Evagorou et al., 2016).

Dissemination

Dissemination of pharmacotherapy for postpartum mental health disorders, such as PPD, requires ongoing worldwide initiatives. Although some countries, such as Australia, have made strides into creating programs for women with PPD, others fall behind. The countries that leave the care of the mother and infant to the family have rightly identified the need for support and rest, but much needs to be done to recognize PPD as a serious illness. Once PPD takes its place among serious psychiatric illness, the dissemination of pharmacological treatment will follow suit. Education of new mothers about the risks/benefits will be essential.

Case of Woman With Postpartum Depression

Ms. S is a 29-year-old mother. She delivered her first child one month ago following a difficult labor although the baby was born healthy. She has been trying to breastfeed him, but the baby is fussy and will not latch easily. She began developing symptoms almost immediately

---

after birth including depressed mood, anxiety with ruminations, frequent tearfulness, indecision, guilt that she is a poor mother, insomnia, and suicidal ruminations. Her symptoms are bewildering, as she has never experienced them before. After a visit to her postpartum care provider, she has been diagnosed with PPD and advised to start antidepressant medication. She is reluctant to start, as she wants to breastfeed but acknowledges that she can barely cope with the baby being fussy and having to try to breastfeed around the clock. Nights are the worst time, she said, as the baby has a "witching hour" and she lays awake, waiting for it. This experience is not at all what she expected, and although she could not wait to deliver as she was so excited, now she looks at the baby almost indifferently. At times, she feels anger toward the baby but realizes that he is helpless. She has had fantasies of running away, and once, she did pack a bag, and when the baby cried, she left the room and then sat in front of the television as the baby continued to cry. She often wondered if he would be better off if she were dead but each time the thought stopped when she thought of her husband whom she then felt sorry for.

This mother has depression of moderate severity. It is concerning that she has suicidal ruminations, has had escape fantasies, and has left the baby crying. She is not bonding with the baby, and if left untreated, she may not care for him in a sensitive manner. It would be very important to make sure she does not have psychotic nor manic symptoms, as these conditions affect the decision as to whether an antipsychotic or mood stabilizer will be needed. Given she has not been depressed in the past, we do not have guidance of previous response, so the drugs with more information on breastfeeding, sertraline or escitalopram, seem appropriate. The latter drug does not have many dose changes, so it has an advantage there. We would need to educate her on the potential side effects of the antidepressant and that low levels (below the 10% threshold) have been reported in breastmilk. We would not advise her to time the feeds, but rather, we would educate her on the importance of getting more sleep, accepting support, and taking breaks from looking after the baby. Pumping breastmilk may help her keep up her supply but may also cause unnecessary burden and stress. She needs to be reassured that formula is an adequate replacement and that it will be important to allow someone else to do some of the night feedings. She would be expected to respond in a few weeks, but we may need to increase the dose before she starts to feel better. Once she feels back to her normal self (likely in few weeks to two months), she will need to continue using the drug for about another six to nine months. We would also educate her on her elevated risk for developing PPD with a subsequent delivery.

Conclusions and Future Directions

The evidence for pharmacotherapy is not vast. Not only are more studies needed, but we also need to understand which treatments would work best for which women. Are there specific drugs that are superior in efficacy, as well as with fewer side effects specifically for women who are postpartum? Risk-benefit decisions continue to remain individualized, but much more information is required to inform the discussions. RCTs with large numbers of women across cultures are needed. Time-to-response is particularly sensitive for postpartum women, given that they need to focus on mothering. Although rapidly acting treatments are being developed, their cost remains prohibitive for many. Until these treatments are affordable, such as by being subsidized by government, they will not be viable. Brain stimulation treatments at home appear promising.

Acknowledgments

We would like to thank Needi Sharma, BSc, for her assistance with the manuscript. There was no funding for this manuscript. Sophie Grigoriadis received support from the Department of Psychiatry, Sunnybrook Health Sciences Centre.

Conflict of Interest Statement

Grigoriadis report royalties from UpToDate Inc for materials on perinatal depression, royalties from the Canadian Pharmacists Association for materials on depression and Norton for materials on psychotherapy for depression. None of the other authors report any potential conflicts.

References

ACOG. (2008). ACOG Practice Bulletin: Clinical management guidelines for obstetrician-gynecologists number 92, April 2008 (replaces practice bulletin number 87, November 2007). Use of psychiatric medications during pregnancy and lactation. *Obstetrics & Gynecology, 111*(4), 1001–1020. https://doi.org/10.1097/AOG.0b013e31816fd910

Akman, I., Kuşçu, K., Ozdemir, N., Yurdakul, Z., Solakoglu, M., Orhan, L., Karabekiroglu, A., & Ozek, E. (2006). Mothers' postpartum psychological adjustment and infantile colic. *Archives of Disease in Childhood, 91*(5), 417–419. https://doi.org/10.1136/adc.2005.083790

American Psychiatric Association. (2022). *Diagnostic and statistical manual of mental disorders* (5th ed., text rev.). American Psychiatric Association. https://doi.org/10.1176/appi.books.9780890425787

Anderson, E. L., & Reti, I. M. (2009). ECT in pregnancy: A review of the literature from 1941 to 2007. *Psychosomatic Medicine, 71*(2), 235–242. https://doi.org/10.1097/PSY.0b013e318190d7ca

Anderson, P. O. (2021). Antidepressants and breastfeeding. *Breastfeeding Medicine, 16*(1), 5–7. https://doi.org/10.1089/bfm.2020.0350

Appleby, L., Warner, R., Whitton, A., & Faragher, B. (1997). A controlled study of fluoxetine and cognitive-behavioural counselling in the treatment of postnatal depression. *British Medical Journal, 314*(7085), 932–936. https://doi.org/10.1136/bmj.314.7085.932

Austin, M.P., Highet, N., & the Expert Working Group. (2017). *Mental health care in the perinatal period: Australian clinical practice guideline*. Centre of Perinatal Excellence.

Bang, K. S., Lee, I., Kim, S., Yi, Y., Huh, I., Jang, S. Y., Kim, D., & Lee, S. (2020). Relation between mother's *taekyo*, prenatal and postpartum depression, and infant's temperament and colic: A longitudinal prospective approach. *International Journal of Environmental Research and Public Health, 17*(20), 7691. doi: 10.3390/ijerph17207691

Berle, J. O., & Spigset, O. (2011). Antidepressant use during breastfeeding. *Current Women's Health Review, 7*(1), 28–34. https://doi.org/10.2174/157340411794474784

Biederman, J., Joshi, G., Mick, E., Doyle, R., Georgiopoulos, A., Hammerness, P., Kotarski, M., Williams, C., & Wozniak, J. (2010). A prospective open-label trial of lamotrigine monotherapy in children and adolescents with bipolar disorder. *CNS Neuroscience and Therapeutics, 16*(2), 91–102. https://doi.org/10.1111/j.1755-5949.2009.00121.x

Bina, R. (2008). The impact of cultural factors upon postpartum depression: A literature review. *Health Care for Women International, 29*(6), 568–592.

Bloch, M., Meiboom, H., Lorberblatt, M., Bluvstein, I., Aharonov, I., & Schreiber, S. (2012). The effect of sertraline add-on to brief dynamic psychotherapy for the treatment of postpartum depression: A randomized, double-blind, placebo-controlled study. *Journal of Clinical Psychiatry, 73*(2), 235–241. https://doi.org/10.4088/JCP.11m07117

Blume, W. T. (2003). Diagnosis and management of epilepsy. *Canadian Medical Association Journal*, *168*(4), 441–448. www.ncbi.nlm.nih.gov/pubmed/12591787

Bolwig, T. G. (2011). How does electroconvulsive therapy work? Theories on its mechanism. *Canadian Journal of Psychiatry*, *56*(1), 13–18. https://doi.org/10.1177/070674371105600104

Briggs, G. G., Ambrose, P. J., Ilett, K. F., Hackett, L. P., Nageotte, M. P., & Padilla, G. (2009). Use of duloxetine in pregnancy and lactation. *Annals of Pharmacotherapy*, *43*(11), 1898–1902. https://doi.org/10.1345/aph.1M317

Brock, D. G., Demitrack, M. A., Groom, P., Holbert, R., Rado, J. T., Gross, P. K., . . . Weeks, H. R. (2016). Effectiveness of NeuroStar transcranial magnetic stimulation (TMS) in patients with major depressive disorder with postpartum onset. *Brain Stimulation*, *9*(5), e7. https://doi.org/10.1016/j.brs.2016.06.023

Brodaty, H., Berle, D., Hickie, I., & Mason, C. (2001). "Side effects" of ECT are mainly depressive phenomena and are independent of age. *Journal of Affective Disorders*, *66*(2–3), 237–245. https://doi.org/10.1016/s0165-0327(00)00314-1

Brown, J. V. E., Wilson, C. A., Ayre, K., Robertson, L., South, E., Molyneaux, E., . . . Khalifeh, H. (2021). Antidepressant treatment for postnatal depression. *Cochrane Database Systemic Review*, *2*, CD013560. https://doi.org/10.1002/14651858.CD013560.pub2

Burt, V. K., Suri, R., Altshuler, L., Stowe, Z., Hendrick, V. C., & Muntean, E. (2001). The use of psychotropic medications during breast-feeding. *American Journal of Psychiatry*, *158*(7), 1001–1009. https://doi.org/10.1176/appi.ajp.158.7.1001

Calvi, A., Fischetti, I., Verzicco, I., Belvederi Murri, M., Zanetidou, S., Volpi, R., Coghi, P., Tedeschi, S., Amore, M., & Cabassi, A. (2021). Antidepressant drugs effects on blood pressure. *Frontiers in Cardiovascular Medicine*, *8*, 704281. https://doi.org/10.3389/fcvm.2021.704281

Chaudron, L. H., & Schoenecker, C. J. (2004). Bupropion and breastfeeding: A case of a possible infant seizure. *Journal of Clinical Psychiatry*, *65*(6), 881–882. https://doi.org/10.4088/jcp.v65n0622f

Chibanda, D., Shetty, A. K., Tshimanga, M., Woelk, G., Stranix-Chibanda, L., & Rusakaniko, S. (2014). Group problem-solving therapy for postnatal depression among HIV-positive and HIV-negative mothers in Zimbabwe. *Journal of the International Association of Providers of AIDS Care*, *13*(4), 335–341. www.ncbi.nlm.nih.gov/pubmed/25513030

Cohen, D., & Monden, M. (2013). White blood cell monitoring during long-term clozapine treatment. *American Journal of Psychiatry*, *170*(4), 366–369. https://doi.org/10.1176/appi.ajp.2012.12081036

Cohen, L. S., Viguera, A. C., Bouffard, S. M., Nonacs, R. M., Morabito, C., Collins, M. H., & Ablon, J. S. (2001). Venlafaxine in the treatment of postpartum depression. *Journal of Clinical Psychiatry*, *62*(8), 592–596. https://doi.org/10.4088/jcp.v62n0803

Collin-Lévesque, L., El-Ghaddaf, Y., Genest, M., Jutras, M., Leclair, G., Weisskopf, E., Panchaud, A., & Ferreira, E. (2018). Infant exposure to methylphenidate and duloxetine during lactation. *Breastfeeding Medicine*, *13*(3), 221–225. https://doi.org/10.1089/bfm.2017.0126

Cox, E. Q., Killenberg, S., Frische, R., McClure, R., Hill, M., Jenson, J., Pearson, B., & Meltzer-Brody, S. E. (2020). Repetitive transcranial magnetic stimulation for the treatment of postpartum depression. *Journal of Affective Disorders*, *264*, 193–200. https://doi.org/10.1016/j.jad.2019.11.069

Dalal, P. G., Bosak, J., & Berlin, C. (2014). Safety of the breast-feeding infant after maternal anesthesia. *Pediatric Anesthesis*, *24*(4), 359–371. https://doi.org/10.1111/pan.12331

Davis, M. F., Miller, H. S., & Nolan, P. E. (2009). Bupropion levels in breast milk for 4 mother-infant pairs: More answers to lingering questions. *Journal of Clinical Psychiatry*, *70*(2), 297–298. https://doi.org/10.4088/jcp.07l03133

Dyer, O. (2019). Postpartum depression: New drug will be monitored at approved sites. *British Medical Journal*, *364*, 1400.

Eberhard-Gran, M., Eskild, A., & Opjordsmoen, S. (2006). Use of psychotropic medications in treating mood disorders during lactation: Practical recommendations. *CNS Drugs*, *20*(3), 187–198. https://doi.org/10.2165/00023210-200620030-00002

Edinoff, A. N., Odisho, A. S., Lewis, K., Kaskas, A., Hunt, G., Cornett, E. M., Kaye, A. D., Kaye, A., Morgan, J., Barrilleaux, P. S., Lewis, D., Viswanath, O., & Urits, I. (2021). Brexanolone, a GABA(A) modulator, in the treatment of postpartum depression in adults: A comprehensive review. *Frontiers in Psychiatry*, *12*, 699740. https://doi.org/10.3389/fpsyt.2021.699740

Evagorou, O., Arvaniti, A., & Samakouri, M. (2016). Cross-cultural approach of postpartum depression: Manifestation, practices applied, risk factors and therapeutic interventions. *Psychiatric Quarterly*, *87*, 129–154. https://doi.org/DOI 10.1007/s11126-015-9367-1

Food and Drug Administration. (2021). *sNDA 211371 S-007 multi-disciplinary review and evaluation ZULRESSO (brexanolone) injection, for intravenous use.* www.accessdata.fda.gov/drugsatfda_docs/label/201 9/211371

Fortinguerra, F., Clavenna, A., & Bonati, M. (2009). Psychotropic drug use during breastfeeding: A review of the evidence. *Pediatrics, 124*(4), e547–e556. https://doi.org/10.1542/peds.2009-0326

Garcia, K. S., Flynn, P., Pierce, K. J., & Caudle, M. (2010). Repetitive transcranial magnetic stimulation treats postpartum depression. *Brain Stimulation, 3*(1), 36–41. https://doi.org/10.1016/j.brs.2009.06.001

Gentile, S. (2004). Clinical utilization of atypical antipsychotics in pregnancy and lactation. *Annals of Pharmacotherapy, 38*(7–8), 1265–1271. https://doi.org/10.1345/aph.1D485

Gentile, S. (2014). Tricyclic antidepressants in pregnancy and puerperium. *Expert Opinion on Drug Safety, 13*(2), 207–225. https://doi.org/10.1517/14740338.2014.869582

Gold, A. K., & Sylvia, L. G. (2016). The role of sleep in bipolar disorder. *Nature and Science of Sleep, 8*, 207–214. https://doi.org/10.2147/NSS.S85754

Gressier, F. R. S., Rotenberg, S., Cazas, O., & Hardy, P. (2015). Postpartum electroconvulsive therapy: A systematic review and case report. *General Hospital Psychiatry, 37*(4), 310–314.

Grigoriadis, S., Robinson, G. E., Fung, K., Ross, L. E., Chee, C., Dennis, C. L., & Romans, S. (2009). Traditional postpartum practices and rituals: Clinical implications. *Canadian Journal of Psychiatry, 54*(12), 834–840.

Hantsoo, L., Ward-O'Brien, D., Czarkowski, K. A., Gueorguieva, R., Price, L. H., & Epperson, C. N. (2014). A randomized, placebo-controlled, double-blind trial of sertraline for postpartum depression. *Psychopharmacology (Berlin), 231*(5), 939–948. https://doi.org/10.1007/s00213-013-3316-1

Hebel, T., Schecklmann, M., & Langguth, B. (2020). Transcranial magnetic stimulation in the treatment of depression during pregnancy: A review. *Archives of Women's Mental Health, 23*(4), 469–478. https://doi.org/10.1007/s00737-019-01004-z

Howard, L. M., Molyneaux, E., Dennis, C. L., Rochat, T., Stein, A., & Milgrom, J. (2014). Nonpsychotic mental disorders in the perinatal period. *The Lancet, 384*(9956), 1775–1788. https://doi.org/10.1016/S0140-6736(14)61276-9

Ilett, K. F., Kristensen, J. H., Hackett, L. P., Paech, M., Kohan, R., & Rampono, J. (2002). Distribution of venlafaxine and its O-desmethyl metabolite in human milk and their effects in breastfed infants. *British Journal of Clinical Pharmacology, 53*(1), 17–22. https://doi.org/10.1046/j.0306-5251.2001.01518.x

Kanes, S. J., Colquhoun, H., Doherty, J., Raines, S., Hoffmann, E., Rubinow, D. R., & Meltzer-Brody, S. (2017). Open-label, proof-of-concept study of brexanolone in the treatment of severe postpartum depression. *Human Psychopharmacology, 32*(2). https://doi.org/10.1002/hup.2576

Kanes, S., Colquhoun, H., Gunduz-Bruce, H., Raines, S., Arnold, R., Schacterle, A., Doherty, J., Epperson, C. N., Deligiannidis, K. M., Riesenberg, R., Hoffmann, E., Rubinow, D., Jonas, J., Paul, S., & Meltzer-Brody, S. (2017). Brexanolone (SAGE-547 injection) in post-partum depression: A randomised controlled trial. *The Lancet, 390*(10093), 480–489. https://doi.org/10.1016/S0140-6736(17)31264-3

Kelly, L. E., Poon, S., Madadi, P., & Koren, G. (2012). Neonatal benzodiazepines exposure during breastfeeding. *Journal of Pediatrics, 161*(3), 448–451. https://doi.org/10.1016/j.jpeds.2012.03.003

Khan, S. J., Fersh, M. E., Ernst, C., Klipstein, K., Albertini, E. S., & Lusskin, S. I. (2016). Bipolar disorder in pregnancy and postpartum: Principles of management. *Current Psychiatry Reports, 18*(2), 13. https://doi.org/10.1007/s11920-015-0658-x

Kim, D. R., Epperson, C. N., Weiss, A. R., & Wisner, K. L. (2014). Pharmacotherapy of postpartum depression: An update. *Expert Opinion on Pharmacotherapy, 15*(9), 1223–1234. https://doi.org/10.1517/14656566.2014.911842

Klinger, G., Stahl, B., Fusar-Poli, P., & Merlob, P. (2013). Antipsychotic drugs and breastfeeding. *Pediatric Endocrinology Reviews, 10*(3), 308–317. www.ncbi.nlm.nih.gov/pubmed/23724438

Kristensen, J. H., Ilett, K. F., Rampono, J., Kohan, R., & Hackett, L. P. (2007). Transfer of the antidepressant mirtazapine into breast milk. *British Journal of Clinical Pharmacology, 63*(3), 322–327. https://doi.org/10.1111/j.1365-2125.2006.02773.x

Kronenfeld, N., Berlin, M., Shaniv, D., & Berkovitch, M. (2017). Use of psychotropic medications in breastfeeding women. *Birth Defects Research, 109*(12), 957–997. https://doi.org/10.1002/bdr2.1077

Lanza di Scalea, T., & Wisner, K. L. (2009). Antidepressant medication use during breastfeeding. *Clinical Obstetrics and Gynecology, 52*(3), 483–497. https://doi.org/10.1097/GRF.0b013e3181b52bd6

Leader, L. D., O'Connell, M., & VandenBerg, A. (2019). Brexanolone for postpartum depression: Clinical evidence and practical considerations. *Pharmacotherapy, 39*(11), 1105–1112. https://doi.org/10.1002/phar.2331

Lee, H. J., Kim, S. M., & Kwon, J. Y. (2021). Repetitive transcranial magnetic stimulation treatment for peripartum depression: Systematic review & meta-analysis. *BMC Pregnancy Childbirth, 21*(1), 118. https://doi.org/10.1186/s12884-021-03600-3

MacQueen, G. M., Frey, B. N., Ismail, Z., Jaworska, N., Steiner, M., Lieshout, R. J., Kennedy, S. H., Lam, R. W., Milev, R. V., Parikh, S. V., Ravindran, A. V., & Group, C. D. W. (2016). Canadian Network for Mood and Anxiety Treatments (CANMAT) 2016 clinical guidelines for the management of adults with major depressive disorder: Section 6. Special populations: Youth, women, and the elderly. *Canadian Journal of Psychiatry, 61*(9), 588–603. https://doi.org/10.1177/0706743716659276

Mammen, O., Shear, K., Greeno, C., Wheeler, S., & Hughes, C. (1997). Anger attacks and treatment nonadherence in a perinatal psychiatry clinic. *Psychopharmacology Bulletin, 33*(1), 105–108. www.ncbi.nlm.nih.gov/pubmed/9133759

McAllister-Williams, R. H., Baldwin, D. S., Cantwell, R., Easter, A., Gilvarry, E., Glover, V., Green, L., Gregoire, A., Howard, L. M., Jones, I., Khalifeh, H., Lingford-Hughes, A., McDonald, E., Micali, N., Pariante, C. M., Peters, L., Roberts, A., Smith, N. C., Taylor, D., . . . Psychopharmacology, E. b. T. B. A. F. (2017). British Association for Psychopharmacology consensus guidance on the use of psychotropic medication preconception, in pregnancy and postpartum 2017. *Journal of Psychopharmacology, 31*(5), 519–552. https://doi.org/10.1177/0269881117699361

McLafferty, L. P., Spada, M., & Gopalan, P. (2018). Pharmacologic treatment of sleep disorders in pregnancy. *Sleep Medicine Clinics, 13*(2), 243–250.

Meltzer-Brody, S., Colquhoun, H., Riesenberg, R., Epperson, C. N., Deligiannidis, K. M., Rubinow, D. R., Li, H., Sankoh, A. J., Clemson, C., Schacterle, A., Jonas, J., & Kanes, S. (2018). Brexanolone injection in post-partum depression: Two multicentre, double-blind, randomised, placebo-controlled, phase 3 trials. *The Lancet, 392*(10152), 1058–1070. https://doi.org/10.1016/S0140-6736(18)31551-4

Milgrom, J., Gemmill, A. W., Ericksen, J., Burrows, G., Buist, A., & Reece, J. (2015). Treatment of postnatal depression with cognitive behavioural therapy, sertraline and combination therapy: A randomised controlled trial. *Australia and New Zealand Journal of Psychiatry, 49*(3), 236–245. https://doi.org/10.1177/0004867414565474

Misri, S., Reebye, P., Corral, M., & Milis, L. (2004). The use of paroxetine and cognitive-behavioral therapy in postpartum depression and anxiety: A randomized controlled trial. *Journal of Clinical Psychiatry, 65*(9), 1236–1241. https://doi.org/10.4088/jcp.v65n0913

Misri, S., Reebye, P., Milis, L., & Shah, S. (2006). The impact of treatment intervention on parenting stress in postpartum depressed mothers: A prospective study. *American Journal of Orthopsychiatry, 76*(1), 115–119. https://doi.org/10.1037/0002-9432.76.1.115

Misri, S., & Sivertz, K. (1991). Tricyclic drugs in pregnancy and lactation: A preliminary report. *International Journal of Psychiatry in Medicine, 21*(2), 157–171. https://doi.org/10.2190/JDTX-BYC3-K3VP-LWAH

Moretti, M. E., Koren, G., Verjee, Z., & Ito, S. (2003). Monitoring lithium in breast milk: An individualized approach for breast-feeding mothers. *Therapeutic Drug Monitoring, 25*(3), 364–366. https://doi.org/10.1097/00007691-200306000-00017

Myczkowski, M. L., Dias, A. M., Luvisotto, T., Arnaut, D., Bellini, B. B., Mansur, C. G., . . . Marcolin, M. A. (2012). Effects of repetitive transcranial magnetic stimulation on clinical, social, and cognitive performance in postpartum depression. *Neuropsychiatric Disease and Treatment, 8*, 491–500.

Nager, A., Sundquist, K., Ramírez-León, V., & Johansson, L. M. (2008). Obstetric complications and postpartum psychosis: A follow-up study of 1.1 million first-time mothers between 1975 and 2003 in Sweden. *Acta Psychiatrica Scandinavia, 117*(1), 12–19. https://doi.org/10.1111/j.1600-0447.2007.01096.x

National Institute for Health and Care Excellence. (2014). *Antenatal and postnatal mental health: Clinical management and service guidance: Updated edition. NICE clinical guideline 192.* www.nice.org.uk/guidance/cg192

Neuman, G., Colantonio, D., Delaney, S., Szynkaruk, M., & Ito, S. (2014). Bupropion and escitalopram during lactation. *Ann Pharmacother, 48*(7), 928–931. https://doi.org/10.1177/1060028014529548

Newmark, R. L., Bogen, D. L., Wisner, K. L., Isaac, M., Ciolino, J. D., & Clark, C. T. (2019). Risk-benefit assessment of infant exposure to lithium through breast milk: A systematic review of the literature. *Internatinal Review of Psychiatry, 31*(3), 295–304. https://doi.org/10.1080/09540261.2019.1586657

Newport, D. J., Pennell, P. B., Calamaras, M. R., Ritchie, J. C., Newman, M., Knight, B., Viguera, A. C., Liporace, J., & Stowe, Z. N. (2008). Lamotrigine in breast milk and nursing infants: Determination of exposure. *Pediatrics, 122*(1), e223–e231. https://doi.org/10.1542/peds.2007-3812

Newport, D. J., Ritchie, J. C., Knight, B. T., Glover, B. A., Zach, E. B., & Stowe, Z. N. (2009). Venlafaxine in human breast milk and nursing infant plasma: Determination of exposure. *Journal of Clinical Psychiatry, 70*(9), 1304–1310. https://doi.org/10.4088/JCP.08m05001

Nonacs, R. M., Soares, C. N., Viguera, A. C., Pearson, K., Poitras, J. R., & Cohen, L. S. (2005). Bupropion SR for the treatment of postpartum depression: A pilot study. *International Journal of Neuropsychopharmacology, 8*(3), 445–449. https://doi.org/10.1017/S1461145705005079

O'Hara, M. W., Pearlstein, T., Stuart, S., Long, J. D., Mills, J. A., & Zlotnick, C. (2019). A placebo controlled treatment trial of sertraline and interpersonal psychotherapy for postpartum depression. *Journal of Affective Disorders, 245*, 524–532. https://doi.org/10.1016/j.jad.2018.10.361

Okanović, M. Z. O. (2016). Valproate, bipolar disorder and polycyctic ovarian syndrome. *Medicinski Pregled, 69*(3–4), 121–126. https://doi.org/10.2298/mpns1604121o

Orsolini, L. B. C. (2015). Serotonin reuptake inhibitors and breastfeeding: A systematic review. *Human Psychopharmacology, 30*, 4–20.

Pacchiarotti, I., León-Caballero, J., Murru, A., Verdolini, N., Furio, M. A., Pancheri, C., Valentí, M., Samalin, L., Roigé, E. S., González-Pinto, A., Montes, J. M., Benabarre, A., Crespo, J. M., de Dios Perrino, C., Goikolea, J. M., Gutiérrez-Rojas, L., Carvalho, A. F., & Vieta, E. (2016). Mood stabilizers and antipsychotics during breastfeeding: Focus on bipolar disorder. *European Neuropsychopharmacology, 26*(10), 1562–1578. https://doi.org/10.1016/j.euroneuro.2016.08.008

Payne, J. L., & Meltzer-Brody, S. (2009). Antidepressant use during pregnancy: Current controversies and treatment strategies. *Clinical Obstetrics and Gynecology, 52*(3), 469–482. https://doi.org/10.1097/GRF.0b013e3181b52e20

Pearlstein, T., Howard, M., Salisbury, A., & Zlotnick, C. (2009). Postpartum depression. *American Journal of Obstetrics and Gynecology, 200*(4), 357–364. https://doi.org/10.1016/j.ajog.2008.11.033

Perucca, E. (2002). Pharmacological and therapeutic properties of valproate: A summary after 35 years of clinical experience. *CNS Drugs, 16*(10), 695–714. https://doi.org/10.2165/00023210-200216100-00004

Pons, G., Francoual, C., Guillet, P., Moran, C., Hermann, P., Bianchetti, G., Thiercelin, J. F., Thenot, J. P., & Olive, G. (1989). Zolpidem excretion in breast milk. *European Journal of Clinical Pharmacology, 37*(3), 245–248. https://doi.org/10.1007/BF00679778

Ray, S., & Stowe, Z. N. (2014). The use of antidepressant medication in pregnancy. *Best Practice in Research in Clinical Obstetrics and Gynaecology, 28*(1), 71–83. https://doi.org/10.1016/j.bpobgyn.2013.09.005

Robakis, T. K., & Williams, K. E. (2013). Biologically based treatment approaches to the patient with resistant perinatal depression. *Archives of Women's Mental Health, 16*(5), 343–351. https://doi.org/10.1007/s00737-013-0366-7

Rommel, A.-S., Bergnik, V., Liu, X., Munk-Olsen, T., & Molenaar, N. M. (2020). Long-term effects of intrauterine exposure to antidepressants on physical, neurodevelopmental, and psychiatric outcomes: A systematic review. *Journal of Clinical Psychiatry, 81*(3), 19r12965.

Rossi, S., Antal, A., Bestmann, S., Bikson, M., Brewer, C., Brockmöller, J., Carpenter, L. L., Cincotta, M., Chen, R., Daskalakis, J. D., Di Lazzaro, V., Fox, M. D., George, M. S., Gilbert, D., Kimiskidis, V. K., Koch, G., Ilmoniemi, R. J., Lefaucheur, J. P., Leocani, L., . . . Hallett, M. (2021). Safety and recommendations for TMS use in healthy subjects and patient populations, with updates on training, ethical and regulatory issues: Expert Guidelines. *Clinical Neurophysiology, 132*(1), 269–306. https://doi.org/10.1016/j.clinph.2020.10.003

Royal Australian and New Zealand College of Psychiatrists Clinical Practice Guidelines Team for Bipolar Disorder. (2004). Australian and New Zealand clinical practice guidelines for the treatment of bipolar disorder. *Australian and New Zealand Journal of Psychiatry, 38*(5), 280–305. https://doi.org/10.1080/j.1440-1614.2004.01356.x

Rundgren, S., Brus, O., Bave, U., Landen, M., Lundberg, J., Nordanskog, P., & Nordenskjold, A. (2018). Improvement of postpartum depression and psychosis after electroconvulsive therapy: A population-based study with a matched comparison group. *Journal of Affective Disorders, 235,* 258–264.

Sachs, H. C., & the Committee on Drugs. (2013). The transfer of drugs and therapeutics into human breastmilk: An update on selected topic. *Pediatrics, 132,* e796.

Sackeim, H. A. (2017). Modern electroconvulsive therapy: Vastly improved yet greatly underused. *JAMA Psychiatry, 74*(8), 779–780. https://doi.org/10.1001/jamapsychiatry.2017.1670

Schoretsanitis, G., Augustin, M., Saßmannshausen, H., Franz, C., Gründer, G., & Paulzen, M. (2019). Antidepressants in breast milk; comparative analysis of excretion ratios. *Archives of Women's Mental Health, 22*(3), 383–390. https://doi.org/10.1007/s00737-018-0905-3

Sharma, V., Sharma, P., & Sharma, S. (2020). Managing bipolar disorder during pregnancy and the postpartum period: A critical review of current practice. *Expert Review of Neurotherapeutics, 20*(4), 373–383. https://doi.org/10.1080/14737175.2020.1743684

Sharp, D. J., Chew-Graham, C., Tylee, A., Lewis, G., Howard, L., Anderson, I., . . . Peters, T. J. (2010). A pragmatic randomised controlled trial to compare antidepressants with a community-based psychosocial intervention for the treatment of women with postnatal depression: The RESPOND trial. *Health Technology Assessment, 14*(43), iii–iv, ix–xi, 1–153. https://doi.org/10.3310/hta14430

So, M., Bozzo, P., Inoue, M., & Einarson, A. (2010). Safety of antihistamines during pregnancy and lactation. *Canadian Family Physician, 56*(5), 427–429.

Stewart, D. E., & Vigod, S. N. (2019). Postpartum depression: Pathophysiology, treatment, and emerging therapeutics. *Annual Review of Medicine, 70,* 183–196. https://doi.org/10.1146/annurev-med-041217-011106

Stowe, Z. N. (2007). The use of mood stabilizers during breastfeeding. *Journal of Clinical Psychiatry, 68*(Suppl. 9), 22–28. www.ncbi.nlm.nih.gov/pubmed/17764381

Stowe, Z. N., Casarella, J., Landry, J., & Nemeroff, C. B. (1995). Sertraline in the treatment of women with postpartum major depression. *Depression, 3,* 49–55.

Uguz, F., & Sharma, V. (2016). Mood stabilizers during breastfeeding: A systematic review of the recent literature. *Bipolar Disorders, 18*(4), 325–333. https://doi.org/10.1111/bdi.12398

Wisner, K. L., Hanusa, B. H., Perel, J. M., Peindl, K. S., Piontek, C. M., Sit, D. K., Findling, R. L., & Moses-Kolko, E. L. (2006). Postpartum depression: A randomized trial of sertraline versus nortriptyline. *Journal of Clinical Psychopharmacology, 26*(4), 353–360. https://doi.org/10.1097/01.jcp.0000227706.56870.dd

World Health Organization. (2019). *International statistical classification of diseases and related health problems* (11th ed.). https://icd.who.int/ (Online version January 2023).

Yatham, L. N., Kennedy, S. H., Parikh, S. V., Schaffer, A., Bond, D. J., Frey, B. N., Sharma, V., Goldstein, B. I., Rej, S., Beaulieu, S., Alda, M., MacQueen, G., Milev, R. V., Ravindran, A., O'Donovan, C., McIntosh, D., Lam, R. W., Vazquez, G., Kapczinski, F., . . . Berk, M. (2018). Canadian Network for Mood and Anxiety Treatments (CANMAT) and International Society for Bipolar Disorders (ISBD) 2018 guidelines for the management of patients with bipolar disorder. *Bipolar Disorders, 20*(2), 97–170. https://doi.org/10.1111/bdi.12609

Yonkers, K. A., Lin, H., Howell, H. B., Heath, A. C., & Cohen, L. S. (2008). Pharmacologic treatment of postpartum women with new-onset major depressive disorder: A randomized controlled trial with paroxetine. *Journal of Clinical Psychiatry, 69*(4), 659–665. https://doi.org/10.4088/jcp.v69n0420

Yonkers, K. A., Wisner, K. L., Stewart, D. E., Oberlander, T. F., Dell, D. L., Stotland, N., Ramin, S., Chaudron, L., & Lockwood, C. (2009). The management of depression during pregnancy: A report from the American Psychiatric Association and the American College of Obstetricians and Gynecologists. *General Hospital Psychiatry, 31*(5), 403–413. https://doi.org/10.1016/j.genhosppsych.2009.04.003

Yoshida, K., Smith, B., Craggs, M., & Kumar, R. C. (1997). Investigation of pharmacokinetics and of possible adverse effects in infants exposed to tricyclic antidepressants in breast-milk. *Journal of Affective Disorders, 43*(3), 225–237. https://doi.org/10.1016/s0165-0327(97)01433-x

22

COGNITIVE BEHAVIORAL THERAPY FOR PERINATAL MENTAL HEALTH DISORDERS

Amy Wenzel

Cognitive behavioral therapy (CBT) is a versatile, semi-structured, and time-sensitive approach to psychotherapy. It was developed in the 1960s and 1970s by Aaron T. Beck (1967, 1972, 1975; A. T. Beck et al., 1979) as an alternative to psychoanalysis, with the rationale that a more active and targeted approach to addressing the core components of pathology (in the early years, depression) would result in faster and more effective remission than psychoanalysis and would work at least as well as psychotropic medications. Although it took some time for the psychiatric community to acknowledge and embrace CBT (cf. Rosner, 2018; Shorter, 1997), currently, it is viewed by countless mental health providers as the psychotherapy of choice for a vast array of mental health disorders and clinical conditions that have mental health sequelae or implications (Knapp et al., 2015).

CBT is frequently viewed as an ideal mental health intervention by perinatal clients and perinatal mental health experts alike. It has a massive evidence supporting its efficacy and effectiveness (e.g., Butler et al., 2006; Hofmann et al., 2012), which instills great confidence that it will be helpful to people in need, including parents or future parents. Its active and time-sensitive nature is often attractive to perinatal clients, who are juggling multiple demands on their time, sleep deprivation, and childcare challenges, and who are simply looking for an intervention that will bring relief as quickly as possible. Moreover, CBT, as practiced in its contemporary form, is customized to the unique life circumstances of each client and places much emphasis on the development of a warm, supportive therapeutic relationship (Kazantzis et al., 2017; Wenzel, in press), which some have advocated as being particularly important for postpartum women (Kleiman, 2017).

In this chapter, I describe CBT for perinatal mental health disorders. First, I present CBT's central tenets and main components. It is in this section that I introduce a perinatal case study (a compilation of clients who I have treated in my own practice), and I illustrate many of these tenets and components in light of this case. Next, I provide a brief overview of the literature on the efficacy and effectiveness of CBT interventions and prevention programs, focused mainly on perinatal depression and anxiety. I follow with considerations of cultural adaptations and the dissemination of CBT for perinatal mental health disorders. Finally, I end the chapter with conclusions that can be drawn from the scholarly literature and clinical practice of CBT for perinatal mental health disorders to date, proposing a specific agenda for future research.

DOI: 10.4324/9781003206903-27

Central Tenets and Main Interventions: Description and Illustration

CBT is based on a foundation of core tenets that pervade the course of treatment, as well as underlie the specific interventions that are delivered. Above all, cognitive behavioral therapists are *strategic*, in that they deliver interventions in a way that (a) follow from the customized case formulation of the client's clinical presentation; (b) are decided upon collaborative by themselves and their client; (c) advance treatment in a way that something tangible and meaningful emerges from the session, often to be implemented for "therapy homework" in between sessions; and (d) commit to seeing the intervention through in its entirety and then evaluating its effectiveness, rather than abandoning it outright if they or their client get "cold feet" (Wenzel, 2013). Moreover, CBT is delivered in a way that balances relative equal attention between the delivery of strategic cognitive behavioral interventions and the development and enhancement of the therapeutic relationship, which can be an agent of change in and of itself (Wenzel, in press).

Central Tenets

CBT is a therapy that encompasses collaboration, the solicitation of feedback from the client, and transparency in building the therapeutic relationship, instilling hope, and allowing for the development of client self-efficacy. *Collaboration* means that the therapist and client work together to agree upon the treatment goals, the most fruitful issues to address in session, and the intervention strategy that has the potential to be the best "match" with the client's needs and preferences at the time. Notice that the definition of collaboration involves *both* the therapist and client; although it is very true that therapists do *not* dictate the agenda or focus of treatment in CBT, neither do clients, lest the therapist inadvertently reinforce client avoidance of issues that very much need to be addressed, or even aspects of the very pathology that the client hopes to overcome in treatment. Thus, cognitive behavioral therapists bring their knowledge of the scholarly literature and clinical experience, and clients bring their intimate knowledge of their life circumstances, their preferences, and their view of what works for them, to the table in deciding upon a course of action.

One way to reinforce this collaborative stance is to regularly obtain *feedback* from clients on whether the specific approach taken in session is sensible and seems promising to them, whether the intervention that was delivered and discussion associated with it ultimately made a difference in their lives between sessions, and whether anything about the session bothered them (which could have implications for their therapeutic relationship, and in turn engagement in therapy). Moreover, cognitive behavioral therapists get feedback, often in the form of quantitative ratings (e.g., 0–10 Likert-type scales, completion of brief self-report inventories like the *Edinburgh Perinatal Depression Scale* [EPDS; Cox et al., 1987]) on clients' symptoms so that they can decide, collaboratively, whether the direction that they are taking in therapy is making a noticeable impact on their clinical presentation.

The tenet of *transparency* means that cognitive behavioral therapists are fully open with their clients about the rationale behind their suggestions, making sure that clients agree after hearing the rationale and can internalize the cognitive behavioral principle encapsulated in the suggestion so that, ultimately, they need not rely on therapists to coach them on implementing the principles and strategies in their lives outside of session. Often, transparency incorporates the provision of *psychoeducation*, or information to help clients understand, cope with, and overcome their mental health problem. Psychoeducation equips clients with knowledge about processes of change so that they can become empowered and ultimately own their recovery from their mental health disorder. With perinatal women, psychoeducation can encompass standard information about CBT that is shared with all clients, ways in which perinatal clients have adapted the knowledge to meet their needs, and information about typical adjustment experiences of perinatal women.

Another important feature of CBT is the use of *Socratic dialogue*, or a style of questioning by the therapist that allows the client to grapple with many different ways of thinking about a situation, ultimately drawing their own conclusion. This principle was inspired by the Greek philosopher and teacher, Socrates, who often encouraged his students to argue multiple points of view so that they could truly understand them and arrive upon their own conclusion, rather than being told what to think (Kazantzis et al., 2018). Cognitive behavioral therapists adopt the same stance with their clients, in that that their stance is that it is not their jobs to simply tell a client what is "right" or what is the "best" way of viewing a situation—in fact, doing so would be seen as presumptuous and invalidating because the cognitive behavioral therapist is *not* living in the client's shoes and experiencing all that the client is experiencing in their life outside of session. This being said, when cognitive behavioral therapists apply Socratic questioning, they do so from a gentle, inquisitive standpoint, rather than one in which clients are "put on the spot" and feel "backed into a corner" to defend their logic (Wenzel, in press). Socratic questioning helps clients to learn how to question their own thoughts in a helpful, productive, and compassionate way, as well as to enhance the therapeutic relationship because it demonstrates therapists' willingness to trust that their clients will embrace the process and their investment in clients' ultimate well-being (Kazantzis et al., 2014).

While this notion of Socratic dialogue seems respectful and enriching, I have had reactions from many perinatal mental health providers who practice outside of the CBT framework that sleep-deprived postpartum parents simply want to be told what to do to feel better. That is, these providers are skeptical that the artful application of Socratic dialogue that we might deliver to the highest functioning of clients would apply here. If this is the case, such that an individual client has difficulty engaging in Socratic questioning, the client's well-being is the priority. The therapist still does not take the stance of telling the client what to do, but the therapist would pose the Socratic question in a digestible way for the client, such as giving the client a "menu" of two or three choices, from which she can choose the option that feels right or that best suits their situation.

The aspect of therapy "homework" is almost synonymous with the definition of CBT, as it is hypothesized that much of the "work" of CBT is completed in between sessions, in clients' lives outside of therapy (Dobson, 2022). The idea underlying homework is that cognitive behavioral therapists want their clients to feel better as quickly as possible, and between-session homework is a straightforward way for clients to bring therapy with them to their lives and do something differently that will improve their mood or life circumstances. I have encountered a similar reaction from many perinatal mental health providers who practice outside of the CBT framework about homework as I do about Socratic dialogue. Specifically, I have fielded concerns that homework is not a good match for new parents—and, in fact, is even inappropriate to suggest to new parents—because it puts too much pressure on perinatal clients who are already overwhelmed, sleep-deprived, and juggling multiple demands in their lives. As will be illustrated in the descriptions of many of the main interventions, cognitive behavioral homework exercises are custom tailored to each person and their life situation. This customization includes not only what the homework targets but also how it is enacted and practiced. In my clinical experience, I find that perinatal clients are grateful for a customized homework exercise that has the potential to bring relief to unrelenting depression and anxiety.

A final fundamental tenet of CBT is the central role played by the *case formulation*, or the intricate application of cognitive behavioral theory to understand the precipitating and maintaining factors for the client's mental health problem, as well as relevant targets for treatment (Kuyken et al., 2006; Persons, 2008). A sophisticated case formulation allows both the therapist and client to understand the key life experiences that have shaped the way in which clients view themselves, others, and the world, as well as ways that they cope with or compensate for painful beliefs or rigid rules and assumptions about how they should live their lives or how the world works. It also helps clients to understand the basis for ways of responding that are seemingly maladaptive, which can bring about a sense of self-compassion. Perinatal clients, in particular, often identify entrenched beliefs about marriage, family, and parenting that either foster or hinder adaptation to the transition to parenthood.

The following case description introduces the client (and the accompanying case formulation) who will be followed throughout the remainder of this chapter.

"Jade" is a 38-year-old Caucasian woman who gave birth to her son ten weeks before she reached out for therapy. She is a single mother by choice who conceived via intrauterine insemination. She presented for treatment for "paralyzing anxiety" and resultant depression, wondering if she had made a "huge mistake" in pursuing single motherhood. At the time of her intake session, she described herself as "nonfunctional," having barely slept, and as relying on her parents to take care of her newborn son.

Jade lives in a duplex a few miles from her parents and also from her brother, and she works for her mother in her mother's business. Initially, Jade described herself as having an extremely close, healthy relationship with her parents and brother. However, as the conversation progressed, it appeared that these relationships caused her great distress at times, as she simultaneously depended on her parents for financial and emotional support and was petrified of their disapproval and disappointment in her. She also reported a sense of obligation that she had to "jump" every time her mother asked something of her and that, if she did not comply, her mother could give her the "cold shoulder," which was intolerable for her. Jade noted that she had the tendency to sulk and "shut down" when it felt as if she were the butt of family jokes. In reflecting on recently becoming a mother, she noted, "I knew my parents didn't think I could do it, and now I've just proven them right."

When cognitive behavioral therapists think conceptually about their clients to develop cognitive behavioral case formulations, much of what they identify are hypotheses to be tested in collaboration with the client. For example, Jade's therapist hypothesized that Jade carried the core belief (i.e., a fundamental belief about the self, others, the world, or the future) that she was incapable of handling life's challenges on her own, without her family. The therapist also suspected that Jade held rigid beliefs about what was and was not acceptable behavior within her family (e.g., "I cannot upset my parents, or it will be awful" and "I must do whatever my parents ask, or there will be consequences"). As a result of these beliefs, Jade's therapist speculated that Jade overcompensated by rushing to please her parents, subjugating her own needs and opinions, and the therapist wondered if Jade never fully differentiated from her family of origin, depriving herself of the opportunity to submit herself to an age-appropriate partner relationship and to develop life skills for functioning as an adult who is independent of one's parents.

Together, Jade and her therapist developed a series of targets for treatment. The first order of business was relief from her "paralyzing anxiety." Although Jade had been prescribed alprazolam by her obstetrician, she did not believe that it was "making a dent in her anxiety," and she hoped to develop strategies for more effectively managing the surges of anxiety that she experienced, particularly in moments when she was alone with her son. More generally, Jade and her therapist hoped to shift Jade's core belief of being incapable of handling life without the help of her parents. The therapist proposed that they could work systematically on developing a sense of being capable through increasingly significant demonstrations of effective parenting. Jade also expressed that, once she had more confidence in her ability to manage her anxiety and care for her son, she would like to shift the long-standing interactional patterns that had developed between her and the other members of her family of origin.

Main Interventions

This section describes many of the main interventions that are used in CBT in general, and particularly with perinatal women. They are described in the rough order in which they were introduced to Jade in treatment. Readers should note that there is no "prescribed" order in which CBT interventions are introduced (and no CBT intervention that absolutely must be introduced in all cases). Rather, interventions are selected on the basis of the emerging case formulation, the needs of the client, and the preferences that the client expresses when they are making treatment decisions in collaboration with their therapist. The astute reader will also observe that, in many cases, the aims of multiple interventions can be achieved simultaneously.

It should be noted here that the reader who is familiar with CBT might notice that many of the strategies described next are associated with CBT as it has, historically or traditionally been practiced (i.e., cognitive restructuring, behavioral activation, problem solving, communication skills training, exposure, relapse prevention), whereas a few of the others might be viewed as more central to "third-wave" evidence-based psychotherapies (i.e., distress tolerance, emotion regulation, cognitive defusion, mindfulness). To date, many scholars who conduct meta-analyses evaluating the efficacy of CBT for perinatal mental health disorders (perinatal depression in particular) exclude interventions incorporating these strategies from consideration (e.g., Pettman et al., 2023). The rationale for the broad inclusion of strategies in this section is that they represent the contemporary practice of CBT, which is an integrated approach in which the cognitive behavioral therapist, informed by relevant theory and data, works collaboratively with the client to develop a customized course of CBT that fits the client's case formulation. In the contemporary practice of CBT, there is often a relative equal balance in the delivery of acceptance- and change-based strategies (Wenzel, 2017), Thus, contemporary cognitive behavioral therapists are heavily influenced by the "third-wave" evidence-based psychotherapies that have their roots in traditional CBT, but that have expanded with the times. As the reader will see in my comments in the concluding section, studies examining "third-wave" and contemporary CBT are just beginning to receive attention in the empirical literature, and I believe that much scholarship will be devoted to their evaluation in the next decade.

Distress Tolerance

The construct of *distress tolerance* was popularized by Marsha Linehan in the context of her innovative cognitive behavioral treatment, *dialectical Behavior therapy* (DBT; Linehan, 1993, 2015). It refers to a person's ability to withstand significant emotional distress or upset and to emerge from it without having done something self-defeating (e.g., self-harm, excessive alcohol or drug use, extreme avoidance). When clients apply strategies and tools in the spirit of distress tolerance, they often learn that they *can* get through difficult times and that they *are* resilient. Jade's therapist strategically reasoned that the practicing of distress tolerance tools in the early stage of therapy would (a) bring Jade some relief from her unrelenting anxiety (which corresponding to her first treatment goal); (b) give her the first taste of evidence that she is, indeed, capable of doing something difficult (in this case, tolerating emotional distress, which corresponded to her second treatment goal); and (c) move her toward a better place at which she could address parenting a newborn and shifting relationship dynamics within her family (which corresponded to her third treatment goal)

Distress tolerance skills help a person to get through moments of upset; this means that they are short-term solutions, rather than long-term "cures." Nevertheless, it is my clinical experience that many clients are especially attracted to learning about and implementing distress tolerance skills because they are the closest to the kinds of "coping strategies" that clients so desperately need and want to acquire in treatment. Examples of distress tolerance skills include distraction, self-soothing (i.e., activating one or more of the five senses in a pleasurable manner, such as listening to music or petting a cat), muscle relaxation, controlled breathing, giving oneself encouragement, and conducting a pro-con analysis of make a poor decision because of emotional distress (e.g., self-harm behavior).

Jade enthusiastically embraced the notion of distress tolerance when her therapist explained to her what it is and provided some examples (i.e., through the provision of psychoeducation). Because she became particularly distressed when her son was crying, and she perceived that she was unable to soothe him, she identified self-soothing options that had the potential to be soothing to both herself and her son. In particular, she was very drawn to the lullabies played by a gadget that attached to her son's crib, which she had been gifted at her baby shower. When she and her son were agitated, she began to go into his bedroom, dim the lights, play the lullaby machine, and rock him in a glider. Jade also developed a plan for distress tolerance when she experienced unbearable anxiety outside of the times in which her son was crying (and when he was under the supervision of a family member), which included going into her bedroom and laying under a weighted blanket with a scented candle lighted and some soothing music playing.

Emotion Regulation

Emotion regulation is another construct that gained increased attention in Marsha Linehan's DBT (1993, 2015), although there is a rich literature examining the importance of emotion regulation for mental health and skills for achieving it outside of the DBT literature (e.g., Gross, 2014). It refers to a person's ability to moderate and "even out" their emotional reactivity over the long-term, in contrast to distress tolerance, which is a person's ability to "survive" an upsetting situation in the short term. I tell my clients that the goal of emotion regulation is to achieve a state of equanimity regardless of the challenges that life presents, so that they are not overcome by maladaptive emotional distress at a time when a sense of centeredness is in order. Thus, when a person implements regular practices to achieve emotion regulation, the likelihood decreases that they would experience excessive emotional distress in times of challenge, disappointment, upset, or transition (and, therefore, would need to rely less on distress tolerance skills). Examples of emotion regulation skills include doing the opposite action as the urge that the unwanted emotion is prompting, accumulating the benefits of positive emotions, building mastery by doing things that give us a sense of enjoyment or accomplishment, "coping ahead" to know how we will handle future challenges, and taking care of ourselves through exercise, nutrition, sleep, and necessary medical care.

Jade's therapist observed that Jade's sleep was even more dysregulated than her typical perinatal client, and that Jade was doing very little else to take care of herself, to the point that she was so depleted that she could not bear to think about caring for her son. Thus, the therapist reasoned that Jade would benefit from psychoeducation about the strong foundation that emotion regulation skills can create in adjusting to the transition to parenthood, to obtain Jade's buy-in so that she would be motivated to make some changes in this area. Jade and her therapist started with basic self-care behaviors of having regular meals, getting good sleep (as much as is possible with a newborn), and getting regular exercise. Jade set alarms on her phone to remind her to have something to eat at breakfast, lunch, and dinner, and the family members who were helping her made sure to stock her refrigerator and cupboards with food that did not require preparation or advance planning. She gave herself permission to nap when the baby napped, and she accepted her brother's girlfriend's offer to spend occasional nights at her residence so that she could sleep when her son woke up. Moreover, she committed to a walk with her son around the neighborhood once a day, and she was pleasantly surprised at how empowered this made her feel. Together, the implementation of both distress tolerance skills and emotion regulation skills began to prompt an important cognitive shift in Jade, in that she no longer viewed herself as completely incapable of handling emotional distress.

Cognitive Restructuring

Cognitive restructuring is a key strategy in CBT, emphasized in the early manifestations of CBT by Aaron T. Beck, in which clients gain skill in recognizing aspects of their thinking that is exacerbating emotional distress, evaluating the degree to which their thinking is accurate and helpful, and if necessary reshaping their thinking into an alternative, more balanced way of viewing an upsetting situation so as to reduce the amount of emotional distress that it brings on. In other words, the goal of cognitive restructuring is to help clients shift from unhelpful thinking that worsens emotional distress to more helpful thinking that is accurate, balanced, and problem-focused, which is expected to soften emotional distress. Although cognitive restructuring is often included in discussions as a key emotion regulation strategy (and often referred to as cognitive reappraisal; Gross, 2002), it is included here as a separate strategy because it is a foundational strategy in CBT practice.

The aims of cognitive restructuring can be achieved either formally or informally. From a formal perspective, there are many resources available that guide clinicians in, very systematically, instilling the process of cognitive restructuring with their clients (e.g., J. S. Beck, 2021; Wenzel, 2017). Oftentimes, "formal" cognitive restructuring involves clients writing out (either handwritten or via the notes function of their phone) their thoughts and the ways in which they questioned their thoughts to arrive upon an alternative. I do agree with my perinatal mental health colleagues who practice outside of the CBT framework, who question whether this is feasible for a new mother who has much "on her plate." However, rather than viewing cognitive restructuring as a strategy that lacks relevance for perinatal women, I would, instead, argue that it can be adapted to the life circumstances of new parents. Some of my perinatal clients access cognitive restructuring through mobile phone applications (e.g., MoodKit) that they can easily access in many settings. I once had a perinatal client practice cognitive restructuring when her newborn had fallen asleep for the night in her arms. Other perinatal clients prefer to work through cognitive restructuring in session and then put the adaptive, balanced thinking that emerged from the exercise on a *coping card*, such as an index card that they can hang in their refrigerator, or a virtual coping card in their phones. Still other perinatal parents craft a mantra that they can remember in times of distress, such as recognition of a cognitive distortion (e.g., fortune telling or catastrophizing) or a statement of their values by which they are living even if they are feeling awful and burned out.

Jade recognized that her thinking could quickly spiral, resulting in what she had described as "paralyzing anxiety" or even panic attacks. For example, if her son did not nap well during the day, she anticipated that she would not get a wink of sleep at night and that the consequences of this would be intolerable (interestingly, she had the same thoughts if her son slept especially well during the day, as well). However, Jade expressed the strong preference not to do "formal" cognitive restructuring using standard CBT worksheets and templates because she found the notion to be too overwhelming for her. Thus, her therapist educated her about the principle underlying cognitive restructuring (which Jade bought into wholeheartedly) and considered ways in which Jade could apply these principles when she noticed the first warning signs that her thinking was beginning to spiral. Together, Jade and her therapist devised a plan in which Jade would first apply a distress tolerance tool (e.g., controlled breathing), then recognize that she was falling into the trap of catastrophic thinking, then consider what, realistically would be the worst-case outcome (e.g., a couple of hours of sleep, but very unlikely not one wink of sleep), and finally, then plan for how she would adjust her routine the next day in light of sleep deprivation.

Cognitive Defusion

In many instances, there is a grain of truth (or more than a grain of truth) in clients' thinking (e.g., a new mother probably will, indeed, be very tired the next day if she only gets a few hours of sleep), and in other instances, clients are fixated on unpleasant facts of life (e.g., "I only got four hours of sleep last night, and I am dead tired."). Oftentimes, cognitive restructuring is not indicated in these types of scenarios because the client's thinking is relatively accurate. In still other instances, clients fixate on thoughts that are riddled with negative judgment, but for which there is not an objective metric readily available to assess the degree to which the thought has validity (e.g., "I'm a failure as a mother"). In this latter instance, cognitive behavioral therapists often find that they get into a "boxing match" with their clients when they apply cognitive restructuring, such that when they gently attempt to supply evidence to the contrary of the unhelpful thought, the client responds with a "yeah but" statement that, in turn, has the potential to disrupt the therapeutic alliance. In general, although cognitive behavioral therapists rely on cognitive restructuring as a fundamental strategy of CBT, they are very mindful of not forcing it upon their clients in a way that could be experienced by the client as invalidating or controlling.

Fortunately, an alternative approach to intervening with unhelpful thoughts has been developed by Steven Hayes within the context of acceptance and commitment therapy approach (ACT; Hayes et al., 1999, 2012). *Cognitive defusion* is a strategy that mobilizes specific techniques for helping clients to get distance from their thoughts and to live their lives the way that it is important for them to do so regardless of whether the thoughts are present. This approach is in contrast to the crux of cognitive restructuring, which is changing thoughts. Even attaching a simple phrase such as "I'm having the thought that . . ." before the expression of the actual upsetting thought creates enough distance from the content of the thought that clients often have the realization that a thought is just a thought, and it does not have to be reality and it need not dictate the way in which they live their lives. Other specific techniques for achieving cognitive defusion include using Google translator to translate the thought into a different language and reading the translation out loud (so that clients recognize that these are just words that need not carry meaning), singing the thought out loud, and saying the thought out loud using a goofy voice. It is not difficult to imagine a perinatal client achieving the aim of cognitive defusion as she sings her unhelpful thoughts to the tune of a lullaby!

Jade took well to the simple tactic of saying "I'm having the thought that . . ." before she expressed the thoughts that were plaguing her. She realized that it was her "modus operandi" to catastrophize about the worst possible outcome and to label herself as a "failure" or a "bad mother" without fully realizing that she was falling into these traps. When she prefaced her thoughts with "I'm having the thought that," she was able to adopt the alternative viewpoint that her anxiety was driving her thinking, rather than the reality of the situation. Thus, paradoxically, Jade achieved an aim of cognitive restructuring not by directly questioning and reshaping her thoughts, but by achieving some distance from them. Importantly, the distance that she achieved from her unhelpful thinking helped her to maintain a sense of calm, which in turn allowed for more seamless care of her newborn and for the accumulation of evidence that she was indeed, capable as a parent.

Behavioral Activation

Behavioral activation is a broad strategy, used on its own or in combination with other CBT strategies, that helps clients to become more actively engaged in their environment, which is expected to, in turn, increase the rate positive reinforcement that provides an antidepressant effect (Dimidjian et al., 2011; Martell et al., 2010). The theoretical rationale underlying behavioral activation is that depression is proposed to result, in part, from a lack of response-contingent positive reinforcement, which further amplifies depressed mood, anhedonia, and fatigue, thereby decreasing the likelihood even further that people with depression will initiate activities that serve as sources of accomplishment, joy, pleasure, meaning, or connection with others. When a cognitive behavioral therapist implements behavioral activation, they work with their clients to (a) identify particularly low times of their day, where they might be in most need of behavioral activation; (b) consider their personal values and the types of activities that would bring them the most antidepressant benefit; and (c) determine ways to work valued activities into their day and observe the degree to which their mood, indeed, improves.

In my clinical experience, I find that women with postpartum depression (PPD), in particular, are in great need of behavioral activation. Many women with PPD describe early motherhood as a time when one day bleeds into the next, with not a lot of activity other than nursing, soothing, and changing diapers. Moreover, it is rare to see a new mother in therapy who has more than the tiniest chunk of time for herself. Thus, behavioral activation is implemented with creativity with postpartum depressed women. Many women resonate with the rationale underlying behavioral activated when they are presented with psychoeducation, and from there, they can identify one or two activities (perhaps on their own, or likely with their babies) that would likely provide a sense of joy or pleasure. Examples of activities identified by my previous clients with PPD include taking walks with their babies in a special location (e.g., a park with beautiful scenery), attending a mommy-infant yoga class, and listening to a podcast or audiobook on low while the baby is sleeping (and they are either relaxing themselves or doing light housework).

Although Jade was more anxious than depressed in her postpartum period, she believed that she could benefit from behavioral activation because she felt so "cooped up" in her house that she viewed herself as going "stir crazy" (which she believed exacerbated her anxiety). The walks that she had been taking for the purpose of emotion regulation were helpful, although she did not view them as especially pleasurable because she was merely walking around her neighborhood, which was located in a densely populated area that was not particularly soothing. Jade was encouraged to identify activities and outings that would be especially likely to enhance her mood, bringing a reprieve from her anxiety. Jade chose one activity that she could do at home while the baby was napping (i.e., crochet), and she chose one activity outside the home (i.e., visiting with a close friend whose child was 18 months old, whom she had not seen since she gave birth). Jade was pleasantly surprised that her mood, indeed, improved when she engaged in these activities, bringing her hope that life would not stay as it is forever.

Problem Solving

Problem solving is a process that is embedded in many of the other strategies in this chapter. As has been mentioned throughout the chapter, perinatal women who present for mental health treatment are usually exhausted, overwhelmed, and struggling to function, so it often takes creative problem solving to discern ways to implement cognitive behavioral principles, techniques, and tools in a way that enhances their lives and relieves stress, rather than serving as a burden. An essential aspect of problem solving is the brainstorming of possible solutions to problems. In point of fact, Jade and her therapist used problem solving to arrive upon (a) ways to self-soothe, (b) ways to achieve basic emotion regulation, (c) an approach for implementing the principles underlying cognitive restructuring "in real time" without having to sequester time for therapy homework, and (d) ways to enact behavioral activation both inside and outside the home.

In my previous writing, I have cautioned cognitive behavioral therapists against solving problems for their clients, or against spending only a few minutes on problem solving without systematically coaching clients in the acquisition of specific problem-solving skills (e.g., operationally defining the problem, brainstorming all possible solutions without judgment, decision analysis, skills for implementing the solution, debriefing on the solution at the time of the next session; Wenzel, 2019, in press). With perinatal women who are scared, exhausted, and overwhelmed, I allow for more leeway with this suggestion, as at times, they indicate that they (understandably) simply do not have the bandwidth to engage in systematic problem-solving coaching. Instead, cognitive behavioral therapists who use problem solving with their clients might abide by the principle of *satisficing*, such that they work collaboratively with their client to solve a problem by focusing on the implementation of the first satisfactory solution that they arrive upon in their discussion of the problem, so that the client is sure to leave the session with a concrete action plan. At a time in their lives that seems especially unpredictable and out of their control, having an action plan can relieve anxiety and instill hope that therapy is effective and that their lives can be different as a result of mental health intervention.

Communication Skills

Communication skills coaching often goes hand-in-hand with problem solving, as in many instances, communication with others is required to enact a solution to life problems. Assertiveness practice is certainly a major aim of communication skills coaching, but that need not be the only skills that are practiced. As Linehan (1993, 2015) has outlined in the context of DBT, at times, skill is required to enact communication aimed at repairing, maintaining, or enhancing a relationship, and at other times, skill is required to enact communication that is aimed at preserving the client's own self-respect. During the course of therapy, many perinatal women describe challenges and conflicts with spouses/partners, their own parents, their in-laws, nannies/day care providers, and their obstetricians/gynecologists. Cognitive behavioral therapists can work collaboratively with their clients to apply problem solving to arrive upon a suggested solution to a problem (e.g., division of household labor while the mother is consumed with caring for a newborn) and discern an effective way of discussing this with the spouse, partner, and others who provide childcare.

After the first eight sessions of CBT, focused on distress tolerance, emotion regulation, cognitive restructuring, and behavioral activation, Jade was feeling more centered and balanced. Although she continued to experience a great deal of anxiety when she was faced with something new in her son's behavior, or when she was called upon to provide some sort of care that was new to her, she was regularly enacting the strategies that had been the focus of previous sessions. It was at this point that she wanted some space from her mother, who, while vitally helpful during the early postpartum period, was now beginning to wear on her. Specifically, Jade experienced her mother as disregarding Jade's wishes regarding feeding and nap times, remarking that Jade was too rigid and that she has more parenting wisdom than Jade does because she raised two children. Jade and her therapist worked together to clarify boundaries that were important for Jade to enact with her mother, as well as an interpersonally effective approach to communicating those to her mother. Jade remarked that she was grateful to focus on this work in therapy, as she had struggled throughout her life to set boundaries with her mother, and she suspected that if she did not set them early on in her child's life that she would continue to be "steamrolled" by her mother's dominant personality. The enactment of communication skills coaching helped Jade to move toward her third treatment goal, which was to shift the dynamic in the relationship with members of her family of origin.

Exposure

Exposure is the systematic contact with a feared stimulus or situation, which is typically implemented on its own or within a comprehensive course of CBT to address anxiety and avoidance that causes life interference and/or personal distress. Perhaps the most powerful form of exposure is *in vivo exposure*, which is "real life" exposure to actual feared stimuli and situations. For example, if a new mother is fearful of driving with her newborn in a car, and her associated avoidance is causing life interference (e.g., missed well visit appointments), her cognitive behavioral therapist could work with her to gain practice in driving with her newborn by taking on longer and longer distances from home. Other types of anxiety do not lend themselves well to in vivo exposure; for example, a new mother who had a traumatic childbirth would not intentionally be subjected to the same situation. Rather, her therapist with work with her using *imaginal exposure* and construct vivid narratives of the childbirth experience that the client would review repeatedly. Exposure works by two mechanisms: (a) habituation, such that the client's emotional and physiological reactivity can acclimate to the feared stimulus or situation; and (b) even in cases in which habituation is achieved, new learning occurs, such that the client learns that she can tolerate the distress associated with contact with the feared stimulus or situation (Wenzel, 2017). Although clinicians sometimes draw the premature conclusion that exposure is not safe for pregnant women due to the excessive stress and anxiety that they believe it will cause, guidelines for exposure safety during pregnancy have been well-established for some time (Arch et al., 2012).

Perhaps the most common target of exposure in perinatal women is for the intrusive, "scary" thoughts that the majority of new parents experience following childbirth (Kleiman et al., 2021). It is estimated that up to 90% of new parents experience intrusive thoughts of harm coming to their newborn (or even more specifically, causing harm to their babies) (Abramowitz et al., 2003). Cognitive behavioral therapists who use exposure never subject their clients to any more than everyday levels of risk (Abramowitz et al., 2019). However, they can harness the power of imaginal exposure to imagine scenarios in which harm might inadvertently come to their newborn. Although such an approach might appear counterintuitive to the average person, it is this component that is the key factor in treating new parents with such intrusive thoughts of harm (Gershkovich, 2019), as it allows them to develop a tolerance for the possibility that harm might come to their children and that safety cannot be guaranteed.

Fortunately, when she first presented for treatment, Jade's anxiety was centered more on anticipatory anxiety associated with her baby being unable to be soothed while crying, her baby not sleeping through the night, and her inability to cope with caring for a newborn than on intrusive thoughts about intentionally causing harm to her child. The interventions described to this point were effective in helping her tolerate her son's crying and lack of sleep, as well as her ability to cope with the transition to parenthood. As her son got older, Jade hoped to enroll her son in "Waterbabies" swim classes and a sing-along music class. In fact, she initially viewed participation in such classes as achieving the goals of behavioral activation. However, when she was about to enroll in the class, Jade experienced a surge of social anxiety, worrying that she would be judged by other mothers for her choice to be a single (and somewhat older) mother and for what she perceived as her inability to soothe her son as well as she thought she should be able to do at this point during motherhood. Although the principles of cognitive restructuring were applied to soften her harsh predictions that she would be judged negatively, Jade still had difficulty bringing herself to sign up for classes. Jade and her therapist decided to use exposure to acclimate Jade to being in the presence of other mothers of infants. Jade started by bringing her son to the park, then by talking with one other mother at the park, then by talking with multiple mothers at the park, and then by stopping by a drop-in mother's group (without signing up for multiple classes). As Jade progressed through this sequence, she began to feel more comfortable around other mothers and learned that most mothers have their own unique struggles that they shy away from sharing with others. Finally, Jade chose what she viewed as the "easier" class for her to participate in—the music class, as a music class did not require her to wear a bathing suit. Completion of these exposure exercises also reinforced the belief that she is, indeed, a capable parent.

Mindfulness

Mindfulness is "the awareness that emerges through paying attention on purpose, in the present moment, and nonjudgmentally to the unfolding of experience moment by moment: (Kabat-Zinn, 2003, p. 145). Although mindfulness has been practiced by Buddhists to facilitate their spiritual practice for over 2,500 years, at the end of the 20th century, it was integrated into traditional cognitive therapy as an intervention to prevent relapse in people with chronic depression (defined as having a history of three of more episodes of depression; Segal et al., 2002, 2013). The practice of mindfulness ranges from "formal" practices, such as an intentional focus on breathing or sounds in one's environment, often guided by a soothing voice on an audio track, to informal practices, such as being slow and intentional while eating to notice the smell, taste, and texture of the food one is eating. Many people find that mindfulness helps them step out of a frantic mode of multitasking or of an "automatic pilot" mode, in which they are going through the motions of life, not fully registering what they are doing or what is going on in their surroundings. Moreover, many people find that they achieve a sense of calm after participating in a mindfulness exercise, although it is important to recognize that a sense of calm may or may not manifest after any particular mindfulness exercise, and that this outcome is okay. Indeed, even if a person has not achieved a sense of calm, it is likely that they have gained increasing awareness of subtle sensations in their bodies that might signify an increase in depression and anxiety, and on the basis of this awareness, the person can take skillful action, such as applying one of the other CBT strategies described in this chapter.

Many perinatal women indeed describe themselves as frantically multitasking or as being numb and in "automatic pilot" mode; thus, mindfulness has the potential to be an ideal match for the needs of this population. Although many perinatal women report that they have difficulty working in "formal" meditation practices during the day (maybe of which average between 10 and 15 minutes in length, though one particular mindfulness exercise, the body scan, can last up to 45 minutes), they find that they can, indeed, work in a few moments to focus on their breath and body in times of distress, or that they enjoy mindfully nursing or rocking their babies to sleep at night. Moreover, in my clinical experience, the aspect of mindfulness that resonates most with perinatal women is the quality of being non-judgmental, as many women with perinatal depression and/or anxiety are extremely hard on themselves and view themselves as a failure or as a bad mother. Thus, the intentional suspension of judgment, in the spirit of mindfulness practice, that can be applied to their self-flagellating thoughts, can be powerful in facilitating distancing from their thoughts.

Jade proactively inquired about mindfulness to her therapist, as she had a friend who had participated in a Mindfulness-Based Stress Reduction course and raved about her experience. When she was provided with psychoeducation about the components and practice of mindfulness, as well as its benefits, Jade was eager to experiment with it, remarking that she has always been an "overthinker" and that she is "stuck" in her head to such a degree that she believes she is often not present for important moments in her life. Jade opted to listen to a mindfulness audio track through a mobile phone application after she put her son down to bed, as she was falling asleep herself. She observed that this practice helped to focus on her breathing rather than on her thoughts and that it reduced her heart rate, making it much easier for her to fall asleep. Because lack of sleep was one of Jade's primary "triggers" for anxiety when she first presented for treatment, she was pleasantly surprised that this practice contributed to improved sleep, in addition to a more general nonjudgmental, present-focused approach to her life. Regarding the latter point, Jade began to see that assuming a nonjudgmental stance about her own parenting helped to soften self-flagellating thoughts about being incapable.

Core Belief Work

According to cognitive behavioral theory and as noted previously, a core belief is a fundamental belief that people hold about the self, others, the world, or the future. These core beliefs often fuel rigid rules and assumptions by which people live their lives, as well as unique strategies to mitigate the pain associated with particularly negative core beliefs. In many instances, the particular thoughts that a person experiences when they are faced with a challenge or stressor are reminiscent of their core beliefs. Many cognitive behavioral therapists believe that the greatest gains that clients make in CBT occur when they shift unhelpful core beliefs to beliefs that are more balanced and adaptive (Wenzel, 2012). Some of the same strategies described in this section can be applied to the shifting of core beliefs (e.g., cognitive restructuring, behavioral activation and exposure to provide different life experiences to clients than those that have shaped unhelpful core beliefs). However, core beliefs are typically not shifted simply by applying one particular strategy—in reality, a combination of strategies over time accumulates in powerful shifts in core belief. J. S. Beck (2021) has described additional strategies that are especially potent in achieving a shift in underlying beliefs.

As Jade's mood began to stabilize, and she began to have parenting successes, Jade shifted the focus to beliefs that she held about being incapable of functioning without the help of her parents, to assumptions that she held about what it would be like to upset her parents or go against their wishes, and to her compensatory strategies of subjugating her own needs and rushing to please her parents. Jade was able to use the evidence that was accumulating across the course of therapy (both in terms of parenting successes, and also in being able to overcome postpartum anxiety and depression) to shift her belief that she was incapable to one of being just as capable as the next person. She also implemented "behavioral experiments" consisting of expressing dissenting opinions to her parents, setting boundaries, and, when necessary, asking them politely to change their behavior with her son. Not only did these behavioral experiments allow her to gain much practice in social problem solving and effective communication, but they also demonstrated to her that there were no dire consequences if she stood up to her parents. In fact, she was pleasantly surprised that her father, in particular, seemed to understand her point of view when she enacted these experiments and responded with kindness, compassion, and reasonableness.

Relapse Prevention

Cognitive behavioral therapists approach treatment with the idea that there will be an eventual end to therapy, such that clients will have acquired the principles and strategies necessary to manage emotional distress and life's challenges, as well as prevent a relapse or recurrence of a mental health disorder that has abated during the course of CBT. After clients have achieved a stable reduction in symptoms, have demonstrated the ability to apply CBT strategies in their lives, and have largely met their treatment goals, they usually move into a ending phase of treatment focused on relapse prevention. *Relapse prevention* involves (a) the consolidation of the learning that has occurred throughout the course of treatment; (b) a consideration of the warning signs that might signal relapse or recurrence; (c) the anticipation of the cognitive behavioral principles and strategies that the client will invoke, on their own, when they notice these warning signs; and (d) the delineation of criteria that will guide the client in reaching out to a mental health professional for help (Wenzel, 2019). After sessions focused on relapse prevention, clients often leave therapy with a relapse prevention plan that they can consult when they are faced with an exacerbation of emotional distress or a new difficulty in their lives. If and when a client chooses to return for more sessions (often referred to by clients as a "tune-up"), it is not viewed as a treatment failure, but rather it is viewed as a choice that is adaptive and wise on the basis of the symptoms and challenges they are observing in their lives (O'Donohue & Cucciare, 2008).

Jade ended treatment when her son was approximately 18 months old. She expressed great delight about the "transformation" that she achieved in CBT, noting that not only did it help her to overcome the paralyzing anxiety, but that she felt more centered and sure of herself than she had ever felt in her life. Although her relationship with her family of origin continued to be challenging, particularly with her mother, she observed that she was applying the principles of problem solving and effective communication in a consistent manner and that she was able to disengage with much less guilt and angst than she had in the past when her family did not respect her boundaries.

Jade resumed treatment with her cognitive behavioral therapist many years later, when her son was nine years old. She was pleased to report that she had kept top-of-mind many of the "pearls of wisdom" that she had attained for managing emotional distress and dealing with her family of origin. In fact, the reason that brought her back to treatment was an increase in social anxiety now that her son was active and engaged in many extracurricular activities (e.g., baseball, orchestra) and requesting play dates and sleepovers with his friends. To address this need, Jade participated in eight additional sessions of exposure-based therapy for social anxiety, geared toward these activities and had experienced "victories" by being active in her son's organizations and by hosting social events.

Perinatal Conditions Treated With CBT: Evidence of Efficacy and Effectiveness

As will be noted in the following sections, the vast majority of the empirical research that has evaluated the efficacy and effectiveness of CBT for perinatal mental health disorders has focused on depression during pregnancy and/or the postpartum period. Moreover, over the past several years, an increasing amount of attention has been devoted to the treatment of perinatal anxiety and anxiety-related disorders. The CBT approaches for these perinatal mental health conditions are similar to the approaches that have been evaluated for people in the general population who have been diagnosed with depression and anxiety disorders, albeit with the content being geared to unique concerns associated with the transition to parenthood.

In contrast, there is a significant paucity of research that has evaluated the efficacy and effectiveness of CBT for other mental health disorders that present in the perinatal period, including eating disorders, substance use disorders, bipolar disorder and psychosis. However, there is nothing inherent about CBT for these mental health disorders that would be precluded in their delivery to perinatal women. Psychotherapists working with perinatal women with these mental health disorders can consult the following CBT manuals for guidance: (a) eating disorders: Fairburn (2008); (b) substance use disorders: Liese and Beck (2022); (c) bipolar disorder: Basco and Rush (2007); and (d) psychosis: A. T. Beck et al. (2011) and A. T. Beck et al. (2021).

In the following sections, I provide highlights of the empirical research that has evaluated the efficacy of CBT for the two most commonly studied perinatal mental health conditions—depression and anxiety.

Depression

Despite the fact that countless studies have established the impressive efficacy of CBT for depression for adult clients (e.g., Butler et al., 2006), evidence for the efficacy of CBT for perinatal depression was decided mixed through the mid-2010s. For example, several studies found that CBT was no more efficacious than a control psychotherapy, such as supportive psychotherapy (e.g., Cooper et al., 2003; Milgrom et al., 2011; Milgrom et al., 2005), or that it did not enhance the efficacy of selective serotonin reuptake inhibitors (Appleby et al., 1997; Misri et al., 2004). Moreover, meta-analyses conducted during this time period found effect sizes favoring interpersonal psychotherapy (IPT) over CBT (Bledsoe & Grote, 2006; Sockol et al., 2011. Authors of meta-analyses focused exclusively on CBT reported that the majority, but not all individual studies found evidence for CBT's efficacy and that the state of the literature was hampered by significant variability in methodological quality (Sockol, 2015).

In my critical evaluation of the literature on CBT or perinatal depression to date during this time period, I and my colleagues observed that many, if not most, of the CBT protocols evaluated contained elements that were inconsistent with the "spirit" of CBT advanced by Aaron T. Beck (Wenzel et al., 2016). Specifically, many of the CBTs evaluated in studies that were included in meta-analyses were very structured and prescribed session-by-session protocols, which is different than the "Beckian" case formulation-driven treatment approach that is typically implemented in clinical settings and that is described in this chapter. Furthermore, some of the CBT protocols actually advanced constructs or practices that are contraindicated in CBT as it is contemporarily delivered, such as including direct advice or reassurance-seeking (Appleby et al., 1997) or even psychodynamic components (e.g., recognition of Oedipal conflicts; Chabrol et al., 2002).

Since that time, research examining the efficacy and effectiveness of CBT for perinatal depression has yielded more consistent positive results. Meta-analyses conducted by Huang et al. (2018) and Li et al. (2022) demonstrated that CBT, relative to control conditions (i.e., treatment as usual, enhanced treatment as usual, no treatment, waitlist controls), has both short-term efficacy (defined as the difference in symptoms from baseline to immediately post-intervention) and long-term efficacy (defined as the difference in symptoms from baseline to the end of a follow-up period). This pattern of results was obtained regardless of modality (e.g., individual, group, inclusion of partners, in-home, telephone-based, Internet, workbook) and provider who delivered the treatment (i.e., specialist or nonspecialist).

Moreover, subgroup analyses conducted by Li et al. indicated efficacy of CBT delivered during pregnancy to prevent postpartum depression, as well as the efficacy of treatment specifically for low-income women.

The most updated meta-analysis at the time of the writing of this chapter was conducted by Pettman et al. (2023), who aimed to update the literature by including the proliferation of randomized controlled trials (RCTs) examining CBT for perinatal depression and by focusing specifically on evidence-based protocols for the treatment (rather than prevention) of perinatal depression. They included CBT protocols that focused on cognitive restructuring, behavioral activation, and/or problem solving, excluding protocols that included "third-wave" elements, and that were compared to a control group (e.g., no treatment, waitlist control, treatment as usual, nonspecific factors component control, specific factors component control, and active competitor). Meta-analytic results for the primary outcome (i.e., depression) yielded a Hedge's g of −0.53 (95% confidence interval; [CI] = 0.65 to −0.40), indicative of a medium effect size and roughly in line with the most heavily cited meta-analysis on psychological treatments, overall, for perinatal depression, which found Hedge's g of 0.67 (95% CI = 0.45–0.89; Cuijpers et al., 2021). Results from moderator analyses indicated that effects were higher when CBT was compared to waitlist control or treatment-as-usual (vs. an active treatment), when a full CBT package or problem solving was delivered (vs. behavioral activation) and when treatment was delivered by a mental health or healthcare provider (vs. a nonspecialist provider). A small effect size was obtained for reduction in anxiety (Hedge's g = −0.44; 95% CI = −0.55 to −0.33), a medium effect size was obtained for reduction in stress (Hedge's g = −0.56; 95% CI = −0.80 to −0.32), a small effect size was found for improvement in social support, (Hedge's g = 0.25; 95% CI = −0.14 to 0.36), a nonsignificant effect size was found for perceived parenting stress, and a large effect size was found for improvement in self-reported parenting (Hedge's g = 0.94; 95% CI = −0.01 to 1.88).

These meta-analytic findings establish that CBT is efficacious for the treatment of perinatal depression. However, the moderate (rather than large) effect size for the main outcome variable—depression—begs the question as to whether there is room for improvement in the potency of CBT for this population. Authors of meta-analyses examining the efficacy of CBT in adults with major depressive disorder, more generally, have reported Hedge's gs of 0.71 (95% CI = 0.62–0.79; Cuijpers et al., 2013) and 0.75 (95% CI = 0.64–0.87; Cuijpers et al., 2016), remarking that effect sizes were lower in higher-quality studies. The degree to which these effect sizes are statistically and clinically significantly higher than the effect sizes obtained for samples of women with perinatal depression is unclear. Nevertheless, this pattern of results raises the possibility that work can still be done to optimize the efficacy and effectiveness of CBT in this population (cf. Waqas et al., 2023). In the final section of this chapter, I share ideas for ways to achieve this lofty aim.

Anxiety

Studies examining the efficacy of CBT for perinatal anxiety have been published in increasing numbers over the last several years. Li et al.'s (2022) meta-analysis demonstrated that CBT for anxiety has both short- and long-term efficacy relative to an array of nonspecific control groups. However, the overall positive finding for the short-term efficacy of CBT for perinatal anxiety was driven by in-person group formats but not in-person individual formats, which could be explained by the fact that general practitioners delivered control treatments in the studies examining individual formats, thereby rendering the control conditions particularly potent.

Perhaps the most systematically studied CBT protocol for perinatal anxiety is cognitive behavioral group treatment (CBGT), developed by Sheryl Green, Randi McCabe, and their colleagues out of Canada (Green et al., 2020; Green et al., 2015). The CBGT evaluated in these studies consists of six weekly sessions of two hours each, incorporating a focus on psychoeducation, cognitive restructuring, consideration of productive (vs. unproductive) worry, behavioral experiments, behavioral activation, and assertiveness. Participants who participated CBGTs reported a significant reduction of anxious and depressive symptoms by the end of the six-week period, as well as "good" or "excellent" satisfaction (Green et al., 2015). Moreover, the gains that they achieved through treatment were maintained three months after treatment ended and continued to be significantly greater than those found in a waitlist control condition (Green et al., 2020). Subgroup analyses indicated that women with generalized anxiety disorder (GAD), in particular, reported a decrease in worry, avoidance, and safety behaviors after participation in CBGT (Green et al., 2021). Moreover, changes in intolerance of uncertainty, self-oriented parenting perfectionism, and societal-prescribed parenting perfectionism emerged as possible mechanisms of change in the reduction of anxiety following this treatment (Donegan et al., 2022).

Another CBT-based program that deserves highlight in this chapter is that developed by Kiara Timpano, Jonathan Abramowitz and their colleagues to prevent the onset of postpartum obsessive-compulsive disorder (OCD; Timpano et al., 2011). In their evaluation, women in the second or third trimester of pregnancy were randomly assigned to a childbirth education program (the control group) or to childbirth education plus prevention. The prevention condition involved psychoeducation about obsessive-compulsive symptoms and the cognitive behavioral model of OCD, practice in cognitive restructuring, tips for developing behavioral experiments and exposures to test out beliefs. Results indicated that women in the prevention condition endorsed significantly fewer obsessive and compulsive symptoms than women in the control condition at one, three, and six months postpartum, as well as fewer beliefs about the importance and control of intrusive thoughts. Given the ubiquity of intrusive thoughts in new parents (Abramowitz et al., 2003), providers developing childbirth education programs would be wise to take lessons from this research and consider integrating psychoeducation about postpartum obsessive-compulsive symptoms into their curriculum.

Cultural Considerations

CBT lends itself well to cross-cultural application due to its manualized intervention strategies and its ability to be culturally adapted (Dixon & Dantas, 2017). Although empirical research demonstrates that CBT is generally effective for ethnic minority individuals, some statistical analyses yield nonsignificant trends, suggesting that the relative effectiveness is weaker for ethnic minority individuals than for White individuals (Huey et al., 2023). Thus, it behooves researchers to be thoughtful in their adaptations of any intervention approach, including CBT, for specific populations, to evaluate their efficacy through empirical research rather than assuming that the intervention applies to particular ethnic minority clients, and to obtain feedback from those clients to ensure that the adaptation is relevant, respectful, helpful, and well-received.

Perhaps the most comprehensive CBT intervention approach to be delivered in across the globe is the *Thinking Healthy Programme* (WHO, 2015), an intervention that was developed in Pakistan (Rahman et al., 2008) and then later applied in many Global South counties (e.g., India; Atif et al., 2017; Vanobberghen et al., 2020). It is an intervention that can be delivered by community health workers and paraprofessionals in areas in which there is a shortage of specialists and uses psychoeducation (communicated through supportive and empathetic conversation, through images, and through practice of simple exercises) about helpful and unhelpful thinking as applied to the relationship with the baby, self-care, and social support. Outcome data for the program are impressive—participation in this program not only has been shown to significantly reduce depressive symptoms at 6 and 12 months postpartum relative to enhanced usual care (Rahman et al., 2008; Vanobberghen et al., 2020), but also have some positive associations with infant health (e.g., fewer diarrheal episodes, increased rate of immunization; Rahman et al., 2008).

The *Mothers and Babies Course* is another well-established CBT-based approach that is implemented from a prevention standpoint to low-income women seeking services at a public sector women's clinic who are at risk for PPD (Muñoz et al., 2004; Muñoz et al., 2007). It is a 12-week group course that consists of three modules: (a) engagement in pleasant activities; (b) recognition of unhelpful thought patterns; and (c) utilization of social support and is delivered in both English and Spanish. In addition, the intervention's aims are to increase awareness of stress and moods, develop an adaptive mother–infant attachment bond, and learn effective parenting strategies. Research by Muñoz and his colleagues has found that participants find the content of the group to be helpful and applicable, that the majority of participants (91%) are retained throughout the program, and that it reduces the incidence of postpartum major depressive disorder (Le et al., 2011; Muñoz et al., 2007; Tandon et al., 2011) and promotes growth in emotion regulation (Mendelson et al., 2013). The course has been adapted for other ethnically diverse individuals, such as African American adolescent mothers (Lieberman et al., 2023), urban Spanish mothers (Le et al., 2020), and mothers in Kenya and Tanzania (Le et al., 2023).

Dissemination

Over the past two decades, there has been increasing attention devoted to the dissemination of CBT so that it has the potential to reach every individual around the world who is struggling with a mental health disorder (Taylor & Chang, 2008). In the United States, for example, the Beck Institute for Cognitive Behavior Therapy was founded in 1994 by Aaron T. Beck and Judith S. Beck as a nonprofit organization with the mission of "improving lives worldwide through excellence and innovation in Cognitive Behavior Therapy" (https://beck-institute.org/about/). Providers from all over the world have traveled to the Beck Institute for in-person training, participate in webinars, and receive intensive supervision to achieve competency in CBT. Moreover, there are countless initiatives to bring CBT to agencies who work with low-income and ethnically diverse clients, such as the Penn Beck Community Initiative to bring CBT to community mental health centers in the Philadelphia area and beyond (Creed et al., 2016). Treatment of perinatal mental health disorders, specifically, is one area that is emphasized by the Beck Institute and by the Penn Beck Community Initiative.

In addition, dissemination is an important end goal for the developers of the two CBT-based programs described in the previous section on cultural considerations. The fact that the Thinking Healthy Programme can be implemented by paraprofessionals and even peers

(Vanobberghen et al., 2020) contributes to its potential to be implemented in widely in Global South countries. In fact, the Thinking Healthy Programme is now being integrated as a universal group intervention in routine prenatal care in Turkey (Boran et al., 2023). In addition, Le et al. (2015) described thoughtful consideration of the dissemination of the Mothers and Babies course, emphasizing that relevant manuals are available for free online, as are monitoring and evaluation tools.

Finally, the use of Internet-based treatments can help to reach more perinatal women in need of cognitive behaviorally based treatment. Research has demonstrated the efficacy of CBT delivered via that synchronous Internet groups, and psychoeducation in the format of a Zoom workshops (Van Lieshout et al., 2021) in the treatment of perinatal depression. Moreover, Nishi et al. (2023) demonstrated that Internet-based CBT is an efficacious approach in the prevention of postpartum depression. Countless CBT-based Internet programs are being evaluated, many of which are described by Loughnan and Grierson's chapter in this volume. Internet-based treatments have the potential to be an especially good match for perinatal women who often have difficulty with regular in-person attendance due to difficulties with childcare, overwhelm with many doctor's appointments, and sleep deprivation (Wenzel et al., 2016).

Conclusion and Future Directions

CBT is a system of psychotherapy that has an abundance of research supporting its efficacy in the treatment of adults with mental health disorders and its efficacy and effectiveness in the treatment of women with perinatal depression and anxiety. It is being disseminated widely through cultural adaptations, training of paraprofessional and even peer providers, and its availability in Internet-based formats. In the past, it might have been viewed as a treatment that is a bit cold and clinical for perinatal women—feedback that I have received in the past when I was in conversation with non-CBT providers of treatment to perinatal women! At present, its desirability for perinatal women is clear by the amount of randomized controlled trials that have been conducted to evaluate it, as well as the number of requests that are made for training in its adaptation for perinatal women.

This being said, I believe there is still room for its optimization, as evidenced by effect sizes achieved in meta-analyses that are small-to-moderate in size, rather than moderate to large in size. "Third-wave" cognitive behavioral therapies are just now starting to be evaluated for perinatal women (Agako et al., 2022) or included in meta-analyses (Waqas et al., 2023). Clinically, I have witnessed that a contemporary CBT approach that balances the delivery of change-based strategies (e.g., cognitive restructuring, behavioral activation, exposure, problem solving) with acceptance-based strategies (e.g., mindfulness) is received especially well by clients and contributes to an especially strong therapeutic relationship (Wenzel, 2017, in press). It will be important to test this clinical observation in empirical research.

Moreover, I continue to believe that, when feasible, the delivery of a customized CBT package based on the individual client's case formulation is optimal. Many of the CBT packages for perinatal mental health disorders continue to be a bit prescribed, such that there are particular topics that are to be covered in particular sessions. This setup is to be expected in group settings, such as those developed by Green, McCabe, and their colleagues and the Mothers and Babies Course developed by Muñoz and his colleagues, and when paraprofessionals (who do not have advanced training in psychology or psychiatry) are delivering the intervention. However, when a clinician is treating a perinatal client in individual psychotherapy in an office setting, the case formulation approach would lend itself to the possibility of the optimization of treatment for the client's unique needs and preferences. This, also, is a notion that will be extremely important to evaluate with empirical research.

Thus, I have specified two important areas for future research: (a) the evaluation of "third-wave" CBT protocols for perinatal mental health disorders (or the evaluation of broad CBT packages that include elements and strategies from "third-wave" protocols); and (b) the evaluation of the efficacy of case formulation–based CBT relative to a pre-scribed package of CBT. I call on researchers to examine two additional issues in the future. First, it is vital that CBT is evaluated for mental health disorders other than perinatal depression and anxiety—the astute research will notice that CBT for perinatal eating disorders, alcohol and drug use disorders, bipolar disorder, and psychosis were not discussed at length in this chapter, and this is because there is a noticeable paucity of research in these areas. Second, it will be important to move beyond standard out-come measures of symptomatology and move toward other meaningful measurements of changes, as researchers are just beginning to do in work that has been published in the past few years (e.g., emotion regulation [Agako et al., 2021]; maternal self-efficacy, psychological flexibility, self-compassion [Branquinho et al., 2022]).

Great gains have been made in the cognitive behavioral treatment of perinatal women since the time of my previous reviews (Wenzel, 2015; Wenzel et al., 2016). The future seems even brighter. It is my great hope that the mission of cognitive behavioral therapists—for CBT to be disseminated to people in need around the world—can be realized for the popu-lation of perinatal women, who can benefit so greatly from it.

References

Abramowitz, J. S., Deacon, B. J., & Whiteside, S. P. H. (2019). *Exposure therapy for anxiety: Principles and practice* (2nd ed.). Guilford Press.

Abramowitz, J. S., Schwartz, S. A., Moore, K. M., & Luenzmann, K. R. (2003). Obsessive-compulsive symptoms in pregnancy and the puerperium: A review of the literature. *Journal of Anxiety Disorders, 17*, 461–478.

Agako, A., Burckell, L., McCabe, R. E., Frey, B. N., Barrett, E., Silang, K., & Green, S. M. (2022). A pilot study examining the effectiveness of a short-term DBT informed skills group for emotion dysregulation during the perinatal period. *Psychological Services, 20*, 697–707.

Agako, A., Donegan, E., McCabe, R. E., Frey, B. N., Streiner, D., & Green, S. (2021). The role of emotion dysregulation in cognitive behavioural group therapy for perinatal anxiety: Results from a randomized controlled trial and routine clinical care. *Journal of Affective Disorders, 292*, 517–525.

Appleby, L., Warner, R., Whitton, A., & Faragher, B. (1997). A controlled study of fluoxetine and cognitive-behavioural counselling in the treatment of postnatal depression. *British Medical Journal, 314*, 932–936.

Arch, J. J., Dimidjian, S., & Chessick, C. (2012). Are exposure-based cognitive behavioral therapies safe during pregnancy? *Archives of Women's Mental Health, 15*, 445–457.

Atif, N., Krishna, R. N., Sikander, S., Lazatus, A., Nisar, A., Ahmad, I., . . . Rahman, A. (2017). Mother-to-mother therapy in India and Pakistan: Adaptation and feasibility evaluation of the peer-delivered Thinking Healthy Programme. *BMC Psychiatry, 17*, 79.

Basco, M. R., & Rush, A. J. (2007). *Cognitive behavioral therapy for bipolar disorder* (2nd ed.). Guilford Press.

Beck, A. T. (1967). *The diagnosis and management of depression.* University of Pennsylvania Press.

Beck, A. T. (1972). *Depression: Causes and treatment.* University of Pennsylvania Press.

Beck, A. T. (1975). *Cognitive therapy and the emotional disorders.* International Universities Press.

Beck, A. T., Grant, P., Inverso, E., Brinen, A. P., & Perivoliotis, D. (2021). *Recovery-oriented cognitive therapy for serious mental health conditions.* Guilford Press.

Beck, A. T., Rector, N. A., Stolar, N., & Grant, P. (2011). *Schizophrenia: Cognitive theory, research, and therapy*. Guilford Press.

Beck, A. T., Rush, A. J., Shaw, B. F., & Emery, G. (1979). *Cognitive therapy of depression*. Guilford Press.

Beck, J. S. (2021). *Cognitive behavior therapy: Basics and beyond* (3rd ed.). Guilford Press.

Bledsoe, S. E., & Grote, N. K. (2006). Treating depression during pregnancy and the postpartum: A preliminary meta-analysis. *Research on Social Work Practice, 16*, 109–120.

Boran, P., Dönmez, M., Bariş, E., Us, M. C., Altaş, Z. M., Nisar, A., . . . Rahman, A. (2023). Delivering the Thinking Health Programme as a universal group intervention integrated into routine antenatal care: A randomized-controlled pilot study. *BMC Psychiatry, 23*, 14.

Branquinho, M., Canavarro, M. C., & Fonseca, A. (2022). A blended cognitive-behavioral intervention for the treatment of postpartum depression: A case study. *Clinical Case Studies, 21*, 438–456.

Butler, A. C., Chapman, J. E., Forman, E. M., & Beck, A. T. (2006). The empirical status of cognitive-behavioral therapy: A review of meta-analyses. *Clinical Psychology Review, 26*, 17–31.

Chabrol, H., Teissedre, F., Saint-Jean. M., Teisseyre, N., Rogé, B., & Mullet, E. (2002). Prevention and treatment of post-partum depression: A controlled randomized study on women at risk. *Psychological Medicine, 32*, 1039–1047.

Cooper, P. J., Murray, L., Wilson, A., & Romaniuk, H. (2003). Controlled trial of the short- and long-term effect of psychological treatment of post-partum depression. I. Impact on maternal mood. *British Journal of Psychiatry, 182*, 412–419.

Cox, J. L., Holden, J. M., & Sagovsky, R. (1987). Detection of postnatal depression: Development of the 10-item Edinburgh Postnatal Depression Scale. *British Journal of Psychiatry, 150*, 782–786.

Creed, T. A., Frankel, S. A., German, R., Green, K. L., Jager-Hyman, S., Pontoski, K., . . . Beck, A. T. (2016). Implementation of transdiagnostic cognitive therapy in diverse community settings: The beck community initiative. *Journal of Consulting and Clinical Psychology, 84*, 1116–1126.

Cuijpers, P., Berking, M., Andersson, G., Quigley, L., Kleiboer, A., & Dobson, K. S. (2013). A meta-analysis of cognitive behavioural therapy for adult depression, alone or in combination with other treatments. *Canadian Journal of Psychiatry, 58*, 376–385.

Cuijpers, P., Cristea, I. A., Karyotaki, E., Reijanders, M., & Huibers, M. J. H. (2016). How effective are cognitive behavior therapies for major depression and anxiety disorders? A meta-analytic update of the evidence. *World Psychiatry, 15*, 245–258.

Cuijpers, P., Franco, P., Ciharvoa, M., Miguel, C., Segre, L. Quero, S., & Karyotaki, E. (2021). Psychological treatment of perinatal depression: A meta-analysis. *Psychological Medicine, 53*, 2596–2608.

Dimidjian, S., Barrera, Jr., M., Martell, C., Muñoz, R. F., & Lewinsohn, P. M. (2011). The origins and current status of behavioral activation treatments for depression. *Annual Review of Clinical Psychology, 7*, 1–38.

Dixon, S., & Dantas, J. A. R. (2017). Best practice for community-based management of postnatal depression in developing countries: A systematic review. *Health Care for Women International, 38*, 118–143.

Dobson, K. S. (2022). Therapeutic relationship. *Cognitive and Behavioral Practice, 29*, 541–544.

Donegan, E., Frey, B. N., McCabe, R. E., Streiner, D. L., & Green, S. M. (2022). Intolerance of uncertainty and perfectionistic beliefs about parenting as cognitive mechanisms of symptom change during cognitive behavior therapy for perinatal anxiety. *Behavior Therapy, 53*, 738–750.

Fairburn, C. G. (2008). *Cognitive behavior therapy and eating disorders*. Guilford Press.

Gershkovich, M. (2019). Exposure and response prevention for postpartum obsessive compulsive disorder. *Journal of Cognitive Psychotherapy: An International Quarterly, 33*, 174–184.

Green, S. M., Donegan, E., McCabe, R. E., Streiner, D. L., Agako, A., & Frey, B. N. (2020). Cognitive behavioral therapy for perinatal anxiety: A randomized controlled trial. *Australian and New Zealand Journal of Psychiatry, 54*, 423–432.

Green, S. M., Donegan, E., McCabe, R. E., Streiner, D. L., Furtado, M., Noble, L., . . . Frey, B. N. (2021). Cognitive behavior therapy for women with generalized anxiety disorder in the perinatal period: Impact on problematic behaviors. *Behavior Therapy, 52*, 907–916.

Green, S. M., Haber, E., Frey, B. N., & McCabe, R. E. (2015). Cognitive behavioral group treatment for perinatal anxiety: A pilot study. *Archives of Women's Mental Health, 18*, 631–638.

Gross, J. J. (2002). Emotion regulation: Affective, cognitive, and social consequences. *Psychophysiology, 39*, 281–291.

Gross, J. J. (Ed.). (2014). *Handbook of emotion regulation* (2nd ed.). Guilford Press.

Hayes, S. C., Strosahl, K. D., & Wilson, K. G. (1999). *Acceptance and commitment therapy: An experiential approach to behavior change.* Guilford Press.

Hayes, S. C., Strosahl, K. D., & Wilson, K. G. (2012). *Acceptance and commitment therapy: The process and practice of mindful change* (2nd ed.). Guilford Press.

Hofmann, S. G., Asnaani, A., Vonk, I. J. J., Sawyer, A. T., & Fang, A. (2012). The efficacy of cognitive behavioral therapy: A review of meta-analyses. *Cognitive Therapy and Research, 36,* 427–440.

Huang, L., Zhao, Y., Qiang, C., & Fan, B. (2018). Is cognitive behavioral therapy a better choice for women with postnatal depression? A systematic review and meta-analysis. *PLoS One, 13,* e0205243.

Huey, S. J., Jr., Park, A. L., Galán, C. A., & Wang, C. X. (2023). Culturally responsive cognitive behavioral therapy for ethnically diverse populations. *Annual Review of Clinical Psychology, 19,* 51–78.

Kabat-Zinn, J. (2003). Mindfulness-based interventions in context: Past, present and future. *Clinical Psychology: Science and Practice, 10,* 144–156.

Kazantzis, N., Beck, J. S., Clark, D. A., Dobson, K. S., Hofmann, S. G., Leahy, R. L., & Wong, C. W. (2018). Socratic dialogue and guided discovery in cognitive behavioral therapy: A modified Delphi panel. *International Journal of Cognitive Therapy, 11,* 140–157.

Kazantzis, N., Dattilio, F. M., & Dobson, K. S. (2017). *The therapeutic relationship in cognitive behavioral therapy: A clinician's guide.* Guilford Press.

Kazantzis, N., Fairburn, C. G., Padesky, C. A., Reinecke, M., & Teesson, M. (2014). Unresolved issues regarding the research and practice of cognitive behavior therapy: The case of guided discovery using Socratic questioning. *Behaviour Change, 31,* 1–17.

Kleiman, K. (2017). *The art of holding: An essential intervention for postpartum depression and anxiety.* Routledge.

Kleiman, K., Wenzel, A., Waller, H., & Adler, A. (2021). *Dropping the baby and other scary thoughts: Breaking the cycle of negative unwanted thoughts in motherhood* (2nd ed.). Routledge.

Knapp, P., Kieling, C., & Beck, A. T. (2015). What do psychotherapists do? A systematic review and meta-regression of surveys. *Psychotherapy and Psychosomatics, 84,* 377–378.

Kuyken, W., Padesky, C. A., & Dudley, R. (2006). *Collaborative case conceptualization: Working effectively with clients in cognitive behavioral therapy.* Guilford Press.

Le, H.-N., McEwan, E., Kapiyo, M., Muthoni, F., Opiyo, T., Rabemananjara, K. M., . . . Hembling, J. (2023). Preventing perinatal depression Cultural adaptation of the Mothers and Babies Course in Kenya and Tanzania. *International Journal of Environmental Research and Public Health, 20,* 6811.

Le, H.-N., Perry, D. F., Mendelson, T., Tandon, S. D., & Muñoz, R. F. (2015). Preventing perinatal depression in high risk women: Moving the Mothers and Babies Course from clinical trials to community implementation. *Maternal and Child Health Journal, 19,* 2102–2110.

Le, H.-N., Perry, D. F., & Stuart, E. A. (2011). Evaluating a preventive intervention for perinatal depression in high-risk Latinas. *Journal of Consulting and Clinical Psychology, 79,* 135–141.

Le, H.-N., Rodríguez-Muñoz, M. F., Soto-Balbuena, C., Olivares Crespo, M. E., Izquierdo Méndez, N., & Marcos-Nájera, R. (2020). Preventing perinatal depression in Spain: A pilot evaluation of *Mamás y Bebés. Journal of Reproductive and Infant Psychology, 38,* 546–559.

Li, X., Laplante, D. P., Paquin, V., Lafortune, S., Elgbeili, G., & King, S. (2022). Effectiveness of cognitive behavioral therapy for perinatal maternal depression, anxiety, and stress: A systematic review and meta-analysis of randomized controlled trials. *Clinical Psychology Review, 92,* 102219.

Lieberman, K., Le, H.-N., Perry, D. F., & Julian, M. (2023). Cultural adaptation and a pilot study of the mothers and babies course for perinatal African American adolescents. *Journal of Child and Family Studies.*

Liese, B. S., & Beck, A. T. (2022). *Cognitive behavioral therapy of addictive disorders.* Guilford Press.

Linehan, M. M. (1993). *Cognitive behavioral treatment of borderline personality disorder.* Guilford Press.

Linehan, M. M. (2015). *DBT skills training handouts and worksheets* (2nd ed.). Guilford Press.

Martell, C. R., Dimidjian, S., & Herman-Dunn, R. (2010). *Behavioral activation for depression: A clinician's guide.* Guilford Press.

Mendelson, T., Leis, J. A., Perry, D. F., Suart, E. A., & Tandon, S. D. (2013). Impact of a preventive intervention for perinatal depression on mood regulation, social support, and coping. *Archives of Women's Mental Health, 16,* 211–218.

Milgrom, J., Holt, C. J., Gemmill, A. W., Ericksen, J., Broncyn, L., . . . Schembri, C. (2011). Treating postnatal depressive symptoms in primary care: A randomized controlled trial of GP management with and without adjunctive counselling. *BMC Psychiatry, 11,* 95.

Milgrom, J., Negri, L. M., Gemmill, A. W., McNeil, M., & Martin, P. R. (2005). A randomized controlled trial of psychological interventions for postnatal depression. *British Journal of Clinical Psychology, 44*, 529–542.

Misri, S., Reebye, P., Corral, M., & Milis, L. (2004). The use of paroxetine and cognitive-behavioral therapy in postpartum depression and anxiety: A randomized controlled trial. *Journal of Clinical Psychiatry, 65*, 1236–1241.

Muñoz, R. F., Le, H.-N., Ghosh-Ippen, C., Diaz, M. A., Urizar, Jr., G. G., & Lieberman, A. F. (2004). *Mother and babies course: Instructor's manual, activities module.* University of California/San Francisco General Hospital. https://i4health.paloaltou.edu/downloads/MBRM_Instructor_English.pdf

Muñoz, R. F., Le, H.-N., Ghosh-Ippen, C., Diaz, M. A., Urizar, Jr., G. G., Soto, J., Mendelson, T., . . . Lieberman, A. F. (2007). Prevention of postpartum depression in low-income women: Development of *Mamás y Bebés*/Mothers and Babies Course. *Cognitive and Behavioral Practice, 14*, 70–83.

Nishi, D., Imamura, K., Wantanabe, K., Obikane, E., Sasaki, N., Yasuma, N., . . . Matsuyama, Y. (2023). The preventive effect of Internet-based cognitive behavioral therapy for prevention of depression during pregnancy and in the postpartum period (iPDP): A large scale randomized controlled trial. *Psychiatry and Clinical Neurosciences, 76*, 570–578.

O'Donohue, W. T., & Cucciare, M. A. (Eds.). (2008). *Terminating psychotherapy: A clinician's guide.* Routledge.

Persons, J. B. (2008). *The case formulation approach to cognitive behavior therapy.* Guilford Press.

Pettman, D., O'Mahen, H., Blomberg, O., Svanberg, A. S., von Essen, L., & Woodward, J. (2023). Effectiveness of cognitive behavioural therapy-based interventions for maternal perinatal depression: A systematic review and meta-analysis. *BMC Psychiatry, 23*, 208.

Rahman, A., Malik, A., Sikander, S., Roberts, C., & Creed, F. (2008). Cognitive behavior therapy-based intervention by community health workers for mothers with depression and their infants in rural Pakistan: A cluster-randomised trial. *The Lancet, 372*, 902–909.

Rosner, R. I. (2018). Three myths and truths about Beck's early years. In R. L. Leahy (Ed.), *Science and practice in cognitive therapy: Foundations, mechanisms, and applications* (pp. 13–28). Guilford Press.

Segal, Z. V., Williams, J. M. G., & Teasdale, J. D. (2002). *Mindfulness-based cognitive therapy for depression.* Guilford Press.

Segal, Z. V., Williams, J. M. G., & Teasdale, J. D. (2013). *Mindfulness-based cognitive therapy for depression* (2nd ed.). Guilford Press.

Shorter, E. (1997). *A history of psychiatry: From the era of the asylum to the age of Prozac.* John Wiley and Sons.

Sockol, L. E. (2015). A systematic review of the efficacy of cognitive behavioral therapy for treating and preventing perinatal depression. *Journal of Affective Disorders, 177*, 7–21.

Sockol, L. E., Epperson, C. N., & Barber, J. P. (2011). A meta-analysis of treatments for perinatal depression. *Clinical Psychology Review, 31*, 839–849.

Tandon, S. D., Mendelson, T., Kemp, K., Leis, L., & Perry, D. F. (2011). Preventing perinatal depression in low-income home visiting clients: A randomized controlled trial. *Journal of Consulting and Clinical Psychology, 79*, 707–712.

Taylor, C. B., & Chang, V. Y. (2008). Issues in the dissemination of cognitive behavior therapy. *Nordic Journal of Psychiatry, 62*(Suppl 47), 37–44.

Timpano, K. R., Abramowitz, J. S., Mahaffey, B. L., Mitchell, M. A., & Schmidt, N. B. (2011). Efficacy of a prevention program for postpartum obsessive compulsive symptoms. *Journal of Psychiatric Research, 45*, 1511–1517.

Van Lieshout, R. J., Layton, H., Savoy, C. D., Brown, J. S. L., Ferro, M. A., Streiner, D. L., . . . Hanna, S. (2021). Effect of online 1-day cognitive behavioral therapy-based workshops plus usual care versus usual care alone for postpartum depression. *JAMA Psychiatry, 78*, 1–8.

Vanobberghen, F., Weiss, H. A., Huhr, D. C., Sikander, S., Afonso, E., Ahmad, I., . . . Rahman, A. (2020). Effectiveness of the Thinking Healthy Programme for perinatal depression delivered through peers: Pooled analysis of two randomized controlled trials in India and Pakistan. *Journal of Affective Disorders, 265*, 660–886.

Waqas, A., Zafar, S. W., Akhtar, P., Naveed, S., & Rahman, A. (2023). Optimizing cognitive and behavioral approaches for perinatal depression: A systematic review and meta-regression analysis. *Cambridge Prisms: Global Mental Health, 10*, e22, 1–14.

Wenzel, A. (2012). Modification of core beliefs in cognitive therapy. In I. R. de Oliveira (Ed.), *Cognitive behavioral therapy* (pp. 17–34). Intech. www.intechopen.com

Wenzel, A. (2013). *Strategic decision making in cognitive behavioral therapy*. American Psychological Association.

Wenzel, A. (2015). *Cognitive behavioral therapy for perinatal distress*. Routledge.

Wenzel, A. (2017). *Innovations in cognitive behavioral therapy: Strategic interventions for creative practice*. Routledge.

Wenzel, A. (2019). *Cognitive behavioral therapy for beginners: An experiential approach*. Routledge.

Wenzel, A. (in press). *Therapeutic relationship-focused cognitive behavioral therapy*. American Psychological Association.

Wenzel, A., Stuart, S., & Koleva, H. (2016). Psychotherapy for psychopathology during pregnancy and the postpartum period. In A. Wenzel (Ed.), *The Oxford handbook of perinatal psychology* (pp. 341–365). Oxford University Press.

World Health Organization. (2015). *Thinking healthy: A manual for psychosocial management of perinatal depression: WHO generic field-trial version 1.0*. Series on Low-Intensity Psychological Interventions. World Health Organization. https://iris.who.int/bitstream/handle/10665/152936/WHO_MSD_MER_15.1_eng.pdf?sequence=1

23

INTEGRATIVE INTERPERSONAL PSYCHOTHERAPY FOR PERINATAL MENTAL HEALTH DISORDERS

Sharon Ben Rafael

In memory of Prof. Josh Lipsitz, who supervised my training and sparked my love for IPT.

> Aaron enters the house at the end of his workday exhausted and hungry, imagining how he will sink into the sofa with his dinner and watch television. Miriam is pacing back and forth in the living room with a crying four-month-old in her arms, relieved that Aaron is back, hoping to get some time off. When Aaron enters, she wants to tell him how happy she is to see him, but before she opens her mouth, he says he is hungry and asks if there is anything to eat. She angrily shoves baby John into his arms and goes to the bedroom, closing the door. Aaron has become accustomed to this scenario, though he was hoping that maybe just for once, Miriam would think about him. He feels disappointed with her and contemplates his decision to marry her. This is a familiar scenario in many homes, where in the context of a role transition of becoming new parents, conflicting gender-based expectations and needs lead to misunderstandings and marital discord. In addition, Miriam is depressed. In the past, she would have resolved this conflict with ease, but her depression is now interfering with her ability to negotiate these recurring situations. Every misunderstanding causes her to feel alone and neglected. Aaron has his work and his life, and she feels as if she has lost everything, including herself. Aaron is feeling regret for starting a family. Although this was a planned pregnancy, Miriam has changed immensely since their son, John, was born. They are both overwhelmed, angry, and irritated, hardly looking at one another and certainly not showing any affection.

The link between stressful life events and depression is well established (Brown & Harris, 1978; Normann & Buttenschøn, 2019; Paykel, 2003; Su et al., 2022). For Miriam, it may have been the transition to motherhood that precipitated her depression. However, her

DOI: 10.4324/9781003206903-28

current difficulty with Aaron is a maintaining factor for the disorder. In three longitudinal studies spanning a course of 15 years, four major themes illustrated key issues in women's depression. All themes demonstrate an association between depression and interpersonal functioning: (a) parent–child vicious cycle in which behaviors of both parties affect each other in negative ways; (b) martial/romantic relationship conflicts; (c) stressful life events (especially interpersonal); and (d) enduring social problems and interpersonal difficulties (Hammen & Brennan, 2002).

Interpersonal psychotherapy (IPT) addresses these themes through four problem areas: role transitions, role disputes, grief, and interpersonal deficits (also referred to as loneliness/social isolation) (World Health Organization and Columbia University, 2016), which provide a focus for intervention. IPT is based on the recognition that the onset or worsening of some mental health disorders for vulnerable individuals is chronologically linked to the client's stressful life events and circumstances in these areas; that social support is important for mental health; and that solving problems in these interpersonal areas and social functioning may help improve symptoms (Markowitz & Weissman, 2004, 2012; Ravitz et al., 2019; Weissman, 2006). IPT is a manualized, time-limited empirically derived psychotherapy that focuses on current interpersonal relationships while recognizing the underlying role of genetic, developmental, biochemical, and personality factors (Klerman et al., 1984; Weissman et al., 2000).

IPT follows the footsteps of Harry Stack Sullivan and John Bowlby, who stressed the importance of relationships in emotional well-being and mental health. In some respects, it also continues the work of Fonagy (1989) by using mentalization as an underlying process (Law et al., 2022; Markowitz et al., 2019). According to the interpersonal theory of Harry Stack Sullivan (Sullivan, 1953), interpersonal relationships are viewed as basic human needs and personality as shaped by relationships with others. He stressed the importance of recognizing real experiences and interactions in addition to unconscious processes. Emotional well-being, in his view, requires healthy relationships with supportive, close others, and the wider social milieu, as well as a good balance between needs for satisfaction and needs for security. Sullivan's theory was a shift from classical Freudian drive theory to a more relational view of the importance of the here and now, current interpersonal relationships.

John Bowlby's attachment theory saw the need to form a close bond with a caregiver as an innate, biologically determined survival system common to all mammals. He proposed that the attachment to caregivers provides a "secure base" from which the infant can safely explore, learn, and develop. Through this secure base, individuals create "internal working models" (Bowlby, 1973) related to expectations of others, and "attachment styles" or patterns of relating in times of need or stress, that guide them in relationships throughout life (Ainsworth et al., 2015; Ravitz et al., 2010). Fonagy et al. (1991) discussed the caregiver's capacity for mentalization as a predictor of attachment in children and the use of mentalizing in therapy as a way of establishing epistemic trust (Fonagy & Allison, 2014).

The state of "primary maternal preoccupation," coined by Winnicott (2016 [1956]), perfectly describes the state many women experience during the last weeks of pregnancy and the first few weeks postpartum: a state of heightened sensitivity with intense attunement and preoccupation with the infant, quickly responding to their needs (pp. 300–305). Expanding on this notion, Stern (1995) referred to "the motherhood constellation" as a psychic shift in the woman's attention to infant development, connection to the infant, the mother's support system, and her identity as a mother, that takes place in the transition to motherhood (pp. 171–190). This state of devoted attention is crucial for the infant, considering the significance of attachment and the influence of the caregiver's responses on the development of the infant (Bowlby, 1973). To maintain this state, perinatal women (who choose the role of being a primary caregiver or are required to take it due to cultural or familial circumstances) need help and support from others and relative freedom from symptoms that impair functioning or the capacity for emotional relatedness.

The goals of IPT enable this by decreasing depressive symptoms, enhancing social support, decreasing interpersonal stress, processing emotions, improving interpersonal skills (Lipsitz & Markowitz, 2013), promoting adaptation to the new social role as a parent, as well as by promoting mentalization (Markowitz et al., 2019). These mechanisms of change extend the important pillars of IPT: instilling hope and expectations for change, creating a new narrative, externalizing the current problem, decreasing guilt, increasing motivation for change, and validating distress (Lipsitz & Markowitz, 2013).

The diathesis-stress model (Simpson & Rholes, 2012) shows how distress that is triggered by external and internal events evokes specific attachment behaviors, guided by the individual's internal working model. The response of the attachment figures to secure, avoidant, or anxious attachment behaviors may further influence coping, adjustment, and the responses of others. For example, a woman with an anxious attachment style may become obsessively dependent on her partner. In time, this may exhaust the partner who withdraws, and his response may trigger a sense of rejection that may further distress the woman and intensify the obsessive, help-seeking behaviors. In contrast, a woman with an avoidant attachment style might not confide in or signal to others that she needs help, thus not eliciting needed social support or even extinguishing the interest of others whose help she rejects, leaving her alone in her suffering. IPT enables us to work with the woman's attachment behaviors and modes of communication and focus on problems especially related to grief, role transitions, and role disputes that are highly appropriate for the difficulties perinatal women face (Stuart & Robertson, 2012).

IPT was originally developed to treat major depressive disorder (Klerman et al., 1984) and later modified and tested to treat bulimia nervosa (Fairburn et al., 1993), dysthymia (Markowitz et al., 2005), social phobia (Lipsitz et al., 1999, 2008), bipolar disorder (Frank et al., 2007), posttraumatic stress disorder, (Bleiberg & Markowitz, 2005; Markowitz et al., 2015; Proença et al., 2022; Rafaeli & Markowitz, 2011) and panic disorder (Lipsitz et al., 2006), among others. IPT has also been adapted and studied for different populations across the lifespan from pre-adolescence (Dietz, 2020) and adolescence (Mufson et al., 1994), to women during pregnancy or postpartum (Spinelli & Endicott, 2003; Stuart & O'Hara, 1995) and in late life (Reynolds et al., 1999).

IPT is considered a first-line treatment for mild to moderate postpartum depression (PPD). The transition to parenthood is an impactful and, at times, stressful life event. It may start with the wish to start a family, attempts to conceive, fertility treatments, pregnancy, pregnancy losses, and eventually birth and parenthood. Parents must cope with difficult decisions, novel challenges, social role transitions, and changes in interpersonal, family, and work circumstances. During this stage, women seek or are referred to therapy for various reasons, including (but not limited to) difficulty adjusting to the new situation, interpersonal difficulties, inner conflict, marital conflict, early trauma, depression, and anxiety. The focus of IPT on real-life situations and current distressing relational events from the past week and the relaxed, supportive, and collaborative therapeutic stance are also good fits for treating perinatal women with depression and anxiety (Stuart & Robertson, 2012). IPT was extended for the treatment of prenatal depression with higher efficacy than a parenting education program in reducing symptoms of depression (Spinelli & Endicott, 2003). This adaptation includes an additional problem area termed "complicated pregnancy," which addresses problems related to gestation: undesired pregnancy, multiple births, and congenital animalities as well as obstetrical and medical complications associated with pregnancy. Spinelli's (2017) focus on issues related to pregnancy brought their importance to attention and stressed the significance of assessing and focusing on these issues when they are relevant. It is important to consider and assess these factors in the formulation and they can also be covered within the role transitions problem area (e.g., the role transition to an undesired, unplanned pregnancy).

In 1995, Stuart and O'Hara reported positive results in a small clinical trial of IPT for postpartum depression (PPD), such that they described how conceptualizing the postpartum period as "role overload" is aligned with the IPT focal area of social role transitions. In a later randomized controlled trial (RCT) for PPD, O'Hara et al. (2000) showed that IPT was associated with significant improvements in depressive symptoms as compared to a waitlist control (WLC). Forty-eight postpartum women who completed a course of 12-session IPT were compared to 51 women in a WLC group. IPT resulted in a statistically significant reduction of depressive symptoms (19.4 to 8.3) relative to WLC (19.8 to 16.8) as measured on the *Hamilton Rating Scale for Depression* (Hamilton, 1967) and (23.6 to 10.6 vs. 23 to 19.2) on the *Beck Depression Inventory* (Beck et al., 1961). At the end of treatment, only 12.5% of the woman who received IPT met DSM-IV criteria for a major depressive episode, versus 68.6% of the women in the WLC group at the 12-week assessment. Women in the treatment group also showed statistically significant improvements relative to WLC in their psychosocial functioning on the *Social Adjustment Scale—Self-Report* (Weissman, 1976) and the *Postpartum Adjustment Questionnaire* (O'Hara et al., 1992).

Other randomized studies also showed that 12 to 16 sessions of IPT is efficacious for perinatal depression (Grote et al., 2009; Lenze & Potts, 2017; Miniati et al., 2014; Sockol, 2018; Spinelli & Endicott, 2003; Spinelli et al., 2013). Other adaptations of IPT for perinatal depression include a group format (Mulcahy et al., 2010; Zlotnick et al., 2001); IPT-B, an eight-session brief format (Swartz et al., 2014); and a culturally adapted format for low-income women in the United States during pregnancy and up to six months postpartum. IPT-B has been associated with significant reductions in depression and improvement in social functioning when compared to enhanced usual care (Grote et al., 2009). IPT has also been adapted for trained nurses, or midwives as nonmental health specialist providers, of telephone-based IPT to postpartum women, with significant improvements in depressive symptoms compared to treatment as usual or a control group referred to mental health professionals (Dennis et al., 2020; Guille & Douglas, 2017; Posmontier et al., 2016). IPT is also recommended for the prevention of depression during pregnancy by the U.S. Preventive Services Task Force (O'Conner et al., 2019) and for the treatment of postpartum depression (National Health Information, n.d.; National Institute of Mental Health, n.d.). Altogether, there is a strong evidentiary base for IPT as a treatment for perinatal depression. Furthermore, because relationship conflicts that are common postpartum negatively affect the emotional well-being of both the woman and her partner, IPT offers a conjoint treatment (Carter et al., 2010).

A recent systematic review of 45 studies evaluating the efficacy of IPT in treating or preventing perinatal psychological distress (from conception to 12 months postpartum) included 25 RCTs, ten quasi-experimental studies, eight open trials, and two single cases. Forty percent of the studies were evaluated as strong overall, 14% as moderate, and 13% as weak. Of the 13 prevention studies, 5 showed a significant reduction in symptoms with small-to-moderate effect sizes. The results of the treatment studies were better, with 26 of 32 studies reporting significant improvement in symptoms of depression, with moderate-to-large effect sizes. Six of 11 treatment studies also reported a significant reduction in anxiety symptoms with a moderate effect size (Bright et al., 2020).

This chapter begins by describing the use of IPT for treating perinatal depression and continues by proposing an adaptation for comorbid perinatal disorders that include obsessive ruminations and compulsions. Integration of behavior therapy (BT) and IPT has yielded a contemporary treatment called interpersonal behavior psychotherapy (IBPT).

IPT Protocol Description

IPT as described in several books (Klerman et al., 1984; Stuart & Robertson, 2012; Weissman et al., 2018) is a well-established, consensus guideline recommended and evidence-supported depression treatment. IPT for perinatal depressed women (IPT-P) is described in detail by Spinelli (2017). The IPT therapeutic process that follows is based on these textbooks and on clinical experience treating perinatal women.

IPT consists of three phases; a beginning, middle, and end delivered within a set time frame of 8–16 sessions.

Phase 1

It is best to divide this phase into two parts: (a) thorough assessment, with the establishment of a therapeutic alliance, aimed at discerning if this woman may benefit from IPT and if this is the best available treatment for her, and (b) evaluation of interpersonal relationships and the identification of a major interpersonal problem area related to the onset or worsening of the current depression.

The first assessment session consists of open-ended and direct questions aimed at understanding the woman's unique situation and discerning if IPT is a good fit. This is achieved by diagnosing the disorder while differentiating normal pregnancy and postpartum discomforts from depressive symptoms; understanding precipitating factors of previous episodes and their resolution; understanding the circumstances of conception and pregnancy; inquiring about safety, trauma history, and domestic violence; and assessing differential diagnosis and suitability for IPT. Eventually, a diagnosis is provided and explained. A formulation and treatment plan are described, and the woman is offered the "sick role," meaning that for a time-limited period, such as a few weeks, she can excuse herself from social obligations and certain responsibilities and receive help and support from others while working toward recovery (Spinelli, 2017).

Stuart and Robertson (2012) suggested basing the IPT formulation on a bio-psycho-social/cultural/spiritual model that explains psychological difficulties as the specific individual's response to a unique stressor. This model brings attention to cultural and spiritual factors and their relevance to understanding the individual who is seeking help. Their model is an expansion of the bio-psycho-social model (Engel, 1977) and the bio-psycho-social-spiritual (BPSS) model (Wright et al., 1996).

IPT focuses on current problems in interpersonal domains of life including conflicts within close relationships, bereavement, life changes, and isolation. While stressing the connection between distress and social problems, it posits that the resolution of interpersonal difficulties or circumstances linked with current distress will result in symptom reduction. Thus, the second part of the initial phase of treatment is assessing the interpersonal world of the client.

The *interpersonal inventory*, an extended psychosocial assessment, is a collaborative process designed to structure information gathering of social supports and guide the identification of problem areas. This is usually completed during the second and third sessions. This can be done verbally (Weissman et al., 2018) or using a paper-and-pencil tool known as the interpersonal circle (Mufson, 2004) to help facilitate discussion. Thinking about relationships and placing them in circles (see Figure 23.1) initiates the process of introspection about interpersonal relationships and their association with current distress.

Using a figure like that depicted in Figure 23.1, the woman is asked to imagine that she is in the center and write down the names of people in her life, according to her perceived emotional closeness to them. The therapist can say something like, "This can be a map of the relationships in your life. Imagine yourself in the middle. You can place the people in your life anywhere you want on this page, in one word tell me who this person is, and we will explore some of these relationships later." The instructions are minimal and nonjudgmental to enable openness, flexibility, and freedom. Asking to briefly describe the people and the relationships she has with those whom she places on the circles invites collaboration, reflection, and mentalizing, although some women are more comfortable delving into this alone and "handing in" the page once they are finished. There is no right or wrong way for filling out the domains represented in these circles. Once she is finished, the therapist and client begin examining this map together. Adding arrows to demonstrate movement within or out of the diagram and marking close others who may be deceased in any way she deems appropriate (spiritually, culturally, or personally) helps visualize the interpersonal changes relating to the current crisis. Some women choose to place their unborn fetus, their children, and their infants, and some write themselves in the circles. It is up to the woman to decide.

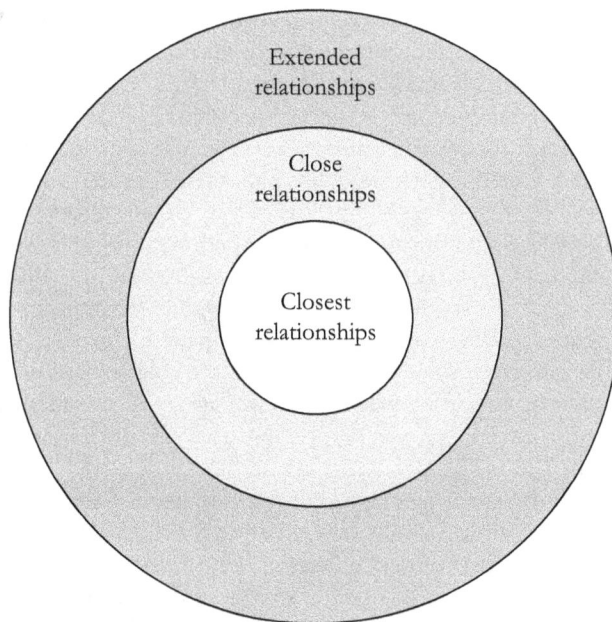

Figure 23.1 Interpersonal circles, a map of the woman's relationships

The interpersonal inventory is continued using this as a foundation. The therapist and client discuss the relationships most relevant to the present life crisis, with the therapist asking open-ended and direct questions to understand her social network and determine the relationships that may become the focus of treatment. It is important to inquire about individuals relevant to the current crisis even if they do not appear in the circles. Therapists gather information about the nature of the relationship, frequency of contact, positive and negative aspects of the relationship, expectations of each party, what has changed during or before the current crisis, what type of support is provided, and in what ways she would like to change the relationship. Moreover, therapists are encouraged to ask for examples of specific incidents, to get a more experience-near view on assessing communication.

Through this examination of her support network, the therapist and client begin identifying patterns in relationships, expectations, and communications, which help to set goals for the second phase of treatment. When working with perinatal women, the relationship with the baby's father, present or absent, should be an area of focus. The current relationship with her parents or in-laws frequently changes and may also become a focus during the current crisis. Therapists should also be prepared to openly and nonjudgmentally address negative feelings about the fetus, infant, and older children in the household. Eventually, therapists collaborate with the client to understand the problems and relationships that are relevant to the acute distress, as well as to choose the IPT problem area(s) (i.e., role disputes, role transitions, grief, social isolation) of focus for the middle phase of treatment.

Phase 2

During the intermediate phase of therapy, the focus is on the acute problem areas. Treatment strategies are derived from the goals and tasks of the specific problem area or areas chosen during phase 1.

Role transitions are life changes that require a role change. Facilitating the transition by grieving the old role and relinquishing it are some of the role transitions tasks (see Closeup 1). For Miriam, introduced at the beginning of the chapter, the initial transition to motherhood was easy, as Aaron was off from work, and they cooperated on caring for John. She did not feel depressed then. It took eight additional weeks of being alone with baby John, with no opportunities for a break in her role, when she started feeling overwhelmed, losing her sense of identity and independence. Symptoms of depression quickly followed, decreasing her ability to negotiate the relationship with Aaron, illuminating their nonreciprocal expectations, and creating repetitive arguments and conflicts. In therapy, Miriam felt understood, she was able to talk about her old life, before the baby and grieve the loss of her old, relaxed self, her independence, and her romantic relationship with Aaron. Relinquishing the old role and expressing affect are some of the tasks of the role transitions problem area (see Closeup 1). Miriam was happy with John but was angry at the fact that Aaron's career and social life continued just as it was before, and that her life as she knew it had halted. She remembered why she fell in love with Aaron, but felt that they were both very young and did not understand what it meant to have an infant. In Miriam's community, where gender-based roles are common (e.g., it was expected for the mother to stay home with her infant for at least six months and for the father to return to work). However, in her family of origin, this was not the case, and she did not expect Aaron to blindly follow this norm. This was a source of many of their arguments. By the time Miriam arrived in therapy, an additional problem area of role disputes was relevant.

Closeup 1 Goals, Strategies, and Techniques

Problem Area	Role Disputes	Role Transitions	Grief	Social Isolation
Description	Conflict with a close support that is relevant to the current crisis (disputes with a partner, family members, close friends, colleagues, supervisors, etc., difficulties with a child or children, and difficulties with the infant).	Life changes that require a role change and are relevant to the current crisis (pregnancy, birth, fertility treatments, loss of fertility, loss of health, move, immigration, etc.).	The recent or past death of a close support, relative, friend, or other that is related to the current crisis (including pregnancy loss, stillbirth, and death of a newborn).	A history of social impoverishment; lack of lasting relationships and extreme social isolation. (This problem area most often refers to long-lasting personality deficits rather than a temporal crisis).
Tasks	1. Identifying the dispute 2. Choosing a plan of action 3. Improving interpersonal communications 4. Reassessing expectations.	1. Relinquishing the old role 2. Expressing affect 3. Acquiring new skills 4. Developing new attachments and support	1. Facilitating the grief process 2. Expressing affect 3. Reestablishing interests 4. Modifying existing relationships or developing new relationships	1. Reviewing past relationships that had significance for the client 2. Examining repetitive problems in these relationships 3. Discussing feelings in therapeutic relationship and parallels in other relationships
Strategies	1. Examining difficulties and nonreciprocal expectations in the relationship as well as parallels in other relationships 2. Exploring the connection between interpersonal disputes and current symptoms 3. Identifying the stage of the dispute and the therapeutic tasks relevant to the stage 4. Facilitating conflict resolution and decision-making regarding the relationship	1. Examining the relation between the transition and current symptoms 2. Facilitating evaluation of the old and new role 3. Encouraging emotional expression 4. Developing social skills for the new role 5. Establishing new interpersonal relationships	1. Examining the relation between grief and current symptoms 2. Examining the significance of the loss, the events surrounding the death, and the complexities of the relationship 3. Encouraging emotional expression 4. Sharing the experience of the loss with others 5. Reestablishing new interests 6. Establishing new interpersonal relationships or modifying existing ones	1. Examining positive and negative experiences in childhood relationships with family members and other significant relationships 2. Examining perceptions and expectations in relationships 3. Identifying positive experiences that could be models for new attachments 4. Focusing on the client-therapist relationship as a source of information about ways of relating 5. Establishing new interpersonal relationships and modifying current ones

Problem Area	Role Disputes	Role Transitions	Grief	Social Isolation
Techniques	*Exploratory* techniques—general, open-ended questions, nondirective techniques such as silence, repeating keywords, paraphrasing with summative comments to provide the client with an experience of being understood and to foster reflecting on relational experiences, nodding or providing other comments aimed at encouraging the individual to keep talking and specific purposeful questions			
	Behavior change techniques—educating, advising, modeling, practical help, decision analysis, role-play			
	Encouragement of affect—acceptance with attenuation of painful effects, use of affect in relationships, acknowledging and identifying suppressed affect, naming affects to improve communication and model empathic understanding			
	Clarification—repeating and rephrasing communications, pointing out assumptions, contradictions, and unhelpful beliefs			
	Communication analysis—examining communications word-by-word to reflect on and understand the emotional reactions and responses of the parties involved, identifying ambiguous or indirect communication, incorrect assumptions, misunderstandings, nonshared expectations, and other communication problems that affect interpersonal relationships			
	Use of the therapeutic relationship—examining perceptions about the therapist and the therapeutic relationship to learn about characteristic ways of feeling and behaving in other relationships, modeling and fostering experiential repair of misunderstandings or tensions, identifying and therapeutically repairing problems in the therapeutic relationship (*Note this is generally reserved when the focus in on interpersonal deficits or sensitivities)			

524

Role disputes are related to conflicts and nonreciprocal expectations within a meaningful relationship. Tasks of this problem area include identifying the dispute, choosing a plan of action: improving interpersonal communications; reassessing expectations (see Closeup 1). Determining the stage of the dispute may help plan a strategy for working toward change. For example, *renegotiation* suggests that both parties are interested in working out the difficulties; *impasse* suggests that the relationship has halted and there is little communication; and *dissolution* implies that there are no attempts at communicating and no interest in negotiation or in continuing the relationship. Miriam and Aaron were in the stage of renegotiation. They were interested in resolving the conflict and working on their differing views. In this case, there would be a heavy emphasis on communication analysis (see Closeup 2), problem solving, and role-play. This involves taking occurrences such as the one described and analyzing the explicit and implicit expectations, the content of communication, the expressed emotion, and the latent emotion, identifying problems in communication, brainstorming solutions, selecting a course of action, role-playing different options, and practicing the chosen solution.

Closeup: 2 Communication Analysis

Communication Analysis

Therapist: Let's look at what happened. Could you describe in detail how each of you acted and what each of you said?

Miriam: I was at home waiting for Aaron to come back, I've been alone with John all day, and he was very cranky. I didn't have any adult talks, and I was just waiting to tell Aaron about my day and to take some time off. I was so relieved when I heard his car in the driveway. John was crying when he entered and instead of taking him, Aaron said he was starving and asked if there was anything to eat. I didn't answer, I shoved John in his arms and stormed out to the bedroom."

Therapist: It sounds very frustrating. Let's go back and look at the interaction. You were waiting for Aaron, wanting to tell him about your day and to get some time off. You were relieved when you heard him approaching. When he walked in, he said he was starving and asked if there was anything to eat. What did you feel then?

Miriam: I felt angry; he is so self-involved. He goes out to work, hangs out with his pals for lunch, and then comes home wanting dinner while I'm here all day, taking care of a crying infant, hardly able to take time off to eat.

Therapist: What do you feel now?

Miriam: I feel frustrated and alone, I feel sad. I never expected it to be this way.

Therapist: What would you like Aaron to understand?

Miriam: I want him to experience what it is like to be at home all day every day with John so he can understand how I feel at the end of the day and why dinner is not waiting on the table when he enters. I want him to be ready to help when he comes home from work.

Therapist: Let's brainstorm on *how you might have a future conversation with him about this.*

The third problem area is that of *grief*, which frequently entails the death of a close support, pregnancy loss, or the death of her child. Tasks of this problem area are like those of the role transition problem area and include facilitating the grief process; expressing effect; reestablishing interests; and modifying existing relationships or developing new relationships (see Closeup 1). Nonjudgmental openness to the patient's subjective experience about the loss facilitates the grieving process and enables the expression of difficult emotions including feelings of guilt and shame about one's responsibility that are common in pregnancy and infant loss. In many cultures, losing a pregnancy, especially early on, is a very lonely experience. Other people accept the loss as a natural occurrence and do not understand the attachment of the mother to her fetus. Enlisting close support to help process the loss characterizes IPT. The perinatal period can also trigger distress related to unresolved grief over previous losses (e.g., parents, partner, previous pregnancy loss) even if they occurred years earlier.

The fourth problem area, *social isolation*, refers to a lack of lasting or meaningful social relationships that may sometimes be due to deficits in social or communication skills. Depression in individuals with this problem area may be more persistent and chronic. These are long-standing difficulties that may exacerbate the difficulties associated with stressful experiences and life events and, thus, complicate the treatment of IPT problem areas. For new mothers with interpersonal deficits, the transition to parenthood may be more difficult due to heightened isolation and minimal connection with social support. In addition, infant attachment may be negatively impacted by the mother's insecure attachment patterns of relating, unresolved developmental trauma, difficulties with mentalizing, and inability to understand and respond to the infant's internal states (Zeegers et al., 2017). The tasks of treatment in this problem area are aligned with promoting mentalization (Law et al., 2022), examining the relationship history to find patterns in relationships, working together to resolve interpersonal problems, and helping the client to become less isolated, furthermore working to enrich the social network by establishing new relationships and modifying existing ones.

Another way to explore communication and relationship patterns is to learn from the therapeutic relationship and to apply this to other relationships in her life. In IPT, the use of transference is not a central intervention as it is in psychodynamic psychotherapy. Interpersonal psychotherapists do not interpret the transference or dynamic conflicts appearing in the therapeutic relationship. However, they do identify repetitive problems in relationships, discuss parallels in the therapeutic relationship if they are apparent, and provide a model for resolving these problems. Stuart and Robertson (2012) regarded interpersonal deficits (social isolation) as an attachment style related to avoidance rather than an acute interpersonal problem area. When in addition to the acute problems the client exhibits social isolation or deficits, this may complicate and prolong treatment, so it is important to assess this early in treatment.

Based on the information described earlier, chart on p. 523 (Closeup 1) provides a description and details the goals and strategies of the various problem areas.

Perinatal Intrusive Thoughts and Obsessive-Compulsive Symptoms

Perhaps the most common mental health occurrence in the postpartum is harm-related unwanted intrusive thoughts, images, and urges. Between 68% and 90% of new mothers in clinical and nonclinical samples experience normal harm-related intrusions with similar rates for fathers (Abramowitz et al., 2003, 2006, 2010). Abramowitz et al. (2010) also found that 74.5% of new mothers endorsing intrusive thoughts also had depression as measured on the *Edinburgh Postnatal Depression Scale* [EPDS] > 11, (Cox et al., 1987) and 38% had clinically significant obsessive-compulsive symptoms (OCS) as measured on the *Yale-Brown Obsessive-Compulsive Scale* [Y-BOCS] > 8 (Goodman et al., 1989). Rates of postpartum obsessive-compulsive disorder (OCD) range from 2.7% to 16.9% depending on the population, the time of measurement, and the scales used (Fairbrother et al., 2021; Uguz et al., 2007; Wenzel et al., 2005; Zambaldi et al., 2009). When assessed at several time points after birth, with both questionnaires and interviews, rates of postpartum OCD in nonclinical samples are substantially higher (9% and 16.9%) than when assessed with questionnaires at one-time point (Fairbrother et al., 2021; Zambaldi et al., 2009).

The perinatal period is the only specific life event that correlates with OCD onset and exacerbation consistently across studies (Miller & O'Hara, 2020). Several reasons may explain this specific vulnerability, including the high responsibility of caring for a helpless newborn (Fairbrother & Abramowitz, 2007); misinterpretation of normal harm-related intrusive thoughts as threatening (Abramowitz et al., 2006; Ojalehto et al., 2021); experiential avoidance that exacerbates the symptoms (Ojalehto et al., 2021), and elevated levels of oxytocin. Elevated oxytocin is correlated with parent-infant attachment (Gordon et al., 2010) and with OCD severity (Leckman et al., 1994).

The distinct clinical features of postpartum OCS and OCD include aggressive obsessions (toward the infant) and checking and reassurance compulsions (Starcevic et al., 2020). The content of intrusions included suffocation, sudden infant death syndrome (SIDS), accidents, intentional harm, losing the baby, illness, contamination, and sexual intrusions (Abramowitz et al., 2003). An additional obsessive-compulsive spectrum disorder that shares features with OCD is illness anxiety (McElroy et al., 1994). Similar to OCD, it is characterized by a preoccupation with thoughts about newborn illness and fears that the disease is overlooked may cause obsessive thoughts, checking, and reassurance behaviors called illness anxiety by proxy (Moreira & Moreira, 1999; Thorgaard et al., 2017).

OCD strongly impacts relationships. It can be all-consuming and lead to social isolation, and it can seriously impact relationships within the family. Conversely, close dysfunctional relationships can exacerbate symptoms of OCD (Abramowitz et al., 2013). These occur in three primary ways, either separately or occurring all together: (a) symptom accommodation—partners or other intimate supports "help" reduce suffering by participating in rituals, facilitating avoidance, assuming the patient's responsibilities, or helping resolve problems; (b) relationship distress and conflict caused by anxiety; and, (c) relationship distress that is unrelated to OCD (Abramowitz et al., 2013). Moreover, communication problems and disputes may cause adverse psychotherapy outcomes, whereas positive communication and relationship patterns correlate with improved exposure and response prevention (ERP) outcomes (Chambless & Steketee, 1999; Abramowitz et al., 2013). Thus, during the perinatal period, stable and supporting relationships with the closest supports are crucial for navigating the challenges of this time.

Abramowitz et al. (2010) suggested that given the high rates of intrusive thoughts, it is crucial to assess anxiety and OCS alongside depressive symptoms in the perinatal period. They recommended viewing intrusive thoughts, anxiety, and depression as part of a broad-spectrum perinatal psychiatric illness. Since harmful intrusive thoughts during this time are very distressing, it is important to educate women and their partners about these thoughts and teach strategies from ERP and cognitive behavioral therapy (CBT) for coping with intrusive thoughts (Abramowitz et al., 2006; Abramowitz et al., 2010).

ERP and exposure-based CBT specifically adapted for OCD are considered the "gold standard," first-line treatment for OCD (Hezel & Simpson, 2019; McKay et al., n.d.;

Sookman et al., 2021). However, these protocols do not specifically target relationship issues that may exacerbate OCD. Furthermore, when there are additional comorbid psychiatric conditions that interfere with ERP, such as severe depression, it may be necessary to treat that condition before engaging in ERP for OCD (Yadin et al., 2012).

IPT, on the other hand, can potentially help alleviate the depressed mood that accompanies OCD (McKay et al., n.d.). Its target is the interpersonal context of the disorder, rather than symptoms, thoughts, and behaviors particular to each disorder. The foundation and strategies of IPT can remain consistent while treating a differing diagnosis (Lipsitz & Markowitz, 2013). However, it has not been tested for the treatment of OCD and does not possess the exposure interventions deemed important for the treatment of OCD, thus, it should not be used as a stand-alone treatment for OCD (McKay et al., n.d.). Taking into account the perinatal period with all its challenges and difficulties as a major life event that predisposes some women to obsessive-compulsive spectrum disorders, the association between relationship distress and OCD, its grave effect on relationships at a time when they are needed most, and the high comorbidity of depression and OCD, it seems fitting that an integration of IPT and exposure-based therapy would be used for treating perinatal difficulties/depression comorbid with obsessive-compulsive spectrum disorders.

There are a few published exposure treatment protocols for anxiety in the perinatal period (Ben-Rafael et al., 2022; Christian & Storch, 2009; Gershkovich, 2019), and it is recognized that exposure-based therapies can be safe during pregnancy (Arch et al., 2012). However, these existing protocols do not focus on the interrelation between anxiety symptoms and interpersonal and role transitional difficulties relating to the perinatal stage. Wenzel and Kleiman (2015) published a comprehensive guide for treating perinatal women with CBT. They devoted a chapter to communication skills training and discuss difficulties in relationships with partners, family members, and friends. The book elaborates on the treatment of anxiety and distress, but it is more cognitively focused on the treatment of anxiety, as opposed to the exposure-based interventions required for OCD. Another book by the same authors is intended for mothers experiencing obsessive thoughts. It thoroughly discusses the importance of a support system to help cope with scary thoughts in the postpartum (Kleiman et al., 2021).

To create a beneficial link between exposure-based CBT/ERP, the best available treatments for obsessive-compulsive spectrum disorders, and IPT, a first-line treatment for perinatal depression focusing on life events, an integration of the two is proposed in the next section of this chapter.

Interpersonal Behavior Psychotherapy (IBPT) for Comorbid Perinatal Disorders

The following pages propose a theoretical integration (Norcross & Goldfried, 2005) of IPT with exposure-based behavior therapy (BT) for the treatment of comorbid depression and OCD/OCS perinatal disorders. This novel theoretical integration was presented at several conferences (Ben-Rafael, 2015, 2017, 2019) for the treatment of postpartum major depressive disorder (PMDD) comorbid with OCD. It relies on the best available treatments for mood disorders and OCD and is in clinical use. However, it has not been empirically tested and is presented as a general guide for integration.

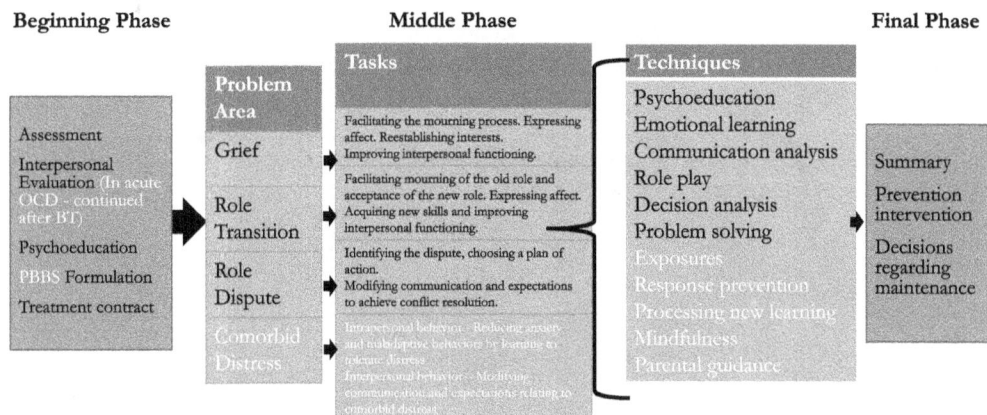

| Beginning Phase | Middle Phase | | | Final Phase |

Beginning Phase

Assessment
Interpersonal Evaluation (In acute OCD - continued after BT)
Psychoeducation
PBBS Formulation
Treatment contract

Middle Phase

Problem Area / Tasks / Techniques

Grief — Facilitating the mourning process. Expressing affect. Reestablishing interests. Improving interpersonal functioning.

Role Transition — Facilitating mourning of the old role and acceptance of the new role. Expressing affect. Acquiring new skills and improving interpersonal functioning.

Role Dispute — Identifying the dispute, choosing a plan of action. Modifying communication and expectations to achieve conflict resolution.

Comorbid Distress — Intrapersonal behavior - Reducing anxiety and maladaptive behaviors by learning to tolerate distress. Interpersonal behavior - Modifying communication and expectations relating to comorbid distress.

Techniques:
Psychoeducation
Emotional learning
Communication analysis
Role play
Decision analysis
Problem solving
Exposures
Response prevention
Processing new learning
Mindfulness
Parental guidance

Final Phase

Summary
Prevention intervention
Decisions regarding maintenance

Figure 23.2 Interpersonal behavior psychotherapy (IBPT) framework

*Listed in black are the congruent elements of IPT and IBPT, the elements specific to IBPT are listed in white.

IPT can be adapted with ease to cater to various populations and disorders (Frank et al., 2014). IBPT extends the theoretical framework of IPT (Figure 23.2) to include the effect of maladaptive thoughts and behaviors on interpersonal functioning with the addition of a *comorbid distress* problem area. Like other IPT adaptations that added a new problem area (Cyranowski et al., 2005; Spinelli, 2017), comorbid distress joins the crisis-oriented problem areas of grief, role transition, and role disputes. The comorbid distress goals are related to the overarching IPT goal of resolving the current interpersonal crisis, relieving symptoms, and mobilizing social support. This is similar to classic IPT, such that treatment attends to interpersonal patterns and tendencies only if they interfere with problem resolution (Lipsitz & Markowitz, 2013). In IBPT, behavioral issues are attended to only if they are interfering with the resolution of the current crisis.

During conception or early pregnancy, comorbid distress is chosen when current behavioral symptoms of avoidance, compulsions, safety behaviors, and the associated interpersonal behaviors interfere with the perinatal transitions (e.g., transition to pregnancy or parenthood, loss of fertility, pregnancy loss) and with the resolution of interpersonal difficulties. The focus on behavioral interventions within the comorbid distress problem area is based on multiple findings that behavioral interventions produce most, if not all, the changes of therapeutic intervention for these comorbidities (Abramowitz et al., 2005; Anholt et al., 2014; Deacon & Abramowitz, 2004; McLean et al., 2001; Vogel et al., 2004). Furthermore, exposures indirectly promote the goal of providing data to challenge erroneous beliefs.

Models of psychotherapy integration emphasize the individual and adapt the therapy to the client's characteristics and needs (Norcross & Goldfried, 2005). The theoretical integration of IPT and BT is based on a proposed psychological, biological, behavioral, and social model (PBBS; Ben-Rafael, 2024) for understanding the woman, her current unique circumstances, and her current crisis (Figure 23.3). This builds upon earlier models of perinatal mental health (Stuart & Robertson, 2012; Wenzel, 2011).

Psychological/spiritual

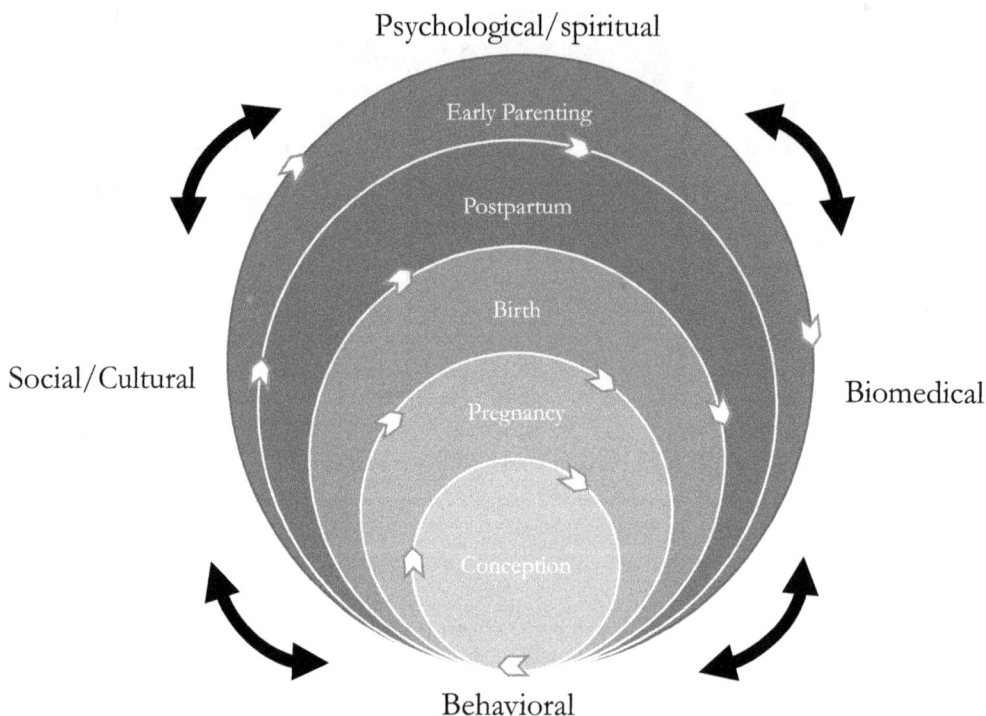

Social/Cultural   Biomedical

Behavioral

Figure 23.3 The PBBS (psychological/spiritual, biomedical, behavioral, social/cultural) circular
model of perinatal mental health

During assessment, the information that will provide a basis for the formulation is
organized in the PBBS realms. Some of the information may only become apparent later in
treatment. The formulation summarizes the reciprocal interactions between the realms, the
interrelated factors the woman arrives with to the current crisis, the changes relating to the
crisis, and the problem areas relevant for each woman at the current stage of the perinatal
cycle. Another important facet is the temporal dynamics between the pre-crisis baseline and
the changes relating to the current crisis. Conceptualizing these changes and identifying
baseline factors may help us understand the current situation, direct us toward therapeutic
targets, normalize and validate the woman's experience, and mobilize motivation for treatment. Some diathesis factors (marked with a star) within the realms, such as age and environmental factors. present strengths or vulnerabilities that have unidirectional interactions
with the factors in the other realms. Figure 23.4 can be used as a guide for information we
may want to include in the assessment.

This is a theoretical model that forms the basis for integration of IPT and exposure-based
BT. There are three main differences between this model and the Stuart and Robertson (2012)
model. First, to maintain a parsimonious model, the cultural and spiritual factors are included
in the PBBS model under the social and psychological realms, respectively. Second, there is an
emphasis on changes relating to the current crisis within each realm. Finally, there is an addition of a behavioral realm as a focal point of intervention both for interpersonal behaviors
and for maladaptive behaviors, enabling a smooth transition between two modalities.

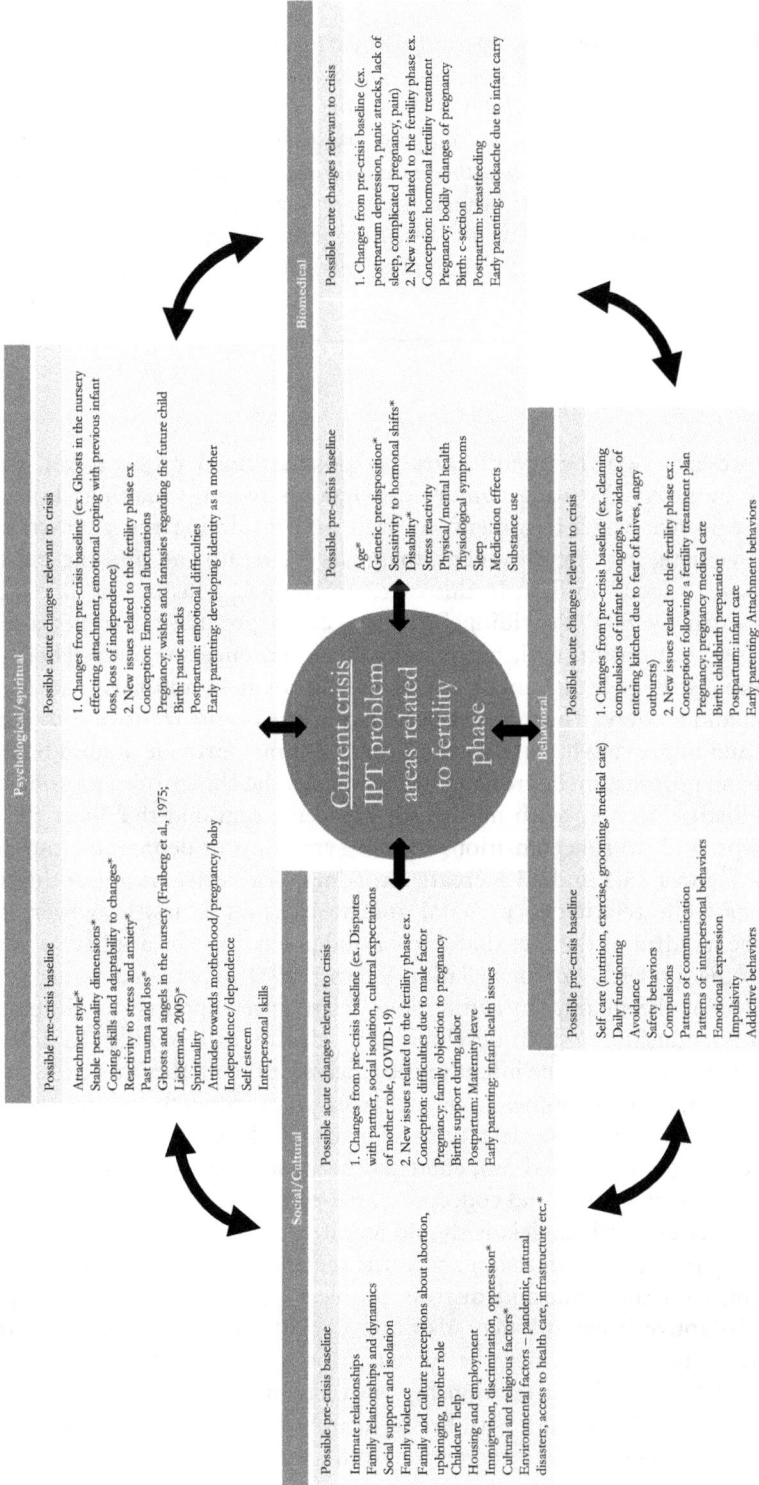

Figure 23.4 The PBBS (psychological/spiritual, biological, behavioral, social/cultural) case formulation

The following composite case (described in *italics*) of Amelia illustrates the use of IBPT. *Amelia started having concerns about the health of her newborn, Roi. This was associated with maladaptive behaviors, such as examining him several times a day for signs of an illness; touching and pressing on different areas of his body; searching the Internet for health-related information; and reassurance-seeking behaviors including doctor visits, unnecessary medical examinations, and excessive questioning. Her husband, Barack, and her mother had frequent arguments with her about this. She felt isolated and alone and this intensified her pre-existing transition-related depression.*

This case presents two therapeutic targets—postpartum depression and comorbid illness anxiety by proxy. Treating comorbid diagnoses requires making choices about the indicated evidence-based treatment, as well as considering the characteristics of the individual woman, her circumstances, the goals for treatment, and the most urgent therapeutic focus to focus on first. In this case, Amelia had a history of illness anxiety, successfully treated by ERP. Providing ERP now could provide fast relief and enable her to repair her relationship with her family. However, once she finds relief, she may continue to exhaust herself at home without asking for help and this may perpetuate her depression and anxiety. Thus, choosing IPT to focus on the transition to mothering four children and improving her ability to ask for help may provide a good balance and lasting relief from postpartum depression. IBPT enables the choice of two problem areas: (a) comorbid distress to help with her health preoccupation and the effect this has on her relationships, and (b) role transitions to ease symptoms of depression and adjust to the transition. Figures 23.5 and 23.6 create a roadmap for decisions about the sequence of interventions while relating to prenatal and postpartum issues. However, it is also important to be mindful of the fact that clinical judgment must be applied as well.

The shift to the motherhood constellation (Stern, 1995) requires achieving four main tasks: (a) caring for the infant, (b) getting help from close supports, (c) developing the mother–infant relationship, and (d) developing the identity as a mother. To achieve this, there is an urgency to attend to the infant's needs, decrease the mother's distress, and assess for safety (Figure 23.5). If the mother is suicidal or shows potential for self-injury behaviors or if her children suffer abuse or neglect, this will take precedence, and an appropriate treatment or referral (e.g., emergency room, child protective services, social worker) should be implemented. During pregnancy and conception, self-care and access to healthcare are also important issues about which clinicians should inquire.

After assessing for safety, a decision about the sequence of interventions is taken. For Amelia, starting with the comorbid distress problem area and teaching her strategies to prevent maladaptive behaviors may also improve attachment and infant care. Once basic and attachment needs are met, the current crisis is considered. What is causing the greatest distress for her? Is it her relationship with a family member? Is she experiencing obsessive thoughts? Collaborating with her to identify her main sources of distress may help us decide on the sequence of interventions and may contribute to her motivation for treatment.

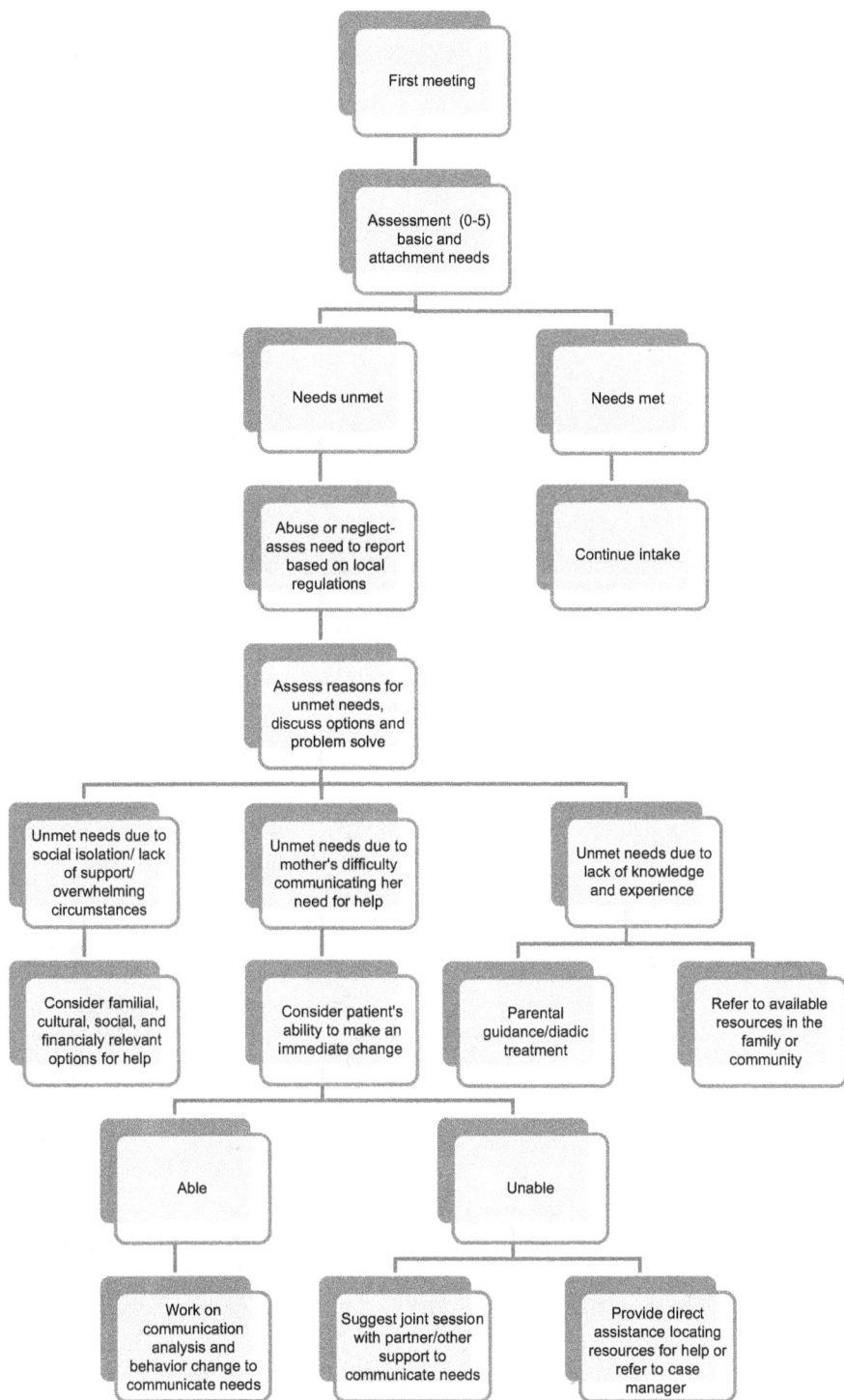

Figure 23.5   Decision map for assessing child needs during the intake session

OCD and illness anxiety can be lifelong disorders with manageable symptoms that the woman has learned to live with or that are treated successfully with medications. When there is no worsening or change of content and these comorbid disorders do not contribute to the current crisis, we may choose to continue with the problem areas of classic IPT. When these symptoms begin or worsen during the perinatal period or cause increased distress, we may choose the comorbid distress problem area (Figure 23.6).

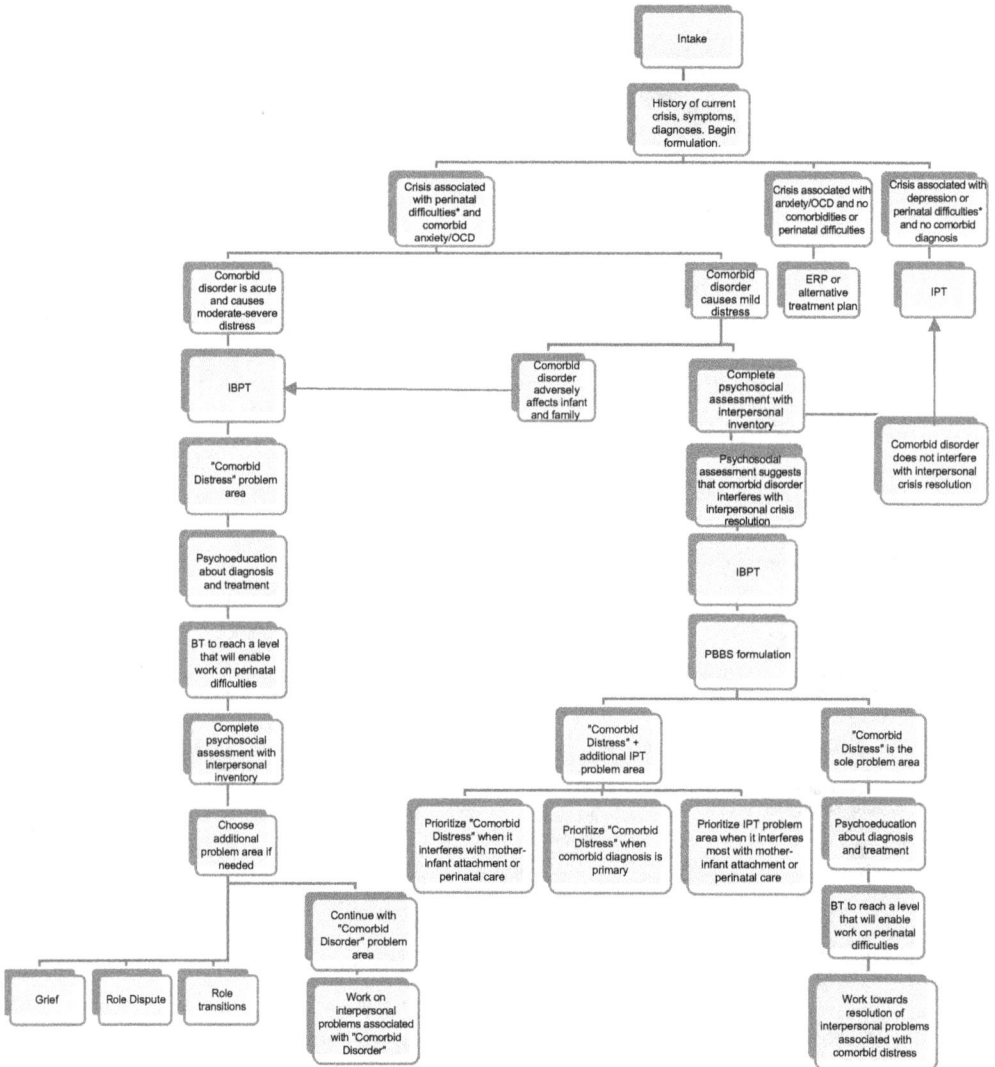

Figure 23.6 Decision map for treatment choices

* Perinatal difficulties include but are not limited to health issues, body image, miscarriage, stillbirth, adjustment difficulties, interpersonal difficulties, lack of support, inner conflict relating to the transition, subsyndromal anxiety, and so on.

For Amelia, the trigger for her depression was the transition to being a "supermom" of four young children. However, at the point in which she arrived at therapy, she identified her main distress as the fear that Roi has an undiagnosed illness. She agreed with the proposed plan to start with the comorbid distress problem area and implement the strategies that have worked for her in the past.

IBPT Treatment Phase 1 (Sessions 1–2)

The first phase of treatment is like IPT's first phase and includes an evaluation of symptoms and history, an explanation of diagnoses, and a detailed exploration of significant relationships and their connection to the current crisis. If, after evaluation, it is decided to treat the acute distress by working on the comorbid distress problem area, the therapist may postpone the completion of the interpersonal inventory and return to finish it once anxiety decreases (the number of sessions for "phase one" can range from 2 to 4, depending on completion of the interpersonal inventory). During the initial phase, the therapist gathers information using the PBBS realms as a guide. This can provide a basis for the case formulation explained to the client.

Case formulation: "I want to summarize what we have been talking about and suggest how therapy can help you feel better. We talked about your life before the current crisis and the changes that occurred in different areas of your life since Roi was born. Your pregnancy and labor were relatively easy, so you continued to be a supermom, not taking time for yourself, and not asking for help. You exhausted yourself and started feeling depressed (note that this is a role transitions problem area). The fears about Roi having an illness caught you off guard. You didn't identify it as illness anxiety because it was so different from your former anxiety occurrences, so you devoted yourself to finding out what was wrong with Roi (note that this is a comorbid distress problem)."

Amelia: "Yes, that's exactly what happened"

"I want to suggest that we concentrate on two interrelated problems. One is the transition to being a mother of four and the other is the distress caused by your illness anxiety. In the past, you responded well to behavioral strategies for illness anxiety. We may start by working in the same way. Once you can use the strategies that have worked for you before, we can turn to the transition that you are going through and try to identify what you need and are willing to accept from your partner and mother and how to communicate your needs to them. What are your thoughts about this plan?"

In IBPT, we look at the changes in the PBBS formulation and intervene in factors that are strongly connected with the current crisis. Changing the woman's circumstances can make a substantial difference in her capacity to cope with perinatal difficulties and solve the current crisis (Spinelli, 2017).

To help Amelia in the process of healing and to enable active participation in exposure home-work, it was obvious that she needed to receive emotional and physical support. She examined this with her therapist, and, using decision analysis, and they discussed the advantages and disadvantages of the different solutions. Amelia decided that she would ask her 12-year-old niece to come to play with the children in the evenings and help with showers and that she will speak with her husband and mother. She role-played different options and decided to say, "I have been very worried about Roi, and I am starting to realize that it's my illness anxiety again. I returned to my therapist, and we are working on it like we did last time. It's probably going to take a few weeks before there is any improvement, and it will help me if you could be patient with me during this time. When we fight, I feel really bad, and it affects my ability to cope with the anxiety." Talking to Barack and her mother helped ease some of the tension at home and her daily calls with her mother offer relief.

Following the formulation, Amelia received psychoeducation about IBPT, her active role in therapy, and the treatment contract. The treatment contract included (a) twice-a-week meetings for six to eight sessions to work on the comorbid distress problem area; (b) completion of the interpersonal inventory before moving to the role transitions problem area; and (c) work on the transition and relationship difficulties in a once-a-week format (i.e., the role transitions problem area).

IBPT Intermediate Phase of Treatment

Similar to IPT, the intermediate phase of IBPT involves work on the chosen problem areas. There is flexibility around the number of sessions. However, considering the benefits of time-limited therapy, an approximate number of sessions are decided upon with the client during the first few sessions, after the evaluation and treatment plan.

Comorbid Distress Problem Area (Sessions 3–9)

The first phase of the intermediate sessions includes a focus on the chosen problem area of comorbid distress. As described previously, this includes psychoeducation, exposure, response prevention, and processing to solidify the new learning that occurred. In addition, attention is given to Amelia's relationship with her husband and mother. Before exposure, psychoeducation is provided including a request to refrain as much as possible from rituals, safety and avoidance behaviors during her daily activities. For Amelia, psychoeducation consisted of simply reminding her of what she already knows, which makes acceptance and motivation for treatment easier to establish.

Therapist: "You remember how, in the past, you had fears that you might develop cancer and how acute it seemed then? You felt there was imminent danger and were compelled to check yourself and visit many doctors urgently. It seems that the same thing is happening now with Roi and your behaviors of urgently seeking answers are intensifying the fear and your social distancing from your partner, mother, and friend."

In the next sessions, Amelia and her therapist developed a hierarchy of anxiety-evoking situations, thoughts, sensations, and consequences and tackled the first scenes on the list with imaginal exposure. One of them was a scene of Roi having red spots on his skin that turn out to be a chronic condition like atopic dermatitis. Imaginal exposure is used as a tool for exposures that cannot be done in vivo; the purpose of this imaginal exposure is to promote the reduction of thoughts and images and tolerance of distressing emotions (Foa et al., 2012). The following imaginal exposure tapped into her underlying fear that because of her negligence, Roi will suffer all his life:

> I see the red spots around his skin and tell myself they are normal. I miss that they have now turned into a chronic condition. Roi now has Atopic dermatitis, and I don't treat him because I am careless and irresponsible. He starts scratching them and they become these horrific broken skin wounds that get infected and have repulsive yellow puss dripping out just like I saw in the pictures. I still overlook them because I am too preoccupied with being a supermom. By the time I take Roi to the doctor, there is nothing that can be done. Because of me, Roi will have scars for the rest of his life.

This imaginal exposure produced a Subjective Units of Distress (SUDS) rating of 70 when she first started the exposures. Processing her expectations and the actual consequence of the exposure is an important part of solidifying new learning. Before the exposure, she thought that she would have a panic attack during exposure, and she expected that her SUDS would be higher at the end of the exposure. In reality, the opposite was true: after 20 minutes of listening to the recording of the imaginal exposure, her SUDS reduced to 50, and she did not have a panic attack. Amelia continued listening to a recording of this exposure at home and, by the next session, her SUDS had reduced to 30 and she was ready for the next exposure.

In the next sessions, Roi accompanied Amelia, and exposures were continued with him. During in vivo exposure, Amelia and her therapist talked and played with Roi while she looked at his lymph nodes without checking them. At first, she was compelled to get some reassurance from the therapist, but, ultimately, she agreed to continue the exposure in the absence of reassurance. Throughout the session, her anxiety dropped from 90 to 40 with no safety behaviors. It was agreed that she would continue practicing this exposure every time she takes off his diaper and, in addition, dedicate 20 minutes a day for exposures—playing with him while looking at his lymph nodes and refraining from doing anything in response to her fear. During the ninth session, Amelia reported decreased distress at home and a relative "return to normal." At the end of the session, the plan for the next few weeks was discussed. At that point, Amelia was ready to start working on the interpersonal changes in her life relating to the current crisis, while still reporting her illness anxiety at the beginning of each session to make sure she is on track.

Role Transitions Problem Area (Sessions 10–14)

After completing the interpersonal inventory, Amelia's transition and her old role were examined. She remembered the good feeling of complete control. Her busy afternoons with three kids were good for her, and she did not expect anything from Barack, so their relationship was very pleasant. When she did ask barrack for help, he always had reasons why he could not help at that time, so she gave up on asking him. She recounted more difficult incidents with Barack, and she realized that when she feels needy, and he refuses, she quickly retreats. She identified anger and a feeling of disappointment and sadness that he does not see or understand her.

Amelia and her therapist examined some patterns of communication and behaviors relating to her expectations that people will not be available if she needs them: (a) taking everything upon herself without asking for help;(b) asking for help only when there is no other option but giving up quickly at the first sign of refusal; (c) doing more than she can handle and exhausting herself; and (d) isolating herself when in distress so others will not see signs of weakness. This discussion reminded Amelia of times when her parents were preoccupied with her sister, and she wanted to be perfect and to not require anything from them.

Amelia continued examining the transition to becoming a mother of four (two of them infants). During this time, she required more help than she needed in the past and expected Barack to realize this and help without her having to ask. During the sessions, Amelia expressed an understanding that Barack was accustomed to her doing everything alone and that she did not display any needs until her illness anxiety kicked in. She realized that her illness anxiety offered her the possibility to receive help while she took Roi to different doctors, and this was acceptable for her at the time. She stated, "I see now how ironic this was. Responding to my anxiety is in fact losing control, not controlling my thoughts and actions. It's the worst situation for me because I hate feeling weak. It's worse than asking for help. I'm so ready to change that."

Amelia's new role as a mother of four required new communication skills, and during the eleventh and twelfth sessions, she addressed her communication with Barack. Through a process of decision analysis, she laid out the problem and evaluated possible solutions. Amelia wanted Barack to be more involved in the home, but this wish represented a sign of weakness for her, and she was afraid to lose his love if he discovers she has needs. After considering several options, Amelia decided to talk to Barack openly about her fears in the evening after the kids fall asleep. The therapist offered to role-play this exchange, and Amelia asked to play herself. During the role-play, she was very explicit and able to say everything she wanted to express, and she left the session feeling good about the exercise. However, during the next session, she admitted that the execution of communication with Barack was much harder than she imagined. She noted that the two of them were not used to having conversations like this, as their relationship had always been "light." She reported that she set out to have this conversation several times, but that she was unable to start. Eventually, Amelia did try to talk with Barack, but it did not go as she planned. To examine this communication, the therapist asks her to describe exactly how it unfolded and what each of them said. This process is called communication analysis.

Amelia:	"I planned to talk with him last night, I tried several times before but didn't say anything and I knew that today we had our session, so I decided I have to do it. The kids were asleep, and we were sitting together eating on the sofa. I said, 'These past few months have been difficult for me.' He hugged and kissed me and said, 'I'm so happy that you are back to being yourself' and that was it."
Therapist	(Amelia is tearing up and since this is not a usual sight, decides to pursue it): "How are you feeling now?"
Amelia	(tears in her eyes): "I'm so disappointed in myself."
Therapist:	(conveying by her silence that this expression of affect is acceptable)

Amelia:	"I also feel sad and hurt. He doesn't really want to see me. He has this ideal image in his mind and for him, I'm back to being his super wife."
Therapist:	"What are you feeling now?"
Amelia:	"I feel neglected and alone."
Therapist:	"Do you think he is aware of these feelings?"
Amelia:	"No. I just had that 'emotional wash' we talked about. It's automatic. The moment I feel weakness I get 'washed' by emotions, and I just back off and retreat. It's like you said, my brain keeps responding like I did when I was a child, even though I know this situation is different." Amelia decided to try again tonight after role-playing different response options and how she will handle them. During one of the role-plays, she felt this 'emotional wash' she had been describing, and she retreated.
Amelia	(playing herself): "I want to talk with you, I know we don't usually have serious talks, but I feel that a lot has been building up in me and I have to say it."
Therapist	(playing Barack in defensive mode): "What are you talking about? We always talk, I know that you had a really rough time with Roi. I listen every time you talk about your anxieties."
Amelia	(backing off)
Therapist:	"What are you feeling now?"
Amelia:	"I don't know."
Therapist:	(gives her a moment) "Is it similar to what you felt yesterday with Barack?"
Amelia:	(tearing) "I don't know."
	They sat in silence for a few minutes, again conveying that her feelings are acceptable.
Amelia:	"It's that emotional wash. I just want to disappear."
Therapist:	"What did you hear me saying that caused this emotional wash?"
Amelia:	"I don't know. I felt I was needy."
Therapist:	"I was playing Barack saying 'I listen every time you talk about your anxieties'"
Amelia:	"Yes. It's hard to continue talking now."
Therapist:	"I understand, I see how hard it is for you now. Is this what happened with Barack yesterday?"
Amelia:	"Yes, this happens every time."
Therapist:	"Thank you for sharing this with me. I understand better now. How are you feeling now?"
Amelia:	"Better now. It's easier because you understand what I'm feeling, and I don't think you will leave me if I cry."

The discussion turned to ways to help Barack to understand what Amelia is feeling so that she can continue talking once this emotional wave passes and not retreat. Several options and possible consequences were considered. For example, Amelia indicated that she wanted Barack to know in advance that she might cry and feel weak, worrying that she will sense his alarm and back off again. Eventually, she decided to text him: "I want to talk tonight and explain what I have been discussing in therapy. It's really hard for me to talk about it and I might cry so please don't be alarmed, I'm doing much better and it's part of my healing process. I just need you to listen."

Amelia arrived at the next session and immediately remarked "this time it worked!" She spoke with Barack, saying she understands that she will need his help now and that trying to do everything alone was the trigger for her depression and illness anxiety. They discussed how Barack could help and decided that their niece will be with him two evenings a week while Amelia goes to the gym. They also divided some chores that Barack could do early in the morning before he leaves for work, including taking the older children to school. Amelia was surprised at how easy it went.

In session 14, Amelia reported that she and Barack started implementing the new plan and that she has been to the gym twice. The original plan was for mornings to be Barack's shift, such that he would get the kids ready and take them to school while Amelia continues sleeping because she is still breastfeeding at night. However, Amelia admitted that she feels energetic and wants to see the kids, so she gets them ready and takes them to school. Amelia and her therapist considered the possible consequences of decision, discussing her regained feelings of control and being back on track, alongside her natural inclination to do everything and exhaust herself. As a result of this discussion, Amelia agreed to talk with Barack to suggest they take the morning shift together.

IBPT Final Phase of Acute Treatment (Sessions 15–16)

The last two sessions are dedicated to concluding the acute phase of treatment. Some clients wish to continue meeting in a different format, usually bimonthly, to gain confidence in their ability to cope before ending treatment, to prevent relapse, or to work on other issues. For others, knowing they can always return to the same therapist who they know and trust, as Amelia did, provides the confidence to leave. This option is not possible in all settings and might be most feasible in private practice. During these final sessions, Amelia and her therapist discussed therapeutic gains, as well as the strategies that helped her achieve change. Feelings about the ending of treatment and relapse prevention were also considered.

In IBPT, exposures are used during the intermediate phase of acute treatment to achieve greater control over behavioral symptoms. The aim is not to achieve remission, but instead to achieve symptom reduction that will enable interpersonal work related to the current crisis. In this case, Amelia had experience with BT and great trust in the therapeutic relationship, so implementation was straightforward. In some cases, it may take several more sessions to achieve symptom reduction and move toward interpersonal goals.

For the purpose of this chapter, the acute phase of treatment was presented. Some women wish to continue beyond the acute phase of treatment and address other goals. This is not part of the classic IPT but was discussed in Stuart and Robertson (2012). Following IBPT acute treatment, the client may choose to continue with BT in an attempt to achieve remission of the comorbid diagnosis. She may also choose to continue with an interpersonal focus when social isolation is a factor. Continuing therapy with an interpersonal focus beyond the acute phase may provide additional opportunities to learn from the therapeutic relationship and make decisions on how to use learned behaviors and information to enrich and improve relationships in the woman's life.

Cultural Considerations

To provide culturally responsive psychotherapy in this globalized world, it is important to understand the effect a certain culture has on one's values, traditions, beliefs, patterns of behavior, social and family ties, and lifestyle. UNESCO defines culture as "the set of distinctive, material, intellectual and emotional features of a society or a social group." It encompasses in addition to art and literature the "lifestyles, ways of living together, value systems, traditions and beliefs" (UNESCO, 2008, https://policytoolbox.iiep.unesco.org/glossary/cultures/).

When providing evidence-based therapy, therapists should educate themselves about their client's culture and religion (Naeem et al., 2019). However, they should be careful of biased and stereotyped representations (Kleinman, 2016) and not assume that by understanding the culture and religion they understand the unique individual. This is true when therapists are working in a country that is different from their own and when working with immigrants and expats. Different levels of acculturation, cross-cultural marriage, influences from other cultures, and westernization in the home country are some factors that might determine the individual's cultural influences. In addition to culture and religion, it is important to consider spirituality, communication barriers, and healthcare accessibility (Naeem et al., 2019). IPT's biopsychosocial-cultural-spiritual (Stuart & Robertson, 2012) and IBPT's PBBS formulation enable the exploration of the client's subjective experience and cultural influences and their reciprocal influence on current psychological distress and the integration of these understandings into the treatment plan.

Grote et al. (2009) added an ethnographic interview to adapt IPT to the specific cultural needs of low-income postpartum women. This included open-ended questions about sociocultural aspects of the woman's life and her views on issues relevant to treatment engagement. The topics covered include: "building trust and addressing the practical, psychological, and cultural barriers to care experienced by individuals who are socioeconomically disadvantaged." (Grote et al., 2009, p. 315). Following the interview, the therapist provides psychoeducation that is specifically tailored to each woman's needs.

Dissemination

IPT was developed in the 1970s at Yale University as part of a randomized controlled trial (RCT) for the maintenance treatment of depression (Weissman, 2020). The first IPT manual was published in 1984 (Klerman et al., 1984) and has been translated into ten languages (Weissman, 2020, p. 5). An updated version was published in 2018 (Weissman et al., 2008) and a new book on IPT global dissemination was recently published (Mootz & Weissman, 2024). By 2014, IPT has been tested in 90 RCTs (Cuijpers et al., 2016) and 1,119 publications on the topic by 2017 (Ravitz et al., 2019). In the past year, dissemination efforts have increased due to the activities of the International Society of Interpersonal Psychotherapy (ISIPT), including a new certification program for therapists, trainers, and supervisors. ISIPT is a noncommercial organization dedicated to advancing worldwide research, training, and dissemination of IPT. It holds an international IPT conference every two years and lists worldwide IPT training and virtual workshops. There are special interest groups (SIG), including an active perinatal SIG, established and led by the author of this chapter, that holds monthly meetings alternating between professional presentations on topics of perinatal IPT and a peer supervision group. The ISIPT website lists worldwide IPT research in 32 countries and contact information of 17 regional IPT groups (https://interpersonalpsychotherapy.org/about-isipt/chapters/) as well as a list of North American University Affiliated IPT Training opportunities including those with a perinatal focus http://interpersonalpsychotherapy.org/wp-content/uploads/2016/09/NA_IPT_Traning_Groups.pdf

Conclusion and Future Directions

IPT is a time-limited, feasible, acceptable, and effective treatment for perinatal mood disorders and anxiety. It is included in treatment guidelines for perinatal depression around the world and has been tested in a variety of populations and settings. The 12 to 16 session IPT protocol has shown efficacy in treating perinatal mood and anxiety in at least 45 RCTs and an eight-session protocol, IPT-B, has also been empirically validated as effective for perinatal women. Future studies may compare classic IPT to IPT-B to test if the length of treatment correlates with outcomes.

The presenting problem in IPT is defined as a medical illness that has a cure, mobilizing the patient to work in treatment and between sessions to achieve fast symptom relief and syndrome remission. The focus of the sessions on the "here and now," and the supportive therapeutic relationship is very suitable for the interpersonal difficulties associated with perinatal transitions and losses. In the future, comparing IPT to other evidence-based therapies such as CBT, to evaluate the efficacy of each modality for different populations (e.g., low-income, minorities, women with a comorbid diagnosis, women with anxiety, women with partner difficulties, and women with insecure attachment) and to test their long-term effects on symptoms, attachment, and interpersonal outcomes. Future studies might also test the adapted posttraumatic stress disorder protocol for perinatal loss and birth-related trauma and compare it to CBT in efficacy and acceptability.

Since the perinatal period is a specific life event that correlates with intrusive thoughts and OCD onset, it is important to account for these instances when providing psychotherapy in clinical settings. Integrating IPT with an exposure-based treatment is one alternative to tackling comorbid depression and obsessive-compulsive spectrum disorders. IBPT offers guidelines for a theoretical integration based on a psychological-biological-behavioral-social formulation. The PBBS case formulation helps achieve a seamless explanation for the woman's problems, uniform interpersonal goals for treatment, and behavioral interventions aimed at achieving these goals.

Future research might test the integration between IPT and exposure-based BT. The proposed integration relies on research supporting the efficacy of IPT for depression and BT for OCD. However, further research is required to test the efficacy of the integration on the symptoms of both disorders as well as other anxiety disorders such as Panic Disorder, birth-related trauma and Specific Phobias and on relationship outcomes. Issues that need to be substantiated or validated include the superiority of the integrative protocol over the use of separate protocols, the sequencing of interventions, the length of treatment for each intervention and the acceptability of changing treatment modality. I suggest that following one protocol that integrates both treatments is more efficient and acceptable than using two health providers with specific specialties. Changing therapists midway through therapy is problematic for the therapeutic alliance and difficult for women having to adjust to a new therapist, develop trust and tell their story over again. Future studies can also test if the length of each section of the intervention (IPT and BT) is related to attachment styles.

Acknowledgments

I would like to thank Prof Paula Ravitz, Prof. Elna Yadin, Prof. Gideon Anholt, Dr. Naomi Epel, and Dr. Alexandra Klein Rafaeli for reading and providing constructive feedback.

References

Abramowitz, J. S., Baucom, D. H., Wheaton, M. G., Boeding, S., Fabricant, L. E., Paprocki, C., & Fischer, M. S. (2013). Enhancing exposure and response prevention for OCD: A couple-based approach. *Behavior Modification, 37*(2), 189–210. https://doi.org/10.1177/0145445512444596

Abramowitz, J. S., Khandker, M., Nelson, C. A., Deacon, B. J., & Rygwall, R. (2006). The role of cognitive factors in the pathogenesis of obsessive-compulsive symptoms: A prospective study. *Behaviour Research and Therapy, 44*(9), 1361–1374. https://doi.org/10.1016/j.brat.2005.09.011

Abramowitz, J. S., Meltzer-Brody, S., Leserman, J., Killenberg, S., Rinaldi, K., Mahaffey, B. L., & Pedersen, C. (2010). Obsessional thoughts and compulsive behaviors in a sample of women with postpartum mood symptoms. *Archives of Women's Mental Health, 13*(6), 523–530. https://doi.org/10.1007/s00737-010-0172-4

Abramowitz, J. S., Schwartz, S. A., & Moore, K. M. (2003). Obsessional thoughts in postpartum females and their partners: Content, severity, and relationship with depression. *Journal of Clinical Psychology in Medical Settings, 10*(3), 157–164. https://doi.org/10.1023/A:1025454627242

Abramowitz, J. S., Taylor, S., & McKay, D. (2005). Potentials and limitations of cognitive treatments for obsessive-compulsive disorder. *Cognitive Behaviour Therapy, 34*(3), 140–147. https://doi.org/10.1080/16506070510041202

Ainsworth, M. D. S., Blehar, M. C., Waters, E., & Wall, S. N. (2015). *Patterns of attachment: A psychological study of the strange situation* (1st ed.). Psychology Press. https://doi.org/10.4324/9780203758045

Anholt, G. E., & Kalanthroff, E. (2014). Do we need a cognitive theory for obsessive-compulsive disorder? *Clinical Neuropsychiatry: Journal of Treatment Evaluation, 11*(6), 194–196.

Arch, J. J., Dimidjian, S., & Chessick, C. (2012). Are exposure-based cognitive behavioral therapies safe during pregnancy? *Archives of Women's Mental Health, 15*, 445–457. https://doi.org/10.1007/s00737-012-0308-9

Beck, A. T., Ward, C. H., Mendelson, M., Mock, J., & Erbaugh, J. (1961). An inventory for measuring depression. *Archives of General Psychiatry, 4*(6), 561–571. https://doi.org/10.1001/archpsyc.1961.01710120031004

Ben-Rafael, S. (2015, August 31–September 3). *Integrating CBT and IPT for complicated perinatal disorders – A case study* [Paper presentation]. 45th Annual EABCT Congress. https://isas.co.il/wp-content/uploads/2020/05/eabct-2015-brochure.pdf

Ben-Rafael, S. (2017, July 12–15). *Integrating CBT and IPT for complex perinatal disorders.* 30th Annual PSI Conference. https://postpartumny.org/wp-content/uploads/2017/07/psi-conference-2017-i-1.pdf

Ben-Rafael, S. (2019, November 8–9). *Integrating CBT and IPT for complex perinatal disorders.* The 8th Conference of the International Society of Interpersonal Psychotherapy. https://isipt2019.congressline.hu/wp-content/uploads/ISIPT-AGENDA_web-1.pdf

Ben-Rafael, S. (2024, March 13–15). *Clinical formulation for integrating IPT with Behavioral Therapy for complex perinatal disorders* [Conference presentation]. The 10th ISIPT international conference. https://www.isiptcon2024.com/meeting-dates–events.htm

Ben-Rafael, S., Bloch, M., & Aisenberg-Romano, G. (2022). Dual-session tokophobia intervention, a novel ultrashort cognitive behavioral therapy protocol for women suffering from tokophobia in the third term of pregnancy. *Cognitive and Behavioral Practice.* Advance online publication. https://doi.org/10.1016/j.cbpra.2022.02.015

Bleiberg, K. L., & Markowitz, J. C. (2005). A pilot study of interpersonal psychotherapy for post-traumatic stress disorder. *The American Journal of Psychiatry, 162*(1), 181–183. https://doi.org/10.1176/appi.ajp.162.1.181

Bowlby, J. (1973). *Attachment and loss. Vol. 2: Separation: Anxiety and anger.* Basic Books.

Bright, K. S., Charrois, E. M., Mughal, M. K., Wajid, A., McNeil, D., Stuart, S., . . . Kingston, D. (2020). Interpersonal psychotherapy to reduce psychological distress in perinatal women: A systematic review. *International Journal of Environmental Research and Public Health, 17*(22), 8421. https://doi.org/10.3390/ijerph17228421

Brown, G. W., & Harris, T. (1978). *Social origins of depression: A study of psychiatric disorders in women.* Tavistock.

Carter, W., Grigoriadis, S., Ravitz, P., & Ross, L. E. (2010). Conjoint IPT for postpartum depression: Literature review and overview of a treatment manual. *American Journal of Psychotherapy, 64*(4), 373–392. https://doi.org/10.1176/appi.psychotherapy.2010.64.4.373

Chambless, D. L., & Steketee, G. (1999). Expressed emotion and behavior therapy outcome: A prospective study with obsessive-compulsive and agoraphobic outpatients. *Journal of Consulting and Clinical Psychology, 67*(5), 658–665. https://doi.org/10.1037/0022-006X.67.5.658

Christian, L. M., & Storch, E. A. (2009). Cognitive behavioral treatment of postpartum onset. *Clinical Case Studies, 8*(1), 72–83. https://doi.org/10.1177/1534650108326974

Cox, J. L., Holden, J. M., & Sagovsky, R. (1987). Detection of postnatal depression. *British Journal of Psychiatry, 150*(6), 782–786. https://doi.org/10.1192/bjp.150.6.782

Cuijpers, P., Donker, T., Weissman, M. M., Ravitz, P., & Cristea, I. A. (2016). Interpersonal psychotherapy for mental health problems: A comprehensive meta-analysis. *American Journal of Psychiatry, 173*(7), 680–687.

Cyranowski, J. M., Frank, E., Shear, M. K., Swartz, H., Fagiolini, A., Scott, J., & Kupfer, D. J. (2005). Interpersonal psychotherapy for depression with panic spectrum symptoms: A pilot study. *Depression and Anxiety, 21*(3), 140–142. https://doi.org/10.1002/da.20069

Deacon, B. J., & Abramowitz, J. S. (2004). Cognitive and behavioral treatments for anxiety disorders: A review of meta-analytic findings. *Journal of Clinical Psychology, 60*(4), 429–441. https://doi.org/10.1002/jclp.10255

Dennis, C. L., Grigoriadis, S., Zupancic, J., Kiss, A., & Ravitz, P. (2020). Telephone-based nurse-delivered interpersonal psychotherapy for postpartum depression: Nationwide randomised controlled trial. *British Journal of Psychiatry, 216*(4), 189–196. https://doi.org/10.1192/bjp.2019.275

Dietz, L. J. (2020). Family-based interpersonal psychotherapy: An intervention for preadolescent depression. *American Journal of Psychotherapy, 73*(1), 22–28. https://doi.org/10.1176/appi.psychotherapy.20190028

Engel, G. L. (1977). The need for a new medical model: A challenge for biomedicine. *Science, 196*(4286), 129–136. https://doi.org/10.1126/science.847460

Fairbrother, N., & Abramowitz, J. S. (2007). New parenthood as a risk factor for the development of obsessional problems. *Behaviour Research and Therapy, 45*(9), 2155–2163. https://doi.org/10.1016/j.brat.2006.09.019

Fairbrother, N., Collardeau, F., Albert, A. Y. K., Challacombe, F. L., Thordarson, D. S., Woody, S. R., & Janssen, P. A. (2021). High prevalence and incidence of obsessive-compulsive disorder among women across pregnancy and the postpartum. *Journal of Clinical Psychiatry, 82*(2), 20m13398. https://doi.org/10.4088/JCP.20m13398

Fairburn, C. G., Jones, R., Peveler, R. C., Hope, R. A., & O'Connor, M. (1993). Psychotherapy and bulimia nervosa. Longer-term effects of interpersonal psychotherapy, behavior therapy, and cognitive behavior therapy. *Archives of General Psychiatry, 50*(6), 419–428. https://doi.org/10.1001/archpsyc.1993.01820180009001

Foa, E. B., Yadin, E., & Lichner, T. K. (2012). *Exposure and response (ritual) prevention for obsessive-compulsive disorder: Therapist guide* (2nd ed.). Oxford University Press. https://doi.org/10.1093/med:psych/9780195335286.001.0001

Fonagy, P. (1989). On tolerating mental states: Theory of mind in borderline personality. *Bulletin of the Anna Freud Centre, 12*(2), 91–115.

Fonagy, P., & Allison, E. (2014). The role of mentalizing and epistemic trust in the therapeutic relationship. *Psychotherapy (Chicago, Ill.), 51*(3), 372–380. https://doi.org/10.1037/a0036505

Fonagy, P., Steele, M., Steele, H., Moran, G. S., & Higgitt, A. C. (1991). The capacity for understanding mental states: The reflective self in parent and child and its significance for security of attachment. *Infant Mental Health Journal, 12*(3), 201–218. https://doi.org/10.1002/1097-0355(199123)12:3<201::AID-IMHJ2280120307>3.0.CO;2-7

Frank, E., Ritchey, F. C., & Levenson, J. C. (2014). Is interpersonal psychotherapy infinitely adaptable? A compendium of the multiple modifications of IPT. *American Journal of Psychotherapy, 68*(4), 385–416. https://doi.org/10.1176/appi.psychotherapy.2014.68.4.385

Frank, E., Swartz, H. A., & Boland, E. (2007). Interpersonal and social rhythm therapy: An intervention addressing rhythm dysregulation in bipolar disorder. *Dialogues in Clinical Neuroscience, 9*(3), 325–332. https://doi.org/10.31887/DCNS.2007.9.3/efrank

Gershkovich, M. (2019). Exposure and response prevention for postpartum obsessive-compulsive disorder. *Journal of Cognitive Psychotherapy*, 33(3), 174–184. https://doi.org/10.1891/0889-8391.33.3.174

Goodman, W. K., Price, L. H., Rasmussen, S. A., Mazure, C., Fleischmann, R. L., Hill, C. L., . . . Charney, D. S. (1989). The Yale-Brown Obsessive Compulsive Scale. I: Development, use, and reliability. *Archives of General Psychiatry*, 46(11), 1006–1011. https://doi.org/10.1001/archpsyc.1989.01810110048007

Gordon, I., Zagoory-Sharon, O., Leckman, J. F., & Feldman, R. (2010). Oxytocin and the development of parenting in humans. *Biological Psychiatry*, 68(4), 377–382. https://doi.org/10.1016/j.biopsych.2010.02.005

Grote, N. K., Swartz, H. A., Geibel, S. L., Zuckoff, A., Houck, P. R., & Frank, E. (2009). A randomized controlled trial of culturally relevant, brief interpersonal psychotherapy for perinatal depression. *Psychiatric Services*, 60(3), 313–321. https://doi.org/10.1176/ps.2009.60.3.313

Guille, C., & Douglas, E. (2017). Telephone delivery of interpersonal psychotherapy by certified nurse-midwives may help reduce symptoms of postpartum depression. *Evidence-Based Nursing*, 20(1), 12–13. https://doi.org/10.1136/eb-2016-102513

Hamilton, M. (1967). Development of a rating scale for primary depressive illness. *British Journal of Social and Clinical Psychology*, 6(4), 278–296. https://doi.org/10.1111/j.2044-8260.1967.tb00530.x

Hammen, C., & Brennan, P. A. (2002). Interpersonal dysfunction in depressed women: Impairments independent of depressive symptoms. *Journal of Affective Disorders*, 72(2), 145–156. https://doi.org/10.1016/S0165-0327(01)00455-4

Hezel, D. M., & Simpson, H. B. (2019). Exposure and response prevention for obsessive-compulsive disorder: A review and new directions. *Indian Journal of Psychiatry*, 61(Suppl 1), S85–S92. https://doi.org/10.4103/psychiatry.IndianJPsychiatry_516_18

Kleinman, A. (2016). Foreword. In R. Lewis-Fernández, N. K. Aggarwal, L. Hinton, D. E. Hinton, & L. J. Kirmayer (Eds.), *DSM-5 handbook on the cultural formulation interview* (pp. xvii–xix). American Psychiatric Publishing.

Kleiman, K., Wenzel, A., Waller, H., & Adler, A. (2021). *Dropping the baby and other scary thoughts: Breaking the cycle of unwanted thoughts in parenthood* (2nd ed.). Routledge. https://doi.org/10.4324/9780429274657

Klerman, G. L., Weissman, M. M., Rounsaville, B. J., & Chevron, E. (1984). *Interpersonal psychotherapy of depression*. Basic Books.

Law, R., Ravitz, P., Pain, C., & Fonagy, P. (2022). Interpersonal psychotherapy and mentalizing-synergies in clinical practice. *American Journal of Psychotherapy*, 75(1), 44–50. https://doi.org/10.1176/appi.psychotherapy.20210024

Leckman, J. F., Goodman, W. K., North, W. G., Chappell, P. B., Price, L. H., Pauls, D. L., . . . Barr, L. C. (1994). The role of central oxytocin in obsessive compulsive disorder and related normal behavior. *Psychoneuroendocrinology*, 19(8), 723–749. https://doi.org/10.1016/0306-4530(94)90021-3

Lenze, S. N., & Potts, M. A. (2017). Brief Interpersonal Psychotherapy for depression during pregnancy in a low-income population: A randomized controlled trial. *Journal of Affective Disorders*, 210, 151–157. https://doi.org/10.1016/j.jad.2016.12.029

Lipsitz, J. D., Gur, M., Miller, N. L., Forand, N., Vermes, D., & Fyer, A. J. (2006). An open pilot study of interpersonal psychotherapy for panic disorder (IPT-PD). *The Journal of Nervous and Mental Disease*, 194(6), 440–445. https://doi.org/10.1097/01.nmd.0000221302.42073.a1

Lipsitz, J. D., Gur, M., Vermes, D., Petkova, E., Cheng, J., Miller, N., . . . Fyer, A. J. (2008). A randomized trial of interpersonal therapy versus supportive therapy for social anxiety disorder. *Depression and Anxiety*, 25(6), 542–553. https://doi.org/10.1002/da.20364

Lipsitz, J. D., & Markowitz, J. C. (2013). Mechanisms of change in interpersonal therapy (IPT). *Clinical Psychology Review*, 33(8), 1134–1147. https://doi.org/10.1016/j.cpr.2013.09.002

Lipsitz, J. D., Markowitz, J. C., Cherry, S., & Fyer, A. J. (1999). Open trial of interpersonal psychotherapy for the treatment of social phobia. *American Journal of Psychiatry*, 156(11), 1814–1816. https://doi.org/10.1176/ajp.156.11.1814

Markowitz, J. C., Kocsis, J. H., Bleiberg, K. L., Christos, P. J., & Sacks, M. (2005). A comparative trial of psychotherapy and pharmacotherapy for "pure" dysthymic patients. *Journal of Affective Disorders*, 89(1–3), 167–175. https://doi.org/10.1016/j.jad.2005.10.001

Markowitz, J. C., Milrod, B., Luyten, P., & Holmqvist, R. (2019). Mentalizing in interpersonal psychotherapy. *American Journal of Psychotherapy*, 72(4), 95–100. https://doi.org/10.1176/appi.psychotherapy.20190021

Markowitz, J. C., Petkova, E., Neria, Y., Van Meter, P. E., Zhao, Y., Hembree, E., . . . Marshall, R. D. (2015). Is exposure necessary? A randomized clinical trial of interpersonal psychotherapy for PTSD. *American Journal of Psychiatry*, 172(5), 430–440. https://doi.org/10.1176/appi.ajp.2014.14070908

Markowitz, J. C., & Weissman, M. M. (2004). Interpersonal psychotherapy: Principles and applications. *World Psychiatry*, 3(3), 136–139.

Markowitz, J. C., & Weissman, M. M. (2012). Interpersonal psychotherapy: Past, present and future. *Clinical Psychology & Psychotherapy*, 19(2), 99–105. https://doi.org/10.1002/cpp.1774

McElroy, S. L., Phillips, K. A., & Keck, P. E., Jr. (1994). Obsessive compulsive spectrum disorder. *The Journal of Clinical Psychiatry*, 55(Suppl), 33–51.

McKay, D., Abramowitz, J., & Storch, E. (n.d.). *Ineffective and potentially harmful psychological interventions for obsessive-compulsive disorder*. International OCD Foundation. Retrieved November 14, 2022, from https://iocdf.org/expert-opinions/ineffective-and-potentially-harmful-psychological-interventions-for-obsessive-compulsive-disorder/

McLean, P. D., Whittal, M. L., Thordarson, D. S., Taylor, S., Söchting, I., Koch, W. J., . . . Anderson, K. W. (2001). Cognitive versus behavior therapy in the group treatment of obsessive-compulsive disorder. *Journal of Consulting and Clinical Psychology*, 69(2), 205–214. https://doi.org/10.1037/0022-006X.69.2.205

Miller, M. L., & O'Hara, M. W. (2020). Obsessive-compulsive symptoms, intrusive thoughts and depressive symptoms: A longitudinal study examining relation to maternal responsiveness. *Journal of Reproductive and Infant Psychology*, 38(3), 226–242. https://doi.org/10.1080/02646838.2019.1652255

Miniati, M., Callari, A., Calugi, S., Rucci, P., Savino, M., Mauri, M., & Dell'Osso, L. (2014). Interpersonal psychotherapy for postpartum depression: A systematic review. *Archives of Women's Mental Health*, 17(4), 257–268. https://doi.org/10.1007/s00737-014-0442-7

Moreira, E. C., & Moreira, L. A. (1999). Hypochondriasis by proxy in children: Report of two cases. *Jornal de Pediatria*, 75(5), 373–376. https://doi.org/10.2223/JPED.333

Mufson, L. (Ed.). (2004). *Interpersonal psychotherapy for depressed adolescents*. Guilford Press.

Mufson, L., Moreau, D., Weissman, M. M., Wickramaratne, P., Martin, J., & Samoilov, A. (1994). Modification of interpersonal psychotherapy with depressed adolescents (IPT-A): Phase I and II studies. *Journal of the American Academy of Child and Adolescent Psychiatry*, 33(5), 695–705. https://doi.org/10.1097/00004583-199406000-00011

Mulcahy, R., Reay, R. E., Wilkinson, R. B., & Owen, C. (2010). A randomised control trial for the effectiveness of group interpersonal psychotherapy for postnatal depression. *Archives of Women's Mental Health*, 13(2), 125–139. https://doi.org/10.1007/s00737-009-0101-6

Naeem, F., Phiri, P., Rathod, S., & Ayub, M. (2019). Cultural adaptation of cognitive – behavioural therapy. *BJPsych Advances*, 25(6), 387–395. https://doi.org/10.1192/bja.2019.15

National Health Information. N. H. S. (n.d.). Postnatal depression symptoms and treatment. *Illnesses & Conditions | NHS Inform*. Retrieved November 27, 2022, from www.nhsinform.scot/illnesses-and-conditions/mental-health/postnatal-depression#treatment

National Institute of Mental Health (Ed.). (n.d.). *Perinatal depression*. National Institute of Mental Health. Retrieved November 27, 2022, from www.nimh.nih.gov/health/publications/perinatal-depression

Norcross, J. C., & Goldfried, M. R. (Eds.). (2005). *Handbook of psychotherapy integration*. Oxford University Press.

Normann, C., & Buttenschøn, H. N. (2019). Gene-environment interactions between HPA-axis genes and stressful life events in depression: A systematic review. *Acta Neuropsychiatrica*, 31(4), 186–192. https://doi.org/10.1017/neu.2019.16

O'Connor, E., Senger, C. A., Henninger, M. L., Coppola, E., & Gaynes, B. N. (2019). Interventions to prevent perinatal depression. *Journal of the American Medical Association*, 321(6), 588–601. https://doi.org/10.1001/jama.2018.20865

O'Hara, M. W., Hoffman, J. G., Philipps, L. H., & Wright, E. J. (1992). Adjustment in childbearing women: The postpartum adjustment questionnaire. *Psychological Assessment*, 4(2), 160–169. https://doi.org/10.1037/1040-3590.4.2.160

O'Hara, M. W., Stuart, S., Gorman, L. L., & Wenzel, A. (2000). Efficacy of interpersonal psychotherapy for postpartum depression. *Archives of General Psychiatry, 57*(11), 1039–1045. https://doi.org/10.1001/archpsyc.57.11.1039

Ojalehto, H. J., Hellberg, S. N., Butcher, M. W., Buchholz, J. L., Timpano, K. R., & Abramowitz, J. S. (2021). Experiential avoidance and the misinterpretation of intrusions as prospective predictors of postpartum obsessive-compulsive symptoms in first-time parents. *Journal of Contextual Behavioral Science, 20*, 137–143. https://doi.org/10.1016/j.jcbs.2021.04.003

Paykel, E. S. (2003). Life events and affective disorders. *Acta Psychiatrica Scandinavica. Supplementum, 108*, 61–66. https://doi.org/10.1034/j.1600-0447.108.s418.13.x

Posmontier, B., Neugebauer, R., Stuart, S., Chittams, J., & Shaughnessy, R. (2016). Telephone-administered interpersonal psychotherapy by nurse-midwives for postpartum depression. *Journal of Midwifery & Women's Health, 61*(4), 456–466. https://doi.org/10.1111/jmwh.12411

Proença, C. R., Markowitz, J. C., Coimbra, B. M., Cogo-Moreira, H., Maciel, M. R., Mello, A. F., & Mello, M. F. (2022). Interpersonal psychotherapy versus sertraline for women with posttraumatic stress disorder following recent sexual assault: A randomized clinical trial. *European Journal of Psychotraumatology, 13*(2), 2127474. Advance online publication. https://doi.org/10.1080/20008066.2022.2127474

Rafaeli, A. K., & Markowitz, J. C. (2011). Interpersonal psychotherapy (IPT) for PTSD: A case study. *American Journal of Psychotherapy, 65*(3), 205–223. https://doi.org/10.1176/appi.psychotherapy.2011.65.3.205

Ravitz, P., Maunder, R., Hunter, J., Sthankiya, B., & Lancee, W. (2010). Adult attachment measures: A 25-year review. *Journal of Psychosomatic Research, 69*(4), 419–432. https://doi.org/10.1016/j.jpsychores.2009.08.006

Ravitz, P., Watson, P., Lawson, A., Constantino, M. J., Bernecker, S., Park, J., & Swartz, H. A. (2019). Interpersonal psychotherapy: A scoping review and historical perspective (1974–2017). *Harvard Review of Psychiatry, 27*(3), 165–180. https://doi.org/10.1097/HRP.0000000000000219

Reynolds, C. F., III, Frank, E., Perel, J. M., Imber, S. D., Cornes, C., Miller, M. D., . . . Kupfer, D. J. (1999). Nortriptyline and interpersonal psychotherapy as maintenance therapies for recurrent major depression: A randomized controlled trial in patients older than 59 years. *Journal of the American Medical Association, 281*, 39–45. https://doi.org/10.1001/jama.281.1.39

Simpson, J. A., & Rholes, W. S. (2012). Adult attachment orientations, stress, and romantic relationships. In *Advances in experimental social psychology* (pp. 279–328). https://doi.org/10.1016/b978-0-12-394286-9.00006-8

Sockol, L. E. (2018). A systematic review and meta-analysis of interpersonal psychotherapy for perinatal women. *Journal of Affective Disorders, 232*, 316–328. https://doi.org/10.1016/j.jad.2018.01.018

Sookman, D., Phillips, K. A., Anholt, G. E., Bhar, S., Bream, V., Challacombe, F. L., . . . Veale, D. (2021). Knowledge and competency standards for specialized cognitive behavior therapy for adult obsessive-compulsive disorder. *Psychiatry Research, 303*, 113752. https://doi.org/10.1016/j.psychres.2021.113752

Spinelli, M. G. (2017). *Interpersonal psychotherapy for perinatal depression: A guide for treating depression during pregnancy and the postpartum period (IPT-P)*. CreateSpace Independent Publishing.

Spinelli, M. G., & Endicott, J. (2003). Controlled clinical trial of interpersonal psychotherapy versus parenting education program for depressed pregnant women. *American Journal of Psychiatry, 160*(3), 555–562. https://doi.org/10.1176/appi.ajp.160.3.555

Spinelli, M. G., Endicott, J., Leon, A. C., Goetz, R. R., Kalish, R. B., Brustman, L. E., . . . Schulick, J. L. (2013). A controlled clinical treatment trial of interpersonal psychotherapy for depressed pregnant women at 3 New York City sites. *Journal of Clinical Psychiatry, 74*(4), 393–399. https://doi.org/10.4088/JCP.12m07909

Starcevic, V., Eslick, G. D., Viswasam, K., & Berle, D. (2020). Symptoms of obsessive-compulsive disorder during pregnancy and the postpartum period: A systematic review and meta-analysis. *Psychiatric Quarterly, 91*(4), 965–981. https://doi.org/10.1007/s11126-020-09769-8

Stern, D. N. (1995). *The motherhood constellation: A unified view of parent-infant psychotherapy* (1st ed.). Routledge. https://doi.org/10.4324/9780429482489

Stuart, S., & O'Hara, M. W. (1995). Interpersonal psychotherapy for postpartum depression: A treatment program. *Journal of Psychotherapy Practice and Research, 4*(1), 18–29.

Stuart, S., & Robertson, M. (2012). *Interpersonal psychotherapy: A clinician's guide.* Arnold.

Su, Y. Y., D'Arcy, C., Li, M., O'Donnell, K. J., Caron, J., Meaney, M. J., & Meng, X. (2022). Specific and cumulative lifetime stressors in the aetiology of major depression: A longitudinal community-based population study. *Epidemiology and Psychiatric Sciences, 31,* e3. https://doi.org/10.1017/S2045796021000779

Sullivan, H. S. (1953). *The interpersonal theory of psychiatry.* WW Norton & Co.

Swartz, H. A., Grote, N. K., & Graham, P. (2014). Brief Interpersonal Psychotherapy (IPT-B): Overview and review of evidence. *American Journal of Psychotherapy, 68*(4), 443–462. https://doi.org/10.1176/appi.psychotherapy.2014.68.4.443

Thorgaard, M. V., Frostholm, L., Walker, L., Jensen, J. S., Morina, B., Lindegaard, H., . . . Rask, C. U. (2017). Health anxiety by proxy in women with severe health anxiety: A case control study. *Journal of Anxiety Disorders, 52,* 8–14. https://doi.org/10.1016/j.janxdis.2017.09.001

Uguz, F., Gezginc, K., Zeytinci, I. E., Karatayli, S., Askin, R., Guler, O., . . . Gecici, O. (2007). Course of obsessive-compulsive disorder during early postpartum period: A prospective analysis of 16 cases. *Comprehensive Psychiatry, 48*(6), 558–561. https://doi.org/10.1016/j.comppsych.2007.05.010

UNESCO. (2008). Cultures – IIEP policy toolbox. *Cultures.* Retrieved November 26, 2022, from https://policytoolbox.iiep.unesco.org/glossary/cultures/

Vogel, P. A., Stiles, T. C., & Götestam, K. G. (2004). Adding cognitive therapy elements to exposure therapy for obsessive compulsive disorder: A controlled study. *Behavioural and Cognitive Psychotherapy, 32*(3), 275–290. https://doi.org/10.1017/S1352465804001353

Weissman, M. M. (1976). Assessment of social adjustment by patient self-report. *Archives of General Psychiatry, 33*(9), 1111. https://doi.org/10.1001/archpsyc.1976.01770090101010

Weissman, M. M. (2006). A brief history of interpersonal psychotherapy. *Psychiatric Annals, 36*(8), 00485713–20060801-03. Advance online publication. https://doi.org/10.3928/00485713-20060801-03

Weissman, M. M. (2020). Interpersonal psychotherapy: History and future. *American Journal of Psychotherapy, 73*(1), 3–7. https://doi.org/10.1176/appi.psychotherapy.20190032

Weissman, M. M., Markowitz, J. C., & Klerman, G. L. (2000). *Comprehensive guide to interpersonal psychotherapy.* Basic Books.

Weissman, M. M., Markowitz, J. C., & Klerman, G. L. (2018). *The guide to interpersonal psychotherapy: Updated and expanded edition.* Oxford University Press.

Weissman, M. M., & Mootz, J. (2024). *Interpersonal psychotherapy: A global reach.* Oxford University Press.

Wenzel, A. (2011). *Anxiety in childbearing women: Diagnosis and treatment.* APA Books.

Wenzel, A., Haugen, E. N., Jackson, L. C., & Brendle, J. R. (2005). Anxiety symptoms and disorders at eight weeks postpartum. *Journal of Anxiety Disorders, 19*(3), 295–311. https://doi.org/10.1016/j.janxdis.2004.04.001

Wenzel, A., & Kleiman, K. R. (2015). *Cognitive behavioral therapy for perinatal distress.* Routledge.

Winnicott, D. W., Caldwell, L., & Robinson, H. T. (2016 [1956]). *The collected works of D.W. Winnicott. volume 5 1955–1959.* Oxford University Press. Retrieved November 10, 2023, from https://search.ebscohost.com/login.aspx?direct=true&scope=site&db=nlebk&db=nlabk&AN=2116571

World Health Organization and Columbia University. (2016). *Group Interpersonal Therapy (IPT) for depression (WHO generic field-trial version 1.0).* WHO.

Wright, L. M., Watson, W. L., & Bell, J. M. (1996). *Beliefs: The heart of healing in families and illness.* Basic Books.

Yadin, E., Foa, E. B., & Lichner, T. K. (2012). *Treating your OCD with exposure and response (ritual) prevention workbook.* Oxford University Press, USA.

Zambaldi, C. F., Cantilino, A., Montenegro, A. C., Paes, J. A., de Albuquerque, T. L., & Sougey, E. B. (2009). Postpartum obsessive-compulsive disorder: Prevalence and clinical characteristics. *Comprehensive Psychiatry, 50*(6), 503–509. https://doi.org/10.1016/j.comppsych.2008.11.014

Zeegers, M., Colonnesi, C., Stams, G., & Meins, E. (2017). Mind matters: A meta-analysis on parental mentalization and sensitivity as predictors of infant-parent attachment. *Psychological Bulletin, 143*(12), 1245–1272. https://doi.org/10.1037/bul0000114

Zlotnick, C., Johnson, S. L., Miller, I. W., Pearlstein, T., & Howard, M. (2001). Postpartum depression in women receiving public assistance: Pilot study of an interpersonal-therapy-oriented group intervention. *American Journal of Psychiatry, 158*(4), 638–640. https://doi.org/10.1176/appi.ajp.158.4.638

24

INTEGRATIVE PSYCHODYNAMIC THERAPY FOR PERINATAL TRAUMA

Deana Stevens

In the parenting groups people ask you "What's your birth story?" Do they want to hear about how I almost died? About all the surgeries? . . . How do I compress all that? It's not just what happened. It's who I am (Allegra, age 28).

The period around conception and birth is a time of great activity and expansion, marking a new phase of development for the birthing parent. Physical changes are expected and naturally, are the focus of many people's attention. Though less apparent to the world outside, it is also a time of ongoing psychological activation and reorganization for the pregnant/birthing person. Navigating this complex, at times chaotic internal experience can be isolating and deeply painful. Pregnant and birthing people are vulnerable in many ways and sometimes have devastating experiences. *Perinatal trauma* is any trauma that occurs during the perinatal period thereby disturbing the developmental shift in a meaningful way. This might include trauma related to conception, pregnancy, birth and postpartum, or unrelated traumatic events that occur contemporaneously, as well as the re-emergence of developmental trauma.

This chapter offers a window into an integrative psychodynamic approach to the treatment of perinatal trauma sequelae in birthing parents. I write as a White, cisgender woman of multi-national European heritage with two children. I share my perspective from the United States as a parent and a clinical psychologist who has experienced pregnancy loss and other perinatal trauma. Here, I refer to birthing people to make room for those of diverse gender and sexual identities. At the same time, I use the term "mothering" to refer to the unique form of intimate care a birthing parent provides to their infant. Two cases of psychodynamic therapy are presented, in which EMDR was utilized at a key point in the treatment. Clinical factors and client preferences guided decisions about when and how EMDR was utilized. Differences between the two cases and implications are also discussed.

Traumatic Experience in the Perinatal Period

Effective treatment of a birthing parent requires nuanced understanding of the sensitivities of this time of life. Jaffe and Diamond (2011) established the importance of the

DOI: 10.4324/9781003206903-29

reproductive story, defined as the "sometimes conscious but largely unconscious narrative of what they believe their children will be like, and what they themselves will be like as parents" (Jaffe, 2017, p. 380). Originating in our own experiences of being parented as an infant, this narrative is entirely unique, and for some it may even include the wish not to become a parent. The framework of the reproductive story also takes into account the developmental tasks relevant to new parents, as outlined by Erikson (1982). Forming a cohesive social identity, creating intimate bonds with others, and contributing to society in a lasting way become central aims from late adolescence into middle adulthood, or the reproductive phase of life. The reproductive story guides therapeutic work with people in the perinatal period, encompassing themes of identity, intimacy, and generativity, as well as ways in which the present does and does not embody what the client has imagined and expected would come to be.

What happens when the reproductive story does not unfold as expected? Stein and Davis (2022) used the term *perinatal crisis* for a parent's experience of threat to their infant's well-being during pregnancy, birth, or early infancy. Perinatal crisis encompasses fertility challenges; pregnancy complications, and unwanted pregnancies; pregnancy loss and stillbirth; medical diagnosis or injury prior to, during and/or after delivery; unexpected induction, intervention and surgical birth, neonatal intensive care unit (NICU) admission, and bringing home a baby who has conditions that require ongoing specialized care. Additionally, a parent might experience intimate partner violence, postpartum mood and anxiety disorders, psychosis, physical injury or illness, and the loss of expected caregivers or other family members. The list of possibilities is long.

Horesh et al. (2021) proposed that childbearing trauma belongs in a category unto itself. They cited four key factors that contribute to the unique experience of the person experiencing birth trauma. First, unlike other potentially traumatizing occurrences, the birth of a baby is a highly anticipated positive event; it is quite common to hear family members, friends and birthing parents themselves say some version of, "Well at least the baby is healthy. That's what counts," particularly in cases where the birth process was prolonged, complicated, or downright terrifying. Second, the sensory and physiological intensity of the event and the trauma are entirely within the body. Finally, whereas "the effects of traumatic childbirth are . . . felt throughout the family," the directly exposed (adult) survivor is always the birthing parent (Horesh et al., 2021, p. 222). This unique status is isolating and can lead to further strain when the nongestational partner does not understand the nature of trauma or why the birthing parent is not doing well emotionally.

Up to 45% of birthing parents report that they experienced birth trauma (Beck et al., 2018). About 8% of birthing people develop clinical posttraumatic stress disorder (PTSD) related to their perinatal trauma. Among racially marginalized and low-income birthing parents, that rate goes up to 14% (Seng et al., 2009; Seng et al., 2011). Furthermore, many birthing parents have a history of trauma that complicates their experience of perinatal care and intervention. For instance, one in five women in the United States has been the victim of an attempted or completed rape in her lifetime, and 43.6% of women experience some form of contact sexual violence in their lifetime; 24.8% of men in the United States. experience some form of contact sexual violence in their lifetime (Smith et al., 2018). Data show that these rates are the same or higher for members of LGBTQIA+ communities and are particularly elevated for transgender individuals (Walters et al., 2013). Rates of sexual violence have also been found to be elevated for individuals who identify as a racial minority and are particularly elevated for people who identify as indigenous (Black et al.,

2011). Racial trauma—not yet in the *Diagnostic and Statistical Manual of Mental Disorders* (DSM) and, therefore, not represented in quantitative research—encompasses both discrete, violent acts as well as the chronic stress of racist microaggressions, representing another significant source of distress and suffering among BIPOC communities.

Although reproductive trauma is an injury unto itself, it can also reignite trauma from early life. Both types of injuries have implications for the present parent–child relationship. In their seminal paper, "Ghosts in the Nursery," Fraiberg et al. (1975) illustrated how the developmental shift into embodied parenthood can include the emergence of the parent's unresolved childhood injuries, which have significant implications for the baby before it is even born. Early relationships shape our ability to form future relationships. Monk et al. (2008) found that pregnant women's attachment styles were associated with their appraisal of their pregnancy experience, as well as with their concurrent and postpartum mood. Pregnant women who were more fearful and less secure with respect to relationships in general reported greater pregnancy distress. People who are diagnosed with PTSD as adults often have histories of trauma in childhood. It is important to address the birthing parent's suffering for their own sake and for the sake of their child who needs a parent to survive. Howard and Khalifeh (2020) identified "impaired attachment" as a key mechanism for transmission of risk to infants" that is related more to "mothers' experience of early trauma (including emotional neglect) than to specific maternal diagnoses" (p. 316). At a time when everyone's focus is on the new baby, memories of the past can feel particularly disorienting and unwelcome. Birthing parents are highly motivated to move forward and the people around them often echo this wish for a fresh start.

Trauma is not a discrete event but what our minds and bodies do with threatening experiences to prioritize survival. The legacies of traumatic events are not always easily recognized. As van der Kolk illuminates in his book, *The Body Keeps the Score* (2014), trauma is first and foremost a bodily experience. Pregnancy, prenatal care, and childbirth are literally the most intrusive experiences one can have. Birthing people often come through pregnancy, labor, and delivery with significant ambivalence about their bodies. In cases of physical injury and loss, this is most certainly the case. When the traumatic events occur within the body itself, it can feel like a very dangerous place to focus one's attention. Sensations accompanying normal fetal development, labor, delivery, postpartum recovery, breastfeeding, diapering, bathing, cuddling, subsequent pregnancies, medical care, and even sexual activity are all potential links to implicit memories of childbearing trauma (Horesh et al., 2021) and earlier trauma. It can be challenging to make sense of it all, let alone find words to explain it to someone else. The widely accepted phase model of trauma treatment outlined by Judith Herman (1997) first calls for stabilization and the establishment of safety in the moment, followed by accessing and working through traumatic material, and finally, a focus on integration and growth. Defenses, the ways we have of protecting ourselves from psychic overwhelm and fragmentation, have survival value. People who have experienced trauma are not always ready to know what they do not want to know about that experience. It is important to use the therapeutic relationship as a gauge for determining the timing and type of interventions.

Psychodynamic Treatment

Contemporary psychodynamic therapy is built on the understanding that the past contains the seeds of current distress. The approach involves creating space for emotion, desire, imagination, uncertainty, and reflection on lived experience in the presence of an attuned other. The therapeutic relationship becomes the container for that which is difficult to tolerate and make sense of on our own, as well as the parts of ourselves and our lives that feel vibrant and healthy. Psychodynamic psychotherapy is used to treat a wide range of conditions, including anxiety, depression, relationship distress, attachment issues, personality disorders, and trauma. Treatment begins with history taking that considers family of origin, constellation of relationships, significant achievements and losses, as well as the trajectory of the distress being experienced. Presenting symptoms are often associated with a sense of "stuckness" that comes with relying on ingrained patterns of response that do not always fit the situation and can become not only obstructive but destructive. A psychodynamic approach seeks to engage the client's conscious and unconscious experience thereby increasing awareness of formative experiences, feelings, and core beliefs so the client can be a more deliberate actor in their own life. Resolving emotionally laden intrapsychic conflicts about real-life experience makes it possible for people to rework their characteristic way of being in the world. With greater affect tolerance and more flexibility in responding to oneself, it becomes possible to connect more fully to the present, to learn new skills, and to build more mutually satisfying relationships with others.

McWilliams (2004) described psychodynamic treatment as an approach that is grounded in openness and honesty with the goal of reaching an expanded experience of oneself. "Being aware of disavowed aspects of our psychology will relieve us of time and effort required to keep them unconscious. Thus, more of our attention and energy can be liberated" (McWilliams, 2004, p. 2). Expectant and new parents often find it surprisingly difficult to be honest about what they are feeling (or not feeling). Many feel inadequate, afraid, and angry at times. This is not what they were taught to expect and not what they imagined, and it can be scary, shameful, or even like a betrayal of one's faith. Being in direct contact, hour after hour, with the infant's needs and attempting to meet them can stir awareness of one's own needs and how they are not or have not been similarly met. Many a birthing parent opines about the obliviousness of the people they hope will care for them. "How can my partner not see that I need help?" Simply having such unwelcome feelings recognized by others can bring substantial relief. Furthermore, awareness of these feelings serves to link current suffering to aspects of a birthing person's own experience of being parented that were painful, confusing, or harmful.

In treatment, the client may experience the therapist as being "just like" someone from their past. *Transference* is the phenomenon of displacing unconscious feelings about primary attachment figures, such as mothers, fathers, or siblings, onto another person in the present. This happens in daily life and in therapy as well. The therapist's felt experience of being with the client, the *countertransference*, complements our understanding of the client's experience. A unique aspect of psychodynamic therapy is the direct exploration of transference and countertransference between client and therapist. Working in the transference means therapist and client together considering the possibility that old patterns are being reenacted in the therapeutic relationship (as well as in other current relationships). Therapeutic intervention consists of recognizing how the old scenario is both similar to and different from the current relational situation, allowing the client to move between perspectives and their associated feelings and ideas about self and others. It creates opportunities for repair in the therapy and other key relationships. This work expands the client's insight and as a result enhances their agency to make new choices in relationships with others.

Birthing parents who feel vulnerable and helpless often insist on prioritizing the needs of the baby to the exclusion of their own. Blum (2007) suggested that this counterdependent attitude often prevents new parents from seeking treatment in the first place. Similarly, Stern (1995) suggested that the "fear of being found inadequate as a mother, of being judged unable to keep the baby alive and healthy and sane" (p. 161) embodied in the transference is the greatest threat to effective treatment. Consequently, a warm and actively supportive stance is required in establishing a sense of safety within the therapeutic relationship. It is also helpful to acknowledge at the outset of treatment the motivation and courage of the birthing parent who asks for therapeutic help.

Importance of the Therapeutic Relationship

Because we grow through our experiences with key people in our lives, the therapeutic relationship is a potential space for growth. Many treatments for emotional distress are informed by the medical model and view treatment from a one-person perspective, which does not incorporate an understanding of the relational nature of psychotherapy. From its inception, psychodynamic therapy has been concerned with the process of the interaction between client and therapist. Furthermore, reflecting the influences of object relations theory, interpersonal psychoanalysis, self-psychology, and attachment theory, contemporary psychodynamic thinking has grown to include the subjectivity of the client and the therapist, focusing attention on processes of mutual influence in development and in treatment. These theories embrace the centrality of the therapeutic relationship and the complexity of the intersubjective process (Greenberg & Mitchell, 1983). The therapeutic dyad consists of two subjective beings, each with minds and bodies engaging in the co-creation of meaning. Rather than locating expertise solely in the therapist, the client is understood to bring knowledge to the process that no one else can. The therapist's contributions are also extended beyond the objective, planned interventions.

This expanded understanding of the therapeutic process is supported by developmental neuroscience mapping of an implicit self (Schore, 2011). Research has identified that attachment experiences in the earliest stages of life are critical for development of the right-brain, home to neurological systems that impact one's capacity for "processing of emotion, modulation of stress, self-regulation, and . . . the bodily-based implicit self" (Schore & Schore, 2008, p. 10). Schore's work integrates neurobiological studies of the human brain and nervous system, including in early stages of development. He applied this body of literature to the therapy context, arguing that the emotional survival systems dominated by the right hemisphere/emotional brain, "are dominant in relational contexts at all stages of the lifespan, including the intimate context of psychotherapy" (Schore, 2009, p. 114). Thus, the therapeutic relationship operates on multiple levels simultaneously. In addition to the explicit verbalized exchange between client and therapist, communication, connection, and, thus, change are all understood to be unfolding, in part, through unconscious, right-brain-to-right-brain interaction. "Through visual—facial, auditory—prosodic, and tactile—gestural communication, caregiver and infant" (Schore, 2009, p. 116) like therapist and client co-create a relational experience and can aid in the client's ability to develop capacities for co-regulation, mentalization about themselves and others, and positive self-esteem. This body of research has led Schore to conclude that "psychotherapy is not the "talking cure" but the affect communicating and regulating cure" (Schore, 2009, p. 128).

Psychodynamic therapy is a fitting approach to perinatal work because it recognizes the interaction of two beings who are both necessary collaborators in determining the structure of the relationship, as in the parent-infant dyad. Bucci's (2011) description of the choreography of the therapeutic relationship captures the fluid quality of engagement. It assumes a degree of uncertainty and unexpected experience for both the client and the therapist. This dialectical understanding provides a stability to the treatment, with the therapist serving as an experienced figure who is not surprised when something surprising or difficult happens. The flow of the therapeutic process, while supported by a mutually understood frame, is not planned or organized by a set agenda. Throughout, the psychodynamic therapist is prepared to provide the very caring stance that we ask the "mothering" parent to provide (Winnicott, 1965): to hold one's own subjectivity in abeyance while prioritizing a receptive, warm, curious stance. At the same time, the psychodynamic therapist strives to remain aware of her own feelings and impulses, such as to save, solve, redirect or warn, reserving them until it is clear they are needed. In response to the client, the therapist may try on different ways of being, such as by offering information, teaching skills, playing, acknowledging conflict and remorse, and also celebrating growth and achievement. Shifting between different modes serves to co-regulate the dyad.

As previously discussed, establishing a sense of safety in the therapeutic relationship is the first step in trauma treatment. Over the course of treatment, as emotionally charged material is worked through, what the client needs to feel physically and emotionally safe may require renegotiation within the therapeutic relationship. Therapists cannot assume that because their intention is to be helpful in a given moment that they will be experienced that way. When viewed as interpersonal enactments of the client's intrapsychic experience, therapeutic impasses provide an opportunity to reduce tension, resolve conflicts, and move the treatment forward in unexpected ways. If the therapist, like a "good-enough parent" (Winnicott, 1953), serves as a secure base, enactments and collaboratively decoding them can be new experiences that strengthen that base by allowing for the presence of conflict. The client no longer has to preserve the security of the relationship by minimizing or denying thoughts and feelings that are felt to threaten the connection with the therapist. This allows for deeper self-awareness, greater understanding of others' perspectives, and improved communication of emotional experience.

Culture in Relationship

Psychodynamic therapy's emphasis on intersubjectivity also serves as an existing pathway for connection of the cultural and the personal. Both therapist and client have complex culturally embedded experiences to unpack in order for treatment to fully address the birthing person's experience. How the developmental shift into parenthood is recognized within a culture varies greatly. Furthermore, many people live at the intersection of multiple cultures. The explicit inclusion of race, gender, culture, spirituality, and class in our reproductive stories allows for an expanded sense of identity that incorporates universal and deeply personal meanings. For instance, in her paper *What Women Want*, Grill (2019) asserted, "the conflation of feminine, woman, and motherhood serves to negate female subjectivity, limiting the possibilities for other creative pursuits" (p. 65). The culturally supported assumption that women "must be, and want to be, mothers" (Grill, 2019, p. 67) precludes consideration of the desire to not be a mother, and, furthermore, excludes the reproductive desires of adults who do not identify as women. Disentangling motherhood from gender creates room for all those who wish to be parents to imagine the fulfillment of their (pro)creative dream without prescribing that women must desire motherhood and that others must not.

Race, culture, migration status, and class are considered within psychodynamic work as active ingredients (Tummala-Narra, 2014) in need of acknowledgement and respectful (non-colonizing) exploration to value the uniqueness of the client's experience. Akhtar (2018) traced the growing awareness since the Nazi Holocaust of the bidirectional association between culture and psyche. In order to be helpful to the client trying to make sense of their perinatal experience, we must consider their existing worldview. Systemic racism continues to impact people's mental and physical health in dramatic ways. In the United States, for example, childbirth-associated mortality rates are three to four times higher for people of color than for White people (MacDorman et al., 2021). How is a legacy that includes serial traumatic experiences intertwined with the experience of birth trauma for the individual? For instance, what does a microaggression during a prenatal visit mean to the pregnant person whose family history includes discrimination and traumatic loss? It is increasingly apparent that practitioners must make explicit our interest in and understanding of these influences. Otherwise, we may willfully dissociate important aspects of the birthing parent's identity and experience, thereby limiting understanding of particular sources of both threat and support in a client's life, or worse, replicating the experience in our offices.

Cultural norms and rituals of childbirth shape expectations of what needs can be acknowledged and what support can be made available. Similarly, therapists have their own unconscious culturally informed dynamics to examine. Community, multicultural, and psychoanalytic psychologists have all emphasized the importance of self-examination (Tummala-Narra, 2014), a practice that is at the heart of psychodynamic work. Attending to *countertransference*, the therapist's own internal experience of the client, is a critical dimension of assessing and guiding interventions throughout the treatment. Furthermore, because of the inclusion of an explicit focus on the therapeutic relationship, such self-examination can be shared in ways that are directly witnessed by the client. To see, hear and feel the therapist's own lived experience of social factors can stimulate the treatment in unexpected ways which may prove to be healing.

Finally, it bears repeating that therapists have their own reproductive stories. Many birthing people seeking treatment request therapists who specialize in reproductive mental health. At the same time, many therapists choose to build expertise with these issues precisely because they have had some personal experiences with infertility, birth trauma, perinatal mood and anxiety disorders, and pregnancy and infant loss. The pull for self-disclosure can be great, particularly when identifying with the client comes so easily. It is important for the therapist to consider the context in which one feels compelled to share and how self-disclosure intended to add something of consciously perceived value might simultaneously have an unconscious impact for the client, such as feeling pressure to care for or protect the therapist, or conversely, to express admiration for the therapist's capacity to endure and prevail. Therapists self-disclose in many ways indirectly. When aspects of the therapist's subjectivity come into the foreground of treatment, it is valuable to cultivate a genuine sense of curiosity about the client's experience of these disclosures in the context of their own reproductive story. Knowledge of the therapist's subjective experience can be burdensome, or it can be validating and comforting; it is important to inquire about the possibility of both.

Common Themes in Perinatal Treatment

For each birthing person, the anticipation of parenthood activates expectations about how to care and be cared for. Brain structures that drive and accommodate social connectedness, such as the hippocampus, the reward system, and the amygdala, all mature within the first year of life (Chambers, 2017). Given that the right hemisphere of the brain (sometimes referred to as the emotion brain) develops first, largely during the first three years of life (Chiron et al., 1997), our first lessons in love come well before our capacity for language develops (housed in the left brain). We learn in and from relationships in ways that are not always conscious (Fosshage, 2011). The earliest experiences of being cared for are, therefore, both formative and enduring. In other words, what it felt like to be cared for as an infant has implications for what it feels like to care for an infant. Some people have very clear ideas about what they plan to do as parents. Yet, the road to parenthood contains many surprises, including previously unimaginable experiences and newly relevant internal expectations that are largely unspoken and unthought, nonverbal, and embodied. The changes associated with pregnancy and birth can be physically and emotionally jarring, occurring with startling rapidity and force and often are more prolonged than expected. Bodies feel different; daily life is transformed. For many, even their sense of time is altered. Birthing people are often unprepared for the sense of loss they experience. There is a largely unconscious expectation that the baby will add dimensionality to life without taking anything away. Similar to adolescence, this phase of development is disruptive in ways that are impossible to anticipate fully.

Birthing parents expect to manage the tasks of caring for a newborn and to still feel the same about themselves. Yet, as the transactions of giving and receiving care establish in the infant a mental system of a self-separate from and in need of the other, these interactions also spur growth in the parent's sense of self in relationship to the child (Benedek, 1959). This requires a shift from one's (largely unconscious) identification as a child to identification with the parent and back again as these are not static or linear states. This unfamiliar territory is often associated with not-me experiences. "I don't know who I am anymore" and "I don't feel like myself" are common expressions of new parents in therapy. Identification with the parent from one's own childhood can be particularly disconcerting for the client who is consciously determined not to be anything like their own parent(s). In her work with perinatal depression Menken (2008) emphasized the centrality of addressing identifications and counter-identifications with one's own parents in constructing a conscious parental identity: "Helping her to mother from a conscious place that is her own choice, not to repeat the way she was mothered, nor to mother in opposition to the ways she was mothered, but rather to find her own authentic identity as a mother is key" (Menken, 2008, p. 315). This task is particularly complex when such relationships have been fraught, abusive, or altogether absent. Many birthing parents strive simply to reject those early experiences out of hand. Yet all new parents need feedback about what they are doing, particularly what they are doing well. Therapists support the client's exploration of how they are and are not like their own parents, with an emphasis on identifying the genuine "mothering" abilities they already possess.

Another frequent theme in treatment of postpartum depression noted by Blum (2007) is the inhibition of anger and guilt about its expression. Birthing parents who have experienced trauma have good reason to feel anger, yet fear the consequences of expressing it. The perinatal period is one of great vulnerability, and people are reluctant to act in ways that will cause others to recoil from them or worse become hostile in return. Consequently, there is motivation to minimize angry feelings or deny them altogether. Providing a safe space to give voice to anger can help birthing parents to learn through experience that their anger will not destroy them or their child. Misunderstandings and moments in which the client feels let down or annoyed with the therapist are invitations to work in the transference, an explicit effort at co-regulation. Acknowledging and committing to working through interpersonal conflict allows the client to experience that their feelings can be tolerated by others, thus increasing the client's tolerance for their own anger, expanding their sense of agency in the context of feeling. Making the traumatized birthing parent's affective knowledge explicit can reduce their suffering, increase their confidence in the parental role, and prevent transmission of implicit conflicts to the child entering the world (Howard & Khalifeh, 2020).

Ultimately, the goal of treatment is to help the client be more open to a greater range of ways their reproductive story might unfold. With very few exceptions, there is no singularly right way to build a family or to parent a child. The work of the psychodynamic therapist is to discover with the birthing parent which experiences have shaped their sense of self either directly or inversely. It is not about choosing one or another but finding ways to authentically integrate the multiple aspects of self that become known to us through each of our key relationships, including the therapeutic relationship into a parental identity that is authentic and sustainable.

Integrating EMDR Into the Treatment

Many therapists identify their approach as integrative (Boswell et al., 2019; Zarbo et al., 2016). The multifaceted nature of trauma's impact requires it (van der Kolk, 2014). Therapists who work extensively with traumatized people keep an open mind about possible ways to relieve suffering while keeping the client safely engaged. When it comes to maintaining the therapeutic relationship, flexibility may be just as important as treatment fidelity (Fonagy & Luyten, 2019), if not more so. *Assimilative integration* is one form of psychotherapy integration, in which the primary therapeutic model, in this case psychodynamic therapy, is augmented by ideas and interventions from another established treatment approach (Messer, 1992). Incorporating a different technique allows for both fidelity to the primary theory and flexibility in the service of the client.

Stricker and Gold's Assimilative Psychodynamic Therapy (2019) is one model for engaging multiple tiers of experience with techniques not endemic to the approach. Stricker and Gold identified three tiers of experience that can be impaired and are necessary to engage to help people to heal: (a) behavioral and interpersonal; (b) cognitive, emotional and perceptual; and (c) the psychodynamic. In addition to the primary interventions of clarification, confrontation, and interpretation, specific interventions grounded in other theories may be used to engage a particular tier of experience in support of the overall goals of increasing self-awareness, self-understanding, and the integration of that new understanding and experiences associated with it.

Similarly, the model of treatment proposed in this chapter incorporates EMDR into a psychodynamic framework to expand the tiers of experience addressed in treatment. *Eye Movement Desensitization and Reprocessing*, widely known as EMDR, was originally intended as a transtheoretical application of neuroscientific trauma research to existing psychological treatments (Shapiro, 2001). The approach is grounded in the *Adaptive Information Processing* (AIP) theory. According to the AIP model, present difficulties are informed by past experiences that have been inadequately processed and maladaptively stored in the nervous system. As in psychodynamic therapy, the interplay between past and present is a central dimension of the work. The EMDR eight-phase protocol addresses past, present, and future experiences and the connections between them. The objective of the protocol is to establish links between affectively charged memories and beliefs and internal resources that could not be made when the trauma occurred. When the client is able to be in contact with distress and the resource simultaneously, the brain's natural tendency toward resolution can proceed unimpeded.

Table 24.1 briefly describes the activities that comprise each of the eight phases. Although the therapist makes key decisions about the timing of each activity, EMDR is a collaborative process that requires the active consent of the client at multiple points along the way.

A key component of the EMDR standard protocol involves identifying the client's habitual responses to their own physiological arousal; this occurs in the Preparation phase and is revisited as needed. In many cases, learning new ways to soothe and ground oneself is a necessary part of the process for creating such linkages. Particularly with complex clinical presentations as are seen in cases of developmental trauma, it is necessary to spend some time incorporating and increasing access to positive memories and affect states. This is consistent with the psychodynamic work of exploring formative experiences, with an emphasis on what was nurturing. Birthing parents can be encouraged to identify memories of adults who they felt cared for them and things that were pleasurable in their own childhood, as

Table 24.1 Eight Phases of EMDR Standard Protocol

Eight Phases of EMDR Standard Protocol

Phase	*Collaborative Aims and Activities*
1. History taking	Gather information about client's history, identity, trauma exposure (including the target event), current triggers, goals, and strengths to determine if EMDR is appropriate.
2. Preparation	Establish a working alliance and clear expectations of the EMDR process. Identify and expand client's existing coping resources to regulate reactions to trauma processing.
3. Assessment	Review target event, associated images, beliefs, feelings, and sensations. Assess current level of distress to establish the client's baseline. Introduce scales to track shifts in client's distress (SUD = subjective units of distress) affect tolerance and resonance with new perspectives (VOC = validity of cognition).
4. Desensitization	Connect to trauma memory while engaging in bilateral stimulation (e.g., side-to-side eye movements, sounds, taps). Observe new thoughts or images that emerge in subsequent rounds of processing and bilateral stimulation. Continue until distress reduces and the target event is integrated into narrative memory.
5. Installation	Identify positive beliefs or strengths regarding the event and reinforce these associations until they feel true for the client.
6. Body Scan	Seek somatic feedback about the thoughts being expressed. Change in internal states is noted. Remaining distress is targeted and reprocessed as needed (see phase 4).
7. Closure	Guide client in returning to a state of safety and calmness in the present moment to end the session.
8. Reevaluation	Reflect on the trauma memory to ensure that distress remains low, and the positive beliefs are strong. Future targets may be identified.

well as to recognize what is going well in the present as they care for their own child. The therapeutic dyad is another place where positive experiences can be located and elaborated. Psychodynamic therapists generally express curiosity about the client's experience of the interaction. "What is it like to share this with me right now?" And, "How does it feel for me to respond to you in this way?" Positive responses from the client can be explored and elaborated through dialogue. With EMDR, such feeling states can also be established as internal resources the client can call upon in future moments of distress. The objective is to help the client know a good thing when they feel it so that they can appreciate what is going well and begin to cultivate more of that feeling in their life.

The first three phases of EMDR lead to the identification of a target which may be a memory, a current situation, or a desired future state. Processing involves directing attention to the target and all its dimensions (i.e., visual, cognitive, emotional, sensory) and intensity while engaging in *bilateral stimulation*, via saccadic eye movements or auditory, tactile stimuli or a combination of them. Bilateral stimulation serves to engage multiple areas of the brain in both hemispheres simultaneously, which allows for memories to be processed and stored adaptively, thereby desensitizing the negative or disturbing aspects of the associated experience. This is reflected by decreasing SUD scores, observable changes in the client's sympathetic nervous system arousal, and when possible, verbal self-report. Once the target can be revisited without the previous disturbance, the positive associations can be installed and elaborated. This is done through a similar set of procedures. The client rates the positive associations as credible and resonant with their felt experience, as evidence by increased VOC. Paying attention to the somatic aspects of this process via the Body Scan is a fundamental part of the protocol that yields information some clients find is not usually available to them. It is an explicit opportunity to check for conflicts between thoughts, verbal statements, and somatic feedback.

Because trauma is fundamentally a physiological process, and perinatal trauma is inseparably linked to bodily experience, it is important to engage nonverbal, somatic experience in a more targeted way. EMDR addresses this realm of experience in ways that support the goals of psychodynamic treatment. In particular, it recognizes that experience is organized along associative chains that are emotional in nature. Experiences that might not appear to be connected are experienced as such in the body. Psychodynamic therapy has deep roots in considering the role of bodily arousal and energetic attachment (e.g., Freud's [1915] drives and cathexis) to others. EMDR serves as another mechanism for identifying and engaging associative chains between past and present experience so that they can be brought into conscious awareness and integrated with new information and experience. EMDR complements the psychodynamic approach, as both emphasize the importance of affect and its activation in treatment as a component of the healing process and extends the reach of the therapy into non and preverbal experience, the realm of early trauma.

Several authors have shared their efforts to assimilate EMDR into psychodynamic treatment and efforts to identify variables for future study (McCullough, 2002). Leighton (2007) noted that EMDR both brings relief and expands the capacity for self-reflection. Ringel (2014) has written about an integrative psychoanalytic approach to sexual trauma. She described the EMDR protocol as a "scaffolding" that provides a comforting container that imbues a sense of safety in the presence of overwhelming affective and sensory states that have yet to be metabolized. Psychodynamic therapy makes it possible to elaborate "the interpersonal aftermath of trauma through the lens of the patient-therapist relationship" (Ringel, 2014, p. 143). In her book, *Integrating Relational Psychoanalysis and EMDR: Embodied experience and clinical practice*, Arad (2017) suggested that "EMDR may offer the missing link between semblances of bodily connection and the organizing yet desire restricting language" (p. 18) of spoken words. She spoke of maintaining awareness of "minimal cues" (Arad, 2017, p. 7). The repeated use of the body scan in EMDR protocol serves to draw the client's attention to such cues in a way that makes their value clearer. This opens the door to greater awareness of bodily experience without the requirement of explaining that experience verbally. Subsequently, it can be linked to language allowing for more of the implicit to be made explicit.

What Integrated Treatment Looks Like

Psychodynamic psychotherapy is best conducted one or more times weekly in an outpatient setting, with people who are medically stable and not experiencing manic or psychotic symptoms. Sitting face-to-face allows the therapist and client to have the option of a full view of each other. When sessions occur on telehealth platforms, reasonable efforts are made to allow for observation of both proximal and distal phenomena, such as facial expressions, breathing, posture, hands and torso, while allowing for comfortable seating. The ability to observe these processes and shifts in them is part of analytic listening. Decisions about whether the postpartum client's infant is present are ideally made by the client and supported by the therapist. The experience of either arrangement becomes part of the therapeutic exploration, providing visceral information about connection and separation.

The initial therapeutic assessment of the birthing parent involves a detailed inquiry about history of the symptoms, past and present relationships, memories from childhood, ideas about the wished for child, dreams, desires, and fears. Of importance is also the client's own reaction to these feelings. Many clients arrive in treatment acutely aware of how experiences with their own childhood are activated and shaping their present state of mind. Other clients may be highly focused on the present or consumed with worry about the future. Birthing people do not always understand what their distress is about; links to past experiences may only become apparent as the treatment unfolds. It is useful to be curious about relationships with the people from whom the birthing person desires or expects support, as they are in the present and have been in the past. "Who can you talk to about what it's like for you right now?" Education about the impact of traumatic experiences and validation that pregnancy and childbirth are, in fact, challenging experiences for most people is likely to be reassuring, soothing the sense of aloneness that is common among birthing people while offering hope that change is possible.

What each session looks like is determined at the outset by the client's sense of need in the present moment. The greeting reveals information about the client's state of mind and body and is an opportunity to tune in to what it is like to reconnect, including any aspects of the separation. Questions funnel from broad to more specific as needed. Emotional themes and patterns are identified and associations to them are explored together.

EMDR looks and feels like a rather different mode of interacting. While the therapist may seem in some respects more overtly active, providing structured guidance, the therapist's subjective contribution diminishes. In particular, during the processing phases of treatment, Desensitization and Installation, sessions resemble a one-person approach as the therapist's interpretations and efforts to verbalize links between associations are paused until there is an agreement to return to conversational mode. The therapist may "interweave" thoughtful comments (Shapiro, 2001) that reinforce the client's awareness that they are not alone during the process. Thus, EMDR serves as an explicit form of holding (Winnicott, 1965) through which the therapist provides the client time with their own associative flow. Wachtel (2002) noted that although EMDR has clear cognitive behavioral roots (e.g., direct exposure to the memory), it also contains elements that are consistent with the "earliest versions of psychoanalytic practice" namely free association, and the "relatively minimal interference by the therapist, who largely stayed silent while allowing the patient's own material to unfold" (p. 125).

Sessions devoted to EMDR processing may require more time than the typical 45- to 50-minute session. Some therapists regularly plan for 60 to 90 minutes in such cases. When EMDR processing has been the activity of the previous session, questions about what, if any, continuing impacts were felt and observed guide the dyadic decision-making about how to proceed next. EMDR processing for a given target is considered complete when the client consistently reports minimal or absent distress in relation to it. Decisions about whether to identify another target for processing are made collaboratively.

Psychodynamic psychotherapy can be time-limited or open-ended. Completion is usually signaled by the client's recognition that the desired changes have occurred, allowing for a sense of agency in acknowledging the need for both support and autonomy. For perinatal clients, it can be beneficial to engage in serial time-limited episodes of treatment (Stern, 1995) and to normalize this course of treatment. Symptoms may reappear in the context of developmental shifts of the birthing parent and/or the infant, such as changing sleeping arrangements, weaning, returning to work, illness, subsequent pregnancies, or unexpected loss. Clients may return to treatment periodically for a number of sessions or even just one to review previous gains and to address present difficulties. This enduring connection to the therapist as a positive transference object serves as a support to the birthing parent even in the absence of active symptoms, thus validating both the parent's dependency needs and their desire for autonomy and competence.

The following section includes vignettes from my clinical work that illustrate two possible ways of using EMDR in a psychodynamic treatment of birthing people who experienced perinatal trauma and a reemergence of symptoms related to developmental trauma. While each treatment is distinct, these vignettes shed light on how to translate the previously outlined principles into clinical practice. To protect confidentiality, names and other identifying information presented have been altered. Throughout the dialogue sections, "therapist" refers to me, the author.

Case 1: Sam

Sam, a 29-year-old White, queer mother, was referred by another therapist for perinatal trauma-informed treatment specifically to work through her birth experience to prepare for having a second child. She was exhausted, scared, and experiencing intrusive thoughts about "disappearing" herself. Her first pregnancy was marked by daily vomiting for 27 weeks, a bout of shingles and heart palpitations. She made it to full term; yet, when labor was not progressing Sam was faced with what felt like false choices about what was happening to her body—an experience all too familiar—and she protested angrily. The response of the hospital staff was experienced as overpowering, and she "just shut down." She was subsequently sedated, and when she awoke a day later her baby had been moved to the NICU after turning blue. She told me the week her family spent in the NICU was the "worst thing that ever happened to me. And that's saying a lot." She felt an added sense of urgency to "get it together" so that she and her spouse could use their own gametes to conceive another child. Sam's spouse had begun hormone therapy as part of her gender transition that would eventually suppress sperm production to the point that spontaneous conception would be unlikely.

Sam's early history included being sexually assaulted by a babysitter at the age of 5 and spending much of her older childhood caring for her younger siblings, while her mother was away for long periods of time studying and working. Her father's presence in the home complicated Sam's experience, in that he had the appearance and the physical skills of an adult, yet he made unreasonable demands for admiration and coddling. He was prone to infantile outbursts when he did not get what he wanted; on multiple occasions he walked into traffic. Once, after telling a coworker of his plans to jump from a bridge, Sam's father was hospitalized. From a young age, Sam came to feel quite conflicted about her own needs and learned to hide what she could and to minimize what she could not. Her intellectual capacity served her well in solving problems, and she came to rely on it heavily.

During her prolonged perinatal hospital stay, Sam found herself consumed with worry about the safety of the very person she needed to protect her most; her wife's gender transition was unfolding daily, and it added another layer of uncertainty for both of them. Sam was worried that hospital staff would avoid or say something hurtful to her partner. This was painfully reminiscent of Sam's childhood and her continuous efforts to function as a caregiver to her siblings while attempting to cushion her father from any potential injury to his fragile self-esteem. Later, she reflected on the loss of safety and heterosexual privilege associated with her spouse's transition. She grieved the fact that despite being queer, she and her spouse had a much more traditional marriage than she expected to have when it came to the distribution of household tasks.

Sam's general orientation toward taking charge (because she did not expect anyone else to do so) provided us clarity about what she wanted to work on with me. We discussed the possible use of EMDR early in our work together, and our preparations included expanding her repertoire of self-soothing options. Looming was her fear that she would not be able to protect her babies (current and future) as she herself had not been protected. She also carried a sense that doctors could not be trusted to keep them safe, and neither could she. Sam identified targets related to the theme of safety (e.g., "I am not safe;" "I cannot protect myself"; "I cannot trust anyone").

EMDR processing over the course of three sessions led to an increase in Sam's confidence about her ability to advocate for her children and for herself in a healthcare setting. This new "I got this" sense had space for recognizing times when she did not, without the associated feeling of panic. "Sometimes I do need help." Because she was no longer completely overwhelmed with negative affect and shame about her need for help, Sam was able to identify people who had some ability to help her with specific tasks.

The plan we made to try this new way of approaching her suffering also demonstrated to Sam that I heard her cries for help. Her unspeakable pain was now understandable, and in giving it our full attention and effort together, she was relieved of the burden that she had been carrying alone. My ability to bear witness to her birth trauma provided an experience of being seen without judgment that was novel for her. Guiding her through the structured protocol illustrated my ability to take the lead so that she did not have to do so, something Sam longed for proof of. This provided an opening to do some more psychodynamic work on her feelings about the care that she had not received as a child. Being allowed to grieve made it possible for her to continue her reproductive journey. When she became pregnant again, Sam was able to advocate for herself by telling healthcare providers what was important to her and seeing if they met her criteria. She met with her midwife to discuss her birth plan line by line. Sam became more open to the reality that while she could not control how things ended up going, she had done everything within her power to communicate her needs and wishes to people who appeared competent and caring. Despite having an unexpected cesarean section performed by a doctor she did not know, Sam described her second birth as "bad and yet better . . . not traumatic." She was able to feel disappointed in the experience without being harshly critical of herself.

Through the process of asking for help with childbirth preparations, she found that her mother, who had been noticeably absent during her own childhood, was able to be present in uniquely supportive ways now. Sam allowed herself to ask her mother for support, specifically to be her labor doula, and once they were home, to care for Sam's toddler so that Sam could focus on establishing a connection with her new baby. This was a time of celebration and mourning, with Sam alternating between soaking up the care and revisiting how little of this was available to her as a child. The continuing focus of our work was on these relationships.

The following excerpt illustrates an exploration of the relationship between dependency, guilt, and anger. An interpretation was made about her own reaction to her developmentally appropriate need to be taken care of, as a child and as a birthing parent. It was brought to Sam's attention that her conflicted feelings about her own needs led her to overfunction (as she had as a child) and, consequently, to feel resentful and depleted. Inviting her to feel her anger without shutting it down due to fear or guilt, led Sam to recognize her coping, here taking initiative regarding trip-planning, as something positive to pass onto her child rather than a sign that she was checking out, as her own mother had done.

During one session, Sam held her newborn as she often did. She expressed frustration with her wife for not scheduling some pediatric appointments in a time frame that seemed reasonable to Sam.

Sam: I was so frustrated . . . (sounding resigned) I called the pediatrician. I just did it myself. It seems silly but I don't want to ask for help. If I do, people will know how vulnerable I really am . . . . If I don't say anything people won't notice.

Therapist: Does that feel true to you right now?

Sam: No, that's why it's silly. I've got a great group (of supporters).

Therapist: Seems like a hangover from early life with your father. You're taking responsibility for his blindness to your needs. (noticing Sam is quiet as color rushes to her face) What's happening?

Sam: I'm angry again! I know it's a healthy feeling but to me it feels like a "not-allowed" feeling. My dad was so explosive. There were no other examples of anger. I don't know what to do with it.

Therapist: (drawing her attention to her ability to safely express her anger in the moment) You can feel it and hold your tiny baby. A moment ago, you said "Hi" to her while we were talking, and she was resting in your arms. How'd that feel?

Sam:	Warm (smiling, breathing deeply).
Therapist:	And now you can feel angry and still hold her gently. That's a lot you can do.
Sam:	In the past when I felt overwhelmed, in survival mode, I'd plan a trip, usually a camping trip. It helped me to feel in control, gave me something to look forward to, a goal. But I can't do that now. We're not going anywhere for a while.
Therapist:	Hmm there seems like an important part of you in there. Can you get in touch with it? Even if it's a dream about next spring or summer?
Sam:	I feel guilty that I even need it.
Therapist:	All your life your father sent a clear message that your needs were a problem for him. The thing is, you were a kid. Of course you need him . . . perfectly natural.

At this point Sam was crying, saying she felt it was wrong to want to leave her baby who needed her so much. She felt such guilt about her own need to be taken care of that she was not able to see how acknowledging her own needs would also benefit her child. As she was holding her infant, the therapist took the opportunity to help her make this connection using the body awareness that had been established in our use of the EMDR protocol.

Therapist:	(speaking slowly and gently as one would to a distressed child) I have a hunch if you were to start thinking about a trip while holding Fiona, she wouldn't protest. Your body temperature might shift. Your breathing might deepen. Some tension might soften You might even smile . . . I don't think she'd mind that a bit.
Sam:	(giggles) Yeah.
Therapist:	So maybe it's a private thought as you drift off to sleep together, or breastfeed. Or it could be more of a conversation with your daughter. Preparing her to be a future camper . . .
Sam:	It's like that song, "I'm going on a bear hunt and I'm gonna bring . . . " (we laugh together). Yeah, it's like envisioning doing the things we most want to do with our kids.

Reflections on Working With Sam

The introduction of EMDR early in the therapy helped to decrease Sam's hypervigilance and physiological dysregulation, making it somewhat easier to reflect and to plan. Sam's glimpse of the future shared above soothed her in the moment and allowed her to rely on an established way of caring for herself without repeating the abandonment that she had experienced. Not only could she express her momentary desire to be in contact with some other aspects of herself with less fear and less guilt, Sam was able to connect to a felt sense of playfulness with me and with her daughter. Her language also reflects some identification with me, who she knows to be a parent and someone who has observed and attended to her emotional needs. This was a strategy Sam continued to make use of that felt familiar and yet uniquely hers, no longer shadowed by her own mother's absences from her. She was freed to focus on figuring out who she wanted to be in her queer family. Sam's reproductive story included several traumatic events, as well as some tragic ones, that she felt able to distinguish from one another and from the present by the end of the treatment.

Case 2: Maritza

Maritza sought treatment the week before her 32nd birthday because she was "having a hard time adjusting to [her] new life" as a mother. She had been working from home following the birth of her first child—an arrangement she thought would last about a year. When the COVID pandemic hit, she was grateful to have steady employment and simultaneously panicked at the thought that she might never be able to leave her home again. Maritza described herself as "a workaholic since the age of 15 . . . Still I'm always the caretaker. My family doesn't get it. Work is a distraction from the pain, but lately I've got no motivation." She was depressed, not eating, and not doing things she had enjoyed in the past like baking treats that would "put a smile on someone's face." At times she was overwhelmed with anxiety which was accompanied by dizziness and gastrointestinal distress. In addition, she experienced frequent muscle tension and back pain.

Her parents' marriage had been a silent source of tension since her father opened a business when Maritza was a young child. As a result of his dedication and hard work, the business quickly became quite successful and pulled for more and more of his time. From Maritza's point of view this was not entirely a positive development. She felt proud and admired his ambition as she felt he admired hers; her mother's reaction was rather different. "As soon as we had money, my mother became greedy." Maritza's mother had a chronic medical condition and was prone to explosive outbursts, verbally and physically punishing behavior, and episodes of depression during which she would withdraw from the demands of running the house. In her father's absence, her mother's physical and emotional state soon pulled for more and more of young Maritza's time. Twice her mother attempted suicide at home. Other members of the family, including Maritza's father, left Maritza in charge of getting her mother to the hospital. Maritza had just started college.

Despite what she described as a "toxic relationship" with her mother, Maritza anticipated that having a child of her own would bring them closer together. She understood the importance of her new role as a mother because "family values," such as devotion to one's mother, were made explicit in her Dominican community. Marianismo, the traditional female role of virtue, passivity, and priority of other over oneself has been associated in some studies with postpartum depression, whereas religiosity has been found to offer some protection (Lara-Cinisomo et al., 2019). Unfortunately, Maritza did not have much in the way as a buffer against the depleting nature of habitual self-sacrifice. In fact, rather than being praised for her efforts as a mother, she often felt criticized.

On some level Maritza hoped that in becoming a mother she would be positioned to be on the receiving end of some version of that preferential care. Instead, her newborn spent the first week of her life in the NICU. Maritza found herself alone, while her husband returned to work.

At home with her new baby, Maritza's anxiety skyrocketed. She arranged with her husband to care for their newborn daughter so she could have a few days to herself at a relative's vacation house. Maritza's mother was horrified. She made this known at the time and periodically for years afterward. Once when Maritza asked her mother if she would not miss seeing her granddaughter while she was away on an extended vacation, her mother replied, "Well did you miss your newborn daughter when you abandoned her for three days?" Maritza told me, "My anxiety went up to my throat." It soon became apparent that her body was doing the talking because she had no other way to express her emotions. Her tendency was to talk about feelings in an intellectualized way while her body was left holding the distress, such as through back pain, headaches, gastrointestinal upset, and elevated blood pressure. I regularly invited Maritza to do something quite different from her usual approach of "Keep it moving," meaning "stay busy caring for others and don't look inward."

Several months into treatment, Maritza reported that she continued to feel trapped in her house and in her marriage. She mused what her life would have been like if her husband had married "one of those White girls he dated before me." While the importance of her "Spanish" identity was regularly acknowledged by us both, her description of "all the other girls" as White brought to the fore my own Whiteness and otherness in relation to Maritza. It was apparent from the outset of treatment that Maritza had come in search of a therapist with perinatal expertise. In this moment, I felt that my racial and cultural difference (from her) was of some yet to be understood value as well. Sharing my sense of that with her, I asked if she had ever thought her husband was drawn to her because she, too, was different in some way. Did she feel like an outsider? "Oh yes! I've got six years of college under my belt. No one in my family has that." She lamented that her parents did not attend her college graduation and had not even given her a card when she earned her master's degree. This was a wound that continued to throb. "I'm going to be the mother who celebrates everything. Because I didn't have that." Her efforts to be different than her own mother inadvertently compounded her suffering. Maritza would exhaust herself by hosting elaborate events for her young child, finding it nearly impossible to involve others in the work. Ironically, Maritza's tendency to "go all out with the decorating and details" when hosting others was something she felt she "got" from her mother. At the same time, she felt she was never on the receiving end of her mother's welcoming embrace.

In the wake of the added demands of motherhood, Maritza was struggling to reconcile her desire to be cared for with her well-worn independent stance. Her conscious identification with her father and counter-identification with her mother were toppled when she gave birth to a child of her own. The part of herself that felt the most alive and resonant with her core identity was also at odds with the cultural expectation that a daughter sees motherhood as the greatest achievement and by extension, her own mother as the greatest. At home with her own child, Maritza felt cut off from the world of work she had always embraced with great vigor. She began to feel that she was in fact very much like her own mother after all, anxious, afraid, and "abandoning."

The following example illustrates how inviting her emotional experience and exploring its meaning in our relationship helped Maritza deepen her sense that she was safe with me. At the same time, our interaction helped her to see that the habits she relies on to shield herself from feelings about interacting with her mother, to think her way through (intellectualize), to "keep it moving" and do for others, also get in the way of people knowing that she wants to be taken care of.

One day Maritza came to a session in no apparent distress. She calmly asked if I had heard the news about a celebrity who committed suicide.

Maritza: I love him! I used to watch him faithfully every day when he was on that talk show. He always put a smile on my face. And then actually the day before I heard about him, I found out that my cousin back in the DR also committed suicide. It touched me.

Therapist: (struck by her continued composure) In what way did it touch you?

Maritza: Well, being in the healthcare field, it bothers me. I mean other people say "(gasps) Oh that's terrible! How could someone do that?" I worry that I don't have enough of a reaction because you know . . . we deal with this.

Therapist: And you certainly have had to deal with it, with your mother . . . (Noticing her breathing speed up) Is there a gasp! Somewhere in you right now? What's happening? If you give it your attention right now, what do you notice?

Maritza: (after a moment) I am so used to not feeling anything . . . I'm thinking about my dad and how it's weird between us now since we had that falling out. I don't know what happened.

Therapist: What theories do you have? About what happened between you two?

Maritza: Since he lost his mother, he's not the same. Have I told you about my grandmothers? They should be sainted! I can't imagine the void that must leave. They always had a kind word, always doing for others. I don't know what they feel but . . . . I'll bring you pictures next time.

Therapist: I would love to see those pictures. Because they're already here, with us, with you. You're measuring yourself against them. But you don't know what they felt. Nobody did. Nobody asked. And here you are living as a daughter and as a mother and sometimes the only thing you're aware of is that you have feelings, and nobody knows what they are

Maritza: Nobody knows that about me really.

Therapist: So how is it that you have gotten this far with me? That I am allowed the privilege of knowing you in this way?

Maritza: Since the first time I talked with you, you didn't just tell me everything was going to be okay. I felt heard by you. And I wanted someone who would challenge me . . . a little (laughs)

Therapist: And have I done that? Challenged you in some way?

Maritza: Well, yes. In this way. By getting me to slow down and see if I'm feeling something

In Maritza's case, her trauma symptoms were largely somatic as opposed to cognitive. The connection between her physical distress and her emotions was unconscious. Over the course of a few months, I introduced EMDR as another way for Maritza to make sense of different dimensions of her affective experience, including cognitions, emotions and perceptions. Because she was prone to intellectualizing and found it hard to be in touch with her emotions, I thought she would benefit from more "scaffolding" (Ringel, 2014)—here the integration of the structured Standard Protocol into the organic and mutually directed flow of treatment. The initial target stemmed from her tendency to devalue and dismiss her own reactions to painful interactions with people "It's just my anxiety." Current interactions with her husband, mother and other family members were triggering traumatic responses, including somatic symptoms that interrupted her ability to function. Maritza identified targets related to the theme of power and control (e.g., "I cannot stand up for myself"; I cannot get what I want"; "I cannot let it out"). The explicit framework of EMDR guided her attention inward, making it possible for her to find words for what no one around her was able to speak about. In one of the EMDR sessions, Maritza connected some of her anxiety sensations to experiences in her childhood, including her own suicide attempt as a teenager. Through EMDR processing, she was able to recognize these physical sensations as memories and to reconnect with the associated emotions (i.e., rage and fear) while simultaneously staying in touch with abilities she now possesses as an adult. As her own distress became more understandable and tolerable to her, it began to decrease.

As we returned to the exploratory mode of our work, Maritza came to understand her feelings as something other than a weakness. Noticing her growing ability to survive the emotional turbulence that followed most interactions with her mother, Maritza began to envision her own path as a mother without being so confined by a mandate to be nothing like her. This brought her closer to the maternal figures in her family that she did feel warmly toward and made it easier to tolerate the idea that she could have conflictual feelings for her own daughter at some point.

Reflections on Working With Maritza

In some cases, birthing parents seek treatment to address birth trauma, a discrete traumatic event as with Sam. In others, it may be necessary to take more time to build the therapeutic alliance and establish a firm sense of trust. In Maritza's case, it took many months for her to trust that I could tolerate her vulnerability without retaliating. It was necessary to explore what makes it hard for her to "get emotional" in front of people in general, and with me in particular. EMDR was subsequently used as a means of helping her to develop a greater appreciation for the connection between her sensory and emotional experience. In fact, what she was feeling in her body could be represented in another way, talking about her anger, sadness, and fear.

In Maritza's case, a more active approach at the outset would likely have felt like an effort to change her when what she wanted most was to be recognized and celebrated for what she had already done well. Once her trust in me and a mutual sense of admiration was established, Maritza could begin to acknowledge her vulnerabilities and her longing to be cared for by her family.

Together, these cases are a reminder that events that are traumatic for one person may be unremarkable for another. For Sam, her NICU experience was the worst in a line of many devastations. In Maritza's case, the time that her daughter spent in the NICU was frightening, and she wishes it had never happened. However, she was not traumatized by the experience itself. Rather, it brought to the fore a lifetime of suffering in relation to her mother which became the main focus of the therapy. The meaning of a given event is highly personal and, thus, attempts to help people recover must include a genuine appreciation of the individual's ways of making meaning. We do not know where it hurts most until we ask.

Support for the Approach

Evidence-based practice is grounded in more than empirical support (Messer, 2004). It "is the integration of the best available research with clinical expertise in the context of patient characteristics, culture and preferences" (American Psychological Association, 2006, p. 273). There is ample evidence that psychodynamic therapy has a beneficial impact on people who engage in it (Steinert et al., 2017; Leichsenring et al., 2015). Shedler (2010) conducted a systematic review that established psychodynamic therapy to be as effective as other therapies considered to be empirically supported and evidence based, with effect sizes ranging from 0.69–1.80. Barber et al. (2021) recently examined an extensive array of meta-analyses demonstrating efficacy of psychodynamic treatment compared to control groups with many common mental disorders, including PTSD. After reviewing 17 studies of psychodynamic treatments for anxiety and trauma disorders, psychodynamic therapies were significantly more effective than control conditions with a large effect size (0.94) (Barber et al., 2021). Multiple meta-analyses have identified a pattern of increasing effect sizes at post-treatment follow-ups, suggesting that gains made during psychodynamic treatment not only are retained but establish in the client the potential for continued change and growth (Barber et al., 2021; Shedler, 2010). For instance, Shedler's systematic review found that for patients with moderate psychopathology, the effect size of symptom improvement after psychodynamic treatment was 0.78 at the end of treatment and increased to 0.94 at long-term follow-up, after about three years. For patients who presented with severe personality pathology, effect sizes grew from 0.94 at the end of treatment to 1.02 at long-term follow-up, after about five years (Shedler, 2010).

The effectiveness of long-term psychodynamic treatment has also been demonstrated (Leichsenring & Rabung, 2008). Researchers found that overall effectiveness, target problems, and personality functioning were all enhanced by long-term psychodynamic psychotherapy compared to short-term therapies and found that the benefit of longer treatment was particularly relevant for patients who presented with more complex difficulties (effect size: 1.8). Patients in the long-term psychodynamic treatment group were functioning significantly better than 96% of patients in the control group (Leichsenring & Rabung, 2008). This may offer hope for phase-oriented or serial short-term treatments seen in postpartum populations, particularly with patients who may have pre-existing histories of psychological difficulties or who may present with multiple psychological challenges. Efforts to evaluate the efficacy/effectiveness of psychodynamic treatment for birthing people have mainly focused on perinatal (Sockol et al., 2011) and postpartum depression (Cramer et al., 1990; Cooper et al., 2003) in cisgender women. There are some positive findings that indicate these interventions can effectively reduce depression symptomatology and can even improve behavioral interactions between parent and infant (reducing parental intrusiveness, enhancing infant cooperation and responsiveness to parent). Other studies have established the benefits of trauma-focused psychodynamic treatment in populations with complex challenges. In a naturalistic study of patients in a particular treatment facility, Sachsse et al. (2006) found a trauma-focused psychodynamic treatment that integrated an EMDR protocol offered lasting benefits for women experiencing complex PTSD and personality pathology, including reduction in trauma-specific symptoms (dissociation, intrusion, avoidance) and improvements in psychiatric stability (reduced distress, self-harm behavior, and number of hospitalizations (effect size 2.88).

EMDR has demonstrated its potential to alleviate symptoms and support posttraumatic growth of adults who have experienced recent trauma as well as symptoms related to developmental trauma (Bisson & Andrew, 2007; Shapiro & Maxfield, 2019). For instance, one meta-analysis found that EMDR was significantly better than being on a waitlist or receiving care as usual, with a large effect size of –1.51 (Bisson & Andrew, 2007). This review found that EMDR reliably reduced PTSD symptoms as well as associated depression and anxiety symptoms. The benefits of EMDR have been replicated with patient samples of diverse cultural backgrounds, and the treatment is considered to be cost-effective given its ability in some cases to achieve symptom relief through limited sessions (Wilson et al., 2018). Although there has been far less research on psychotherapy integration than psychotherapy as a whole, new research is beginning to close this gap. Assimilative integration offers researchers an opportunity to study the relative contributions of different techniques without reinventing a preferred treatment paradigm (Castonguay et al., 2015).

Sharing Ideas

Psychodynamic training is available at the graduate level and more widely for licensed mental health providers from a variety of training backgrounds at the post-graduate level. Proficiency with the EMDR standard protocol requires formal training which usually includes an experiential component, followed by supervised practice. In addition to training, the integration of therapeutic approaches requires collaboration with others, particularly in terms of teaching, supervising and consulting with perinatal care professionals. Assessing the effectiveness of these integrative efforts is another way for professionals to interact with different models of change. While we all have our own reproductive stories, it is incumbent upon us to recognize the unique needs of birthing people and their families with cultural curiosity and humility. Specialized training is increasingly available thanks to some teaching hospitals and family advocacy groups. Ideally, curricula addressing this developmental phase, including common psychological complications and varied methods of care will become a standard component in professional programs, doctoral level psychology externships, medical and psychiatry residencies and advanced practice nursing placements.

Future Possibilities

Given what we know about the nature of trauma—it is often misunderstood, it can be difficult to speak and hear about, and it is transmissible from parent to child—coupled with the immense neuropsychological vulnerability of the infant in the first year of life (Chambers, 2017) it is necessary to actively seek to identify higher risk parents-to-be as early as possible. Howard and Khalifeh (2020) discuss preconception intervention from a public health perspective. This is likely to be appreciated by people seeking to have children. Many a parent has lamented, "No one told me anything like this could happen." As cultural and systemic support for perinatal mental health interventions become more visible and less stigmatized, some birthing people will feel less conflicted about seeking help when they need it. Empirical research and case studies will be strengthened by including gender diverse parents with a variety of racial and cultural identities.

In this chapter the Standard Protocol EMDR was briefly described and applied to the cases presented. A number of scripted EMDR protocols have been developed to address specific perinatal issues that impact quality of life and potentially bonding and attachment, for example, hyperemesis gravidarum in pregnancy (Kavakci, 2019), fear of childbirth (Baas et al., 2020), recent birth trauma (Chiorino et al., 2020), and breastfeeding difficulties (Chiorino et al., 2019). It might be useful to compare specialized protocols to the standard protocol within the context of psychodynamic treatment. The timing of EMDR usage might also be a variable to consider in more detail. If the traumatic material is more recent, occurring within the perinatal period would it make sense to engage in EMDR earlier in the treatment to reduce reactivity, thereby increasing openness to current support, as in the case of Sam. If the client identifies unresolved developmental and attachment trauma as the presenting concern, it might be more helpful to explore the client's psychodynamics first as they present in the therapeutic relationship, introducing EMDR later, as in the case of Maritza.

Due to the rich contextual nature of an individual treatment, it can be useful to consider other ways to refine our knowledge base through ongoing dialogue with other therapists. Pragmatic Case Studies in Psychotherapy is a peer-reviewed, open-access journal and database. It provides innovative, quantitative and qualitative knowledge about psychotherapy process and outcome. PCSP is published by the National Register of Health Service Psychologists (nationalregister.org).

Conclusion

Psychodynamic psychotherapy is applicable to a broad range of issues that can impede the developmental process. It is an approach that is trauma-informed at its core and at times becomes actively trauma-focused. It is well-suited for use during the perinatal period in that it explicitly values the subjective experience of the birthing parent, appreciates the complexity of factors that shape it, and recognizes the development of parental identity as a process of expansion across the lifespan. Psychodynamic therapy is compatible with other forms of support that may be relevant based on the needs of the birthing parent, including peer support, self-help groups, pharmacological, holistic, and spiritual interventions. In the context of psychodynamic psychotherapy clients can explore their feelings about various forms of care and what it means to accept or decline them and at times to move ahead without them. Van der Kolk (2014) refers to self-leadership as the moment when the frontal cortex is functioning in a way that our capacity for planning and communicating is available for use in responding to our own distress and the situations that lead to it. This is the objective of psychodynamic work, to support parents in recognizing their own competence in the face of so many novel tasks, new relationships and intense emotions.

References

Akhtar, S. (2018). *Mind, culture, and global unrest: Psychoanalytic reflections*. Routledge. https://doi.org/10.4324/9780429466960

American Psychological Association, Presidential Task Force on Evidence-Based Practice. (2006). Evidence-based practice in psychology. *American Psychologist, 61*(4), 271–285. https://doi.org/10.1037/0003-066X.61.4.271

Arad, H. (2017). *Integrating relational psychoanalysis and EMDR: Embodied experience and clinical practice*. Routledge. https://doi.org/10.4324/9781315159775

Baas, M., van Pampus, M. G., Braam, L., Stramrood, C., & de Jongh, A. (2020). The effects of PTSD treatment during pregnancy: Systematic review and case study. *European Journal of Psychotraumatology, 11*(1), 1762310. https://doi.org/10.1080/20008198.2020.1762310

Barber, J., Muran, C., McCarthy, K., Keefe, J., & Zilcha-Mano, S. (2021). Research on dynamic therapies. In M. Barkham, W. Lutz, & L. G. Castonguay (Eds.), *Bergin and Garfield's handbook of psychotherapy and behavior change* (pp. 387–419). Wiley.

Beck, C. T., Watson, S., & Gable, R. K. (2018). Traumatic childbirth and its aftermath: Is there anything positive? *The Journal of Perinatal Education*, 27(3), 175–184. https://doi.org/10.1891/1058-1243.27.3.175

Benedek, T. (1959). Parenthood as a developmental phase: A contribution to the libido theory. *Journal of the American Psychoanalytic Association*, 7, 389–417. https://doi.org/10.1177/000306515900700301

Bisson, J., & Andrew, M. (2007). Psychological treatment of post-traumatic stress disorder (PTSD). *The Cochrane Database of Systematic Reviews*, (3), CD003388. https://doi.org/10.1002/14651858.CD003388.pub3

Black, M., Basile, K., Breiding, M., Smith, S., Walters, M., Merrick, M., . . . Stevens, M. (2011). *National intimate partner and sexual violence survey: 2010 summary report*. National Center for Injury Prevention and Control, Centers for Disease Control and Prevention.

Blum, L. D. (2007). Psychodynamics of postpartum depression. *Psychoanalytic Psychology*, 24(1), 45–62. https://doi.org/10.1037/0736-9735.24.1.45

Boswell, J., Newman, M., & McGinn, L. (2019). Outcome research on psychotherapy integration. In J. C. Norcross, J. & M. Goldfried (Eds.), *Handbook of psychotherapy integration* (3rd ed., online ed.). Oxford Academic. https://doi.org/10.1093/medpsych/9780190690465.003.0019. Retrieved September 28, 2022.

Bucci, W. (2011). The interplay of subsymbolic and symbolic processes in psychoanalytic treatment: It takes two to tango – but who knows the steps, who's the leader? The choreography of the psychoanalytic interchange. *Psychoanalytic Dialogues*, 21(1), 45–54. https://doi.org/10.1080/10481885.2011.545326

Castonguay, L. G., Eubanks, C. F., Goldfried, M. R., Muran, J. C., & Lutz, W. (2015). Research on psychotherapy integration: Building on the past, looking to the future. *Psychotherapy Research*, 25(3), 365–382. https://doi.org/10.1080/10503307.2015.1014010

Chambers, J. (2017). The neurobiology of attachment: From infancy to clinical outcomes. *Psychodynamic Psychiatry*, 45(4), 542–563. https://doi.org/10.1521/pdps.2017.45.4.542

Chiorino, V., Cattaneo, M. C., Macchi, E. A., Salerno, R., Roveraro, S., Bertolucci, G. G., . . . Fernandez, I. (2020). The EMDR recent birth trauma protocol: A pilot randomised clinical trial after traumatic childbirth. *Psychology & Health*, 35(7), 795–810. https://doi.org/10.1080/08870446.2019.1699088

Chiorino, V., Roveraro, S., Cattaneo, M. C., Salerno, R., & Fernandez, I. (2019). The breastfeeding and bonding EMDR protocol. In M. Luber (Ed.), *Treating trauma in somatic and medical-related conditions: EMDR therapy: Scripted protocols and summary sheets* (pp. 427–454). Springer Publishing Company.

Chiron, C., Jambaque, I., Nabbout, R., Lounes, R., Syrota, A., & Dulac, O. (1997). The right brain hemisphere is dominant in infants. *Brain*, 120, 1057–1065.

Cooper, P., Murray, L., Wilson, A., & Romaniuk, H. (2003). Controlled trial of the short- and long-term effect of psychological treatment of post-partum depression: I. Impact on maternal mood. *British Journal of Psychiatry*, 182(5), 412–419. https://doi.org/10.1192/bjp.182.5.412

Cramer, B., Robert-Tissot, C., Stern, D. N., Serpa-Rusconi, S., De Muralt, M., Besson, G., . . . D'Arcis, U. (1990). Outcome evaluation in brief mother-infant psychotherapy: A preliminary report. *Infant Mental Health Journal*, 11(3), 278–300. https://doi.org/10.1002/1097-0355(199023)11:3<278::aid-imhj2280110309>3.0.co;2-h

Erikson, E. (1982). *The life cycle completed*. Norton & Company.

Fonagy, P., & Luyten, P. (2019). Fidelity vs. flexibility in the implementation of psychotherapies: Time to move on. *World Psychiatry: Official Journal of the World Psychiatric Association (WPA)*, 18(3), 270–271. https://doi.org/10.1002/wps.20657

Fosshage, J. L. (2011). How do we "know" what we "know" and change what we "know?". *Psychoanalytic Dialogues*, 21(1), 55–74.

Fraiberg, S., Adelson, E., & Shapiro, V. (1975). Ghosts in the nursery: A psychoanalytic approach to the problems of impaired infant-mother relationships. *Journal of the American Academy of Child Psychiatry*, 14(3), 387–421. https://doi.org/10.1016/S0002-7138(09)61442-4

Freud, S. (1915). *Instincts and their vicissitudes*. Hogarth.

Greenberg, J. R., & Mitchell, S. A. (1983). *Object relations in psychoanalytic theory*. Harvard University Press.

Grill, H. (2019). What women want: A discussion of "childless." *Psychoanalytic Dialogues, 29*(1), 59–68. https://doi.org/10.1080/10481885.2018.1560867

Herman, J. L. (1997). *Trauma and recovery.* Basic Books.

Horesh, D., Garthus-Niegel, S., & Horsch, A. (2021). Childbirth-related PTSD: Is it a unique post-traumatic disorder? *Journal of Reproductive and Infant Psychology, 39*(3), 221–224. https://doi.org/10.1080/02646838.2021.1930739

Howard, L. M., & Khalifeh, H. (2020). Perinatal mental health: A review of progress and challenges. *World Psychiatry: Official Journal of the World Psychiatric Association (WPA), 19*(3), 313–327. https://doi.org/10.1002/wps.20769

Jaffe, J. (2017). Reproductive trauma: Psychotherapy for pregnancy loss and infertility clients from a reproductive story perspective. *Psychotherapy, 54*(4), 380–385.

Jaffe, J., & Diamond, M. O. (2011). *Reproductive trauma: Psychotherapy with infertility and pregnancy loss clients.* American Psychological Association. https://doi.org/10.1037/12347-000

Kavakci, O. (2019). EMDR therapy, nausea and vomiting in pregnancy (NVP) and hyperemesis gravidarum in pregnant women. In M. Luber (Ed.), *Treating trauma in somatic and medical-related conditions: EMDR therapy: Scripted protocols and summary sheets* (pp. 355–370). Springer Publishing Company.

Lara-Cinisomo, S., Wood, J., & Fujimoto, E. M. (2019). A systematic review of cultural orientation and perinatal depression in Latina women: Are acculturation, Marianismo, and religiosity risks or protective factors? *Archives of Women's Mental Health, 22*(5), 557–567. https://doi.org/10.1007/s00737-018-0920-4

Leichsenring, F., Luyten, P., Hilsenroth, M. J., Abbass, A., Barber, J. P., Keefe, J. R., . . . Steinert, C. (2015). Psychodynamic therapy meets evidence-based medicine: A systematic review using updated criteria. *The Lancet, Psychiatry, 2*(7), 648–660. https://doi.org/10.1016/S2215-0366(15)00155-8

Leichsenring, F., & Rabung, S. (2008). Effectiveness of long-term psychodynamic psychotherapy: A meta-analysis. *Journal of the American Medical Association, 200,* 1551–1565. https://doi.org/10.1001/jama.300.13.1551

Leighton, J. (2007). Enhancing psychoanalysis: A case of integrating EMDR. *Psychoanalytic Perspectives, 5*(1), 105–125. https://doi.org/10.1080/1551806X.2007.10473015

MacDorman, M., Thoma, M., Declcerq, E., & Howell, E. (2021). Racial and ethnic disparities in maternal mortality in the United States using enhanced vital records, 2016–2017. *American Journal of Public Health, 111*(9), 1673–1681. https://doi.org/10.2105/AJPH.2021.306375

McCullough, L. (2002). Exploring change mechanisms in EMDR applied to "small-t trauma" in short-term dynamic psychotherapy: Research questions and speculations. *Journal of Clinical Psychology, 58,* 1531–1544.

McWilliams, N. (2004). *Psychoanalytic psychotherapy: A practitioner's guide.* Guilford Press.

Menken, A. E. (2008). A psychodynamic approach to treatment for postpartum depression. In S. D. Stone & A. E. Menken (Eds.), *Perinatal and postpartum mood disorders: Perspectives and treatment guide for the health care practitioner* (pp. 309–320). Springer Publishing Co.

Messer, S. B. (1992). A critical examination of belief structures in integrative and eclectic psychotherapy. In J. C. Norcross & M. R. Goldfried (Eds.), *Handbook of psychotherapy integration* (pp. 130–165). Basic Books.

Messer, S. B. (2004). Evidence-based practice: Beyond empirically supported treatments. *Professional Psychology: Research and Practice, 35*(6), 580–588. https://doi.org/10.1037/0735-7028.35.6.580

Monk, C., Leight, K. L., & Fang, Y. (2008). The relationship between women's attachment style and perinatal mood disturbance: Implications for screening and treatment. *Archives of Women's Mental Health, 11*(2), 117–129. https://doi.org/10.1007/s00737-008-0005-x

Ringel, S. (2014). An integrative model in trauma treatment: Utilizing eye movement desensitization and reprocessing and a relational approach with adult survivors of sexual abuse. *Psychoanalytic Psychology, 31*(1), 134–144. https://doi.org/10.1037/a0030044

Sachsse, U., Vogel, C., & Leichsenring, F. (2006). Results of psychodynamically oriented trauma-focused inpatient treatment for women with complex posttraumatic stress disorder (PTSD) and borderline personality disorder (BPD). *Bulletin of the Menninger Clinic, 70*(2), 125–144. https://doi.org/10.1521/bumc.2006.70.2.125

Schore, A. N. (2009). Right brain affect regulation: An essential mechanism of development, trauma, dissociation, and psychotherapy. In D. Fosha, D. Siegel, & M. Solomon (Eds.), *The healing power of emotion: Affective neuroscience, development, & clinical practice* (pp. 112–144). W. W. Norton.

Schore, A. N. (2011). The right brain implicit self lies at the core of psychoanalysis. *Psychoanalytic Dialogues, 21*(1), 75–100. https://doi.org/10.1080/10481885.2011.545329

Schore, J. R., & Schore, A. N. (2008). Modern attachment theory: The central role of affect regulation in development and treatment. *Clinical Social Work Journal, 36*, 9–20. https://doi.org/10.1007/s10615-007-0111-7

Seng, J. S., Kohn-Wood, L. P., McPherson, M. D., & Sperlich, M. (2011). Disparity in posttraumatic stress disorder diagnosis among African American pregnant women. *Archives of Women's Mental Health, 14*(4), 295–306. https://doi.org/10.1007/s00737-011-0218-2

Seng, J. S., Low, L. K., Sperlich, M., Ronis, D. L., & Liberzon, I. (2009). Prevalence, trauma history, and risk for posttraumatic stress disorder among nulliparous women in maternity care. *Obstetrics and Gynecology, 114*(4), 839–847. https://doi.org/10.1097/AOG.0b013e3181b8f8a2

Shapiro, E., & Maxfield, L. (2019). The efficacy of EMDR early interventions. *Journal of EMDR Practice and Research, 13*(4), 291–301. https://doi.org/10.1891/1933-3196.13.4.291

Shapiro, F. (2001). *Eye movement desensitization and reprocessing: Basic principles, protocols, and procedures* (2nd ed.). Guilford Press.

Shedler, J. (2010). The efficacy of psychodynamic psychotherapy. *The American Psychologist, 65*(2), 98–109. https://doi.org/10.1037/a0018378

Smith, S. G., Zhang, X., Basile, K. C., Merrick, M. T., Wang, J., Kresnow, M., & Chen, J. (2018). *The national intimate partner and sexual violence survey: 2015 data brief – updated release.* Centers for Disease Control and Prevention.

Sockol, L. E., Epperson, C. N., & Barber, J. P. (2011). A meta-analysis of treatments for perinatal depression. *Clinical Psychology Review, 31*(5), 839–849. https://doi.org/10.1016/j.cpr.2011.03.009

Stein, M., & Davis, D. (2022). Perinatal crisis and traumatic bereavement. In A. Dempsey, J. Cole, & S. Saxton (Eds.), *Behavioral health services with high-risk infants and families: Meeting the needs of patients, families, and providers in fetal, neonatal intensive care unit, and neonatal follow-up settings* (pp. 245–260). Oxford Academic. https://doi.org/10.1093/med-psych/9780197545027.003.0016

Steinert, C., Munder, T., Rabung, S., Hoyer, J., & Leichsenring, F. (2017). Psychodynamic therapy: As efficacious as other empirically supported treatments? A meta-analysis testing equivalence of outcomes. *The American Journal of Psychiatry, 174*(10), 943–953. https://doi.org/10.1176/appi.ajp.2017.17010057

Stern, D. (1995). *The motherhood constellation: A unified view of parent-infant psychotherapy.* Routledge.

Stricker, G., & Gold, J. (2019). Assimilative psychodynamic psychotherapy. In J. C. Norcross & M. R. Goldfried (Eds.), *Handbook of psychotherapy integration* (pp. 207–227). Oxford University Press.

Tummala-Narra, P. (2014). Cultural competence as a core emphasis of psychoanalytic psychotherapy. *Psychoanalytic Psychology, 32*(2). https://doi.org/10.1037/a0034041

van der Kolk, B. A. (2014). *The body keeps the score: Brain, mind, and body in the healing of trauma.* Viking.

Wachtel, P. (2002). EMDR and psychoanalysis. In F. Shapiro (Ed.), *EMDR as an integrative psychotherapy approach* (pp. 123–150). American Psychological Association.

Walters, M. L., Chen, J., & Breiding, M. J. (2013). *The national intimate partner and sexual violence survey (NISVS): 2010 findings on victimization by sexual orientation.* National Center for Injury Prevention and Control, Centers for Disease Control and Prevention.

Wilson, G., Farrell, D., Barron, I., Hutchins, J., Whybrow, D., & Kiernan, M. D. (2018). The use of eye-movement desensitization reprocessing (EMDR) therapy in treating post-traumatic stress disorder-A systematic narrative review. *Frontiers in Psychology, 9*, 923.

Winnicott, D. W. (1953). Transitional objects and transitional phenomena: A study of the first not-me possession. *The International Journal of Psycho-Analysis, 34*(2), 89–97.

Winnicott, D. W. (1965). *The maturational processes and the facilitating environment: Studies in the theory of emotional development.* International Universities Press.

Zarbo, C., Tasca, G. A., Cattafi, F., & Compare, A. (2016). Integrative psychotherapy works. *Frontiers in Psychology, 6.* https://doi.org/10.3389/fpsyg.2015.02021

25

MINDFULNESS-BASED INTERVENTIONS FOR PERINATAL MENTAL HEALTH DISORDERS

Anne Fritzson, Laurel E. Kordyban, Caitlin McKimmy, Laurel M. Hicks, and Sona Dimidjian

Current research estimates that 15–20% of pregnant and postpartum individuals experience perinatal depression and 25% report high levels of anxiety (Hall et al., 2009; Marcus, 2009). These rates of perinatal depression and anxiety are important to address because perinatal mental health conditions are associated with risk for adverse biological and psychosocial outcomes for all members of the family, including poor infant development and preterm delivery, in addition to underutilization of health services and increased risk of substance use among parents (Luca et al., 2020; Marcus, 2009). Furthermore, up to 50% of patients decline pharmacological treatment for perinatal mental health due to concerns about adverse impacts to the infant in utero or during chestfeeding (Cohen et al., 2006), and perinatal individuals demonstrate a preference to discontinue antidepressants and other psychiatric medications while pregnant (Hayes et al., 2012). Effective interventions to reduce symptoms of depression and anxiety in the perinatal period are crucial to prevent the deleterious effects of untreated mental illness on the parent, infant, and developing dyad relationship. Mindfulness-based interventions (MBIs) provide an alternative to pharmacological interventions to manage depression and anxiety symptoms during the perinatal period (Dimidjian & Goodman, 2014). MBIs were designed initially to prevent depressive relapse, rather than to address acute symptomatology; however, they have been used for the purpose of intervention and have been shown to be effective in managing symptoms of depression and anxiety in general adult populations (Hofmann et al., 2010; Kuyken et al., 2008). MBIs also have been shown to be effective in reducing symptom burden during the perinatal period, and research on acceptability has found MBIs to be both acceptable and feasible for this population (Davis et al., 2015; Dimidjian & Goodman, 2014). In this chapter, we review the two primary MBIs that have been studied widely and adapted specifically for the perinatal period: *Mindfulness-Based Stress Reduction (MBSR)* and *Mindfulness-Based Cognitive Therapy (MBCT)*.

Description and Main Components

One of the most cited definitions of mindfulness is that it is "the awareness that emerges through paying attention on purpose, in the present moment, and nonjudgmentally to the

DOI: 10.4324/9781003206903-30

unfolding of experience moment by moment" (Kabat-Zinn, 2003, p. 145). In this definition, which serves as a foundation for many contemporary MBIs, Kabat-Zinn draws from his experience practicing meditation in an Asian Buddhist framework (Anālayo, 2019; Kabat-Zinn, 2003, 2011; Wilson, 2014). Numerous cultural traditions draw upon the power of present-moment awareness, such as the Indian practice of yoga (Salmon et al., 2009), Indigenous North American contemplative ceremonies (Proulx et al., 2018), and forms of prayer in multiple other religious traditions (Holmes, 2017; Wahbeh et al., 2018).

Mindfulness has increasingly been adapted as a secular practice that can be understood through a scientific lens (McMahan, 2009). It is challenging to articulate a definitive definition of mindfulness, as what we know as "mindfulness" captures a variety of psychological states and skills. A need for clarity in defining mindfulness is a prevalent concern in contemporary scientific literature (Van Dam et al., 2018). Mindfulness has been studied in psychological science as a multidimensional construct that often includes nonjudgment, awareness of the present moment, and self-regulation of attention (Baer, 2019). Furthermore, it is common for mindfulness to connote an attitude of compassion, including self-compassion and compassion toward others (Grossman, 2019). Despite the challenges in operationalizing the construct of mindfulness, research has shown that MBIs have great potential for supporting mental health and wellness across the lifespan (Goldberg et al., 2022; Zoogman et al., 2015).

MBIs reviewed in this chapter are implementations, derivatives, and adaptations of two evidence-based interventions, *MBSR* and *MBCT*. These programs and their adaptations for perinatal populations are described next.

Mindfulness-Based Stress Reduction (MBSR) and Adaptation for the Perinatal Period

The first established and manualized MBI, *MBSR*, was developed in 1979 by Jon Kabat-Zinn at the University of Massachusetts Medical Center (Kabat-Zinn, 2003). *MBSR* was designed to employ intensive meditation skills for medical patients to cope with pain, illness, and stress (Kabat-Zinn, 2003). *MBSR* consists of eight weekly sessions that last up to 2.5 hours, with at-home practice activities assigned between sessions. In addition to the eight-week group sessions, there is often a six-hour meditation retreat offered in the sixth week, which participants are strongly encouraged to attend (Kabat-Zinn, 1982). In the weekly group sessions, participants learn formal meditation practices, such as: (a) awareness of breathing, which is paying attention to your breath rather than trying to change or control it; (b) body scan, the practice of bringing attention across one's body noticing sensations, tension, pain, etc.; (c) automatic pilot, in which individuals notice when they are disconnected from awareness of the present moment (on "autopilot"); (d) three-minute breathing space, which is a short, three-minute practice that focuses on one's sensations, thoughts, and emotions and can also be referred to as "mindfulness of breathing"; (e) the sitting meditation, which makes space for non-doing and brings attention to the sensation of sitting; and (f) mindful movement, which is the act of bringing attention to the breath and bodily sensations while engaging in movement, as exhibited through the practice of yoga. Informal practices, specifically "mindfulness in everyday activities," are also taught to bring mindful attention to everyday experiences (e.g., mindfully eating, walking, listening, and talking). Mindful inquiry is employed by the teacher to evoke a sense of curiosity about the experience in an open and accepting way (Kabat-Zinn, 1982). The teacher also cultivates seven foundational attitudes: nonjudging, patience, beginner's mind, trust, nonstriving, acceptance, and letting go (Kabat-Zinn, 2003). Nonjudging describes an open-hearted and compassionate attitude, while patience is an attitude of calmly tolerating difficulty. Beginner's mind is the practice of bringing the wonder of a child to one's practice, so attending to things as if it is the first time doing so in one's life. Trust is an attitude of believing one's own senses and feelings, while nonstriving is embracing an intention to relax and just be with oneself, or engage in "nondoing." Lastly, acceptance is willingness to observe and accept things as they are in the present moment, and letting go is the practice of learning to release attachments to what one is attending to.

This eight-week secular program has been studied widely, with evidence to date supporting its use among adults suffering from chronic pain (Kabat-Zinn, 1982), anxiety (Hofmann et al., 2010), depression (Hofmann et al., 2010), posttraumatic stress disorder (PTSD; Earley et al., 2014; Goulao & MacLennan, 2016), and cancer (Grossman et al., 2004). A variety of adaptations of *MBSR* have been developed for individuals suffering from specific conditions, including major depressive disorder, substance abuse disorders, and chronic illness. For example, the *Mindfulness-Based Childbirth and Parenting* (MBCP) group intervention is a childbirth and parenting program adapted from *MBSR* by Nancy Bardacke. MBCP uses formal and informal mindfulness practices to address fear and anxiety around childbirth and manage the ups and downs of the postpartum period. *MBCP* is designed for couples to attend together; however, pregnant individuals may also attend alone. The program typically enrolls participants in the second half of pregnancy, either in the late second trimester or early in the third trimester. However, Bardacke also recommends that those with complicated current or previous pregnancies can engage with the program at any time (Bardacke, 2012, pp. 300–301). The standard course of *MBCP* involves a three-hour class for nine weeks, one full-day silent retreat, daily 30-minute home practice, and a reunion class after childbirth. The *MBCP* program begins with present-centered awareness practices, including the Body Scan, in which participants focus their attention on individual body parts from their feet to their head. Participants are directed to refocus their attention to the scan if their minds wander. Beginning in session three, mindfulness practices shift to center on the experience of childbirth (Bardacke, 2012, p. 305; Duncan & Bardacke, 2010). One of the unique practices that MBCP developed is a meditation focused around "Being with Baby." This practice guides the parent to focus on their baby in their womb and to bring attention to the subtle sensations of the baby beginning to move. (Duncan & Bardacke, 2010). Later sessions teach practices to move through and with pain during childbirth. Ice cubes are used to generate unpleasant, but unharmful, sensations while participants engage "non-reactive, concentrated, calm, and focused state[s] of mind" to move through painful sensations with present-centered awareness (Duncan & Bardacke, 2010). Additional programmatic focus on planning, expectations, and response to daily stress work to prepare participants for childbirth and reduce anxiety or fear around the experience.

Mindfulness-Based Cognitive Therapy (MBCT) *and*
Adaptation for the Perinatal Period

MBCT is an eight-week program that was adapted from the *MBSR* curriculum and initially developed to prevent depression relapse (Segal et al., 2002, 2012). *MBCT* also consists of eight sessions, which include elements of formal and informal mindfulness practice, inquiry, and home practice to address specific session themes. Some common *MBCT* session themes include awareness of automatic pilot, mindfulness of breath, allowing and accepting one's experiences, and decentering. Examples of formal mindfulness practices include the body scan, sitting meditation, and the three-minute breathing space, which are done in sessions for a total of 30 to 45 minutes. Informal practices include "mindfulness in everyday activities." Additionally, activities from cognitive behavioral therapy are incorporated to support clients in working effectively with difficult thoughts and emotions. Specific cognitive behavioral therapy techniques utilized in *MBCT* include psychoeducation about depression, automatic thought tracking, and activity tracking. Delivered typically in a group context, *MBCT* facilitators are mental health professionals with specific training in *MBCT* program elements, such as how to engage in curious inquiry with clients (Segal et al., 2002, 2012).

A growing body of evidence demonstrates that *MBCT* is effective for individuals across the lifespan, and can be helpful for people struggling with substance abuse, perinatal depression and anxiety, hypochondriasis, chronic fatigue syndrome, tinnitus, auditory hallucinations, insomnia, major depressive disorder, social phobia, generalized anxiety disorder, panic disorder, PTSD, and cancer (Dimidjian et al., 2015; Felder et al., 2018; King et al., 2013; Miklowitz et al., 2015; Shulman et al., 2018).

Up to 45% of new mothers report experiencing traumatic birth experiences (Beck et al., 2018) and rates of PTSD are higher among perinatal populations than general samples of women (Seng et al., 2009), highlighting the prevalence of trauma history among perinatal individuals. Although *MBCT* has been utilized with individuals suffering from PTSD (King et al., 2013), Segal and colleagues (2012) advise that care be taken when working with clients who suffer from unresolved trauma. *MBCT* was initially developed as a program that does not involve the clients sharing their "story." Instead, clients share their experiences of the mindfulness exercises. If a client has acute PTSD, they may not be able to regulate strong and triggering emotions that can surface during group practice. In addition, *MBCT* group sessions are recommended for clients who are not in an acute state of depression or anxiety, as clients experiencing severe symptoms could require more attention during the group or find the exercises too challenging (Segal et al., 2012).

MBCT was adapted by Dimidjian, Goodman, and colleagues (2015) for perinatal individuals (named *MBCT-PD*) to prevent relapse of depression during the perinatal period. The eight-week *MBCT-PD* course is a group intervention involving a weekly two-hour, group meeting and assigned home practice activities. Modifications from the standard implementation of *MBCT* include a shorter duration of meditations, inclusion of a loving-kindness meditation, a heightened focus on self-care and self-acceptance practices, and an emphasis on strengthening social support. Meditations specifically focused on being with one's baby are also included. The "Being with Baby" meditation builds on the prenatal focused meditation developed by Nancy Bardacke in the *MBCP* program. The parent is guided to bring a curiosity and present-focused awareness to carrying the baby either in utero or in one's arms. The parent is invited to notice the physical sensations such as weight, any movement of the baby, the sensation of touch, and sounds of the baby (Dimidjian et al., 2015). To further expand dissemination and reach, Segal and Dimidjian developed a web-based, self-guided course for both *MBCT* (Segal et al., 2020) and *MBCT-PD* (in preparation) called *Mindful Mood Balance* (MMB) and *Mindful Mood Balance for Moms*. The courses follow a similar curriculum as in-person *MBCT*; however, they include interactive components suitable for different styles of learning, videos of group inquiry, as well as space for reflection.

The *Coping with Anxiety through Living Mindfully* (CALM) pregnancy group intervention was also adapted from *MBCT*, although specifically to target perinatal anxiety. *CALM* pregnancy intervention teaches skills to manage anxiety symptoms, including mindfulness techniques, cognitive therapy approaches, psychoeducation about anxiety and depression, and utilization of home practice to encourage the use of mindfulness in everyday life (Goodman et al., 2014).

Potharst and colleagues (2017) created *Mindful with your baby*, a program based on *MBCT* and *MBSR* to address parenting skills in the perinatal period. *Mindful with your baby* is a group intervention that consists of eight weekly two-hour sessions, with a follow-up session eight weeks following program completion. Sessions are conducted with babies present and consist of a formal mindfulness practice (e.g., body scan), inquiry, baby-specific mindfulness practices, and discussions of home practice. An example of baby-specific mindfulness practice is "mindful seeing with attention to the baby," in which parents focus friendly attention and curiosity on their baby, notice their internal reactions, and practice taking the perspective of their baby.

Additionally, Abatemarco et al. (2021) developed an MBI called *Mindfully in Pregnancy* (*MIP*) based on *MBSR* and *MBCP* that was explicitly developed for perinatal people who have increased stress due to race, poverty, homelessness, substance use treatment, and other comorbid health risks. Researchers adapted the curriculum with respect to cultural context, metaphors, concepts, goals, and language. Examples of adaptations include: offering the program for free and providing transportation reimbursement, increased emphasis on loving-kindness meditation, and "identifying a physician champion" at the clinic to foster familiarity and trust with obstetric clinic providers. *MIP* is a group intervention that consists of six, two-hour sessions that occur once per week at a local OB/GYN office. These group sessions utilize seated and moving meditations, gentle yoga postures, and discussions around stress during the perinatal period. Structured session time is dedicated to group discussion to facilitate social bonding and shared learning among clients. Sessions are taught by trained *MBSR* teachers and trained yoga instructors. Examples of meditations used in *MIP* include a "being with baby" meditation and loving-kindness meditation. Clients were provided with mp3 players with meditation recordings and paper forms of session content to facilitate at-home practice (Abatemarco et al., 2021).

Perinatal Conditions to Which MBIs Are Applied

Historically, MBIs were designed to help patients cope with pain, illness, and stress (Kabat-Zinn, 2003). Research on MBIs for perinatal mental health have similarly targeted pain and stress (Perez-Blasco et al., 2013; Timlin & Simpson, 2017; Zhang et al., 2019), with the addition of anxiety and depression symptoms (Dhillon et al., 2017; Hall et al., 2016; Lever Taylor et al., 2016). In fact, research on MBIs has demonstrated benefits for perinatal individuals with a history of depression or anxiety, and individuals with elevated depressive and anxiety symptom burden at the time of program enrollment (Dimidjian et al., 2015, 2016; Dunn et al., 2012; Goodman et al., 2014; Guo et al., 2020; Lönnberg et al., 2020, 2018). In addition to reducing symptom severity in patients with a history of depression or anxiety, MBIs reduce perceived stress, anxiety, and depressive symptoms for perinatal individuals without histories of mental illness (Buttner et al., 2015; Kinser et al., 2021; Pan et al., 2019; Shulman et al., 2018). Furthermore, MBI studies have been used to support perinatal individuals experiencing trauma or loss, with evidence for reductions in posttraumatic stress symptoms (Huberty et al., 2018); however, studies have found that attendance is challenging in this work (Roberts &

Montgomery, 2015) and it is advised that clients not be in an acute state of depression or anxiety or discuss unresolved experiences of trauma when engaging in MBIs, as clients experiencing more acute symptoms could find the exercises too challenging or have difficulty regulating strong and triggering emotions (Segal et al., 2012). In the evidence of efficacy and effectiveness section, we provide more detailed information about the outcomes of depression, anxiety, stress, and trauma in research on perinatal MBIs.

Case Illustration

When utilizing MBIs in clinical practice, many clinicians follow the group curriculum for individual treatment. Both group and individual MBCT are shown to be feasible and effective (Schroevers et al., 2016; Paterniti et al., 2022). Although it may appear as if following the curriculum of an MBI may suffice, it is imperative for the clinician to embody a mindful stance when working with a client. A mindful stance is typically cultivated through personal practice with mindfulness and is observed as present-focused, openness, acceptance, nonjudgment, curiosity and compassion in sessions. This case study illustrates the experience of Riley, a client with a history of perinatal depression and anxiety, as she engages in individual therapy to stay mentally well in her current perinatal period. We will examine how the clinician utilizes a mindful stance in sessions and Riley's experience and reflections following engagement in *MBCT*.

Intake

During the intake, the clinician explored Riley's previous experiences with mindfulness, meditation and yoga. Riley acknowledged severe difficulties in practicing mindfulness in the past. For Riley, the idea and practice of focusing on breathing, being still, and relaxing ironically evoked symptoms of anxiety and stress. Riley explained a specific scenario where she was asked to practice a 20-minute mindfulness meditation exercise focused on paying attention to the breath. She stated that *"the whole time, I was just overwhelmed and crying, and I needed to get out of that class."* She reflected that she had felt trapped and did not have the foundational coping skills needed to sit with her anxiety for long periods of time. This previous experience created an expectation of anxiety around future guided meditation.

The clinician inquired about Riley's willingness to practice mindfulness again, to which Riley expressed openness to trying and stated that it would be important for the clinician to offer an "out" so that she does not feel trapped. Riley also described her difficulty in attending group meditation and yoga classes: *"You can't really speak out during that deep breathing and relaxation at the end of class (savasana). Whenever I've tried yoga in the past, I would just skip that part (savasana), and I would roll up my mat and sneak out early. But I think that working individually may feel safer, especially if I know I can stop when I want to."* Riley's insights into her anxiety about mindfulness highlight the importance of creating a safe place when considering MBIs for clients and of customizing interventions for specific client needs and preferences.

In planning the treatment sessions, the clinician adapted practices to often offer choice so that Riley would not feel trapped. The clinician also oriented Riley to the arc of mindfulness practice in evidence-based MBIs, which generally start from more concrete and tangible objects of attention. Thus, the clinician assured Riley that the practices could be calibrated to her skill level and confidence. Additionally, the clinician planned for dedicated session time focused on building foundational skills of distress tolerance and emotion regulation as needed. The clinician and Riley discussed what internal signals (i.e., feeling trapped, increased heart rate, panic) she experiences when moving out of her window of tolerance, which empowered the client to identify her warning signs and feel comfortable expressing if a practice was eliciting distress.

Treatment

The clinician used aspects of *Mindfulness-Based Cognitive Therapy for Postpartum Depression* (*MBCT-PD*; Dimidjian et al., 2015) in treatment with the client due to her history of perinatal depression and her worries about experiencing postpartum depression again. Each week, the sessions started with a meditation aligned with the main theme of the session. For example, the clinician started with leading Riley through practicing mindfulness with an object of her choosing and engaged in mindful inquiry afterward, asking "what did you notice?" and "how is this different from how you would normally pay attention." Riley reflected that *"with a toddler at home, it feels like I barely pay attention to such small things and I feel like I am missing out on so much. I would really love to be more present with my daughter, but it's so hard when I'm tired, working and her main caregiver at home."* Riley reported appreciating the concrete focus of the practice and the direct links to her concerns about mood and parenting. Following Riley's reflection, the patient and clinician collaboratively decided her daily home practice activity, which was to practice mindfulness in one everyday activity. Riley chose washing her hands and also extended this to helping her daughter wash her hands.

When Riley returned the following week, she reported that she forgot a few days of home practice, but did practice a few times with her daughter. She explained, *"It was really wonderful, it gave me a moment to slow down, and connect with my daughter. I realized that she is so present all the time. When I asked her what she noticed, she surprised me by noticing so much, down to the bubbles forming on her hands."*

As the sessions progressed, the clinician introduced new mindfulness practices at the beginning of each session, including body scans, mindfulness of the breath, the three-minute breathing space, and walking meditation. Riley began to notice and recognize her internal physical sensations and emotions that arise during both pleasant and unpleasant moments.

At session five, the clinician guided Riley in a mindfulness practice purposefully focused on a minor difficulty that had recently occurred, such as being stuck in traffic. This practice is often challenging for clients, as it is common to want to avoid difficult situations rather than embrace them. Riley reflected, *"during the practice, I could feel my entire body tense up and I had the urge to run away from it. Then you led me to pay attention to the tension. I noticed that I always try to just make the tension go away. But today, I really focused on the tension in my jaw and neck, and found that as I noticed it, I naturally started to soften. I then had a thought that, of course I was tense, I had so much to do and had no time to deal with this difficulty. I then began to feel some compassion for myself, which was quite different for me. I am so hard on myself typically. I really wish I could be more kind to myself in general."* Throughout each session the clinician asked inquiry questions that tied Riley's awareness back to how this may help her stay well. Riley began to realize that the ups and downs of being a new mom are to be expected, and she started to accept her experience from a nonjudgmental stance.

Final Session

In the final session, the clinician and Riley worked toward creating a relapse prevention plan. Throughout the previous weeks, Riley began to identify her own "signature of depression" and gained awareness of her warning signs. She determined that she wanted to improve at adjusting her expectations and asking for support from others in this postpartum period. Riley identified specific practices and tools that she found helpful and asked supportive people in her life to remind her of her skills to stay well in her pregnancy and postpartum period.

Evidence of Efficacy and Effectiveness

MBIs were initially designed for the purpose of prevention, especially in regard to depressive relapse (Fjorback et al., 2011), rather than to address acute symptomatology; however, MBIs have also been utilized for the purpose of intervention, with a strong evidence base supporting the efficacy and effectiveness of MBIs for mental health symptomatology in the perinatal period (Dhillon et al., 2017; Hall et al., 2016; Lever Taylor et al., 2016). In this section, we report the literature on effectiveness of *MBSR* and *MBCT*, as they are two primary MBIs that have been studied widely and adapted into a variety of MBIs for the perinatal period. Then, we discuss the major reviews that have been published on the use of MBIs in the perinatal period, with the majority highlighting impact on depression, anxiety, and stress.

MBSR *Evidence Base*

Although not specific to perinatal individuals, a wide breadth of research on *MBSR* supports its use among adults suffering from chronic pain (Kabat-Zinn, 1982), anxiety (Hofmann et al., 2010; Khoury et al., 2015), depression (Hofmann et al., 2010; Khoury et al., 2015), PTSD (Earley et al., 2014; Goulao & MacLennan, 2016), and cancer (Grossman et al., 2004). It has also been found to be effective in reducing depressive relapse (Fjorback et al., 2011) and reducing stress (Khoury et al., 2015). Furthermore, a review of ten studies of remote delivery of *MBSR* found that *MBSR* can be effective at improving mental health when delivered over video conference (Moulton-Perkins et al., 2022).

Specific to perinatal populations, research on the Mindful with Your Baby parenting class based on *MBSR* and *MBCT* enrolled 44 postpartum mothers (84% with clinical diagnoses of depression or anxiety) and found that participation in the intervention was associated with significant improvement in mindfulness, self-compassion, and mindful parenting, with medium and large effect sizes at post-intervention and longitudinal follow-ups. Participants also reported significant improvement in parental well-being and psychopathology across the study, with small effects at post-intervention, medium effects at eight-week follow-up, and large effects at one-year follow-up (Potharst et al., 2017). Additionally, the *MBCP* course adapted by Duncan and Bardacke (2010) enrolled 27 pregnant women who demonstrated significant reductions in perinatal anxiety ($d = .81$) and negative affect ($d = .74$) from pre- to post-intervention, with large effect sizes for both outcomes. Participants also experienced improvements in mindfulness, nonjudging, nonreactivity, and positive affect. Qualitative feedback from program participants indicated that the skills taught through the program were perceived as beneficial for pregnant people and their partners (Duncan & Bardacke, 2010). More research on *MBSR* for perinatal individuals is needed, as preliminary evidence is promising.

MBCT *Evidence Base*

Research on the effectiveness of *MBCT* shows that it is effective in supporting individuals with substance abuse disorder, auditory hallucinations, insomnia, major depressive disorder, social phobia, generalized anxiety disorder, panic disorder, PTSD, and chronic medical conditions (Dimidjian et al., 2015; Felder et al., 2018; Ghahari et al., 2020; King et al., 2013; Miklowitz et al., 2015; Shulman et al., 2018). *MBCT* has also been found to be effective in reducing depressive relapse and symptoms of depression (Fjorback et al., 2011; MacKenzie et al., 2018; Musa et al., 2020).

For perinatal individuals with risk for depression relapse, Dimidjian and colleagues (2015) assessed MBCT-PD for perinatal depressive relapse prevention and reported that participants experienced a significant reduction in depressive symptoms ($d = .84$; large effect sizes) from pre- to post-intervention, while rates of depressive relapse/recurrence in this sample were 18.37% at six-month follow-up.

Research on the utility of *MBCT* as an intervention to improve mental health in perinatal individuals has found that it is effective in reducing both depression and anxiety symptoms (Abatemarco et al., 2021; Dimidjian et al., 2015; Goodman et al., 2014). For example, an RCT of *MBCT* with individuals diagnosed with perinatal depression or anxiety found that participation in the intervention was associated with trending reductions in symptoms of depression ($i = .84$) and anxiety ($d = .83$), with moderate effect sizes for these outcomes (Shulman et al., 2018). Another study implemented *MBCT* with pregnant and postpartum individuals with a history of major depressive disorder and found that participants reported significant improvements in depression ($d = .52$) at post-treatment, indicating a moderate effect size (Miklowitz et al., 2015). Additionally, a pilot study of the *CALM* intervention based on *MBCT* enrolled 23 perinatal women and showed a significant reduction in depression ($d = .56$) and anxiety ($d = .36$) symptoms among program completers, with small-to-moderate effect sizes for these outcomes (Goodman et al., 2014). Furthermore, a large randomized clinical trial of Mindful Mood Balance (MMB), a web-based application that delivers MBCT (Noggin, 2020), was assessed with 460 participants experiencing residual depressive symptoms and findings support the effectiveness of remote MBCT in reducing depression symptom burden (Segal et al., 2020). Thus, research to date supports the effectiveness of *MBCT* in improving depression and anxiety symptoms among perinatal populations in both in-person and remote delivery settings.

Summary

Narrative and meta-analytic reviews support the findings of the specific studies of MBIs reviewed earlier. Specifically, seven reviews have examined impacts of MBIs on depression, nine on anxiety, and four on stress outcomes. In addition, reviews of the literature identified that participation in MBIs was associated with improvements in the following outcomes for perinatal individuals: self-compassion (Matvienko-Sikar et al., 2016), mindfulness skills (Lever Taylor et al., 2016), management of pain (Hughes et al., 2009), childbirth self-efficacy (Matvienko-Sikar et al., 2016), and ability to attend to one's baby (Hughes et al., 2009). Specific findings with respect to mental health outcomes are described in detail next.

Among the seven reviews that assessed impact on depression symptoms, two were meta-analyses that reviewed 14 to 17 studies, primarily with pregnant people, including both RCTs and non-RCTs, and indicated that participation in MBIs during the perinatal period was associated with significant improvements in depression symptoms with small to medium effect sizes (Dhillon et al., 2017; Lever Taylor et al., 2016). Of the remaining reviews, three were systematic reviews that found that mindfulness interventions in the perinatal period reduced levels of depression symptoms with moderate-to-large effect sizes ($d = .38$ to 2.26; Hall et al., 2016;

Lucena et al., 2020; Matvienko-Sikar et al., 2016). Lastly, two reviews of nonpharmacologic approaches for improving perinatal mental health also highlighted that participation in MBIs is linked to improvements in depression symptoms (Lavender et al., 2016; Traylor et al., 2020). The majority of MBI studies focused on depression have identified eligible participants with mild to moderate self-report depressive symptom burden, as assessed with surveys such as the *Edinburgh Postnatal Depression Scale* (EPDS; Cox et al., 1987) and the *Patient Health Questionnaire-9* (PHQ-9; Kroenke et al., 2001). MBI studies that have recruited perinatal individuals who meet diagnostic criteria of major depressive disorder have required participants to be engaging in SSRI treatment during their time in the study (Ahmadpanah et al., 2018).

Of the nine reviews focused on anxiety symptoms, two were meta-analyses that reviewed a range of 14 to 17 studies, primarily among pregnant people, including both RCTs and non-RCTs, and indicated that participation in MBIs during the perinatal period was associated with significant improvements in anxiety symptoms (Dhillon et al., 2017; Lever Taylor et al., 2016). Of the remaining reviews, four were systematic reviews that found that mindfulness interventions in the perinatal period were viewed as acceptable and satisfactory and reduced levels of anxiety symptoms (Evans et al., 2020; Hall et al., 2016; Lucena et al., 2020; Matvienko-Sikar et al., 2016). Lastly, two reviews of nonpharmacologic approaches for improving perinatal mental health also highlighted that participation in MBIs is linked to improvements in anxiety symptoms (Lavender et al., 2016; Traylor et al., 2020).

Stress, along with depression and anxiety, has known negative consequences on perinatal people and infants, including obstetric complications, nausea, and preterm birth (Dipietro, 2012). Importantly, individuals may identify more with feeling stressed than depressed or anxious, due to the stigma associated with mental health. Of the four reviews that assessed impact on stress, two were meta-analyses that reviewed a range of 14 to 17 studies, including both RCTs and non-RCTs, and indicated that participation in MBIs during the perinatal period was associated with significant reductions in stress (Dhillon et al., 2017; Lever Taylor et al., 2016). The remaining reviews were systematic reviews that found that mindfulness interventions in the perinatal period reduced stress levels in participants (Hall et al., 2016; Lucena et al., 2020).

Thus, the evidence base on MBIs for perinatal individuals found that participation in MBIs was associated with reductions in stress, anxiety, and depression (Dhillon et al., 2017; Hall et al., 2016; Lever Taylor et al., 2016). However, many reviews noted a need for greater rigor in research methodology and larger sample sizes for this topic (Evans et al., 2020; Hall et al., 2016). Researchers reported difficulties with varying gestational characteristics for participants across studies, which can be a confound in perinatal research (Evans et al., 2020; Hall et al., 2016). Also, the majority of research on perinatal MBIs has focused on intervention in pregnancy, rather than the postpartum period. Furthermore, reviews often did not report if patients met clinical thresholds of major depressive disorder or anxiety disorder, making it difficult to understand if results are generalizable to individuals experiencing higher severity symptoms. Future research should highlight MBIs in the postpartum period, increase scientific rigor in research methodology through usage of RCTs and larger sample sizes, and report differences between individuals who meet clinical thresholds of major depressive disorder or anxiety disorders compared to patients who do not meet clinical criteria.

Cultural Considerations

A common and valid critique of MBIs is that white, Westernized culture has been disproportionately overrepresented in secular mindfulness research and practice (Fleming et al., 2022;

Eichel et al., 2021). Disregarding lived experience and replicating harmful dynamics in the therapeutic process is a significant barrier to care for underserved populations (Sue, 2015). Thus, when implementing MBIs among communities who have endured systemic oppression, providers must bring a culturally competent lens to their work (Proulx et al., 2018).

Little research has been done into whether MBIs effectively reduce depression, stress, and anxiety for people who experience structural racism and social inequality. Garfield and Watson-Singleton (2021) discuss the significant health disparities among African American perinatal individuals due to increased stress, including racism, and suggest that MBIs have potential to serve as a culturally responsive intervention approach (Garfield & Watson-Singleton, 2021). Despite limited research on the efficacy of MBIs with historically marginalized communities, there is support for the acceptance and feasibility of these programs among this population. For example, the aforementioned *MIP* program adapted MBI curriculum with respect to cultural context, metaphors, concepts, goals, and language for utilization with pregnant people with minoritized identities and health risks. Research on *MIP* reported that participants viewed it as acceptable and demonstrated decreases in depression, perceived stress, and anxiety up to seven months following intervention completion (Abatemarco et al., 2021). Another study, conducted by Goodman et al. (2013), found that in a sample of 60 pregnant African American women, behavioral health interventions, including MBIs, were preferred over pharmacological intervention for the treatment and management of depression and stress. Furthermore, participants indicated that both traditional, interpersonal therapy, and MBIs were viewed as equally acceptable (Goodman et al., 2013).

Training clinicians to be culturally competent diversifying the clinical workforce, and adapting interventions to be culturally sensitive are promising options to increase relatability and adherence to MBIs during pregnancy and the postpartum period. As a central tenet of MBIs is present-centered awareness and acceptance, MBIs are well positioned to be oriented to the lived experiences of clients and the real and negative health impacts of social inequality and structural and interpersonal racism on individuals' well-being. Garfield and Watson-Singleton (2021) provide recommendations to develop culturally adaptive and responsive mindfulness-based programs, including openly acknowledging the distinct lived experiences of African American women, recognizing oppression, and providing mindfulness courses taught by African American women (Garfield & Watson-Singleton, 2021). Additional cultural adaptations for MBIs for historically underserved communities include incorporating story-telling, spirituality, faith, recognition of discrimination and inequitable access to healthcare, and acknowledgement of the potential for meditation to trigger trauma responses in clients (Ponting et al., 2020). Lastly, given the history of mistreatment of African Americans by the U.S. medical system, partnering with local and community-based organizations could promote higher treatment adherence among historically marginalized communities, rather than operating in hospital settings (Ponting et al., 2020).

Dissemination

There are a variety of barriers to care in the perinatal period. A study surveying over 600 perinatal individuals found that only 13% of perinatal individuals sought help, highlighting that help-seeking is a difficulty in the perinatal period. Furthermore, participants identified barriers to care, including a lack of knowledge about mental health conditions and symptoms, lack of knowledge about treatment options, lack of financial resources, lack of time, transportation difficulties, and fear of stigma (Fonseca et al., 2015). These identified barriers hinder perinatal individuals from utilizing traditional mental healthcare options; however, MBIs are promising as they may overcome some barriers to care and promote dissemination of treatment among this population.

Knowledge About Mental Health

It is common for perinatal individuals to have a lack of knowledge about signs and symptoms of depression and anxiety (Fonseca et al., 2015). It is imperative that knowledge about mental health is shared with this population and that effort is put into identifying individuals in need. The *Edinburgh Postnatal Depression Scale* (EPDS) has been frequently used to identify individuals with elevated depression symptoms, as it is a well-known depression scale used among perinatal populations. Current calls across the United States for universal screening at all prenatal appointments highlight the accuracy, brevity, and simplicity of administering the EPDS ("ACOG Committee Opinion No. 757: Screening for Perinatal Depression," 2018). Standard use of the EPDS at prenatal visits could be a feasible method by which clinicians identify perinatal individuals who could benefit from MBIs.

Knowledge of MBIs Among Patients and Practitioners

Although mindfulness has become more well-known in recent years, patients may not have knowledge about the different types of mindfulness-based treatment options and the empirical support for these interventions. Mental health providers can provide their perinatal clients with information on the research supporting MBIs. MBIs should be facilitated by trained, knowledgeable mindfulness practitioners (Crane et al., 2010; Crane et al., 2012). Due to the lack of accreditation and ethical process required for training facilitators for MBIs (Kenny et al., 2020), some researchers have developed mindfulness-based training programs for individuals to learn how to be *MBCT* or *MBSR* teachers. A typical requirement for training is for trainees to have at least three years of personal mindfulness-based practice to begin learning to teach mindfulness-based techniques (Crane et al., 2012). Crane et al. (2010) document a training process that they have used for *MBCT* and *MBSR* teachers, which includes basic teachers training (e.g., cultivate personal mindfulness practice; experience *MBCT* or *MBSR*; learn theory and research underpinning mindfulness practice) and advanced training (e.g., teaching a mindfulness-based course; supervision; continued professional development). For individuals new to the mindfulness field, one can begin by cultivating a personal mindfulness practice, such as by taking meditation classes, using a mindfulness app, or engaging in formal training in *MBCT* or *MBSR*.

Time

One of the most common barriers for engaging in MBIs during the perinatal period is time. As described earlier, *MBSR* and *MBCT* typically consist of eight 90- to 120-minute sessions with dedicated daily home practice (Kabat-Zinn, 1982; Segal et al., 2002, 2012). Basso and colleagues conducted an RCT of non-perinatal adult nonexperienced meditators and results suggested that brief, daily meditation (13 minutes per day) can significantly improve mood, anxiety, attention, and memory when compared to listening to a daily 13-minute podcast (Basso et al., 2019). Research on formal versus informal mindfulness with non-perinatal adult mindfulness practitioners indicated that frequency, rather than duration, was important to outcomes and that more informal practice was associated with increased psychological flexibility and positive well-being (Birtwell et al., 2019). A study of non-perinatal adult women similarly found that consistency of engaging in MBI treatment was important, as their results showed a significant positive association between *MBCT* session attendance and reduction in depression scores (Elices et al., 2022). Research has not assessed the effectiveness of short mindfulness practices compared to long mindfulness practices, so more research is needed on this topic.

Transportation and Geographic Location

Geographic accessibility and transportation can be significant barriers to access. Mindfulness-based practices have been adapted to remote formats to overcome the lack of access. For example, a randomized clinical trial ($n = 460$) of *MMB*, a web-based application based on *MBCT* (Noggin, 2020; Segal et al., 2020), found that remote delivery was effective in reducing depression symptom burden when compared to a usual care control (Segal et al., 2020). Effectiveness of the *MMB* program is being assessed with perinatal individuals by Dimidjian and colleagues, as it improves accessibility of mental health resources to this population. *Headspace*, *Smiling Mind*, and *Calm* are smartphone apps for mindfulness techniques that have empirical support for their usability (Mani et al., 2015) and effectiveness (Economides et al., 2018; Huberty et al., 2019), although research on these smartphone apps has not focused on perinatal individuals. Overall, research on remote delivery of mindfulness-based interventions indicates that digital mindfulness interventions can be effective in improving a range of outcomes, including stress, depression, and anxiety. However, experts (or investigators) highlight the need for more research and active comparison of remote delivery to in-person delivery (Mrazek et al., 2019; van Emmerik et al., 2020). Also, it is important to remember that many individuals have experienced "digital fatigue" following the shift to remote care during the COVID-19 pandemic (Döring et al., 2022). Additional challenges to remote interventions include low engagement and retention, shallow learning, and technological frustrations (Mrazek et al., 2019). It will be important for future studies and design of digital interventions to address such possible barriers.

Finances

Many MBIs have become more financially accessible in different settings and numerous accessible options are in the research and development phase. For example, the web-based application MMB (Noggin, 2020) has been rigorously studied as an intervention to reduce depression symptomatology and improve mental health (Segal et al., 2020), with specific research on this program focused on perinatal individuals. Smartphone apps have also become an important tool for affordable dissemination, as they offer various mindfulness apps, often for free. Research has highlighted *Headspace* (Economides et al., 2018; Mani et al., 2015), *Smiling Mind* (Mani et al., 2015), and *Calm* (Huberty et al., 2019) as affordable, high-quality app options to use in collaboration with mental health clinicians. In addition to personal financial responsibility to participate in MBIs, healthcare systems may offer reimbursement through insurance (e.g., Medicaid) to improve the affordability of these programs.

Stigma

The stigma around mental health treatment is a barrier to intervention engagement. MBIs have potential to bypass barriers of stigma due to cultural relevance and adaptability. Mindfulness originates from Buddhist traditions and may be more acceptable to individuals for whom Buddhist traditions or meditation are relevant or valuable (Anālayo, 2019; Wilson, 2014). Furthermore, various researchers have pursued adaptations of mindfulness practices to be culturally responsive to specific communities, such as African American (Watson-Singleton et al., 2019), Asian (Thapaliya et al., 2018), and Hispanic (Castellanos et al., 2020) individuals. However, as previously mentioned, practitioners must engage in culturally sensitive practice when using mindfulness techniques with individuals who endure systemic oppression (Proulx et al., 2018).

Conclusion and Future Directions

A strong evidence base supports the efficacy and effectiveness of MBIs for the perinatal period in preventing depressive relapse (Fjorback et al., 2011) and reducing symptoms of depression, anxiety, and stress (Dhillon et al., 2017; Hall et al., 2016; Lever Taylor et al., 2016). Much research on MBIs for the perinatal period has been conducted with individuals who have a history of perinatal depression or anxiety, or are currently experiencing elevated depression or anxiety symptoms. Research has also demonstrated that MBIs can be effective among perinatal people without elevated symptoms or history of mental health conditions, highlighting the role of MBIs in primary prevention. Adaptations to standard *MBSR* and *MBCT* programs for the perinatal period included adapting practices and session themes to focus on the struggles and experiences of new and expecting parents or including baby in the practices.

Continued work is needed in the perinatal MBI field to strengthen our knowledge on ideal duration and essential components of MBIs for perinatal populations. Many reviews of perinatal MBIs highlighted a need for greater rigor in research methodology and larger sample sizes to strengthen takeaways from this research (Evans et al., 2020; Hall et al., 2016), so future research should utilize RCT methodology, recruit larger samples, and collect longitudinal data. To additionally strengthen results, future research should standardize gestational characteristics for participants across studies, as this can be a confound in perinatal research (Evans et al., 2020; Hall et al., 2016). Next, the majority of perinatal MBI research focuses on intervention in pregnancy, so future research should also highlight postpartum interventions and experiences. Lastly, studies should report differences between individuals who meet clinical thresholds of major depressive disorder or anxiety disorders compared to patients who do not meet clinical criteria, as this may shed light on the utility of MBIs for prevention versus intervention.

Further research on cultural adaptations and implementations of MBIs for perinatal individuals is also imperative to increase accessibility of MBIs to historically marginalized communities, and future work should document these adaptation details to help community members adapt MBIs in an empirically supported manner. Future research must also prioritize diversifying the sample of individuals engaged in perinatal MBIs so that study results have a wider range of generalizability. Additional important expansions of MBI research include implementing MBIs with clients' partners in the intervention and expansion to perinatal people who identify as gender or sexual minorities.

References

Abatemarco, D. J., Gannon, M., Short, V. L., Baxter, J., Metzker, K. M., Reid, L., & Catov, J. M. (2021, December). Mindfulness in pregnancy: A brief intervention for women at risk. *Maternal and Child Health Journal, 25*(12), 1875–1883. https://doi.org/10.1007/s10995-021-03243-y

ACOG committee opinion no. 757: Screening for perinatal depression. (2018, November). *Obstetrics & Gynecology, 132*(5), e208–e212. https://doi.org/10.1097/aog.0000000000002927

Ahmadpanah, M., Nazaribadie, M., Aghaei, E., Ghaleiha, A., Bakhtiari, A., Haghighi, M., . . . Brand, S. (2018, February). Influence of adjuvant detached mindfulness and stress management training compared to pharmacologic treatment in primiparae with postpartum depression. *Archives of Women's Mental Health, 21*(1), 65–73. https://doi.org/10.1007/s00737-017-0753-6

Anālayo, B. (2019, August). Adding historical depth to definitions of mindfulness. *Current Opinion in Psychology, 28*, 11–14. https://doi.org/10.1016/j.copsyc.2018.09.013

Baer, R. (2019). Assessment of mindfulness by self-report. *Current Opinion in Psychology, 28*, 42–48. https://doi.org/10.1016/j.copsyc.2018.10.015

Bardacke, N. (2012). *Mindful birthing: Training the mind, body, and heart for childbirth and beyond* (1st ed., pp. 299–315). HarperCollins Publishers.

Basso, J. C., McHale, A., Ende, V., Oberlin, D. J., & Suzuki, W. A. (2019, January 1). Brief, daily meditation enhances attention, memory, mood, and emotional regulation in non-experienced meditators. *Behavioural Brain Research, 356*, 208–220. https://doi.org/10.1016/j.bbr.2018.08.023

Beck, C. T., Watson, S., & Gable, R. K. (2018). Traumatic childbirth and its aftermath: Is there anything positive? *The Journal of Perinatal Education, 27*(3), 175–184. https://doi.org/10.1891/1058-1243.27.3.175

Birtwell, K., Williams, K., van Marwijk, H., Armitage, C. J., & Sheffield, D. (2019). An exploration of formal and informal mindfulness practice and associations with wellbeing. *Mindfulness, 10*(1), 89–99. https://doi.org/10.1007/s12671-018-0951-y

Buttner, M. M., Brock, R. L., O'Hara, M. W., & Stuart, S. (2015, May). Efficacy of yoga for depressed postpartum women: A randomized controlled trial. *Complementary Therapies in Clinical Practice, 21*(2), 94–100. https://doi.org/10.1016/j.ctcp.2015.03.003

Castellanos, R., Yildiz Spinel, M., Phan, V., Orengo-Aguayo, R., Humphreys, K. L., & Flory, K. (2020, February 1). A systematic review and meta-analysis of cultural adaptations of mindfulness-based interventions for Hispanic populations. *Mindfulness, 11*(2), 317–332. https://doi.org/10.1007/s12671-019-01210-x

Cohen, L. S., Altshuler, L. L., Harlow, B. L., Nonacs, R., Newport, D. J., Viguera, A. C., . . . Stowe, Z. N. (2006, February 1). Relapse of major depression during pregnancy in women who maintain or discontinue antidepressant treatment. *JAMA, 295*(5), 499–507. https://doi.org/10.1001/jama.295.5.499

Cox, J. L., Holden, J. M., & Sagovsky, R. (1987, June). Detection of postnatal depression: Development of the 10-item Edinburgh Postnatal Depression Scale. *British Journal of Psychiatry, 150*, 782–786.

Crane, R. S., Kuyken, W., Hastings, R. P., Rothwell, N., & Williams, J. M. (2010, June). Training teachers to deliver mindfulness-based interventions: Learning from the UK experience. *Mindfulness, 1*(2), 74–86. https://doi.org/10.1007/s12671-010-0010-9

Crane, R. S., Kuyken, W., Williams, J. M., Hastings, R. P., Cooper, L., & Fennell, M. J. (2012, March). Competence in teaching mindfulness-based courses: Concepts, development and assessment. *Mindfulness, 3*(1), 76–84. https://doi.org/10.1007/s12671-011-0073-2

Davis, K., Goodman, S. H., Leiferman, J., Taylor, M., & Dimidjian, S. (2015, August). A randomized controlled trial of yoga for pregnant women with symptoms of depression and anxiety. *Complementary Therapies in Clinical Practice, 21*(3), 166–172. https://doi.org/10.1016/j.ctcp.2015.06.005

Dhillon, A., Sparkes, E., & Duarte, R. V. (2017). Mindfulness-based interventions during pregnancy: A systematic review and meta-analysis. *Mindfulness, 8*(6), 1421–1437. https://doi.org/10.1007/s12671-017-0726-x

Dimidjian, S., & Goodman, S. H. (2014, March). Preferences and attitudes toward approaches to depression relapse/recurrence prevention among pregnant women. *Behaviour Research and Therapy, 54*, 7–11. https://doi.org/10.1016/j.brat.2013.11.008

Dimidjian, S., Goodman, S. H., Felder, J. N., Gallop, R., Brown, A. P., & Beck, A. (2015, February). An open trial of mindfulness-based cognitive therapy for the prevention of perinatal depressive relapse/recurrence. *Archives of Women's Mental Health*, *18*(1), 85–94. https://doi.org/10.1007/s00737-014-0468-x

Dimidjian, S., Goodman, S. H., Felder, J. N., Gallop, R., Brown, A. P., & Beck, A. (2016, February). Staying well during pregnancy and the postpartum: A pilot randomized trial of mindfulness-based cognitive therapy for the prevention of depressive relapse/recurrence. *Journal of Consulting and Clinical Psychology*, *84*(2), 134–145. https://doi.org/10.1037/ccp0000068

Dipietro, J. A. (2012, August). Maternal stress in pregnancy: Considerations for fetal development. *Journal of Adolescent Health*, *51*(2 Suppl), S3–S8. https://doi.org/10.1016/j.jadohealth.2012.04.008

Döring, N., Moor, K., Fiedler, M., Schoenenberg, K., & Raake, A. (2022, February 12). Videoconference fatigue: A conceptual analysis. *International Journal of Environmental Research and Public Health*, *19*(4). https://doi.org/10.3390/ijerph19042061

Duncan, L. G., & Bardacke, N. (2010, April). Mindfulness-based childbirth and parenting education: Promoting family mindfulness during the perinatal period. *Journal of Child and Family Studies*, *19*(2), 190–202. https://doi.org/10.1007/s10826-009-9313-7

Dunn, C., Hanieh, E., Roberts, R., & Powrie, R. (2012, April). Mindful pregnancy and childbirth: Effects of a mindfulness-based intervention on women's psychological distress and well-being in the perinatal period. *Archives of Women's Mental Health*, *15*(2), 139–143. https://doi.org/10.1007/s00737-012-0264-4

Earley, M. D., Chesney, M. A., Frye, J., Greene, P. A., Berman, B., & Kimbrough, E. (2014, October). Mindfulness intervention for child abuse survivors: A 2.5-year follow-up. *Journal of Clinical Psychology*, *70*(10), 933–941. https://doi.org/10.1002/jclp.22102

Economides, M., Martman, J., Bell, M. J., & Sanderson, B. (2018). Improvements in stress, affect, and irritability following brief use of a mindfulness-based smartphone app: A randomized controlled trial. *Mindfulness*, *9*(5), 1584–1593. https://doi.org/10.1007/s12671-018-0905-4

Eichel, K., Gawande, R., Acabchuk, R. L., Palitsky, R., Chau, S., Pham, A., . . . Britton, W. (2021, November 1). A retrospective systematic review of diversity variables in mindfulness research, 2000–2016. *Mindfulness*, *12*(11), 2573–2592. https://doi.org/10.1007/s12671-021-01715-4

Elices, M., Pérez-Sola, V., Pérez-Aranda, A., Colom, F., Polo, M., Martín-López, L. M., & Gárriz, M. (2022, February 1). The effectiveness of mindfulness-based cognitive therapy in primary care and the role of depression severity and treatment attendance. *Mindfulness*, *13*(2), 362–372. https://doi.org/10.1007/s12671-021-01794-3

Evans, K., Spiby, H., & Morrell, J. C. (2020, February). Non-pharmacological interventions to reduce the symptoms of mild to moderate anxiety in pregnant women: A systematic review and narrative synthesis of women's views on the acceptability of and satisfaction with interventions. *Archives of Women's Mental Health*, *23*(1), 11–28. https://doi.org/10.1007/s00737-018-0936-9

Felder, J. N., Laraia, B., Coleman-Phox, K., Bush, N., Suresh, M., Thomas, M., . . . Prather, A. A. (2018, November–December). Poor sleep quality, psychological distress, and the buffering effect of mindfulness training during pregnancy. *Behavioral Sleep Medicine*, *16*(6), 611–624. https://doi.org/10.1080/15402002.2016.1266488

Fjorback, L. O., Arendt, M., Ornbøl, E., Fink, P., & Walach, H. (2011, August). Mindfulness-based stress reduction and mindfulness-based cognitive therapy: A systematic review of randomized controlled trials. *Acta Psychiatrica Scandinavica*, *124*(2), 102–119. https://doi.org/10.1111/j.1600-0447.2011.01704.x

Fleming, C. M., Womack, V. Y., & Proulx, J. (Eds.). (2022). *Beyond white mindfulness: Critical perspectives on racism, well-being and liberation* (1st ed.). Routledge, Taylor & Francis Group.

Fonseca, A., Gorayeb, R., & Canavarro, M. C. (2015, December). Women's help-seeking behaviours for depressive symptoms during the perinatal period: Socio-demographic and clinical correlates and perceived barriers to seeking professional help. *Midwifery*, *31*(12), 1177–1185. https://doi.org/10.1016/j.midw.2015.09.002

Garfield, L., & Watson-Singleton, N. N. (2021, March). Culturally responsive mindfulness interventions for perinatal African-American women: A call for action. *Western Journal of Nursing Research*, *43*(3), 219–226. https://doi.org/10.1177/0193945920950336

Ghahari, S., Mohammadi-Hasel, K., Malakouti, S. K., & Roshanpajouh, M. (2020, June). Mindfulness-based cognitive therapy for generalised anxiety disorder: A systematic review and meta-analysis. *East Asian Archives of Psychiatry*, *30*(2), 52–56. https://doi.org/10.12809/eaap1885

Goldberg, S. B., Riordan, K. M., Sun, S., & Davidson, R. J. (2022, Jane). The empirical status of mindfulness-based interventions: A systematic review of 44 meta-analyses of randomized controlled trials. *Perspectives on Psychological Science, 17*(1), 108–130. https://doi.org/10.1177/1745691620968771

Goodman, J. H., Guarino, A., Chenausky, K., Klein, L., Prager, J., Petersen, R., . . . Freeman, M. (2014, October). CALM pregnancy: Results of a pilot study of mindfulness-based cognitive therapy for perinatal anxiety. *Archives of Women's Mental Health, 17*(5), 373–387. https://doi.org/10.1007/s00737-013-0402-7

Goodman, S. H., Dimidjian, S., & Williams, K. G. (2013). Pregnant African American women's attitudes toward perinatal depression prevention. *Cultural Diversity and Ethnic Minority Psychology, 19*, 50–57. https://doi.org/10.1037/a0030565

Goulao, B., & MacLennan, G. S. (2016, January 5). Mindfulness-based stress reduction for veterans with PTSD. *JAMA, 315*(1), 87–88. https://doi.org/10.1001/jama.2015.15170

Grossman, P. (2019). On the porosity of subject and object in "mindfulness" scientific study: Challenges to "scientific" construction, operationalization and measurement of mindfulness. *Current Opinion in Psychology, 28*, 102–107. https://doi.org/10.1016/j.copsyc.2018.11.008

Grossman, P., Niemann, L., Schmidt, S., & Walach, H. (2004, July). Mindfulness-based stress reduction and health benefits: A meta-analysis. *Journal of Psychosomatic Research, 57*(1), 35–43. https://doi.org/10.1016/s0022-3999(03)00573-7

Guo, L., Zhang, J., Mu, L., & Ye, Z. (2020, February). Preventing postpartum depression with mindful self-compassion intervention: A randomized control study. *Journal of Nervous and Mental Disease, 208*(2), 101–107. https://doi.org/10.1097/nmd.0000000000001096

Hall, H. G., Beattie, J., Lau, R., East, C., & Anne Biro, M. (2016, February). Mindfulness and perinatal mental health: A systematic review. *Women and Birth, 29*(1), 62–71. https://doi.org/10.1016/j.wombi.2015.08.006

Hall, W. A., Hauck, Y. L., Carty, E. M., Hutton, E. K., Fenwick, J., & Stoll, K. (2009, September–October). Childbirth fear, anxiety, fatigue, and sleep deprivation in pregnant women. *Journal of Obstetric, Gynecologic, & Neonatal Nursing, 38*(5), 567–576. https://doi.org/10.1111/j.1552-6909.2009.01054.x

Hayes, R. M., Wu, P., Shelton, R. C., Cooper, W. O., Dupont, W. D., Mitchel, E., & Hartert, T. V. (2012, July). Maternal antidepressant use and adverse outcomes: A cohort study of 228,876 pregnancies. *American Journal of Obstetrics and Gynecology, 207*(1), 49.e41–49. https://doi.org/10.1016/j.ajog.2012.04.028

Hofmann, S. G., Sawyer, A. T., Witt, A. A., & Oh, D. (2010, April). The effect of mindfulness-based therapy on anxiety and depression: A meta-analytic review. *Journal of Consulting and Clinical Psychology, 78*(2), 169–183. https://doi.org/10.1037/a0018555

Holmes, B. A. (2017). *Joy unspeakable: Contemplative practices of the Black church.* Fortress Press.

Huberty, J., Green, J., Cacciatore, J., Buman, M. P., & Leiferman, J. (2018, November). Relationship between mindfulness and posttraumatic stress in women who experienced stillbirth. *Journal of Obstetric, Gynecologic, & Neonatal Nursing, 47*(6), 760–770. https://doi.org/10.1016/j.jogn.2018.09.002

Huberty, J., Green, J., Glissmann, C., Larkey, L., Puzia, M., & Lee, C. (2019, June 25). Efficacy of the mindfulness meditation mobile app "calm" to reduce stress among college students: Randomized controlled trial. *JMIR mHealth and uHealth, 7*(6), e14273. https://doi.org/10.2196/14273

Hughes, A., Williams, M., Bardacke, N., Duncan, L. G., Dimidjian, S., & Goodman, S. H. (2009, October 1). Mindfulness approaches to childbirth and parenting. *British Journal of Midwifery, 17*(10), 630–635. https://doi.org/10.12968/bjom.2009.17.10.44470

Kabat-Zinn, J. (1982, April). An outpatient program in behavioral medicine for chronic pain patients based on the practice of mindfulness meditation: Theoretical considerations and preliminary results. *General Hospital Psychiatry, 4*(1), 33–47. https://doi.org/10.1016/0163-8343(82)90026-3

Kabat-Zinn, J. (2003). Mindfulness-based interventions in context: Past, present, and future. *Clinical Psychology: Science and Practice, 10*(2), 144–156. https://doi.org/10.1093/clipsy.bpg016

Kabat-Zinn, J. (2011). Some reflections on the origins of MBSR, skillful means, and the trouble with maps. *Contemporary Buddhism, 12*(1), 281–306. https://doi.org/10.1080/14639947.2011.564844

Kenny, M., Luck, P., & Koerbel, L. (2020). Tending the field of mindfulness-based programs: The development of international integrity guidelines for teachers and teacher training. *Global Advances in Health and Medicine, 9*, 2164956120923975. https://doi.org/10.1177/2164956120923975

Khoury, B., Sharma, M., Rush, S. E., & Fournier, C. (2015, June). Mindfulness-based stress reduction for healthy individuals: A meta-analysis. *Journal of Psychosomatic Research*, 78(6), 519–528. https://doi.org/10.1016/j.jpsychores.2015.03.009

King, A. P., Erickson, T. M., Giardino, N. D., Favorite, T., Rauch, S. A., Robinson, E., Kulkarni, M., & Liberzon, I. (2013, July). A pilot study of group mindfulness-based cognitive therapy (MBCT) for combat veterans with posttraumatic stress disorder (PTSD). *Depress Anxiety*, 30(7), 638–645. https://doi.org/10.1002/da.22104

Kinser, P. A., Thacker, L. R., Rider, A., Moyer, S., Amstadter, A. B., Mazzeo, S. E., . . . Starkweather, A. (2021, March–April 1). Feasibility, acceptability, and preliminary effects of "mindful moms": A mindful physical activity intervention for pregnant women with depression. *Nursing Research*, 70(2), 95–105. https://doi.org/10.1097/nnr.0000000000000485

Kroenke, K., Spitzer, R. L., & Williams, J. B. (2001, September). The PHQ-9: Validity of a brief depression severity measure. *Journal of General Internal Medicine*, 16(9), 606–613.

Kuyken, W., Byford, S., Taylor, R. S., Watkins, E., Holden, E., White, K., . . . Teasdale, J. D. (2008, December). Mindfulness-based cognitive therapy to prevent relapse in recurrent depression. *Journal of Consulting and Clinical Psychology*, 76(6), 966–978. https://doi.org/10.1037/a0013786

Lavender, T. J., Ebert, L., & Jones, D. (2016, October). An evaluation of perinatal mental health interventions: An integrative literature review. *Women and Birth*, 29(5), 399–406. https://doi.org/10.1016/j.wombi.2016.04.004

Lever Taylor, B., Cavanagh, K., & Strauss, C. (2016). The effectiveness of mindfulness-based interventions in the perinatal period: A systematic review and meta-analysis. *PLoS One*, 11(5), e0155720. https://doi.org/10.1371/journal.pone.0155720

Lönnberg, G., Jonas, W., Unternaehrer, E., Bränström, R., Nissen, E., & Niemi, M. (2020, February 1). Effects of a mindfulness based childbirth and parenting program on pregnant women's perceived stress and risk of perinatal depression-results from a randomized controlled trial. *Journal of Affective Disorders*, 262, 133–142. https://doi.org/10.1016/j.jad.2019.10.048

Lönnberg, G., Nissen, E., & Niemi, M. (2018, December 3). What is learned from mindfulness based childbirth and parenting education? – Participants' experiences. *BMC Pregnancy Childbirth*, 18(1), 466. https://doi.org/10.1186/s12884-018-2098-1

Luca, D. L., Margiotta, C., Staatz, C., Garlow, E., Christensen, A., & Zivin, K. (2020, June). Financial toll of untreated perinatal mood and anxiety disorders among 2017 births in the United States. *American Journal of Public Health*, 110(6), 888–896. https://doi.org/10.2105/ajph.2020.305619

Lucena, L., Frange, C., Pinto, A. C. A., Andersen, M. L., Tufik, S., & Hachul, H. (2020, November). Mindfulness interventions during pregnancy: A narrative review. *Journal of Integrative Medicine*, 18(6), 470–477. https://doi.org/10.1016/j.joim.2020.07.007

MacKenzie, M. B., Abbott, K. A., & Kocovski, N. L. (2018). Mindfulness-based cognitive therapy in patients with depression: Current perspectives. *Neuropsychiatric Disease and Treatment*, 14, 1599–1605. https://doi.org/10.2147/ndt.S160761

Mani, M., Kavanagh, D. J., Hides, L., & Stoyanov, S. R. (2015, August 19). Review and evaluation of mindfulness-based iPhone apps. *JMIR mHealth and uHealth*, 3(3), e82. https://doi.org/10.2196/mhealth.4328

Marcus, S. M. (2009, Winter). Depression during pregnancy: Rates, risks and consequences – Motherisk update 2008. *Canadian Journal of Clinical Pharmacology*, 16(1), e15–e22.

Matvienko-Sikar, K., Lee, L., Murphy, G., & Murphy, L. (2016, December). The effects of mindfulness interventions on prenatal well-being: A systematic review. *Psychology & Health*, 31(12), 1415–1434. https://doi.org/10.1080/08870446.2016.1220557

McMahan, D. L. (2009). *The making of Buddhist modernism*. Oxford University Press. https://doi.org/10.1093/acprof:oso/9780195183276.001.0001

Miklowitz, D. J., Semple, R. J., Hauser, M., Elkun, D., Weintraub, M. J., & Dimidjian, S. (2015, October). Mindfulness-based cognitive therapy for perinatal women with depression or bipolar spectrum disorder. *Cognitive Therapy and Research*, 39(5), 590–600. https://doi.org/10.1007/s10608-015-9681-9

Moulton-Perkins, A., Moulton, D., Cavanagh, K., Jozavi, A., & Strauss, C. (2022). Systematic review of mindfulness-based cognitive therapy and mindfulness-based stress reduction via group videoconferencing: Feasibility, acceptability, safety, and efficacy. *Journal of Psychotherapy Integration*, 32, 110–130. https://doi.org/10.1037/int0000216

Mrazek, A. J., Mrazek, M. D., Cherolini, C. M., Cloughesy, J. N., Cynman, D. J., Gougis, L. J., . . . Schooler, J. W. (2019). The future of mindfulness training is digital, and the future is now. *Current Opinion in Psychology*, *28*, 81–86. https://doi.org/10.1016/j.copsyc.2018.11.012

Musa, Z. A., Kim Lam, S., Binti Mamat @ Mukhtar, F., Kwong Yan, S., Tajudeen Olalekan, O., & Kim Geok, S. (2020). Effectiveness of mindfulness-based cognitive therapy on the management of depressive disorder: Systematic review. *International Journal of Africa Nursing Sciences*, *12*, 100200. https://doi.org/10.1016/j.ijans.2020.100200

Noggin, M. (2020). *Mindful mood balance*. Retrieved November 21, 2022, from https://mindfulnoggin.com/about/

Pan, W.-L., Chang, C.-W., Chen, S.-M., & Gau, M.-L. (2019). Assessing the effectiveness of mindfulness-based programs on mental health during pregnancy and early motherhood – a randomized control trial. *BMC Pregnancy and Childbirth*, *19*(1), 346. https://doi.org/10.1186/s12884-019-2503-4

Paterniti, S., Raab, K., Sterner, I., Collimore, K. C., Dalton, C., & Bisserbe, J. C. (2022). Individual mindfulness-based cognitive therapy in major depression: A feasibility study. *Mindfulness*, *13*(11), 2845–2856.

Perez-Blasco, J., Viguer, P., & Rodrigo, M. F. (2013, June). Effects of a mindfulness-based intervention on psychological distress, well-being, and maternal self-efficacy in breast-feeding mothers: Results of a pilot study. *Archives of Women's Mental Health*, *16*(3), 227–236. https://doi.org/10.1007/s00737-013-0337-z

Ponting, C., Mahrer, N. E., Zelcer, H., Dunkel Schetter, C., & Chavira, D. A. (2020). Psychological interventions for depression and anxiety in pregnant Latina and Black women in the United States: A systematic review. *Clinical Psychology & Psychotherapy*, *27*(2), 249–265. https://doi.org/10.1002/cpp.2424

Potharst, E. S., Aktar, E., Rexwinkel, M., Rigterink, M., & Bögels, S. M. (2017). Mindful with your baby: Feasibility, acceptability, and effects of a mindful parenting group training for mothers and their babies in a mental health context. *Mindfulness*, *8*(5), 1236–1250. https://doi.org/10.1007/s12671-017-0699-9

Proulx, J., Croff, R., Oken, B., Aldwin, C. M., Fleming, C., Bergen-Cico, D., . . . Noorani, M. (2018). Considerations for research and development of culturally relevant mindfulness interventions in American minority communities. *Mindfulness*, *9*(2), 361–370. https://doi.org/10.1007/s12671-017-0785-z

Roberts, L. R., & Montgomery, S. B. (2015, March). Mindfulness-based intervention for perinatal grief after stillbirth in Rural India. *Issues in Mental Health Nursing*, *36*(3), 222–230. https://doi.org/10.3109/01612840.2014.962676

Salmon, P., Lush, E., Jablonski, M., & Sephton, S. E. (2009). Yoga and mindfulness: Clinical aspects of an ancient mind/body practice. *Cognitive and Behavioral Practice*, *16*, 59–72. https://doi.org/10.1016/j.cbpra.2008.07.002

Schroevers, M. J., Tovote, K. A., Snippe, E., & Fleer, J. (2016). Group and individual mindfulness-based cognitive therapy (MBCT) are both effective: A pilot randomized controlled trial in depressed people with a somatic disease. *Mindfulness*, *7*, 1339–1346.

Segal, Z. V., Dimidjian, S., Beck, A., Boggs, J. M., Vanderkruik, R., Metcalf, C. A., . . . Levy, J. (2020). Outcomes of online mindfulness-based cognitive therapy for patients with residual depressive symptoms: A randomized clinical trial. *JAMA Psychiatry*, *77*(6), 563–573. https://doi.org/10.1001/jamapsychiatry.2019.4693

Segal, Z. V., Williams, J. M. G., & Teasdale, J. D. (2002). *Mindfulness-based cognitive therapy for depression: A new approach to preventing relapse*. Guilford Press.

Segal, Z. V., Williams, J. M. G., & Teasdale, J. D. (2012). *Mindfulness-based cognitive therapy for depression* (2nd ed.). Guilford Press.

Seng, J., Kane Low, L. M., Sperlich, M. I., Ronis, D. L., & Liverzon, I. (2009). Trauma history and risk for PTSD among nulliparous women in maternity care. *Obstetrics & Gynaecology*, *114*, 839–847.

Shulman, B., Dueck, R., Ryan, D., Breau, G., Sadowski, I., & Misri, S. (2018). Feasibility of a mindfulness-based cognitive therapy group intervention as an adjunctive treatment for postpartum depression and anxiety. *Journal of Affective Disorders*, *235*, 61–67. https://doi.org/10.1016/j.jad.2017.12.065

Sue, D. W. (2015). Therapeutic harm and cultural oppression. *The Counseling Psychologist, 43*(3), 359–369. https://doi.org/10.1177/0011000014565713

Thapaliya, S., Upadhyaya, K. D., Borschmann, R., & Kuppili, P. (2018). Mindfulness based interventions for depression and anxiety in Asian population: A systematic review. *Journal of Psychiatrists' Association of Nepal, 7.* https://doi.org/10.3126/jpan.v7i1.22933

Timlin, D., & Simpson, E. E. (2017, March). A preliminary randomised control trial of the effects of Dru yoga on psychological well-being in Northern Irish first time mothers. *Midwifery, 46,* 29–36. https://doi.org/10.1016/j.midw.2017.01.005

Traylor, C. S., Johnson, J. D., Kimmel, M. C., & Manuck, T. A. (2020, November). Effects of psychological stress on adverse pregnancy outcomes and nonpharmacologic approaches for reduction: An expert review. *American Journal of Obstetrics & Gynecology MFM, 2*(4), 100229. https://doi.org/10.1016/j.ajogmf.2020.100229

Van Dam, N. T., van Vugt, M. K., Vago, D. R., Schmalzl, L., Saron, C. D., Olendzki, A., . . . Meyer, D. E. (2018, January). Mind the hype: A critical evaluation and prescriptive agenda for research on mindfulness and meditation. *Perspectives on Psychological Science, 13*(1), 36–61. https://doi.org/10.1177/1745691617709589

van Emmerik, A., Keijzer, R., & Schoenmakers, T. (2020). Integrating mindfulness into a routine schedule: The role of mobile-health mindfulness applications. In (pp. 217–222). https://doi.org/10.1007/978-3-030-30892-6_15

Wahbeh, H., Sagher, A., Back, W., Pundhir, P., & Travis, F. (2018, January–February). A systematic review of transcendent states across meditation and contemplative traditions. *Explore (NY), 14*(1), 19–35. https://doi.org/10.1016/j.explore.2017.07.007

Watson-Singleton, N. N., Black, A. R., & Spivey, B. N. (2019, February). Recommendations for a culturally-responsive mindfulness-based intervention for African Americans. *Complementary Therapies in Clinical Practice, 34,* 132–138. https://doi.org/10.1016/j.ctcp.2018.11.013

Wilson, J. (2014). *Mindful America: The mutual transformation of Buddhist meditation and American culture.* Oxford University Press. https://doi.org/10.1093/acprof:oso/9780199827817.001.0001

Zhang, J. Y., Cui, Y. X., Zhou, Y. Q., & Li, Y. L. (2019, January). Effects of mindfulness-based stress reduction on prenatal stress, anxiety and depression. *Psychology, Health & Medicine, 24*(1), 51–58. https://doi.org/10.1080/13548506.2018.1468028

Zoogman, S., Goldberg, S. B., Hoyt, W. T., & Miller, L. (2015, April 1). Mindfulness interventions with youth: A meta-analysis. *Mindfulness, 6*(2), 290–302. https://doi.org/10.1007/s12671-013-0260-4

26

INTERNET INTERVENTIONS FOR PERINATAL MENTAL HEALTH DISORDERS

Siobhan A. Loughnan and Ashlee B. Grierson

Perinatal mental health concerns commonly remain underdiagnosed and undertreated in many countries in both women and men. Despite continued improvements in the implementation of routine screening in primary care and availability of effective evidence-based treatments, fewer than half of parents that are identified as anxious and/or depressed will seek help or receive evidence-based treatment (Austin, 2004; Cox et al., 2016; Earls et al., 2019; Goodman & Tyer-Viola, 2010; Kingston, Austin, et al., 2015; Woolhouse et al., 2009). The COVID-19 global pandemic has further amplified help-seeking and treatment barriers, with widespread disruptions to maternity care, reduced access to and provision of mental health services, and other psychosocial barriers such as social isolation (Lebel et al., 2020).

Over the past 30 years, digital technologies have greatly improved routine screening and mental health assessment (Martin-Key et al., 2021) and have increased the availability and accessibility of perinatal mental health support. Digital technologies in the form of Internet-based interventions help meet health system and clinician needs for standardized, scalable, and cost-effective treatment options, as well as support parents' needs for anonymity and privacy, convenience, and affordability (Andersson et al., 2014; Andrews et al., 2018; Carlbring et al., 2018). Currently available Internet-based interventions for perinatal populations range from Internet-based cognitive behavioral therapy (iCBT) and behavioral activation (iBA) programs to mindfulness-based and stress-reduction interventions. These Internet interventions are designed to mirror face-to-face treatments in terms of content and length and can be delivered with high fidelity while minimizing therapist drift (Carlbring et al., 2018; Lau et al., 2021).

Internet interventions can also be delivered in a variety of formats, including web-based services, smart phone applications, and email programs, and can be accessed in both self-guided and clinician-guided formats. Clinician-guided interventions include a varying degree of coaching or supervision, usually provided remotely via phone or email, and either can be offered as part of the program delivery (e.g., MindSpot, Australia; Titov et al., 2018, 2015) or require the user to nominate their own clinician to support their treatment progression (e.g., THIS WAY UP, Australia; Newby et al., 2021; Williams et al., 2014). In contrast, self-guided Internet interventions require no coaching or assistance by a health professional to be completed, with all support functions automated and delivered digitally (Andersson et al., 2019).

DOI: 10.4324/9781003206903-31

Suitability of Internet-Based Interventions for Perinatal Populations

A range of factors influence individual help-seeking behaviors in perinatal populations, including positive beliefs about treatment and confidence about individual change, which help increase treatment uptake and adherence (O'Mahen & Flynn, 2008). Yet even when positive treatment beliefs are expressed, other attitudinal and practical barriers can limit access and engagement with existing treatment services, including perceived stigma about disclosing mental health concerns, uncertainty around whether symptoms are normal or abnormal, time constraints, out-of-pocket costs, and logistical issues such as childcare arrangements (Kingston, Janes-Kelley, et al., 2015). Of these, the "cost to attend" face-to-face therapy is one of the greatest barriers to treatment identified by perinatal women and men (Anderson et al., 2016).

Internet-based interventions can help overcome many of these attitudinal and practical barriers for perinatal populations, providing parents with a mental health support option that is both accessible and effective. Internet-based interventions can be easily accessed at a convenient time and place (e.g., at home, while feeding, between sleep schedules), helping to avoid difficulties in committing to the time requirements of a treatment during a particularly time-poor time of life. In contrast to traditional treatment protocols, which can require up to 16 regularly scheduled face-to-face sessions (Austin et al., 2008), Internet interventions are typically delivered in 6–8 treatment sessions (i.e., lessons or modules; Milgrom et al., 2016), and can even be delivered effectively in as little as three lessons (Loughnan, Butler, et al., 2019; Loughnan, Sie, et al., 2019). Additionally, Internet interventions can provide a greater degree of anonymity and privacy to parents by opening pathways to self-refer to and complete treatment without the need to access care through a clinician. This can help minimize reluctance to disclose symptoms due to the perceived social stigma associated with anxiety and depression as a parent, which is often discordant with societal expectations that the perinatal period is a time of immense joy and happiness (Biaggi et al., 2016). Internet interventions also help remove geographical barriers to treatment (i.e., proximity to services), reaching parents residing in communities who may otherwise not receive treatment at all, such as rural and remote communities (Dennis & Chung-Lee, 2006; Goodman, 2009; Thompson et al., 2004).

Importantly, Internet interventions can be accessed at no or low-to-moderate cost by both parents and clinicians. This is due to a marked reduction in clinician time required in delivering treatments via the Internet (Carlbring et al., 2018), and when Internet programs are used as an adjunct to face-to-face appointments. For self-guided Internet interventions, no additional clinical resources are required once an intervention is accessed from a publicly available web-based service or smartphone application. Internet interventions are also a cost-effective option for health systems due to their long-term impact on health improvements and recovery, as well as their capacity for large-scale dissemination and integration into current healthcare systems (Richards et al., 2020).

Structure and Components of Internet-Based Interventions for Perinatal Populations

Internet-based interventions for perinatal populations are delivered in the form of a structured program or course consisting of modules, lessons, or workbooks. Users commonly progress through the content in a sequential pre-determined order (i.e., lesson approach) or in a flexible modular approach with users deciding their preferred order of completion. On average, most Internet interventions consist of 6–8 modules or lessons delivered over the course of two to three months (Milgrom et al., 2016) with some interventions delivering treatment in as little as three lessons (one to three hours each) over four weeks (e.g., Loughnan, Butler, et al., 2019; Loughnan, Sie, et al., 2019). Individual modules or lessons focus on key topics for perinatal mental health, such as psychoeducation on perinatal emotional and physical symptoms, how to tackle maladaptive cognitions and behaviors, stress management and relaxation, and strategies for increasing pleasant activities and self-care. Internet interventions such as iCBT, iBA, and mindfulness-based interventions explore these key topics within a traditional cognitive behavioral therapy, behavioral activation, and mindfulness framework. For example, maladaptive cognitions are explored alongside evidenced techniques such as cognitive restructuring or reframing, and becoming aware of existing thoughts, emotions, and sensations to cultivate acceptance of each moment. Intervention content is delivered in the form of text, video, and/or audio, with all forms commonly integrated in a multimodal style of delivery. Some interventions utilize graphically illustrated parent stories to deliver treatment content and show dialogue between characters and health professionals as they learn skills and strategies to identify and manage symptoms. See Table 26.1 for program characteristics of a selected range of Internet interventions that have been evaluated in a randomized controlled trial (RCT) and demonstrated efficacy and acceptability in treating anxiety, depression and/or posttraumatic stress symptoms in perinatal women.

Table 26.1 A Selected Range of Evidence-Based Internet Interventions for Perinatal Mental Health

Targeted Mental Health Issue	*Program Name and Country*	*Program Characteristics*	
		Format	*Content*
Prenatal anxiety and depression	THIS WAY UP Pregnancy program; Australia (Loughnan, Sie, et al., 2019; Mahoney et al., 2023)	Three lessons accessed sequentially over four weeks; available as clinician-guided and self-guided for Australian users; available only as clinician-guided for international users.	• CBT-based content: psychoeducation, self-care practices, controlled breathing, progressive muscle relaxation, thought challenging, structured problem solving, activity planning, graded exposure, assertive communication, and relapse prevention. • Each lesson consists of a set of lesson slides (character stories), brief lesson summary, and action plan. • Extensive range of extra resources.

(Continued)

Table 26.1 (Continued)

Targeted Mental Health Issue	Program Name and Country	Program Characteristics	
		Format	*Content*
Prenatal anxiety and depression	China (Yang et al., 2019)	Four sessions delivered over eight weeks; evaluated as therapist-guided with support provided by nurses who contacted participants via video or telephone	• Mindfulness-based therapy content: paying attention to the intended target and discriminating present experiences; adopting an accepting attitude toward physical and emotional experiences. • Each session consisted of a review of previous session, introduction to central theme of current mindfulness practice, and assignment of homework for upcoming week. • All sessions were recorded and uploaded to platform including additional text, pictures, and audio for review
Prenatal depression	Sweden (Forsell et al., 2017)	Seven to ten modules delivered over ten weeks; evaluated as clinician-guided with support provided by CBT-trained therapist via online platform	• CBT-based content: psychoeducation, behavioral activation, cognitive restructuring, relationships, summary and relapse prevention. • Optional modules for anxiety and worry, and sleep problems. • Each module consists of reading material, assessments, homework and worksheets
Prenatal depression	United States (Kelman et al., 2018)	Initial 45-minute didactic course to introduce course materials, followed by 14 days of follow-up materials presented via email	• Compassion-focused content: finding ourselves here in the flow of life, old brain/new brain, affect regulation, and cultivating the compassionate self. Audio meditations as follow-up materials. • iCBT program: thoughts, activities, assertiveness, and sleep. CBT exercises as follow-up materials.

(Continued)

Table 26.1 (Continued)

Targeted Mental Health Issue	Program Name and Country	Program Characteristics	
		Format	Content
Childbirth-related posttraumatic stress	Sweden (Nieminen, Berg et al., 2016)		• Trauma-focused CBT content: psychoeducation, anxiety coping methods and skill training, imaginary and *in vivo* exposure, cognitive restructuring. • 8 modules consisting of written information including homework activities
Postpartum anxiety and depression	THIS WAY UP postpartum program, Australia (Loughnan, Butler, et al., 2019; Mahoney et al., 2023)	Three sequential lessons delivered over six weeks; available as clinician-guided and self-guided for Australian users; only available as clinician-guided for international users	• CBT-based content: psychoeducation, self-care practices, controlled breathing, progressive muscle relaxation, thought challenging, structured problem solving, activity planning, graded exposure, assertive communication, and relapse prevention. • Each lesson consists of a set of lesson slides (character stories), brief lesson summary and action plan; range of supplementary resources • Extensive range of extra resources available.
Postpartum depression	Maternal Depression Online, Canada (Pugh et al., 2016)	Seven sequential modules delivered over seven weeks; evaluated as clinician-guided with support provided weekly by clinical psychology doctoral students via email	• CBT-based content relevant to mothers of young infants • Delivered via a range of media (e.g., text, graphics, animation, audio, video), including check-in questions at the start of each module and homework exercises at end of each module.

(Continued)

Table 26.1 (Continued)

Targeted Mental Health Issue	Program Name and Country	Program Characteristics	
		Format	Content
Postpartum depression	NetMums/ NetMumsHWD, United Kingdom (O'Mahen et al., 2014, 2013)	NetMums (original): 11 sessions delivered over 15 weeks NetMumsHWD (modified): 12 sessions consisting of five core modules and a relapse prevention module with an additional six optional modules; evaluated as clinician-guided with support provided weekly via telephone.	• BA-based content: self-monitoring, role of avoidance, goal-oriented behaviors, problem solving, contingency planning, communication strategies, addressing support needs, rumination strategies, and relapse prevention. • Sessions presented via multimedia with interactive in-session and homework exercises. • Additional local peer support available, including online chat room.
Postpartum depression	MomMoodBooster, United States; MumMoodBooster, Australia (Danaher et al., 2013; Milgrom et al., 2016)	Six sequential sessions delivered over 6–12 weeks; evaluated as clinician-guided with support provided weekly via telephone by graduate research assistants or research psychologists	• CBT-based content: getting started, managing mood, increasing pleasant activities, managing negative thoughts, increasing positive thoughts, and planning for the future. • Each session opens with a video with content delivered on webpages as text. • Additional peer-based web forum and partner support website.

Interventions are commonly accessed using an Internet platform to deliver and manage the intervention, including assessment instruments to monitor progress, and technology to facilitate clinician guidance or support. Most Internet interventions also include in-built automated notifications and reminders to assist with treatment engagement and completion. Automated email and SMS notifications can help increase adherence and completion rates by reminding users to login and complete their next module when available, or to complete unfinished modules. Automated functions are also used to provide crisis referral information (e.g., national mental health services and helplines), which are particularly important for users completing self-report assessments throughout the program (e.g., prior to each lesson) who indicate severe symptoms of distress, depression, and/or suicidality.

Reliable and built-in risk management protocols are important factors for health professionals and self-referring parents when using Internet interventions as a stand-alone or adjunct treatment for perinatal mental health concerns.

Effectiveness and Efficacy of Internet Interventions for Perinatal Populations

Overall, there is good support for the use of Internet interventions for perinatal mental health disorders, namely in the treatment of clinically significant symptoms, as well as some support for the use of preventive and general well-being programs. Several reviews have now synthesized the evidence base of interventions available across a range of perinatal mental health concerns, primarily in depression and anxiety (Ashford et al., 2016; Lau et al., 2021; Loughnan, Butler, et al., 2019). Other RCTs and pilot studies have also been completed in the areas of stress management, fear of childbirth (Nieminen, Andersson, et al., 2016), posttraumatic stress after childbirth (Nieminen, Berg, et al., 2016), and complicated grief after pregnancy loss (Kersting et al., 2013). Importantly, Internet interventions such as iCBT have shown efficacy and acceptability in treating depression and anxiety in the perinatal period across both clinician-guided (i.e., clinician guidance or therapist coaching provided) and self-guided formats (Lau et al., 2021; Loughnan, Joubert, et al., 2019) with growing evidence of their effectiveness in routine care (Mahoney et al., 2023).

Perinatal Depression

For depression during pregnancy and postpartum, most studies have investigated the utility of interventions based on CBT (i.e., iCBT), which has been demonstrated to be an efficacious Internet-based treatment for depression in the general adult population (Andrews et al., 2010). Two meta-analytic studies showed superiority of Internet interventions for depression outcomes compared to control condition with a moderate mean between-group effect size at post-intervention (Hedge's $g = -0.56$, 95% CI: -0.85, -0.27, $n = 15$ studies, Lau et al., 2021; $g = 0.55$ (adjusted), 95% CI: 0.38, 0.71, $n = 5$ studies; Loughnan, Joubert, et al., 2019). Subgroup analyses by Lau and colleagues (2021) found effect sizes were greater among postpartum women ($g = -0.78$, 95% CI: -1.19, -0.37) than prenatal women ($g = -0.22$, 95% CI: -0.55, 0.11; Lau et al., 2021).

It is unclear if positive effects continue long-term as few studies include follow-up assessments. Meta-analysis showed a small between-group effect size at follow-up for depression outcomes ($g = -0.28$; 95% CI: -0.60, 0.04; $p = 0.08$; $n = 5$ studies; Lau et al., 2021). At an individual study level, several interventions delivered in a clinician-guided format have demonstrated reductions in perinatal depressive symptoms that were sustained for one to six months post-treatment (Ashford et al., 2018; Forsell et al., 2017; Kim et al., 2014; Milgrom et al., 2016). Self-guided iCBT programs have identified similar effects, where RCTs have demonstrated large effect size reductions in depression that were sustained for one month (Loughnan, Butler, et al., 2019; Loughnan, Sie, et al., 2019). In a meta-analysis by Lau and colleagues (2021), subgroup analyses explored effect sizes based on intervention characteristics, where interventions delivered over six weeks or longer ($g = -0.75$, 95% CI: -1.32, -0.18) and consisting of eight or more sessions demonstrated greater effect size reduction in symptoms of depression compared with other intervention types ($g = -0.68$; 95% CI: -1.05, -0.30). Furthermore, interventions which included CBT and other therapeutic components ($g = -0.82$, 95% CI: -1.99, 0.35) showed greater effect sizes than those including only behavioral activation ($g = -0.59$, 95% CI: -0.78, -0.40) or CBT alone ($g = -0.42$, 95% CI: -0.72. -0.13; Lau et al., 2021).

Little research has focused on preventive Internet interventions for perinatal mental health; however preliminary findings appear promising. In Norway, an RCT was conducted to assess the effectiveness of a self-guided preventive Internet intervention which specifically targets risk and protective factors for depressive symptoms from pregnancy through to postpartum (44 sessions over 11.5 months; Haga et al., 2019). Mothers that received the intervention (alongside usual perinatal care at a Norwegian well-baby clinic) demonstrated significantly lower depressive symptoms at gestational week 37 (-0.65, 95% CI: -1.13, -0.17) and at six weeks postpartum (-0.56, 95% CI: -1.07, -0.05), compared to the control condition. However no significant differences were observed at three and six months postpartum.

Internet interventions for fathers have also received little attention in both the prevention and treatment of perinatal mental health. In Australia, a web-based text messaging intervention, *SMS4dads*, was developed as an early depression prevention program for fathers and has shown promise as an acceptable and feasible intervention to support men in their transition to fatherhood (Fletcher et al., 2017). In a feasibility study ($n = 520$ fathers recruited over eight months), the average duration of intervention use was 21 weeks (range $= 0$ to 45 weeks) with 63% of fathers clicking at least one link and 20.5% responding to mood tracker questions. Longitudinal analysis ($n = 240$ fathers) showed the probability of reporting worse mood scores on the mood tracker decreased over time (odds ratio (OR) $= 0.95$, $p = 0.0295$). Fathers who self-reported higher distress scores at baseline (>13 on six-item *Kessler Psychological Distress Scale* (K6)) had increased odds of having worse mood tracking scores (OR $= 2.79$, $p = 0.0004$), compared to those who had lower baseline distress scores (score of 0–13 on K6); yet there was no significant difference in trends over time between these two groups (OR $= 0.97$, $p = 0.6459$). Follow-up assessment ($n = 101$) showed the impact of the intervention was positive with fathers reporting that the messages helped them in their experience of becoming a new father (92.8%) and helped develop a strong relationship with their baby (54.9%) and partner (79%).

In 2019, a process evaluation of the text-messaging intervention was conducted with 40 Australian fathers to explore mechanisms of impact. Fathers were enrolled between 16 weeks' gestation and 12 weeks postpartum; and demonstrated post-program reductions in feelings of social isolation, and improvements in transitioning to their role as a new dad and in their relationship with their partner (Fletcher et al., 2019). The mechanisms by which the program was found to work were both structural and psychological, including syncing information to needs, normalization of emotions and thoughts, the provision of a safety net, boosting of confidence, and a sense of being connected. *SMS4dads* highlights the benefits of tailored interventions for parents in the perinatal period, where personalized and accessible treatment approaches should be the focus of future perinatal Internet intervention research (Fletcher et al., 2019).

Perinatal Anxiety

Compared to depression, perinatal anxiety has received significantly less attention in the context of Internet-based interventions, with few programs designed to directly address anxiety symptomology with or without depressive symptoms. As anxiety and depression commonly co-occur in perinatal populations, transdiagnostic programs have shown promise in this population (Loughnan, Butler, et al., 2019; Loughnan, Sie, et al., 2019), and could be expected to reduce the risk of relapse and need for additional anxiety or depression treatment. One RCT of an prenatal-specific iCBT intervention targeting anxiety and depression demonstrated superior improvements in anxiety symptoms for the intervention group compared to a usual care control group, with a moderate-to-large effect size at four-week follow-up ($g = 0.76$; 95% CI: 0.17, 1.35), yet no significant difference observed between groups at post-intervention (Loughnan, Sie, et al., 2019). A second RCT of a postpartum-specific iCBT intervention targeting anxiety and depression demonstrated a moderate-to-large effect size reduction in anxiety symptoms at post-intervention ($g = 0.78$; 95% CI: 0.36, 1.19) and sustained at four-week follow-up ($g = 1.14$; 95% CI: 0.66, 1.62; Loughnan, Butler, et al., 2019).

Anxiety outcomes for interventions addressing depression, but not anxiety specifically, have been mixed, with some studies demonstrating large and significant improvements in anxiety (postpartum sample: Cohen's $d = -0.59$, 95% CI: -1.11, -0.07; O'Mahen et al., 2014) and others small and nonsignificant differences at post-intervention compared to control conditions (prenatal sample: $g = 0.63$, 95% CI: -0.84, 2.10; Forsell et al., 2017; postpartum sample: $d = 0.18$, 95% CI: -0.42, 0.78; Milgrom et al., 2016). However, when all perinatal internet interventions are pooled using meta-analysis, a small-to-moderate effect on anxiety symptoms at post-treatment has been indicated ($g = 0.54$; 95% CI: 0.24, 0.85, $n = 4$ studies, Loughnan, Joubert, et al., 2019; $g = -0.30$, 95% CI: -0.44, -0.17, $n = 11$ studies, Lau et al., 2021).

Mindfulness-based and compassion-focused Internet interventions have also shown similar promise for perinatal anxiety and depression (Kelman et al., 2018; Yang et al., 2019). One RCT was conducted to evaluate the efficacy and acceptability of an Internet-based mindfulness training intervention. Pregnant women with elevated depressive or anxiety symptoms were recruited from a hospital in China and randomized to an eight-week mindfulness Internet intervention (four sessions based on mindfulness principles of attention monitoring and acceptance) or a routine care control condition (Yang et al., 2019). Women in the mindfulness training group showed greater reductions in depressive and anxious symptoms at post-intervention compared with those in the control group (depression symptoms: $t = -5.212$, $p < .001$; anxiety symptoms: $t = -4.853$, $p < .001$, Yang et al., 2019). Participants also demonstrated a significant improvement in mindfulness at post-intervention ($t = 4.501$, $p < .001$). In a pilot RCT, pregnant and postpartum women and women intending to become pregnant were randomized to a brief compassionate mind training Internet intervention (including information on finding ourselves here in the flow of life; old brain and new brain; the three circles of affect regulation and pregnancy; and cultivating the compassionate self) or a brief iCBT program (including information on cognitions, behavioral activation, interpersonal effectiveness, and sleep hygiene). Both groups received 45-minute didactic programs with follow-up materials provided via email following course completion. Women who received the compassionate mind training program showed greater reductions in depression ($F(1, 82) = 4.88$, $p = .03$) and anxiety symptoms ($F(1, 82) = 4.42$, $p = .04$) at two weeks post-completion of the course, compared to women who received the 45-minute didactic iCBT course (Kelman et al., 2018). Other mindfulness-based Internet interventions (e.g., *mindmom*) are currently being trialed to evaluate their effectiveness in reducing pregnancy-related depression for women (Müller et al., 2020). In addition, Internet interventions for stress management for women experiencing pregnancy complications have been evaluated. In an RCT, a self-guided stress management focused iCBT program for women experiencing premature labor was compared to a usual care control condition with both groups demonstrating significant symptom reductions in stress and anxiety from pre- to post-intervention (Scherer et al., 2016).

Engagement and Adherence to Internet-Based Interventions

iCBT appears to be an acceptable method of treatment delivery with RCTs showing high adherence rates to programs delivered in the prenatal period (self-guided: 76%, Loughnan, Sie, et al., 2019; clinician-guided: 82–83%, Forsell et al., 2017; Kim et al., 2014) and moderate to high adherence rates to programs delivered postpartum (self-guided: 75%, Loughnan, Butler, et al., 2019; clinician-guided: 60%–97%, Lau et al., 2017). Similarly, high rates of adherence have been reported for online mindfulness training for pregnant women, where 84% of women completed at least three lessons (Yang et al., 2019). iBA has also shown moderate rates of program adherence with women completing an average of five Internet sessions and a mode of 12 telephone sessions (O'Mahen et al., 2014; O'Mahen et al., 2013).

As could be expected, intensive iCBT programs with the largest number of treatment sessions (e.g., more than six modules) and longest treatment period (e.g., 15 weeks) report the lowest adherence rates and participant satisfaction in this population. A limited number of studies have investigated other correlates of adherence to Internet-based interventions in a perinatal population, with some evidence suggesting that lower perceived social support, working or studying, higher work and social impairment, and lower socioeconomic status are predictive of poorer adherence (O'Mahen et al., 2014).

Whilst iCBT for perinatal anxiety and depression are promising under research conditions, limited research has been published evaluating the effectiveness of perinatal iCBT programs when delivered in routine care. Broader iCBT research for anxiety and depression in the general adult population has found adherence to iCBT to be lower in routine care compared to RCT settings (Mahoney et al., 2021; Newby et al., 2013) and most markedly for self-guided programs that receive no clinician support (Morgan et al., 2017). Recent studies have sought to close this gap and investigate the effectiveness of iCBT in routine care. For example, Mahoney and colleagues (2023) evaluated the effectiveness of two brief iCBT programs for pregnant and postpartum women when delivered in a self-guided or clinician-guided format via an online clinic based in Australia. Participants included women who were experiencing anxiety and depressive symptoms across the full spectrum of severity with 30–40% self-reporting subthreshold symptom severity (most RCTs only include participants experiencing clinical threshold symptoms). The mean number of lessons completed for the clinician-guided versus self-guided programs was similar (pregnancy: $M(SD)$ = 1.93(0.88); postpartum: $M(SD)$ = 2.07(0.87)) with approximately 35% and 42% of women completing all lessons. Program completion rates were lower in this study compared to previous RCTs, though they were consistent with rates observed for iCBT programs disseminated in routine care which range from 14% to 47% (Hobbs et al., 2017, 2018; Morgan et al., 2017; Grierson et al., 2020). When delivered in routine care, both the pregnancy and postpartum iCBT programs were associated with medium pre- to post-treatment effect size reductions in symptoms of generalized anxiety (pregnancy: g = 0.63, 95% CI: 0.50, 0.75; postpartum: g = 0.71, 95% CI: 0.62, 0.80), depression (pregnancy: g = 0.58, 95% CI: 0.46, 0.70; postpartum: g = 0.64, 95% CI: 0.55, 0.74), and psychological distress (pregnancy: g = 0.52, 95% CI: 0.40, 0.64; postpartum: g = 0.60, 95% CI: 0.51, 0.69). Consistent with prior research, women in the clinician-guided intervention experienced slightly greater improvements in symptom severity compared to participants who completed the program as self-guided (Mahoney et al., 2023). Additional investigation is justified to clarify the impact of patient-related and contextual factors on therapy effectiveness, as well as factors that may moderate or mediate outcomes across treatment settings. For example, approximately half of women included in this study were recommended their perinatal program by a health professional (Mahoney et al., 2023), where it could be important for future research to examine factors driving the uptake of Internet programs and how these variables impact program effectiveness.

Case Study

Cherie is a new mum with a four-month-old baby. She has always been very driven and successful both at school and in her working life. She has been looking forward to this stage in her life since she married her husband and they decided they would have a child when she turned 30 years old and a little more financially secure. So, when she became a mum, Cherie couldn't understand all the powerful feelings of being overwhelmed and inadequate. She finds she worries her baby doesn't like her as he cries all the time when she has him on her own. She feels she is not good at being a mother and maybe she just shouldn't have had a child, but she is so ashamed of these thoughts she feels she can't tell anyone.

One day, Cherie searches online for information about her feelings and she comes across an Internet-based program created to help parents manage feelings of anxiety and low mood during pregnancy and postpartum. This online program is free and has a self-help option, so Cherie signs up straight away. She likes the idea that she can access the program immediately and doesn't need a referral from her doctor, so she can keep her thoughts and feelings confidential for now. The program recommends completing a module each week, which Cherie thinks is manageable. Cherie receives automatic emails every week from the online program, which help remind her to log back in and encourage her to read through the content.

Over the next few weeks, Cherie manages to snatch 10- to 15-minute blocks of time between her son's naps and other household tasks. She likes that she can do bits and pieces of the program when it suits and that she doesn't need to organize for a babysitter like if she would to attend a face-to-face appointment. Cherie particularly likes the audio mindfulness meditations in the program to calm herself and her son down when she is putting him down for his naps. She has also been finding the program helpful in tackling unhelpful behaviors like avoiding going out, such as going to the grocery store or to mother's group and has found the information helpful in learning how to accept uncertainty. One behavior that Cherie has been able to change which has been powerful for her is going out of the house on her own with her baby. Previously, she was so worried that if he cried while she was out that it meant she was not a good mother, so she just avoided go out. By reading the online program information and practicing some of the strategies, Cherie has been able to reframe this thought from "I'm failing as a mother" to "All babies cry sometimes, and I can change my plans and come home to accommodate his needs if necessary." Sometimes during the night, when Cherie finds her thoughts are keeping her from sleeping, she will get up and practice parts of the online program on her phone or laptop. She can select the modules and topics that are relevant to her at the time, such as practicing ways to manage her thoughts so she can get back to sleep. It's also helpful to remind herself of some sleep hygiene strategies that she can prioritize before bed. Cherie particularly likes the Progressive Muscle Relaxation exercise for those times at night.

By using the program, Cherie starts to understand that the feelings she has been having are much more common than she thought and that just because she thinks something, it doesn't mean it's necessarily true (e.g., that she is a bad mum). At her next doctor's appointment, Cherie is asked how she has been coping with a new baby. For the first time, Cherie tells her doctor about the online program she has been using and the things she has learned about her thoughts and worries. The doctor reinforces to Cherie that lots of parents have similar feelings and that there is additional face-to-face support available for new parents just like her. Cherie feels the online program is enough at this stage but feels comfortable talking with her doctor and asking for help in the future if she needs.

Internet-Based Interventions for Other Perinatal-Related Concerns

It is also important to establish whether Internet-based interventions can offer benefit to parents beyond reductions in anxiety, depression, and distress. Few studies of Internet-based interventions have extended their investigations to focus on other outcomes related to parent well-being that may be improved through Internet-based interventions. In studies of Internet-based interventions for perinatal depression and anxiety, emerging evidence has found iCBT to significantly improve other outcomes not directly targeted in treatment content, including maternal bonding with the infant, parenting confidence, and maternal quality of life (Loughnan, Butler, et al., 2019; Loughnan, Sie, et al., 2019). These are interesting and important findings for future research and suggest that mental health interventions presented in an online format may be worthwhile investigating for other perinatal-related concerns.

Internet-Based Interventions and Posttraumatic Stress

After childbirth, up to 34% of women report moderate to severe symptoms of acute stress (Soet et al., 2003). At one month postpartum, about 3% of women meet diagnostic criteria for posttraumatic stress disorder (PTSD; Wijma, 2006). Childbirth-related PTSD has severe consequences with long-lasting adverse effects on the emotional and social well-being of the mother, partner, and child (Ayers et al., 2006). One study has investigated trauma-focused clinician-guided iCBT for the treatment of posttraumatic stress symptoms following childbirth (Nieminen, Berg et al., 2016). Mothers were provided with eight web-based modules to complete over eight weeks and were guided by a clinician. Trauma-focused iCBT showed large effect size reductions in posttraumatic stress symptoms, as well as large effect size reductions in comorbid depression and anxiety, and improvements in quality of life. Further studies are needed to examine the long-term effects of trauma-focused iCBT for childbirth-related posttraumatic stress symptoms, however preliminary investigations are encouraging and suggest that Internet-based interventions may have some utility in the treatment of perinatal posttraumatic stress.

Internet-Based Interventions and Perinatal Grief

The death of a baby during pregnancy or soon after birth is a devastating outcome, with long-lasting psychological, social, and economic consequences on parents and families extending into subsequent pregnancies (Ellis et al., 2016; Flenady et al., 2016; Heazell et al., 2016). Perinatal loss increases a woman's risk for major depressive disorder (Johnson et al., 2016; Klier et al., 2002) with 60–70% of women meeting diagnostic criteria for grief-related depression up to one year after their baby's death, and 50% of those experiencing depression for at least four years post-loss (Heazell et al., 2016; Kersting et al., 2013). There are also adverse impacts on other family members, particularly spouse and siblings, following stillbirth or neonatal death, and significant economic impacts in terms of both personal impact (e.g., inability to work, loss of income) and societal costs (e.g., increased welfare payment, lost income-tax; Heazell et al., 2016; Murphy & Cacciatore, 2017; Schofield et al., 2006).

Internet-delivered supports, including courses and programs, are one option to increase accessibility to evidence-based and effective perinatal bereavement and mental health support for both bereaved parents during a time which many find difficult to access evidence-based support, both attitudinally and logistically (Loughnan et al., 2022). This is important considering many parents will become pregnant again within a year of the death of their baby (Mills et al., 2016; Wojcieszek et al., 2018) and often experience conflicted emotions, including intense anxiety, fear, depression, and may not bond with their baby as a coping mechanism (Heazell et al., 2019; Mills et al., 2014). Furthermore, parents who have experienced the tragedy of stillbirth are five times more likely to have a stillborn baby in their next pregnancy and are at increased risk for other adverse pregnancy outcomes such as pre-term birth (Lamont et al., 2015). Despite these risks, this group remain under-represented in the research concerning types of psychosocial support required to best meet the needs of bereaved parents at the time of loss and in subsequent pregnancies (Koopmans et al., 2013; Wojcieszek, Shepherd, et al., 2018).

Future Directions for Internet Interventions in Perinatal Populations

Given the significant and long-term health, economic, and intergenerational impacts of perinatal mental health concerns, further research on scalable and cost-effective treatments such as Internet interventions is justified. This is particularly true for gaps identified in the perinatal literature, including Internet interventions for other perinatal-related mental health concerns, as well as for underexplored populations such as fathers, parents residing in rural and remote communities, and cultural and linguistically diverse populations.

Paternal perinatal depression and anxiety is slowly being recognized as an important public health priority, with up to 10% of fathers experiencing significant symptoms (Rodrigues et al., 2022). Nonetheless, few evidence-based interventions are currently available, and only a small portion of depressed or anxious fathers typically engage with support (Fletcher et al., 2023; Rodrigues et al., 2022; Rominov et al., 2018). To date, most Internet interventions have focused solely on mothers. However, some Internet interventions have shown promise in reaching fathers, particularly for prevention of mental health problems. In Australia, a novel web-based text messaging intervention, *SMS4dads* has shown effectiveness in providing parenting information to support men in their transition to fatherhood (Fletcher et al., 2017); and demonstrated feasibility in identifying distressed fathers living in rural areas (Fletcher et al., 2023). Couple-based interventions may also be feasible for prevention of perinatal mental health concerns. Pilkington and colleagues (2017) published their formative work on the development of a web-based intervention (i.e., *Partners to Parents website*) for both mothers and fathers to prevent perinatal anxiety and depression. Content included parenthood, connection, teamwork, health, mood, and further options for support, where user testing showed parents appreciated the personalization of the website and simple design. Utilizing Internet interventions to prevent perinatal mental health difficulties and optimize parental well-being from a couples-based approach is a key area for future research.

Furthermore, most interventions have been evaluated in Western and high-income countries. Of these samples, most parents resided within metropolitan areas with widespread access to technology. Some caution is therefore warranted in evaluating program efficacy, as it is unknown whether these interventions would be as effective in other countries, and especially in rural and remote communities where there may be inequitable access to digital services and resources. It is also important to acknowledge the existing digital divide, namely the inequity of access to digital technology and disparities in technological health literacy for many parents, including in culturally and linguistically diverse communities (Titov et al., 2019). Most systematic reviews and meta-analyses have reviewed studies with participants from English-speaking countries and communities, which limits the generalizability of these findings. One systematic review has examined six studies of technology-based interventions for perinatal depression and anxiety in Latina and African American women (Lara-Cinisomo et al., 2021), demonstrating high patient satisfaction and promise for symptom management. If we are to increase perinatal mental health screening and treatment uptake with those most in need, it is important for researchers to continue to evaluate whether Internet interventions are acceptable and effective in different cultural, ethnic, and socioeconomic contexts. Future research should also investigate mental health knowledge or literacy influences help-seeking behavior and its impact on treatment engagement with Internet interventions outside Western countries, and how these factors can be improved by tailoring programs to culturally and linguistically diverse communities.

Conclusion

The delivery of accessible and evidence-based mental health support for parents throughout the perinatal period is a worldwide public health priority. Internet-based interventions have been shown to be effective and acceptable in perinatal populations and have the potential to overcome attitudinal and practical barriers to care. Internet interventions also have the potential to be integrated into current healthcare systems for perinatal populations, with many interventions already being used as an adjunct to face-to-face therapy and in usual community care. The shifting landscape of mental health treatment in the digital age has been demonstrated through the rapidly growing engagement of parents with digital resources for mental health support such as Internet-based programs, social media, forum-based support groups, and podcasts. This has been particularly evident during the COVID-19 pandemic, with face-to-face delivery of mental health support services either being limited or otherwise unavailable parallel to an increased volume of users demanding access to digital health services (e.g., Mahoney et al., 2021; Palmer et al., 2021). While further studies are needed to evaluate the effectiveness of Internet interventions in diverse communities and other perinatal health concerns, Internet interventions represent an effective and scalable treatment option that can be integrated into existing healthcare systems, and one which will help increase the accessibility and availability of evidence-based mental healthcare for parents during this critical period of life.

References

Anderson, R., Wong, N., Newby, J. M., & Andrews, G. (2016). The non-medical out-of-pocket costs to attend a free anxiety disorders treatment clinic in Australia. *Australasian Psychiatry, 24*(3), 261–263.

Andersson, G., Cuijpers, P., Carlbring, P., Riper, H., & Hedman, E. (2014). Guided Internet-based vs. face-to-face cognitive behavior therapy for psychiatric and somatic disorders: A systematic review and meta-analysis. *World Psychiatry, 13*(3), 288–295.

Andersson, G., Titov, N., Dear, B. F., Rozental, A., & Carlbring, P. (2019). Internet-delivered psychological treatments: From innovation to implementation. *World Psychiatry, 18*(1), 20–28.

Andrews, G., Basu, A., Cuijpers, P., Craske, M. G., McEvoy, P., English, C. L., & Newby, J. M. (2018). Computer therapy for the anxiety and depression disorders is effective, acceptable and practical health care: An updated meta-analysis. *Journal of Anxiety Disorders, 55*, 70–78.

Andrews, G., Cuijpers, P., Craske, M. G., McEvoy, P., & Titov, N. (2010). Computer therapy for the anxiety and depressive disorders is effective, acceptable and practical health care: A meta-analysis. *PloS One, 5*(10), e13196.

Ashford, M. T., Olander, E. K., & Ayers, S. (2016). Computer-or web-based interventions for perinatal mental health: A systematic review. *Journal of Affective Disorders, 197*, 134–146.

Ashford, M. T., Olander, E. K., Rowe, H., Fisher, J. R., & Ayers, S. (2018). Feasibility and acceptability of a web-based treatment with telephone support for postpartum women with anxiety: Randomized controlled trial. *JMIR Mental Health, 5*(2), e9106.

Austin, M.-P. (2004). Antenatal screening and early intervention for "perinatal" distress, depression and anxiety: Where to from here? *Archives of Women's Mental Health, 7*(1), 1–6.

Austin, M.-P., Frilingos, M., Lumley, J., Hadzi-Pavlovic, D., Roncolato, W., Acland, S., . . . Parker, G. (2008). Brief antenatal cognitive behaviour therapy group intervention for the prevention of postnatal depression and anxiety: A randomised controlled trial. *Journal of Affective Disorders, 105*(1), 35–44.

Ayers, S., Eagle, A., & Waring, H. (2006). The effects of childbirth-related post-traumatic stress disorder on women and their relationships: A qualitative study. *Psychology, Health & Medicine, 11*(4), 389–398.

Biaggi, A., Conroy, S., Pawlby, S., & Pariante, C. M. (2016). Identifying the women at risk of antenatal anxiety and depression: A systematic review. *Journal of Affective Disorders, 191*, 62–77.

Carlbring, P., Andersson, G., Cuijpers, P., Riper, H., & Hedman-Lagerlöf, E. (2018). Internet-based vs. face-to-face cognitive behavior therapy for psychiatric and somatic disorders: An updated systematic review and meta-analysis. *Cognitive Behaviour Therapy, 47*(1), 1–18.

Cox, E., Sowa, N., Meltzer-Brody, S., & Gaynes, B. N. (2016). The perinatal depression treatment cascade: Baby steps towards improving outcomes. *Journal of Clinical Psychiatry, 77*(9), 1189–1200.

Danaher, B. G., Milgrom, J., Seeley, J. R., Stuart, S., Schembri, C., Tyler, M. S., . . . Lewinsohn, P. (2013). MomMoodBooster web-based intervention for postpartum depression: Feasibility trial results. *Journal of Medical Internet Research, 15*(11), e242.

Dennis, C. L., & Chung-Lee, L. (2006). Postpartum depression help-seeking barriers and maternal treatment preferences: A qualitative systematic review. *Birth, 33*(4), 323–331.

Earls, M. F., Yogman, M. W., Mattson, G., Rafferty, J., Baum, R., Gambon, T., . . . Committee on Psychosocial Aspects of Child and Family Health. (2019). Incorporating recognition and management of perinatal depression into pediatric practice. *Pediatrics, 143*(1).

Ellis, A., Chebsey, C., Storey, C., Bradley, S., Jackson, S., Flenady, V., . . . Siassakos, D. (2016). Systematic review to understand and improve care after stillbirth: A review of parents' and healthcare professionals' experiences. *BMC Pregnancy and Childbirth, 16*, 1–19.

Flenady, V., Wojcieszek, A. M., Middleton, P., Ellwood, D., Erwich, J. J., Coory, M., . . . Goldenberg, R. L. (2016). Stillbirths: Recall to action in high-income countries. *The Lancet, 387*(10019), 691–702.

Fletcher, R., Kay-Lambkin, F., May, C., Oldmeadow, C., Attia, J., & Leigh, L. (2017). Supporting men through their transition to fatherhood with messages delivered to their smartphones: A feasibility study of SMS4dads. *BMC Public Health, 17*(1), 1–10.

Fletcher, R., Knight, T., Macdonald, J. A., & St George, J. (2019). Process evaluation of text-based support for fathers during the transition to fatherhood (SMS4dads): Mechanisms of impact. *BMC Psychology, 7*(1), 1–11.

Fletcher, R., Regan, C., Leigh, L., Dizon, J., & Deering, A. (2023). Online mental health screening for rural fathers over the perinatal period. *Australian Journal of Rural Health, 31*(5), 796–804.

Forsell, E., Bendix, M., Holländare, F., von Schultz, B. S., Nasiell, J., Blomdahl-Wetterholm, M., . . . Kaldo, V. (2017). Internet delivered cognitive behavior therapy for antenatal depression: A randomised controlled trial. *Journal of Affective Disorders, 221,* 56–64.

Goodman, J. H. (2009). Women's attitudes, preferences, and perceived barriers to treatment for perinatal depression. *Birth, 36*(1), 60–69.

Goodman, J. H., & Tyer-Viola, L. (2010). Detection, treatment, and referral of perinatal depression and anxiety by obstetrical providers. *Journal of Women's Health, 19*(3), 477–490.

Grierson, A. B., Hobbs, M. J., & Mason, E. C. (2020). Self-guided online cognitive behavioural therapy for insomnia: A naturalistic evaluation in patients with potential psychiatric comorbidities. *Journal of Affective Disorders, 266,* 305–310.

Haga, S. M., Drozd, F., Lisøy, C., Wentzel-Larsen, T., & Slinning, K. (2019). Mamma Mia – A randomized controlled trial of an Internet-based intervention for perinatal depression. *Psychological Medicine, 49*(11), 1850–1858.

Heazell, A. E., Siassakos, D., Blencowe, H., Burden, C., Bhutta, Z. A., Cacciatore, J., . . . Downe, S. (2016). Stillbirths: Economic and psychosocial consequences. *The Lancet, 387*(10018), 604–616.

Heazell, A. E., Wojcieszek, A., Graham, N., & Stephens, L. (2019). Care in pregnancies after stillbirth and perinatal death. *International Journal of Birth and Parent Education, 6*(2), 23–28.

Hobbs, M. J., Joubert, A. E., Mahoney, A. E., & Andrews, G. (2018). Treating late-life depression: Comparing the effects of internet-delivered cognitive behavior therapy across the adult lifespan. *Journal of Affective Disorders, 226,* 58–65.

Hobbs, M. J., Mahoney, A. E., & Andrews, G. (2017). Integrating iCBT for generalized anxiety disorder into routine clinical care: Treatment effects across the adult lifespan. *Journal of Anxiety Disorders, 51,* 47–54.

Johnson, J. E., Price, A. B., Kao, J. C., Fernandes, K., Stout, R., Gobin, R. L., & Zlotnick, C. (2016). Interpersonal psychotherapy (IPT) for major depression following perinatal loss: A pilot randomized controlled trial. *Archives of Women's Mental Health, 19,* 845–859.

Kelman, A. R., Evare, B. S., Barrera, A. Z., Muñoz, R. F., & Gilbert, P. (2018). A proof-of-concept pilot randomized comparative trial of brief Internet-based compassionate mind training and cognitive-behavioral therapy for perinatal and intending to become pregnant women. *Clinical Psychology & Psychotherapy, 25*(4), 608–619.

Kersting, A., Dölemeyer, R., Steinig, J., Walter, F., Kroker, K., Baust, K., & Wagner, B. (2013). Brief Internet-based intervention reduces posttraumatic stress and prolonged grief in parents after the loss of a child during pregnancy: A randomized controlled trial. *Psychotherapy and Psychosomatics, 82*(6), 372–381.

Kim, D. R., Hantsoo, L., Thase, M. E., Sammel, M., & Epperson, C. (2014). Computer-assisted cognitive behavioral therapy for pregnant women with major depressive disorder. *Journal of Women's Health, 23*(10), 842–848.

Kingston, D., Austin, M.-P., Heaman, M., McDonald, S., Lasiuk, G., Sword, W., . . . Biringer, A. (2015). Barriers and facilitators of mental health screening in pregnancy. *Journal of Affective Disorders, 186,* 350–357.

Kingston, D., Janes-Kelley, S., Tyrrell, J., Clark, L., Hamza, D., Holmes, P., . . . Austin, M.-P. (2015). An integrated web-based mental health intervention of assessment-referral-care to reduce stress, anxiety, and depression in hospitalized pregnant women with medically high-risk pregnancies: A feasibility study protocol of hospital-based implementation. *JMIR Research Protocols, 4*(1), e4037.

Klier, C. M., Geller, P. A., & Ritsher, J. B. (2002). Affective disorders in the aftermath of miscarriage: A comprehensive review. *Archives of Women's Mental Health, 5*(4), 129–149. https://doi.org/10.1007/s00737-002-0146-2

Koopmans, L., Wilson, T., Cacciatore, J., & Flenady, V. (2013). Support for mothers, fathers and families after perinatal death. *Cochrane Library,* (6). https://doi.org/10.1002/14651858.CD000452.pub3

Lamont, K., Scott, N. W., Jones, G. T., & Bhattacharya, S. (2015). Risk of recurrent stillbirth: Systematic review and meta-analysis. *BMJ, 350.* https://doi.org/10.1136/bmj.h3080

Lara-Cinisomo, S., Ramirez Olarte, A., Rosales, M., & Barrera, A. Z. (2021). A systematic review of technology-based prevention and treatment interventions for perinatal depression and anxiety in Latina and African American women. *Maternal and Child Health Journal, 25*(2), 268–281. https://doi.org/10.1007/s10995-020-03028-9

Lau, Y., Htun, T., Wong, S., Tam, W., & Klainin-Yobas, P. (2017). Therapist-supported internet-based cognitive behavior therapy for stress, anxiety, and depressive symptoms among postpartum women: A systematic review and meta-analysis. *Journal of Medical Internet Research, 19*(4), e138. https://www.jmir.org/2017/4/e138/

Lau, Y., Yen, K. Y., Wong, S. H., Cheng, J. Y., & Cheng, L. J. (2021). Effect of digital cognitive behavioral therapy on psychological symptoms among perinatal women in high income-countries: A systematic review and meta-regression. *Journal of Psychiatric Research, 146*, 234–248. https://doi.org/10.1016/j.jpsychires.2021.11.012

Lebel, C., MacKinnon, A., Bagshawe, M., Tomfohr-Madsen, L., & Giesbrecht, G. (2020). Elevated depression and anxiety symptoms among pregnant individuals during the COVID-19 pandemic. *Journal of Affective Disorders, 277*, 5–13. https://doi.org/10.1016/j.jad.2020.07.126

Loughnan, S. A., Boyle, F. M., Ellwood, D., Crocker, S., Lancaster, A., Astell, C., . . . Flenady, V. (2022). Living with loss: Study protocol for a randomized controlled trial evaluating an Internet-based perinatal bereavement program for parents following stillbirth and neonatal death. *Trials, 23*(1), 1–15. https://doi.org/10.1186/s13063-022-06363-0

Loughnan, S. A., Butler, C., Sie, A. A., Grierson, A. B., Chen, A. Z., Hobbs, M. J., . . . Newby, J. M. (2019). A randomised controlled trial of "MUMentum postnatal": Internet-delivered cognitive behavioural therapy for anxiety and depression in postpartum women. *Behaviour Research and Therapy, 116*, 94–103. https://doi.org/10.1016/j.brat.2019.03.001

Loughnan, S. A., Joubert, A. E., Grierson, A. B., Andrews, G., & Newby, J. M. (2019). Internet-delivered psychological interventions for clinical anxiety and depression in perinatal women: A systematic review and meta-analysis. *Archives of Women's Mental Health, 22*, 737–750. https://doi.org/10.1007/s00737-019-00961-9

Loughnan, S. A., Sie, A. A., Hobbs, M. J., Joubert, A. E., Smith, J., Haskelberg, H., . . . Newby, J. M. (2019). A randomized controlled trial of "MUMentum pregnancy": Internet-delivered cognitive behavioral therapy program for antenatal anxiety and depression. *Journal of Affective Disorders, 243*, 381–390. https://doi.org/10.1016/j.jad.2018.09.057

Mahoney, A. E., Elders, A., Li, I., David, C., Haskelberg, H., Guiney, H., & Millard, M. (2021). A tale of two countries: Increased uptake of digital mental health services during the COVID-19 pandemic in Australia and New Zealand. *Internet Interventions, 25*, 100439. https://doi.org/10.1016/j.invent.2021.100439

Mahoney, A. E., Shiner, C. T., Grierson, A. B., Sharrock, M., Loughnan, S. A., Harrison, V., & Millard, M. (2023). Online cognitive behaviour therapy for maternal antenatal and postnatal anxiety and depression in routine care. *Journal of Affective Disorders, 338*, 121–128. https://doi.org/10.1016/j.jad.2023.06.008

Mahoney, A. E., Li, I., Haskelberg, H., Millard, M., & Newby, J. M. (2021). The uptake and effectiveness of online cognitive behaviour therapy for symptoms of anxiety and depression during COVID-19. *Journal of Affective Disorders, 292*, 197–203. https://doi.org/10.1016/j.jad.2021.05.116

Martin-Key, N. A., Spadaro, B., Schei, T. S., & Bahn, S. (2021). Proof-of-concept support for the development and implementation of a digital assessment for perinatal mental health: Mixed methods study. *Journal of Medical Internet Research, 23*(6), e27132. https://www.jmir.org/2021/6/e27132

Milgrom, J., Danaher, B. G., Gemmill, A. W., Holt, C., Holt, C. J., Seeley, J. R., . . . Ericksen, J. (2016). Internet cognitive behavioral therapy for women with postnatal depression: A randomized controlled trial of MumMoodBooster. *Journal of Medical Internet Research, 18*(3), e54. https://doi.org/10.2196/jmir.4993

Mills, T. A., Ricklesford, C., Cooke, A., Heazell, A. E. P., Whitworth, M., & Lavender, T. (2014). Parents' experiences and expectations of care in pregnancy after stillbirth or neonatal death: A metasynthesis. *BJOG: An International Journal of Obstetrics & Gynaecology, 121*(8), 943–950. https://doi.org/10.1111/1471-0528.12656

Mills, T. A., Ricklesford, C., Heazell, A. E. P., Cooke, A., & Lavender, T. (2016). Marvellous to mediocre: Findings of national survey of UK practice and provision of care in pregnancies after stillbirth or neonatal death. *BMC Pregnancy and Childbirth, 16*(1), 1–10. https://doi.org/10.1186/s12884-016-0891-2

Morgan, C., Mason, E., Newby, J. M., Mahoney, A. E., Hobbs, M. J., McAloon, J., & Andrews, G. (2017). The effectiveness of unguided Internet cognitive behavioural therapy for mixed anxiety and depression. *Internet Interventions, 10*, 47–53. https://doi.org/10.1016/j.invent.2017.10.003

Müller, M., Matthies, L. M., Goetz, M., Abele, H., Brucker, S. Y., Bauer, A., . . . Wallwiener, S. (2020). Effectiveness and cost-effectiveness of an electronic mindfulness-based intervention (eMBI) on maternal mental health during pregnancy: The mindmom study protocol for a randomized controlled clinical trial. *Trials*, 21(1), 1–11. https://doi.org/10.1186/s13063-020-04873-3

Murphy, S., & Cacciatore, J. (2017). The psychological, social, and economic impact of stillbirth on families. *Seminars in Fetal and Neonatal Medicine*, 22(3), 129–134. https://doi.org/10.1016/j.siny.2017.02.002

Newby, J. M., Mackenzie, A., Williams, A. D., McIntyre, K., Watts, S., Wong, N., & Andrews, G. (2013). Internet cognitive behavioural therapy for mixed anxiety and depression: A randomized controlled trial and evidence of effectiveness in primary care. *Psychological Medicine*, 43(12), 2635–2648. https://doi.org/10.1017/s0033291713000111

Newby, J. M., Mason, E., Kladnistki, N., Murphy, M., Millard, M., Haskelberg, H., . . . Mahoney, A. (2021). Integrating Internet CBT into clinical practice: A practical guide for clinicians. *Clinical Psychologist*, 25(2), 164–178. https://doi.org/10.1080/13284207.2020.1843968

Nieminen, K., Andersson, G., Wijma, B., Ryding, E.-L., & Wijma, K. (2016). Treatment of nulliparous women with severe fear of childbirth via the Internet: A feasibility study. *Journal of Psychosomatic Obstetrics & Gynecology*, 37(2), 37–43. https://doi.org/10.3109/0167482X.2016.1140143

Nieminen, K., Berg, I., Frankenstein, K., Viita, L., Larsson, K., Persson, U., . . . Wijma, K. (2016). Internet-provided cognitive behaviour therapy of posttraumatic stress symptoms following childbirth – a randomized controlled trial. *Cognitive Behaviour Therapy*, 45(4), 287–306. https://doi.org/10.1080/16506073.2016.1169626

O'Mahen, H. A., & Flynn, H. A. (2008). Preferences and perceived barriers to treatment for depression during the perinatal period. *Journal of Women's Health*, 17(8), 1301–1309. https://doi.org/10.1089/jwh.2007.0631

O'Mahen, H. A., Richards, D. A., Woodford, J., Wilkinson, E., McGinley, J., Taylor, R. S., & Warren, F. C. (2014). Netmums: A phase II randomized controlled trial of a guided Internet behavioural activation treatment for postpartum depression. *Psychological Medicine*, 44(8), 1675–1689. https://doi:10.1017/S0033291713002092

O'Mahen, H. A., Woodford, J., McGinley, J., Warren, F. C., Richards, D. A., Lynch, T. R., & Taylor, R. S. (2013). Internet-based behavioral activation – Treatment for postnatal depression (Netmums): A randomized controlled trial. *Journal of Affective Disorders*, 150(3), 814–822. https://doi.org/10.1016/j.jad.2013.03.005

Palmer, K. R., Tanner, M., Davies-Tuck, M., Rindt, A., Papacostas, K., Giles, M. L., . . . Hodges, R. J. (2021). Widespread implementation of a low-cost telehealth service in the delivery of antenatal care during the COVID-19 pandemic: An interrupted time-series analysis. *The Lancet*, 398(10294), 41–52. https://doi.org/10.1016/S0140-6736(21)00668-1

Pilkington, P. D., Rominov, H., Milne, L. C., Giallo, R., & Whelan, T. A. (2017). Partners to parents: Development of an online intervention for enhancing partner support and preventing perinatal depression and anxiety. *Advances in Mental Health*, 15(1), 42–57. https://doi.org/10.1080/18387357.2016.1173517

Pugh, N. E., Hadjistavropoulos, H. D., & Dirkse, D. (2016). A randomised controlled trial of therapist-assisted, Internet-delivered cognitive behavior therapy for women with maternal depression. *PloS One*, 11(3), e0149186. https://doi.org/10.1371/journal.pone.0149186

Richards, D., Enrique, A., Eilert, N., Franklin, M., Palacios, J., Duffy, D., . . . Timulak, L. (2020). A pragmatic randomized waitlist-controlled effectiveness and cost-effectiveness trial of digital interventions for depression and anxiety. *NPJ Digital Medicine*, 3(1), 85. https://doi.org/10.1038/s41746-020-0293-8

Rodrigues, A. L., Ericksen, J., Watson, B., Gemmill, A. W., & Milgrom, J. (2022). Interventions for perinatal depression and anxiety in fathers: A mini-review. *Frontiers in Psychology*, 12, 744921. https://doi.org/10.3389/fpsyg.2021.744921

Rominov, H., Giallo, R., Pilkington, P. D., & Whelan, T. A. (2018). "Getting help for yourself is a way of helping your baby:" Fathers' experiences of support for mental health and parenting in the perinatal period. *Psychology of Men & Masculinity*, 19(3), 457. http://dx.doi.org/10.1037/men0000103

Scherer, S., Alder, J., Gaab, J., Berger, T., Ihde, K., & Urech, C. (2016). Patient satisfaction and psychological well-being after Internet-based cognitive behavioral stress management (IB-CBSM) for women with preterm labor: A randomized controlled trial. *Journal of Psychosomatic Research*, 80, 37–43. https://doi.org/10.1016/j.jpsychores.2015.10.011

Schofield, P., Carey, M., Bonevski, B., & Sanson-Fisher, R. (2006). Barriers to the provision of evidence-based psychosocial care in oncology. *Psycho-Oncology: Journal of the Psychological, Social and Behavioral Dimensions of Cancer, 15*(10), 863–872. https://doi.org/10.1002/pon.1017

Soet, J. E., Brack, G. A., & DiIorio, C. (2003). Prevalence and predictors of women's experience of psychological trauma during childbirth. *Birth, 30*(1), 36–46. https://doi.org/10.1046/j.1523-536X.2003.00215.x

Thompson, A., Hunt, C., & Issakidis, C. (2004). Why wait? Reasons for delay and prompts to seek help for mental health problems in an Australian clinical sample. *Social Psychiatry and Psychiatric Epidemiology, 39*, 810–817. https://doi.org/10.1007/s00127-004-0816-7

Titov, N., Dear, B. F., Nielssen, O., Staples, L., Hadjistavropoulos, H., Nugent, M., . . . Kaldo, V. (2018). ICBT in routine care: A descriptive analysis of successful clinics in five countries. *Internet Interventions, 13*, 108–115. https://doi.org/10.1016/j.invent.2018.07.006

Titov, N., Dear, B. F., Staples, L. G., Bennett-Levy, J., Klein, B., Rapee, R. M., . . . Nielssen, O. B. (2015). MindSpot clinic: An accessible, efficient, and effective online treatment service for anxiety and depression. *Psychiatric Services, 66*(10), 1043–1050. https://doi.org/10.1176/appi.ps.201400477

Titov, N., Hadjistavropoulos, H. D., Nielssen, O., Mohr, D. C., Andersson, G., & Dear, B. F. (2019). From research to practice: Ten lessons in delivering digital mental health services. *Journal of Clinical Medicine, 8*(8), 1239. https://doi.org/10.3390/jcm8081239

Wijma, K. (2006). Post-traumatic stress disorder and childbirth. In *Psychiatric disorders and pregnancy* (pp. 170–205). CRC Press.

Williams, A. D., O'Moore, K., Mason, E., & Andrews, G. (2014). The effectiveness of Internet cognitive behaviour therapy (iCBT) for social anxiety disorder across two routine practice pathways. *Internet Interventions, 1*(4), 225–229. https://doi.org/10.1016/j.invent.2014.11.001

Wojcieszek, A. M., Boyle, F. M., Belizan, J. M., Cassidy, J., Cassidy, P., Erwich, J. J. H. M., . . . Flenady, V. (2018). Care in subsequent pregnancies following stillbirth: An international survey of parents. *BJOG: An International Journal of Obstetrics and Gynaecology, 125*(2), 193–201. http://dx.doi.org/10.1111/1471-0528.14424

Wojcieszek, A. M., Shepherd, E., Middleton, P., Lassi, Z. S., Wilson, T., Murphy, M. M., . . . Flenady, V. (2018). Care prior to and during subsequent pregnancies following stillbirth for improving outcomes. *Cochrane Database of Systematic Reviews*, (12). http://dx.doi.org/10.1002/14651858.CD012203.pub2

Woolhouse, H., Brown, S., Krastev, A., Perlen, S., & Gunn, J. (2009). Seeking help for anxiety and depression after childbirth: Results of the maternal health study. *Archives of Women's Mental Health, 12*, 75–83. https://doi.org/10.1007/s00737-009-0049-6

Yang, M., Jia, G., Sun, S., Ye, C., Zhang, R., & Yu, X. (2019). Effects of an online mindfulness intervention focusing on attention monitoring and acceptance in pregnant women: A randomized controlled trial. *Journal of Midwifery & Women's Health, 64*(1), 68–77. https://doi.org/10.1111/jmwh.12944

Acknowledgments

Shannon Loughnan and Ann Lancaster.

PART V

Special Issues and Populations

27

FATHERS' PERINATAL MENTAL HEALTH

John R. Holmberg and M. Laura Pappa

The power to transform oneself and the possibilities presented by becoming a dad—for the first or the tenth time—are vast. Fatherhood influences every part of a man's life—biological, emotional, social, partnered relationship, and relationships with extended family—just to name a few. Research shows that men's lifestyles, bodies, and brains undergo important changes during the "perinatal period" or from the point when they learn they are expecting a baby until around the child's first birthday (Chin et al., 2011). Shifting hormones, such as testosterone, oxytocin, vasopressin, and cortisol stimulate fathers' instincts to care for and nurture their infants (Gordon et al., 2017). When fathers spend time nurturing and caring for their infants, their brains literally change (i.e., structure, complexity, functioning) to support baby bonding (Abraham et al., 2014). What's more, this is not new news! Many of the world's indigenous cultures have long understood that fathers naturally undergo biological changes, including mood shifts and weight gain, as they prepare for the birth of their baby (Powis, 2022; Tylor, 1865). Fathers' social, psychological, and lifestyle changes, such as growth in parenting skills and development of communication rhythms with their infants, can be exhilarating and lead to feelings of deep joy and love (Cabrera, 2020).

The perinatal period is challenging and, for most fathers, associated with a wide range of lifestyle changes that contribute to unexpected experiences of sadness, worry, exhaustion, emotional distance from partners, increased relationship conflicts, and many other changes (Bakermans-Kranenburg et al., 2019). Birth-related changes bring new stress and appear to exacerbate previously existing difficulties which increases the need for professional and natural sources of support for dads (Fisher, 2017). Increasingly, it is clear that the transition to parenthood starts a period of prolonged risk for physical (Garfield et al., 2022; Torche & Rauf, 2021) and mental health problems for fathers, relative to nonparenting males (Fisher et al., 2021). Mental health screening studies find that a third to nearly half (i.e., 48.9%) of new dads exceeded a threshold for referral to clinical mental health services (Dudley et al., 2001; Molgora et al., 2017). When these stressful experiences are intense and long-standing, a father is likely experiencing one of the conditions that are collectively referred to as perinatal mental health disorders or PMHDs (Fisher et al., 2021). Awareness of the prevalence and impact of PMHDs for fathers is increasingly shedding light on the previously taboo idea that fathers, like mothers, suffer from intense emotions

DOI: 10.4324/9781003206903-33

and psychopathology following the birth of their babies. The impact of PMHDs on fathers was recently highlighted in the film *Daddy Blues* which portrayed one father's perinatal journey through depression, panic, and anxiety; until, ultimately, he found recovery, healing, and growth. This chapter summarizes key knowledge developed to date about the ways in which birth can result in mental health difficulties for men, the associated risk and protective factors, impacts of these difficulties on children, couples, and families, as well as the emerging intervention approaches to address paternal psychopathology to benefit child and family outcomes.

Paternal Perinatal Mental Health Disorders and Rates of Prevalence

Mental distress and disorder emerging from fathers' adjustment during pregnancy and through the first year after birth is very common (Howard et al., 2014), and these interrelated mental health conditions are collectively referred to as Paternal—perinatal mental health disorders or P-PMHDs, formerly perinatal mood and anxiety disorders or PMADs (Moyer & Kinser, 2021). The most well-known P-PMHD disorders are depression and generalized anxiety disorder (Leiferman et al., 2021; Paulson & Bazemore, 2010), panic disorder, posttraumatic stress disorder, obsessive-compulsive disorder, alcohol and substance misuse, bipolar disorder, and death (e.g., by overdose, suicide) which all evidence elevations among fathers in the perinatal period (Amaral Tavares Pinheiro et al., 2011; Clemans-Cope et al., 2019; Cirillo et al., 2014; Etheridge & Slade, 2017; Fisher, 2017; Hanley & Williams, 2020; Inglis et al., 2016; Richardson et al., 2021; Yoshida et al., 2005).

Box 27.1 Fathers' Voices of Perinatal Psychological Distress

"Claustrophobic"
"You cannot sleep"
"You cannot relax"
"Living a life other than you had expected"
"Like a robot with no choices or happiness"
"You have nothing to fall back on"

"Everything is falling apart"
"Life is a treadmill, I constantly run"
"(partner) relationship becomes difficult and strenuous"
"Dark thoughts"
"Everything will be hard"

Paternal—Perinatal Depression (P-PD) includes lasting mood and anxiety symptoms such as sadness, fatigue, poor focus, low moods, irritability, hopelessness, persistent worry and preoccupying fears, rumination, bodily symptoms (e.g., nausea, knots in the stomach), irritability, restlessness and feeling on-edge, social isolation, and withdrawal from enjoyable activities, insomnia, alcohol or substance misuse, and thoughts and behaviors related to suicidality and self-harm. Box 27.1 lists some of the ways that dads describe their experience of birth-related mental health distress (Edhborg et al., 2016).

Researchers have been exploring the possibility that men with depression experience some mental health symptoms that are seldom seen in women (a.k.a., Masculine Subtype Depression) such as (a) frequent anger, rage, or aggressive behavior, (b) increased alcohol or substance misuse, (c) hyper engagement at work and recreational activities (e.g., online games or chatting, gambling) to avoid experiencing their negative emotions around the family; or (d) impulsive or risk-taking behavior such as extramarital affairs or making unplanned expenditures (Baldoni & Giannotti, 2020; Oliffe et al., 2019; Rice et al., 2019, 2020). Perinatal depression is estimated to affect around 20% of mothers and 8.5–11% of fathers across the world (Cameron et al., 2016; Giallo et al., 2013; Paulson et al., 2006; Paulson & Bazemore, 2010). Levels of depression symptoms vary considerably across the perinatal period (Vänskä et al., 2017) but there are indications that the most common period of elevated rates occur from child age three to six months, where around 25% of had significant symptoms (Paulson & Bazemore, 2010). For fathers with moderate to high depression symptoms, their difficulties may change little by child age 2 years (Kiviruusu et al., 2020), by school entry (Garfield et al., 2014), and even persist into adolescence (Garfield et al., 2016; Reeb et al., 2015). While far less well understood, depressive disorders in fathers that include periods of elevated, pressured or hypomanic episodes, manic mood states, or mixed mood states are likely experiencing one of the bipolar disorders which appear to evidence exacerbations in the perinatal period (Amaral Tavares Pinheiro et al., 2011).

Paternal—Perinatal Anxiety Disorders (P-PAD) include experiences of high and persistent worry, anxiety, rumination, sleep problems, difficulty with focus and concentration, physical symptoms such as nausea or gastrointestinal distress, intrusive repetitive thoughts that are difficult to quiet, restlessness, irritability, and sense of panic. Prevalence rates for P-PAD in mothers fall between 18% and 25%, with the highest rates a few months after birth (Dennis et al., 2017). Prevalence rates for fathers are about 11–15%, on average, during this period but there is inconsistent data (i.e., some studies find pregnancy rates to be highest) as to a unique period of elevated symptoms (Leiferman et al., 2021).

Typically classified as one of the anxiety disorders, paternal perinatal obsessive-compulsive disorder (P-POCD) includes experiences of intrusive difficulty with focus and concentration, intrusive repetitive thoughts (i.e., obsessions), and behaviors (i.e., compulsions) that persist at high-frequency and are highly difficult to slow or quiet. The preoccupying and intrusive thoughts of perinatal parents often relate to harm befalling the baby. Excessive and repetitive cleaning, checking and re-checking for safety, exhaustively researching potentially scary issues, and restriction of activities to avoid potential upset or harm are all common compulsive behaviors for fathers in the perinatal period. Individuals struggling with P-POCD often report great distractibility when trying to accomplish tasks and significant interference with their ability to complete daily activities as well as experiences of unrelenting restlessness and irritability. Paternal POCD has been studied little but found to occur in about 6% of fathers (Coelho et al., 2014).

When fathers witness or experience exceptionally stressful circumstances, it can result in *Paternal—Perinatal Post-Traumatic Stress Disorder* (P-PPTSD). P-PPTSD results from personal experience with or witnessing a life-threatening event. Some examples, from the perinatal period, include fathers witnessing spontaneous pregnancy loss, the mother or child experiencing birth-related trauma, having a premature or low-weight birth baby, or children having to face life-threatening medical conditions and procedures. Due to the heightened sense of vulnerability to self, partner, and the baby, non-birth-related events such as the worldwide pandemic, community violence, civil unrest and rioting, natural disasters, transportation accidents, crime, or warfare experienced by the family may also be an antecedent to perinatal PTSD (e.g., Fisher, 2017; Vignato et al., 2017). Symptoms of P-PTSD include chronic and easily evoked high anxiety, hyper-arousal, difficulty establishing and maintaining calm states, sudden and persistent intrusive memories (i.e., including dreams), irritability and low mood, helplessness, repetitive behaviors thought to avoid a repetition of the event or stimulating intrusive memories associated with the trauma. Fathers with PTSD often describe being cognitively aware that the threat or danger has passed, and their current levels of distress and anxiety are not rational; still, the dissonance between their cognitive and emotional experiences is highly distressing. The degree of distress fathers experience may be linked to masculine beliefs related to men being good problem solvers who stay calm in a crisis but they lost those abilities during traumatic events (Daniels et al., 2020). Fathers often describe, in palpable detail, the helplessness experienced in unexpected situations (Hollywood & Hollywood, 2011; B. Lindberg et al., 2007, 2008; Provenzi & Santoro, 2015). Birth-related medical crises can be particularly difficult for fathers. Fathers often do not know what is happening medically to the mother and baby, which contributes greatly to their sense of being overwhelmed (I. Lindberg & Engström, 2013). Of the few available prevalence studies on P-PPTSD, most in the context of birth trauma or NICU admission, 3% to 5% of fathers develop PTSD which is roughly equivalent to maternal rates (Daniels et al., 2020; Inglis et al., 2016; Parfitt et al., 2013). For some fathers, PTSD symptoms are long-lasting (Binder et al., 2011) and reinforced by recurring life-threatening stressors such as infant health crises. For example, in families facing repeated NICU admissions, PTSD was evident for almost half the dads (i.e., 47%) (Aftyka et al., 2017).

Despite the fact that there has been very little study of paternal perinatal alcohol and substance abuse and overdose (Benoit & Magnus, 2017), suicidal ideation and behavior (Quevedo et al., 2011), or intimate partner violence (Giallo et al., 2021; Kristin Håland et al., 2016; Stewart et al., 2017), each is likely to exhibit a pattern of elevation like those in paternal mood and anxiety disorders.

The previously described prevalence rates of paternal mental health disorders are by themselves cause for significant concern; but, there is evidence that current rates grossly underestimate the actual degree of suffering faced by fathers. For example, perinatal fathers report feeling marginalized by healthcare providers (Hodgson et al., 2021; Lever Taylor et al., 2018) and avoid mental health services (Scholz et al., 2017) due to strongly held mental health stigma and masculinity-linked beliefs (Cameron et al., 2017; Chatmon, 2020; Mniszak et al., 2020). Men also may experience mental health symptoms (e.g., irritability, impulsivity) in ways that differ from women (Oliffe & Phillips, 2008). Men are more likely to use avoidant or numbing coping strategies rather than acknowledge emotional distress (Giallo et al., 2018). The Covid-19 Pandemic may have had a unique impact on perinatal fathers, relative to fathers with nonpandemic births, due to further restricted access to medical providers and social support services (Menzies, 2021). Early in the pandemic, mental health services were limited since treatment was largely being conducted exclusively virtually. Concerns about the newly offered telehealth treatment modality were common, and many opted out of needed treatment in hopes that regular, in-person treatment, would soon resume. Support groups were particularly impacted during the pandemic, given the high risk for confidentiality violations and use of unfamiliar technology. These factors contributed to increasing the number of barriers and worsening access to care for fathers. However, there is now a growing body of literature showing equivalent effectiveness of virtual treatment as compared with in-person (Sullivan et al., 2020).

Thus far, we have reviewed the most common P-PMHDs, their symptoms and prevalence. Boxes 27.2.1, 27.2.2 and 27.2.3 introduce you (in three parts) to a clinical a case that illustrates common elements of a P-PMHD presentation, risk factors, engagement and course of treatment. In subsequent sections the case will be further reviewed as related to content discussed in this chapter.

Box 27.2.1 Introduction to Case Review—A Father's Journey From Frozen to Warmth

The patient in this vignette gave us permission to share his experience and we further protect his privacy through use of a pseudonym ("Zane").

Zane, a 29-year-old cis-gendered White male, presented for treatment with significant hesitance about engaging mental health treatment. He was the second oldest of five brothers. Originally from Serbia, Zane's desire for greater economic security led to him to take a new job in the United States, working on satellite programming for a government contractor. At the time of entry to treatment, Zane had only been in the United States for a few years. He met his wife, at church, shortly after immigrating and they were married and expecting within that year. Zane reported that despite exceptional work performance his first few years, he had been experiencing symptoms of prolonged distractibility that was difficulty to control, persistent anxiety, nightmares and sleep problems, fear that something was wrong in his brain, recurrent headaches, panic episodes including difficulty controlling his body temperature during these episodes, increased problems in his relationship with his wife, difficulty engaging parenting behaviors with his daughters, atypical spiritual concerns such as God no longer listening to his prayers and none really seemed related to his actual life circumstances. Zane sought support from his pastor and his supervisor at work; ultimately, they both recommended he get medical intervention. Zane's primary care provider suggested he try psychotherapy prior to starting medications.

Genetic, Biological, and Psychosocial Risk Factors

Like many disorders, paternal PMHDs result from an interaction of factors such as genetic, biological, environmental (e.g., social adversity), relationship, cognitive, and behavioral factors. *Genetic Factors*—Currently, there is little know about genetic variations that potentiate or protect against developing paternal PMHDs. Heritability estimates for life span depression are reported in the 40–50% range (Edvardsen et al., 2009) and considerable work continues to specify the specific genetic influences (Arnau-Soler Id et al., 2018; Bogdan et al., 2013). As with other complex disorders, the genetic contribution is likely a range of individual and cumulative predispositions that result in susceptibilities (i.e., stress reactivity or negative affectivity) or resiliencies that interact with or are activated by life stresses in the perinatal period resulting in high symptoms in fathers (Caspi & Moffitt, 2006). Many gene—environment interactional mechanisms have been explored as being involved in maternal depression (Nemoda & Szyf, 2017) but paternal focused work has lagged well behind.

Biological Factors

In Western cultures, it was previously thought that only mothers experienced hormonal changes in the perinatal period; that belief has been debunked (Rilling & Mascaro, 2017). Studies show a wide range of paternal changes at the level of hormones (i.e., bonding hormones like oxytocin, prolactin, and vasopressin, stress hormones like cortisol, and sex hormones such as testosterone and estrogen) (Gettler et al., 2011; Saltzman & Ziegler, 2014; Swain et al., 2014). Fathers undergo shifts in brain region activation seen on functional brain scans (Kim et al., 2014) and even neuroanatomical or brain structure changes (Sethna et al., 2019). For dads, these changes start in pregnancy (Diaz-Rojas et al., 2021) and occur in response to nurturing and caregiving experiences (Kim et al., 2014). The most widely acknowledged biological changes observed in fathers appear to contribute to the expression of Couvade Syndrome or sympathetic pregnancy (Bruno et al., 2020). The complex interaction of stressors, cycles of rewards (e.g., bonding), and how they protect or potentiate paternal PMHDs will continue to be important areas of study.

Socioeconomic and Family Demographic Factors

Social determinants of health also influence paternal mental health difficulties and point to vulnerable populations with limited personal, family, and community supports. The family's degree of economic self-sufficiency represents important indicators or risk factors for paternal PMADS. Young or teen fathering, low educational attainment, unmarried parenting, unemployment, legal barriers to employment, limited interpersonal skills, incarceration history, and low formal social supports are linked to increased rates of paternal psychopathology (Bergström, 2013; Bronte-Tinkew et al., 2007; Davé et al., 2010; Gao et al., 2009; Paulson et al., 2020; Poh et al., 2014). While low-income status is associated with increased paternal PMHDs, higher-range socioeconomic status has not been found to be additionally protective relative to average financial resources (Cameron et al., 2016).

Despite the available evidence suggesting higher rates of depression among low-income fathers of color (Bronte-Tinkew et al., 2007; S. J. Lee et al., 2009; Roubinov et al., 2014; Simonovich et al., 2021), most paternal PMHDs research has focused on convenience samples of White middle-class fathers (Philpott et al., 2019, 2020). In a complementary study to the perinatal follow-up of the Fragile Families study, Sinkewicz and Lee (2010) found the prevalence of depression among Black fathers to be 1.5 times higher than nonparenting African American men of similar age. Although there is limited available data for Latinx fathers, one recent study of perinatal fathers found exceptionally high endorsement of depression and anxiety symptoms (i.e., 81% had >10 on the EPDS) and reinforces the need to prioritize engagement of services for and more research with fathers from nonmajority groups (Roubinov et al., 2014).

Personal History and Behavioral Factors

Fathers with preexisting health and mental health difficulties are known to be at risk of experiencing a PMHD (Fisher & Garfield, 2016; P. G. Ramchandani et al., 2008). History of previous perinatal loss, traumatic birth, and highly stressful perinatal circumstances such as NICU admission, caring for a baby with very low birth weight, or raising infants facing chronic medical conditions are also associated with increased rates of paternal PMHDs (Demontigny et al., 2013; Helle et al., 2018). In something of a mutually reinforcing cycle, prenatal anxiety is a predictor of infant fussiness which is a predictor of paternal PMHD symptoms (Bamishigbin et al., 2020). Parental sleep is almost always impacted by caring for a baby and poor sleep is associated with increased paternal mental health symptoms (Gallaher et al., 2018). At the transition to parenthood, many fathers are engaging in multiple health risk behaviors (i.e., alcohol misuse, tobacco use, poor diets, very low activity rates coupled with high body mass) (Everett et al., 2006). For men, the perinatal period is associated with rapid accumulation of body fat (Garfield et al., 2016). These health difficulties are likely to persist as fathers are less likely to access healthcare compared to mothers (Isacco et al., 2016; Salvesen von Essen et al., 2021).

Box 27.2.2 Introduction to Case Review—Risk and Protective Factors

Several risk and protective factors became evident during the intake interview with Zane. While not his native language, Zane communicated well in English, self-identified as White, and had a household income in the average range. He had advanced education and a secure job with opportunity for advancement. The culture at his place of work was to put in long hours, so as to produce products with very few problems so as to maintain their government contracts. In his late teens, with financial support from his uncle, Zane studied computer science in England.

While he certainly longed for greater connection with his mother and siblings, who were still in Europe, they spoke regularly. Zane reported his father died in an industrial accident when he was young, but alcoholism may have been a contributing factor. Zane found a church community that was supportive but not as tight knit as his home church in Serbia. His experience with healthcare providers in Serbia was limited, unless the condition was dire, most people turned to traditional and nutritional treatments or they used prayer to restore health.

Zane arranged for his mother-in-law to join them in the United States shortly after the birth, but they did not have a plan for her self-sufficiency in the United States or return to her family in Croatia. Zane reported feeling very close to wife, but they rarely had time alone with such a busy household. Zane felt left out when his partner and mother-in-law spoke in Croatian, which the children were also learning to speak.

Paternal PMHDs Links With Maladaptive Outcomes in Relationship, Parenting, and Child Development

While current data indicates that rates of PMHDs are higher in women, evidence of paternal mental health disorders adds significantly to the segment of families who are in need of professional and extra-familial support. Since most parents are each other's primary sources of support (i.e., dads are the primary support for mothers around their health and mental health and vice versa), when one or both parents are struggling with a PMHD, profound and lasting negative influences are exerted on parental relationships, parenting behaviors, and child development (Paulson et al., 2020).

A regularly cited impact of paternal mental health problems is the reduction in interpersonal resources to support the mothers (Rowe et al., 2013). Relying heavily on co-paternal support is encouraged in many cultures and data indicates high paternal support is typically linked with reduction of maternal postpartum depressive symptoms (Fagan & Lee, 2010). When fathers with PMHDs are struggling, they often report low support from partners, high rates of partner relationship problems, and marital distress (Don & Mickelson, 2012; Gawlik et al., 2014; Salcuni et al., 2016; Zhang et al., 2016). When dads are struggling with PMHDs, high rates of difficulties like coparenting problems (Bradley & Slade, 2011; Bronte-Tinkew et al., 2007) and high parenting stress (Skjothaug et al., 2018) commonly occur. The clear link between parents' respective mental health symptoms (Paulson et al., 2016, 2020) having a reciprocal negative impact on parental relationship and their parenting processes led to the development of a theoretical model of the etiology of perinatal PMHDs, where interpersonal distress is a core influence in the emergence of the disorder. We present an adapted version of

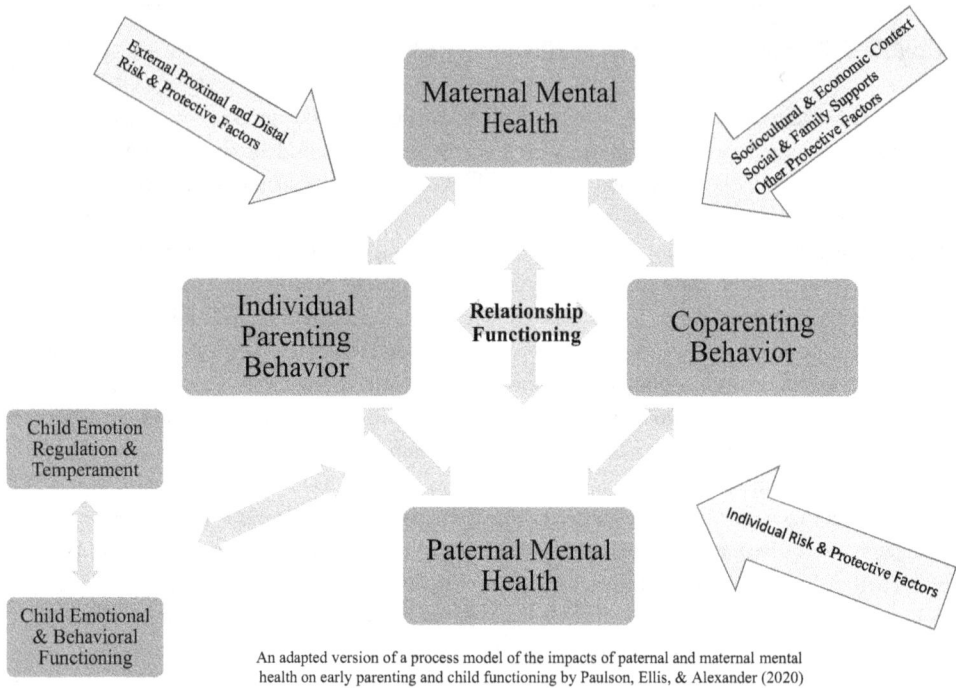

An adapted version of a process model of the impacts of paternal and maternal mental health on early parenting and child functioning by Paulson, Ellis, & Alexander (2020)

Figure 27.1 Influences on paternal and maternal mental health which impact early parenting and child functioning

Source: Adapted from Paulson et al. (2020).

the Paulson et al. (2020) Interpersonal Process Model for perinatal depression which illustrates the centrality of reciprocal parental relationship functioning as impacting parental mental health and child outcomes and extends the model to include influence by individual risk and protective as well as cultural and socioeconomic factors.

In terms of parenting outcomes, paternal PMHDs are associated with maladaptive perceptions of self and the infant as well negative shifts in parenting behaviors. Fathers with PMHDs experience cognitive dysfunctions such as low parenting self-efficacy (Philpott et al., 2019; Skjothaug et al., 2018), greater likelihood of holding negative attributions about their babies (Hart et al., 1997), and viewing their infants as being rejecting, unpredictable, and not bonded with them (Edhborg et al., 2005). Perinatal fathers with mental health difficulties engage in more frequent dysfunctional parenting behaviors (e.g., spanking, negative utterances, hostility, high reactivity, or unresponsiveness) and less participation in enriching activities (e.g., playfulness, expressing warmth, reading together, reflecting on child's experience, and singing to the child) as compared with their psychologically average counterparts (Davis et al., 2011; Demontigny et al., 2013; Paulson et al., 2006; Paulson & Bazemore, 2010; Sethna et al., 2015; Thapa et al., 2020; Wee et al., 2011; Wilson & Durbin, 2010).

The negative child outcomes associated with paternal PMHDs are among the most compelling and replicated findings, showing the importance of fathers' mental health as one of several key factors in child cognitive, emotional, and behavioral functioning. Given the previously described correlations between paternal PMHDs and dysfunctional parenting, seeing that lack of positive input correlated with developmental delays (e.g., expressive vocabulary) is, perhaps, expectable (Paulson et al., 2009). Links between paternal PMHDs and child outcomes are evident in the prenatal and postpartum periods, across childhood, and seen in adolescence to at least child age 20 years (Gutierrez-Galve et al., 2019; Paulson et al., 2009; Sweeney & MacBeth, 2016). Thus far, no studies have maintained longitudinal samples where associations between paternal PMHDs and early adult functioning or second-generation parenting could be assessed.

Children's developmental difficulties associated with paternal PMHDs include cognitive and language delays, self-regulation difficulties such as higher infant crying and lower acquisition of academic readiness skills (R. J. Fletcher et al., 2011; Kaplan et al., 2007; Sweeney & MacBeth, 2016; M. P. Van Den Berg et al., 2009). A number of studies report and replicate associations between PMHDs and poor child social, emotional, and behavioral outcomes (i.e., externalizing symptoms such as oppositional behavior, attention-deficit disorders, and conduct problems as well as internalizing symptoms such as depression and anxiety) resulting in about a doubled risk of psychopathology relative to children without perinatally affected fathers (Barker et al., 2017; Capron et al., 2015; R. J. Fletcher et al., 2011; Kvalevaag et al., 2013; P. Ramchandani et al., 2008; P. Ramchandani & Psychogiou, 2009; Sweeney & MacBeth, 2016).

Healthy father support for mothers and babies has been found to even moderate (or disconnect) the association between maternal depression and poor child outcomes (e.g., Boyce et al., 2006). Additionally, Boyce and colleagues found that paternal involvement had a main effect in the prediction of children's mental wellness above and beyond that of mother care. Low paternal caregiving in infancy was significantly associated with greater symptom severity at follow-up a decade later. In the same study, healthy paternal caregiving was found to moderate risks associated with child biobehavioral or temperamental reactivity (i.e., heart rate, cortisol level, arterial pressure) on later child behavior problems. Children with an early onset of low father involvement, often characteristic of P-PMHD, were significantly more likely to develop mental illness related to their sensitivity to social stressors.

Child gender has been proposed to be an important factor in predicting negative outcomes associated with paternal PMHDs but that data is mixed (sometimes greater impact on boys, other times girls) (R. J. Fletcher et al., 2011; Gutierrez-Galve et al., 2019; Hanington et al., 2010). The pathways, mediators, and moderators through which paternal PMHDs exert a teratogenic effect on child development (e.g., impacting the amount of time in caregiving, amount of child exposure to the father, greater maladaptive and less adaptive parenting behavior, taxing the other parent's interpersonal and emotional resources, facilitating parental and household conflict) continue to be explored but those are complex and interrelated influences to untangle (Barker et al., 2017; Sweeney & MacBeth, 2016).

Lastly but not of least importance, paternal PMHDs have an important economic impact. Fathers' mental health symptoms impact occupational, family, and parental functioning which likely requires some degree of external support to remedy. The cost estimate for the mental health treatment alone, in the United Kingdom's single payer model, is estimated to be about $1,100 GBP per father per year. The cascading financial impacts related to fathers' employment (i.e., given the traditional gender divisions related to family income and disequity in pay for men, relative to women in many nations), plus the child development and family functioning outcomes likely represent costs to families and societies in the tens of millions of dollars per year within highly industrialized nations. To date, precise economic estimates have only been established for maternal perinatal depression and only in select countries (Center of Perinatal Excellence: COPE, 2014; Edoka et al., 2011).

Interventions and Treatments

In this section, we organize the discussion of mental health interventions according to the broadly defined intervention categories (Misra et al., 2003; Mrazek & Haggerty, 1994) of *primary prevention* (i.e., universally available, targeting fathers before a disorder is present or identified), *secondary prevention* (i.e., interventions for individuals who by their social or other circumstance are at high-risk for developing a disorder and/or are already exhibiting difficulties beyond the normal range), and *direct care or tertiary intervention* (i.e., traditional treatments for individuals with diagnosable symptoms and impact on functioning).

Primary Prevention Strategies

Currently, there are no universal interventions focused on engaging fathers to prevent or reduce mental health problems before they occur. This is not surprising as there is little education or socially established traditions (e.g., baby showers) to help males gain caregiving experience (e.g., expectations to babysit) or prepare for parenthood (Bakermans-Kranenburg et al., 2019).

Social policies, while not technically an intervention, impact both parents' mental health in the perinatal period (Fagan & Pearson, 2020; Teti et al., 2017). It has been suggested that paternal family leave policies could universally affect paternal PMHDs (Bamishigbin et al., 2020). Minimum paid parental leave is directly influenced by governmental policies and the United States is the only high-income nation without universal paid parental leave (Bakermans-Kranenburg et al., 2019; Kornfeind & Sipsma, 2018; Teti et al., 2017). The United States is an outlier, relative to 22 other high-income countries, in degree of disproportionately high distress reported by parents (a.k.a., happiness penalty associated with parenting) as compared to nonparenting age-mates in that country (Glass et al., 2016). Although not yet assessed in fathers, longer parental leave is associated with reduced maternal postpartum depression (Dagher et al., 2014; Van Niel et al., 2020). Furthermore, longer paternal leave (i.e., >14 days) is correlated with reduced paternal postpartum stress, increased support for partners, greater caregiving and paternal infant bonding, and adaptive work-family balance (Conde et al., 2021; Feldman et al., 2004; Séjourné et al., 2012; Tanaka & Waldfogel, 2007).

Another potential, as of yet unexplored, universal preventive strategy could be public health advertisements or health marketing campaigns targeting perinatal fathers. Two nationwide initiatives in the United States have been the National Institute of Mental Health's Real Men, Real Depression (RMRD) and the Public Broadcast System's Men Get Depression (MGD) projects. Other countries, such as Canada and Australia and individual states such as Colorado, have developed male-specific mental health awareness campaigns (e.g., www.ManTherapy.org). The goals of these initiatives are to increase men's self-awareness of symptoms, reduce stigma, and decrease hesitance to seek treatment (Hammer & Vogel, 2010; Rochlen et al., 2005; Rochlen & Hoyer, 2005; Watts, 2008) which are important because men's awareness of perinatal mental health problems is lower than it is for women (Schumacher et al., 2008). Unfortunately, outside of some initial preference studies showing that men prefer the gender-specific approach to mental health messaging, little is known about the impact of such initiatives or how adaptations for the perinatal period might be received (Erentzen et al., 2018).

Secondary Prevention—Screening Strategies

Targeted or universal screening of fathers would represent a potential intervention to detect and address paternal PMHDs (Allport et al., 2018). Obstetric, pediatric, and primary care providers have many opportunities to engage fathers and screen for mental health symptoms. Ideally, obstetricians would screen men early in the course of prenatal care and pediatricians could repeat screenings across the child's first year, when mental health symptom prevalence may be higher (Kiviruusu et al., 2020; Leiferman et al., 2021; Paulson & Bazemore, 2010). Pediatricians are currently charged to engage fathers in well-baby care (Coleman & Garfield, 2004) so they are well-positioned to screen fathers postnatally (Gjerdincjen et al., 2009). If such an approach were implemented, both obstetric and pediatric providers would need to implement a systematic outreach to reach at-risk fathers, since the fathers who attend well-baby visits typically have fewer risks than those who do not (Walsh et al., 2020a). Initial studies suggest that fathers are open to universal screening but they would best be part of an integrated model where stigma is addressed, the purpose of screening is clear, and access to a continuum of care is assured, should difficulties be identified (Schuppan et al., 2019).

In the previous sections, we reviewed estimates for how many fathers were determined to have reached a threshold of symptoms and/or severity to represent a likely "positive case" or that with further assessment likely would result in a diagnosis. Healthcare providers working with individual fathers can use screening tools such as those used in prevalence studies to better understand the experience of individual fathers. Table 27.1 lists mental health screening tools used with fathers and indicates which mental health symptoms are assessed, the number of total items, symptom counts or item totals indicative of a father in need of clinical attention and an example citation, where the tool was used with fathers. Of course, fathers with scores even approaching the thresholds used to identify a "case" are likely to need and benefit from professional services, when that level of distress is acknowledged.

While the research work to identify reliable, valid, and efficient methods to screen fathers for mental health problems has progressed, a larger set of challenges relates to how to reach and engage fathers so that they can be screened (Fisher & Garfield, 2016). Unlike mothers, fathers avoid and under-utilize health and mental health services (O'Brien et al., 2005; Schuppan et al., 2019). Stigma, traditional masculine values, low expectations for benefit, and lack of service awareness are barriers to men's healthcare service engagements (Addis & Mahalik, 2003; Berger et al., 2013; Mansfield et al., 2003) where routine screening could occur. For many years, the American Academy of Pediatrics has published statements encouraging providers to outreach to and invite fathers to their children's well-child visits (Allport, Johnson, et al., 2018; Yogman & Garfield, 2016). Those visits have been identified as a priority opportunity to broadly screen fathers and identify those who may be facing PMHDS (A. R. Berg & Ahmed, 2016).

Table 27.1 lists a wide range of screeners successfully used with fathers, but the most commonly used tool is the *Edinburgh Postnatal Depression Scale* (EPDS) (Kennedy & Munyan, 2021). The EPDS has been adapted for multiple cultures and translated into many languages. The EPDS collects information about symptoms present in the past week, relative

Table 27.1 Measures of Paternal Distress and Mental Health Problems

Measure name	Condition(s) assessed	Number of items	Positive case (i.e., referral or clinical threshold)	Citations
Mood Disorder Tools				
Beck Depression Inventory—2nd edition	Depression, self-harm ideation	21	Total ≥ 20 = Case	Psouni et al. (2017)
Center for Epidemiological Studies—Depression (CES-D)	Depression	20	Total ≥ 16 = Case	Field et al. (2006)
Composite International Diagnostic Interview Short Form—Major Depressive Episode (MDE)	Depression	2	Total ≥ 1 = Case	Davis et al. (2011)
Depression-Anxiety Stress Scale (DASS-21)	Depression, anxiety, emotional distress	21	Depression ≥ 9 = Case anxiety ≥ 6 = Case Distress ≥ 12 = Case Total ≥ 27 = Case	Nasreen et al. (2018)
Edinburgh Postnatal Depression Scale (EPDS)[a]	Depression, anxiety, self-harm ideation	10	Total ≥ 10 = Case	Edmondson et al. (2010)
Edinburgh-Gotland Depression Scale (EGDS)	Depression, anxiety, self-harm ideation	12	Total ≥ 11 = Case	Psouni et al. (2017)
General Health Questionnaire	Somatic (bodily) symptoms, anxiety, social dysfunction, depression	28	Total ≥ 24 = Case	Boyce et al. (2007)
Male Depression Risk Scale (MDRS)	Depression (with irritable and impulsive symptoms)	22	Total ≥ 51 = Case	Rice et al. (2020)
Mood Disorder Questionnaire (MDQ)	Hypomanic (with impulsivity, pressured activity), depression (with irritable symptoms)	17	Section I ≥ 7 = Case, when Section II = Yes Section III = Yes	Fisher and Garfield (2016)
Goldberg Depression and Anxiety Scales (GMDAS)	Depression, anxiety	18	Depression Total ≥ 2 = Case Anxiety Total ≥ 5 = Case	Leach et al. (2016)
Gotland Male Depression Scale (GMDS)	Depression	13	Total > 13 = Case	Carlberg et al. (2018)
Physician Health Questionnaire (PHQ-2)	Depression	2	Total ≥ 3 = Case	Kroenke et al. (2003)
Physician Health Questionnaire (PHQ-9)	Depression, self-harm ideation	9	Total ≥ 10 = Case	Lai et al. (2010)

Table 27.1 (Continued)

Anxiety Tools

State/Trait Anxiety Inventory (STAI)[a]	Current or state anxiety level (S-subscale)	20	State total ≥ 40 = Case	Charandabi et al. (2017)
Generalized Anxiety Disorder Scale (GAD—7)	Persistent worry, anxiety, restlessness	7	Total > 10 = Case	Zacher et al. (2022)
HADS-A: Hospital Anxiety and Depression Scale	Anxiety, depression (flat affect, lost interest)	7	Total ≥ 10 = Case	Tohotoa et al. (2012)
Perinatal Anxiety Screening Scale (PASS)	Acute anxiety and detachment; general and specific worries; perfectionism, control, and trauma; social anxiety	31	Total ≥ 26 = Case	Cameron et al. (2020)
Symptom Checklist 90 Revised—Anxiety Subscale	Worry, Anxiety, Panic	10	Total ≥ 10 = Case	Don et al. (2014)

Posttraumatic Stress Disorder (PTSD) Tools

Birmingham Interview of Maternal Mental Health (BIMMH)	Posttraumatic stress	1	Total ≥ 1 = Case	Parfitt et al. (2013)
City Birth Trauma Scale (City BiTS)	Evident stressor, re-experiencing, avoidance, negative cognitions and mood, hyperarousal, symptom duration, impairment, exclusion of other causes	29	Case = yes for trauma, when subsequent symptoms evident for re-experiencing, avoidance, negative cognition or mood, hyperarousal	Webb et al. (2021)
Perinatal PTSD Questionnaire (PPQ)	Trauma, invasive memories or feelings, avoidance, hypervigilance	14	Total ≥ 6 = Clinical	Koliouli et al. (2016)
Posttraumatic Stress Disorder Impact of Events Scale (PTSD-IES)	Intrusion, avoidance	15	Total ≥ 20 = Clinical	Ayers et al. (2007)
Posttraumatic Stress Disorder Questionnaire (PTSD-Q)	Intrusion, avoidance, hyperarousal	17	Symptoms occur "commonly" for Intrusion (1), Avoidance (3), and Hyperarousal (2) items	Bradley et al. (2008)
The Posttraumatic Stress Diagnostic Scale (PDS)	Intrusive thoughts, avoidant behaviors, hyperarousal symptoms	17	Total ≥ 28 = Clinical	Parfitt & Ayers (2014)

[a]Most frequently used screening tool in that diagnostic category

to other times in the person's life. Questions reflect cognitive or thinking issues, somatic or bodily expressions of stress, and mood symptoms typical of depression, worry, panic, and anxiety symptoms as well as self-harm ideation (Matthey et al., 2001). Identifying what level of symptoms best represents a "case" on this measure, representing clinically significant distress or a diagnosable paternal PMHD, is still being clarified. Many cut points (i.e., the score at which or above represents clinical significance) have been studied but reviews of the EPDS suggests a score of 10 or more is justification for further mental health assessment and intervention among fathers (Walsh et al., 2020b). Alternate versions of this tool have been developed that augment the EPDS with additional anxiety, irritability, and impulsive symptoms to see if the adapted tool better capture the PMHDs experiences of struggling fathers (Carlberg et al., 2018; Mangialavori et al., 2021).

Secondary Prevention—Prenatal Classes and Home-Visiting Strategies

While a few services and targeted interventions are available for economically at-risk fathers in the perinatal period (e.g., perinatal classes with paternal augmentations, coparenting interventions, home-visiting programs), they have seldom been developed for or tested in relation to reducing or preventing perinatal mental health disorders.

Prenatal (e.g., childbirth, baby care, infant first aid) and coparenting (i.e., how parents work together to manage child and household care) classes have been successful in engaging fathers to a variable degree, more so when specifically tailoring services and recruitment strategies for fathers but findings in terms of mental health outcomes are mixed (Aponte Johnson et al., 2019; Friedewald et al., 2005; Matthey & Barnett, 1999). Initial studies of perinatal class approaches did not detect impacts on paternal depression or anxiety (Feinberg & Kan, 2008; Hung et al., 1996; Linville et al., 2017; Melnyk et al., 2006; Shorey et al., 2017). Other prenatal class interventions, while not finding intervention effects on mental health symptoms, did have impacts on correlates of paternal PMHDS such as distress, parenting well-being, confidence, self-efficacy, and reduced family stressors (Daley-McCoy et al., 2015; Eira Nunes et al., 2021; Goldstein et al., 2020; J. Y. Lee et al., 2018; Mihelic et al., 2018; Suto et al., 2016).

One co-parenting focused prenatal class (i.e., Family Foundations) found an impact on paternal depression in one of the two trials of the program (i.e., impact only seen in the replication trial, not the initial trial). Why those trials found differing effects on paternal depression has not fully been disentangled (Feinberg et al., 2016). Two additional studies of prenatal class interventions showed beneficial impacts on paternal PMHD symptoms (Charandabi et al., 2017; Tohotoa et al., 2012). The first study (Tohotoa et al., 2012) found an impact of reduced paternal anxiety pre- versus post-test for the intervention group with no change for the control group. Unfortunately, that study evidenced nearly twice as many intervention fathers relative to control with high anxiety at baseline (i.e., 24 (7%) vs. 13 (2%), respectively), leaving open the question as to a floor effect being evident for the control group which may have skewed the results (Tohotoa et al., 2012). A second study of prenatal classes, conducted in an urban city in Iran (i.e., Bukan), found impacts on paternal depression and anxiety later in pregnancy (eight weeks after the class) which were maintained at six weeks after the birth (Charandabi et al., 2017).

A few additional preventive interventions, though not specifically focused on paternal mental health, were found to beneficially impacts paternal psychopathology symptoms (see Goldstein et al., 2020). A father-tailored augmentation of home visitation found beneficial impacts on fathers' perceived stress levels and a statistical trend toward improved levels of depression (Tandon et al., 2021). A quasi-experimental home-visitation study (Castel et al., 2016) of parents with babies born prematurely (i.e., 28–35 weeks' gestation at birth) found beneficial impacts on paternal parenting stress and mental health symptoms (i.e., on the EPDS), relative to control parents who were raising like-aged full term children. A program teaching skin-to-skin father-newborn caregiving found that infants fared better and intervention fathers rated their anxiety and mood symptoms lower than treatment as usual comparison dads (Huang et al., 2019). Studies of classes teaching infant bathing and/ or infant massage showed secondary impacts on paternal depression and anxiety (Samuels et al., 1992) as did teaching fathers massage therapy techniques to use with their partners (Field et al., 2008).

Direct Care and Tertiary Prevention Strategies

For more than two decades (Areias et al., 1996), a wide range of direct intervention approaches have been suggested as potentially helpful for fathers with perinatal mental health disturbances (e.g., group therapy, individual therapy using multiple approaches, couples' therapy, family therapy, group-based therapies, medications) (Freitas et al., 2016; Freitas & Fox, 2015; Wittenborn et al., 2012). Fathers report preferring individual and couples therapy approaches as compared with individual and tend to be most hesitant to consider psychiatric medications (Cameron et al., 2017). No matter which treatment approach is implemented, research suggests that services need to directly address paternal barriers to accessing care. Furthermore, interventions are encouraged to directly address stigma and degree to which highly traditional or hegemonic masculine beliefs impact parenting and relationships. It is recommended that interventions be tailored to fathers' perspectives and needs, emphasizing the universally stressful nature of the perinatal period, and making adaptations to ensure multicultural and diversity issues are addressed (Rominov et al., 2018).

Recent studies that comprehensively reviewed the literature for interventions seeking to impact paternal mental health (O'Brien et al., 2017; Philpott et al., 2019; Rominov et al., 2016) found no published studies testing treatment efficacy for fathers with PMHD symptoms. Those reviews found the previous indirect interventions such as perinatal classes, massage skills training, and coparenting programs to have secondary paternal PMHDs impacts. Nonetheless, few of those studies demonstrated beneficial mental health impacts for fathers (e.g., Field et al., 2008; Li et al., 2009; Tohotoa et al., 2012).

To date, only two tertiary intervention studies specifically addressing paternal symptoms in the perinatal period have been reported. One study tested group-based psychoeducation for fathers to address parenting adjustment and found a significant reduction in anxiety symptoms for the intervention group, at a four-week follow-up (Mohammadpour et al., 2021). In a second study, fathers with depression symptoms were recruited to a perinatal and early childhood parenting intervention that infused paternal specific coping skills, child responsive play techniques, and mental health content (Cognitive Behavioral Therapy). Conducted with fathers in the social context of extreme poverty in Pakistan, the pilot evaluation of (i.e., *n* = 18) found change in repeated measures of depression symptoms (i.e., *Edinburgh Postnatal Depression Scale, Hamilton Depression Scale*), parenting stress, and paternal ratings of social support (Husain et al., 2021). Interventions such as these, which frame the intervention as impacting child development and including a normalizing aspect of the group-based approach, use strategies to explicitly focus on recruitment and engagement of fathers and likely those efforts contributed to beneficial outcomes.

As treatments for fathers are developed, they likely to need to modify conventional therapies (e.g., cognitive behavioral therapy, interpersonal psychotherapy, psychodynamic psychotherapy) to address men's barriers to treatment (i.e., stigma, hegemonic masculinity) and gender-specific tendencies to avoid health interventions and providers as well as limited provider awareness of men's treatment needs (Rominov et al., 2018). Men are found to maintain higher levels of stigma relative to women (i.e., beliefs about and fears of disapproving judgment of people with mental health difficulties, assumptions of a mental health problems as having an origin in personal or moral failings, as well as the desire to avoid being seen as one of or similar to the ostracized) (Addis & Hoffman, 2017; Berger et al., 2013; Chatmon, 2020). For men, stigma is often interrelated with internalization of rigid and traditional (a.k.a., hegemonic) masculine beliefs (e.g., valuing independence, toughness, and low affective expression) (Rochlen & Hoyer, 2005; Seidler et al., 2020). Stigma and masculine beliefs reinforce other barriers such as men's beliefs related to prioritizing their contributions family financial well-being over their health (Parent et al., 2018; Schuppan et al., 2019; Vogel et al., 2011). While providers may believe they can deliver universal or nonpaternal specific mental healthcare and get analogous outcomes, there is no data support this contention (Isacco et al., 2016; Molloy & Pierro, 2020; Panter-Brick et al., 2014). Rather, treatment adaptations related to the intersection of masculinity, race/ethnicity, and culture are likely needed (Cokley et al., 2013; Mellinger & Liu, 2006; Vogel et al., 2011). Other systemic barriers will also need to be addressed to facilitate access to care for fathers (e.g., not having health insurance, no pediatric electronic medical record capability for a separate treatment file for the father) (Affleck et al., 2018; Whitley, 2021).

Some factors cited to be motivating for fathers to engage services include their perceived need for parenting information (i.e., infant development, baby care skills), desire for validation of parenting efficacy, and preference for using strengths-based and directive techniques (Domoney et al., 2020; R. Fletcher et al., 2008; Kilmartin, 2005; Levant et al., 2009; S. A. Madsen, 2009; Mniszak et al., 2020; O'Brien et al., 2017; Rowe et al., 2013). Similarly fathers prefer emphasis on content for relationship enhancement (i.e., offering concrete techniques to support distressed partners and conceptualizing treatment from a holistic or family-focused as opposed to individual treatment perspective (O'Brien et al., 2017).

The cascading impacts of paternal depression (i.e., partner, parenting behavior, child development) indicate potential benefits from implementing multi-modal approaches, based on symptom acuity (Habib, 2012; Madsen, 2009). Thematic review of past psychotherapy case studies with fathers reported the importance of including nontraditional mood symptoms as an aspect of treatment (i.e., male-subtype depression). Given the disproportionate completion of suicide by males, routine risk assessment is likely warranted (R. Fletcher et al., 2020). As compared to insight based approaches, the relatively concrete approach of cognitive behavioral therapy with its emphasis on the present time and relationship dynamics, provision of psychoeducation, use of practical exercises, and addressing underlying masculine-linked beliefs related to fatherhood has also been prioritized in work with men (Domoney et al., 2020; Primack et al., 2010). Men often report a preference for group-based workshops and interventions, due to those approaches allowing them to share experiences and coping strategies with other fathers (Addis & Mahalik, 2003). Tailoring psychotherapy further for critical cultural and context (e.g., age, economic, legal) influences are also important to engage and help struggling fathers (Allan et al., 2021; Bronte-Tinkew et al., 2007; Cole et al., 2018; Mniszak et al., 2020; Ramos & Chavira, 2022). Telehealth may be an important strategy for fathers in psychotherapy due to the increased degree of accessibility relative to in-office sessions (Geller et al., 2021; Paul et al., 2022). While evidence shows contradictory findings in studies of father's stated treatment preferences, the most common form of treatment according to treatment utilization review (i.e., in the context of universal healthcare) was primary care delivery of psychiatric medications (K. B. Madsen et al., 2022).

Box 27.2.3 Introduction to Case Review—Engagement in Treatment

After the intake meeting, Zane appeared less apprehensive about starting treatment. He previously shared with his pastor how he feared his wife might not make it through childbirth. His wife of only 11 months had developed pregnancy complications one month prior to the birth. In the birthing room of the hospital, her physical situation quickly became acute. The birth process seemed incredibly fast and Zane's twin daughters were tiny and frail in appearance, due to their degree of prematurity.

He only gained a glimpse of their miniature bodies before the pair was whisked away to the neonatal intensive care area. A female doctor in the room tried to be reassuring, "it's going to be alright after the procedures." Zane didn't know what the "procedures" were or why this was all happening. He was consumed with the real potential of his greatest fear—losing his wife and his daughters. He recalled asking himself, "How can I, alone, parent these two tiny babies?"

The following session, Zane recalled how his next memory was learning that his wife underwent a successful, but stressful, surgery. The babies had minor procedures as well, Zane was told. Zane went on to share that his wife returned home to recuperate, after just a couple of days. The infants' journey through the Neonatal Intensive Care Unit or NICU was rocky and turbulent. Nonetheless, Zane was incredibly thankful for the care and support from the medical team. Liya, the older of the twins, was strong and growing at discharge. Dani needed daily in-home nursing care after discharge; but soon, she was making slow and steady progress.

Zane recalled a pediatrician visit a few months later was more hopeful. Their daughters were still small for their age and not quite hitting their developmental milestones (e.g., rolling over, sitting up, making noises, and responding to voices). As his daughters continued to recover and gain strength, Zane remembered how he felt encouraged and began to let his emotional guard down. He felt confident that the family was on the right track, everyone and that would be ok.

As his daughters' birthday approached, Spring was in bloom and the family was thriving, Zane was jarred awake by a huge weight pressing down on his chest. He couldn't breathe and didn't know why. Was something wrong with his heart or his lungs? Although he couldn't make the connection at the time, the therapist asked if a seemingly forgotten experience on the floor of the delivery room—feeling overwhelmed, confused, panicked, and terrified—might have come home from the hospital with him. Tears began to roll down his face as he shook his head to indicate his agreement. The ghost of that traumatic birth experience even found him during the day, in the form of unpredictable panic attacks.

Zane recalled how the babies were sleeping well, but he just couldn't rest. Worries swirled through his mind day and night. Even though Zane was an exceptionally kind, thoughtful and polite man, he found himself becoming irritable and lashing out at others. He recalled fearing that he had been abandoned by God and mortified with shame regarding his short temper.

"Breathe. Allow Your Lungs to Take in the Deep Breath"

Early in the course of psychotherapy, the psychologist often had to step in and interrupt Zane when he was overwhelmed by his reaction to a memory evoked by the treatment. The therapist repeatedly reassured Zane that he was safely in the office and not stuck as the frozen or "statuesque" version of himself, watching his wife and twin daughters being whisked away. During treatment, Zane and his therapist revisited the traumatic birth to help him reflect, better understand, and ultimately work through his experience of the trauma.

Over time, the treatment started to help. The therapist offered lessons on how to maintain awareness of his emotional unrest and when to use grounding or de-escalation strategies to unpack the seemingly frozen thoughts, observations, and experiences of that moment. Zane again felt comfortable at church and was reassured by his nightly prayer routines. In a handful of treatment visits followed by some booster sessions (e.g., follow-up sessions after the therapy has ended), the symptoms dissipated. Zane's ability to work and enjoy family life returned. Zane was back to feeling like himself.

Conclusion

Most fathers do not have a clear sense of what to expect from the transition to parenthood. Birth-related adjustments bring unanticipated lifestyle changes and stressors, which place fathers in the unexperienced place of needing natural and professional support (Fisher, 2017). Research is clarifying the perinatal period as a window of prolonged risk for physical (Garfield et al., 2022; Torche & Rauf, 2021) and mental health problems for fathers, relative to nonparenting age-mates (Fisher et al., 2021); but, this transition also represents a time when men may be more open to support and making changes to become the type of father they want to be. Mental health screening studies find a third to nearly a half (i.e., 48.9%) of new dads exceeded mental distress to the level justifying referral to services (Dudley et al., 2001; Molgora et al., 2017). While some commonly identified risk factors (e.g., previous episodes of mental health problems, social determinants of health disparities, interpersonal risks due to having a partner struggling with mental wellness) have been studied in fathers, much more work is needed to clarify risk and protective factors. Building from the more broadly studied outcomes associated with maternal mental health difficulties in the perinatal period, impacts of paternal PMHDs on individual, couple, family and parenting functioning as well as the long cascading risks of these difficulties on child development make a strong case for the need of more intervention work with fathers.

Little established knowledge is currently available to guide naturally existing and professional support intervention for fathers in the perinatal period. A number of potentially complementary approaches could be elaborated to better support fathers with particular needs to aid fathers from disenfranchised, marginalized, or otherwise compounded adverse circumstances. Some example strategies at the primary prevention level are family supportive policy changes and public information campaigns. Secondary interventions, or those made available on a selective and higher need basis, include father focused prenatal classes and in-community interventions like home visiting as well as systems of screening fathers as part of obstetric, pediatric, and primary care. So far, there are few studies of tertiary preventive interventions or effective treatments for struggling fathers. While this doesn't necessarily mean the currently available treatments do not work for men, decades of clinical research have highlighted some important cornerstones to prioritize as outcome studies are more widely implemented.

References

Abraham, E., Hendler, T., Shapira-Lichter, I., Kanat-Maymon, Y., Zagoory-Sharon, O., & Feldman, R. (2014). Father's brain is sensitive to childcare experiences. *PNAS, 111*(27), 9792–9797. https://doi.org/10.1073/pnas.1402569111

Addis, M. E., & Hoffman, E. (2017). Men's depression and help-seeking through the lenses of gender. *The Psychology of Men and Masculinities*, 171–196. https://doi.org/10.1037/0000023-007

Addis, M. E., & Mahalik, J. R. (2003). Men, Masculinity, and the contexts of help seeking. *American Psychologist, 58*(1), 5–14. https://doi.org/10.1037/0003-066X.58.1.5

Affleck, W., Carmichael, V., & Whitley, R. (2018). Men's mental health: Social determinants and implications for services. *Canadian Journal of Psychiatry, 63*(9), 581–589. https://doi.org/10.1177/0706743718762388

Aftyka, A., Rybojad, B., Rosa, W., Wróbel, A., & Karakuła-Juchnowicz, H. (2017). Risk factors for the development of post-traumatic stress disorder and coping strategies in mothers and fathers following infant hospitalization in the neonatal intensive care unit. *Journal of Clinical Nursing, 26*(23–24), 4436–4445. https://doi.org/10.1111/jocn.13773

Allan, J. A., Herron, R. V., Ahmadu, M. E., Waddell, C., & Roger, K. (2021). "I never wanted my children to see their father the way I've seen mine": Caring masculinities and fathering on the Prairies. *NORMA, 16*(1), 23–37. https://doi.org/10.1080/18902138.2020.1866322

Allport, B. S., Johnson, S., Aqil, A., Labrique, A. B., Nelson, T., Carabas, Y., & Marcell, A. V. (2018). Promoting father involvement for child and family health. *Academic Pediatrics, 18*(7), 746–753. https://doi.org/10.1016/J.ACAP.2018.03.011

Amaral Tavares Pinheiro, K., Monteiro da Cunha Coelho, F., de Ávila Quevedo, L., Jansen, K., de Mattos Souza, L., Pierre Oses, J., . . . Tavares Pinheiro, R. (2011). Paternal postpartum mood: Bipolar episodes? Depressão paterna: Episódio bipolar? *Journal of Brazilian Psychiatry Revista Brasileira de Psiquiatria, 33*(3), 283–286.

Aponte Johnson, C., Fournakis, N., Anderson Thomas, M., & Hartsock, T. (2019, November 2). Boot camp for new dads: Equipping dads-to-be with male-centered support and education in their transition to fatherhood. *APHA's Annual Meeting and Expo*. https://apha.confex.com/apha/2019/meetingapi.cgi/Paper/437758?filename=2019_Abstract437758.html&template=Word

Areias, M. E. G., Kumar, R., Barros, H., & Figueiredo, E. (1996). Correlates of postnatal depression in mothers and fathers. *British Journal of Psychiatry, 169*(1), 36–41. https://doi.org/10.1192/bjp.169.1.36

Arnau-Soler Id, A., Adams, M. J., Hayward, C., & Thomson, P. A. (2018). *Genome-wide interaction study of a proxy for stress-sensitivity and its prediction of major depressive disorder, Generation Scotland*. Major Depressive Disorder Working Group of the Psychiatric Genomics Consortium Report. https://doi.org/10.1371/journal.pone.0209160

Ayers, S., Wright, D. B., & Wells, N. (2007). Symptoms of post-traumatic stress disorder in couples after birth: Association with the couple's relationship and parent-baby bond. *Journal of Reproductive and Infant Psychology, 25*(1), 40–50. https://doi.org/10.1080/02646830601117175

Bakermans-Kranenburg, M. J., Lotz, A., Alyousefi-van Dijk, K., & van IJzendoorn, M. (2019). Birth of a father: Fathering in the first 1,000 days. *Child Development Perspectives, 13*(4), 247–253. https://doi.org/10.1111/cdep.12347

Baldoni, F., & Giannotti, M. (2020). Perinatal distress in fathers: Toward a gender-based screening of paternal perinatal depressive and affective disorders. *Frontiers in Psychology, 11*(1892), 1–5. https://doi.org/10.3389/fpsyg.2020.01892

Bamishigbin, O. N., Wilson, D. K., Abshire, D. A., Mejia-Lancheros, C., & Dunkel Schetter, C. (2020). Father involvement in infant parenting in an ethnically diverse community sample:

Predicting paternal depressive symptoms. *Frontiers in Psychiatry, 11*(578688), 1–28. https://doi. org/10.3389/fpsyt.2020.578688

Barker, B., Iles, J. E., & Ramchandani, P. G. (2017). Fathers, fathering and child psychopathology. *Current Opinion in Psychology, 15*, 87–92. https://doi.org/10.1016/J.COPSYC.2017.02.015

Benoit, C., & Magnus, S. (2017). "Depends on the father": Defining problematic paternal substance use during pregnancy and early parenthood. *Canadian Journal of Sociology, 42*(4), 379–402. https://www.jstor.org/stable/pdf/90018218.pdf

Berg, A. R., & Ahmed, A. H. (2016). Clinical case report paternal perinatal depression: Making a case for routine screening. *The Nurse Practitioner*, 1–5. https://doi.org/10.1097/01. NPR.0000499558.20110.82

Berger, J. L., Addis, M. E., Green, J., Mackowiak, C., & Goldberg, V. (2013). Men's reactions to mental health labels, forms of help-seeking, and sources of help-seeking advice. *Psychology of Men and Masculinity, 14*(4), 433–443.

Bergström, M. (2013). Depressive symptoms in new first-time fathers: Associations with age, sociodemographic characteristics, and antenatal psychological well-being. *Birth, 40*(1), 32–38. https://doi. org/10.1111/birt.12026

Binder, W. S., Zeltzer, L. K., Simmons, C. F., Mirocha, J., & Pandya, A. (2011). The father in the hallway: Posttraumatic stress reactions in fathers of NICU babies. *Psychiatric Annals, 41*(8), 396–402. https://doi.org/10.3928/00485713-20110727-05

Bogdan, R., Nikolova, Y. S., & Pizzagalli, D. A. (2013). Neurogenetics of depression: A focus on reward processing and stress sensitivity. *Neurobiology of Disease, 52*, 12–23. https://doi. org/10.1016/J.NBD.2012.05.007

Boyce, P., Condon, J., Barton, J., & Corkindale, C. (2007). First-time fathers' study: Psychological distress in expectant fathers during pregnancy. *Australian and New Zealand Journal of Psychiatry, 41*(9), 718–725. https://doi.org/10.1080/00048670701517959

Boyce, W. T., Essex, M. J., Alkon, A., Goldsmith, H. H., Kraemer, H. C., & Kupfer, D. J. (2006). Early father involvement moderates biobehavioral susceptibility to mental health problems in middle childhood. *Journal of the American Academy of Child and Adolescent Psychiatry, 45*(12), 1510–1520. https://doi.org/10.1097/01.CHI.0000237706.50884.8B

Bradley, R., & Slade, P. (2011). A review of mental health problems in fathers following the birth of a child. *Journal of Reproductive and Infant Psychology, 29*(1), 19–42. https://doi.org/10.1080/02 646838.2010.513047

Bradley, R., Slade, P., & Leviston, A. (2008). Low rates of PTSD in men attending childbirth: A preliminary study. *British Journal of Clinical Psychology, 47*(3), 295–302. https://doi. org/10.1348/014466508X279495

Bronte-Tinkew, J., Moore, K. A., Matthews, G., & Carrano, J. (2007). Symptoms of major depression in a sample of fathers of infants: Sociodemographic correlates and links to father involvement. *Journal of Family Issues, 28*(1), 61–99. https://doi.org/10.1177/0192513X06293609

Bruno, A., Celebre, L., Mento, C., Rizzo, A., Silvestri, M. C., De Stefano, R., . . . Muscatello, M. R. A. (2020). When fathers begin to falter: A comprehensive review on paternal perinatal depression. *International Journal of Environmental Research and Public Health, 17*(4). MDPI AG. https://doi. org/10.3390/ijerph17041139

Cabrera, N. J. (2020). Father involvement, father-child relationship, and attachment in the early years. *Attachment and Human Development, 22*(1), 134–138. https://doi.org/10.1080/1461673 4.2019.1589070

Cameron, E. E., Hunter, D., Sedov, I. D., & Tomfohr-Madsen, L. M. (2017). What do dads want? Treatment preferences for paternal postpartum depression. *Journal of Affective Disorders, 215*, 62–70. https://doi.org/10.1016/j.jad.2017.03.031

Cameron, E. E., Joyce, K. M., Rollins, K., & Roos, L. E. (2020). Paternal depression & anxiety during the COVID-19 pandemic. *PsyArVix, Preprint*, e01–e17. https://doi.org/10.31234/OSF. IO/DRS9U

Cameron, E. E., Sedov, I. D., & Tomfohr-Madsen, L. M. (2016). Prevalence of paternal depression in pregnancy and the postpartum: An updated meta-analysis. *Journal of Affective Disorders, 206*, 189–203. https://doi.org/10.1016/J.JAD.2016.07.044

Capron, L. E., Glover, V., Pearson, R. M., Evans, J., O'Connor, T. G., Stein, A., . . . Ramchandani, P. G. (2015). Associations of maternal and paternal antenatal mood with offspring anxiety disorder at age 18 years. *Journal of Affective Disorders*, *187*, 20–26. https://doi.org/10.1016/j.jad.2015.08.012

Carlberg, M., Edhborg, M., & Lindberg, L. (2018). Paternal perinatal depression assessed by the Edinburgh Postnatal Depression Scale and the Gotland Male Depression Scale: Prevalence and possible risk factors. *American Journal of Men's Health*, *12*(4), 720–729. https://doi.org/10.1177/1557988317749071

Caspi, A., & Moffitt, T. E. (2006). Gene–environment interactions in psychiatry: Joining forces with neuroscience. *Nature Reviews Neuroscience*, *7*(7), 583–590. https://eds.s.ebscohost.com/abstract?site=eds&scope=site&jrnl=1471003X&asa=Y&AN=21553646&h=o6De1%2Fb0yv7NF0FqTGv4QbQVUsUkTnU5vG%2B%2FVXbgw8DGdBPmcTNriUbeWCZ5Fj%2FtaKqnFMr4n4zvSaOK34FIcg%3D%3D&crl=f&resultLocal=ErrCrlNoResults&resultNs=Ehost&crlhashurl=login.aspx%3Fdirect%3Dtrue%26profile%3Dehost%26scope%3Dsite%26authtype%3Dcrawler%26jrnl%3D1471003X%26asa%3DY%26AN%3D21553646

Castel, S., Beunard, A., Creveuil, C., Blaizot, X., Proia, N., & Guillois, B. (2016). Effects of an intervention program on maternal and paternal parenting stress after preterm birth: A randomized trial. *Early Human Development*, *103*, 17–25. https://doi.org/10.1016/J.EARLHUMDEV.2016.05.007

Center of Perinatal Excellence: COPE. (2014). Valuing perinatal mental health. In *Valuing perinatal mental health: The consequences of NOT treating perinatal depression and anxiety*. Center of Perinatal Excellence. https://cope.org.au/wp-content/uploads/2013/12/PWC-2013_Final3.pdf.

Charandabi, S. M. A., Mirghafourvand, M., & Sanaati, F. (2017). The effect of life style based education on the fathers' anxiety and depression during pregnancy and postpartum periods: A randomized controlled trial. *Community Mental Health Journal*, *53*(4), 482–489. https://doi.org/10.1007/S10597-017-0103-1/TABLES/2

Chatmon, B. N. (2020). Males and mental health stigma. *American Journal of Men's Health*, *14*(4).

Cirillo, P., Passos, R., Lpez, J., Nardi, A., Coelho, F., da Silva, R., de Quevedo, L., Souza, L., Pinheiro, K., Pinheiro, R., Lowenthal, R., Zaqueu, L., Rohde, L., Mari, J., Paula, C., Medeiros, G., Sampaio, D., Sampaio, S., & Lotufo-Neto, F. (2014). Obsessive-compulsive disorder in fathers during pregnancy and postpartum. *Brazilian Journal of Psychiatry*, *36*(3), 272. https://doi.org/10.1590/1516-4446-2013-1312

Clemans-Cope, L., Lynch, V., Epstein, M., & Kenney, G. M. (2019). Opioid and substance use disorder and receipt of treatment among parents living with children in the United States, 2015–2017. *The Annals of Family Medicine*, *17*(3), 207–211. https://doi.org/10.1370/AFM.2389

Coelho, F., da Silva, R., de Quevedo, L., Souza, L., Pinheiro, K., Pinheiro, R., Lowenthal, R., Zaqueu, L., Rohde, L., Mari, J., Paula, C., Medeiros, G., Sampaio, D., Sampaio, S., & Lotufo-Neto, F. (2014). Obsessive-compulsive disorder in fathers during pregnancy and postpartum. *Brazilian Journal of Psychiatry*, *36*(3), 272. https://doi.org/10.1590/1516-4446-2013-1312

Cokley, K., McClain, S., Enciso, A., & Martinez, M. (2013). An examination of the impact of minority status stress and impostor feelings on the mental health of diverse ethnic minority college students. *Journal of Multicultural Counseling and Development*, *41*(2), 82–95. https://doi.org/10.1002/J.2161-1912.2013.00029.X

Cole, B. P., Petronzi, G. J., Singley, D. B., & Baglieri, M. (2018). Predictors of men's psychotherapy preferences. *Counseling & Psychotherapy Research*, *19*, 45–56.

Coleman, W. L., & Garfield, C. (2004). Fathers and pediatricians: Enhancing men's roles in the care and development of their children. *Pediatrics*, *113*(5 I), 1406–1411. https://doi.org/10.1542/PEDS.113.5.1406

Conde, A., De Stasio, S., Kokkinaki, T., Garthus-Niegel, S., Schaber, R., Kopp, M., . . . Kress, V. (2021). Paternal leave and father-infant bonding: Findings from the population-based cohort study DREAM. *Frontiers in Psychology | Www.Frontiersin.Org*, *1*, 668028. https://doi.org/10.3389/fpsyg.2021.668028

Dagher, R. K., McGovern, P. M., & Dowd, B. E. (2014). Maternity leave duration and postpartum mental and physical health: Implications for leave policies. *Journal of Health Politics, Policy and Law*, *39*(2), 369–416. https://watermark.silverchair.com/369.pdf?token=AQECAHi208BE49Ooan9kkhW_Ercy7Dm3ZL_9Cf3qfKAc485ysgAAAtAwggLMBgkqhkiG9w0BBwagggK-9MIICuQIBADCCArIGCSqGSIb3DQEHATAeBglghkgBZQMEAS4wEQQMPk8ly6MDqmfG9tuAAgEQgIICg2c0sY1SrQZwYw32-SW1zCjNWT5BEdBnzFnEBPArR9b4ROLpeWQ

Daley-McCoy, C., Rogers, M., & Slade, P. (2015). Enhancing relationship functioning during the transition to parenthood: A cluster-randomised controlled trial. *Archives of Women's Mental Health, 18*(5), 681–692. https://doi.org/10.1007/S00737-015-0510-7

Daniels, E., Arden-Close, E., & Mayers, A. (2020). Be quiet and man up: A qualitative questionnaire study into fathers who witnessed their Partner's birth trauma. *BMC Pregnancy and Childbirth, 20*(1). https://doi.org/10.1186/s12884-020-02902-2

Davé, S., Petersen, I., Sherr, L., & Nazareth, I. (2010). Incidence of maternal and paternal depression in primary care: A cohort study using a primary care database. *Archives of Pediatrics & Adolescent Medicine, 164*(11), 1038–1044. https://doi.org/10.1001/ARCHPEDIATRICS.2010.184

Davis, R. N., Davis, M. M., Freed, G. L., & Clark, S. J. (2011). Fathers' depression related to positive and negative parenting behaviors with 1-year-old children. *Pediatrics, 127*(4), 612–618. https://publications.aap.org/pediatrics/article/127/4/612/65166/Fathers-Depression-Related-to-Positive-and

Demontigny, F., Girard, M. E., Lacharité, C., Dubeau, D., & Devault, A. (2013). Psychosocial factors associated with paternal postnatal depression. *Journal of Affective Disorders, 150*(1), 44–49. https://doi.org/10.1016/j.jad.2013.01.048

Dennis, C. L., Falah-Hassani, K., & Shiri, R. (2017). Prevalence of antenatal and postnatal anxiety: Systematic review and meta-analysis. *British Journal of Psychiatry, 210*(5), 315–323. https://doi.org/10.1192/bjp.bp.116.187179

Diaz-Rojas, F., Matsunaga, M., Tanaka, Y., Kikusui, T., Mogi, K., Nagasawa, M. & Myowa, M. (2021). Development of the paternal brain in expectant fathers during early pregnancy. *NeuroImage, 225*. https://doi.org/10.1016/j.neuroimage.2020.117527

Domoney, J., Trevillion, K., & Challacombe, F. L. (2020). Developing an intervention for paternal perinatal depression: An international Delphi study. *Journal of Affective Disorders Reports, 2*(100033), 1–32. https://doi.org/10.1016/j.jadr.2020.100033

Don, B. P., Chong, A., Biehle, S. N., Gordon, A., & Mickelson, K. D. (2014). Anxiety across the transition to parenthood: Change trajectories among low-risk parents. *27*(6), 633–649. https://doi.org/10.1080/10615806.2014.903473

Don, B. P., & Mickelson, K. D. (2012). Paternal postpartum depression: The role of maternal postpartum depression, spousal support, and relationship satisfaction. *Couple and Family Psychology Research and Practice*, e01–e12. https://doi.org/10.1037/a0029148

Dudley, M., Roy, K., Kelk, N., & Bernard, D. (2001). Psychological correlates of depression in fathers and mothers in the first postnatal year. *Journal of Reproductive and Infant Psychology, 19*(3), 187–202. https://doi.org/10.1080/02646830124397

Edhborg, M., Carlberg, M., Simon, F., & Lindberg, L. (2016). "Waiting for better times": Experiences in the first postpartum year by Swedish fathers with depressive symptoms. *American Journal of Men's Health, 10*(5), 428–439. https://doi.org/10.1177/1557988315574740

Edhborg, M., Matthiesen, A. S., Lundh, W., & Widström, A. M. (2005). Some early indicators for depressive symptoms and bonding 2 months postpartum: A study of new mothers and fathers. *Archives of Women's Mental Health, 8*(4), 221–231. https://doi.org/10.1007/s00737-005-0097-5

Edmondson, O. J. H., Psychogiou, L., Vlachos, H., Netsi, E., & Ramchandani, P. G. (2010). Depression in fathers in the postnatal period: Assessment of the Edinburgh Postnatal Depression Scale as a screening measure. *Journal of Affective Disorders, 125*(1–3), 365–368. https://doi.org/10.1016/j.jad.2010.01.069

Edoka, I. P., Petrou, S., & Ramchandani, P. G. (2011). Healthcare costs of paternal depression in the postnatal period. *Journal of Affective Disorders, 133*(1–2), 356–360. https://doi.org/10.1016/j.jad.2011.04.005

Edvardsen, J., Torgersen, S., Røysamb, E., Lygren, S., Skre, I., Onstad, S., & Øien, P. A. (2009). Unipolar depressive disorders have a common genotype. *Journal of Affective Disorders, 117*(1–2), 30–41. https://doi.org/10.1016/J.JAD.2008.12.004

Eira Nunes, C., de Roten, Y., El Ghaziri, N., Favez, N., & Darwiche, J. (2021). Co-parenting programs: A systematic review and meta-analysis. *Family Relations, 70*(3), 759–776. https://doi.org/10.1111/FARE.12438

Erentzen, C., Quinlan, J. A., & Mar, R. A. (2018). Sometimes you need more than a wingman: Masculinity, femininity, and the role of humor in men's mental health help-seeking campaigns. *Journal of Social and Clinical Psychology, 37*(2), 128–157. https://ca.movember.com/mens-health/

Etheridge, J., & Slade, P. (2017). "Nothing's actually happened to me.": The experiences of fathers who found childbirth traumatic. *BMC Pregnancy and Childbirth*, *17*(1), 80. https://doi.org/10.1186/s12884-017-1259-y

Everett, K. D., Bullock, L., Gage, J. D., Longo, D. R., Geden, E., & Madsen, R. (2006). Health risk behavior of rural low-income expectant fathers. *Public Health Nursing*, *23*(4), 297–306. https://doi.org/10.1111/J.1525-1446.2006.00565.X

Fagan, J., & Lee, Y. (2010). Perceptions and satisfaction with father involvement and adolescent mothers' postpartum depressive symptoms. *Journal of Youth and Adolescence*, *39*(9), 1109–1121. https://doi.org/10.1007/s10964-009-9444-6

Fagan, J., & Pearson, J. (2020). Fathers' dosage in community-based programs for low-income fathers. *Family Process*, *59*(1), 81–93. https://doi.org/10.1111/FAMP.12416

Feinberg, M. E., Jones, D. E., Hostetler, M. L., Roettger, M. E., Paul, I. M., & Ehrenthal, D. B. (2016). Couple-focused prevention at the transition to parenthood, a randomized trial: Effects on coparenting, parenting, family violence, and parent and child adjustment. *Prevention Science*, *17*(6), 751–764. https://doi.org/10.1007/S11121-016-0674-Z

Feinberg, M. E., & Kan, M. L. (2008). Establishing family foundations: Intervention effects on coparenting, parent/infant well-being, and parent-child relations. *Journal of Family Psychology*, *22*(2), 253–263. https://doi.org/10.1037/0893-3200.22.2.253

Feldman, R., Sussman, A. L., & Zigler, E. (2004). Parental leave and work adaptation at the transition to parenthood: Individual, marital, and social correlates. *Journal of Applied Developmental Psychology*, *25*(4), 459–479. https://doi.org/10.1016/j.appdev.2004.06.004

Field, T., Diego, M., Hernandez-Reif, M., Figueiredo, B., Deeds, O., Contogeorgos, J., & Ascencio, A. (2006). Prenatal paternal depression. *Infant Behavior and Development*, *29*(4), 579–583. https://doi.org/10.1016/j.infbeh.2006.07.010

Field, T., Figueiredo, B., Hernandez-Reif, M., Diego, M., Deeds, O., & Ascencio, A. (2008). Massage therapy reduces pain in pregnant women, alleviates prenatal depression in both parents and improves their relationships. *Journal of Bodywork and Movement Therapies*, *12*(2), 146–150. https://doi.org/10.1016/J.JBMT.2007.06.003

Fisher, S. D. (2017). Paternal mental health: Why is it relevant? *American Journal of Lifestyle Medicine*, *11*(3), 200–211. https://doi.org/10.1177/1559827616629895

Fisher, S. D., Cobo, J., Figueiredo, B., Fletcher, R., Garfield, C. F., Hanley, J., Ramchandani, P., & Singley, D. B. (2021). Expanding the international conversation with fathers' mental health: Toward an era of inclusion in perinatal research and practice. *Archives of Women's Mental Health*, *24*(5), 841–848. https://doi.org/10.1007/S00737-021-01171-Y

Fisher, S. D., & Garfield, C. (2016). Opportunities to detect and manage perinatal depression in men. *American Family Physician*, *93*(10). www.aafp.org/afp/2010/1015/p926.

Fletcher, R. J., Feeman, E., Garfield, C., & Vimpani, G. (2011). The effects of early paternal depression on children's development. *Medical Journal of Australia*, *195*(11), 685–689. https://doi.org/10.5694/MJA11.10192

Fletcher, R., St George, J., Newman, L., & Wroe, J. (2020). Male callers to an Australian perinatal depression and anxiety help line–understanding issues and concerns. *Infant Mental Health Journal*, *41*(1), 145–157. https://doi.org/10.1002/IMHJ.21829

Fletcher, R., Vimpani, G., Russell, G., & Sibbritt, D. (2008). Psychosocial assessment of expectant fathers. *Archives of Women's Mental Health*, *11*(1), 27–32. https://doi.org/10.1007/s00737-008-0211-6

Freitas, C. J., & Fox, C. A. (2015). Fathers matter: Family therapy's role in the treatment of paternal peripartum depression. *Contemporary Family Therapy*, *37*(4), 417–425. https://doi.org/10.1007/s10591-015-9347-5

Freitas, C. J., Williams-Reade, J., Distelberg, B., Fox, C. A., & Lister, Z. (2016). Paternal depression during pregnancy and postpartum: An international Delphi study. *Journal of Affective Disorders*, *202*, 128–136. https://doi.org/10.1016/j.jad.2016.05.056

Friedewald, M., Fletcher, R., & Fairbairn, H. (2005). All-male discussion forums for expectant fathers: Evaluation of a model. *The Journal of Perinatal Education*, *14*(2), 8–18. https://doi.org/10.1624/105812405X44673

Gallaher, K. G. H., Slyepchenko, A., Frey, B. N., Urstad, K., & Dørheim, S. K. (2018). The role of Circadian rhythms in postpartum sleep and mood. *Sleep Medicine Clinics*, *13*(3), 359–374. https://doi.org/10.1016/J.JSMC.2018.04.006

Gao, L. L., Chan, S. W. C., & Mao, Q. (2009). Depression, perceived stress, and social support among first-time Chinese mothers and fathers in the postpartum period. *Research in Nursing and Health*, 32(1), 50–58. https://doi.org/10.1002/nur.20306

Garfield, C. F., Duncan, G., Gutina, A., Rutsohn, J., McDade, T. W., Adam, E. K., . . . Chase-Lansdale, P. L. (2016). Longitudinal study of body mass index in young males and the transition to fatherhood. *American Journal of Men's Health*, 10(6), N158–N167. https://doi.org/10.1177/1557988315596224

Garfield, C. F., Duncan, G., Rutsohn, J., McDade, T. W., Adam, E. K., Coley, R. L., & Chase-Lansdale, P. L. (2014). A longitudinal study of paternal mental health during transition to fatherhood as young adults. *Pediatrics*, 133(5), 836–843. https://doi.org/10.1542/PEDS.2013-3262

Garfield, C. F., Simon, C. D., Stephens, F., Castro Román, P., Bryan, M. I., Smith, R. A., Kortsmit, K., Salvesen von Essen, B., Williams, L., Kapaya, M., Dieke, A., Barfield, W., Warner, L., Castro Romá, P., Bryan, M. I., Smith, R. A., Kortsmit, K., Salvesen von Essen, B., Williams, L., & Warner, L. (2022). Pregnancy risk assessment monitoring system for dads: A piloted randomized trial of public health surveillance of recent fathers' behaviors before and after infant birth. *PLoS One*, 17(1), e0262366. https://doi.org/10.1371/journal.pone.0262366

Gawlik, S., Müller, M., Hoffmann, L., Dienes, A., Wallwiener, M., Sohn, C., . . . Reck, C. (2014). Prevalence of paternal perinatal depressiveness and its link to partnership satisfaction and birth concerns. *Archives of Women's Mental Health*, 17(1), 49–56. https://doi.org/10.1007/S00737-013-0377-4

Geller, P. A., Spiecker, N., Cole, J. C. M., Zajac, L., & Patterson, C. A. (2021). The rise of tele-mental health in perinatal settings. *Seminars in Perinatology*, 45(5), 151431. https://doi.org/10.1016/J.SEMPERI.2021.151431

Gettler, L. T., McDade, T. W., Agustin, S. S., & Kuzawa, C. W. (2011). Short-term changes in fathers' hormones during father-child play: Impacts of paternal attitudes and experience. *Hormones and Behavior*, 60(5), 599–606. https://doi.org/10.1016/j.yhbeh.2011.08.009

Giallo, R., D'Esposito, F., Cooklin, A., Mensah, F., Lucas, N., Wade, C., & Nicholson, J. M. (2013). Psychosocial risk factors associated with fathers' mental health in the postnatal period: Results from a population-based study. *Social Psychiatry and Psychiatric Epidemiology*, 48(4), 563–573. https://doi.org/10.1007/S00127-012-0568-8

Giallo, R., Evans, K., & Williams, L. A. (2018). A pilot evaluation of 'working out dads': Promoting father mental health and parental self-efficacy. *Journal of Reproductive and Infant Psychology*, 36(4), 421–433. https://doi.org/10.1080/02646838.2018.1472750

Giallo, R., Seymour, M., Treyvaud, K., Christensen, D., Cook, F., Feinberg, M., Brown, S., & Cooklin, A. (2021). Interparental conflict across the early parenting period: Evidence from fathers participating in an Australian population-based study. *Journal of Family Issues*, 0192513X2110300. https://doi.org/10.1177/0192513X211030042

Gjerdincjen, D., Crow, S., McGovern, P., Miner, M., & Center, B. (2009). Postpartum depression screening at well-child visits: Validity of a 2-question screen and the PHQ-9. *The Annals of Family Medicine*, 7(1), 63–70. https://doi.org/10.1370/AFM.933

Glass, J., Simon, R. W., & Andersson, M. A. (2016). Parenthood and happiness: Effects of work-family reconciliation policies in 22 OECD countries. *American Journal of Sociology*, 122(3), 886–929. https://doi.org/10.1086/688892/ASSET/IMAGES/LARGE/FG2.JPEG

Goldstein, Z., Rosen, B., Howlett, A., Anderson, M., & Herman, D. (2020). Interventions for paternal perinatal depression: A systematic review. *Journal of Affective Disorders*, 265, 505–510. https://doi.org/10.1016/j.jad.2019.12.029

Gordon, I., Pratt, M., Bergunde, K., Zagoory-Sharon, O., & Feldman, R. (2017). Testosterone, oxytocin, and the development of human parental care. *Hormones and Behavior*, 93, 184–192. https://doi.org/10.1016/j.yhbeh.2017.05.016

Gutierrez-Galve, L., Stein, A., Hanington, L., Heron, J., Lewis, G., Ramchandani, P. G., & Author, C. (2019). Association of maternal and paternal depression in the postnatal period with offspring depression at age 18 years supplemental content. *JAMA Psychiatry*, 76(3), 290–296. https://doi.org/10.1001/jamapsychiatry.2018.3667

Habib, C. (2012). Paternal perinatal depression: An overview and suggestions towards an intervention model. *Journal of Family Studies*, 18(1), 4–16. https://doi.org/10.5172/jfs.2012.18.1.4

Håland, K., Lundgren, I., & Eri, T. S. (2016). Fathers' experiences of being in change during pregnancy and early parenthood in a context of intimate partner violence. *International Journal of Qualitative Studies on Health and Well-Being, 11*(1), 1–10. https://doi.org/10.3402/qhw.v11.30935

Hammer, J. H., & Vogel, D. L. (2010). Men's help seeking for depression: The efficacy of a male-sensitive brochure about counseling. *The Counseling Psychologist, 38*(2), 296–313. https://doi.org/10.1177/0011000009351937

Hanington, L., Ramchandani, P., & Stein, A. (2010). Parental depression and child temperament: Assessing child to parent effects in a longitudinal population study. *Infant Behavior and Development, 33*(1), 88–95. https://doi.org/10.1016/j.infbeh.2009.11.004

Hanley, J., & Williams, M. (2020). Fathers' perinatal mental health. *British Journal of Midwifery, 28*(2), 84–85. https://doi.org/10.12968/bjom.2020.28.2.84

Hart, S., Field, T., Stern, M., & Jones, N. (1997). Depressed fathers' stereotyping of infants labeled "depressed". *Infant Mental Health Journal, 18*(4), 436–445. https://doi.org/10.1002/(SICI)1097-0355(199724)18:4

Helle, N., Barkmann, C., Ehrhardt, S., & Bindt, C. (2018). Postpartum posttraumatic and acute stress in mothers and fathers of infants with very low birth weight: Cross-sectional results from a controlled multicenter cohort study. *Journal of Affective Disorders, 235*, 467–473. https://doi.org/10.1016/j.jad.2018.04.013

Hodgson, S., Painter, J., Kilby, L., Hirst, J., Moran, J. M., & Mohamed, A.-L. (2021). The experiences of first-time fathers in perinatal services: Present but invisible. *Healthcare (Switzerland), 9*(2), 1–12. https://doi.org/10.3390/healthcare9020161

Hollywood, M., & Hollywood, E. (2011). The lived experiences of fathers of a premature baby on a neonatal intensive care unit. *Journal of Neonatal Nursing, 17*(1), 32–40. https://doi.org/10.1016/j.jnn.2010.07.015

Howard, L. M., Molyneaux, E., Dennis, C. L., Rochat, T., Stein, A., & Milgrom, J. (2014). Non-psychotic mental disorders in the perinatal period. *The Lancet, 384*(9956), 1775–1788. https://doi.org/10.1016/S0140-6736(14)61276-9

Huang, X., Chen, L., & Zhang, L. (2019). Effects of paternal skin-to-skin contact in newborns and fathers after Cesarean delivery. *Journal of Perinatal and Neonatal Nursing, 33*(1), 68–73. https://doi.org/10.1097/JPN.0000000000000384

Hung, C., Chung, H., Medical, Y. C.-K. J. of, & 1996, U. (1996). The effect of child-birth class on first-time fathers' psychological responses. *Kaohsiung Journal of Medical Science, 12*, 248–255. http://ir.kmu.edu.tw/retrieve/5019/735009-2.pdf

Husain, M. I., Chaudhry, I. B., Khoso, A. B., Wan, M. W., Kiran, T., Shiri, T., . . . Husain, N. (2021). A group parenting intervention for depressed fathers (LTP + Dads): A feasibility study from Pakistan. *Children, 8*(1), 26. https://doi.org/10.3390/CHILDREN8010026

Inglis, C., Sharman, R., & Reed, R. (2016). Paternal mental health following perceived traumatic childbirth. *Midwifery, 41*, 125–131. https://doi.org/10.1016/J.MIDW.2016.08.008

Isacco, A., Hofscher, R., & Molloy, S. (2016). An examination of fathers' mental health help seeking: A brief report. *American Journal of Men's Health, 10*(6), N33–N38. https://doi.org/10.1177/1557988315581395

Kaplan, P. S., Sliter, J. K., & Burgess, A. P. (2007). Infant-directed speech produced by fathers with symptoms of depression: Effects on infant associative learning in a conditioned-attention paradigm. *Infant Behavior and Development, 30*(4), 535–545. https://doi.org/10.1016/J.INFBEH.2007.05.003

Kennedy, E., & Munyan, K. (2021). Sensitivity and reliability of screening measures for paternal postpartum depression: An integrative review. *Journal of Perinatology : Official Journal of the California Perinatal Association, 41*(12), 2713–2721. https://doi.org/10.1038/S41372-021-01265-6

Kilmartin, C. (2005). Depression in men: Communication, diagnosis and therapy. *Journal of Men's Health and Gender, 2*(1), 95–99. https://doi.org/10.1016/J.JMHG.2004.10.010

Kim, P., Rigo, P., Mayes, L. C., Feldman, R., Leckman, J. F., & Swain, J. E. (2014). Neural plasticity in fathers of human infants. *Social Neuroscience, 9*(5), 522–535. https://doi.org/10.1080/17470919.2014.933713

Kiviruusu, O., Pietikäinen, J. T., Kylliäinen, A., Pölkki, P., Saarenpää-Heikkilä, O., Marttunen, M., . . . Paavonen, E. J. (2020). Trajectories of mothers' and fathers' depressive symptoms from pregnancy to 24 months postpartum. *Journal of Affective Disorders, 260,* 629–637. https://doi. org/10.1016/j.jad.2019.09.038

Koliouli, F., Gaudron, C. Z., & Raynaud, J. P. (2016). Stress, coping, and post-traumatic stress disorder of French fathers of premature infants. *Newborn and Infant Nursing Reviews, 16*(3), 110–114. https://doi.org/10.1053/J.NAINR.2016.08.003

Kornfeind, K. R., & Sipsma, H. L. (2018). Exploring the link between maternity leave and postpartum depression. *Women's Health Issues, 28*(4), 321–326. https://doi.org/10.1016/J.WHI.2018.03.008

Kroenke, K., Spitzer, R. L., & Williams, J. B. W. (2003). The patient health questionnaire-2: Validity of a two-item depression screener. *Medical Care, 41*(11), 1284–1292. https://doi.org/10.1097/01. MLR.0000093487.78664.3C

Kvalevaag, A. L., Ramchandani, P. G., Hove, O., Assmus, J., Eberhard-Gran, M., & Biringer, E. (2013). Paternal mental health and socioemotional and behavioral development in their children. *Pediatrics, 131*(2). https://doi.org/10.1542/PEDS.2012-0804

Lai, B. P. Y., Tang, A. K. L., Lee, D. T. S., Yip, A. S. K., & Chung, T. K. H. (2010). Detecting postnatal depression in Chinese men: A comparison of three instruments. *Psychiatry Research, 180*(2–3), 80–85. https://doi.org/10.1016/J.PSYCHRES.2009.07.015

Leach, L. S., Poyser, C., Cooklin, A. R., & Giallo, R. (2016). Prevalence and course of anxiety disorders (and symptom levels) in men across the perinatal period: A systematic review. *Journal of Affective Disorders, 190,* 675–686. https://doi.org/10.1016/J.JAD.2015.09.063

Lee, J. Y., Knauer, H. A., Lee, S. J., MacEachern, M. P., & Garfeld, C. F. (2018). Father-inclusive perinatal parent education programs: A systematic review. *Pediatrics, 142*(1), 2021. https://doi. org/10.1542/peds.2018-0437

Lee, S. J., Bellamy, J. L., & Guterman, N. B. (2009). Fathers, physical child abuse, and neglect: Advancing the knowledge base. *Child Maltreatment, 14*(227), 227–231. https://doi. org/10.1177/1077559509339388

Leiferman, J. A., Farewell, C. V, Jewell, J., Lacy, R., Walls, J., Harnke, B., & Paulson, J. F. (2021). *Anxiety among fathers during the prenatal and postpartum period: A meta-analysis.* https://doi. org/10.1080/0167482X.2021.1885025

Levant, R. F., Wimer, D. J., Williams, C. M., Smalley, K. B., & Noronha, D. (2009). The relationships between masculinity variables, health risk behaviors and attitudes toward seeking psychological help. *International Journal of Men's Health, 8*(1), 3–21. https://doi.org/10.3149/ JMH.0801.3

Lever Taylor B, Billings J, Morant N, Johnson S. (2018). How do women's partners view perinatal mental health services? A qualitative meta-synthesis. *Clin Psychol Psychother, 25,* 112–129. https:// doi.org/10.1002/cpp.2133

Li, H.-T., Lin, K.-C., Chang, S.-C., Kuo, S.-C., Liu, C.-Y., & Kuo, S.-C. (2009). A birth education program for expectant fathers in Taiwan: Effects on their anxiety. *Birth, 36*(4), 289–296. https:// doi.org/10.1111/J.1523-536X.2009.00356.X

Lindberg, B., Axelsson, K., & Öhrling, K. (2007). The birth of premature infants: Experiences from the fathers' perspective. *Journal of Neonatal Nursing, 13*(4), 142–149. https://doi.org/10.1016/J. JNN.2007.05.004

Lindberg, B., Axelsson, K., & Öhrling, K. (2008). Adjusting to being a father to an infant born prematurely: Experiences from Swedish fathers. *Scandinavian Journal of Caring Sciences, 22*(1), 79–85. https://doi.org/10.1111/J.1471-6712.2007.00563.X

Lindberg, I., & Engström, Å. (2013). A qualitative study of new fathers' experiences of care in relation to complicated childbirth. *Sexual and Reproductive Healthcare, 4*(4), 147–152. https://doi. org/10.1016/J.SRHC.2013.10.002

Linville, D., Todahl, J., Brown, T., Terrell, L., & Gau, J. (2017). Healthy nests transition to parenthood program: A mixed-methods study. *Journal of Couple and Relationship Therapy, 16*(4), 346–361. https://doi.org/10.1080/15332691.2016.1270867

Madsen, K. B., Mægbæk, M. L., Thomsen, N. S., Liu, X., Eberhard-Gran, M., Skalkidou, A., . . . Munk-Olsen, T. (2022). Pregnancy and postpartum psychiatric episodes in fathers: A population-based study on treatment incidence and prevalence. *Journal of Affective Disorders, 296,* 130–135.

Madsen, S. A. (2009). Men's mental health: Fatherhood and psychotherapy. *The Journal of Men's Studies, 17*(1), 15–30. https://doi.org/10.3149/jms.1701.15

Mangialavori, S., Giannotti, M., Cacioppo, M., Spelzini, F., & Baldoni, F. (2021). Screening for early signs of paternal perinatal affective disorder in expectant fathers: A cluster analysis approach. *Journal of Personalized Medicine*, 11(1), 1–15. https://doi.org/10.3390/jpm11010010

Mansfield, A., Addis, M., & Mahalik, J. (2003). "Why won't he go to the doctor?": The psychology of men's help seeking. *International Journal of Men's Health*, 2(2), 93–109. https://doi.org/10.3149/JMH.0202.93

Matthey, S., & Barnett, B. (1999). Parent–infant classes in the early postpartum period: Need and participation by fathers and mothers–Matthey–1999–Infant Mental Health Journal–Wiley Online Library. *Infant Mental Health Journal*, 20(3), 287–290. https://onlinelibrary.wiley.com/doi/pdf/10.1002/(SICI)1097-0355(199923)20:3%3C278::AID-IMHJ5%3E3.0.CO;2-I

Matthey, S., Barnett, B., Kavanagh, D. J., & Howie, P. (2001). Validation of the Edinburgh Postnatal Depression Scale for men and comparison of item endorsement with their partners. *Journal of Affective Disorders*, 64(2–3), 175–184. https://doi.org/10.1016/s0165-0327(00)00236-6

Mellinger, T. N., & Liu, W. M. (2006). Men's issues in doctoral training: A survey of counseling psychology programs. *Professional Psychology: Research and Practice*, 37(2), 196–204. https://doi.org/10.1037/0735-7028.37.2.196

Melnyk, B. M., Feinstein, N. F., Alpert-Gillis, L., Fairbanks, E., Crean, H. F., Sinkin, R. A., . . . Gross, S. J. (2006). Reducing premature infants' length of stay and improving parents' mental health outcomes with the Creating Opportunities for Parent Empowerment (COPE) neonatal intensive care unit program: A randomized, controlled trial. *Pediatrics*, 118(5), e1414–e1427. https://doi.org/10.1542/PEDS.2005-2580

Menzies, J. (2021). Forgotten fathers: The impact of service reduction during Covid-19. *Journal of Health Visiting*, 9(4), 150–153. https://doi.org/10.12968/JOHV.2021.9.4.150

Mihelic, M., Morawska, A., & Filus, A. (2018). Does a perinatal parenting intervention work for fathers? A randomized controlled trial. *Infant Mental Health Journal*, 39(6), 687–698. https://doi.org/10.1002/IMHJ.21748

Misra, D. P., Guyer, B., & Allston, A. (2003). Integrated perinatal health framework: A multiple determinants model with a life span approach. *American Journal of Preventive Medicine*, 25(1), 65–75. https://doi.org/10.1016/S0749-3797(03)00090-4

Mniszak, C., O'Brien, H. L., Greyson, D., Chabot, C., & Shoveller, J. (2020). "Nothing's available": Young fathers' experiences with unmet information needs and barriers to resolving them. *Information Processing & Management*, 57(2), 102081. https://doi.org/10.1016/j.ipm.2019.102081

Mohammadpour, M., Mohammad-Alizadeh Charandabi, S., Malakouti, J., Mohammadi, M. N., & Mirghafourvand, M. (2021). The effect of counseling on fathers' stress and anxiety during pregnancy: A randomized controlled clinical trial. *BMC Psychiatry*, 21(1). https://doi.org/10.1186/s12888-021-03217-y

Molgora, S., Fenaroli, V., Malgaroli, M., & Saita, E. (2017). Trajectories of postpartum depression in Italian first-time fathers. *American Journal of Men's Health*, 11(4), 880–887. https://doi.org/10.1177/1557988316677692

Molloy, S., & Pierro, A. (2020). "It's not girly": Rural service providers' perceptions of fathering, masculinities, and intersectionality. *Children and Youth Services Review*, 115. https://doi.org/10.1016/J.CHILDYOUTH.2020.105095

Moyer, S. W., & Kinser, P. A. (2021). A comprehensive conceptual framework to guide clinical practice and research about mental health during the perinatal period. *Journal of Perinatal and Neonatal Nursing*, 35(1), 46–56. https://doi.org/10.1097/JPN.0000000000000535

Mrazek, P. J., & Haggerty, R. J. (1994). Reducing risks for mental disorders: Frontiers for preventive intervention research. In *Reducing risks for mental disorders*. https://doi.org/10.17226/2139

Nasreen, H. E., Rahman, J. A., Rus, R. M., Kartiwi, M., Sutan, R., & Edhborg, M. (2018). Prevalence and determinants of antepartum depressive and anxiety symptoms in expectant mothers and fathers: Results from a perinatal psychiatric morbidity cohort study in the east and west coasts of Malaysia. *BMC Psychiatry*, 18(1), 195. https://doi.org/10.1186/s12888-018-1781-0

Nemoda, Z., & Szyf, M. (2017). Epigenetic alterations and prenatal maternal depression. *Birth Defects Research*, 109(12), 888–897. https://doi.org/10.1002/BDR2.1081

O'Brien, A. P., McNeil, K. A., Fletcher, R., Conrad, A., Wilson, A. J., Jones, D., & Chan, S. W. (2017). New fathers' perinatal depression and anxiety–treatment options: An integrative review. *American Journal of Men's Health*, 11(4), 863–876. https://doi.org/10.1177/1557988316669047

O'Brien, R., Hunt, K., & Hart, G. (2005). It's caveman stuff, but that is to a certain extent how guys still operate: Men's accounts of masculinity and help seeking. *Social Science & Medicine (1982)*, 61(3), 503–516. https://doi.org/10.1016/j.socscimed.2004.12.008

Oliffe, J. L., & Phillips, M. J. (2008). Men, depression and masculinities : A review and recommendations. *Journal of Men's Health*, 5(3), 194–202; 1–9.

Oliffe, J. L., Rossnagel, E., Seidler, Z. E., Kealy, D., Ogrodniczuk, J. S., & Rice, S. M. (2019). Men's depression and suicide. *Current Psychiatry Reports*, 21(103), e01–e06. https://doi.org/10.1007/s11920-019-1088-y

Panter-Brick, C., Burgess, A., Eggerman, M., McAllister, F., Pruett, K., & Leckman, J. F. (2014). Practitioner review: Engaging fathers–recommendations for a game change in parenting interventions based on a systematic review of the global evidence. *Journal of Child Psychology and Psychiatry and Allied Disciplines*, 55(11), 1187–1212. https://doi.org/10.1111/JCPP.12280

Parent, M. C., Hammer, J. H., Bradstreet, T. C., Schwartz, E. N., & Jobe, T. (2018). Men's mental health help-seeking behaviors: An intersectional analysis. *American Journal of Men's Health*, 12(1), 64–73. https://doi.org/10.1177/1557988315625776

Parfitt, Y., & Ayers, S. (2014). Transition to parenthood and mental health in first-time parents. *Infant Mental Health Journal*, 35(3), 263–273. https://doi.org/10.1002/imhj.21443

Parfitt, Y., Pike, A., & Ayers, S. (2013). The impact of parents' mental health on parent-baby interaction: A prospective study. *Infant Behavior and Development*, 36(4), 599–608. https://doi.org/10.1016/j.infbeh.2013.06.003

Paul, J. J., Dardar, S., River, L. M., & St. John-Larkin, C. (2022). Telehealth adaptation of perinatal mental health mother–infant group programming for the COVID-19 pandemic. *Infant Mental Health Journal*, 43(1), 85–99. https://doi.org/10.1002/IMHJ.21960

Paulson, J. F., & Bazemore, S. D. (2010). Prenatal and postpartum depression in fathers and its association with maternal depression: A meta-analysis. *JAMA–Journal of the American Medical Association*, 303(19), 1961–1969. https://doi.org/10.1001/JAMA.2010.605

Paulson, J. F., Bazemore, S. D., Goodman, J. H., & Leiferman, J. A. (2016). The course and interrelationship of maternal and paternal perinatal depression. *Arch Womens Ment Health*, 19(4), 655–663. https://doi.org/10.1007/s00737-016-0598-4

Paulson, J. F., Dauber, S., & Leiferman, J. A. (2006). Individual and combined effects of postpartum depression in mothers and fathers on parenting behavior. *Pediatrics*, 118(2), 659–668. https://doi.org/10.1542/PEDS.2005-2948

Paulson, J. F., Ellis, K. T., & Alexander, R. L. (2020). Paternal prenatal and postpartum depression. In *Handbook of fathers and child development*, 229–244. https://doi.org/10.1007/978-3-030-51027-5_15

Paulson, J. F., Keefe, H. A., & Leiferman, J. A. (2009). Early parental depression and child language development. *Journal of Child Psychology and Psychiatry and Allied Disciplines*, 50(3), 254–262. https://doi.org/10.1111/J.1469-7610.2008.01973.X

Philpott, L. P., Savage, E., Fitzgerald, S. M., & Leahy-Warren, P. (2019). Anxiety in fathers in the perinatal period: A systematic review. *Midwifery*, 76, 54–101. https://doi.org/10.1016/j.midw.2019.05.013

Philpott, L. P., Savage, E., Leahy-Warren, P., & Fitzgerald, S. (2020). Paternal perinatal depression: A narrative review. *International Journal of Men's Social and Community Health*, 3(1), e01–e15. www.ijmsch.com/index.php/IJMSCH/article/view/22/17

Poh, H. L., Koh, S. S. L., & He, H. G. (2014). An integrative review of fathers' experiences during pregnancy and childbirth. *International Nursing Review*, 61(4), 543–554. https://doi.org/10.1111/INR.12137

Powis, R. (2022). From covade to "men's involvement": Sociocultural perspectives of expectant fatherhood. In S. Han & C. Tomori (Eds.), *The Routledge handbook of anthropology and reproduction* (pp. 410–421). Routledge.

Primack, J. M., Addis, M. E., Syzdek, M., & Miller, I. W. (2010). The men's stress workshop: A gender-sensitive treatment for depressed men. *Cognitive and Behavioral Practice*, 17(1), 77–87. https://doi.org/10.1016/J.CBPRA.2009.07.002

Provenzi, L., & Santoro, E. (2015). The lived experience of fathers of preterm infants in the neonatal intensive care unit: A systematic review of qualitative studies. *Journal of Clinical Nursing*, 24(13–14), 1784–1794. https://doi.org/10.1111/JOCN.12828

Psouni, E., Agebjörn, J., & Linder, H. (2017). Symptoms of depression in Swedish fathers in the postnatal period and development of a screening tool. *Scandinavian Journal of Psychology, 58*(6), 485–496. https://doi.org/10.1111/sjop.12396

Quevedo, L., Da Silva, R. A., Coelho, F., Pinheiro, K. A. T., Horta, B. L., Kapczinski, F., & Pinheiro, R. T. (2011). Risk of suicide and mixed episode in men in the postpartum period. *Journal of Affective Disorders, 132*(1–2), 243–246. https://doi.org/10.1016/J.JAD.2011.01.004

Ramchandani, P. G., & Psychogiou, L. (2009). Paternal psychiatric disorders and children's psychosocial development. In *The Lancet* (Vol. 374, Issue 9690, pp. 646–653). Elsevier B.V. https://doi.org/10.1016/S0140-6736(09)60238-5

Ramchandani, P. G., Stein, A., O'Connor, T. G., Heron, J., Murray, L., & Evans, J. (2008). Depression in men in the postnatal period and later child psychopathology: A population cohort study. *Journal of the American Academy of Child and Adolescent Psychiatry, 47*(4), 390–398. https://doi.org/10.1097/CHI.0b013e31816429c2

Ramos, G., & Chavira, D. A. (2022). Use of technology to provide mental health care for racial and ethnic minorities: Evidence, promise, and challenges. *Cognitive and Behavioral Practice, 29*(1), 15–40. https://doi.org/10.1016/J.CBPRA.2019.10.004

Reeb, B. T., Wu, E. Y., Martin, M. J., Gelardi, K. L., Chan, S. Y. S., & Conger, K. J. (2015). Long-term effects of fathers' depressed mood on youth internalizing symptoms in early adulthood. *Journal of Research on Adolescence, 25*(1), 151–162. https://doi.org/10.1111/JORA.12112

Rice, S. M., Kealy, D., Seidler, Z. E., Oliffe, J. L., Levant, R. F., & Ogrodniczuk, J. S. (2020). Male-type and prototypal depression trajectories for men experiencing mental health problems. *International Journal of Environmental Research and Public Health, 17*(7322), e01–e15. https://doi.org/10.3390/ijerph17197322

Rice, S. M., Ogrodniczuk, J. S., Kealy, D., Seidler, Z. E., Dhillon, H. M., & Oliffe, J. L. (2019). Validity of the male depression risk scale in a representative Canadian sample: Sensitivity and specificity in identifying men with recent suicide attempt. *Journal of Mental Health, 28*(2), 132–140. https://doi.org/10.1080/09638237.2017.1417565

Richardson, C., Robb, K. A., & O'Connor, R. C. (2021). A systematic review of suicidal behaviour in men: A narrative synthesis of risk factors. *Social Science & Medicine, 276*, 113831. https://doi.org/10.1016/J.SOCSCIMED.2021.113831

Rilling, J. K., & Mascaro, J. S. (2017). The neurobiology of fatherhood. *Current Opinion in Psychology, 15*, 26–32. https://doi.org/10.1016/j.copsyc.2017.02.013

Rochlen, A. B., & Hoyer, W. D. (2005). Marketing mental health to men: Theoretical and practical considerations. *Journal of Clinical Psychology, 61*(6), 675–684. https://doi.org/10.1002/JCLP.20102

Rochlen, A. B., Whilde, M. R., & Hoyer, W. D. (2005). The real men: Real depression campaign: Overview, theoretical implications, and research considerations. *Psychology of Men and Masculinity, 6*(3), 186–194. https://doi.org/10.1037/1524-9220.6.3.186

Rominov, H., Giallo, R., Pilkington, P. D., & Whelan, T. A. (2018). "Getting help for yourself is a way of helping your baby": Fathers' experie . . .: EBSCOhost. *Psychology of Men & Masculinity, 19*(3), 457–468. https://web.a.ebscohost.com/ehost/pdfviewer/pdfviewer?vid=0&sid=070affcc-f2ed-4cea-bae6-217a2ea85ba3%40sdc-v-sessmgr01

Rominov, H., Pilkington, P. D., Giallo, R., & Whelan, T. A. (2016). A systematic review of interventions targeting paternal mental health in the perinatal period. *Infant Mental Health Journal, 37*(3), 289–301. https://doi.org/10.1002/IMHJ.21560

Roubinov, D. S., Luecken, L. J., Crnic, K. A., & Gonzales, N. A. (2014). Postnatal depression in Mexican American fathers: Demographic, cultural, and familial predictors. *Journal of Affective Disorders, 152–154*(1), 360–368. https://doi.org/10.1016/j.jad.2013.09.038

Rowe, H. J., Holton, S., & Fisher, J. R. W. (2013). Postpartum emotional support: A qualitative study of women's and men's anticipated needs and preferred sources. *Australian Journal of Primary Health, 19*(1), 46–52. https://doi.org/10.1071/PY11117

Salcuni, S., Sharpe, D., Candelori, C., Vismara, L., Rollè, L., Agostini, F., . . . Tambelli, R. (2016). *Perinatal parenting stress, anxiety, and depression outcomes in first-time mothers and fathers: A 3- to 6-months postpartum follow-up study.* https://doi.org/10.3389/fpsyg.2016.00938

Saltzman, W., & Ziegler, T. E. (2014). Functional significance of hormonal changes in mammalian fathers. In *Journal of Neuroendocrinology* (Vol. 26, Issue 10, pp. 685–696). Blackwell Publishing Ltd. https://doi.org/10.1111/jne.12176

Salvesen von Essen, B., Kortsmit, K., D'Angelo, D. V., Warner, L., Smith, R. A., Simon, C., . . . Vargas Bernal, M. I. (2021). Opportunities to address men's health during the perinatal period–Puerto Rico, 2017. *MMWR. Morbidity and Mortality Weekly Report, 69*(5152), 1638–1641. https://doi.org/10.15585/mmwr.mm695152a2

Samuels, C. A., Scholz, K., & Edmundson, S. (1992). The effects of baby bath and massage by fathers on the family system: The Sunraysia Australia Intervention Project. *Early Development and Parenting, 1*(1), 39–49. https://doi.org/10.1002/EDP.2430010109

Schumacher, M., Zubaran, C., & White, G. (2008). Bringing birth-related paternal depression to the fore. In *Women and Birth* (Vol. 21, Issue 2, pp. 65–70). https://doi.org/10.1016/j.wombi.2008.03.008

Schuppan, K. M., Roberts, R., & Powrie, R. (2019). Paternal perinatal mental health: At-risk fathers' perceptions of help-seeking and screening. *Journal of Men's Studies, 27*(3), 307–328. https://doi.org/10.1177/1060826519829908

Seidler, Z. E., Rice, S. M., Kealy, D., Oliffe, J. L., & Ogrodniczuk, J. S. (2020). What gets in the way? Men's perspectives of barriers to mental health services. *International Journal of Social Psychiatry, 66*(2), 105–110. https://doi.org/10.1177/0020764019886336

Séjourné, N., Vaslot, V., Beaumé, M., Goutaudier, N., & Chabrol, H. (2012). The impact of paternity leave and paternal involvement in child care on maternal postpartum depression. *30*(2), 135–144. https://doi.org/10.1080/02646838.2012.693155

Sethna, V., Murray, L., Netsi, E., Psychogiou, L., & Ramchandani, P. G. (2015). Paternal depression in the postnatal period and early father–infant interactions. *Parenting, 15*(1), 1–8. https://doi.org/10.1080/15295192.2015.992732

Sethna, V., Siew, J., Pote, I., Wang, S., Gudbrandsen, M., Lee, C., . . . McAlonan, G. M. (2019). Father-infant interactions and infant regional brain volumes: A cross-sectional MRI study. *Developmental Cognitive Neuroscience, 40*, 100721. https://doi.org/10.1016/J.DCN.2019.100721

Shorey, S., Dennis, C. L., Bridge, S., Chong, Y. S., Holroyd, E., & He, H. G. (2017). First-time fathers' postnatal experiences and support needs: A descriptive qualitative study. *Journal of Advanced Nursing, 73*(12), 2987–2996. https://doi.org/10.1111/jan.13349

Simonovich, S. D., Nidey, N. L., Gavin, A. R., Piñeros-Leaño, M., Hsieh, W.-J., Sbrilli, M. D., . . . Tabb, K. M. (2021). Meta-analysis of antenatal depression and adverse birth outcomes in US populations, 2010–20. *Health Affairs, 40*(10), 1560–1565. https://doi.org/10.1377/HLTHAFF.2021.00801

Sinkewicz, M., & Lee, R. (2010). Prevalence, comorbidity, and course of depression among black fathers in the United States. *Research on Social Work Practice, 21*(3), 289–297. https://doi.org/10.1177/1049731510386497

Skjothaug, T., Smith, L., Wentzel-Larsen, T., & Moe, V. (2018). Does fathers' prenatal mental health bear a relationship to parenting stress at 6 months? *Infant Mental Health Journal, 39*(5), 537–551. https://doi.org/10.1002/IMHJ.21739

Stewart, D. E., Vigod, S. N., Macmillan, H. L., Chandra, P. S., Han, A., Rondon, M. B., Macgregor, J. C. D., & Riazantseva, E. (2017). Current reports on perinatal intimate partner violence. *Current Psychiatry Reports, 19*(26), 1–10. https://doi.org/10.1007/s11920-017-0778-6

Sullivan, A. B., Kane, A., Roth, A. J., Davis, B. E., Drerup, M. L., & Heinberg, L. J. (2020). The COVID-19 crisis: A mental health perspective and response using telemedicine. *Journal of Patient Experience, 7*(3), 295–301. https://doi.org/10.1177/2374373520922747

Suto, M., Takehara, K., Yamane, Y., & Ota, E. (2016). Effects of prenatal childbirth education for partners of pregnant women on paternal postnatal mental health: A systematic review and meta-analysis protocol. *Systematic Reviews, 5*(1), 1–4. https://doi.org/10.1186/S13643-016-0199-3

Swain, J. E., Dayton, C. J., Kim, P., Tolman, R. M., & Volling, B. L. (2014). Progress on the paternal brain: Theory, animal models, human brain research, and mental health implications. *Infant Mental Health Journal, 35*(5), 394–408. https://doi.org/10.1002/imhj.21471

Sweeney, S., & MacBeth, A. (2016). The effects of paternal depression on child and adolescent outcomes: A systematic review. *Journal of Affective Disorders, 205*, 44–59. https://doi.org/10.1016/j.jad.2016.05.073

Tanaka, S., & Waldfogel, J. (2007). Effects of parental leave and work hours on fathers' involvement with their babies. *Community, Work and Family, 10*(4), 409–426. https://doi.org/10.1080/13668800701575069

Tandon, S. D., Hamil, J., Gier, E. E., & Garfield, C. F. (2021). Examining the effectiveness of the fathers and babies intervention: A pilot study. *Frontiers in Psychology, 12*. https://doi.org/10.3389/FPSYG.2021.668284

Teti, D. M., Cole, P. M., Cabrera, N., Goodman, S. H., & McLoyd, V. C. (2017). Supporting parents: How six decades of parenting research can inform policy and best practice. *SRCD Social Policy Report, 30*(5), 1–34. https://eric.ed.gov/?id=ED581662

Thapa, S. B., De Prisco, M., Kingstone, T., Thiel, F., Pittelkow, M.-M., Wittchen, H.-U., & Garthus-Niegel, S. (2020). The relationship between paternal and maternal depression during the perinatal period: A systematic review and meta-analysis. *Frontiers in Psychiatry | Www.Frontiersin.Org, 11*, 563287. https://doi.org/10.3389/fpsyt.2020.563287

Tohotoa, J., Maycock, B., Hauck, Y. L., Dhaliwal, S., Howat, P., Burns, S., & Binns, C. W. (2012). Can father inclusive practice reduce paternal postnatal anxiety? A repeated measures cohort study using the hospital anxiety and depression scale. *BMC Pregnancy and Childbirth, 12*(1), 1–8. https://doi.org/10.1186/1471-2393-12-75/TABLES/3

Torche, F., & Rauf, T. (2021). The transition to fatherhood and the health of men. *Journal of Marriage and Family, 83*(2), 446–465. https://doi.org/https://doi.org/10.1111/jomf.12732

Tylor, E. B. (1865). *Researches into the early history of mankind and the development of civilization*. John Murray. https://archive.org/details/researchesintoea65tylo

Van Den Berg, M. P., Van Der Ende, J., Crijnen, A. A. M., Jaddoe, V. W. V., Moll, H. A., Mackenbach, J. P., . . . Verhulst, F. C. (2009). Paternal depressive symptoms during pregnancy are related to excessive infant crying. *Pediatrics, 124*(1). https://doi.org/10.1542/peds.2008-3100

Van Niel, M. S., Bhatia, R., Riano, N. S., De Faria, L., Catapano-Friedman, L., Ravven, S., . . . Mangurian, C. (2020). The impact of paid maternity leave on the mental and physical health of mothers and children: A review of the literature and policy implications. *Harvard Review of Psychiatry, 28*(2), 113–126. https://doi.org/10.1097/HRP.0000000000000246

Vänskä, M., Punamäki, R.-L. L., Tolvanen, A., Lindblom, J., Flykt, M., Unkila-Kallio, L., Tulppala, M., & Tiitinen, A. (2017). Paternal mental health trajectory classes and early fathering experiences: Prospective study on a normative and formerly infertile sample. *International Journal of Behavioral Development, 41*(5), 570–580. https://doi.org/10.1177/0165025416654301

Vignato, J., Georges, J. M., Bush, R. A., & Connelly, C. D. (2017). Post-Traumatic Stress Disorder (PPTSD) in the perinatal period: A concept analysis. *Journal of Clinical Nursing, 26*(23–24), 3859. https://doi.org/10.1111/JOCN.13800

Vogel, D. L., Heimerdinger-Edwards, S. R., Hammer, J. H., & Hubbard, A. (2011). "Boys don't cry": Examination of the links between endorsement of masculine norms, self-stigma, and help-seeking attitudes for men from diverse backgrounds. *Journal of Counseling Psychology, 58*(3), 368–382. https://doi.org/10.1037/A0023688

Walsh, T. B., Davis, R. N., & Garfield, C. (2020a). A call to action: Screening fathers for perinatal depression. *Pediatrics, 145*(1). https://doi.org/10.1542/PEDS.2019-1193

Walsh, T. B., Davis, R. N., & Garfield, C. (2020b). A call to action: Screening fathers for perinatal depression. *Pediatrics, 145*(1), e20191193. https://doi.org/10.1542/peds.2019-1193

Watts, G. (2008). *Men get depression guide*. www.mengetdepression.com/incl/men_get_depression.pdf

Webb, R., Smith, A. M., Ayers, S., Wright, D. B., & Thornton, A. (2021). Development and validation of a measure of birth-related PTSD for fathers and birth partners: The city birth trauma scale (partner version). *Frontiers in Psychology, 12*. https://doi.org/10.3389/FPSYG.2021.596779

Wee, K. Y., Skouteris, H., Pier, C., Richardson, B., & Milgrom, J. (2011). Correlates of ante- and postnatal depression in fathers: A systematic review. *Journal of Affective Disorders, 130*(3), 358–377. https://doi.org/10.1016/j.jad.2010.06.019

Whitley, R. (2021). Why do men have low rates of formal mental health service utilization? An analysis of social and systemic barriers to care and discussion of promising male-friendly practices. *Men's Issues and Men's Mental Health*, 127–149. https://doi.org/10.1007/978-3-030-86320-3_6

Wilson, S., & Durbin, C. E. (2010). Effects of paternal depression on fathers' parenting behaviors: A meta-analytic review. *Clinical Psychology Review, 30*(2), 167–180. https://doi.org/10.1016/J.CPR.2009.10.007

Wittenborn, A. K., Culpepper, B., Liu, T., Wittenborn, A. K., Culpepper, Á. B., & Liu, T. (2012). Treating depression in men: The role of emotionally focused couple therapy. *Contemporary Family Therapy, 34*(1), 89–103. https://doi.org/10.1007/S10591-012-9176-8

Yogman, M., & Garfield, C. F. (2016). Fathers' roles in the care and development of their children: The role of pediatricians. *Pediatrics, 138*(1). https://doi.org/10.1542/PEDS.2016-1128

Yoshida, T., Taga, C., Matsumoto, Y., & Fukui, K. (2005). Paternal overprotection in obsessive-compulsive disorder and depression with obsessive traits. *Psychiatry and Clinical Neurosciences, 59*(5), 533–538. https://doi.org/10.1111/j.1440-1819.2005.01410.x

Zacher, M., Sauer, C., Haßdenteufel, K., Wallwiener, S., Wallwiener, M., & Maatouk, I. (2022). *Prenatal paternal depression, anxiety, and somatic symptom burden in different risk samples: An explorative study.* https://doi.org/10.21203/rs.3.rs-1275875/v1

Zhang, Y.-P., Zhang, L.-L., Wei, H.-H., Zhang, Y., Zhang, C.-L., & Porr, C. (2016). Post partum depression and the psychosocial predictors in first-time fathers from northwestern China. *Midwifery, 35*, 47–52. https://doi.org/10.1016/j.midw.2016.01.005

28

2SLGBTQ+ INDIVIDUALS AND PERINATAL MENTAL HEALTH DISORDERS

Michelle W. Y. Tam, Jennifer M. Goldberg,
Zafiro Andrade-Romo, and Lori E. Ross

Many Two-Spirit, lesbian, gay, bisexual, transgender, and queer (2SLGBTQ+) people have children or desire to have children. There are various pathways for 2SLGBTQ+ parents to form families, including gestational parenting, adoption, or co-parenting. Advancements in legal protections and assisted reproductive technologies such as in vitro fertilization, insemination, and surrogacy have assisted many 2SLGBTQ+ people to have biologically related children. The experiences associated with pregnancy for 2SLGBTQ+ people are informed by biological, legal, and social factors associated with sexuality, gender, and family formation. Whichever route for family expansion is chosen, there are additional decisions and challenges that 2SLGBTQ+ people may face compared to their heterosexual and cisgender counterparts, such as homophobia, transphobia, and biphobia, as well as economic and legal burdens. Thus, navigating legal and medical systems alongside discriminatory social ideologies presents unique challenges to 2SLGBTQ+ people which can impact their mental health.

How Many 2SLGBTQ+ People Are There?

Globally, the estimate of adults identifying as LGBT has significantly increased over the years and is projected to continue to increase (Ipsos, 2021; Jones, 2021; Office for National Statistics, 2022; Gates, 2011). In the United States, 2020 data estimate that 5.6% of adults identify as LGBT, an increase from 4.5% in 2017 (Jones, 2021). An estimated 0.39%–0.6% of the U.S. adult population identifies as transgender (Flores et al., 2016; Meerwijk & Sevelius, 2017). Canada is the first country to collect and publish national census data on gender diversity. In Canada, 0.33% of the population over the age of 15 identifies as transgender or nonbinary (Statistics Canada, 2022), and 3.3% of the population over the age of 15 identifies as lesbian, gay, or bisexual (LGB), with a younger average age compared to the heterosexual population (Statistics Canada, 2021). Mexico's first national survey on sexual and gender diversity showed that 4.8% of people over the age of 15 identify as LGB+ and 0.9% as trans (INEGI, 2022). In the United Kingdom, 3.1% of the population identified as LGB in 2020, an increase from 2.7% in 2019 (Office for National Statistics, 2022). Across the United States, Canada, Mexico, and the United Kingdom, younger people are more likely to identify as LGBT compared to their older counterparts.

DOI: 10.4324/9781003206903-34

649

It is essential to highlight that these population-based data likely provide underestimates. Globally, estimates of the size of 2SLGBTQ+ populations are challenging to determine, since few population-based surveys collect data on sexual orientation or gender identity. Furthermore, an international survey conducted by Pachankis and Bränström (2019) estimates that 83% of sexual minorities in the world conceal their sexual orientation (although analogous data for gender identity are not available, we would estimate concealment rates to be as high or higher). This finding is critical, both as it pertains to our interpretation of the available population-based data, and also in that concealment of sexual orientation can have consequences for the mental and physical health of 2SLGBTQ+ people (Ramos et al., 2021; Pachankis et al., 2020; Ruben & Fullerton, 2018; Pachankis & Bränström, 2018; Pachankis et al., 2015). In practice, this means that there will likely be patients in clinical encounters that will not disclose their sexual and gender minority status (Ruben & Fullerton, 2018; Goldberg et al., 2017; Malterud & Bjorkman, 2016; Durso & Meyer, 2013).

Considering perinatal mental health in particular, it is notable that the legal and social context of 2SLGBTQ+ parenting varies widely globally, both between countries and within state and provincial jurisdictions. For these reasons, this chapter will focus on regions where there are human rights protections for sexual and gender minority people and at least some available research on 2SLGBTQ+ parenting. As a result, this chapter is limited by the significant gaps in knowledge and legal protections for 2SLGBTQ+ parents internationally. However, we would argue that it is still important for clinicians around the world to consider the perinatal mental health of 2SLGBTQ+ people, whether their identities are visible or not, and to avoid making assumptions about people's sexual and gender identities.

How Many 2SLGBTQ+ Parents Are There?

Studies from the United States, Canada, Taiwan, Israel, Portugal, the United Kingdom, Iceland, and the Netherlands have found that many 2SLGBTQ+ people desire to become parents (Bos et al., 2003; Chan et al., 2022; Dierckx et al., 2016; Digoix, 2020; Jeffries et al., 2020; Pyne et al., 2015; Shenkman et al., 2021; Tornello & Bos, 2017). Studies in Canada and the United States show that between 24% and 49% of trans people are parents (Dierckx et al., 2016; Grant et al., 2011; Pyne et al., 2015). A survey by The Family Equality Council, a national nonprofit organization in the United States, found that 77% of LGBTQ adults aged 18–35 years are already parents or are considering becoming parents (Harris & Hopping-Winn, 2019). Conversely, 33% of LGBTQ adults aged 55 years and older either already have children or are considering becoming parents. Additionally, the survey reported that 3.8 million LGBTQ adults aged 18–35 years are considering expanding their families in the next few years and 2.9 million were already actively doing so. As young adults make up the highest 2SLGBTQ+ population, and this proportion is projected to grow, perinatal mental health must be prioritized to support 2SLGBTQ+ family formation and expansion.

2SLGBTQ+ Family Formation

In vitro fertilization and *insemination* are family expansion pathways used by lesbian women, bisexual women, and trans and nonbinary people. Insemination is used to achieve pregnancy by placing sperm in a person's uterus (*intrauterine insemination*) or near the cervical opening (*intracervical*). Insemination can be done with known or anonymous donor sperm depending on jurisdictional laws. There may be legal concerns when choosing to use a known donor such as legal insecurity or potential legal custody challenges (Shapiro, 2020; Abelsohn et al., 2013). *In vitro fertilization* is another procedure where an egg and sperm are combined in a high-technology laboratory to form embryos outside of the body. The developed embryo(s) is then placed in the uterus of the person carrying the pregnancy. In reciprocal IVF, one partner's egg is used to create the embryo and then the embryo is transferred to be carried by another partner.

Another family formation pathway used by 2SLGBTQ+ people is surrogacy. A surrogate is a person who carries and delivers a baby for an intended parent or parents. Among 2SLGBTQ+ people, surrogacy has been most studied with cisgender gay men who desire to become parents. There are two types of surrogacy arrangements: traditional and gestational. In traditional surrogacy, a surrogate's egg is fertilized by sperm using insemination. In this case, the surrogate is genetically related to the baby. In *gestational surrogacy*, an embryo is created using a donor egg combined with sperm (i.e., IVF). The embryo is then transferred into the uterus of the surrogate who will carry and deliver the baby. In this case, the surrogate is not genetically related to the baby. Although gestational surrogacy often costs more than traditional surrogacy, gestational surrogacy is the preferred type of surrogacy due to legal custody and emotional concerns (Blake et al., 2017; Berkowitz, 2020). In countries where surrogacy is legal, depending on jurisdictional contexts, the surrogate may be compensated (i.e., receive a fee for carrying and delivering a baby) or uncompensated (i.e., altruistic, only be reimbursed for fees associated with the pregnancy) (Ross & Goldberg, 2016).

Lastly, 2SLGBTQ+ parents may also have children in heterosexual or heterosexual-passing contexts. For example, 2SLGBTQ+ people may choose to have children or co-parent with a different sex partner or may have had children with a different sex partner. 2SLGBTQ+ people may also choose to have other kinship arrangements such as donating sperm or eggs to couples and sharing co-parenting roles.

Our Approach to This Chapter

The aim of this chapter is to inform scholars, practitioners, and policymakers about the context of 2SLGBTQ+ parenting and perinatal mental health, to enable appropriate and effective care during the perinatal period and inform further research with these communities. We provide an overview of the prevalence of perinatal mental health disorders (PMHD), correlates and risk factors among 2SLGBTQ+ communities, including the effects on nonbirthing partners. We then provide treatment recommendations for practitioners and discuss considerations for an intersectional anti-oppression approach toward addressing PMHD in 2SLGBTQ+ individuals. We have woven a case study throughout the chapter to add dimension and context to these points. Finally, we close with conclusions and recommendations for future directions.

Language and Terminology

Research on 2SLGBTQ+ health consistently reports on the importance of inclusive, affirmative, and culturally competent language by service providers (Rossi & Lopez, 2017; Fredriksen-Golsen et al., 2014; Ross et al., 2006). In this section, we provide a note on language usage in this chapter, as well as a brief glossary of key terms that are used in this chapter and terminologies that are relevant in working with 2SLGBTQ+ people. We recognize that language is dynamic, shifting, and changes over time and geography. As we offer brief definitions of terms used in the chapter, this glossary is not meant to be exhaustive. There are many more terminologies that individuals and communities use internationally. As services providers, it is important to respect how a client or patient self-identifies and use the language they use to describe themselves.

In this chapter, the acronym 2SLGBTQ+ is used. We consider the acronym 2SLGBTQ+ to be the most contemporary and inclusive acronym. We place 2S at the beginning of the acronym to recognize that Indigenous sexual and gender minority people were in North America (where the authors are located) before settler LGBTQ+ people. In some instances, different acronyms such as LGBT, 2SLGBTQ+, LGBTQI, and LGBTQIA2 are used to reflect the specific research being cited.

Terms	Definition
Asexual	A person who experiences little to no sexual attraction to others, regardless of gender. Unlike celibacy, which is a choice to abstain from sexual activity, this term refers to an intrinsic part of identity, just like other sexual orientations.
Biphobia	Prejudice and discrimination against bisexual people. Can include erasure of bisexual identity, or the belief that bisexuality is not real, or temporary.
Bisexual	A person who is emotionally, physically, spiritually and/or sexually attracted to people of more than one gender, though not necessarily at the same time.
Cisgender	Someone who identifies as the sex they were assigned at birth. It is recommended to use this term instead of saying "bio," "real," or "genetic," as these suggest that trans people's gender identities are less authentic or natural.
Cisnormative	A system of attitudes, bias and discrimination in favor of cisgender people that marginalizes and renders invisible trans people and treats their needs and identities as less important than those of cisgender people, who are considered to exist within social normalcy.
Cissexism	The assumption that all people are cisgender, and that cisgender people are "normal" and trans people are "abnormal," as well as normative assumptions about bodies (all women have vaginas, someone with a penis is male).
Gay	A man who is emotionally, physically, spiritually and/or sexually attracted to men. Can also refer to women, though some women prefer other terms such as "lesbian" or "queer." This term is sometimes used as an umbrella term for the 2SLGBTQ community.
Gender Expression	How a person expresses or presents their gender. Can include things like dress, voice, make-up, hair, jewelry, and so on.
Homophobia	Negative attitudes, discrimination, erasure, and violence toward lesbian, bisexual, gay, and queer people at individual and systemic levels. Can also be a form of gender-based discrimination (e.g., feminine men are often presumed gay and discriminated against for not aligning with expectations of what it means to be a heterosexual man).
Heteronormativity	A system of regulation and normalization that ascribes power, privilege, and normative status to heterosexuality.

(Continued)

Terms	Definition
Heterosexism	A system of attitudes, bias, and discrimination in favor of heterosexual sexuality and relationships. This includes the assumption that everyone is, or should be, heterosexual and that heterosexuality is inherently superior to queerness. It also refers to organizational discrimination against people who are not heterosexual, or against behaviors not stereotypically heterosexual.
Lesbian	A woman who is emotionally, physically, spiritually and/or sexually attracted to women.
Nonbinary	Someone who identifies outside the gender binary of male/masculine and female/feminine, refers to people who are both, neither, in between, and/or without reference to male/female, masculine/feminine.
Racialization	A process of ascribing racial identity to a social group based on historical and present structures of power and domination (e.g., White supremacy, colonialism, nationalism). The social construction of different racial groups give rise to racial hierarchies that place power and privilege to groups perceived as dominant over the groups perceived as nondominant.
Racialized	Describes a person or group that is ascribed a racial identity based on the processes of racialization. For example, in the Canadian context, a racialized person or racialized communities commonly refers to people that are non-White.
Transgender	Someone who does not identify with the sex they were assigned at birth and who may or may not transition, socially (name, pronouns, legal gender markers), physically (hair, clothes, binding, tucking etc.), or medically (hormones, surgery) access medical means of transition.
Transphobia	Negative attitudes, feelings and an aversion toward trans people. This can take the form of disparaging jokes, rejection, exclusion, denial of services, employment discrimination, name-calling and violence.
Two-Spirit	A term used by many Indigenous communities on Turtle Island (typically known as Canada and the United States) to describe people with diverse gender identities, gender expressions, gender roles, and sexual orientations, who were included and respected in most Indigenous communities, sometimes considered sacred and highly revered. They often took on important roles as healers, mediators, and warriors. One of the devastating impacts of colonization was the theft and attempted erasure of this way of being in Indigenous societies.
Queer	A term that has been used as an insult, which has been reclaimed and used proudly. For many it also signifies resistance to the idea that there are binary genders and sexualities. This term is sometimes used as an umbrella term for the 2SLGBTQ community.

Adapted from www.buildingcompetence.ca/resources.php

B.B. is a 32-year-old racialized trans man who delivered his second baby with midwives six weeks ago and is chest-feeding. B.B. gave birth in Edmonton, Alberta, Canada. He is presenting for a routine discharge visit with his baby, together with his wife and their three-year-old. B.B uses he/him pronouns and identifies as bisexual; his partner, C.C., identifies as a White queer cisgender woman and uses she/her pronouns.

During the visit, B.B. starts to cry and talks about experiencing symptoms of postpartum depression. He explains that he is not sleeping well, not feeling happy, and feels irritable all the time. He feels that he has no patience and is snapping with his toddler because of anxiety. B.B.'s wife has been as supportive as possible, limited by the fact that she hasn't been able to take parental leave.

Prevalence of Mental Health Disorders

Multiple studies have found disparities in mental health in the 2SLGBTQ+ population compared to their cisgender heterosexual peers (Pitman et al., 2021; Tan et al., 2021; Chaudhry & Reisner, 2019; Gonzales & Henning-Smith, 2017; Pakula et al., 2016; Bolton & Sareen, 2011; Dilley et al., 2010). A nationally representative study in the United Kingdom found that lesbians, gays, and bisexuals were more likely to have a common mental disorder, hazardous alcohol use and illicit drug use than their heterosexual peers (Pitman et al., 2021). In a national probability study of adults in the United States, compared to their heterosexual peers, lesbian and bisexual women had a higher prevalence of a lifetime major depressive episode (16%, 22.5%, and 35.8%, respectively); and during the past 12 months a higher prevalence of a major depressive episode (8.21%, 11.6%, 24.4%), alcohol abuse or dependence (3.98%, 7.5%, 12.7%) and illicit drug abuse (1.6%, 4.36%, 7.53%). Compared to their heterosexual peers, gay and bisexual men also had a higher prevalence of a lifetime major depressive episode (9.16%, 20.9%, 30.8%); and during the past 12 months, a higher prevalence of a major depressive episode (4.16%, 9.89%, 22%), alcohol abuse or dependence (8.35%, 14%, 9.13%) and illicit drug abuse or dependence (3.61%, 12.5%, 7.11%) (Chaudhry & Reisner, 2019). A study using data from the Canadian Community Health Survey found that compared to their heterosexual peers, bisexuals had nearly four times the rates of anxiety, mood, and combined anxiety and mood disorders; and twice the rates compared to their lesbian and gay peers (Pakula et al., 2016). A nationally representative sample in Canada also found a higher prevalence of lifetime mental disorders (i.e., mood, anxiety, personality, substance use disorders, schizophrenia, psychotic illness, or episode) in lesbian, gay and bisexual people compared to their heterosexual counterparts and higher odds of lifetime suicide attempt (Bolton & Sareen, 2011).

A nationally representative study in New Zealand found that people of diverse genders and sexualities had three times the risk of considering self-harm and suicide compared to their cisgender and heterosexual peers (22% vs. 5%) (Tan et al., 2021). Compared to their cisgender counterparts, substantial evidence has shown that transgender people report worse physical and mental health outcomes (Budge et al., 2013; Seelman et al., 2017; McNeil et al., 2012; Motmans et al., 2012; Warren et al., 2016; Veale et al., 2017). For example, a community-engaged online survey study in Nebraska, found that among transgender (n = 91) and non-transgender individuals (n = 676), 53.9% of transgender respondents reported experiencing depressive symptoms in the past week, as compared to 33.4% of non-transgender respondents (Su et al., 2016). In the same study, 37.7% of transgender respondents reported attempting suicide in their lifetime compared to 15.9% of non-transgender respondents (Su et al., 2016). It is estimated that the lifetime prevalence of depression among transgender and gender nonconforming individuals is as high as 50% to 67% (Carmel & Erickson-Schroth, 2016; Nuttbrock et al., 2010; Rotondi et al., 2012).

Most studies about 2SLGBTQ+ perinatal mental health have been carried out in the global north on sexual minority women (Kirubarajan et al., 2022; Marsland et al., 2022; Flanders et al., 2016; Alang & Fomotar, 2015; Khajehei et al., 2012; Maccio & Pangburn, 2011; Ross et al., 2005, 2012; Maccio & Pangburn, 2012; Goldberg & Smith, 2008; Ross et al., 2007; Trettin et al., 2006; Ross, 2005). However, studies that estimate the prevalence of 2SLGBTQ+ perinatal mental health issues are still scarce. The most recent study found that among 194 sexual minority women in the United States and Australia, recruited online through social media pages aimed at sexual minority and perinatal communities, 35.6% scored above the cutoff for probable clinical depression in the perinatal period; defined as the period from birth until two years after. In the same study, 29.4% of the women reported thoughts of self-harm within the past week. Compared to lesbians, more bisexual women (49.2% vs. 27%) scored above the clinical cutoff of the *Edinburgh Postnatal Depression Scale* (EPDS) (Cox et al., 1987) and had higher perinatal depression scores (12.81 vs. 9.95) (Marsland et al., 2022).

Marsland et al.'s (2022) study did not have heterosexual women as participants to compare the rates they found in sexual minority women. However, compared to the global pooled prevalence of PPD, which a systematic review, meta-analysis, and meta-regression of 291 studies from 56 countries by Hahn-Holbrook et al. (2018) found to be 17.7%, we can see that in Marsland et al.'s (2022) study, the PPD rate in sexual minority women is more than the double. Regarding thoughts of self-harm, a Canadian study by Palladino et al. (2020) using data from the 2018/2019 Survey on Maternal Health found that the prevalence of thoughts of self-harm among 6,558 respondents was 10.4%.

A Canadian study by Ross et al. (2007) found that compared to heterosexual women (*n* = 149), lesbian and bisexual biological (birth) mothers (*n* = 18) had significantly higher EPDS scores at 16 weeks postpartum (7.39 vs. 4.91). A secondary analysis of the previous study found that among 64 perinatal sexual minority women, bisexuals (*n* = 14) reported significantly lower scores on two subscales of the *Medical Outcomes Study Short-Form General Health Survey (SF-36) Version 2* (Ware & Sherbourne, 1992), the *SF-36 Role-Emotional Scale* and the *SF-36 Mental Health Summary Score*. The study also reported significantly higher state anxiety scores among bisexuals, compared to other minority sexual identities, but no differences regarding depression or substance abuse (Ross et al., 2012). A study in Australia with 16 lesbian participants found that 31.3% of the women indicated symptoms of depression during the first year postpartum (Khajehei et al., 2012).

Regarding transgender and nonbinary people, the prevalence of PMHD is currently unknown (Brandt et al., 2019; Greenfield & Darwin, 2020). However, recent review articles have suggested that transgender and nonbinary people may experience increased vulnerability to perinatal mental health issues given higher rates of mental health challenges generally (Brandt et al., 2019; Greenfield & Darwin, 2020). As further discussed next, the high levels and high risks of depression are associated with discrimination and determinants of health (e.g., poverty, race).

Risk Factors

It is clear from extant research that there are perinatal risk factors and protective factors that correlate with PMHD in 2SLGBTQ+ people that are distinct from non-2SLGBTQ+ populations. Recent literature reviews demonstrate that in addition to stressors faced by the general population, 2SLGBTQ+ people face discrimination, prejudice, cis-heteronormativity, transphobia, biphobia, and homophobia, which add layers of complexity to 2SLGBTQ+ people's risk for PMHD (Kirubarajan et al., 2022; Greenfield & Darwin, 2020). These experiences contribute to chronic high levels of stress that are experienced by many 2SLG-BTQ+ people. Within heteronormative and cisnormative institutions, 2SLGBTQ+ people can experience structural oppression and discrimination, which reframes the risk factors for PMHD that can be encountered within this oppressive system (Kirubarajan et al., 2022). 2SLGBTQ+ people can also experience discrimination within their families, resulting in a lack of social support that impacts their mental health (Ross et al., 2005; Greenfield & Darwin, 2020). Discrimination can both result in trauma and can serve as forms of trauma, in and of itself. Research has shown that in 2SLGBTQ+ populations, experiences of discrimination are strongly associated with poor mental health outcomes such as depression and anxiety (Van Beusekom et al., 2018; Feinstein et al., 2012; Ross et al., 2010).

The major risk factors for PMHD in sexual minority women (i.e., bisexuals and lesbians) include social isolation; invisibility; lack of social support; and negative or harmful experiences with healthcare providers (Ross, 2005; Ross et al., 2007; Goldberg et al., 2020; Marsland et al., 2022). The most important predictors of perinatal depressive symptomology for lesbian and bisexual women include experiences of societal and institutionalized discrimination in the form of social stigma, homo- and biphobia, and heterosexism (Ross et al., 2007). This can negatively impact their healthcare experiences, invisibilize their partners, and contribute to an increased risk for PMHD (Ross et al., 2007).

Within sexual minority women, other risk factors for postpartum depression in childbearing lesbian and bisexual mothers include past medical history of mental disorders (Ross, 2005), lack of acknowledgement of the co-parent, and lack of support—especially from families of origin (Ross, 2005; Ross et al., 2007). Past medical history of mental disorders, prenatal history of depression and anxiety are more common in lesbian mothers than in heterosexual mothers (Maccio & Pangburn, 2011). A study by Ross et al.'s (2005) on perinatal depression among LGBQ women in Ontario, Canada, found that barriers from the legal system were a primary source of stress and a determinant of their mental health.

For bisexual women, distinct risk factors include lack of social support and community, and experiences of invisibility (Rossi & Lopez, 2017; Goldberg et al., 2020; Leal et al., 2021). Compared to lesbians, bisexual women have more risk of perinatal depression and lack of partner and family support (Marsland et al., 2022). Lack of social support correlates with higher symptoms of depression and anxiety prenatally and six months postpartum for bisexual women and sexual minority women partnered with men (Goldberg et al., 2020). Bisexual women and sexual minority women can experience a greater risk of sexual orientation-based discrimination when they are assumed to be heterosexual when presenting to care with a male partner (Marsland et al., 2022), and this invisibility may increase risk for depression (Goldberg et al., 2020).

Within gender minority groups, transgender and nonbinary individuals experience similar PMHD risk factors as sexual minorities, alongside additional complexities. The gender minority stress model considers the multiple ways transgender people experience oppression, discrimination, and stress from cisnormativity and homophobia (Testa et al., 2015). Most studies have examined perinatal experiences of transgender men or transmasculine people. Compared to cisgender women, transgender individuals face increased vulnerability to traumatic birth and PMHD due to (a) provision of healthcare that does not consider the needs of transgender people; (b) social isolation and exclusion; and (c) and gender dysphoria (Greenfield & Darwin, 2020; Hafford-Letchfield et al., 2019; Wolfe-Roubatis & Spatz, 2015; Falck et al., 2020; Obedin-Maliver & Makadon, 2016).

Transgender people can experience a lack of inclusive and affirmative perinatal care and support in the context of perinatal loss, fertility treatment, labor and delivery, and the postpartum period (Obedin-Maliver & Makadon, 2016). Care providers' cis-heteronormative assumptions, incorrect clinical documentation, misgendering, and the refusal of services for transgender patients, all contribute to transgender individuals' negative, and even harmful, experiences of care (Greenfield & Darwin, 2020; Hafford-Letchfield et al., 2019; Pulice-Farrow et al., 2022). Such negative or harmful experiences, whether actual or anticipated, are a risk factor for PMHD in transgender individuals, as this can culminate in traumatic care and birth experiences (Greenfield & Darwin, 2020). Previous experiences or fear of transphobia and misgendering can lead to a trans individual feeling loss of control over their care; this increases their vulnerability, fear of childbirth, and can lead to a traumatic birth experience (Hafford-Letchfield et al., 2019; Greenfield & Darwin, 2020). The association between poor care and birth trauma has been well established—childbearing women who receive dismissive and unresponsive care experience elevated rates of posttraumatic stress symptoms (Beck, 2004; Simpson & Catling, 2016)—yet the impact of this knowledge has not trickled down to trauma-informed perinatal care for transgender people. A previous traumatic birth experience, pre-existing mental health challenges, poor care during labor, and loss of choice and control during birth, all increase the risk of traumatic delivery and postpartum depression for transgender people (Greenfield & Darwin, 2020; Hafford-Letchfield et al., 2019).

Transgender people can experience isolation, invisibility, and lack of social support, which are linked to depression and PMHD. Feelings of social isolation can be worsened within cisnormative healthcare settings where language and images that are trans-inclusive are missing, leading to trans men feeling discomfort, invisible, and vulnerable (Greenfield & Darwin, 2020). Transgender people experiencing loneliness are especially vulnerable to intense distress during the preconception period (Ellis et al., 2015) and experiences of isolation, exclusion and vulnerability can be exacerbated during pregnancy loss (de Castro-Peraza et al., 2019). The need to conceal or hide oneself in social settings to avoid *gender dysphoria* can lead to feelings of loneliness, which impact PMH (Greenfield & Darwin, 2020).

Discrimination and incompetent healthcare can trigger gender dysphoria in transgender people. Gender dysphoria (GD) is a term used to characterize experiences of distress within gender minority people (Davy & Toze, 2018) and does not look the same for every transgender person (Kirczenow MacDonald et al., 2020). In their study, Falck et al. (2020) found that inconsistent use of correct pronouns triggered GD in transgender men. Experiences of pregnancy, childbirth, postpartum, and breast/chestfeeding can all lead to or exacerbate GD due to bodily changes (de Castro-Peraza et al., 2019; Obedin-Maliver & Makadon, 2016; Greenfield & Darwin, 2020). Besse et al. (2020) found that pregnant transgender individuals felt that pregnancy removed their bodily autonomy and experienced a loss of control over their body, triggering GD and impacting their mental health. The direct experience of birthing a baby through the vagina, exposure of genitals, assumptions about the reproductive organs as "female," and the inconsistent use of pronouns, were identified as triggers for GD (Falck et al., 2020; Greenfield & Darwin, 2020; Brandt et al., 2019; Obedin-Maliver & Makadon, 2016). Although GD has been linked to trauma and posttraumatic stress disorder (PTSD) (Kirczenow MacDonald et al., 2020), it has not been found to be a major contributor to depression (Greenfield & Darwin, 2020, p. 212).

Nonbinary individuals are often included under the transgender umbrella, but nonbinary identities can be distinct from transgender identities because they do not present at one end of the gender binary. This may account for the fact that nonbinary people's experiences of GD vary across studies (Fischer, 2020). Due to their rejection of the gender binary, nonbinary people may face higher rates of discrimination compared to binary transgender individuals, and chronic stress due to experiences of invisibility by not accommodating the gender binary (Matsuno & Budge, 2017). Findings from a critical review of the literature on nonbinary identities shows compared their transgender counterparts who identify with a binary gender (i.e., transgender men or transgender women), nonbinary individuals experience greater risk for negative mental health outcomes including higher risk of suicidality, psychological distress, anxiety, and depression (Matsuno & Budge, 2017). Many of the correlates for PMHD in sexual minority and transgender people likely apply to nonbinary people, but there is a need for targeted studies.

Taken together, disparities in mental health of 2SLGBTQ+people are shaped by their experiences of discrimination, lack of inclusive healthcare, and social isolation, all of which can increase their risk of PMHD. However, 2SLGBTQ+ people also benefit from protective factors for PMHD similar to the general population, and protective factors related to their experiences as 2SLGBTQ+ people further decrease their risk for PMHD. Correlates leading to the optimization of perinatal mental health in sexual minority women include social support from families of origin, other LGBQ parents, and the lesbian and gay community (Ross et al., 2005; Kirubarajan et al., 2022). Protective factors leading to positive psychological outcomes for gender minority people depend on perinatal care experiences being inclusive and affirmative (Obedin-Maliver & Makadon, 2016). Control during the birth is important for gender minority well-being, and the connection between the postpartum emotional well-being of trans people and their experiences of birth and the language used by healthcare providers is established (Wolfe-Roubatis & Spatz, 2015).

B.B. and his wife have a history of negative encounters with reproductive healthcare providers. During their last pregnancy, both B.B. and C.C. felt that B.B.'s gender identity was invalidated when healthcare providers learned that he was trans; for example, he was cisgendered (assumed to be a woman) and felt excluded in the clinic where there were only posters of White cisgender women nursing their babies. In their former birthing experience, the birthing unit in the hospital was called the "mother and baby unit," equating pregnancy with motherhood which invisibilizes all pregnant individuals' identities and experiences. These experiences, and B.B.'s pregnancy-related body changes that are perceived to be feminine, contrary to his transmasculine self, have triggered B.B.'s gender dysphoria.

Prior to transitioning and receiving gender-affirming care, B.B. had a history of suicide ideation and depression. B.B. was taking gender-affirming hormones but had to stop taking them when trying to conceive, which caused changes in B.B.'s body and increased his sense of gender dysphoria. B.B. has been successfully chestfeeding his newborn baby and feels comfortable chestfeeding at home and in private spaces. However, B.B. experiences gender dysphoria when chestfeeding in public spaces. Additionally, B.B. and his partner do not have support from their families of origin/biological families due to transphobia. They have support through their communities and chosen families, including trans/nonbinary birthing and parenting support groups.

Impact on Partner

Perinatal Mental Health of Nonbirthing 2SLGBTQ+ Parents

Expecting parents who are not biologically involved in the conception or birthing of their child are often referred to as the nonbirthing, nonbiological, and/or co-parent (Abelsohn et al., 2013; Bergen et al., 2006). As nonbirthing 2SLGBTQ+ parents have a unique experience in parenting, it is also important to consider the mental health of nonbirthing parents and the factors that impact mental health during the transition to parenthood (Abelsohn et al., 2013; Goldberg, 2010; Ross, 2005). Growing research demonstrates that a significant portion of cisgender men in heterosexual relationships experience prenatal and postpartum depression (Rao et al., 2020; Scarff, 2019; Maleki et al., 2018; Paulson & Bazemore, 2010). It is estimated that 10–14% of fathers experience prenatal depression (Rao et al., 2020) and 8–10% of fathers experience postpartum depression (Rao et al., 2020; Paulson & Bazemore, 2010). Additionally, there has been shown to be a moderate positive correlation between paternal and maternal depressive symptoms (meta-analytic estimate, 0.308) (Paulson & Bazemore, 2010). Thus, the mental health of nonbirthing partners should be considered.

There are limited studies on the mental health of nonbirthing 2SLGBTQ+ parents during the perinatal period. Research has mainly focused on the experiences of lesbian, bisexual, and queer nonbirthing parents. Factors that impact LBQ nonbirthing parents have been found to include worries related to their lack of biological relationship, experiences of infertility for parents who want to conceive, social invisibility as a parent, legal issues (e.g., gamete donors changing their minds and desiring a parenting role), lack of legal recognition (e.g., birth certificates), and lack of services for nonbirth parents (Abelsohn et al., 2013). Nonbirthing 2SLGBTQ+ parents face discrimination and invisibility at the hands of family, strangers, and institutions (Dalton & Bielby, 2000; Abelsohn et al., 2013), particularly in healthcare and clinical contexts when there is a lack of acknowledgement of parental status (Abelsohn et al., 2013; Ross et al., 2006).

The legal recognition and treatment of nonbirthing 2SLGBTQ+ parents vary across countries, as well as state and provincial jurisdictions (Paulsen, 2018; Shapiro, 2020; Snow, 2016). Marriage equality does not necessarily mean that an expecting nonbirthing 2SLGBTQ+ parent will have legal recognition of their parental status. In Canada and the United States, although 2SLGBTQ+ people have obtained the legal right to marry, being a legally married partner does not ensure that birth registration includes the nonbirthing or nonbiological parent as a legal parent of their child. This is often due to inconsistencies in family law, birth registration, and noncomprehensive laws around assisted reproduction. Birth registration can be federally, provincially, or state-regulated across countries. In Canada and the United States, birth registration is regulated by state, province, or territory. For example, in recent years, some Canadian provincial courts ruled that intended parents who use sperm donors and other reproductive technologies, often 2SLGBTQ+ people, can be named as parents on their child's birth certificate. However, in other Canadian provinces, same-sex couples, specifically nonbirthing parents, are often required to go through a lengthy and expensive legal process to adopt their own children. This variability means that 2SLGBTQ+ parents and their children will have varying legal protection depending on the location of birth and residence even within the same country. Legal parentage and birth registration are even more complex in countries where same-sex marriage is not recognized.

The lack of legal recognition as a parent has been found to be a major challenge for non-birthing 2SLGBTQ+ parents (Abelsohn et al., 2013; Ross et al., 2005). Although some of the research on the challenges of legal parentage is from older studies, the legal situation at that time still reflects the contemporary situation in many states and provinces. Legal parent status enables parents to make critical decisions about medical care, education, and upbringing impacting the child's health and wellness. In contrast, lack of legal parent status bars parents from making medical decisions for the child during an emergency or visitation of a child in a hospital (Shapiro, 2020). The anticipation of and actual lack of legal recognition are factors that impact the mental health of nonbirthing LGBTQ parents. Conversely, research has also demonstrated that when policies change to permit legal recognition of nonbiological parents (e.g., specifically in the context of the 2010 lifting of an adoption ban in Florida, that had previously prevented same-sex parents from adopting children their partners had birthed) this can significantly reduce levels of anxiety and stress for these parents (Goldberg et al., 2013).

B.B. and C.C. are often assumed to be in a heterosexual relationship, and as a result, C.C. is often presumed to be the birthing parent of their children. Their last healthcare provider asked them questions that they found intrusive about why C.C. didn't give birth to avoid all the "complications" of a trans man giving birth. Their current provider, however, has been affirming and inclusive. As the nonbirthing parent, C.C. has felt fully included in the process and recognized during the prenatal care appointments. Their current provider often asks C.C. about her emotions and acknowledges joint decision-making between B.B. and C.C.

When B.B. and C.C. had their first child, the baby was conceived through insemination with an anonymous sperm donor and the baby was born in Ontario, Canada, where it is legal for both B.B. and C.C. to be named as parents on the birth certificate, and where gender appropriate designations are possible (i.e., B.B. does not have to be named as "mother"). During the second pregnancy, they were living in another province. They conceived through insemination with the same anonymous sperm donor, but the province they reside in now does not recognize C.C. as a legal parent since she is not the biological father, and B.B., as the birth parent, must be designated as "mother." In order to be recognized as her baby's parent, C.C. must go through the process of adopting her own child. This situation has caused both C.C. and B.B. stress, anxiety and financial strain as a result of the legal fees involved.

Intersecting Identities

In the national Trans PULSE Canada survey, more than half of racialized trans and nonbinary people rated their mental health as poor and compared to their nonracialized trans and nonbinary peers, a higher number reported living with a disability (24% vs. 18%), chronic pain (26% vs. 20%) and being a psychiatric survivor or person with a mental illness (48% vs. 42%) (Chih et al., 2020). Also, racialized trans and nonbinary people reported higher levels of violence, discrimination, and harassment as compared to already high levels among nonracialized trans and nonbinary respondents (Chih et al., 2020). In their lifetimes, compared to nonracialized trans and nonbinary people, more racialized trans and non-binary people reported experiencing physical assault (30% vs. 39%), and sexual assault (25% vs. 32%) during the past five years. Regarding the health and well-being of Indigenous Two-Spirit, trans, and nonbinary people, the Tans PULSE Canada survey found that 51% of participants had unmet healthcare needs in the past year, 54% identified themselves as a psychiatric survivor or person with a mental illness, and 19% did not have a primary healthcare provider (Merasty et al., 2021). Reporting on self-rated mental health, 43% rated their mental health as fair and 23% as poor, whereas 41% had contemplated suicide in the past year.

2SLGBTQ+ migrants also face additional challenges that must be considered while receiving care. A scoping review by Lee et al. (2022) found that LGBTQI migrants face structural barriers when accessing health and social services. They also experience racism (Lee et al., 2022) and homophobia/transphobia at workplaces, health and social services, and immigration and/or refugee-specific services (Munro et al., 2013; Yee et al., 2014). Racialized 2SLGBTQ+ migrants also have a higher risk for social isolation (Logie et al., 2016). In addition, LGBTQI migrants who also have undocumented or precarious status may be experiencing increased stress due to constant fear of deportation and might also be exposed to higher discrimination and violence (Lee et al., 2022). Because of the additional levels of violence, discrimination, harassment, housing insecurity and mental health issues that 2SLGBTQ+ people with intersecting identities might be facing, considering this while approaching treatment and care of PMHD is essential.

While B.B. feels that his current perinatal care has been gender-affirming, he has previously experienced feelings of loss of control over healthcare decisions due to healthcare provider attitudes toward his various identities. For example, during his first birth and while in labor, he requested an epidural for pain management multiple times, but his care providers didn't believe he was in enough pain to warrant the intervention. Giving birth without an epidural was a traumatic experience for B.B. since he had wanted to avoid feeling sensations while the baby was being born. B.B. believes this experience was shaped by health providers' racism and transphobia and has contributed to B.B.'s deep distrust of perinatal health services.

During the second pregnancy, when looking for a healthcare provider, B.B. tried to find a racialized and queer/trans-inclusive healthcare provider. However, he was only able to find queer/trans-inclusive midwives in his community who were not racialized. He often feels like he has to choose between two options and is tired of having to choose which of his identities to prioritize.

From a socioeconomic perspective, B.B. and C.C. have struggled financially during this pregnancy. In addition to the financial resources required to conceive through assisted reproduction, there have been legal consultation costs necessary for C.C. to adopt her baby and secure legal parentage. These financial burdens have impacted B.B. and C.C.'s mental health.

Approaches to Treatment and Care

According to Tripathy (2020), approximately half of perinatal women who have anxiety and depression are "not diagnosed or not given proper treatment if diagnosed" (p. 3). Rates of treatment for 2SLGBTQ+ people have not been studied but given barriers to accessing mental healthcare outside of the perinatal period, may be even lower. Treatment for perinatal mental health conditions among 2SLGBTQ+ people will largely follow the same protocols and practices as for heterosexual, cisgender patients; however, the context of widespread societal discrimination and associated risk factors necessitates some particular concerns on the part of mental health service providers.

2SLGBTQ+ Competent Trauma-Informed Care

Trauma-informed care (TIC) is an approach based on understanding the effects of trauma, whereas trauma-specific treatment includes programs, interventions, and therapeutic services that are aimed at decreasing symptoms and problems resulting from traumatizing event(s). Trauma-informed care does not have to be trauma-specific. Research on LGBTQ people who have experienced trauma from intimate partner violence report that a greater perception of overall TIC in services is associated with greater empowerment, greater emotion regulation, and lower social withdrawal (Scheer & Poteat, 2021; Antebi-Gruszka & Scheer, 2021). However, it has been suggested that TIC is most effective when delivered with LGBTQ+ affirmative (or competent) approaches (Antebi-Gruszka & Scheer, 2021; Elze, 2019).

2SLGBTQ+ competent trauma-informed care is a universal approach that recognizes the prevalence of trauma history and the diverse effects of trauma that 2S2SLGBTQ+ people may experience. (Tam et al., 2022; SAMHSA, 2014). Building on the principles of trauma-informed care, this approach is a strengths-based paradigm shift from "What is wrong with you?" to "What happened to you?," where "what happened" includes experiences of ongoing violence, discrimination, and oppression that diverse 2SLGBTQ+ communities experience (Tam et al., 2022). 2SLGBTQ+ competent trauma-informed care works from a strengths-based perspective to recognize people's resilience and that people are coping the best way they can. Thus, 2SLGBTQ+ competent trauma-informed care is aimed at addressing barriers to care and the potential for re-traumatization in service provision.

A recent study has shown how 2SLGBTQ+ competent TIC can be applied at the personal, practice, and organizational levels (Tam et al., 2022; Re:searching for LGBTQ2S+ Health Team, 2019). Briefly, at the personal level, 2SLGBTQ+ competent TIC includes reflecting on one's own assumptions and examining stereotypical beliefs about sexual orientation and gender identities, as well as not assuming a person's sexual orientation, gender, or trauma history based on their appearance. At the practice level, recommendations include recognizing that individuals may be afraid to disclose their gender identity or sexual orientation for various reasons; not making assumptions about how clients/patients identify based on whom their partners are; and noticing if gender and/or sexuality is being brought into the conversation and whether the client believes it is relevant to the discussion. Additionally, there should be a language shift away from a deficit perspective (i.e., what is wrong, disorder, treatment-resistant) and instead, toward a trauma-informed, strengths-based, and non-stigmatizing perspective (i.e., what happened, trauma response, formulation/plan is not meeting the individual's needs). Service providers should also ask patients/clients their pronouns, and if comfortable, share their own pronouns.

At the organizational level, recommendations include ensuring that leadership is actively committed to 2SLGBTQ+ competency and trauma-informed care (e.g., allowing staff time and resources to focus on building organizational capacity and implementing trauma-informed care); ensuring that internal and external organizational documents are inclusive and affirming of 2SLGBTQ+ peoples (e.g., policy and procedures, manuals, promotional materials); and engage people with lived experience in the development and evaluation of policies and procedures (Tam et al., 2022). Organizations should also be aware that trauma can impact anyone, including staff. Lastly, it is important to regard 2SLGBTQ+ identities as healthy and legitimate.

Gender-Affirming Care

Together with a 2SLGBTQ+ competent TIC approach, a crucial part of the treatment for trans, Two-Spirit and gender diverse parents is providing gender-affirming care. Gender-affirming care is not a specific set of goals or protocols but rather a model of care and an approach to the person and their families that actively affirms gender identity (Smith, 2021). According to TRANS Care BC (2021) some of the roles of the healthcare provider while providing gender-affirming care include (a) respecting the patient and partner's right to self-determine their gender identity; (b) using the person and partner's chosen names and pronouns, and (c) "seek[ing] to restore or build capacity [in the patient] where it is diminished" (p. 3) among others.

Gender-affirming care is about finding a way to support the patient and their family in terms of presenting their "true, authentic self from a physical and emotional perspective" (Smith, 2021, p. 1). For example, it is known that for some transgender men who have delivered a baby and decide to chestfeed/nurse, this might provoke gender dysphoria (Brandt et al., 2019). Thus, providing gender-affirming care (e.g., using the patient's preferred language for both the process of chestfeeding/nursing and for the involved body parts, in case the patient was taking hormone therapy talk about concerns or questions, talk about how the person is managing the changes in their appearance and gender expression at their work or school) will be an important part of providing lactation support. Also, according to Brandt et al.'s (2019), for transgender men who recently delivered, more frequent assessments might be beneficial.

The protective effects of gender-affirming care have been shown to improve depression, anxiety, and stress symptoms (Hughto et al., 2020; Seelman et al., 2017). In the United States, gender-affirming care provided to low-income transgender people through public medical insurance (Medicaid) has been associated with a reduction in mental distress (Mann et al., 2022). These protective effects are enhanced over time: the more often gender-affirming care is experienced, the better are mental health outcomes (Hughto et al., 2020; Mann et al., 2022). Advancements in gender-affirming care are not restricted to the Global North: the sustained activism, advocacy, and efforts of transgender communities across the globe have led to establishing gender-affirming care clinics, such as the Mitr Clinic in Hyderabad, India (Keuroghlian et al., 2022).

Referral to 2SLGBTQ+ Community Support

Finally, the literature emphasizes the role of social support in reducing the risk for prenatal mental health concerns in 2SLGBTQ+ people (Alang & Fomotar, 2015; Trettin et al., 2006; Ross et al., 2005; Ross, 2005). A way to support 2SLGBTQ+ people with PMHD involves referring them to 2SLGBTQ+ community support groups, including parenting-specific supports if available in the local community. In-person community support ongoing groups might not be available in the surrounding areas for all patients; thus, it would be key to identify online groups (Alang & Fomotar, 2015) and have those resources updated and available when needed.

Throughout the postpartum period, the midwife has been actively listening to B.B. and C.C. talk about B.B.'s depressive symptoms, financial troubles, experiences of chestfeeding, and lack of support from his family of origin. In discussions with CC and BB, the midwife acknowledges various forms of discrimination that are impacting them. The midwife reflects on her limitations of knowledge about racialized trans communities and is seeking out sources to expand her knowledge. The midwife then proceeds to do a formal assessment for postpartum depression. As part of this, the midwife implements the EPDS, with B.B. scoring over 16. Given this high score, the midwife then assesses him for self-harm ideation and suicidality and determines this is not of current concern.

Seeing that B.B. and C.C. are about to be discharged from care, the midwife collaborates with them on a follow-up care plan for B.B.'s depression. Because B.B. has been experiencing gender dysphoria, and there are few mental health providers in the local community who have experience with both gender dysphoria and perinatal depression, the midwife offers two referrals: the first to a gender-affirming physician who can help plan a timeline for re-introducing gender-affirming hormones, and the second to a community-based perinatal mental health specialist. B.B. requests information about online parenting support groups for trans people, which the midwife has listed on a handout about 2SLGBTQ+ parenting groups in the area. C.C. requests information about nonbirth parent support groups, but the midwife does not know of any such support in their area and tells C.C. that searching on different social media platforms might be a good option. B.B. and C.C. are happy with their care plan. Finally, the midwife reminds B.B. of the importance of attending follow-up visits with his primary care providers in the next two weeks.

Conclusion and Future Directions

2SLGBTQ+ people have unique needs in the context of PMHD, beyond those seen in non-2SLGBTQ+ individuals. Negative, and even harmful, healthcare experiences, and social isolation, are significant factors that contribute to PMHD in this population. Most studies have examined experiences of lesbian and bisexual women, and transgender men; however, as described in recent reviews of the literature, there are important gaps in our knowledge of perinatal mental health among subgroups of 2SLGBTQ+ people.

We strongly recommend that approaches to inquiry be intersectional and consider how racism, classism, migration status, ableism, and other systems oppression, all factor into the perinatal mental health of 2SLGBTQ+ people. Moreover, research about 2SLGBTQ+ communities should be designed with, by, and for the communities that stand to benefit from such research. To this end, our recommendations for future studies include examining:

- Perinatal mental health of populations with limited research, such as transgender and nonbinary individuals
- Mental health outcomes and experiences of transgender women as co-parents and/or partners of gestational parents
- Impact of traumatic birth on 2SLGBTQ+ mental health

- Acceptability and effectiveness of 2SLGBTQ+ competent trauma-informed care with 2SLGBTQ+ parents who are experiencing PMHD
- Role of partner and/or co-parent/s in supporting 2SLGBTQ+ gestational parent's perinatal mental health
- Impact of the lack of legal recognition (in a specified jurisdiction) on the perinatal mental health of nongestational 2SLGBTQ+ parent
- Prevalence and experiences of 2SLGBTQ+ people in countries in the Global South

The provision of affirming and inclusive healthcare and social supports are important starting points for healthcare providers to consider making changes in their own practice. Understanding how structural and systemic forces of oppression (e.g., homo-, bi-, and transphobia, racism, sexism, ableism) contribute to the risk of PMHD in 2SLGBTQ+ parents enables healthcare providers and policymakers to work toward change in their own practices and institutions. Studies to assess the attitudes, behaviors, and practices of healthcare providers across disciplines regarding 2SLGBTQ+ perinatal mental health can inform capacity building programs for healthcare providers who care for 2SLGBTQ+ people in the perinatal period.

All healthcare providers, including those who provide perinatal care (midwives, family doctors, obstetricians) and mental healthcare (therapists, psychologists, psychiatrists) must take the necessary steps to build their capacity to provide care that is tailored to the unique needs of 2SLGBTQ+ individuals to improve their perinatal care experiences, and in so doing, their mental health. Healthcare providers can take tangible first steps toward assessing their own capacity to address 2SLGBTQ+ people's unique needs, and the capacity of their clinic, in several ways. Given that 2SLGBTQ+ specific guidelines are currently not available, healthcare providers should follow regional guidelines about how to treat mental health conditions during the perinatal period and develop clear referral and management protocols that incorporate the specific needs of 2SLGBTQ+ individuals. Healthcare providers should identify and address gaps in knowledge where needed and seek out the support of 2SLGBTQ+ health capacity building training programs. Healthcare providers must acknowledge that they already care for 2SLGBTQ+ people, and that individuals with these identities are not always visible or ready to share those identities with their care providers. Together, we must all work toward being able to provide quality, inclusive, affirming, and safe care to 2SLGBTQ+ communities across all settings where 2SLGBTQ+ people seek perinatal and mental healthcare.

References

Abelsohn, K. A., Epstein, R., & Ross, L. E. (2013). Celebrating the "other" parent: Mental health and wellness of expecting lesbian, bisexual, and queer non-birth parents. *Journal of Gay & Lesbian Mental Health, 17*(4), 387–405. https://doi.org/10.1080/19359705.2013.771808

Alang, S. M., & Fomotar, M. (2015). Postpartum depression in an online community of lesbian mothers: Implications for clinical practice. *Journal of Gay & Lesbian Mental Health, 19*(1), 21–39. https://doi.org/10.1080/19359705.2014.910853

Antebi-Gruszka, N., & Scheer, J. R. (2021). Associations between trauma-informed care components and multiple health and psychosocial risks among LGBTQ survivors of intimate partner violence. *Journal of Mental Health Counseling, 43*(2), 139–156.

Beck, C. T. (2004). Birth trauma: In the eye of the beholder. *Nursing Research, 53*(1), 28–35. https://doi.org/10.1097/00006199-200401000-00005

Bergen, K. M., Suter, E. A., & Daas, K. L. (2006). About as solid as a fish net: Symbolic construction of a legitimate parental identity for nonbiological lesbian mothers. *The Journal of Family Communication, 6*(3), 201–220. https://doi.org/10.1207/s15327698jfc0603_3

Berkowitz, D. (2020). Gay men and surrogacy. In A. E. Goldberg & K. Allen (Eds.), *LGBTQ-parent families: Innovations in research and implications for practice* (pp. 143–160). Springer.

Besse, M., Lampe, N. M., & Mann, E. S. (2020). Focus: Sex & reproduction: Experiences with achieving pregnancy and giving birth among transgender men: A narrative literature review. *The Yale Journal of Biology and Medicine, 93*(4), 517–528.

Blake, L., Carone, N., Raffanello, E., Slutsky, J., Ehrhardt, A. A., & Golombok, S. (2017). Gay fathers' motivations for and feelings about surrogacy as a path to parenthood. *Human Reproduction, 32*(4), 860–867. https://doi.org/10.1093/humrep/dex026

Bolton, S. L., & Sareen, J. (2011). Sexual orientation and its relation to mental disorders and suicide attempts: Findings from a nationally representative sample. *Canadian Journal of Psychiatry, 56*(1), 35–43. https://doi.org/10.1177/070674371105600107

Bos, H. M., Van Balen, F., & Van den Boom, D. C. (2003). Planned lesbian families: Their desire and motivation to have children. *Human Reproduction, 18*(10), 2216–2224. https://doi.org/10.1093/humrep/deg427

Brandt, J. S., Patel, A. J., Marshall, I., & Bachmann, G. A. (2019). Transgender men, pregnancy, and the "new" advanced paternal age: A review of the literature. *Maturitas, 128*, 17–21. https://doi.org/10.1016/j.maturitas.2019.07.004

Budge, S. L., Adelson, J. L., & Howard, K. A. (2013). Anxiety and depression in transgender individuals: The roles of transition status, loss, social support, and coping. *Journal of Consulting and Clinical Psychology, 81*(3), 545. https://doi.org/10.1037/a0031774

Carmel, T. C., & Erickson-Schroth, L. (2016). Mental health and the transgender population. *Journal of Psychosocial Nursing and Mental Health Services, 54*(12), 44–48. https://doi.org/10.3928/02793695-20161208-09

Chan, C. H. Y., Huang, Y. T., So, G. Y. K., Leung, H. T., Forth, M. W., & Lo, P. Y. I. (2022). Examining the demographic and psychological variables associating with the childbearing intention among gay and bisexual men in Taiwan. *Journal of Ethnic & Cultural Diversity in Social Work*, 1–11. https://doi.org/10.1080/15313204.2022.2027313

Chaudhry, A. B., & Reisner, S. L. (2019). Disparities by sexual orientation persist for major depressive episode and substance abuse or dependence: Findings from a national probability study of adults in the United States. *LGBT Health, 6*(5), 261–266. https://doi.org/10.1089/lgbt.2018.0207

Chih, C., Wilson-Yang, J. Q., Dhaliwal, K., Khatoon, M., Redman, N., Malone, R., . . . Persad, Y. on behalf of the Trans PULSE Canada Team. (2020). Health and well-being among racialized trans and non-binary people in Canada, 2, 1–10. https://transpulsecanada.ca/research-type/reports

Cox, J. L., Holden, J. M., & Sagovsky, R. (1987). Detection of postnatal depression: Development of the 10-item Edinburgh Postnatal Depression Scale. *The British Journal of Psychiatry, 150*(6), 782–786. https://doi.org/10.1192/bjp.150.6.782

Dalton, S. E., & Bielby, D. D. (2000). "That's our kind of constellation" lesbian mothers negotiate institutionalized understandings of gender within the family. *Gender & Society, 14*(1), 36–61. https://doi.org/10.1177/089124300014001004

Davy, Z., & Toze, M. (2018). What is gender dysphoria? A critical systematic narrative review. *Transgender Health, 3*(1), 159–169. https://doi.org/10.1089/trgh.2018.0014

De Castro-Peraza, M. E., García-Acosta, J. M., Delgado-Rodriguez, N., Sosa-Alvarez, M. I., Llabrés-Solé, R., Cardona-Llabrés, C., & Lorenzo-Rocha, N. D. (2019). Biological, psychological, social, and legal aspects of trans parenthood based on a real case – a literature review. *International Journal of Environmental Research and Public Health, 16*(6), 925. https://doi.org/10.3390/ijerph16060925

Dierckx, M., Motmans, J., Mortelmans, D., & T'sjoen, G. (2016). Families in transition: A literature review. *International Review of Psychiatry, 28*(1), 36–43. https://doi.org/10.3109/09540261.2015.1102716

Digoix, M. (2020). LGBT Desires in family land: Parenting in Iceland, from social acceptance to social pressure. In *Same-Sex Families and Legal Recognition in Europe* (pp. 117–154). Springer.

Dilley, J. A., Simmons, K. W., Boysun, M. J., Pizacani, B. A., & Stark, M. J. (2010). Demonstrating the importance and feasibility of including sexual orientation in public health surveys: Health disparities in the Pacific Northwest. *American Journal of Public Health, 100*(3), 460–467. https://doi.org/10.2105/AJPH.2007.130336

Durso, L. E., & Meyer, I. H. (2013). Patterns and predictors of disclosure of sexual orientation to healthcare providers among lesbians, gay men, and bisexuals. *Sexuality Research and Social Policy, 10*(1), 35–42. https://doi.org/10.1007/s13178-012-0105-2

Ellis, S. A., Wojnar, D. M., & Pettinato, M. (2015). Conception, pregnancy, and birth experiences of male and gender variant gestational parents: It's how we could have a family. *Journal of Midwifery & Women's Health, 60*(1), 62–69. https://doi.org/10.1111/jmwh.12213

Elze, D. E. (2019). The lives of lesbian, gay, bisexual, and transgender people: A trauma-informed and human rights perspective. In L. D. Butler, F. M. Critelli, & J. Carello (Eds.), *Trauma and human rights: Integrating approaches to address human suffering* (pp. 179–206). Palgrave Macmillan.

Falck, F., Frisén, L., Dhejne, C., & Armuand, G. (2020). Undergoing pregnancy and childbirth as trans masculine in Sweden: Experiencing and dealing with structural discrimination, gender norms and microaggressions in antenatal care, delivery and gender clinics. *International Journal of Transgender Health, 22*(1–2), 42–53. https://doi.org/10.1080/26895269.2020.1845905

Feinstein, B. A., Goldfried, M. R., & Davila, J. (2012). The relationship between experiences of discrimination and mental health among lesbians and gay men: An examination of internalized homonegativity and rejection sensitivity as potential mechanisms. *Journal of Consulting and Clinical Psychology, 80*(5), 917. https://doi.org/10.1037/a0029425

Fischer, O. J. (2020). Non-binary reproduction: Stories of conception, pregnancy, and birth. *International Journal of Transgender Health, 22*(1–2), 77–88. https://doi.org/10.1080/26895269.2020.1838392

Flanders, C. E., Gibson, M. F., Goldberg, A. E., & Ross, L. E. (2016). Postpartum depression among visible and invisible sexual minority women: A pilot study. *Archives of Women's Mental Health, 19*(2), 299–305. https://doi.org/10.1007/s00737-015-0566-4

Flores, A. R., Herman, J., Gates, G. J., & Brown, T. N. (2016). *How many adults identify as transgender in the United States?* https://williamsinstitute.law.ucla.edu/wp-content/uploads/Trans-Adults-US-Aug-2016.pdf

Fredriksen-Goldsen, K. I., Hoy-Ellis, C. P., Goldsen, J., Emlet, C. A., & Hooyman, N. R. (2014). Creating a vision for the future: Key competencies and strategies for culturally competent practice with lesbian, gay, bisexual, and transgender (LGBT) older adults in the health and human services. *Journal of Gerontological Social Work, 57*(2–4), 80–107. https://doi.org/10.1080/01634372.2014.890690

Gates, G. J. (2011). *How many people are lesbian, gay, bisexual and transgender?* https://escholarship.org/uc/item/09h684x2

Goldberg, A. E. (2010). *Lesbian and gay parents and their children: Research on the family life cycle.* American Psychological Association. https://doi.org/10.1037/12055-000

Goldberg, A. E., Moyer, A. M., Weber, E. R., & Shapiro, J. (2013). What changed when the gay adoption ban was lifted? Perspectives of lesbian and gay parents in Florida. *Sexuality Research and Social Policy, 10*(2), 110–124. https://doi.org/10.1007/s13178-013-0120-y

Goldberg, A. E., Ross, L. E., Manley, M. H., & Mohr, J. J. (2017). Male-partnered sexual minority women: Sexual identity disclosure to health care providers during the perinatal period. *Psychology of Sexual Orientation and Gender Diversity, 4*(1), 105–114. https://doi.org/10.1037/sgd0000215

Goldberg, A. E., & Smith, J. Z. (2008) The social context of lesbian mothers' anxiety during early parenthood. *Parenting: Science and Practice, 8*(3), 213–239. https://doi.org/10.1080/15295190802204801

Goldberg, A. E., Smith, J. Z., & Ross, L. (2020). 4. Postpartum depression and anxiety in male-partnered and female-partnered sexual minority women: A longitudinal study. In H. Liu, C. Reczek, & L. Wilkinson (Eds.), *Marriage and health: The well-being of same-sex couples* (pp. 53–70). Rutgers University Press. https://doi.org/10.36019/9781978803527-007

Gonzales, G., & Henning-Smith, C. (2017). Health disparities by sexual orientation: Results and implications from the behavioral risk factor surveillance system. *Journal of Community Health, 42*(6), 1163–1172. https://doi.org/10.1007/s10900-017-0366-z

Grant, J. M., Mottet, L. A., Tanis, J., Harrison, J., Herman, J. L., & Keisling, M. (2011). *Injustice at every turn: A report of the National Transgender Discrimination Survey.* National Center for Transgender Equality and National Gay and Lesbian Task Force. https://bit.ly/3w3r5YI

Greenfield, M., & Darwin, Z. (2020). Trans and non-binary pregnancy, traumatic birth, and perinatal mental health: A scoping review. *International Journal of Transgender Health, 22*(1–2), 203–216. https://doi.org/10.1080/26895269.2020.1841057

Hafford-Letchfield, T., Cocker, C., Rutter, D., Tinarwo, M., McCKormack, K., & Manning, R. (2019). What do we know about transgender parenting? Findings from a systematic review. *Health & Social Care in the Community, 27*(5), 1111–1125. https://doi.org/10.1111/hsc.12759

Hahn-Holbrook, J., Cornwell-Hinrichs, T., & Anaya, I. (2018). Economic and health predictors of national postpartum depression prevalence: A systematic review, meta-analysis, and meta-regression of 291 studies from 56 countries. *Frontiers in Psychiatry, 8*, 248, 1–23. https://doi.org/10.3389/fpsyt.2017.00248

Harris, E., & Hopping-Winn, A. (2019). *LGBTQ family building survey.* www.familyequality.org/wp-content/uploads/2019/02/LGBTQ-Family-Building-Study_Jan2019-1.pdf

Hughto, J. M., Gunn, H. A., Rood, B. A., & Pantalone, D. W. (2020). Social and medical gender affirmation experiences are inversely associated with mental health problems in a US non-probability sample of transgender adults. *Archives of Sexual Behavior, 49*, 2635–2647.

Instituto Nacional de Estadística y Geografía (INEGI). (2022). *Encuesta nacional sobre diversidad sexual y de género (ENDISEG) 2021. [National survey on sexual and gender diversity (ENDISEG) 2021].* www.inegi.org.mx/contenidos/saladeprensa/boletines/2022/endiseg/Resul_Endiseg21.pdf?fbclid=IwAR2iaIvaSFPigWllSTrggUZOh5oSW7igAhPiyhz1K7g7hRRGVGLHcs64XpI&fs=e&s=cl

Ipsos. (2021). *LGBT+ pride 2021 global survey.* www.ipsos.com/sites/default/files/ct/news/documents/2021-06/lgbt-pride-2021-global-survey-ipsos.pdf

Jeffries IV, W. L., Marsiglio, W., Tunalilar, O., & Berkowitz, D. (2020). Fatherhood desires and being bothered by future childlessness among US Gay, bisexual, and heterosexual men–United States, 2002–2015. *Journal of GLBT Family Studies, 16*(3), 330–345. https://doi.org/10.1080/1550428X.2019.1652876

Jones, J. M. (2021). LGBT identification rises to 5.6% in latest US estimate. *Gallup News, 24.* www.optumhealtheducation.com/sites/default/files/LGBT%20Identification%20Rises%20to%205.6%25%20in%20Latest%20U.S.%20Estimate.pdf

Keuroghlian, A. S., Keatley, J., Shaikh, S., & Radix, A. E. (2022). The context, science and practice of gender-affirming care. *Nature Medicine, 28*(12), 2464–2467.

Khajehei, M., Doherty, M., & Tilley, M. (2012). Assessment of postnatal depression among Australian lesbian mothers during the first year after childbirth: A pilot study. *International Journal of Childbirth Education, 27*(4), 49–51.

Kirczenow MacDonald, T., Walks, M., Biener, M., & Kibbee, A. (2020). Disrupting the norms: Reproduction, gender identity, gender dysphoria, and intersectionality. *International Journal of Transgender Health, 22*(1–2), 18–29. https://doi.org/10.1080/26895269.2020.1848692

Kirubarajan, A., Barker, L. C., Leung, S., Ross, L. E., Zaheer, J., Park, B., Abramovich, A., . . . Lam, J. S. H. (2022). LGBTQ2S+ childbearing individuals and perinatal mental health: A systematic review. *BJOG: An International Journal of Obstetrics & Gynaecology.* https://doi.org/10.1111/1471-0528.17103

Leal, D., Gato, J., Coimbra, S., Freitas, D., & Tasker, F. (2021). Social support in the transition to parenthood among lesbian, gay, and bisexual persons: A systematic review. *Sexuality Research and Social Policy,* 1–15. https://doi.org/10.1007/s13178-020-00517-y

Lee, J. J., Leyva Vera, C. A., Ramirez, J. I., Munguia, L., Aguirre Herrera, J., Basualdo, G., . . . Robles, G. (2022). "They already hate us for being immigrants and now for being trans – we have double the fight": A qualitative study of barriers to health access among transgender Latinx immigrants in the United States. *Journal of Gay & Lesbian Mental Health,* 1–21. https://doi.org/10.1080/19359705.2022.2067279

Logie, C. H., Lacombe-Duncan, A., Lee-Foon, N., Ryan, S., & Ramsay, H. (2016). "It's for us–newcomers, LGBTQ persons, and HIV-positive persons. You feel free to be": A qualitative study exploring social support group participation among African and Caribbean lesbian, gay, bisexual and transgender newcomers and refugees in Toronto, Canada. *BMC International Health and Human Rights, 16*(1), 1–10. https://doi.org/10.1186/s12914-016-0092-0

Maccio, E. M., & Pangburn, J. A. (2011). The case for investigating postpartum depression in lesbians and bisexual women. *Women's Health Issues, 21*(3), 187–190. https://doi.org/10.1016/j.whi.2011.02.007

Maccio, E. M., & Pangburn, J. A. (2012). Self-reported depressive symptoms in lesbian birth mothers and comothers. *Journal of Family Social Work, 15*(2), 99–110. https://doi.org/10.1080/10522158.2012.662860

Maleki, A., Faghihzadeh, S., & Niroomand, S. (2018). The relationship between paternal prenatal depressive symptoms with postnatal depression: The PATH model. *Psychiatry Research, 269*, 102–107. https://doi.org/10.1016/j.psychres.2018.08.044

Malterud, K., & Bjorkman, M. (2016). The invisible work of closeting: A qualitative study about strategies used by lesbian and gay persons to conceal their sexual orientation. *Journal of Homosexuality, 63*(10), 1339–1354. https://doi.org/10.1080/00918369.2016.1157995

Mann, S., Campbell, T., & Nguyen, D. H. (2022). *Access to gender-affirming care and transgender mental health: Evidence from medicaid coverage.* SSRN 4164673.

Marsland, S., Treyvaud, K., & Pepping, C. A. (2022). Prevalence and risk factors associated with perinatal depression in sexual minority women. *Clinical Psychology & Psychotherapy, 29*(2), 611–621. https://doi.org/10.1002/cpp.2653

Matsuno, E., & Budge, S. L. (2017). Non-binary/genderqueer identities: A critical review of the literature. *Current Sexual Health Reports, 9*(3), 116–120. https://doi.org/10.1007/s11930-017-0111-8

McNeil, J., Bailey, L., Ellis, S., Morton, J., & Regan, M. (2012). *Trans mental health study 2012.* www.gires.org.uk/assets/Medpro-Assets/trans_mh_study.pdf

Meerwijk, E. L., & Sevelius, J. M. (2017). Transgender population size in the United States: A meta-regression of population-based probability samples. *American Journal of Public Health, 107*(2), e1–e8. https://doi.org/10.2105/AJPH.2016.303578

Merasty, C., Gareau, F., Jackson, R., Masching, S., Dopler, S. on behalf of the Trans PULSE Canada Team. (2021). *Health and well-being among indigenous trans, two-spirit and non-binary people.* https://transpulsecanada.ca/results/report-health-and-well-being-among-indigenous-trans-two-spirit-and-non-binary-people/

Motmans, J., Meier, P., Ponnet, K., & T'Sjoen, G. (2012). Female and male transgender quality of life: Socioeconomic and medical differences. *The Journal of Sexual Medicine, 9*(3), 743–750. https://doi.org/10.1111/j.1743-6109.2011.02569.x

Munro, L., Travers, R., John, A. S., Klein, K., Hunter, H., Brennan, D., & Brett, C. (2013). A bed of roses? Exploring the experiences of LGBT newcomer youth who migrate to Toronto. *Ethnicity and Inequalities in Health and Social Care, 6*(4), 137–150. https://doi.org/10.1108/EIHSC-09-2013-0018

Nuttbrock, L., Hwahng, S., Bockting, W., Rosenblum, A., Mason, M., Macri, M., & Becker, J. (2010). Psychiatric impact of gender-related abuse across the life course of male-to-female transgender persons. *Journal of Sex Research, 47*(1), 12–23. https://doi.org/10.1080/00224490903062258

Obedin-Maliver, J., & Makadon, H. J. (2016). Transgender men and pregnancy. *Obstetric Medicine, 9*(1), 4–8. https://doi.org/10.1177/1753495X15612658

Office for National Statistics. (2022). *Sexual orientation, UK: 2020.* www.ons.gov.uk/peoplepopulationandcommunity/culturalidentity/sexuality/bulletins/sexualidentityuk/2020

Pachankis, J. E., & Bränström, R. (2018). Hidden from happiness: Structural stigma, sexual orientation concealment, and life satisfaction across 28 countries. *Journal of Consulting and Clinical Psychology, 86*(5), 403. https://doi.org/10.1037/ccp0000299

Pachankis, J. E., & Bränström, R. (2019). How many sexual minorities are hidden? Projecting the size of the global closet with implications for policy and public health. *PLoS One, 14*(6), e0218084. https://doi.org/10.1371/journal.pone.0218084

Pachankis, J. E., Hatzenbuehler, M. L., Hickson, F., Weatherburn, P., Berg, R. C., Marcus, U., & Schmidt, A. J. (2015). Hidden from health: Structural stigma, sexual orientation concealment, and HIV across 38 countries in the European MSM Internet Survey. *AIDS (London, England), 29*(10), 1239. https://doi.org/10.1097/QAD.0000000000000724

Pachankis, J. E., Mahon, C. P., Jackson, S. D., Fetzner, B. K., & Bränström, R. (2020). Sexual orientation concealment and mental health: A conceptual and meta-analytic review. *Psychological Bulletin, 146*(10), 831. https://doi.org/10.1037/bul0000271

Pakula, B., Shoveller, J., Ratner, P. A., & Carpiano, R. (2016). Prevalence and co-occurrence of heavy drinking and anxiety and mood disorders among gay, lesbian, bisexual, and heterosexual Canadians. *American Journal of Public Health, 106*(6), 1042–1048. https://doi.org/10.2105/AJPH.2016.303083

Palladino, E., Varin, M., Lary, T., & Baker, M. M. (2020). Thoughts of self-harm and associated risk factors among postpartum women in Canada. *Journal of Affective Disorders, 270*, 69–74. https://doi.org/10.1016/j.jad.2020.03.054

Paulsen, B. S. (2018). A stranger in the eyes of the court: How the judicial system is failing to protect nonbiological LGBTQ parents. *University of Illinois Law Review*, 311–344.

Paulson, J. F., & Bazemore, S. D. (2010). Prenatal and postpartum depression in fathers and its association with maternal depression: A meta-analysis. *JAMA, 303*(19), 1961–1969. http://doi.org/0.1001/jama.2010.605

Pitman, A., Marston, L., Lewis, G., Semlyen, J., McManus, S., & King, M. (2021). The mental health of lesbian, gay, and bisexual adults compared with heterosexual adults: Results of two nationally representative English household probability samples. *Psychological Medicine, 52*(15), 3402–3411.

Pulice-Farrow, L., Lindley, L., & Gonzalez, K. A. (2022). "Wait, what is that? A man or woman or what?": Trans microaggressions from gynecological healthcare providers. *Sexuality Research and Social Policy*, 1–12. https://doi.org/10.1007/s13178-021-00675-7

Pyne, J., Bauer, G., & Bradley, K. (2015). Transphobia and other stressors impacting trans parents. *Journal of GLBT Family Studies*, 11(2), 107–126. https://doi.org/10.1080/1550428X.2014.941127

Ramos, S. R., Lardier Jr, D. T., Opara, I., Turpin, R. E., Boyd, D. T., Gutierrez Jr, J. I., . . . Kershaw, T. (2021). Intersectional effects of sexual orientation concealment, internalized homophobia, and gender expression on sexual identity and HIV risk among sexual minority men of color: A path analysis. *The Journal of the Association of Nurses in AIDS Care*, 32(4), 495. https://doi.org/10.1097%2FJNC.0000000000000274

Rao, W. W., Zhu, X. M., Zong, Q. Q., Zhang, Q., Hall, B. J., Ungvari, G. S., & Xiang, Y. T. (2020). Prevalence of prenatal and postpartum depression in fathers: A comprehensive meta-analysis of observational surveys. *Journal of Affective Disorders*, 263, 491–499. https://doi.org/10.1016/j.jad.2019.10.030

Re:searching for LGBTQ2S+ Health Team. (2019). *Resources: Workshop materials–2SLGBTQ+ competent trauma-informed care, a workshop for service providers. Building competence, building capacity: 2SLGBTQ+ competent trauma-informed care*. www.buildingcompetence.ca/resources.php

Ross, L. E. (2005). Perinatal mental health in lesbian mothers: A review of potential risk and protective factors. *Women & Health*, 41(3), 113–128. https://doi.org/10.1300/J013v41n03_07

Ross, L. E., Dobinson, C., & Eady, A. (2010). Perceived determinants of mental health for bisexual people: A qualitative examination. *American Journal of Public Health*, 100(3), 496–502. https://doi.org/10.2105/AJPH.2008.156307

Ross, L. E., & Goldberg, A. E. (2016). Perinatal experiences of lesbian, gay, bisexual and transgender people. In A. Wenzel (Ed.), *The Oxford handbook of perinatal psychology* (pp. 618–631). Oxford University Press.

Ross, L. E., Siegel, A., Dobinson, C., Epstein, R., & Steele, L. S. (2012). "I don't want to turn totally invisible": Mental health, stressors, and supports among bisexual women during the perinatal period. *Journal of GLBT Family Studies*, 8(2), 137–154. https://doi.org/10.1080/1550428X.2012.660791

Ross, L. E., Steele, L., & Epstein, R. (2006). Service use and gaps in services for lesbian and bisexual women during donor insemination, pregnancy, and the postpartum period. *Journal of Obstetrics and Gynaecology Canada*, 28(6), 505–511. https://doi.org/10.1016/S1701-2163(16)32181-8

Ross, L. E., Steele, L., Goldfinger, C., & Strike, C. (2007). Perinatal depressive symptomatology among lesbian and bisexual women. *Archives of Women's Mental Health*, 10(2), 53–59. https://doi.org/10.1007/s00737-007-0168-x

Ross, L. E., Steele, L., & Sapiro, B. (2005). Perceptions of predisposing and protective factors for perinatal depression in same-sex parents. *Journal of Midwifery & Women's Health*, 50(6), e65–e70. https://doi.org/10.1016/j.jmwh.2005.08.002

Rossi, A. L., & Lopez, E. J. (2017). Contextualizing competence: Language and LGBT-based competency in health care. *Journal of Homosexuality*, 64(10), 1330–1349. https://doi.org/10.1080/00918369.2017.1321361

Rotondi, N. K., Bauer, G. R., Travers, R., Travers, A., Scanlon, K., & Kaay, M. (2012). Depression in male-to-female transgender Ontarians: Results from the Trans PULSE Project. *Canadian Journal of Community Mental Health*, 30(2), 113–133. https://doi.org/10.7870/cjcmh-2011-0020

Ruben, M. A., & Fullerton, M. (2018). Proportion of patients who disclose their sexual orientation to healthcare providers and its relationship to patient outcomes: A meta-analysis and review. *Patient Education and Counseling*, 101(9), 1549–1560. https://doi.org/10.1016/j.pec.2018.05.001

Scarff, J. R. (2019). Postpartum depression in men. *Innovations in Clinical Neuroscience*, 16(5–6), 11. PMCID: PMC6659987

Scheer, J. R., & Poteat, V. P. (2021). Trauma-informed care and health among LGBTQ intimate partner violence survivors. *Journal of Interpersonal Violence*, 36(13–14), 6670–6692. https://doi.org/10.1177/0886260518820688

Seelman, K. L., Colón-Diaz, M. J., LeCroix, R. H., Xavier-Brier, M., & Kattari, L. (2017). Transgender noninclusive healthcare and delaying care because of fear: Connections to general health and mental health among transgender adults. *Transgender Health*, 2(1), 17–28. https://doi.org/10.1089/trgh.2016.0024

Shapiro, J. (2020). The law governing LGBTQ-parent families in the United States. In A. E. Goldberg & K. R. Allen (Eds.), *LGBTQ-parent families: Innovations in research and implications for practice* (2nd ed., pp. 365–382). Springer.

Shenkman, G., Gato, J., Tasker, F., Erez, C., & Leal, D. (2021). Deciding to parent or remain child-free: Comparing sexual minority and heterosexual childless adults from Israel, Portugal, and the United Kingdom. *Journal of Family Psychology*, 35(6), 844. https://psycnet.apa.org/doi/10.1037/fam0000843

Simpson, M., & Catling, C. (2016). Understanding psychological traumatic birth experiences: A literature review. *Women and Birth*, 29(3), 203–207. https://doi.org/10.1016/j.wombi.2015.10.009

Smith, T. M. (2021). *What to know about gender-affirming care for younger patients*. American Medical Association. www.ama-assn.org/print/pdf/node/79151

Snow, D. (2016). Measuring parentage policy in the Canadian provinces: A comparative framework. *Canadian Public Administration*, 59(1), 5–25. https://doi.org/10.1111/capa.12160

Statistics Canada. (2021, March 26). *Socioeconomic profile of the lesbian, gay and bisexual population, 2015 to 2018*. https://www150.statcan.gc.ca/n1/daily-quotidien/210326/dq210326a-eng.htm

Statistics Canada. (2022, April 27). *Canada is the first country to provide census data on transgender and non-binary people*. https://www150.statcan.gc.ca/n1/daily-quotidien/220427/dq220427b-eng.htm

Su, D., Irwin, J. A., Fisher, C., Ramos, A., Kelley, M., Mendoza, D. A. R., & Coleman, J. D. (2016). Mental health disparities within the LGBT population: A comparison between transgender and nontransgender individuals. *Transgender Health*, 1(1), 12–20. https://doi.org/10.1089/trgh.2015.0001

Substance Abuse and Mental Health Services Administration. (2014). *SAMHSA's concept of trauma and guidance for a trauma-informed approach*. https://ncsacw.acf.hhs.gov/userfiles/files/SAMHSA_Trauma.pdf

Tam, M. W., Pilling, M. D., MacKay, J. M., Gos, W. G., Keating, L., & Ross, L. E. (2022). Development and implementation of a 2SLGBTQ+ competent trauma-informed care intervention. *Journal of Gay & Lesbian Mental Health*, 1–25. https://doi.org/10.1080/19359705.2022.2141936

Tan, K. K. H., Wilson, A. B., Flett, J. A. M., Stevenson, B. S., & Veale, J. F. (2021). Mental health of people of diverse genders and sexualities in Aotearoa/New Zealand: Findings from the New Zealand mental health monitor. *Health Promotion Journal of Australia*, 33(3), 580–589. https://doi.org/10.1002/hpja.543

Testa, R. J., Habarth, J., Peta, J., Balsam, K., & Bockting, W. (2015). Development of the gender minority stress and resilience measure. *Psychology of Sexual Orientation and Gender Diversity*, 2(1), 65–77. https://psycnet.apa.org/doi/10.1037/sgd0000081

Tornello, S. L., & Bos, H. (2017). Parenting intentions among transgender individuals. *LGBT Health*, 4(2), 115–120. https://doi.org/10.1089/lgbt.2016.0153

Trans Care BC Provincial Health Services Authority. (2021). *Gender-affirming care for trans, two-spirit, and gender diverse patients in BC: A primary care toolkit*. www.phsa.ca/transcarebc/Documents/HealthProf/Primary-Care-Toolkit.pdf

Trettin, S., Moses-Kolko, E., & Wisner, K. (2006). Lesbian perinatal depression and the heterosexism that affects knowledge about this minority population. *Archives of Women's Mental Health*, 9(2), 67–73. https://doi.org/10.1007/s00737-005-0106-8

Tripathy, P. (2020). A public health approach to perinatal mental health: Improving health and well-being of mothers and babies. *Journal of Gynecology Obstetrics and Human Reproduction*, 49(6), 101747. https://doi.org/10.1016/j.jogoh.2020.101747

Van Beusekom, G., Bos, H. M., Kuyper, L., Overbeek, G., & Sandfort, T. G. (2018). Gender nonconformity and mental health among lesbian, gay, and bisexual adults: Homophobic stigmatization and internalized homophobia as mediators. *Journal of Health Psychology*, 23(9), 1211–1222. https://doi.org/10.1177/1359105316643378

Veale, J. F., Watson, R. J., Peter, T., & Saewyc, E. M. (2017). Mental health disparities among Canadian transgender youth. *Journal of Adolescent Health*, 60(1), 44–49. https://doi.org/10.1016/j.jadohealth.2016.09.014

Ware, J., & Sherbourne, C. D. (1992). The MOS 36-item short-form health survey (SF-36): I. conceptual framework and item selection. *Medical Care, 30*(6), 473–483. https://doi.org/10.1097/00005650-199206000-00002

Warren, J. C., Smalley, K. B., & Barefoot, K. N. (2016). Psychological well-being among transgender and genderqueer individuals. *International Journal of Transgenderism, 17*(3–4), 114–123. https://doi.org/10.1080/15532739.2016.1216344

Wolfe-Roubatis, E., & Spatz, D. L. (2015). Transgender men and lactation: What nurses need to know. *MCN: The American Journal of Maternal/Child Nursing, 40*(1), 32–38. https://doi.org/10.1097/NMC.0000000000000097

Yee, J. Y., Marshall, Z., & Vo, T. (2014). Challenging neo-colonialism and essentialism: Incorporating hybridity into new conceptualizations of settlement service delivery with lesbian, gay, bisexual, trans, and queer immigrant young people. *Critical Social Work, 15*(1), 88–103. https://doi.org/10.22329/csw.v15i1.5910

29

INFERTILITY, PREGNANCY LOSS, AND MENTAL HEALTH DISORDERS

Laura J. Miller

It is hard to know what you are grieving for in a way.

(Meaney et al., 2017, p. 3)

This quote, from a qualitative study of parents' reactions after miscarriage, reflects the confusion sometimes evoked by reproductive loss. Reproductive loss encompasses the loss of a pregnancy or newborn as well as the loss of desired, expected reproductive experiences (Earle et al., 2008). The main types of reproductive losses are defined as follows:

- *Infertility*: Inability to achieve a pregnancy after 12 months or more of regular, unprotected sexual intercourse (World Health Organization, 2023). It may be diagnosed sooner than 12 months based on known factors that reduce fertility, such as age and urogenital injuries. Infertility is classified as *primary* for those who have never been pregnant, and *secondary* for those who have had one or more pregnancies.
- *Miscarriage* and *stillbirth*: Both involve the involuntary, spontaneous loss of a pregnancy. Losses earlier in gestation are termed miscarriages; those later in gestation, or above a certain birth weight, are called stillbirths. The dividing line differs from country to country and sometimes within countries (Boo et al., 2023).
- *Neonatal death*: Death of a liveborn baby within the first 28 days after birth (UNICEF, 2020).
- *Ectopic pregnancy*: Pregnancy that occurs outside of the uterine cavity (Barnhart & Franasiak, 2018).
- *Termination of pregnancy for fetal abnormality*: A decision to end a pregnancy due to prenatal diagnosis of a structural or functional fetal condition that would result in high levels of morbidity or mortality (Heaney et al., 2022).

Each of these reproductive losses can lead to a wide range of reactions and mental health consequences. Some people experience sadness, anger, anxiety, helplessness, and/or guilt (Burden et al., 2016). Some become preoccupied with the loss and a search for its meaning (Ritsher & Neugebauer, 2002; Leith, 2009; Carolan & Wright, 2017). Grief can manifest as

DOI: 10.4324/9781003206903-35

feeling as if one is still pregnant, feeling as though the baby is still inside, dreaming that one is still pregnant, dreaming about the baby, wanting to hold the baby, planning things for the baby, and/or imagining what the baby would look like (Ritsher & Neugebauer, 2002). In addition to this range of normal reactions, some people develop symptoms of depression, anxiety, posttraumatic stress, sexual dysfunction, and/or suicidality after reproductive loss (Burden et al., 2016; Weng et al., 2018; Farren et al., 2020; Westby et al., 2021; Herbert et al., 2022; Ghuman et al., 2021; Kiesswetter et al., 2020; de Castro et al., 2021). In a meta-analysis, perinatal loss was associated with a more than twofold increased risk of depressive disorders and a 1.75-fold increased risk of anxiety disorders (Herbert et al., 2022).

In this chapter, we will explore the mental health effects of infertility and perinatal loss, and mental health interventions that can promote recovery from reproductive losses. In doing so, we will be guided by two cases, one a woman who experienced infertility and the other a woman who experienced a stillbirth. These are composite cases, with no actual personal identifiers.

When she first presented for a mental health evaluation, Ana was a 36-year-old woman who had intense anxiety about an upcoming hysterosalpingogram as part of an infertility workup. She had no children and had been trying to conceive for 15 months. Her husband Jack's testing showed no causes of male infertility. Ana had served in the Marines and was proud of that, but later felt guilty for postponing pregnancy due to deployments. She blamed herself for developing pelvic inflammatory disease (PID) after having multiple sexual partners in her 20s; she thought that caused her infertility. She hadn't told Jack about the sexual partners or the PID and feared he would divorce her when he found out. She identified becoming a mom as her most central life goal.

At the time Leeza was referred for a mental health evaluation, she had recently learned she was pregnant. Her husband Derek was worried about her and their unborn baby. Though Leeza was usually health conscious, she wasn't taking prenatal vitamins and hadn't scheduled a prenatal visit. She said she was happy to be pregnant but didn't look or sound happy. She avoided babies and other pregnant women. Derek suspected this stemmed from Leeza's stillbirth two years prior.

Prevalence of Infertility and Perinatal Loss

Ana is among an estimated one in six people worldwide who experience infertility. Using data from studies published between 1990 and 2021, the World Health Organization estimates that the lifetime prevalence of infertility is 17.5% of the adult population worldwide, whereas the period prevalence (proportion of people with infertility at any given point in time) is 12.6% (World Health Organization, 2023). Rates of infertility are similar across all countries and regions studied.

Like Leeza, many women experience pregnancy loss. Among recognized pregnancies, prevalence estimates range from 1% for stillbirth (Adeyinka et al., 2019) to more than 15% for miscarriage (Quenby et al., 2021). Rates vary considerably from place to place. For example, in a study of the 194 World Health Organization member countries (Adeyinka et al., 2019), stillbirth rates averaged 12.8 per 1,000 total births, ranging from

1.3 per 1,000 total births in Iceland to 43.1 per 1,000 total births in Pakistan. Among many medical and social variables studied, the most influential for stillbirth rate was the gender inequality index.

Correlates and Risk Factors

Reproductive losses are unique stressors (Stanhiser & Steiner, 2018; Kiesswetter et al., 2020). Infertility can feel like a threat to central life goals and expected developmental milestones. It can challenge a person's basic assumptions, such as the ability to choose one's destiny, and can reduce a person's sense of self-efficacy. It is an invisible loss that many women do not discuss outside of their families (Sormunen et al., 2018), which can lead to a unique sense of isolation. Infertility treatment can involve invasive medical procedures, financial strain, time burden, uncertainty, and decisional stress. Treatment decisions many people find wrenching include how many tries they will undergo, how many embryos will be transferred, whether they would consider reduction for a multiple pregnancy, whether it is important for each parent to be genetically related to a child, and/or whether they would consider surrogacy.

An individual's strengths, vulnerabilities, life circumstances and/or past experiences can influence their reactions to reproductive loss. Life satisfaction in the context of infertility has been found to be reduced by higher stress levels, lower partnership quality, and inadequate social support (Kiesswetter et al., 2020). Among people seeking infertility treatments, those who blame themselves for being infertile are more likely to have depressive and anxiety symptoms; women are more likely to blame themselves than men (Péloquin et al., 2018). Adverse mental health consequences also increase with the duration of infertility (Zurlo et al., 2018) and when women do not conceive despite using assisted reproductive technology (Joelsson et al., 2017). That said, some individuals and couples experience reduced distress over time due to successful adaptation.

The relationship between infertility and mental health symptoms can be bidirectional and interactive. Cigarette smoking (Practice Committee of the American Society for Reproductive Medicine, 2018), obesity (Broughton & Moley, 2017), sexual dysfunction (Berger et al., 2016) and some psychotropic medications (Bostwick et al., 2009; Zhang et al., 2016) can impair fertility. Depression reduces initiation of infertility treatment and increases treatment dropout rate (Pedro et al., 2017). Women with prior mental health diagnoses, cigarette smoking, alcohol drinking, body mass index ≥25, and low exercise levels are more likely to develop anxiety and depressive symptoms while infertile, compared to women who are infertile who do not have any of those factors (Joelsson et al., 2017).

Ana's case illustrates some risk factors for mental health challenges in the context of infertility. She experienced infertility as a threat to her most cherished life goal. She blamed herself for infertility due to her prior PID. While PID can anatomically impair fertility, to Ana infertility also felt like a punishment for having had multiple sexual partners in the past. By joining the Marines, Ana had chosen a path that was counter to traditional gender stereotypes. Though she was previously proud of this, infertility caused her to question this choice and feel it interfered with her cultural role as a woman who is expected to bear children.

There are also unique aspects of pregnancy loss that influence emotional reactions. There is a stark emotional contrast between expecting to create life and experiencing a loss. Most pregnant women experience strong attachment to their fetuses, expressed as emotions, internal representations, and protective behaviors (Rich, 2018). Yet grieving a person whom one has not known nor shared experiences with makes it difficult to self-console with meaningful memories. Many perinatal losses are abrupt and associated with traumatic experiences, such as emergency procedures with insufficient information and explanations (LaRivière-Bastien et al., 2019). Unlike other types of loss, usually nothing in parents' lives has prepared them.

Factors associated with developing depressive symptoms after a miscarriage include younger age, lower education level, being unpartnered, having conceived through assisted reproduction, and prior miscarriage (Mutiso et al., 2019). Depressive symptoms also happen more often with more advanced gestational age (Mutiso et al., 2019), though it is posited that depressive symptoms may correlate more with the degree of maternal attachment to the fetus than to gestational age per se. Persistent grief and depression after a miscarriage correlate with remaining childless (deMontigny et al., 2017).

After a stillbirth, a heightened risk of depression has been found when women were not able to be with their babies to the extent that they wished (Surkan et al., 2008). While a subsequent pregnancy sometimes leads to relief, it can also trigger recurrence or exacerbation of depressive, anxiety and posttraumatic symptoms (Burden et al., 2016; Hunter et al., 2017; Gravensteen et al., 2018). During a subsequent pregnancy, reactions to a prior stillbirth can be evoked by changes in fetal movement, ultrasounds, pregnancy milestones, the anniversary of the stillbirth, and/or feelings of attachment to the fetus.

Leeza's experiences illustrate how stillbirth and a subsequent pregnancy can affect maternal mental health. At the time of the stillbirth, she felt emotionally numb and declined to hold her baby, but later came to regret this choice. She developed depressive and posttraumatic stress symptoms, which were undiagnosed and untreated at the time. She coped by staying very busy and avoiding situations that might evoke memories of the stillbirth, such as social gatherings where she might see pregnant women or babies. This coping style was reinforced internally, because it kept intense emotions at bay, and externally, because family members told her how strong she was. When she learned she was pregnant again, she was abruptly flooded with feelings, thoughts and images associated with the stillbirth. Overwhelmed by the intensity of these experiences, she emotionally and behaviorally distanced herself from the pregnancy.

Effects of Perinatal Loss on Partners, Children, and Other Family Members

Partners and Intimate Relationships

For couples, reproductive loss is often a shared stressor or trauma. Whereas this can bring couples closer together, it can also lead to relationship tension and dissolution (Burden et al., 2016). In a U.S. national survey, it was found that parental relationships had a higher risk of dissolving after miscarriage or stillbirth compared to live birth (Gold et al., 2010). Sometimes this stems from both members of a couple experiencing simultaneous mental health challenges. For example, depression symptom intensity of partners struggling with infertility strongly correlate with one another (Ghuman et al., 2021). This reduces the likelihood that partners can help one another by initiating pleasurable or meaningful activities together.

Tension may arise if partners have different styles, expressions, and/or intensity of grief (Burden et al., 2016). Among heterosexual couples, this may be influenced by societal gender role expectations. After stillbirth, fathers have been found to have less intense and shorter duration psychological reactions than mothers but are more likely than mothers to use avoidance coping, including alcohol drinking (Jones et al., 2019). This may be a form of grief suppression, consistent with fathers reporting a perceived need to remain stoic and protect their partners. Tensions can be amplified when partners make assumptions about one another without communicating (Avelin et al., 2013; Burden et al., 2016; Brown-Bowers et al., 2012). A partner who grieves best by talking about feelings might erroneously believe that a quieter partner is not grieving as much.

Leeza and Derek had a strong marriage, but they experienced considerable tension for several months after the stillbirth. Leeza used more avoidant coping strategies than Derek, underscoring that couples don't always follow the more typical pattern. For Derek, having mementoes of the baby helped him grieve. At first, he kept a photo of their stillborn baby on a shelf. Whenever he saw it, he felt connected to the baby and comforted. When Leeza saw it, she experienced horrifying flashbacks. She didn't mention this, choosing instead to avoid that shelf. During that time, Derek was frustrated that Leeza seemed to "just get on with life" as if she never thought about their baby. Leeza was secretly furious that Derek had displayed the picture, but she didn't discuss it because she felt guilty about not wanting to be reminded of their baby. Derek eventually noticed Leeza avoiding the shelf and placed the photo in his clothing drawer.

Navigating infertility together has been shown to strengthen some partnerships and weaken others (Luk & Loke, 2015). One factor in weakened relationships is pressure from extended family members to abandon the partner perceived to be causing the infertility (van Balen & Bos, 2009). Relationships may be strengthened by communication and commitment to one another. *Posttraumatic growth*—the experience of positive psychological change after living through a challenging or traumatic situation—can happen to couples as well as individuals. In the context of infertility, posttraumatic growth in members of a couple correlate with one another (Zhang et al., 2021).

Sexual intimacy, and its associated emotional intimacy, can be adversely affected by infertility (El Amiri et al., 2021). When couples try to conceive in the context of infertility, sex can feel like a chore rather than a means to connect. Among heterosexual couples undergoing infertility treatment, the sexual functioning of male and female members of a couple have been found to strongly correlate with one another (Yeoh et al., 2014). Perinatal loss can also interfere with sexual relationships; sexual intimacy after a loss sometimes triggers guilt and/or disturbing images, thoughts, and feelings (Burden et al., 2016).

In Ana's case, the infertility workup threatened to uncover secrets about her past that she'd kept from Jack. Her fear that Jack would divorce her stopped her from disclosing her prior sexual relationships and PID. Jack felt that Ana was withdrawing from him but didn't know why. He'd inadvertently contributed to Ana's anxiety by repeatedly expressing relief that his part of the infertility workup showed no abnormalities.

Children and Other Family Members

Parents may be faced with helping their children manage a perinatal loss amidst their own distress. Data about children's reactions to perinatal loss, and optimal interventions, are limited. Like adults, children have a wide range of reactions to perinatal loss. Children who have not been told about the loss may notice and react to changes in their parents' moods and behaviors. In qualitative and survey studies of parents (Wilson, 2001; Avelin et al., 2012), participants report that a first step is recognizing their children's grief, which could manifest in various ways (e.g., clinginess, tantrums, regression) or could be more easily expressed through drawings than with words. They note the importance of explaining changes in their children's behavior to others, such as teachers. They recommend answering children's questions honestly and directly in an age-appropriate way, showing their own emotions openly, helping children participate in farewell rituals, and recruiting others to help their children as needed.

Children born after a perinatal loss may also be affected by the loss. Case reports led researchers to posit a "replacement child syndrome" (expecting the new child to be just like the one who died was imagined to be, with the child struggling to live up to expectations) and a "vulnerable child syndrome" (overprotectiveness stemming from excessive fear of losing the child) (Lamb, 2002). While these patterns may be found in some families, studies have not found them to be widespread. However, among women with a history of perinatal loss, experiencing loss later in the gestational period and experiencing multiple perinatal losses have been found to be associated with less positive feelings about parenting and less secure attachment for subsequent children (Côté-Arsenault et al., 2020).

Perinatal losses can affect people throughout the extended family. Leeza and Derek had no living children at the time of their stillbirth. However, their three-year-old niece Keisha had eagerly anticipated the arrival of a cousin. After the stillbirth, Keisha became uncharacteristically quiet. Her preschool teacher noticed and asked her parents whether something had happened at home. Keisha hadn't been told about the stillbirth; everyone had thought she was too young to understand. Her parents now realized she had picked up on the grownups' sadness, so they explained that her cousin had died. They explained it wasn't anyone's fault. They emphasized that Keisha was strong and healthy and wouldn't die. Having previously tried to hide their own reactions, they cried openly. Later, they helped Keisha make table decorations to surround a candle they lit in memory of her cousin.

Cultural Influences

Fertility symbols have figured prominently in many cultures from Paleolithic times onward, reflecting the centrality of concerns about reproduction (Behjati-Ardakani et al., 2016). Current cultures or subcultures vary in the degree to which they are pronatalist—that is, conveying that parenthood and fertility are centrally important contributions (Wells & Heinsch, 2020). Some pronatalist groups or cultures associate femininity, fulfillment, and moral worth more with motherhood than with women's other achievements. Women who are not parents may be stigmatized, ridiculed, harassed, excluded, and devalued (van Balen & Bos, 2009). Many women who experience reproductive loss report a sense of shame and failure, with heightened discomfort in family-focused social settings.

In most cultures, women experience greater blame and ostracism than men for reproductive setbacks (Inhorn, 1994). In some cultures, male infertility is denied altogether (van Balen & Bos, 2009). Reproductive losses may be attributed to a moral flaw in the woman. They may be viewed as a punishment or curse by a deity or spirit. In such contexts, infertility can threaten a woman's status, marriage, and economic security. Reproductive losses can sometimes give men license to abuse, abandon, or kill their wives or take another wife. Some women resort to frightening and/or expensive rituals or purported cures due to the pressure to bear a child.

Ana experienced some of these cultural pressures. She grew up in a Catholic family which strongly valued procreation. Though her parents disapproved of her decision to join the Marines, they remained loving and supportive but now say that her military service interfered with starting a family. She has imbued the cultural insecurity many women face that her husband might reject her if he thinks her behavior led to their inability to bear children. She tacitly believes her infertility is punishment for the sin of having too much sex in the past, consistent with beliefs in many cultures.

In many cultural contexts, the customary rituals and traditions which help people mourn losses are not applied to perinatal losses (Markin & Zilcha-Mano, 2018; Burden et al., 2016). Especially in the case of miscarriage, the loss can remain invisible to others and the grief unrecognized. In the absence of familiar rituals, many people who mean to be supportive inadvertently invalidate parents' grief—for example, saying the loss was for the best and encouraging them to move on and try again. Bereft individuals can experience a cultural taboo against open expression of grief and may feel isolated. Avoiding situations in which they might encounter pregnant women or babies can intensify the isolation.

Leeza and Derek experienced this. After the stillbirth, most of their friends and relatives seemed to feel awkward and didn't talk about it. Derek mentioned to his parents the idea of naming the baby and having a funeral; his parents seemed horrified, so he dropped these plans. Leeza's cousin Tamar brought over meals and did errands for them, but Derek and Leeza were both upset when Tamar kept saying that at least they now knew they could get pregnant and that maybe it just wasn't meant to be yet. Because they appreciated that Tamar was trying to be supportive, they didn't know how to tell her that her comments hurt.

Intervention and Treatment

Acute Interventions

The nurse told me I was going to bleed a lot. But she never said, "There's going to be a fetus that will be expelled, and it will be about the size of a lime. And something will have to be done with it, you'll decide." We didn't talk about that, but it was an important part of the whole process, that I didn't realize until it happened. I didn't know it would happen at home, and I didn't really know what to do, either. I was on the toilet . . . Was I supposed to flush? Would it block the toilet? They didn't explain much to me. There was blood, but there were also bits of the placenta, and of baby . . . It was a fairly traumatic experience.

—From a qualitative study of the experience
of miscarriage (LaRivière-Bastien et al., 2019, p. 673).

There is limited quantitative research on the impact of healthcare personnel interactions on parental mental health after perinatal loss (Rich, 2018). Qualitative studies suggest that recovery-promoting interventions can begin during and immediately after a perinatal loss, in the way healthcare personnel relate to parents. When early pregnancy loss is diagnosed, people are often faced with deciding among expectant management (e.g., miscarrying at home with no intervention), medical interventions (e.g., medications such as mifepristone and/or misoprostol), or procedural interventions (e.g., suction aspiration or dilatation and curettage). This decision may need to be made rapidly, while a woman is in a state of emotional shock. Healthcare providers can reduce the adverse emotional impact by providing clear information about the course of miscarriage, the treatment options, and what to expect with each (LaRivière-Bastien et al., 2019). Promoting patient-centered decisions involves nonjudgmentally eliciting the patient's relationship to her pregnancy, preferences, responsibilities, social supports, and tolerance for pain and bleeding (Schreiber et al., 2016).

At the time of a stillbirth, studies have found that most parents want some form of contact with their stillborn babies, such as seeing, holding, and dressing the baby and/or keeping mementos like a photo or footprint. Even though holding a stillborn baby can be associated with intensified grief, increased anxiety, and subsequent re-experiencing (Redshaw et al., 2016; Wilson et al., 2015), it is rare for parents to regret this choice, and the intensified grief does not translate to worse mental health (Wilson et al., 2015). Many parents report that holding their babies helped them come to terms with the loss (Kingdon et al., 2015).

Qualitative data (Farrales et al., 2020) have identified that what parents want from healthcare providers in the aftermath of a perinatal loss includes:

- Recognizing that the baby is an irreplaceable individual. Parents report feeling invalidated by providers' suggestions that they can just have another baby as a replacement, or by language like "products of conception" instead of "baby." By contrast, they report feeling validated by healthcare providers who ask to see the baby, ask the baby's name, say the baby is beautiful, etc.

- Recognizing how traumatic stillbirth can be, including during the delivery. Some parents report that they were unable to recognize the experience as traumatic themselves at first, because their healthcare providers did not act like it was a trauma and did not explain that it could be traumatic. Parents also describe some healthcare providers being unaware of environmental cues that intensified their trauma, such as pictures of smiling babies throughout the hospital. Parents reported examples of recognition of trauma that felt supportive, such as signage on the door indicating a baby had died so personnel walking in would not default to smiling and congratulations.
- Telling them what to expect, physically and emotionally. For example, some parents report not being told to expect lactation and being shocked when it occurred. Some parents who had not received information about the normal range and expression of grief reactions were left wondering whether their reactions, or those of their partner, were normal.
- Understanding and accepting the intensity and duration of their grief. Parents describe sometimes feeling their grief is minimized or disenfranchised by others, including healthcare professionals. They may also feel pressured to "get over" a perinatal loss quickly, though grief can endure for years.
- Being aware of how painful it can be to see and hear other babies. Examples of supportive interventions by healthcare personnel include closing doors so parents do not hear crying babies, and timing hospital discharge so that parents who have experienced a loss will not see others leaving with live babies.
- Connecting emotionally and interpersonally rather than avoiding them. Some parents describe being treated by healthcare providers in an impersonal manner, solely as patients rather than people. An example of this is a nurse quickly taking vital signs and leaving, with no further interaction. An example of supportive connection is a healthcare provider who cries with the parents.

Leeza recalled her sense of dread when the technician performing her ultrasound appeared tense and wouldn't explain what was going on. An obstetrician she hadn't met before arrived and explained she had had a stillbirth in what felt to Leeza like a detached medical manner, not making direct eye contact. The obstetrician described her options, but Leeza felt dissociated and couldn't take in the information. Derek arrived and stayed with Leeza while the baby was delivered. Leeza recalls her intense feeling of shock when the baby was silent. She experienced an additional shock when she first noticed her breastmilk. No one had told her that might happen. These two experiences—the baby's silence and her breastmilk—recurred repeatedly in the form of vivid flashbacks over the next few months.

Psychotherapy in the Context of Infertility

Psychotherapy for infertility-related distress may be undertaken to alleviate symptoms, improve ability to cope, address contributory factors to infertility (e.g., smoking, sexual difficulties), reduce relationship tension, and help couples think through difficult decisions. Among psychotherapy modalities, evidence for efficacy is strongest for cognitive behavioral therapy (CBT) (Wang et al., 2023a) and mindfulness-based interventions (MBI) (Patel et al., 2020; Wang et al., 2023b). There is also some evidence for efficacy of interpersonal psychotherapy (IPT) (Koszycki et al., 2012), acceptance and commitment therapy (ACT) (Hosseinpanahi et al., 2020), and couples therapy (Soleimani et al., 2015).

Cognitive Behavioral Therapy

A meta-analysis of 16 studies, including a total of 1,102 participants (Wang et al., 2023a), found that CBT led to significant reductions in depressive symptoms, anxiety, perceived stress, psychological distress, and fertility-specific distress. CBT has been found to be effective when delivered individually or in groups. A randomized controlled trial compared therapist-guided Internet-based CBT to face-to-face CBT for women who had adjustment disorders in the context of infertility and found it to be noninferior for reducing depressive and anxiety symptoms (Shafierizi et al., 2023). Despite it clear efficacy for alleviating mental health symptoms, it is less clear whether CBT improves the likelihood of becoming pregnant (Zhou et al., 2021).

In the context of infertility, frequent targets of cognitive interventions include self-blame and feelings of helplessness (Dube et al., 2021). Behavioral interventions often focus on reducing excessive reassurance-seeking and reducing avoidance—for example, of pregnant women and babies—while increasing self-nurturing behaviors (Dube et al., 2021).

Mindfulness-Based Interventions

A meta-analysis of ten randomized controlled trials of mindfulness-based interventions (MBI) for women with infertility (Wang et al., 2023b) found that MBI significantly reduced depressive and anxiety symptoms and improved health-related quality of life. MBI has been posited to be especially relevant for people whose infertility-related distress is strongly influenced by feeling a lack of control. Rather than altering the stress itself, MBI changes the way people relate to the stressor and its associated thoughts and emotions (Patel et al., 2020). When a focus on infertility has led people to disinvest emotionally in their usual activities and relationships, MBI aims to help people experience and cherish their lives for what they are (Patel et al., 2020).

Interpersonal Psychotherapy

In a randomized controlled trial comparing two types of psychotherapy for infertility-linked depression, interpersonal psychotherapy (IPT) led to greater reductions of depressive and anxiety symptoms than the active control intervention of brief supportive therapy (Koszycki et al., 2012). This psychotherapy modality may be especially relevant for those who are facing interpersonal challenges related to infertility, such as relationship tensions and social isolation. IPT can also help people address feelings of infertility-related grief and loss. IPT techniques include actionable ways to increase social supports and connection, such as role-plays to help people figure out whether and how they want to talk to others about infertility.

Acceptance and Commitment Therapy

In a randomized controlled trial (Hosseinpanahi et al., 2020), acceptance and commitment therapy (ACT) delivered in group format to couples experiencing infertility led to reductions in mental health symptoms and improved quality of life compared to control couples receiving no mental health intervention. ACT emphasizes acceptance of thoughts, feelings and circumstances, and commitment to behaviors and activities that stem from one's values. As applied to infertility, ACT can help people accept infertility and its consequences, identify other key values and reasons for self-worth, and re-engage in other valued goals. Sometimes this can be facilitated by identifying values-driven motivators for wanting a child, such as religious beliefs, carrying forward traditions, sharing knowledge and helping to shape the future (Langdridge et al., 2005) and considering additional ways to foster these values.

Couples Therapy

In a small randomized controlled trial (Soleimani et al., 2015), emotionally focused couples therapy (EFT-C) improved marital adjustment and sexual satisfaction for heterosexual married couples experiencing infertility, compared to control couples who did not receive any mental health intervention. In the context of infertility, couples therapy may focus on improving communication, managing conflicts, and navigating different perspectives on infertility treatment decisions (Stammer et al., 2002).

Ana was referred to a psychotherapist when she told her gynecologist she was panicking at the thought of the hysterosalpingogram and wasn't sure she could go through with it. Her psychotherapist helped her reframe self-blaming thoughts and reconsider her belief that infertility was a punishment for her past behaviors. Having done that, Ana realized that given what she knew about Jack, he would be very unlikely to divorce her if she disclosed her PID. After role-playing a conversation in therapy, Ana felt confident enough to tell Jack. He was initially shocked and upset that she had kept this a secret, but he worked through that. They felt closer and better able to support one another through the rest of their infertility journey. They realized they had put too much of the rest of their lives "on hold" and helped one another feel ready to re-engage with friends who had babies.

Psychotherapy After Perinatal Loss

Among psychotherapeutic interventions after perinatal loss, efficacy data are strongest for CBT and MBI (Dolan et al., 2022; Shaohua & Shorey, 2021). With less robust data, efficacy has also been found for IPT (Johnson et al., 2016) and grief counseling (Navidian et al., 2017; Shaohua & Shorey, 2021). Evidence-based couples therapies, such as cognitive behavioral conjoint therapy for posttraumatic stress disorder (Brown-Bowers et al., 2012) and narrative therapy (Romney et al., 2021), have been applied to the context of perinatal loss.

In treating the mental health aspects of perinatal loss, relevant psychotherapeutic modalities may be combined. For example, cognitive behavioral psychotherapists may incorporate mindfulness meditation to foster nonjudgmental awareness, and acceptance to promote understanding that people can lead valued lives despite the presence of upsetting thoughts, feelings, and experiences (Wenzel, 2017).

Cognitive Behavioral Therapy

A systematic review (Dolan et al., 2022) concluded that CBT is effective for reducing symptoms of grief, depression, and posttraumatic stress after perinatal loss. CBT can help people understand what the pregnancy meant to them, to reframe unhelpful beliefs prompted by pregnancy loss, and to engage or re-engage in adaptive behaviors (Wenzel, 2017). Cognitive interventions may focus on beliefs that they could have done something to prevent the loss, adjusting to not having the family for which they had hoped, and experiencing a sense of betrayal. Cognitive restructuring may help reshape catastrophic thoughts such as concerns about never being able to have a successful pregnancy or that the loss is a punishment. Behavioral interventions may focus on self-care, re-engaging in activities that bring joy, and reducing avoidance of reminders of loss. Cognitions and behaviors can be intertwined—for example, when a belief that experiencing joy would be disloyal to the deceased child precludes resuming pleasurable activities.

Mindfulness-Based Interventions

A systematic review (Dolan et al., 2022) concluded that MBI is effective for reducing symptoms of grief, depression, and posttraumatic stress after perinatal loss. Mindfulness techniques that have been applied in the context of perinatal loss include breathing exercises, body scans, attention to sensory experiences, meditation, and focus on gratitude (Jensen et al., 2021; Nasrollahi et al., 2022).

Interpersonal Psychotherapy

A randomized controlled trial (Johnson et al., 2016) found greater reductions in depressive and grief symptoms and improved social support after group IPT adapted for perinatal loss compared to a control condition of group CBT for depression. There were three main IPT adaptations. The first was a focus on coping with others' reactions because there are few social norms about how to grieve a perinatal loss and affected parents may not know how to ask others to react. The second was addressing issues of fault and meaning, because self-blame and a search for meaning can be more prominent after perinatal loss as compared to other types of loss. The third was finding ways to maintain a sense of connection to the lost baby while also re-engaging in meaningful activities and relationships.

Grief Counseling

Little is systematically known about grief counseling after miscarriage. A randomized controlled trial found that group-delivered grief counseling alleviated PTSD symptoms more than routine postpartum care in women who had recently experienced stillbirth (Navidian et al., 2017). Because perinatal loss differs in some respects from other types of loss, grief counseling may need to be modified to encompass these differences (Condon, 1986). This could include eliciting knowledge or fantasies about what the baby was like or would become, discussing in detail the circumstances of the death, identifying strategies parents have used to feel connected to the baby, addressing guilt and self-blame, and understanding changes in self-concept. A cornerstone of grief counseling after perinatal loss is to validate and facilitate a wide range in styles and expressions of grief without pathologizing grief, while accounting for cultural influences and spiritual beliefs (Markin & Zilcha-Mano, 2018).

Couples Therapies

There is a paucity of systematic data about couples therapies after perinatal loss. When evidence-based couples interventions are applied to perinatal loss, psychotherapy goals may include understanding one another's grieving styles, improving conflict management, and enhancing communication skills (Brown-Bowers et al., 2012). Members of a couple can approach feared situations together and help each other increase positive behaviors. Couples can reconfigure their support network by strengthening ties with supportive others and repairing ties when supportive others were inadvertently hurtful. They can consider whether to establish rituals to mark anniversaries of the loss and prepare to conceive again if desired. Narrative couples therapy invites couples to co-construct a narrative of their loss and recovery, with an emphasis on new possibilities (Romney et al., 2021).

Leeza and Derek began cognitive behavioral conjoint therapy (CBCT) (Brown-Bowers et al., 2012). They articulated their coping styles and learned from the therapist that each style was within the norm. They both learned to use slowed breathing and "time outs" for conflict management, and to "channel check" by asking whether their partner wanted to share feelings or problem-solve. They each re-examined previously tacit core beliefs: Derek reconsidered his belief that his job was to "cheerlead" or "fix," and Leeza reconsidered her belief that if she wasn't in total control another disaster was sure to happen. Leeza's symptoms improved, as did their relationship.

Prescribing Psychotropic Medication in the Context of Reproductive Loss

A careful mental health assessment can distinguish grief from major depressive disorder or other mental health conditions warranting consideration for pharmacotherapy. Though large-scale prescribing practices after perinatal loss have not been systematically studied, a survey of parents after perinatal loss (Lacasse & Cacciatore, 2014) revealed that among those who were prescribed psychotropics, 32.2% of prescriptions were issued within 48 hours of the loss, 43.7% within a week of the loss, and 74.7% within a month of the loss. This underscores the importance of taking the time for thorough evaluation and for implementation of nonpharmacologic supportive measures as clinically indicated.

In cases where psychotropic medication is indicated, women who have experienced reproductive loss may be especially concerned about whether medication could cause infertility, miscarriage, or stillbirth. Those who seek information online may find a plethora of material ranging from accurate to outdated and misleading. Published studies differ widely in quality, especially regarding the influence of potential confounds. The most methodologically sounds studies do not find an association between antidepressant use and miscarriage (Ross et al., 2013; Wu et al., 2019), stillbirth (Jimenez-Solem et al., 2013), or female infertility (Sylvester et al., 2019). By contrast, certain antipsychotic medications that raise prolactin levels (Bostwick et al., 2009), or the mood stabilizer valproate that is associated with polycystic ovary syndrome (Zhang et al., 2016), could potentially impair fertility. In the context of perinatal loss, patient-centered decision-making about pharmacotherapy can be promoted by eliciting specific concerns, providing detailed information, and recommending accurate sources for further reading.

Personal and Posttraumatic Growth After Reproductive Loss

Reproductive losses often challenge people's core beliefs, such as tacit assumptions regarding safety and control. For example, women who have experienced a stillbirth have reported a nearly constant awareness of fragility, a sense of how quickly things can change, and difficulty trusting others, particularly doctors (Üstündağ-Budak et al., 2015). While challenges to core beliefs can cause substantial distress, they can also lead to posttraumatic growth, defined as positive psychological or developmental changes after stressful or traumatic experiences. Examples of such growth include greater appreciation of life and of personal strength (Krosch & Shakespeare-Finch, 2017; Shafierizi et al., 2022). Posttraumatic growth has been identified in people who have experienced infertility (Kong et al., 2018) and perinatal loss (Ryninks et al., 2022).

Studies of women who have experienced miscarriage or stillbirth have found that core belief disruption predicts posttraumatic growth after both types of perinatal loss (Krosch & Shakespeare-Finch, 2017; Freedle & Kashubeck-West, 2021). Significantly higher levels of posttraumatic growth have been found in those who experienced stillbirth compared to those who experienced miscarriage (Ryninks et al., 2022); this was associated with greater challenges to core beliefs.

The connection between core belief disruption and posttraumatic growth is mediated by intentional, reflective cognitive work to make meaning out of the loss (Freedle & Kashubeck-West, 2021). By contrast, intrusive, uncontrolled rumination about the loss reduces the likelihood of posttraumatic growth. Along with core belief disruption, other factors that have been found to promote posttraumatic growth after perinatal loss include resilience and social support (Kong et al., 2018).

Ana experienced personal growth as she learned to cope with infertility. She began to realize that she held a tacit core belief that people would only love her if she performed to their expectations. While she wanted a child for several important reasons, one of them was that she felt only a child would love her unconditionally. After identifying this core belief, she was able to challenge it—for example, realizing that her parents still loved her despite her unconventional choices, and Jack still loved her after learning her secrets. Though she still deeply wanted a child, she developed renewed confidence that she could feel worthwhile and lead a meaningful, connected life regardless of whether she became pregnant.

Leeza and Derek also experienced growth, individually and as a couple. They came to understand that they had both viewed Leeza as fragile, despite her external show of strength. Leeza felt she had to protect herself through emotional and behavioral avoidance; Derek felt he had to protect Leeza by hiding his own needs and enabling her avoidance. With psychotherapy, Leeza developed a new appreciation of her strength and resilience. Derek expanded his view of how a husband could be supportive in a way that facilitated recovery, while also fully acknowledging and expressing his own grief.

Conclusion and Future Directions

Reproductive losses are unique stressors that can lead to a wide range of emotional reactions. Infertility and perinatal loss can affect the individuals involved as well as their partners, children, and extended family members. Individual reactions can be affected by cultural context. Pronatalist cultures can increase pressures on those who have experienced perinatal loss while rendering significant others less able to be supportive. Evidence-based psychotherapies can be adapted to the specific concerns of people experiencing reproductive losses. When psychopharmacology is indicated, eliciting a history of reproductive loss can help prescribers understand people's heightened concerns and explain risks and benefits of medication in that context. Mental health interventions can alleviate symptoms, improve functioning, and in many cases promote personal growth.

There are several aspects of reproductive loss for which additional research could be especially helpful. Additional data about protective and vulnerability factors that influence mental health after perinatal loss could pave the way for developing and studying preventive interventions. Considerably more understanding is needed of the effects of perinatal loss on relationships, children, and extended family members, as well as effective couples and family interventions in this context. Among pregnancy losses, the mental health consequences of miscarriage and stillbirth have been better studied than those of ectopic pregnancy, fetal reduction, and termination of pregnancy for fetal abnormality; the particulars of those types of loss need additional illumination. Further clarifying how to best adapt evidence-based psychotherapies to apply to the unique challenges presented by reproductive losses could increase their effectiveness. Research to clarify which parents may benefit from pharmacotherapy after experiencing perinatal loss could shape safer and more effective prescribing practices.

Although Ana, Jack, Leeza, and Derek are composite cases, their experiences are based on those of many real people. On behalf of those people, thank you for reading this chapter and for caring about, and for, those who have experienced reproductive losses.

References

Adeyinka, D. A., Olakunde, B. O., & Muhajarine, N. (2019). Evidence of health inequity in child survival: Spatial and Bayesian network analyses of stillbirth rates in 194 countries. *Scientific Reports*, 9(1), 19755.

Avelin, P., Erlandsson, K., Hildingsson, I., Bremborg, A. D., & Rådestad, I. (2012). Make the stillborn baby and the loss real for the siblings: Parents' advice on how the siblings of a stillborn baby can be supported. *The Journal of Perinatal Education*, 21(2), 90–98.

Avelin, P., Rådestad, I., Säflund, K, Wredling, R., & Erlandsson, K. (2013). Parental grief and relationships after the loss of a stillborn baby. *Midwifery*, 29(6), 668–673.

Barnhart, K. T., & Franasiak, J. M. (2018). ACOG practice bulletin no. 193: Tubal ectopic pregnancy. *Obstetrics & Gynecology*, 131(3), e91–e103.

Behjati-Ardakani, Z., Akhondi, M. M., Mahmoodzadeh, H., & Hosseini, S. H. (2016). An evaluation of the historical importance of fertility and its reflection in ancient mythology. *Journal of Reproduction & Infertility*, 17(1), 2–9.

Berger, M. H., Messore, M., Pastuszak, A. W., & Ramasamy, R. (2016). Associations between infertility and sexual dysfunction in men and women. *Sexual Medicine Reviews*, 4(4), 353–365.

Boo, Y. Y., Gwacham-Anisiobi, U., Thakrar, D. B., Roberts, N., Kurinczuk, J. J., Lakhanpaul, M., & Nair, N. (2023). Facility-based stillbirth review processes used in different countries across the world: A systematic review. *eClinicalMedicine*, 59, 101976.

Bostwick, J. R., Guthrie, S. K., & Ellingrod, V. L. (2009). Antipsychotic-induced hyperprolactinemia. *Pharmacotherapy*, 29(1), 64–73.

Broughton, D. E., & Moley, K. H. (2017). Obesity and female infertility: Potential mediators of obesity's impact. *Fertility and Sterility, 107*(4), 840–847.

Brown-Bowers, A., Fredman, S. J., Wanklyn, S. G., & Monson, C. M. (2012). Cognitive-behavioral conjoint therapy for posttraumatic stress disorder: Application to a couple's shared traumatic experience. *Journal of Clinical Psychology, 68*(5), 536–547.

Burden, C., Bradley, S., Storey, C., Ellis, A., Heazell, A. E. P., Downe, S., . . . Siassakos, D. (2016). From grief, guilt, pain and stigma to hope and pride: A systematic review and meta-analysis of mixed-method research of the psychosocial impact of stillbirth. *BMC Pregnancy and Childbirth, 16*, 9.

Carolan, M., & Wright, R. J. (2017). Miscarriage at advanced maternal age and the search for meaning. *Death Studies, 41*(3), 144–153.

Condon, J. T. (1986). Management of established pathological grief reaction after stillbirth. *The American Journal of Psychiatry, 143*, 987–992.

Côté-Arsenault, D., Leerkes, E. M., & Zhou, N. (2020). Individual differences in maternal, marital, parenting and child outcomes following perinatal loss: A longitudinal study. *Journal of Reproductive and Infant Psychology, 38*(1), 3–15.

de Castro, M. H. M., Mendonça, C. R., Noll, M., de Abreu Tacon, F. S., & do Amaral, W. N. (2021). Psychosocial aspects of gestational grief in women undergoing infertility treatment: A systematic review of qualitative and quantitative evidence. *International Journal of Environmental Research and Public Health, 18*(24), 13143.

deMontigny, F., Verdon, C., Meunier, S., & Dubeau, D. (2017). Women's persistent depressive and perinatal grief symptoms following a miscarriage: The role of childlessness and satisfaction with healthcare services. *Archives of Women's Mental Health, 20*(5), 655–662.

Dolan, N., Grealish, A., Tuohy, T., & Bright, A.-M. (2022). Are mindfulness-based interventions as effective as cognitive behavioral therapy in reducing symptoms of complicated perinatal grief? A systematic review. *Journal of Midwifery & Women's Health, 67*(2), 209–225.

Dube, L., Nkosi-Mafutha, N., Balsom, A. A., & Gordon, J. L. (2021). Infertility-related distress and clinical targets for psychotherapy: A qualitative study. *BMJ Open, 11*(11), e050373.

Earle, S., Foley, P., Komaromy, C., & Lloyd, C. (2008). Conceptualizing reproductive loss: A social sciences perspective. *Human Fertility, 11*(4), 259–262.

El Amiri, S., Brassard, A., Rosen, N. O., Rossi, M. A., Beaulieu, N., Bergeron, S., & Péloquin, K. (2021). Sexual function and satisfaction in couples with infertility: A closer look at the role of personal and relational characteristics. *The Journal of Sexual Medicine, 18*(12), 1984–1997.

Farrales, L. L., Cacciatore, J., Jonas-Simpson, C., Dharamsi, S., Ascher, J., & Klein, M. C. (2020). What bereaved parents want healthcare providers to know when their babies are stillborn: A community-based participatory study. *BMC Psychology, 8*(1), 18.

Farren, J., Jalmbrant, M., Falconieri, N., Mitchell-Jones, N., Bobdiwala, S., Al-Memar, M., . . . Bourne, T. (2020). Posttraumatic stress, anxiety and depression following miscarriage and ectopic pregnancy: A multicenter, prospective, cohort study. *American Journal of Obstetrics & Gynecology, 222*(4), 367.

Freedle, A., & Kashubeck-West, S. (2021). Core belief challenge, rumination, and post-traumatic growth in women following pregnancy loss. *Psychological Trauma: Theory, Research, Practice, and Policy, 13*(2), 157–164.

Ghuman, N. K., Raikar, S., Singh, P., Nebhinani, N., & Kathuria, P. (2021). In it together: A dyadic approach to assessing the health-related quality of life and depression among infertile couples. *Families, Systems, & Health, 39*(4), 576–587.

Gold, K. J., Sen, A., & Hayward, R. A. (2010). Marriage and cohabitation outcomes after pregnancy loss. *Pediatrics, 125*(5), e1202–1207.

Gravensteen, I. K., Jacobsen, E.-M., Sandset, P. M., Helgadottir, L. B., Rådestad, I., Sandvik, L., & Ekeberg, O. (2018). Anxiety, depression and relationship satisfaction in the pregnancy following stillbirth and after the birth of a live-born baby: A prospective study. *BMC Pregnancy and Childbirth, 18*(1), 41.

Heaney, S., Tomlinson, M., & Aventin, A. (2022). Termination of pregnancy for fetal anomaly: A systematic review of the healthcare experiences and needs of parents. *BMC Pregnancy and Childbirth, 22*(1), 441.

Herbert, D., Young, K., Pietrusińska, M., & MacBeth, A. (2022). The mental health impact of perinatal loss: A systematic review and meta-analysis. *Journal of Affective Disorders, 297*, 118–129.

Hosseinpanahi, M., Mirghafourvand, M., Farshbaf-Khalili, A., Esmaeilpour, K., Rezaei, M., & Malakouti, J. (2020). The effect of counseling based on acceptance and commitment therapy on mental health and quality of life among infertile couples: A randomized controlled trial. *Journal of Education and Health Promotion, 9*, 251.

Hunter, A., Tussis, L., & MacBeth, A. (2017). The presence of anxiety, depression and stress in women and their partners during pregnancies following perinatal loss: A meta-analysis. *Journal of Affective Disorders, 223*, 153–164.

Inhorn, M. (1994). Interpreting infertility: Medical anthropological perspectives. *Social Science & Medicine, 39*(4), 459–461.

Jensen, K. H. K., Krog, M. C., Koert, E., Hedegaard, S., Chonovitsch, M., Schmidt, L., . . . Nielsen, H. S. (2021). Meditation and mindfulness reduce perceived stress in women with recurrent pregnancy loss: A randomized controlled trial. *Reproductive Biomedicine Online, 43*(2), 246–256.

Jimenez-Solem, E., Andersen, J. T., Petersen, M., Broedbaek, K., Lander, A. R., Afzal, S., . . . Poulsen, H. E. (2013). SSRI use during pregnancy and risk of stillbirth and neonatal mortality. *The American Journal of Psychiatry, 170*(3), 299–304.

Joelsson, L. S., Tydén, T., Wanggren, K., Georgakis, M. K., Stern, J., Berglund, A., & Skalkidou, A. (2017). Anxiety and depression symptoms among sub-fertile women, women pregnant after infertility treatment, and naturally pregnant women. *European Psychiatry, 45*, 212–219.

Johnson, J. E., Price, A. B., & Kao, J. C. (2016). Interpersonal psychotherapy (IPT) for major depression following perinatal loss: A pilot randomized controlled trial. *Archives of Women's Mental Health, 19*(5), 845–859.

Jones, K., Robb, M., Murphy, S., & Davies, A. (2019). New understandings of fathers' experiences of grief and loss following stillbirth and neonatal death: A scoping review. *Midwifery, 79*, 102531.

Kiesswetter, M., Marsoner, H., Luehwink, A., Fistarol, M., Mahlknecht, A., & Duschek, S. (2020). Impairments in life satisfaction in infertility: Associations with perceived stress, affectivity, partnership quality, social support and the desire to have a child. *Behavioral Medicine, 46*(2), 130–141.

Kingdon, C., Givens, J. L., O'Donnell, E., & Turner, M. (2015). Seeing and holding baby: Systematic review of clinical management and parental outcomes after stillbirth. *Birth, 42*(3), 206–218.

Kong, L., Fang, M., Ma, T., Li, G., Yang, F., Meng, Q., . . . Li, P. (2018). Positive affect mediates the relationships between resilience, social support, and posttraumatic growth of women with infertility. *Psychology, Health & Medicine, 23*(6), 707–716.

Koszycki, D., Bisserbe, J.-C., Blier, P., Bradwejn, J., & Markowitz, J. (2012). Interpersonal psychotherapy versus brief supportive therapy for depressed infertile women: First pilot randomized controlled trial. *Archives of Women's Mental Health, 15*(3), 193–201.

Krosch, D. J., & Shakespeare-Finch, J. (2017). Grief, traumatic stress, and post-traumatic growth in women who have experienced pregnancy loss. *Psychological Trauma: Theory, Research, Practice, and Policy, 9*(4), 425–433.

Lacasse, J. R., & Cacciatore, J. (2014). Prescribing of psychiatric medication to bereaved parents following perinatal/neonatal death: An observational study. *Death Studies, 38*, 589–596.

Lamb, E. H. (2002). The impact of previous perinatal loss on subsequent pregnancy and parenting. *The Journal of Perinatal Education, 11*(2), 33–40.

Langdridge, D., Sheeran, P., & Connolly, K. (2005). Understanding the reasons for parenthood. *Journal of Reproductive and Infant Psychology, 23*(2), 121–133. https://doi.org/10.1080/02646830500129438

LaRivière-Bastien, D., deMontigny, F., & Verdon, C. (2019). Women's experiences of miscarriage in the emergency department. *Journal of Emergency Nursing, 45*(6), 670–676.

Leith, V. M. S. (2009). The search for meaning after pregnancy loss: An autoethnography. *Illness, Crisis & Loss, 17*(3), 201–221.

Luk, B. H., & Loke, A. Y. (2015). The impact of infertility on the psychological well-being, marital relationships, sexual relationships, and quality of life of couples: A systematic review. *Journal of Sex & Marital Therapy, 41*(6), 610–625.

Markin, R. D., & Zilcha-Mano, S. (2018). Cultural processes in psychotherapy for perinatal loss: Breaking the cultural taboo against perinatal grief. *Psychotherapy, 55*(1), 20–26.

Meaney, S., Corcoran, P., Spillane, N., & O'Donahue, K. (2017). Experience of miscarriage: An interpretive phenomenological analysis. *BMJ Open, 7*(3), e011382.

Mutiso, S. K., Murage, A., & Mwaniki, A. M. (2019). Factors associated with a positive depression screen after a miscarriage. *BMC Psychiatry*, 19(1), 8.

Nasrollahi, M., Pour, M. G., Ahmadi, A., Mirzaee, M., & Alidousti, K. (2022). Effectiveness of mindfulness-based stress reduction on depression, anxiety, and stress of women with the early loss of pregnancy in southeast Iran: A randomized control trial. *Reproductive Health*, 19, 233.

Navidian, A., Saravani, Z., & Shakiba, M. (2017). Impact of psychological grief counseling on the severity of post-traumatic stress symptoms in mothers after stillbirth. *Issues in Mental Health Nursing*, 38(8), 650–654.

Patel, A., Sharma, P. S. V. N., & Kumar, P. (2020). Application of mindfulness-based psychological interventions in infertility. *Journal of Human Reproductive Sciences*, 13(1), 3–21.

Pedro, J., Sobral, M. P., Mesquita-Guimarães, J., Leal, C., Costa, M. E., & Martins, M. V. (2017). Couples' discontinuation of fertility treatments: A longitudinal study on demographic, biomedical and psychosocial risk factors. *Journal of Assisted Reproduction and Genetics*, 34(2), 217–224.

Péloquin, K., Brassard, A., Arpin, V., Sabourin, S., & Wright, J. (2018). Whose fault is it? Blame predicting psychological adjustment and couple satisfaction in couples seeking fertility treatment. *Journal of Psychosomatic Obstetrics & Gynecology*, 39(1), 64–72.

Practice Committee of the American Society for Reproductive Medicine. (2018). Smoking and infertility: A committee opinion. *Fertility and Sterility*, 110(4), 611–618.

Quenby, S., Gallos, J. D., Dhillon-Smith, R. K., Podesek, M., Stephenson, M. D., Fisher, J., . . . Coomarasamay, A. (2021). Miscarriage matters: The epidemiological, physical, psychological, and economic costs of early pregnancy loss. *Lancet*, 397(10285), 1658–1667.

Redshaw, M., Hennegan, J. M., & Henderson, J. (2016). Impact of holding the baby following stillbirth on maternal mental health and well-being: Findings from a national survey. *BMJ Open*, 6(8), e010996.

Rich, D. (2018). Psychological impact of pregnancy loss: Best practice for obstetric providers. *Clinical Obstetrics and Gynecology*, 61(3), 628–636.

Ritsher, J. B., & Neugebauer, R. (2002). Perinatal bereavement grief scale: Distinguishing grief from depression following miscarriage. *Assessment*, 9(1), 31–40.

Romney, J., Fife, S. T., Sanders, D., & Behrens, S. (2021). Treatment of couples experiencing pregnancy loss: Reauthoring loss from a narrative perspective. *International Journal of Systemic Therapy*, 32(2), 134–152.

Ross, L. E., Grigoriadis, S., Mamisashvili, L., Vonderporten, E. H., Roerecke, M., Rehm, J., . . . Cheung, A. (2013). Selected pregnancy and delivery outcomes after exposure to antidepressant medication: A systematic review and meta-analysis. *JAMA Psychiatry*, 70(4), 436–443.

Ryninks, K., Wilkinson-Tough, M., Stacey, S., & Horsch, A. (2022). Comparing posttraumatic growth in mothers after stillbirth or early miscarriage. *PLoS One*, 17(8), e0271314.

Schreiber, C. A., Chavez, V., Whittaker, P. G., Ratcliffe, S. J., Easley, E., & Barg, F. K. (2016). Treatment decisions at the time of miscarriage diagnosis. *Obstetrics & Gynecology*, 128(6), 1347–1356.

Shafierizi, S., Faramarzi, M., Esmaelzadeh, S., Khafri, S., & Ghofrani, F. (2022). Does infertility develop posttraumatic growth or anxiety/depressive symptoms? Roles of personality traits, resilience, and social support. *Perspectives in Psychiatric Care*, 58(4), 2017–2028. https://doi.org/10.1111/ppc.13023

Shafierizi, S., Faramarzi, M., Nasiri-Amiri, F., Chehrazi, M., Basirat, Z., Kheirkhah, F., & Pasha, H. (2023). Therapist-guided internet-based cognitive behavioral therapy versus face-to-face CBT for depression/anxiety symptoms in infertile women with adjustment disorders: A randomized controlled trial. *Psychotherapy Research*, 33(6), 803–819.

Shaohua, L., & Shorey, S. (2021). Psychosocial interventions on psychological outcomes of parents with perinatal loss: A systematic review and meta-analysis. *International Journal of Nursing Studies*, 117, 103871.

Soleimani, A. A., Najafi, M., Ahmadi, K., Javidi, N., Kamkar, E. H., & Mahboubi, M. (2015). The effectiveness of emotionally focused couples therapy on sexual satisfaction and marital adjustment of infertile couples with marital conflicts. *International Journal of Fertility & Sterility*, 9(3), 393–402.

Sormunen, T., Aanesen, A., Fossum, B., Karlgren, K., & Westerbotn, M. (2018). Infertility-related communication and coping strategies among women affected by primary or secondary infertility. *Journal of Clinical Nursing*, 27(1–2), e335–344.

Stammer, H., Wischmann, T., & Verres, R. (2002). Counseling and couple therapy for infertile couples. *Family Process*, 41(1), 111–122.

Stanhiser, J., & Steiner, A. Z. (2018). Psychosocial aspects of fertility and assisted reproductive technology. *Obstetrics and Gynecology Clinics of North America*, 45(3), 563–574.

Surkan, P. J., Rådestad, I., Cnattingius, S., Steineck, G., & Dickman, P. W. (2008). Events after still-birth in relation to maternal depressive symptoms: A brief report. *Birth*, *35*(2), 153–157.

Sylvester, C., Menke, M., & Gopalan, P. (2019). Selective serotonin reuptake inhibitors and fertility: Considerations for couples trying to conceive. *Harvard Review of Psychiatry*, *27*(2), 108–118.

UNICEF. (2020). *Neonatal mortality*. Neonatal mortality–UNICEF DATA.

Üstündağ-Budak, A. M., Larkin, M., Harris, G., & Blissett, J. (2015). Mothers' accounts of their stillbirth experiences and of their subsequent relationships with their living infant: An interpretive phenomenological analysis. *BMC Pregnancy and Childbirth*, *15*, 263.

van Balen, F., & Bos, H. M. W. (2009). The social and cultural consequences of being childless in poor resource areas. *Facts, Views & Vision in ObGyn*, *1*(2), 106–121.

Wang, G., Liu, X., & Lei, J. (2023a). Cognitive behavioural therapy for women with infertility: A systematic review and meta-analysis. *Clinical Psychology & Psychotherapy*, *30*(1), 38–53.

Wang, G., Liu, X., & Lei, J. (2023b). Effects of mindfulness-based intervention for women with infertility: A systematic review and meta-analysis. *Archives of Women's Mental Health*, *26*(2), 245–258.

Wells, H., & Heinsch, M. (2020). Not yet a woman: The influence of socio-political constructions of motherhood on experiences of female infertility. *The British Journal of Social Work*, *50*, 890–907.

Weng, S.-C., Chang, J.-C., Yeh, M.-K., Wang, S.-M., Lee, C.-S., & Chen, Y.-H. (2018). Do stillbirth, miscarriage and termination of pregnancy increase risk of attempted and completed suicide within a year? A population-based nested case-control study. *BJOG*, *125*(8), 983–990.

Wenzel, A. (2017). Cognitive behavioral therapy for pregnancy loss. *Psychotherapy (Chic)*, *54*(4), 400–405.

Westby, C. L., Erlandsen, A. R., Nilsen, S. A., Visted, E., & Thimm, J. C. (2021). Depression, anxiety, PTSD, and OCD after stillbirth: A systematic review. *BMC Pregnancy Childbirth*, *21*(1), 782.

Wilson, P. A., Boyle, F. M., & Ware, R. S. (2015). Holding a stillborn baby: The view from a specialist perinatal bereavement service. *Australian and New Zealand Journal of Obstetrics and Gynaecology*, *55*(4), 337–343.

Wilson, R. E. (2001). Parents' support of their other children after a miscarriage or perinatal death. *Early Human Development*, *61*(2), 55–65.

World Health Organization. (2023). *Infertility prevalence estimates, 1990–2021*. World Health Organization.

Wu, P., Velez Edwards, D. R., Gorrindo, P., Sundermann, A. C., Torstenson, E. S., Jones, S. H., . . . Hartmann, K. E. (2019). Association between first trimester antidepressant use and risk of spontaneous abortion. *Pharmacotherapy*, *39*(9), 889–898.

Yeoh, S. H., Razali, R., Sidi, H., Razi, Z. R. M., Midin, M., Jaafar, N. R. N., & Das, S. (2014). The relationship between sexual functioning among couples undergoing infertility treatment: A pair of perfect gloves. *Comprehensive Psychiatry*, *55*(Suppl 1), S1–6.

Zhang, L., Li, H., Li, S., & Zou, X. (2016). Reproductive and metabolic abnormalities in women taking valproate for bipolar disorder: A meta-analysis. *European Journal of Obstetrics & Gynecology and Reproductive Biology*, *202*, 26–31.

Zhang, X., Deng, X., Mo, Y., Li, Y., Song, X., & Li, H. (2021). Relationship between infertility-related stress and resilience with posttraumatic growth in infertile couples: Gender differences and dyadic interaction. *Human Reproduction*, *36*(7), 1862–1870.

Zhou, R., Cao, Y.-M., Liu, D., & Xiao, J.-S. (2021). Pregnancy or psychological outcomes of psychotherapy interventions for infertility: A meta-analysis. *Frontiers in Psychology*, *12*, 643395.

Zurlo, M. C., della Volta, M. F. C., & Vallone, F. (2018). Predictors of quality of life and psychological health in infertile couples: The moderating role of duration of infertility. *Quality of Life Research*, *27*(4), 945–954.

30

NEONATICIDE AND PREGNANCY DENIAL

Tomasz Gruchala and Cara Angelotta

While we recognize that not all individuals capable of pregnancy identify as women, nearly all studies on neonaticide and pregnancy denial use the terms woman or mother to identify an individual who gave birth.

Neonaticide, the act of killing a newborn within 24 hours of birth, is an understudied phenomenon with significant personal, social, and legal ramifications for involved mothers (Barnes, 2022). Psychiatrist Phillip Resnick pioneered early research into neonaticide in the 1970s and 1980s and received credit for coining neonaticide as a term and distinguishing it from filicide and infanticide (Friedman et al., 2005). Filicide is a parent killing a child at any point in life, and infanticide in a parent killing a child between 24 hours and one year of life (Friedman & Resnick, 2007). The cause of death in neonaticide is most often abandonment (due to the neonate's complete reliance on a caregiver) or attempted disposal of the neonate. However, it frequently includes active asphyxiation (strangulation or drowning) and, more rarely, stabbing or blunt trauma (Malmquist, 2013).

The connection between neonaticide and mental illness is debated. Building on Resnick's early work, some authors have found that neonaticide is most often unrelated to underlying psychiatric conditions (Porter & Gavin, 2010). Although cases differ widely based on life circumstances, common threads include chronic life stressors, panic experienced during birth, and regret or grief following the infant's death (Milia & Noonan, 2022). Some women cited being unprepared for motherhood as a contributing factor, especially in cases where the mother did not intentionally kill the baby and instead left it behind. Mental illness is frequently implicated in both infanticide and filicide rather than neonaticide (Kenner & Nicolson, 2015).

Instead, scholars have found a strong connection between neonaticide and the phenomenon of pregnancy denial and dissociative experiences (Spinelli, 2001). *Pregnancy denial* is a term used to describe pregnancy recognition after 20 weeks' gestation. Although there is no standard definition, complete or pervasive pregnancy denial refers to the lack of recognition of pregnancy until intrapartum, meaning the pregnancy is not recognized until the onset of labor or even following delivery. Affective pregnancy denial occurs when a person has

DOI: 10.4324/9781003206903-36

cognitive knowledge of the pregnancy but lacks emotional recognition of the pregnancy. Using the psychological defense of denial, she continues to think, act, and behave as though she is not pregnant despite knowing at some level that she is pregnant. The pregnant person with affective denial does not experience the emotional changes that accompany pregnancy or feel an attachment to the child (Jenkins et al., 2011; Friedman et al., 2007). A published case report describes a 20-year-old woman who recognized fetal movements one month before delivery and believed she was pregnant but did not prepare for the birth, falling into the category of affective pregnancy denial (Neifert & Bourgeois, 2000). Psychotic pregnancy denial occurs when a person has a delusion or fixed false belief that they are not pregnant despite evidence to the contrary (e.g., an ultrasound showing a fetus). Psychotic pregnancy denial is usually associated with chronic mental illnesses like schizophrenia whereas nonpsychotic pregnancy denial may be associated with mood disorders and dissociative symptoms at birth (Barnes, 2022). Among women who committed a neonaticide offense, 53% were diagnosed with pregnancy denial in one study (Beier et al., 2006). Research consistently indicates that pregnancy denial increases the risk of neonaticide (Kenner & Nicolson, 2015; Lee et al., 2006; Stenton & Cohen, 2020; Vellut et al., 2012).

In the last several decades, there has been an increase in research exploring neonaticide and pregnancy denial, but there is still some uncertainty regarding the demographics, risk factors, and conditions surrounding affected women. This chapter will explore the current understanding of neonaticide, pregnancy recognition, and pregnancy denial primarily through English-language literature published after 2000.

Pregnancy recognition plays a vital role in the understanding of neonaticide. The point at which and method by which a woman recognizes she is pregnant varies by individual. For some, a personal conclusion is reached based on physiological symptoms in the context of sexual activity, birth control use, and menstrual cycle tracking. Others may learn they are pregnant with an over-the-counter pregnancy test or by receiving a formal diagnosis by a healthcare professional. Instead of being a binary state between "pregnant" and "not pregnant," pregnancy recognition is a spectrum (Watson & Angelotta, 2022). Not every woman recognizes their pregnancy at the same point, and rarely may not recognize it at all, only coming to a conclusion while giving birth. Barriers to pregnancy recognition include access to medical care and pregnancy tests and the availability of community resources. A woman with low-risk sexual behavior who uses a form of birth control may recognize her pregnancy late by having no reason to suspect pregnancy.

Despite its use in psychiatric literature, the term "pregnancy *denial*" is misleading to lay audiences because it implies a conscious decision to ignore or hide the pregnancy, which may not be the case. *Pregnancy concealment* occurs when a pregnant person is consciously aware of the pregnancy but takes active steps to conceal the pregnancy from others. Pregnancy concealment increases the risk of neonaticide (Murphy-Tighe & Lalor, 2016). In the aftermath of an out-of-hospital death of a newborn, it may be difficult to determine with certainty if the pregnant person was intentionally concealing the pregnancy or experiencing pregnancy denial.

The terms "collective denial" or "consensus of denial" are sometimes used when a woman's social circle is also unaware of a pregnancy. Caution should be used with these terms because the social factors surrounding pregnancy denial can vary widely between women, and they imply varying degrees of blame on both the women and their family or friends without considering individual circumstances. Women with affective pregnancy denial are unlikely to disclose their pregnancy to their family and partner, and some cite fear of abandonment or negative response from others due to personal or cultural factors (Amon et al.,

2012). Those with pervasive pregnancy denial may not give their social circle any reason to suspect pregnancy. For women in relationships who commit neonaticide, their partners are often unaware of the pregnancy (Amon et al., 2012).

Significant physiological and psychological changes accompany pregnancy, so it can be challenging to understand how a woman may experience pregnancy denial. Physiological changes affect every organ system in the body to some degree as the woman prepares to give birth. Throughout the pregnancy, women often experience exhaustion, sleepiness, mood changes, and anxiety, among other feelings and symptoms. Attachment to the baby also begins to occur during the prenatal period. Despite pregnancy denial seeming unlikely in the context of these symptoms, literature in the last two decades highlights many cases of this occurring. For example, a published case report describes a 27-year-old woman who did not recognize her pregnancy for most of the gestation (Nanjundaswamy et al., 2019). She interpreted the lack of menstruation and occasional vaginal spotting as irregularities in her menstrual cycle and her physical changes as weight gain. Mental status exams after delivery and throughout one month of inpatient care revealed no psychiatric symptoms. She reunited with her infant; follow-up studies showed no mental health concerns. Despite no apparent adverse effects on both mother and child in this case, not all cases of pregnancy denial end with a positive outcome. Failure to obtain prenatal care increases the risk of preterm birth, stillbirths, and neonatal death, as well as reduced gestational weight and infection for the infant and morbidity for the mother (Knight et al., 2014; Maupin et al., 2004). Giving birth unexpectedly and experiencing dissociative symptoms as a result of pregnancy denial can also result in the infant's death within 24 hours (Spinelli, 2001). Death may be due to the actions taken by the mother, for example strangulation, or it may be due to inattention at birth or the failure of the mother to recognize that the baby was liveborn. In legal cases where charges are brought against the mother, forensic pathologists may debate whether the baby was stillborn or liveborn or whether the baby died from complications of an unassisted birth or was actively killed by the mother.

Instead of chronic mental illness, a common link between neonaticide and pregnancy denial is the presence of acute dissociative symptoms while giving birth. Women with dissociation at birth after an unrecognized pregnancy commonly report giving birth alone precipitously into a toilet, mistaking labor for needing to have a bowel movement or menstrual pains. Some report a lack of pain during delivery. These circumstances are one factor that can precipitate dissociation, a disruption of normally integrated mental functions like memory, time, sensory perception, and sense of identity. This leads to an inability to respond appropriately to adverse situations (American Psychiatric Association, 2013). In pregnancy denial, dissociative symptoms may include derealization, the sense that the surrounding environment is unreal, and depersonalization, the sense that one is watching oneself from outside one's body (Barnes, 2022). Neonaticide can result from dissociation, especially if the mother incorrectly perceives the baby as stillborn or does not attend to the baby's medical needs after birth. Shock, shame, guilt, and fear tend to be the emotions preceding neonaticide rather than anger or aggression (Barnes, 2022).

Furthermore, physicians or other healthcare providers can accidentally reinforce pregnancy denial by not diagnosing pregnancy or mistaking pregnancy for an alternative condition. In one study, 38% of women with pregnancy denial in the study sample visited a physician's office while pregnant without receiving a pregnancy diagnosis during the visit (Beier et al., 2006). Some studies have even suggested that a woman's firm belief that she is not pregnant can influence a physician's ability to correctly diagnose a pregnancy (Wessel et al., 2003b). One remarkable case report describes a 23-year-old woman who presented to the emergency department after several days of lower back pain and gave birth shortly after; she had seen a physician two days prior to the emergency visit, where she was treated for a urinary tract infection without a diagnosis of pregnancy (Stammers & Long, 2014). Several similar case reports are published, indicating a need for greater awareness and further study of pregnancy denial. Recognition of a woman's pregnancy, in the context of pregnancy denial, is a complex interplay of personal, social, and medical factors.

Rarely, chronic psychotic disorders and mood disorders may be directly involved in some neonaticide cases. A published case report described a woman who experienced prenatal depression with psychotic features (Karakasi et al., 2017). She reached a critical point post-delivery where she believed the baby would be better off dead. She ultimately killed her infant within 24 hours of delivery by stabbing and dropping them from a height. Another published case report described a woman who committed a series of five neonaticides related to her depression and pathological dissociative tendencies (Huchzermeier & Heinzen, 2015).

A lack of clarity about the relation between mental health and neonaticide may affect legal outcomes for these women. Ultimately, mothers who commit neonaticide may be criminally charged for actions taken or not taken during the birth, and legal outcomes are case-specific. In the United States, differences between state laws contribute to varied sentences, even for cases that are similar in how they progressed and the outcome for the baby. The same applies to outcomes for women in different European countries.

The following illustrative case highlights several events and risk factors relevant to many neonaticide cases. However, it does not represent every woman's experience, as neonaticide circumstances can be highly individualized. This case is not based on a real person, but rather is an example to highlight common features of women who experience complete pregnancy denial. While Anna's case is used as a generalized example, every instance of neonaticide presents a unique set of circumstances surrounding the woman's background, social circle, demographics, and access to resources.

Anna was a 37-year-old woman who gave birth to a 5.5-pound baby boy, estimated to be 34 weeks' gestation, in a public bathroom at a mall. She mistook labor pains for menstrual cramps and the delivery for a bowel movement. She reported no awareness of the pregnancy and was shocked when she saw a baby in the bathroom. Anna left the baby in the toilet, who was not crying or making noise and was blue. Another person entered the bathroom stall, called for help, and emergency services provided emergency medical care. The neonatal intensive care unit at a local hospital admitted the baby. Anna had a well-documented history of irregular menses. She had one prior pregnancy not identified until 24 weeks' gestation, followed by an expected spontaneous vaginal delivery in a hospital. Her husband was the biological father of both children and reported no awareness of the pregnancy in the second case. She takes oral contraceptives. Eight weeks prior to the delivery of the baby, Anna went to a primary care physician with complaints of an upset stomach, who diagnosed her with gastroesophageal reflux disease and prescribed a proton pump inhibitor. The pregnancy was not diagnosed at this visit. Following the discovery and treatment of the baby, a court charged Anna with attempted murder.

Incidence of Neonaticide and Pregnancy Denial

Psychiatric and forensic literature includes several case reports exploring individual neonaticide events. Some papers provide information on the causes and risk factors of neonaticide on a population level. However, research on the incidence of neonaticide is lacking; relatively few studies that review neonaticide can provide rates for specific areas. Incidence is difficult to quantify due to the following considerations:

• In studies of a single country, neonaticide rates may vary between urban and rural areas or counties, jurisdictions, and states. For example, one report on neonaticide in Lithuania found that most recorded neonaticides occurred in rural areas, although this is likely influenced by there being large rural populations in Central and Eastern Europe (Stasiuniene et al., 2015). Even if multiple studies analyze neonaticide in the same country, the reported rates can vary in location, period, and population size, so trends are difficult to establish.

• The meaning of neonaticide is not the same between studies despite the recent trend toward a unified definition (death within 24 hours after birth). The authors of several papers consider children to be neonates up to 28 days old, and thus in these papers, the neonaticide rates include children up to this age. Neonaticide beyond 24 hours is less associated with pregnancy denial. Different legal systems may also use this definition of neonaticide, so government-published statistics on neonaticides lack consistency.

• Some neonaticides are not recorded if the mother does not seek medical care or otherwise come forward, especially if a third party does not find the deceased neonate. The actual rates of neonaticide may be higher than what is currently published. An autopsy is frequently used to determine the cause of death in neonaticide cases but is less accurate if the body is found days to weeks later due to decomposition. Some studies have described infrequently used methods to identify death means in neonaticide that may partially circumvent the issue of a decomposing body, including post-mortem computed tomography (Sieswerda-Hoogendoorn et al., 2013).

• Legal issues complicate the reporting of neonaticide cases, resulting in inconsistencies between medical or judicial records and published mortality statistics. In France, a study found that in the proceedings of 26 courts between 1996 and 2000, judicial data indicated a neonaticide rate of 2.1 neonaticides per 100,000 births, whereas official mortality statistics indicated 0.39 per 100,000 (Tursz & Cook, 2011). In Finland, a study analyzed all police-reported neonaticides between 1980 and 2000 to calculate a 0.18 per 100,000 births rate. Not all of the cases went through a court process. If only cases that underwent a complete court process are considered, the rate is 0.07 per 100,000 births (Putkonen et al., 2007).

• Some cases and data may not be available for researchers to access. Personal information laws vary globally; thus, specific data are protected depending on the country.

Of the neonaticide rates that are published, the majority of them are from European countries. Data from less industrialized countries are almost nonexistent. A systematic review by Tanaka et al. (2017) compiled neonaticide rates around the world and concluded that neonaticide has few geographical boundaries and is often seen in high-income countries, although similarly found that most available estimates were from Europe.

Between the 1970s and 1990s, neonaticide estimates exhibit a wide range and France, Finland, and Austria have ample data compared to other countries. In France, estimates range from 0.12 cases per 100,000 births to 2.10 or more (Makhlouf & Rambaud, 2014; Tursz & Cook, 2011). In Finland, two studies over roughly the same period calculated an incidence of 0.78 cases per 100,000 births during 1995–2005 from death certificates from coroner's departments and 1.63 during 1991–2001 from police-reported statistics (Amon et al., 2012; Klier et al., 2012). For many of these incidence estimates, additional context is needed. For example, the study by Klier et al. (2012) analyzed police-reported cases before and after the implementation of an anonymous birth law in Austria; from 1991 to 2001, their estimate was 7.22 cases per 100,000 births, whereas from 2002 to 2009 it was 3.10. Some non-European countries have data but with caveats. Tunisia in North Africa had a rate of 0.42 cases per 100,000 births from 1977 to 2016, but this rate is based on autopsies from a single teaching hospital (Ben Khelil et al., 2019). In the United States, the only available study calculated an incidence of 2.10 cases per 100,000 births from 1985 to 2000 in the state of North Carolina only (Herman-Giddens et al., 2003).

In the last several decades, there have been changes in pregnancy-related laws and attitudes around the world, yet there are relatively few studies calculating neonaticide incidence after the year 2000. In Japan, the rate was 0.96 between 2003 and 2018 (Yoshiba, 2020). A 2015 study by Stasiuniene et al. provided incidence from 2008 to 2012 for Poland (2.40 cases per 100,000 births), Latvia (2.90), Estonia (5.2), and Lithuania (5.80). In Tanzania, in the city of Dar es Salaam, there was an incidence of 27.7 cases per 100,000 births in 2005, although this number includes deaths up to 1 week after birth (Outwater et al., 2010).

Pregnancy denial can also be difficult to quantify, made apparent by a lack of epidemiological studies. A German study of pregnancy denial found that pregnancy is not recognized until after 20 weeks' gestation in 1 in 475 pregnancies (Wessel & Buscher, 2002). A French study determined a rate of 1 in 300 pregnancies (Simermann et al., 2018). Wessel et al. also found that 1 in about 2,500 pregnancies are recognized intrapartum. Most cases of complete pregnancy denial are not associated with neonaticide. Still, the incidence of pregnancy denial needs further exploration to identify factors affecting how frequently it occurs in different countries. The characteristics and classification of pregnancy denial are case-specific, and confusion about the pregnancy recognition spectrum may make it difficult for medical and legal professionals to come to a consensus on whether a pregnant person charged with a neonaticide offense experienced pregnancy denial.

Correlates and Risk Factors

The research on neonaticide and pregnancy denial over the last several decades has yielded a variety of associations and considerations for women at risk. Although many questions remain, this section explores the general demographic profile of affected mothers and the circumstances surrounding neonaticide.

Demographics

Our understanding of the demographics and backgrounds of women who experience pregnancy denial or who commit neonaticide has evolved. Earlier studies in the late 20th century of neonaticidal mothers and mothers who experienced pregnancy denial indicated that demographic factors trend toward a young age, a low level of formal education, and a lack of committed relationships with partners. These formed the overall understanding of neonaticide demographics in psychiatric literature until the 1990s and early 2000s, and still remains prevalent in medicine, law, and popular culture. Recent evidence challenges these trends and suggests that women who commit neonaticide or experience pregnancy denial are more heterogeneous than prior research indicated, demonstrating diversity in demographics, background, and motivation. A 2007 study analyzed 65 women who experienced pregnancy denial. Fifty-four had a stable partner, 56 were at or over the age of 20 with a median of 27 years, and nearly all had completed their secondary education (Wessel et al., 2007). In a different study, most women who committed neonaticide had completed at least their high school education (Friedman et al., 2007). A publication assessing neonaticide and pregnancy denial had similar results; 57% of the women who committed neonaticide were in long-term relationships, and the mean age was 24, ranging from 14 to 39 years (Stenton & Cohen, 2020).

Whereas certain factors are still consistent with older research, including that many mothers who commit neonaticide are in their early or mid-20s, neonaticide and pregnancy denial can occur in a broader population of women than previously believed. However, peer-reviewed contemporary studies exist that support the earlier findings as well. One such paper found a lack of a stable relationship, a lack of a high school diploma, and a history of psychiatric illness to be predictive factors for pregnancy denial and that being older was a protective factor (Delong et al., 2022). The small volume of literature calls for further study better to understand the demographics and backgrounds of affected women. Given the much rarer incidence of neonaticide relative to other perinatal events, most studies have small sample sizes. Cultural factors can also affect results; for example, typical educational attainment for women and marriage attitudes differ between countries, making it challenging to identify widely applicable demographic trends for neonaticide risk.

Circumstances Surrounding the Pregnancy

Beyond demographic and social factors, the specific features of pregnancy can influence the likelihood of pregnancy denial or neonaticide. Likewise, pregnancy denial can influence the outcome of the neonate. Gynecologists and primary care physicians can consider these features when assessing patients who present with pregnancy symptoms.

Although demographic risk factors differ between studies, many have found that women who commit neonaticide tend to be multigravidas (Delong et al., 2022). A lack of prenatal care increases the risk of adverse outcomes for the neonate and the risk of neonaticide. Out-of-hospital delivery is a consistent risk factor for neonaticide. A history of irregular menses is frequently found in those who present with pregnancy denial (Friedman et al., 2007).

Women who have experienced pregnancy denial in the past or had a late recognition of their pregnancy are at greater risk of experiencing it again if they have another pregnancy, relative to women with no pregnancy denial in their past (Delong et al., 2022). Women with pregnancy denial are more likely to give birth preterm, increasing the neonate's morbidity and mortality risk relative to women with no pregnancy denial (Wessel et al., 2002). Births resulting in neonaticide usually occur alone, and many have an unsuspecting third party nearby that may discover whether the neonate is alive or deceased (Shelton et al., 2010). Common settings include the home or a hotel room, and the births are often directly into the toilet (Shelton et al., 2010). There is also a high contraceptive use rate in both single and repeat neonaticide cases (Klier et al., 2019). This rate is higher in the repeat group, and the methods most frequently used include hormonal contraceptives, intrauterine devices, and condoms. Although proper protection prevents pregnancy, it may also increase the likelihood of a woman not believing or knowing she is pregnant. Women who commit successive neo-naticides in multiple pregnancies (repeat neonaticide) tend to be older, more educated, and have more children (Klier et al., 2019).

The sample case introduced at the beginning of the chapter highlights some of these correlates and risk factors in context. Anna is a woman in a long-term relationship with a history of irregular menses who experienced a pervasive pregnancy denial in which she misinterpreted her pregnancy symptoms. The surprise birth resulted in a dissociative reac-tion that caused her to leave her unresponsive neonate in the toilet. Her prior pregnancy that was recognized late and her use of contraceptives are key risk factors for neonaticide. It is also important to note that her social circle lacked awareness of the pregnancy and she experienced misdiagnosis in a healthcare clinic.

Effects on Mothers, Partners, and Children

Although the definition of neonaticide does not exclude killing by a father or partner, it remains an act committed almost exclusively by mothers. Likewise, pregnancy denial can only be experienced by those capable of giving birth, most of whom identify as women. Generally, fathers who kill their children tend to do so when they are significantly older than one year, which is an act of general filicide rather than infanticide or neonaticide (Putkonen et al., 2011). For fathers or partners involved in a neonaticide case, especially if they were unaware of the pregnancy before the event, it is not unreasonable to speculate that they could experience adverse psychological effects following the death. However, at the time of writing, there is little to no research exploring these potential ripple effects of neonaticide. In the illustrative case presented previously, Anna's husband did not receive follow-up mental health inquiries or care. Similarly, little is known about the psychological effects of these events on a mother's other children.

There is ample evidence to conclude that pregnancy denial affects the health of both mothers and children. The primary cause of maternal and child morbidity due to pregnancy denial is a lack of prenatal care (Friedman et al., 2007). Prenatal care is critical to maintain-ing the health of both mother and child. It includes regular check-ups with a physician or healthcare professional who can review lab values, behaviors, diet, and disease. Not receiv-ing care during pregnancy increases the risk to both mother and child of experiencing com-plications during and after birth. Women who experience pregnancy denial and do not seek prenatal care are more likely to experience preeclampsia and eclampsia and are more likely to be admitted to the intensive care unit compared to women without pregnancy denial and who receive timely prenatal care (Schultz & Bushati, 2015). Preeclampsia, in particular, can cause premature birth in infants, leading to further morbidity and mortality.

Similarly, babies born to mothers with pregnancy denial frequently require treatment in the neonatal intensive care unit; common reasons for admission include respiratory distress, nuchal cord (where the umbilical cord is wrapped around the neonate's neck), and apnea (temporary cessation of breathing) (Friedman et al., 2009). They are also at increased risk of prematurity and low birth weight and are more likely to be delivered surgically com-pared to babies born to mothers without pregnancy denial, which carries risks for both mother and child (Wessel et al., 2003a). Cognitive effects are also a concern. Children born to a mother with pregnancy denial appear to have an increased risk of psychomotor developmental issues in the first two years of life (Simermann et al., 2018). They also may be more likely to develop a speech disorder relative to children whose mothers did not have pregnancy denial (Kettlewell et al., 2021). Physicians should be aware of these risks and discuss them with patients who may have experienced pregnancy denial. In Anna's illustrative case, as with many women who experienced pregnancy denial, her child was treated in the neonatal intensive care unit following her dissociative reaction.

Research on the long-term consequences of pregnancy denial on children is lacking. There is an opportunity to explore potential consequences because mothers with pregnancy denial who did not commit neonaticide are still likely to retain custody of their children even if they did not receive prenatal care. Only a minority of mothers with pregnancy denial are referred to child protective services, and even fewer have their cases accepted by these services (Friedman et al., 2009). Circumstances surrounding pregnancy denial are highly case-specific, so making generalizations about the preparedness of mothers for long-term child rearing is difficult. There is yet to be a prospective study that follows babies born to mothers with pregnancy denial beyond the first few years of life. Similarly, there is little research on the long-term mental health impact of pregnancy denial or neonaticide on the mother, especially if it involves intense guilt or regret that could harm her future quality of life.

Prevention of Neonaticide and Pregnancy Denial

Implementing the same prevention strategy in every country will yield differences in success. Cultural differences and beliefs about pregnancy, abortion, child rearing, and neonaticide mean no one-size-fits-all approach exists. As such, most studies on prevention focus on a single country, and extrapolation of findings to other countries needs careful consideration. In high-income countries such as the United States, law and policy change could be a best first step in preventing neonaticide. In lower-income countries such as India, large-scale societal factors that increase risk of neonaticide play an additional role, such as gender biases.

At a case-specific level, prevention of neonaticide could include increasing awareness and identifying women at risk. Primary care physicians, obstetricians or gynecologists, and other professionals involved in pregnancy care should be aware of the risk factors and incorporate that knowledge into their practice. In the context of pregnancy denial, pregnancy should always be considered in the differential diagnosis of women who present with nausea and vomiting, weight gain, and abdominal pain or changes, even if there is a lack of more obvious pregnancy symptoms (Friedman et al., 2007). Unfortunately, healthcare providers are not always aware of the immediate pregnancy status of their patients (Vallone & Hoffman, 2003). They should screen for pregnancy especially in women who are part of higher-risk groups for neonaticide, particularly those with previous pregnancies or pregnancy denials and a history of irregular menses. In teenage populations, school nurses can help prevent neonaticide in students who may be at risk by taking a complete history, promoting safe sex, discussing relationships and social support, and even exploring the student's attitudes toward pregnancy (Platt, 2014). In general, sex education and contraceptive access should be provided to teenagers and young adults to reduce the risk of neonaticide and, more generally, unwanted pregnancy.

However, placing the burden of neonaticide prevention solely on professionals or the women themselves is not an effective long-term strategy. Effective prevention may rely most strongly on changing overarching policy over individual or community-based interventions. For example, the 1973 Roe v. Wade decision in the United States (which protected the right to have an abortion) had an impact on neonaticide rates. In the decade following the decision, neonaticide occurred less frequently across the country compared to the decade prior

(Lester, 1992). Accessible abortion options for women with pregnancy denial or who are at risk for neonaticide may reduce surprise or unwanted pregnancies that then lead to neonaticide. The Dobbs v. Jackson Women's Health Organization decision in 2022 that overturned the precedent set by Roe v. Wade may lead to an increase in neonaticide rates over the next several years.

Another potential way to reduce neonaticide in the United States through policy change is by implementing or extending Safe Haven laws (Friedman & Resnick, 2009). Safe Haven laws allow parents to give up their child for adoption under state-dependent conditions. For example, in Illinois, an infant can be given up without legal consequence if they are less than 30 days old and unhurt. Drop-off locations include most hospitals, emergency care facilities, police stations, and staffed fire stations. Safe Haven laws provide an alternative to neonaticide, and offering a place where an unexpected infant can be safely left may reduce the mother's guilt and confusion about what to do next. More comprehensive implementation would be beneficial. However, most states are not required or permitted to gather statistics about infants given up under these laws, so analyzing the Safe Haven impact on neonaticide prevention is difficult.

Initiatives similar to Safe Haven laws are present outside of the United States. Many European countries, as well as Japan, South Africa, and Pakistan, offer "baby hatches," which are incubators outside hospitals where mothers can drop an infant off for care and eventual adoption. Some countries also offer anonymous delivery, which allows women to give birth in a hospital without legal complications or monetary charge if she agrees to give it up for adoption. The introduction of such an anonymous delivery option in Austria in 2001 correlated with reduced police-reported neonaticides after it went into effect (Klier et al., 2012). As mentioned previously, before the law took effect, the Austrian rate of neonaticide was 7.22 per 100,000 births. The rate became 3.10 per 100,000 births within eight years after implementation. Ultimately, evidence suggests that policies surrounding abortion and pregnancy can significantly impact the frequency of neonaticide.

Cultural Considerations

Regardless of the availability of published statistics, neonaticide is likely to occur in all cultures (Tanaka et al., 2017). Pregnancy denial also occurs worldwide but much more commonly than neonaticide. Culture can significantly affect both the quantitative and qualitative features of neonaticide. As rates differ between countries, so can parent demographics and means of death. Remarkable differences are seen in the treatment of women in criminal justice systems and the legal outcomes of neonaticide.

At the time of writing, there are very few or no published English-language studies analyzing the circumstances of neonaticide in several highly populated countries, including but not limited to Indonesia, Nigeria, Bangladesh, Russia, Mexico, Ethiopia, Philippines, and Thailand. Likewise, there are few or no studies that compare pregnancy denial and neonaticide across cultures. Most studies review neonaticide in Western Europe or the United States; some data is available for select countries in Asia, Africa, and South America.

United States and Europe

In the United States and European countries, several studies have described a relatively heterogeneous group of women who commit neonaticide. However, information on neonate gender and maternal ethnicity or race is minimal. Thus far, one study in the United States found that neonate gender is not a risk factor for neonaticide and that the rates for Black, non-Hispanic White, or Hispanic individuals are not significantly different (Salihu et al., 2021). Conversely, the study found that foreign-born U.S. residents of any ethnicity are nearly four times as likely to commit neonaticide. The authors reasoned that immigrants and those with lower socioeconomic status have inadequate access to medical and community resources, contributing to the risk of pregnancy denial and neonaticide, among many other health concerns.

Around the globe, the means of death tend to be through nonviolent methods. The United States and Europe are no different; passive neglect is common in France, while asphyxiation comprises most neonaticides in Denmark (Makhlouf & Rambaud, 2014; Gheorghe et al., 2011).

Africa

In Africa, there are striking differences in neonaticide frequency between countries. Africa records some of the highest and lowest rates of neonaticide globally. In Tanzania, one study found that the incidence of neonaticide is a remarkably high 27.7 per 100,000 births and that nearly 80% of child homicides, including both filicide and non-filicidal child murder, are neonaticides (Outwater et al., 2010). This study was conducted in Dar es Salaam, a city, and the rates in Tanzania may differ between urban and rural areas as they might in other countries. Suggested factors contributing to this high rate include a lack of abortion access except to save a mother's life and few or no safe zones to give up neonates for adoption. Many Tanzanian people live below the international poverty line with reduced access to medical care and community resources.

Conversely, neonaticide is less common in Tunisia than in most European countries or the United States (Ben Khelil et al., 2019). Similarities include no difference in the gender of neonates and neglect being the most common cause of death. One significant difference is that many bodies are abandoned on public roads instead of the home, public bathrooms, hospitals, or garbage disposal areas, although this proportion is decreasing. The authors suggested that the low proportion of neonaticides found in the mother's home is because women tend to live with their parents until they get married, and thus the body is placed elsewhere for fear of being discovered.

In South Africa, neonaticide more closely reflects the trends in Europe and North America. Mothers commit nearly all cases with a mean age of 23.5 years, there are no significant differences in the gender of deceased neonates, and the most common means of death are abandonment and passive neglect (Abrahams et al., 2016). As of the publication of this chapter, this is the only study on South African neonaticide and identifies a high rate (19.6 per 100,000 births) but defines neonaticide as death within 0–28 days. Data assessing mental health are not available. South Africa has an upper-middle-income economy, and its relatively industrialized status may help explain some of its similarities in neonaticide with wealthier countries.

South America

Data on South American neonaticide are minimal. One study reviewed infanticide and neonaticide (combined into the term filicide) and found that filicidal mothers tended to be single and unemployed, which differs from many other studies (Benitez-Borrego et al., 2013). One factor to consider is the inclusion of infanticide into this finding, which can affect the overall result; the authors also suggested that the high unemployment rate is more so due to the cultural standard of men having paid jobs over women who traditionally tend to household tasks.

Asia (and the Middle East)

Research on neonaticide in Asian countries reflects several notable differences from other countries. Gender plays a much more significant role than in Western countries. In India, neonaticide happens more frequently to female neonates than males, reflecting a broader cultural preference for male children (Mishra et al., 2014). The Prenatal Diagnostic Techniques Act of 1994 attempted to alleviate female filicides by preventing prenatal sex determination and selective abortion. However, the gender preference remains for neonaticide and filicide more generally. Like many other countries, official statistics regarding neonaticide are unavailable, making the event analysis in India difficult. Conversely, in Pakistan, neonaticide victims are more likely to be male than female (Mehmood et al., 2022). The reason behind this difference is unclear, and data on maternal mental health and socioeconomic status is limited.

Japan earned notoriety for infanticide and neonaticide in the late 20th century through "coin-locker babies," or infants abandoned inside coin-operated public storage spaces (Kouno & Johnson, 1995). Today, the leading causes of death are suffocation and strangulation, and there are no gender differences in the rate of neonaticide (Yoshiba, 2020). Japan is notable for having a low birth rate that continues to decline. The fertility rate was below replacement-level fertility as far back as 1974 (Oizumi et al., 2022). Therefore, it would logically follow that neonaticide is less common in Japan than in other countries, which may be the case. However, a study found that the overall neonaticide rate in the last two decades has remained unchanged despite decreasing birth rates (Yoshiba, 2020). The author states that data on each neonaticide case is limited due to personal information laws, making this finding challenging to analyze.

Neonaticide in other parts of Asia is less remarkable than in Japan. In Hong Kong and South Korea, pregnancy denial is commonly a factor in neonaticide, there is a low frequency of mental illness in neonaticidal mothers, and the most common means of death are suffocation or abandonment (Lee et al., 2006; Jung et al., 2020).

Legal Considerations of Neonaticide Cases

The legal treatment of neonaticide and outcomes for convicted mothers varies drastically between countries. The United States and Scotland have never had special regulations for neonaticide or infanticide, while France, Argentina, Western Australia, and Hungary abolished their existing regulations (Kruger, 2015). Legal considerations of neonaticide are further complicated because pregnancy denial is not included in the DSM-5 or ICD-11, which are often referenced by lawyers or medical professionals involved in court cases (American Psychiatric Association, 2013; World Health Organization, 2021). The definition of neonaticide also varies between jurisdictions (sometimes the first 24 hours and others the first 28 days), adding a layer of complexity. Some countries, such as India, have regulations for infanticide but not for neonaticide (Mishra et al., 2014).

A review of the legal outcomes of women who commit neonaticide in the United States concluded that they are often seen as fully responsible for a homicide without considering the unique circumstances of neonaticide and pregnancy denial (Malmquist, 2013).

Convicted mothers receive highly varied punishments ranging from probation to life prison sentences. Courts may see women as having full agency in the death without considering physical or mental circumstances at the time of labor and delivery. Courts may otherwise view pregnancy denial as intentionally concealed pregnancy.

The legal treatment of neonaticide in the United States is in contrast to other countries with legal regulations, where the outcomes for convicted mothers tend to be less severe. In Finland, special regulations exist for neonaticide, and convicted mothers spend a mean of 617 days in prison (Putkonen et al., 2007). Britain has had special regulations since 1938, when the Infanticide Act was passed (Kruger, 2015). In Eastern Croatia, several courts have tried neonaticide without giving prison time to the mother, claiming that the emotional pain and guilt following the death was a suitable punishment (Marcikic et al., 2006). Austria imprisons few convicted offenders, and those who are convicted serve an average sentence of 1.65 years (Amon et al., 2020). The authors of the Austrian study argue that treatment detention, especially for neonaticidal mothers with mental illness, is a better alternative to imprisonment.

Conclusion and Future Directions

Because neonaticide and pregnancy denial are frequently misunderstood, additional research and advocacy are recommended. Although nearly all subtopics discussed in this chapter require additional exploration, the ones particularly in need of study include maternal demographics, incidence between and within countries, maternal risk factors, ripple effects on families, prevention strategies, and cultural differences focused on legal policy. Physicians involved in primary care or pregnancy care should recognize the risk factors for pregnancy denial. Pregnancy, and thus the possibility of pregnancy denial, should be considered in all reproductive-age individuals regardless of contraceptive use, relationship status, or menstrual patterns (Watson & Angelotta, 2022). Medical resources directed toward lawyers that explain the circumstances surrounding neonaticide and pregnancy denial should also be produced.

One of the main concerns regarding the treatment of and legal outcome of women with pregnancy denial is the lack of a formal psychiatric definition for "pregnancy denial." Research studies often fail to differentiate complete pregnancy denial from late pregnancy recognition. Likewise, the definition of neonaticide varies between studies. There have been previous proposals for inclusion of pregnancy denial in diagnostic manuals that suggest categorizing pregnancy denial as an adjustment disorder, dissociative disorder, or disorder of adult personality or behavior (Barnes, 2022; Beier et al., 2006). A lack of standardized information means that women may be more likely to be charged with actions they took or did not take after birth without adequate consideration of their mental state.

The current categorization of neonaticide in specific legal systems further compounds this gap in psychiatric manuals. In the United States, there have been calls for special regulations that distinguish neonaticide and infanticide from homicide, as in several European and Asian countries (Spinelli, 2018). This lack of separation leads to neonaticide frequently being considered a motivated or premeditated crime, and women who experienced dissociation while giving birth that resulted in neonaticide may receive excessive sentences.

Neonaticide and pregnancy denial are important topics in the field of perinatal mental health yet are rarely discussed. Over time, we hope that this special issue will gain greater awareness in the public eye and medical and legal fields through additional study.

References

Abrahams, N., Mathews, S., Martin, L. J., Lombard, C., Nannan, N., & Jewkes, R. (2016). Gender differences in homicide of neonates, infants, and children under 5 y in South Africa: Results from the cross-sectional 2009 national child homicide study. *PLoS Medicine*, *13*(4), e1002003.

American Psychiatric Association. (2013). Glossary of technical terms. In *Diagnostic and statistical manual of mental disorders* (5th ed.). American Psychiatric Association.

Amon, S., Klier, C. M., Putkonen, H., Weizmann-Henelius, G., & Arias, P. F. (2020). Neonaticide in the courtroom–room for improvement? Conclusions drawn from Austria and Finland's register review. *Child Abuse Review*, *29*, 61–72.

Amon, S., Putkonen, H., Weizmann-Henelius, G., Almiron, M. P., Formann, A. K., Voracek, M., . . . Klier, C. M. (2012). Potential predictors in neonaticide: The impact of the circumstances of pregnancy. *Archives of Women's Mental Health*, *15*, 167–174.

Barnes, D. L. (2022). Towards a new understanding of pregnancy denial: The misunderstood dissociative disorder. *Archives of Women's Mental Health*, *25*, 51–59.

Beier, K. M., Wille, R., & Wessel, J. (2006). Denial of pregnancy as a reproductive dysfunction: A proposal for international classification systems. *Journal of Psychosomatic Research*, *61*, 723–730.

Benitez-Borrego, S., Guardia-Olmos, J., & Aliaga-Moore, A. (2013). Child homicide by parents in Chile: A gender-based study and analysis of post-filicide attempted suicide. *International Journal of Law and Psychiatry*, *36*, 55–64.

Ben Khelil, M., Boukthir, I., Hmandi, O., Zhioua, M., & Hamdoun, M. (2019). Trends of infanticides in northern Tunisia: A 40 years study (1977–2016). *Child Abuse & Neglect*, *95*, 104047.

Delong, H., Eutrope, J., Thierry, A., Sutter-Dallay, A. L., Vulliez, L., Gubler, V., . . . Rolland, A.-C. (2022). Pregnancy denial: A complex symptom with life context as a trigger? A prospective case–control study. *British Journal of Obstetrics and Gynaecology*, *129*, 485–492.

Friedman, S. H., Heneghan, A., & Rosenthal, M. (2007). Characteristics of women who deny or conceal pregnancy. *Psychosomatics*, *48*, 117–122.

Friedman, S. H., Heneghan, A., & Rosenthal, M. (2009). Disposition and health outcomes among infants born to mothers with no prenatal care. *Child Abuse & Neglect*, *33*, 116–122.

Friedman, S. H., Horwitz, S. M., & Resnick, P. J. (2005). Child murder by mothers: A critical analysis of the current state of knowledge and a research agenda. *American Journal of Psychiatry*, *162*, 1578–1587.

Friedman, S. H., & Resnick, P. J. (2007). Child murder by mothers: Patterns and prevention. *World Psychiatry*, *6*, 137–141.

Friedman, S. H., & Resnick, P. J. (2009). Neonaticide: Phenomenology and considerations for prevention. *International Journal of Law and Psychiatry*, *32*, 43–47.

Gheorghe, A., Banner, J., Hansen, S. H., Stolborg, U., & Lynnerup, N. (2011). Abandonment of newborn infants: A Danish forensic medical survey 1997–2008. *Forensic Science, Medicine and Pathology*, *7*, 317–321.

Herman-Giddens, M. E., Smith, J. B., Mittal, M., Carlson, M., & Butts, J. D. (2003). Newborns killed or left to die by a parent: A population-based study. *Journal of the American Medical Association*, *289*(11), 1425–1429.

Huchzermeier, C., & Heinzen, H. (2015). A young woman who killed 5 of her own babies: A case of multiple neonaticide. *Journal of Forensic and Legal Medicine*, *35*, 15–18.

Jenkins, A., Millar, S., & Robins, J. (2011). Denial of pregnancy: A literature review and discussion of ethical and legal issues. *Journal of the Royal Society of Medicine*, *104*, 286–291.

Jung, K. H., Kim, H., Lee, E., Choi, I., Lim, H., Lee, B., . . . Hong, H. (2020). Cluster analysis of child homicide in South Korea. *Child Abuse & Neglect*, *101*, 104322.

Karakasi, M., Markopoulou, M., Tentes, I. K., Tsikouras, P. N., Vasilikos, E., & Pavlidis, P. (2017). Prepartum psychosis and neonaticide: Rare case study and forensic-psychiatric synthesis of literature. *Journal of Forensic Sciences*, *62*(4).

Kenner, W. D., & Nicolson, S. E. (2015). Psychosomatic disorders of gravida status: False and denied pregnancies. *Psychosomatics*, *56*, 119–128.

Kettlewell, D., Dujeu, M., & Nicolis, H. (2021). What happens next? Current knowledge and clinical perspective of pregnancy Denial and children's outcome. *Psychiatria Danubina*, *33*(2), 140–146.

Klier, C. M., Amon, S., Putkonen, H., Fernandez Arias, P., & Weizmann-Henelius, G. (2019). Repeated neonaticide: Differences and similarities to single neonaticide events. *Archives of Women's Mental Health*, *22*, 159–164.

Klier, C. M., Grylli, C., Amon, S., Fiala, C., Weizmann-Henelius, G., Pruitt, S. L., & Putkonen, H. (2012). Is the introduction of anonymous delivery associated with a reduction of high neonaticide rates in Austria? A retrospective study. *British Journal of Obstetrics and Gynaecology, 120,* 428–434.

Knight, E., Morris, M., & Heaman, M. (2014). A descriptive study of women presenting to an obstetric triage unit with no prenatal care. *Journal of Obstetrics and Gynaecology Canada, 36*(3), 216–222.

Kouno, A., & Johnson, C. F. (1995). Child abuse and neglect in Japan: Coin-operated-locker babies. *Child Abuse & Neglect, 19*(1), 25–31.

Kruger, P. (2015). Prevalence and phenomenology of neonaticide in Switzerland 1980–2010: A retrospective study. *Violence and Victims, 30*(2), 194–207.

Lee, A. C. W., Li, C. H., Kwong, N. S., & So, K. T. (2006). Neonaticide, newborn abandonment, and denial of pregnancy–newborn victimisation associated with unwanted motherhood. *Hong Kong Medical Journal, 12*(1), 61–64.

Lester, D. (1992). Roe v Wade was followed by a decrease in neonatal homicide. *Journal of the American Medical Association, 267*(22), 3027. [Letter].

Makhlouf, F., & Rambaud, C. (2014). Child homicide and neglect in France: 1991–2008. *Child Abuse & Neglect, 38,* 37–41.

Malmquist, C. P. (2013). Infanticide/neonaticide: The outlier situation in the United States. *Aggression and Violent Behavior, 18,* 399–408.

Marcikic, M., Dumencic, B., Matuzalem, E., Marjanovic, K., Pozgain, I., & Ugljarevic, M. (2006). *Collegium Antropologicum, 30*(2), 437–442.

Maupin, Jr. R., Lyman, R., Fatsis, J., Prystowiski, E., Nguyen, A., Wright, C., . . . Miller, Jr. J. (2004). Characteristics of women who deliver with no prenatal care. *The Journal of Maternal-Fetal & Neonatal Medicine, 16*(1), 45–50.

Mehmood, Q., Yasin, F., & Rasheed Malik, A. (2022). An audit of foeticide, neonaticide and infanticide: A retrospective study in the Department of Forensic Medicine, King Edward Medical University, Lahore. *Medico-Legal Journal, 90*(2), 98–103.

Milia, G., & Noonan, M. (2022). Experiences and perspectives of women who have committed neonaticide, infanticide and filicide: A systematic review and qualitative evidence synthesis. *Journal of Psychiatric and Mental Health Nursing, 29*(6), 813–828.

Mishra, K., Ramachandran, S., Kumar, A., Tiwari, S., Chopra, N., Datta, V., & Saili, A. (2014). Neonaticide in India and the stigma of female gender: Report of two cases. *Paediatrics and International Child Health, 34*(3), 224–226.

Murphy-Tighe, S., & Lalor, J. G. (2016). Concealed pregnancy: A concept analysis. *Journal of Advanced Nursing, 72*(1), 50–61.

Nanjundaswamy, M. H., Gaddapati, S., Thippeswamy, H., Thampy, M., Vaiphei, K., Kashyap, H., . . . Chandra, P. S. (2019). Denial of pregnancy: Psychopathology and clinical management. *Psychopathology, 52,* 271–274.

Neifert, P. L., & Bourgeois, J. A. (2000). Denial of pregnancy: A case study and literature review. *Military Medicine, 165*(7), 566–568.

Oizumi, R., Inaba, H., Takada, T., Enatsu, Y., & Kinjo, K. (2022). Sensitivity analysis on the declining population in Japan: Effects of prefecture-specific fertility and interregional migration. *PLoS One, 17*(9), e0273817.

Outwater, A., Mgaya, E., Campbell, J. C., Becker, S., Kinabo, L., & Menick, D. M. (2010). Homicide of children in Dar es Salaam, Tanzania, 2005. *East African Journal of Public Health, 7*(4), 345–349.

Platt, L. M. (2014). Preventing neonaticide by early detection and intervention in student pregnancy. *NASN School Nurse, 29*(6), 304–308.

Porter, T., & Gavin, H. (2010). Infanticide and neonaticide: A review of 40 years of research literature on incidence and causes. *Trauma, Violence, & Abuse, 11*(3), 99–112.

Putkonen, H., Amon, S., Eronen, M., Klier, C. M., Almiron, M. P., Yourstone Cederwall, J., & Weizmann-Henelius, G. (2011). Gender differences in filicide offense characteristics: A comprehensive register-based study of child murder in two European countries. *Child Abuse & Neglect, 35,* 319–328.

Putkonen, H., Weizmann-Henelius, G., Collander, J., Santtila, P., & Eronen, M. (2007). Neonaticides may be more preventable and heterogeneous than previously thought–neonaticides in Finland 1980–2000. *Archives of Women's Mental Health, 10,* 15–23.

Salihu, H. M., Gonzales, D. N., & Dongarwar, D. (2021). Infanticide, neonaticide, and post-neonaticide: Racial/ethnic disparities in the United States. *European Journal of Pediatrics, 180*, 2591–2598.

Schultz, J. M., & Bushati, T. (2015). Maternal physical morbidity associated with denial of pregnancy. *Australian and New Zealand Journal of Obstetrics and Gynaecology, 55*, 559–564.

Shelton, J. L. E., Muirhead, Y., & Canning, K. E. (2010). Ambivalence toward mothers who kill: An examination of 45 U.S. cases of maternal neonaticide. *Behavioral Sciences and the Law, 28*, 812–831.

Sieswerda-Hoogendoorn, T., Soerdjbalie-Maikoe, V., Maes, A., & van Rijn, R. R. (2013). The value of post-mortem CT in neonaticide in case of severe decomposition: Description of 12 cases. *Forensic Science International, 233*, 298–303.

Simermann, M., Rothenburger, S., Auburtin, B., & Hascoet, J. M. (2018). Outcome of children born after pregnancy denial. *Archives de Pediatrie, 25*, 219–222.

Spinelli, M. G. (2001). A systematic investigation of 16 cases of neonaticide. *American Journal of Psychiatry, 158*(5), 811–813.

Spinelli, M. G. (2018). Infanticide and American criminal justice (1980–2018). *Archives of Women's Mental Health, 22*, 173–177.

Stammers, K., & Long, N. (2014). Not your average birth: Considering the possibility of denied or concealed pregnancy. *BMJ Case Reports 2014*, bcr2014204800.

Stasiuniene, J., Justickis, V., & Jasulaitis, A. (2015). Newborn Murder and its Legal Prevention. *Health Policy and Management, 1*(8), 91–119.

Stenton, S., & Cohen, M. C. (2020). Assessment of neonaticide in the setting of concealed and denied pregnancies. *Forensic Science, Medicine and Pathology, 16*(2), 226–233.

Tanaka, C. T., Berger, W., Valenca, A. M., Coutinho, E. S. F., Jean-Louis, G., Fontenelle, L. F., & Mendlowicz, M. V. (2017). The worldwide incidence of neonaticide: A systematic review. *Archives of Women's Mental Health, 20*, 249–256.

Tursz, A., & Cook, J. M. (2011). A population-based survey of neonaticides using judicial data. *Archives of Disease in Childhood Fetal and Neonatal Edition, 96*, 259–263.

Vallone, D. C., & Hoffman, L. M. (2003). Preventing the tragedy of neonaticide. *Holistic Nursing Practice, 17*(5), 223–228.

Vellut, N., Cook, J. M., & Tursz, A. (2012). Analysis of the relationship between neonaticide and denial of pregnancy using data from judicial files. *Child Abuse & Neglect, 36*, 553–563.

Watson, K., & Angelotta, C. (2022). The frequency of pregnancy recognition across the gestational spectrum and its consequences in the United States. *Perspectives on Sexual and Reproductive Health, 54*(2), 32–27.

Wessel, J., & Buscher, U. (2002). Denial of pregnancy: Population based study. *British Medical Journal, 324*, 458.

Wessel, J., Endrikat, J., & Buscher, U. (2002). Frequency of denial of pregnancy: Results and epidemiological significance of a 1-year prospective study in Berlin. *Acta Obstetricia et Gynecologica Scandinavica, 81*, 1021–1027.

Wessel, J., Endrikat, J., & Buscher, U. (2003a). Elevated risk for neonatal outcome following denial of pregnancy: Results of a one-year prospective study compared with control groups. *Journal of Perinatal Medicine, 31*, 29–35.

Wessel, J., Endrikat, J., & Kastner, R. (2003b). Projective identification and denial of pregnancy–consideration of the reasons and background of unrecognized pregnancy also undiagnosed by a physician. *Zeitschrift für Geburtshilfe und Neonatologie, 207*(2), 48–53. [German].

Wessel, J., Gauruder-Burmester, A., & Gerlinger, C. (2007). Denial of pregnancy–characteristics of women at risk. *Acta Obstetricia et Gynecologica Scandinavica, 86*, 542–546.

World Health Organization. (2021). *International statistical classification of diseases and related health problems* (11th ed.). World Health Organization.

Yoshiba, K. (2020). Neonaticide rate unchanged in Japan despite a decrease in the birth rate. *Paediatrics and International Child Health, 40*(4), 238–241.

31

PERINATAL DEPRESSION IN PEOPLE OF COLOR

Patrece Hairston Peetz, Brooke Dorsey Holliman, and Nathalie Dieujuste

When considering the prevalence, assessment, and treatment of perinatal mood disorders among communities of color, particularly from a global perspective, it's critical to examine the historical and relevant contextual factors that impact individuals, families, and the broader communities in which they live. "Race" as a social construct driven by a supremacy model (whereby the needs, traditions, and cultural values of one group are prioritized over another) has been identified as a critical factor in determining the inequities that exist between groups when it comes to perinatal health outcomes (MacDorman et al., 2021; Leimert & Olson, 2020; Petersen et al., 2019; de Graaf et al., 2013). Despite experiencing perinatal mood disorders at higher rates than White birthing populations, birthers of color are much less likely to be provided access to treatment than their White counterparts (Declercq et al., 2022; Jankovic et al., 2020; Watson et al., 2019; Prady et al., 2016). This inequity exists in predominantly White, Westernized nations across the world (Prady et al., 2021; Salameh et al., 2019; Macedo et al., 2018; Bécares & Atatoa-Carr, 2016). The meaning ascribed to a given racial identity or skin color by the "dominant" cultural group within a society is critical to both understand and explore as a mental health provider, policy maker, or researcher. Although this will vary across cultures, a frequently dominant narrative that emerges is one that places a high value on Whiteness and Eurocentricity. Placing such a high value on the belief systems, physical characteristics, healing practices, language, and history of one group over others permeates all of the systems that exist within a given society; leading to the marginalization, inequitable, and mistreatment of groups that fall outside of White, Eurocentricity. Specifically, communities of color is a broad term that includes groups of individuals that fall outside of Whiteness and may identify as Black, Hispanic or Latino/a, Asian, Native or Indigenous, Aboriginal, or More than one Race. Throughout this chapter, the term *perinatal mood disorders* refers to mood disruptions that occur throughout the perinatal period. This can include during pregnancy and in the years immediately following the birth of a child.

When considering the provision of mental healthcare, it is relevant to simultaneously acknowledge the shared experience of potential marginalization that occurs when an individual has "minority" status within a given society; while also honoring the unique history of a particular group. This means examining how experiences of racism in systems

DOI: 10.4324/9781003206903-37

of care may be both similar and different among individuals from diverse communities of color and how to integrate those experiences when conceptualizing struggles with mental health during the perinatal period. For example, in the United States, individuals who identify as "Black" or African American have long experienced deadly racism, maltreatment, and oppression in culture that is dominated by White Eurocentrism. This has led to devastating economic, social, and health-related outcomes, particularly as it relates to perinatal mental health and infant mortality (Bishop-Royse et al., 2021; Owens-Young & Bell, 2020; Pabayo et al., 2019; Kothari et al., 2016). However, individuals who identify as Indigenous or Native American have also long experienced genocide, erasure, and maltreatment in the United States. Individuals within this community also experience disproportionately negative outcomes in economics, social power and mobility, and health, also having significantly poorer perinatal health outcomes (Dennis, 2019; Dunbar-Ortiz, 2014; Palacios & Portillo, 2009). But each community has a rich and unique history, both before and after the influence of White Europeans and North Americans. So, although these communities share in their experience of being directly impacted by racism, oppression, genocide, and xenophobia; their unique historical stories, traditions, and experienced must be honored.

There are various models and guidelines that have been developed to integrate relevant cultural factors into psychological conceptualization and treatment. However, few have focused exclusively on the interaction between race and gender, a concept that has particular relevance in discussions of racial disparities in perinatal health outcomes. A pioneering legal scholar and critical race theorist in the United States, Kimberle Crenshaw, powerfully defined and outlined the impact of having multiple, overlapping identities that each experience their own unique forms of oppression (e.g., being a woman AND a person of color in a White, Eurocentric society) (Crenshaw et al., 1995; Crenshaw, 1989, 1991). The concept of *intersectionality* builds on earlier theories that have focused on the same complex dynamic, such as "double jeopardy" (Beal, 1970, 2008), "multiple jeopardy," (King, 1988) and "interlocking oppressions" (Combahee River Collective, 1982). Crenshaw pointedly asserted that these identities do not exist independently of one another; they converge and create a complex experience of oppression. When considering how larger sociocultural factors impact individuals in the perinatal period, this complex interaction of factors cannot be ignored and must be considered when conceptualizing and treating perinatal mood disorders. Having access to quality mental healthcare, interacting with healthcare and other related social safety-net systems, creating trust in the therapeutic alliance, safety in utilizing community-based resources, and methods for reducing stigma are all impacted by identity factors (Rivenbark & Ichou, 2020; Stoute, 2020; Budhwani & De, 2019; Medlock et al., 2017; Hoberman, 2012). In this context, "identity factors" refer to unique personal characteristics such as race, gender, or socioeconomic status that are shaped and influenced by sociocultural interactions.

As clinicians, researchers, and policymakers, thinking critically and thoughtfully about incorporating specific identity factors into the development, implementation, and evaluation of interventions for perinatal mood disorders will move toward achieving more effective outcomes. Even the term "communities of color" represents a broad number of experiences that have to be disentangled. Individuals who identify as people of color represent a vast number of unique communities with their own history, values, and experiences within White-dominant cultures. Intersectionality provides a conceptual framework to consider how specific overlapping identities are influenced by social context.

Prevalence

Depression is the most prevalent and commonly studied mood disorder among pregnant women and birthing people worldwide. Global prevalence of depression among perinatal populations ranges between 17% and 28% (Al-abri et al., 2023; Hahn-Holbrook et al., 2017). However, prevalence of perinatal mood disorders in women of color varies greatly across countries and racial/ethnic groups. Varying rates of perinatal mood disorders among mothers and birthers of color may be reflective of differences in cultural expectations, perceptions of parenthoods and mental health, and may be impacted by other contextual factors (e.g., socioeconomic status, access to culturally relevant treatment modalities, acculturation to a White dominant nation) (Howell et al., 2005). This can prevent significant barriers in terms of understanding the nature of perinatal mood disorders among communities of color.

Research examining perinatal depression among women in Nigeria, South Africa, Uganda, Ethiopia, Morocco, The Gambia, Zimbabwe, and Malawi found average incidence rates of 11.3% and 18.3% (Sawyer et al., 2010). Evidence suggests that, globally, the highest prevalence of postpartum depression can be observed in South Africa (Mokwena & Modjadji, 2022; Ramchandani et al., 2009; Stellenberg & Abrahams, 2015). Meta-regression analyses of six studies examining postpartum depression found a 39% prevalence of postpartum depression among South African women (Wang et al., 2021). Among Ethiopian women, estimates of the prevalence of perinatal depression range from approximately 19% to 26%, depending on data instrumentation (e.g., *Beck Depression Inventory-II* (A. T. Beck et al., 1996), *Edinburgh Postnatal Depression Scale* (Cox et al., 1987), *Patient Health Questionnaire* (Kroenke et al., 2001)) and trimester (Al-abri et al., 2023; Ayano et al., 2019; Getinet et al., 2018; Zegeye et al., 2018). For Malawi women, perinatal depression prevalence rates are 17.1% and 19.8%, respectively (Chorwe-Sungani et al., 2022).

Research across 17 Asian countries, including China, Lebanon, Singapore, and the United Arab Emirates, found a wide range of prevalence estimates for perinatal depression, from 3.5% to 63.3% (Klainin & Arthur, 2009). In China, the prevalence of perinatal depression varies among studies and samples. A meta-analysis of postpartum depressive symptoms among Chinese women 0 to 6 months after giving birth found a prevalence of 21% (Mu et al., 2019). Meanwhile, the estimated prevalence of perinatal depression among Chinese women exposed to earthquakes ranges from 7.1% to 35.2% (Khatri et al., 2019). Among Japanese women, the estimated prevalence of postpartum depression is 14.3% (Tokumitsu et al., 2020).

The prevalence of perinatal depression in Turkish women ranges from 9% to 51%, with a pooled prevalence estimate of approximately 24% (Karaçam et al., 2018; Özcan et al., 2017). Among Nepali women, the prevalence of perinatal depression is estimated to be 4.9% among women 2 to 12 weeks after giving birth (Jones & Coast, 2013). In Bangladesh and Pakistan, the prevalence of postpartum depression ranges from 19.8% to 35.6% (Jones & Coast, 2013). In India, the overall prevalence of perinatal depression ranges from 22% to 25%, with higher rates observed in southern regions compared to northern regions (Upadhyay et al., 2017).

Among Middle Eastern Asian countries, the overall incidence of perinatal depression is 27% (Alshikh Ahmad et al., 2021). The incidence rates of perinatal depression among Pakistani women are 37%, whereas perinatal depression is 30% (Atif et al., 2021). The general estimated prevalence of perinatal depression among Iranian women is 41.2%; however, among women in southern Iran, this estimate is as high as 51.7% (Azami et al., 2018). The average prevalence estimates of perinatal depression among Iranian women range from 25% to 28.7% (Veisani et al., 2013; Veisani & Sayehmiri, 2012).

Among Arabic women residing in their native country, such as Lebanon and the United Arab Emirates, rates of perinatal depression range from 10% to 37% (Alhasanat & Giurgescu, 2017). However, Arabic women who have migrated to industrialized countries, such as the United States, Australia, and Taiwan, demonstrate higher rates of postpartum depression, ranging from 11.2% to 60% (Alhasanat & Giurgescu, 2017).

In the United States, it has long been estimates of rates of depression among in perinatal Hispanic women ranges from 18% to 59%, depending on data instrumentation method (Alhasanat & Giurgescu, 2017; C. T. Beck et al., 2005; Heilemann et al., 2004). It is frequently outlined in the literature that women who identify as Black or African American have higher rates of perinatal depression and anxiety than their White counterparts (Pointing et al., 2021; Rich-Edwards et al., 2006; Collins & David, 2005). However, prevalence rates vary from 10% to more than 50% depending on the screening instrument utilized and the specific populations studied (Beeghly et al., 2003; Zayas et al., 2002).

Perinatal depression and other mood disorders significantly impact women and birthers of color across the world at significant rates. Globally, data are indicative of a 9% prevalence (at the low end) up to a 59% prevalence (at the high end); however, it is important to note that several studies identified that screening tool or instrumentation method significantly impacted the data. This is not to suggest that the outlined rates of prevalence should be questioned. On the contrary, this points toward a larger potential implication; one that suggests that clinicians and researchers need to continue to consider the applicability of widely utilized screening protocols, further understand how symptoms present among diverse communities, and examine the most effective way to collect data on perinatal mood disorder symptomatology.

Relevant Correlates and Risk Factors

Globally, evidence suggests that women of color residing in countries with greater income equality, higher maternal and infant mortality rates, and greater working hours among younger mothers are at unique risk of perinatal mood disorders (Hahn-Holbrook et al., 2017).

Among women in Nigeria, South Africa, Uganda, Ethiopia, Morocco, The Gambia, Zimbabwe, and Malawi risk factors for perinatal depression includes high conflict within the marriage and insufficient social support (Sawyer et al., 2010). Among Ethiopian women, risk factors for perinatal depression include a current or past history of pregnancy complications (including previous stillbirth), past depression, exposure to intimate partner violence and lack of social support (Al-abri et al., 2023; Ayano et al., 2019). Additionally, Ethiopian women between the ages of 20 and 29 may also be at increased risk for perinatal depression (Ayano et al., 2019).

In Asian countries, including China, Vietnam, Malaysia, and Indonesia, risk factors for postpartum depression include poor nutrition and vitamin B2 and docosahexaenoic acid (DHA) deficiency, past history of mental illness including past perinatal depression, and traumatic life event exposure (Klainin & Arthur, 2009). Additionally, in these countries lack of previous breastfeeding in multiparous women is also a risk factor for perinatal depression (Klainin & Arthur, 2009). Factors associated with risk for perinatal depression among Chinese women exposed to earthquakes includes spousal conflict and poor social support, parenting stress, and poor coping skills (Khatri et al., 2019).

Risk factors for perinatal depression among Turkish women include a significant history of mental illness prior to pregnancy, past unplanned pregnancies, financial stressors, and spousal conflict (Karaçam et al., 2018). Among Nepali, Bangladeshi, and Pakistani women, risk factors for perinatal depression include low social support (Jones & Coast, 2013). More specifically, Nepali, Bangladeshi, and Pakistani women who reported poor relationships with their spouse or spouse's parents were at increased risk of perinatal depressive symptoms. In India, financial insecurity, interpersonal violence, past mental illness, and marital conflict are risk factors for perinatal depression (Upadhyay et al., 2017).

Among Middle Eastern Asian countries, women exposed to financial stressors, unplanned pregnancy or complications during pregnancy or childbirth are at increased risk of perinatal depression (Alshikh Ahmad et al., 2021). Additional, low education, being a housewife, and formula feeding instead of breast feeding are also risk factors associated with postpartum (Alshikh Ahmad et al., 2021). Pakistani women exposed to intimate partner violence or poor spousal relationships, financial insecurity, and unplanned pregnancy are at increased risk of perinatal depression (Atif et al., 2021).

Regardless of residency status, among Arabic women, evidence suggests that lack of social support, financial stress, and exposure to intimate partner violence are notable risk factors for perinatal depression (Alhasanat & Giurgescu, 2017; Alhasanat et al., 2017). Arabic women who have migrated to industrialized countries face additional stressors which uniquely contribute to risk for perinatal depression, such as immigration stress and lack of healthcare access (Alhasanat & Giurgescu, 2017; Alhasanat et al., 2017). Among Hispanic women in the United States, stress associated with acculturation is linked to higher rates of perinatal depressive symptoms (Alhasanat & Giurgescu, 2017).

In examining risk factors, context becomes critical. Globally, there are certain risk factors that impact women and birthers across cultures, including exposure to intimate partner violence, previous history of mental health struggles, exposure to trauma, and financial stress. Other correlates are representative of specific cultural experiences, such as exposure to ongoing social conflicts, multi-generational family dynamics and expectations that are culturally specific, like poor relationships with family of origin and parental involvement. This only amplifies the need to examine risk factors and correlates within a socioecological framework and ensure that interventions are culturally sensitive and relevant.

Conceptualization of Perinatal Mood Disorders With a Socioecological Lens

Congruent with a contextual lens, the socioecological model provides a way of identifying all of the relevant biological, relational, psychological, and sociocultural factors that may be impacting a woman or birther during the perinatal period. Intersectionality provides a framework for thinking about how those identity factors intersect in ways that are meaningful to the client's experience.

Considering these two models in combination provides a robust overarching framework that accounts for the nuanced interplay of individual factors and the larger sociocultural factors that influence the expression of perinatal mood disorders. Originally developed by Urie Bronfenbrenner (Bronfenbrenner, 1979, 2005), the Ecological Model of Human Development asserts that individuals are impacted by a combination of familial, environmental, and sociocultural factors that are tied to life outcomes. Unlike other psychological theories at the time, which focused exclusively on individual development of psychopathology, Bronfenbrenner recognized that human development depends upon a series of complex interactions between the individual and relevant systems and that these interactions are bi-directional. The bi-directional component of this theory is particularly relevant when discussing the impact of race and culture during the perinatal period, as external characteristics (such as race) have been shown to affect the quality of care that is received during this critical time. The Ecological Model posits that individual characteristics shape how the environment interacts with individuals and thus, an environment that feels safe and affirming for one individual may not feel safe and affirming for another. Research has demonstrated that harmful stereotypes and prejudicial attitudes on the part of clinicians and healthcare providers leads to poorer health outcomes among birthers of color (Waters, 2022; Chambers et al., 2021; Chambers et al., 2020; Alhusen et al., 2016), including an increased risk of maternal death and other complications related to birth.

Despite an increased focus on training and education in cultural humility and the development of culturally competent models of care, women and birthers of color also experience disparate outcomes when it comes to accessing and receiving perinatal mental healthcare in predominantly White countries across the world. Widespread systemic racism, dismissive interactions with healthcare professionals, fragmented healthcare systems, stigma related to cultural expectations, fear of child welfare or justice-system involvement, and lack of adequate providers of color have all be identified as causal factors (Iturralde et al., 2021; Huggins et al., 2020; Takeshita et al., 2020; Watson et al., 2019; Ramsay, 2016; Ertel et al., 2012). As these systemic-level interactions have a significant impact on health outcomes, these must be incorporated into the conceptual model for mental health treatment and intervention during the perinatal period. Conceptualizing from a socioecological approach supports that integration, while also incorporating the biological and psychological factors that are unique to each women or birther.

Other researchers and clinicians have adapted and expanded Bronfenbrenner's original model for specific application to perinatal health (Khan et al., 2021; Chopak-Foss et al., 2020; Noursi et al., 2021; Bingham et al., 2019; Guillfoyle et al., 2014; Alio et al., 2010). One of these models includes a framework adapted by the University of Minnesota Center for Leadership Education in Maternal and Child Health in the United States (Michaels et al., 2022). This fluid, strengths-based model includes six spheres of influence. These include (a) **Individual:** this sphere of influence includes biological or genetic factors, personal characteristics (such as age, race/ethnicity, sexual orientation, education level, economic status, coping and adaptability skills); (b) **Relationships:** this sphere includes formal and informal support networks that include family, friends, neighbors, healthcare providers, etc.; (c) **Organizations:** this sphere includes the relationship between public, private, and nonprofit organizations that include schools, workplaces, agencies, businesses, healthcare, childcare, and faith communities; (d) **Communities:** this sphere includes neighborhoods, and cultural affinity groups, these are the broad settings in which relationships occur; (d) **Policy:** this sphere represents that laws and policies that govern and support health behaviors; and (e) **Society:** this final sphere represents the broad societal factors that influence mental health and behavior, including exposure to societal conflict, racism or marginalization, and the general values, beliefs, customs and practices that influence an individual's health status. All of these spheres of influence can have a direct impact on a women or birther's ability to understand, access, and benefit from psychological interventions in the perinatal period. Recognition of the effect of larger sociocultural conditions often changes the way that assessment, intervention, research and treatment are developed and implemented; which is critical to ensure that women and birthers from communities of color are equally able to benefit from psychological interventions in the perinatal period.

The following case description will demonstrate how to integrate these two theoretical models in clinical practice and how they might inform the development of more holistic approaches to perinatal mental healthcare for communities of color.

Case Description: Sheena A

*Identifying information such as client name have been changed to ensure anonymity.

Sheena* is a 34-year-old, multiracial women with a six-month-old baby. Sheena identifies as heterosexual, describes herself as "religious," and has been married to her spouse, Eli for four years. Sheena works as a public health professional at a large public university in the Mountain West region of the United States. Sheena and her spouse relocated to the Mountain West for job opportunities from Central America. In terms of her racial identity, Sheena's mother is from El Salvador, while her Black/African American father was raised in the Northeast region of the United States. Sheena is bilingual (English and Spanish) and identifies Spanish as her first language. She was born in El Salvador and spoke Spanish exclusively for the first seven years of her life, until emigrating to the United States at age 8 to live with her father and his family.

Initially Sheena meets the mental health provider at a community literacy event for young children. In casual conversation, Sheena discusses being "exhausted but fine" and describes that she's been having headaches, feeling "weak," body aches, and just general lethargy. Once finding out that she's been having a conversation with a mental health provider, she quickly laughs and says "you don't think I'm crazy though, right?" The mental health provider assured that struggling after birth is a common experience for many women and birthing people. Sheena stated that she was interested in spiritual guidance on how to manage this new phase in her life and the mental health provider listened and affirmed. Sheena and the mental health provider exchanged contact information with the mental health provider offering to discuss psychological adjustment in the postpartum period if Sheena was interested in additional support.

Sheena contacted the mental health provider nearly three months later indicating that she was feeling "very stressed" and overwhelmed. In the first session, Sheena indicated that she was continuing to have somatic symptoms (headaches, body aches), sleep disturbances, feelings of detachment from her infant, inability to focus and concentrate at work, feelings of loneliness, and was struggling with feelings of doubt about her caregiving abilities. At the advice of her spiritual leader, Sheena talked with her primary care provider, who dismissed many of her concerns and indicated that she should likely have some bloodwork and testing done but expressed doubt about whether or not she could "afford it" or would follow through. Her primary care provider also asked several questions about drug and alcohol use which Sheena adamantly denied. Her primary care provider also suggested that she speak with the clinic social worker to discuss food, clothing, and diapering needs; even though this was not something that Sheena indicated needing assistance with. Sheena quickly left the clinic without speaking to anyone and did not return. Sheena expressed that she had experienced similar treatment in prior medical settings and found the interactions exhausting and discouraging.

She described intense feelings of isolation and loneliness as she was new to her current geographic community. Sheena also shared that she had attended a few "mommy and baby groups" but did not feel like she belonged or shared affinity with the other mothers and birthers in the groups, Sheena indicated that they had different life experiences and perspectives and that she didn't feel heard or understood.

In the workplace, Sheena described ongoing exposure to verbal, nonverbal, and behavioral microaggressions related to her racial background. She further explained that although the organization was publicly supportive of equity and cultural competency efforts, they blatantly engaged in prejudicial behavior.

Concurrently, Sheena also expressed missing her mom and extended family in El Salvador. Sheena described often feeling "torn" between her understanding of a "good mother" in the United States and the contrast with what she experienced in El Salvador in her early years.

In addition to her somatic symptoms, feelings of loneliness and isolation, cognitive symptoms, sleep challenges, and feelings of detachment from her baby, Sheena described feeling an overwhelming sense of concern for her baby's safety. This accompanies an all-consuming sense of dread that leads to feelings of hopelessness and despair that has been present since her baby's birth. She ends each interaction by expressing that she knows she has a "lot to be grateful for" and that she "must" persevere. She indicates that she knows that she's strong and that everyone is depending on her to take care of everything.

Case Conceptualization: Integration of
Intersectionality and the Socioecological Model

While conceptualizing Sheena's experience, the importance of integrating her identity factors is critical to creating an effective and responsive treatment plan. Utilizing the lens of intersectionality allows for this integration and is congruent with the theoretical underpinnings of the socioecological model. Both of these theoretical models are grounded in the interconnectedness of sociocultural systems and how that relates to unique identity factors. The focus of these theories is not simply on identifying risk factors in isolation; but understanding how spheres of influence or identity factors are meaningful in a given societal context and how they influence an individual's experience in the world. Intersectionality adds a richness and depth to case conceptualization that allows the clinician to have a more holistic view of a client's experience and further identify how that impacts psychological functioning.

Some might argue that utilizing the theories in combination allows neither to be fully realized. However, many conceptual models utilized in psychotherapy offer very little in terms of incorporating identity factors into their core theories. With regard to experiencing oppression, the relationship in psychotherapy cannot be fully realized unless the client perceives that their world and experiences are acknowledged and regarded by the mental health provider. Intersectionality provides a conceptual lens through which to understand a client's unique experience with oppression and support the client in understanding and navigating how those experiences may be contributing to their psychological functioning.

In the case of Sheena, she identifies as a woman and a multiracial person living in a White-dominant nation that has a long and storied history of systemic racism that influences every facet of daily life. Sheena also immigrated to the United States as a child and is bilingual. She describes her experiences with racism and marginalization in the workplace, interacting with a healthcare provider, and attending a community-based group. Although many of her presenting symptoms are consistent with "typical" perinatal depression symptomatology, her experience as a multiracial woman interacting with White-dominant systems creates an additional layer of psychological burden. Dealing with day-to-day experiences of racism have a negative impact on overall health and well-being, both physical and psychological (Stopforth et al., 2022; Stanley et al., 2019; Paradies et al., 2015). Additionally, intersectionality asserts that the experience of women of color represents a unique perspective; different from that of White women and different from that of men of color (Crenshaw, 1989, 2017; Lewis et al., 2017). Integrating this lens into the therapeutic conceptualization allows for a deeper and richer understanding of Sheena's lived experience and the external and societal factors that are influencing her well-being.

With the overarching lens of intersectionality, there are several biological, psychological, and sociocultural factors to consider when conceptualizing her perinatal mood symptoms from a socioecological perspective. Within each sphere of influence, there are relevant considerations. At the **individual** level, being within the postpartum period represents a number of biological and hormonal changes that impact woman and birthers (Schaffir, 2016). In addition to high levels of progesterone during pregnancy that plummet post-birth, there are changes in estradiol, oxytocin, cortisol, and thyroid hormones that create a vulnerable landscape for perinatal mood changes (Trifu et al., 2019; Schiller et al., 2015; Meltzer-Brody, 2011). This represents a point of medical intervention that may be overlooked for many experiencing perinatal mood disorders, particularly women of color who have a history of not being taken seriously by healthcare providers. Sheena's identity factors, her age, race, gender identity and educational level are also important within this sphere of influence. Although higher levels of education and socioeconomic status are typically considered a protective factor in terms of health outcomes, research on morbidity and mortality in the perinatal period in the United States indicate that this is not necessarily the case for women of color (Petersen et al., 2019). For a mental health provider working with Sheena, this is a critical point of understanding. It is also important to note that Sheena presents as an individual with a propensity for resiliency and high levels of adaptability, both significant strengths and should be acknowledged and centered within the therapeutic work.

At the **relationship** level, Sheena has little formal or informal support in the current scenario. Her partner, Eli is her primary source of support within the home, and Sheena still indicates feeling like she has to manage the bulk of the domestic tasks. Her relationships with her extended family are relatively strong, but they live in El Salvador and they have struggled to understand Sheena's need to remain in the workforce. They could not provide practical day-to-day support around childcare or other needs. Additionally, her experience with other potential sources of support, including co-workers or healthcare professionals, was rife with microaggressions. In attempting to connect with community members and other mothers and birthers in her new city, Sheena attended a parent-baby connection group. She described feeling misunderstood and misaligned in the White dominant space. Sheena's support network is fairly minimal during a period of the lifespan where those supports are critical.

With regard to the **communities, policy,** and **societal** spheres of influence, it is important to assess the resource allocation, accessibility, and the lack of supportive structures that exist for mothers and birther in the United States, where Sheena is currently living. According to a report that analyzed family-friendly policies among the world's most affluent nations, the United States was last on the list (Chzhen et al., 2019) as it offers zero weeks of paid time off for new mothers and birthers. Additionally, the United States is lacking in affordable healthcare (Osborn et al., 2016; Schoen et al., 2013), has some of the worst maternal health outcomes among industrialized nations, particularly for mothers and birthers of color, and fails to provide widespread access to doula or midwifery care. Furthermore, although supportive resources vary by community, the United States also lacks any form of high-quality, universal childcare, with the financial burden falling to individual families (Child Care Aware of America, 2019). This is particularly salient for Sheena as she is the financial breadwinner for her family. Although a wage gap exists between men and women in the United States, the wage gap is even greater for women of color (United States Census Bureau, 2020; Institute for Women's Policy Research, 2020). This is another point at which intersectionality becomes particularly salient. When analyzing that data by racial group, White women earned an estimated $0.79 cents to the White man's dollar; whereas Black women earned $0.63 cents and Latina women earned $0.58 cents (United States Government Accountability Office, 2022). Being a woman of color means less overall earning power and thus, less fiscal resources for Sheena and her family in a society that offers little in terms of economic support or other social supports to those raising young children.

In terms of cultural beliefs and values within this individualistic society, mothers and birthing people are often expected to manage work, caregiving, and domestic tasks with very little support from others (Daminger, 2019; Moulding, 2019; Hubert & Aujoulat, 2018; Lachance-Grzela & Bouchard, 2010). Images and stories of post-birth productivity are widespread and prized among media sources and the broader community, who tout that "doing-it-all" is both normative and expected (Adams et al., 2021; Germic et al., 2021; Nippert et al., 2021; Wardrop & Popadiuk, 2013). These beliefs impact the overall social climate for mothers and birthers and can lead to unrealistic and unattainable expectations. Additionally, stigma related to accessing mental health treatment during the perinatal period remains salient and can impact help-seeking among mothers and birthers (Schofield et al., 2023).

Fear of child welfare involvement and reporting also contributes to a lack of help-seeking and disclosures, particularly among mothers and birthers of color. In the United States, child welfare decision-making is significantly impacted by negative stereotypes of certain racial groups around parenting, particularly for mothers that identify as Black or Indigenous (Thomas et al., 2023; Roberts & Sangoi, 2018; Lash, 2017; Krase, 2015; Putnam-Hornstein et al., 2013; Crofoot & Harris, 2012; Font et al., 2012; Wells et al., 2009; Roberts, 2001). For a multiracial woman like Sheena, disclosures of perinatal mood disorders or substance misuse could lead to child welfare involvement as opposed to referrals to treatment or other supportive services (Smith & Roane, 2023; Harp & Bunting, 2020; Roberts & Nuru-Jeter, 2012). Sheena may be forced to make a calculated decision about whether or not there is safety in seeking support from governmental entities and community organizations that have been designed and funded to help mothers, birthers, and their families, but that often penalize families like hers. As a mental health provider, this is another factor that needs to be considered in developing and implementing a treatment plan that is culturally relevant, responsive, and effective for Sheena.

When considering how to most effectively treat perinatal mood disorders, it is critical to integrate contextual information that informs the individual's experience. Identity factors (e.g., race, gender) influence the ways that systems and structures engage with an individual and the nature of that engagement is critical to understanding a client's experience. Intersectionality provides a theoretical lens with which to contextualize an individual's experience; while the socioecological framework provides the mental health provider, researcher, or policymaker with points of engagement on which to intervene. Both are pertinent in supporting mothers and birthers like Sheena in addressing the bio-psycho-social and cultural factors that contribute to the expression of perinatal mood disorders.

Treatment Considerations

In terms of evidence-based treatment modalities for mothers and birthers of color, the empirical literature is significantly lacking. Historically, randomized controlled trials (RCTs) conducted on large samples of White, Eurocentric women with small numbers of women from racially or ethnically diverse backgrounds establish the "gold standard" of standardized treatment modalities. However, generalizability is not always indicated for diverse communities, particularly with regard to psychological interventions in the perinatal period. A recent meta-analysis reviewed the effectiveness of traditional cognitive behavioral therapy (CBT) and interpersonal psychotherapy (IPT), both widely regarded as the most effective psychotherapeutic treatment modalities for perinatal depression. The analysis produced mixed results in decreasing symptoms among women of color (Branquinho et al., 2021; Nillni et al., 2018). For example, although CBT demonstrated general efficacy in reducing perinatal depression among general community samples of women, when examining data among women of color, CBT was not found to be superior to the control group in more instances than not (Branquinho et al., 2021). Similarly, inconsistencies have also been noted in the utilization of IPT among women of color who also low-income. As such, there are multiple facets to consider when examining the available treatment modalities and how to potentially integrate them into a culturally responsive treatment plan.

One pathway for mental health providers to consider is utilizing a culturally adapted and informed version of an existing intervention. Cultural adaptation refers to modifying an intervention protocol to make it consistent with an identified group's cultural beliefs, values, and patterns of behavior (Bernal & Adames, 2017). Research indicates that culturally adapted psychotherapy shows great promise in improving psychological outcomes among individuals of color (Khan et al., 2019; Rathod et al., 2018; Hall et al., 2016; Benish et al., 2011; Smith et al., 2010; Griner & Smith, 2006). A culturally informed adaptation should include more than just a translation of materials; it should include attention to multiple dimensions of culture and should be led or co-led by individuals from the target community (Bernal et al., 2009; Hwang, 2009). If developed and executed with fidelity to the values, beliefs, and traditions of the target community, culturally adapted models show promise in reducing mood symptomatology in the perinatal period. For example, in the United Kingdom, a culturally adapted CBT intervention called the Positive Health Program (PHP) was developed to treat perinatal depression symptoms in British Pakistani and Indian women (Masood et al., 2015; Khan et al., 2019). Cultural adaptation focused on the following three areas based on prior research conducted within the South Asian community: (1) the inclusion of relevant cultural issues and preparation for therapy; (2) adjusting assessment protocols and engagement; and (3) adjustments in therapy that are initiated by obtain relevant cultural information (Naeem et al., 2015). This intervention produced statistically significant improvements in depressive symptoms and health-related quality of life. Depressive symptoms were evaluated by a decrease in scores on the *Hospital Anxiety and Depression-Anxiety Subscale*, decease in reported somatic symptoms on the *Bradford Somatic Inventory*, and a change in symptoms on the *Brief Disability Question-naire*. Additionally, birthers who were assigned to the CaCBT intervention (the culturally adapted treatment group) reported higher satisfaction with treatment.

In the United States, a culturally adapted treatment program utilizing brief interpersonal psychotherapy (IPT-B) showed significant reductions in depressive symptoms among Black women who were economically disadvantaged (Grote et al., 2009). In addition to utilizing culturally relevant materials, there was an emphasis on providing additional wraparound supports to facilitate engagement and make treatment more accessible (e.g., providing childcare, bus passes, access to social services that included food, job training, housing). When mothers could not attend treatment, sessions were conducted over the phone to ensure continuity. The positive effects were observed at six months postpartum. Another study conducted in the United States focused on providing a home-based, culturally rel-evant IPT intervention for Latina mothers who were economically disadvantaged (Beeber et al., 2010). A reduction in perinatal depression symptoms was observed. Additionally, this intervention utilized a home-based approach, skillfully trained Spanish-language interpret-ers, and psychiatric nurse home visitors.

Another potential pathway for mental health providers to consider is utilizing multidisci-plinary approaches that are delivered in a community-sanctioned environment. This could include providing psychotherapy services in a nonclinical setting, intervention as a part of a general health services program or early childhood program, or integrating services with other community-based providers. Considering the lens of intersectionality and the socioeco-logical framework, as referenced earlier, provides an opportunity to involve other relevant systems in the effective treatment of perinatal mood distress. In the case of Sheena, receiving care within a medical or formal psychiatric setting may not have been effective as she reported experiences of racism and microaggressions from her medical provider. Spirituality was also an important aspect of Sheena's identity and her spiritual leader was considered a trusted source for information and guidance. For Sheena and others, this could be an important aspect of her identity to utilize as a part of the treatment process. A review of studies on the use of prayers and faith-based practices for Muslim women across multiple countries demon-strated effectiveness in reducing perinatal depression and anxiety (Simonovich et al., 2022). In addition, this study indicated that reciting parts of the Quran, saying a Dua, and listening to audio recordings of prayers decreased stress, pain, and fear during pregnancy, childbirth, during an unexpected cesarean section, and when experiencing infant loss. As indicated in the earlier referenced study on Latina mothers, home visitation is another option for providing community-based care from a culturally relevant lens. Studies on the efficacy of home visita-tion for treating perinatal mood disorders indicated that interventions that begin during preg-nancy demonstrate more consistent and favorable outcomes (Tabb et al., 2022). Although further study and analysis is needed, a home-based intervention could remove practical and systemic barriers that may be particularly salient for mothers from diverse communities.

Other community-based models include the utilization of trained community health workers, midwives, doulas, or other trusted and trained community members to provide therapeutic interventions. The World Health Organization (WHO) created a "low-inten-sity" perinatally focused psychological intervention, based on evidence-based models, that was intended to be administered by community health workers across the globe (World Health Organization, 2015). This program, called Thinking Healthy, targets perinatal depression and has been adapted to work in low-, middle-, and high-income countries, as access to mental health providers in some parts of the world is scarce. Additionally, a qualitative study among rural mothers in Rwanda demonstrated that mothers placed a high value on community health workers for information support (advice on nutrition, prenatal care, delivery care), emotional support (counseling), and tangible support (assisting mothers in solving practical problems) (Mwendwa, 2018). The ROSE program (Reach Out, Stay Strong, Essentials for mothers of newborns), developed in the United States, is an IPT-focused intervention that can be administered by nurses, community health workers, or other trained community members. It has demonstrated efficacy among economically disadvantaged population and women of color as a preventive tool for perinatal depression (Crockett et al., 2008; Zlotnik et al., 2016). In countries with widespread midwifery-led models of care in the perinatal period, specialist mental health midwives could play a critical role in gaining access to treatment for perinatal mood disorders (Maternal Mental Health Alliance et al., 2018). The midwifery model of care emphasizes community-based care and strong relationships between providers and patients, an approach that produces improved labor and birth outcomes (Kennedy et al., 2020; McRae et al., 2018; Sandall et al., 2016) and could ameliorate the systemic bias and racism that has historically plagued established medical institutions (Julian et al., 2020; Nove et al., 2021).

Furthermore, mental health providers, researchers, and other healthcare professionals that are interacting with women during the perinatal period must be prepared to address their own biases and blind spots that are a result of a privileged identity. Receiving formal and ongoing training on implicit bias, challenging racist or xenophobic policies within White dominant institutions, and approaching the therapeutic process with a lens on power and privilege are methods through which to begin this ongoing process. Power differentials between client and mental health provider also affect a client's ability to fully participate decision-making around their diagnosis and treatment plan (Maharaj et al., 2021; Stoute, 2020; Vasquez, 2007). For communities that have long experienced historical trauma, oppression, racism, sexism, and xenophobia in White-dominant institutions, this is particularly relevant. In a qualitative study conducted in the United States, Black women identified seven themes that hinder relationships with perinatal health providers: (1) provides unequal or differential treatment; (2) expresses biased attitudes; (3) lacks empathy; (4) limits choices; (5) communicates inadequate health information; (6) provides deficient care; and (7) dismisses concerns (Renbarger et al., 2023). Mental health providers frequently describe diverse communities as "difficult to reach" or "hard to treat" or lament that individuals from these communities do not engage in therapy or other mental health interventions. However, as a mental health provider, part of engaging in this work is ensuring that the therapeutic interventions, research protocols, and community-based supports are psychologically safe and accessible. The Cycle to Respectful Care, as developed by the National Birth Equity Collaborative in the United States, provides an actionable, cyclical framework with which to engage in this critical work (Green et al., 2021).

Conclusion and Future Directions

According to the World Health Organization, one in five women globally will experience a perinatal mood disorder (WHO, 2022). As such, the need for evidence-based treatment modalities that are community-informed and culturally responsive is significant.

Throughout this chapter, much of the discussion focused on perinatal depression, as this is the most widely researched and understood mental health condition that presents during the perinatal period. Culturally responsive, community-informed treatment modalities that target other mood disorders during the perinatal period, including perinatal anxiety disorders, perinatal-related posttraumatic stress disorder, perinatal bipolar disorder, postpartum psychosis, and perinatal substance abuse are also significantly lacking. This should be a focus area for researchers, policymakers, and clinicians.

Additionally, there needs to be increased attention to the utilization of community-based participatory research modalities to engage diverse communities in the development of treatment modalities. Community-based participatory research has been discussed extensively in the literature as a paradigm that can bridge the gap between science and practice to promote a broader goal of health equity (Ortiz et al., 2020; Collins et al., 2018; Wallerstein & Duran, 2010). Allowing the inclusion of members from a target community to participate in all aspects of the research design and implementation process could promote the development of treatment modalities that are specific to cultural contexts and thus, have the potential to increase utilization and effectiveness.

References

Adams, M. K., Byrn, M., Penckofer, S., Bryant, F., & Almonte, A. (2021). Expectations of motherhood and quality of life. *MCN: The American Journal of Maternal/Child Nursing, 46*(2), 70–75.

Al-abri, K., Edge, D., & Armitage, C. J. (2023). Prevalence and correlates of perinatal depression. *Social Psychiatry and Psychiatric Epidemiology.* https://doi.org/10.1007/s00127-022-02386-9

Alhasanat, D., Fry-McComish, J., & Yarandi, H. N. (2017). Risk for postpartum depression among immigrant Arabic women in the United States: A feasibility study. *Journal of Midwifery & Women's Health, 62*(4), 470–476. https://doi.org/10.1111/jmwh.12617

Alhasanat, D., & Giurgescu, C. (2017). Acculturation and postpartum depressive symptoms among Hispanic women in the United States: Systematic review. *MCN. The American Journal of Maternal Child Nursing, 42*(1), 21–28. https://doi.org/10.1097/NMC.0000000000000298

Alhusen, J. L., Bower, K. M., Epstein, E., & Sharps, P. (2016). Racial discrimination and adverse birth outcomes: An integrative review. *Journal of Midwifery and Women's Health, 61*(6), 707–720. https://doi.org/10.1111/jmwh.12490

Alio, A. P., Richman, A. R., Clayton, H. B., Jeffers, D. F., Wathington, D. J., & Salihu, H. M. (2010). An ecological approach to understanding Black–White disparities in perinatal mortality. *Maternal and Child Health Journal, 14*, 557–566.

Alshikh Ahmad, H., Alkhatib, A., & Luo, J. (2021). Prevalence and risk factors of postpartum depression in the Middle East: A systematic review and meta-analysis. *BMC Pregnancy and Childbirth, 21*(1), 542. https://doi.org/10.1186/s12884-021-04016-9

Atif, M., Halaki, M., Raynes-Greenow, C., & Chow, C.-M. (2021). Perinatal depression in Pakistan: A systematic review and meta-analysis. *Birth, 48*(2), 149–163. https://doi.org/10.1111/birt.12535

Ayano, G., Tesfaw, G., & Shumet, S. (2019). Prevalence and determinants of antenatal depression in Ethiopia: A systematic review and meta-analysis. *PLoS One, 14*(2), e0211764. https://doi.org/10.1371/journal.pone.0211764

Azami, M., Badfar, G., Shohani, M., Mansouri, A., Soleymani, A., Shamloo, M. B. B., . . . Nasirkandy, M. P. (2018). The prevalence of depression in pregnant Iranian women: A systematic review and meta-analysis. *Iranian Journal of Psychiatry and Behavioral Sciences, 12*(3), Article 3. https://doi.org/10.5812/ijpbs.9975

Beal, F. M. (1970). Double jeopardy: To be Black and female. In R. Morgan (Ed.), *Sisterhood is powerful: An anthology of writing from the women's liberation movement.* Random House and Vintage Paperbacks.

Beal, F. M. (2008). Double jeopardy: To be Black and female. *Meridians, 8*(2), 166–176.

Bécares, L., & Atatoa-Carr, P. (2016). The association between maternal and partner experienced racial discrimination and prenatal perceived stress, prenatal and postnatal depression: Findings from the growing up in New Zealand cohort study. *International Journal for Equity in Health*, *15*(1), 1–12. https://doi.org/10.1186/s12939-016-0443-4

Beck, A. T., Steer, R. A., & Brown, G. K. (1996). *The Beck Depression Inventory: Manual (2nd ed.)*. Psychological Corporation.

Beck, C. T., Froman, R. D., & Bernal, H. (2005). Acculturation level and postpartum depression in Hispanic mothers. *MCN. The American Journal of Maternal Child Nursing*, *30*(5), 299–304. https://doi.org/10.1097/00005721-200509000-00006.

Beeber, L. S., Holditch-Davis, D., Perreira, K., A. Schwartz, T., Lewis, V., Blanchard, H., & Goldman, B. D. (2010). Short-term in-home intervention reduces depressive symptoms in early head start Latina mothers of infants and toddlers. *Research in Nursing & Health*, *33*(1), 60–76. https://doi.org/10.1002/nur.20363

Beeghly, M. J., Olson, K. L., Weinberg, M. K., Pierre, S. C., Downey, N., & Tronick, E. Z. (2003). Prevalence, stability, and socio-demographic correlates of Depressive symptoms in Black mothers during the first 18 months postpartum. *Maternal and Child Health Journal*, *7*(3), 157–168. https://doi.org/10.1023/A:1025132320321

Benish, S. G., Quintana, S., & Wampold, B. E. (2011). Culturally adapted psychotherapy and the legitimacy of myth: A direct-comparison meta-analysis. *Journal of Counseling Psychology*, *58*(3), 279–289. https://doi.org/10.1037/a0023626

Bernal, G., & Adames, C. (2017). Cultural adaptations: Conceptual, ethical, contextual, and methodological issues for working with ethnocultural and majority-world populations. *Prevention Science*, *18*(6), 681–688. https://doi.org/10.1007/s11121-017-0806-0

Bernal, G., Jiménez-Chafey, M. I., & Domenech Rodríguez, M. M. (2009). Cultural adaptation of treatments: A resource for considering culture in evidence-based practice. *Professional Psychology: Research and Practice*, *40*(4), 361. https://doi.org/10.1037/a0016401

Bingham, D., Jones, D. K., & Howell, E. A. (2019). Quality improvement to eliminate disparities in perinatal morbidity and mortality. *Obstetrics and Gynecology Clinics of North America*, *46*(2), 227–238. https://doi.org/10.1016/j.ogc.2019.01.006

Bishop-Royse, J., Lange-Maia, B., Murray, L., Shah, R. C., & DeMaio, F. (2021). Structural racism, socio-economic marginalization, and infant mortality. *Public Health*, *190*, 55–61. https://doi.org/10.1016/j.puhe.2020.10.027

Branquinho, M., Rodriguez-Muñoz, M. F., Maia, B. R., Marques, M., Matos, M., Osma, J., Moreno-Peral, P., Conejo-Cerón, S., Fonseca, A., & Vousoura, E. (2021). Effectiveness of psychological interventions in the treatment of perinatal depression: A systematic review of systematic reviews and meta-analyses. *Journal of Affective Disorders*, *291*, 294–306. https://doi.org/10.1016/j.jad.2021.05.010

Bronfenbrenner, U. (1979). *The ecology of human development: Experiments by nature and design*. Harvard University Press.

Bronfenbrenner, U. (2005). *Making human beings human: Bioecological perspectives on human development*. Sage.

Budhwani, H., & De, P. (2019). Perceived stigma in health care settings and the physical and mental health of people of color in the United States. *Health Equity*, *3*(1), 73–80. https://doi.org/10.1089/heq.2018.0079

Chambers, B. D., Arabia, S. E., Arega, H. A., Altman, M. R., Berkowitz, R., Feuer, S. K., . . . McLemore, M. R. (2020). Exposures to structural racism and racial discrimination among pregnant and early post-partum Black women living in Oakland, California. *Stress and Health*, *36*(2), 213–219. https://doi.org/10.1002/smi.2922

Chambers, B. D., Taylor, B., Nelson, T., Harrison, J., Bell, A., O'Leary, A., . . . McLemore, M. R. (2022). Clinicians' perspectives on racism and Black women's maternal health. *Women's Health Reports*, *3*(1), 476–482. https://doi.org/10.1089/whr.2021.0148

Child Care Aware of America. (2019). *The US and the high price of child care: An examination of a broken system*. www.childcareaware.org/our-issues/research/the-us-and-the-high-price-of-child-care-2019/

Chopak-Foss, J., Harris, K., & Choongo, J. (2020). Applying the socio-ecological model to improving maternal mental health in Georgia. *Eagles Talking about Public Health*, Spring 2020, p. 1–3. http://works.bepress.com/joanne_chopak-foss/132/

Chorwe-Sungani, G., Wella, K., Mapulanga, P., Nyirongo, D., & Pindani, M. (2022). Systematic review on the prevalence of perinatal depression in Malawi. *The South African Journal of Psychiatry, 28*, 1859. https://doi.org/10.4102/sajpsychiatry.v28i0.1859

Chzhen, Y., Gromada, A., & Rees, G. (2019). Are the world's riches countries family friendly? Policy in the OECD and EU. *UNICEF Office of Research*. www.unicef-irc.org/publications/pdf/Family-Friendly-Policies-Research_UNICEF_%202019.pdf

Collins, J. W., & David, R. J. (2005). Pregnancy outcome of Mexican-American women: The effect of generational residence in the United States. *Obstetrical & Gynecological Survey, 60*(3), 147–148.

Collins, S. E., Clifasefi, S. L., Stanton, J., Straits, K. J., Gil-Kashiwabara, E., Rodriguez Espinosa, P., . . . Wallerstein, N. (2018). Community-Based Participatory Research (CBPR): Towards equitable involvement of community in psychology research. *American Psychologist, 73*(7), 884. https://doi.org/10.1037/amp0000167

Combahee River Collective. (1982). A Black feminist statement. In A. Hull, P. B. Scott, & B. Smith (Eds.), *All the women are White, all the Blacks are men, but some of us are brave: Black women's studies*. Feminist Press.

Cox, J. L., Holden, J. M., & Sagovsky, R. (1987). Detection of postnatal depression: Development of the 10-item Edinburgh Postnatal Depression Scale. *The British Journal of Psychiatry, 150*(6), 782–786. https://doi.org/10.1192/bjp.150.6.782

Crenshaw, K. W. (1989). Demarginalizing the intersection of race and sex: A Black feminist critique of antidiscrimination doctrine, feminist theory and antiracist politics. *University of Chicago Legal Forum, 1989*(8), 139.

Crenshaw, K. W. (1991). Mapping the margins: Intersectionality, identity politics, and violence against women of color. *Stanford Law Review, 43*(6), 1241–1299. https://doi.org/10.2307/1229039.

Crenshaw, K. W. (2017). *On intersectionality: Essential writings*. New Press.

Crenshaw, K. W., Gotanda, N., Peller, G., & Thomas, K. (1995). *Critical race theory: The key writings that formed the movement*. New Press.

Crockett, K., Zlotnick, C., Davis, M., Payne, N., & Washington, R. (2008). A depression preventive intervention for rural low-income African-American pregnant women at risk f or postpartum depression. *Archives of Women's Mental Health, 11*, 319–325. https://doi.org/10.1007/s00737-008-0036-3

Crofoot, T. L., & Harris, M. S. (2012). An Indian child welfare perspective on disproportionality in child welfare. *Child and Youth Services Review, 34*, 1667–1674.

Daminger, A. (2019). The cognitive dimension of household labor. *American Sociological Review, 84*(4), 609–633. https://doi.org/10.1177/0003122419859007

Declercq, E., Feinberg, E., & Belanoff, C. (2022). Racial inequities in the course of treating perinatal mental health challenges: Results from listening to mothers in California. *Birth, 49*(1), 132–140. https://doi.org/10.1111/birt.12584

de Graaf, J. P., Steegers, E. A., & Bonsel, G. J. (2013). Inequalities in perinatal and maternal health. *Current Opinion in Obstetrics and Gynecology, 25*(2), 98–108. https://doi.org/10.1097/GCO.0b013e32835ec9b0

Dennis, J. A. (2019). Birth weight and maternal age among American Indian/Alaska Native mothers: A test of the weathering hypothesis. *SSM-Population Health, 7*, 100304. https://doi.org/10.1016/j.ssmph.2018.10.004

Dunbar-Ortiz, R. (2014). *An indigenous peoples' history of the United States* (Vol. 3). Beacon Press.

Ertel, K. A., James-Todd, T., Kleinman, K., Krieger, N., Gillman, M., Wright, R., & Rich-Edwards, J. (2012). Racial discrimination, response to unfair treatment, and depressive symptoms among pregnant Black and African American women in the United States. *Annals of Epidemiology, 22*(12), 840–846. https://doi.org/10.1016/j.annepidem.2012.10.001

Font, S. A., Berger, L. M., & Slack, K. S. (2012). Examining racial disproportionality in child protective services case decision. *Children and Youth Services Review, 34*(11), 2188–2200.

Germic, E. R., Eckert, S., & Vultee, F. (2021). The impact of Instagram mommy blogger content on the perceived self-efficacy of mothers. *Social Media + Society, 7*(3), 1–19. https://doi.org/10.1177/205630512110416

Getinet, W., Amare, T., Boru, B., Shumet, S., Worku, W., & Azale, T. (2018). Prevalence and risk factors for antenatal depression in Ethiopia: Systematic review. *Depression Research and Treatment, 2018*, 3649269. https://doi.org/10.1155/2018/3649269

Green, C. L., Perez, S. L., Walker, A., Estriplet, T., Ogunwole, S. M., Auguste, T. C., & Crear-Perry, J. A. (2021). The cycle to respectful care: A qualitative approach to the creation of an action-able framework to address maternal outcome disparities. *International Journal of Environmental Research and Public Health*, 18(9), 4933. https://doi.org/10.3390/ijerph18094933

Griner, D., & Smith, T. B. (2006). Culturally adapted mental health intervention: A meta ana-lytic review. *Psychotherapy: Theory, Research, Practice, Training*, 43(4), 531–548. https://doi.org/10.1037/0033-3204.43.4.531

Grote, N. K., Swartz, H. A., Geibel, S. L., Zuckoff, A., Houck, P. R., & Frank, E. (2009). A ran-domized controlled trial of culturally relevant, brief interpersonal psychotherapy for perinatal depression. *Psychiatric Services (Washington, DC)*, 60(3), 313–321. https://doi.org/10.1176/ps.2009.60.3.313

Guillfoyle, A. M., La Rosa, A., Botsis, S., & Butler-O'Halloran, B. (2014). Perinatal mental health, ecological systems, and social support: Refugee women and facilitated playgroup. *International Journal of Health, Wellness & Society*, 3(4).

Hahn-Holbrook, J., Cornwell-Hinrichs, T., & Anaya, I. (2017). Economic and health predictors of national postpartum depression prevalence: A systematic review, meta-analysis, and meta-regres-sion of 291 studies from 56 countries. *Frontiers in Psychiatry*, 8, 248. https://doi.org/10.3389/fpsyt.2017.00248

Hall, G. C. N., Ibaraki, A. Y., Huang, E. R., Marti, C. N., & Stice, E. (2016). A meta-analysis of cultural adaptations of psychological interventions. *Behavior Therapy*, 47(6), 993–1014. https://doi.org/10.1016/j.beth.2016.09.005.

Harp, K. L., & Bunting, A. M. (2020). The racialized nature of child welfare policies and the social control of Black bodies. *Social Politics: International Studies in Gender, State & Society*, 27(2), 258–281. https://doi.org/10.1093/sp/jxz039

Heilemann, M., Frutos, L., Lee, K., & Kury, F. S. (2004). Protective strength factors, resources, and risks in relation to depressive symptoms among childbearing women of Mexican descent. *Health Care for Women International*, 25(1), 88–106. https://doi.org/10.1080/07399330490253265

Hoberman, J. (2012). *Black and blue: The origins and consequences of medical racism*. University of California Press.

Howell, E. A., Mora, P. A., Horowitz, C. R., & Leventhal, H. (2005). Racial and ethnic differences in factors associated with early postpartum depressive symptoms. *Obstetrics and Gynecology*, 105(6), 1442–1450. https://doi.org/10.1097/01.AOG.0000164050.34126.37

Hubert, S., & Aujoulat, I. (2018). Parental burnout: When exhausted mothers open up. *Frontiers in Psychology*, 9, 1021. https://doi.org/10.3389/fpsyg.2018.01021

Huggins, B., Jones, C., Adeyinka, O., Ofomata, A., Drake, C., & Kondas, C. (2020). Racial disparities in perinatal mental health. *Psychiatric Annals*, 50(11), 489–493. https://doi.org/10.3928/00485713-20201007-02

Hwang, W. C. (2009). The Formative Method for Adapting Psychotherapy (FMAP): A community-based developmental approach to culturally adapting therapy. *Professional Psychology: Research and Practice*, 40(4), 369. https://doi.org/10.1037/a0016240

Institute for Women's Policy Research. (2020). *Women's median earnings as a percent of men's 1985–2019 (full-time, year-round workers) with projections for pay equity, by race/ethnicity*. Retrieved September, 2022, from https://iwpr.org/iwpr-publications/quick-figure/pay-equity-projection-race-ethnicity-2020/

Iturralde, E., Hsiao, C. A., Nkemere, L., Kubo, A., Sterling, S. A., Flanagan, T., & Avalos, L. A. (2021). Engagement in perinatal depression treatment: A qualitative study of barriers across and within racial/ethnic groups. *BMC Pregnancy and Childbirth*, 21(1), 1–11. https://doi.org/10.1186/s12884-021-03969-1

Jankovic, J., Parsons, J., Jovanović, N., Berrisford, G., Copello, A., Fazil, Q., & Priebe, S. (2020). Dif-ferences in access and utilisation of mental health services in the perinatal period for women from ethnic minorities–a population-based study. *BMC Medicine*, 18, 1–12. https://doi.org/10.1186/s12916-020-01711-w

Jones, E., & Coast, E. (2013). Social relationships and postpartum depression in South Asia: A systematic review. *International Journal of Social Psychiatry*, 59(7), 690–700. https://doi.org/10.1177/0020764012453675

Julian, Z., Robles, D., Whetstone, S., Perritt, J. B., Jackson, A. V., Hardeman, R. R., & Scott, K. A. (2020, August). Community-informed models of perinatal and reproductive health services provision: A justice-centered paradigm toward equity among Black birthing communities. *Seminars in Perinatology*, 44(5), p. 151267. https://doi.org/10.1016/j.semperi.2020.151267

Karaçam, Z., Çoban, A., Akbaş, B., & Karabulut, E. (2018). Status of postpartum depression in Turkey: A meta-analysis. *Health Care for Women International*, 39(7), 821–841. https://doi.org/10.1080/07399332.2018.1466144

Kennedy, H. P., Balaam, M. C., Dahlen, H., Declercq, E., De Jonge, A., Downe, S., . . . Wolfe, I. (2020). The role of midwifery and other international insights for maternity care in the United States: An analysis of four countries. *Birth*, 47(4), 332–345. https://doi.org/10.1111/birt.12504

Khan, M., Brown, H. K., Lunsky, Y., Welsh, K., Havercamp, S. M., Proulx, L., & Tarasoff, L. A. (2021). A socio-ecological approach to understanding the perinatal care experiences of people with intellectual and/or developmental disabilities in Ontario, Canada. *Women's Health Issues*, 31(6), 550–559. https://doi.org/10.1016/j.whi.2021.08.002

Khan, S., Lovell, K., Lunat, F., Masood, Y., Shah, S., Tomenson, B., & Husain, N. (2019). Culturally-adapted cognitive behavioural therapy based intervention for maternal depression: A mixed-methods feasibility study. *BMC Women's Health*, 19(1), 1–11. https://doi.org/10.1186/s12905-019-0712-7

Khatri, G. K., Tran, T. D., & Fisher, J. (2019). Prevalence and determinants of symptoms of antenatal common mental disorders among women who had recently experienced an earthquake: A systematic review. *BMC Psychiatry*, 19(1), 47. https://doi.org/10.1186/s12888-018-1986-2

King, D. (1988). Multiple jeopardy, multiple consciousness: The context of a Black feminist ideology. *Signs: Journal of Women in Culture and Society*, 14(1), 42–72.

Klainin, P., & Arthur, D. G. (2009). Postpartum depression in Asian cultures: A literature review. *International Journal of Nursing Studies*, 46(10), 1355–1373. https://doi.org/10.1016/j.ijnurstu.2009.02.012

Kothari, C. L., Paul, R., Dormitorio, B., Ospina, F., James, A., Lenz, D., . . . Wiley, J. (2016). The interplay of race, socioeconomic status and neighborhood residence upon birth outcomes in a high Black infant mortality community. *SSM-Population Health*, 2, 859–867. https://doi.org/10.1016/j.ssmph.2016.09.011

Krase, K. S. (2015). Child maltreatment reporting by educational personnel: Implications for racial disproportionality in the child welfare system. *Children & Schools*, 37(2), 89–99. https://doi.org/10.1093/cs/cdv005

Kroenke, K., Spitzer, R. L., & Williams, J. B. W. (2001). The PHQ-9: Validity of a brief severity depression measure. *Journal of General Internal Medicine*, 16(9), 606–613. https://doi.org/10.1046/j.1525-1497.2001.016009606.x

Lachance-Grzela, M., & Bouchard, G. (2010). Why do women do the lion's share of housework? A decade of research. *Sex Roles*, 63, 767–780. https://doi.org/10.1007/s11199-010-9797-z

Lash, D. (2017). *"When the welfare people come": Race and class protection in the US child protection system*. Haymarket Books.

Leimert, K. B., & Olson, D. M. (2020). Racial disparities in pregnancy outcomes: Genetics, epigenetics, and allostatic load. *Current Opinion in Physiology*, 13, 155–165. https://doi.org/10.1016/j.cophys.2019.12.003

Lewis, J. A., Williams, M. G., Peppers, E. J., & Gadson, C. A. (2017). Applying intersectionality to explore the relations between gendered racism and health among Black women. *Journal of Counseling Psychology*, 64(5), 475–486. https://doi.org/10.1037/cou0000231

MacDorman, M. F., Thoma, M., Declcerq, E., & Howell, E. A. (2021). Racial and ethnic disparities in maternal mortality in the United States using enhanced vital records, 2016-2017. *American Journal of Public Health*, 111(9), 1673–1681. https://doi.org/10.2105/AJPH.2021.306375

Macedo, D. M., Smithers, L. G., Roberts, R. M., & Jamieson, L. M. (2018). Racism, stress, and sense of personal control among aboriginal Australian pregnant women. *Australian Psychologist*, 55(4), 336–348. https://doi.org/10.1111/ap.12435

Maharaj, A. S., Bhatt, N. V., & Gentile, J. P. (2021). Bringing it in the room: Addressing the impact of racism on the therapeutic alliance. *Innovations in Clinical Neuroscience*, 18(7-9), 39.

Masood, Y., Lovell, K., Lunat, F., Atif, N., Waheed, W., Rahman, A., Mossabir, R., Chaudhry, N., & Husain, N. (2015). Group psychological intervention for postnatal depression: A nested qualitative study with British South Asian women. *BMC Women's Health*, 15(109).

Maternal Mental Health Alliance, The Royal College of Midwives, & The National Society for the Prevention of Cruelty to Children. (2018). *Specialist mental health midwives: What they do and why they matter.* The Royal College of Midwives. Retrieved September 2021 from https://www.rcm.org.uk/publications?pagesize=0

McRae, D. N., Janssen, P. A., Vedam, S., Mayhew, M., Mpofu, D., Teucher, U., & Muhajarine, N. (2018). Reduced prevalence of small-for-gestational-age and preterm birth for women of low socioeconomic position: A population-based cohort study comparing antenatal midwifery and physician models of care. *BMJ Open, 8*(10), e022220. https://doi.org/10.1136/bmjopen-2018-022220

Medlock, M., Weissman, A., Wong, S. S., Carlo, A., Zeng, M., Borba, C., . . . Shtasel, D. (2017). Racism as a unique social determinant of mental health: Development of a didactic curriculum for psychiatry residents. *MedEdPORTAL, 13*, 10618. https://doi.org/10.15766/mep_2374-8265.10618

Meltzer-Brody, S. (2022). New insights into perinatal depression: Pathogenesis and treatment during pregnancy and postpartum. *Dialogues in Clinical Neuroscience, 13*(1), 89–100. https://doi.org/10.31887/DCNS.2011.13.1/smbrody

Michaels, C., Blake, L., Lynn, A., Greylord, T., & Benning, S. (2022, April 18). *Mental health and well-being ecological model.* Center for Leadership Education in Maternal & Child Public Health, University of Minnesota–Twin Cities. Retrieved January 2023, from https://mch.umn.edu/resources/mhecomodel/

Mokwena, K., & Modjadji, P. (2022). A comparative study of postnatal depression and associated factors in Gauteng and Free State provinces, South Africa. *African Journal of Primary Health Care & Family Medicine, 14*(1), e1–e11. https://doi.org/10.4102/phcfm.v14i1.3031

Moulding, N. (2019). "We never quite measure up, do we?": An intersectional approach to mothering, mental health and social inequality. In *Intersections of Mothering* (pp. 168–179). Routledge.

Mu, T.-Y., Li, Y.-H., Pan, H.-F., Zhang, L., Zha, D.-H., Zhang, C.-L., & Xu, R.-X. (2019). Postpartum depressive mood (PDM) among Chinese women: A meta-analysis. *Archives of Women's Mental Health, 22*(2), 279–287. https://doi.org/10.1007/s00737-018-0885-3

Mwendwa, P. (2018). Assessing the demand for community health workers' social support: A qualitative perspective of mothers in rural Rwanda. *Africa Health Agenda International Journal, 1*(4).

Naeem, F., Phiri, P., Munshi, T., Rathod, S., Ayub, M., Gobbi, M., & Kingdon, D. (2015). Using cognitive behaviour therapy with South Asian Muslims: Findings from the culturally sensitive CBT project. *International Review of Psychiatry, 27*(3), 233–246. https://doi.org/10.3109/09540261.2015.1067598.

Nillni, Y. I., Mehralizade, A., Mayer, L., & Milanovic, S. (2018). Treatment of depression, anxiety, and trauma-related disorders during the perinatal period: A systematic review. *Clinical Psychology Review, 66*, 136–148. https://doi.org/10.1016/j.cpr.2018.06.004

Nippert, K. E., Tomiyama, A. J., Smieszek, S. M., & Incollingo Rodriguez, A. C. (2021). The media as a source of weight stigma for pregnant and postpartum women. *Obesity, 29*(1), 226–232. https://doi.org/10.1002/oby.23032

Noursi, S., Saluja, B., & Richey, L. (2021). Using the ecological systems theory to understand Black/White disparities in maternal morbidity and mortality in the United States. *Journal of Racial and Ethnic Health Disparities, 8*, 661–669. https://doi.org/10.1007/s40615-020-00825-4

Nove, A., Friberg, I. K., de Bernis, L., McConville, F., Moran, A. C., Najjemba, M., Homer, C. S. (2021). Potential impact of midwives in preventing and reducing maternal and neonatal mortality and stillbirths: A lives saved tool modelling study. *The Lancet Global Health, 9*(1), e24–e32. https://doi.org/10.1016/S2214-109X(20)30397-1.

Ortiz, K., Nash, J., Shea, L., Oetzel, J., Garoutte, J., Sanchez-Youngman, S., & Wallerstein, N. (2020). Partnerships, processes, and outcomes: A health equity–focused scoping meta-review of community-engaged scholarship. *Annual Review of Public Health, 41*, 177–199. https://doi.org/10.1146/annurev-publhealth-040119-094220

Osborn, R., Squires, D., Doty, M. M., Sarnak, D. O., & Schneider, E. C. (2016). In new survey of eleven countries, US adults still struggle with access to and affordability of health care. *Health Affairs, 35*(12), 2327–2336. https://doi.org/10.1377/hlthaff.2016.1088

Owens-Young, J., & Bell, C. N. (2020). Structural racial inequities in socioeconomic status, urban-rural classification, and infant mortality in US counties. *Ethnicity & Disease, 30*(3), 389. https://doi.org/10.18865/ed.30.3.389

Özcan, N. K., Boyacıoğlu, N. E., & Dinç, H. (2017). Postpartum depression prevalence and risk factors in Turkey: A systematic review and meta-analysis. *Archives of Psychiatric Nursing, 31*(4), 420–428. https://doi.org/10.1016/j.apnu.2017.04.006

Pabayo, R., Ehntholt, A., Davis, K., Liu, S. Y., Muennig, P., & Cook, D. M. (2019). Structural racism and odds for infant mortality among infants born in the United States 2010. *Journal of Racial and Ethnic Health Disparities, 6*, 1095–1106. https://doi.org/10.1007/s40615-019-00612-w

Palacios, J. F., & Portillo, C. J. (2009). Understanding native women's health: Historical legacies. *Journal of Transcultural Nursing, 20*(1), 15–27. https://doi.org/10.1177/1043659608325844

Paradies, Y., Ben, J., Denson, N., Elias, A., Priest, N., Pieterse, A., . . . Gee, G. (2015). Racism as a determinant of health: A systematic review and meta-analysis. *PLoS One, 10*(9), e0138511. https://doi.org/10.1371/journal.pone.0138511

Petersen, E. E., Davis, N. L., Goodman, D., Cox, S., Syverson, C., Seed, K., . . . Barfield, W. (2019). Racial/ethnic disparities in pregnancy-related deaths–United States, 2007–2016. *Morbidity and Mortality Weekly Report, 68*(35), 762–765. https://doi.org/10.15585/mmwr.mm6835a3externalicon

Pointing, C., Mahrer, N. E., Zelcer, H., Schetter, C. D., & Chavira, D. A. (2021). Psychological interventions for depression and anxiety in pregnant Latina and Black women in the United States: A systematic review. *Clinical Psychology & Psychotherapy, 27*(2), 249–265.

Prady, S. L., Endacott, C., Dickerson, J., Bywater, T. J., & Blower, S. L. (2021). Inequalities in the identification and management of common mental disorders in the perinatal period: An equity focused re-analysis of a systematic review. *PLoS One, 16*(3), e0248631. https://doi.org/10.1371/journal.pone.0248631.

Prady, S. L., Pickett, K. E., Gilbody, S., Petherick, E. S., Mason, D., Sheldon, T. A., & Wright, J. (2016). Variation and ethnic inequalities in treatment of common mental disorders before, during and after pregnancy: Combined analysis of routine and research data in the Born in Bradford cohort. *BMC Psychiatry, 16*(1), 1–13. https://doi.org/10.1186/s12888-016-0805-x

Putnam-Hornstein, E., Needell, B., King, B., & Johnson-Motoyama, M. (2013). Racial and ethnic disparities: A population-based examination of risk factors for involvement with child protective services. *Child Abuse & Neglect, 37*(1), 33–46. https://doi.org/10.1016/j.chiabu.2012.08.005

Ramchandani, P. G., Richter, L. M., Stein, A., & Norris, S. A. (2009). Predictors of postnatal depression in an urban South African cohort. *Journal of Affective Disorders, 113*(3), 279–284. https://doi.org/10.1016/j.jad.2008.05.007

Ramsay, G. (2016). Black mothers, bad mothers: African refugee women and the governing of "good" citizens through the Australian child welfare system. *Australian Feminist Studies, 31*(89), 319–335. https://doi.org/10.1080/08164649.2016.1254021

Rathod, S., Gega, L., Degnan, A., Pikard, J., Khan, T., Husain, N., Munshi, T., & Naeem, F. (2018). The current status of culturally adapted mental health interventions: A practice-focused review of meta-analyses. *Neuropsychiatric Disease and Treatment, 14*, 165–178. https://doi.org/10.2147/NDT.S138430

Renbarger, K. M., Phelps, B., & Broadstreet, A. (2023). Provider characteristics that hinder relationships with Black women in the perinatal period. *Western Journal of Nursing Research, 45*(3). https://doi.org/10.1177/01939459221120390

Rich-Edwards, J. W., Kleinman, K., Abrams, A., Harlow, B. L., McLaughlin, T. J., Joffe, H., & Gillman, M. W. (2006). Sociodemographic predictors of antenatal and postpartum depressive symptoms among women in a medical group practice. *Journal of Epidemiology and Community Health, 60*(3), 221–227. https://doi.org/10.1136/jech.2005.039370

Rivenbark, J. G., & Ichou, M. (2020). Discrimination in healthcare as a barrier to care: Experiences of socially disadvantaged populations in France from a nationally representative survey. *BMC Public Health, 20*(1), 1–10. https://doi.org/10.1186/s12889- 019-8124-z

Roberts, D. (2001). *Shattered bonds: The color of child welfare*. Civitas Books.

Roberts, D., & Sangoi, L. (2018). Black families matter: How the child welfare system punishes poor families of color. *The Appeal*. https://theappeal.org/black-families-matter-how-the-child-welfare-system-punishes-poor-families-of-color-33ad20e2882e/

Roberts, S. C., & Nuru-Jeter, A. (2012). Universal screening for alcohol and drug use and racial disparities in child protective services reporting. *The Journal of Behavioral Health Services & Research, 39*(1), 3–16. https://doi.org/10.1007/s11414-011-9247-x

Salameh, T. N., Hall, L. A., Crawford, T. N., Staten, R. R., & Hall, M. T. (2019). Racial/ethnic differences in mental health treatment among a national sample of pregnant women with mental health and/or substance use disorders in the United States. *Journal of Psychosomatic Research, 121,* 74–80. https://doi.org/10.1016/j.jpsychores.2019.03.015

Sandall, J., Soltani, H., Gates, S., Shennan, A., & Devane, D. (2016). Midwife-led continuity models versus other models of care for childbearing women. *Cochrane Database of Systematic Reviews, 4.* https://doi.org/10.1002/14651858.CD004667.pub5

Sawyer, A., Ayers, S., & Smith, H. (2010). Pre- and postnatal psychological wellbeing in Africa: A systematic review. *Journal of Affective Disorders, 123*(1–3), 17–29. https://doi.org/10.1016/j.jad.2009.06.027

Schaffir, J. (2016). Biological changes during pregnancy and the postpartum period. In A. Wenzel (Ed.), *The Oxford handbook of perinatal psychology* (pp. 26–37). Oxford University Press. https://doi.org/10.1093/oxfordhb/9780199778072.013.23

Schiller, C. E., Meltzer-Brody, S., & Rubinow, D. R. (2015). The role of reproductive hormones in postpartum depression. *CNS Spectrums, 20*(1), 48–59. https://doi.org/10.1017/S1092852914000480

Schoen, C., Osborn, R., Squires, D., & Doty, M. M. (2013). Access, affordability, and insurance complexity are often worse in the United States compared to ten other countries. *Health Affairs, 32*(12), 2205–2215. https://doi.org/10.1377/hlthaff.2013.0879

Schofield, C. A., Brown, S., Siegel, I. E., & Moss-Racusin, C. A. (2023). What you don't expect when you're expecting: Demonstrating stigma against women with postpartum psychological disorders. *Stigma and Health.* Advance online publication. https://doi.org/10.1037/sah0000431

Simonovich, S. D., Quad, N., Kanji, Z., & Tabb, K. M. (2022). Faith practices reduce perinatal anxiety and depression in Muslim women: A mixed-methods scoping review. *Frontiers in Psychiatry, 13,* 826769. https://doi.org/10.3389/fpsyt.2022.826769

Smith, D. Y., & Roane, A. (2023). Child removal fears and Black mothers' medical decision-making. *Contexts, 22*(1), 18–23. https://doi.org/10.1177/15365042221142834

Smith, T. B., Domenech Rodríguez, M., & Bernal, G. (2010). Culture. *Journal of Clinical Psychology, 67*(2), 166–175. http://doi.org/10.1002/jclp.20757

Stanley, J., Harris, R., Cormack, D., Waa, A., & Edwards, R. (2019). The impact of racism on the future health of adults: Protocol for a prospective cohort study. *BMC Public Health, 19*(1), 1–10. https://doi.org/10.1186/s12889-019-6664-x

Stellenberg, E. L., & Abrahams, J. M. (2015). Prevalence of and factors influencing postnatal depression in a rural community in South Africa. *African Journal of Primary Health Care & Family Medicine, 7*(1), 874. https://doi.org/10.4102/phcfm.v7i1.874

Stopforth, S., Kapadia, D., Nazroo, J., & Bécares, L. (2022). The enduring effects of racism on health: Understanding direct and indirect effects over time. *SSM-Population Health, 19,* 101217. https://doi.org/10.1016/j.ssmph.2022.101217.

Stoute, B. J. (2020). Racism: A challenge for the therapeutic dyad. *American Journal of Psychotherapy, 73*(3), 69–71. https://doi.org/10.1176/appi.psychotherapy.20200043

Tabb, K. M., Bentley, B., Pineros Leano, M., Simonovich, S. D., Nidey, N., Ross, K., . . . Huang, H. (2022). Home visiting as an equitable intervention for perinatal depression: A scoping review. *Frontiers in Psychiatry, 13,* 315. https://doi.org/10.3389/fpsyt.2022.826673

Takeshita, J., Wang, S., Loren, A. W., Mitra, N., Shults, J., Shin, D. B., & Sawinski, D. L. (2020). Association of racial/ethnic and gender concordance between patients and physicians with patient experience ratings. *JAMA Network Open, 3*(11), e2024583–e2024583. https://doi.org/10.1001/jamanetworkopen.2020.24583

Thomas, M. M. C., Waldfogel, J., & Williams, O. F. (2023). Inequities in child protective services contact between Black and White children. *Child Maltreatment, 28*(1), 42–54. https://doi.org/10.1177/107755952110702

Tokumitsu, K., Sugawara, N., Maruo, K., Suzuki, T., Shimoda, K., & Yasui-Furukori, N. (2020). Prevalence of perinatal depression among Japanese women: A meta-analysis. *Annals of General Psychiatry, 19*(1), 41. https://doi.org/10.1186/s12991-020-00290-7

Trifu, S., Vladuti, A., & Popescu, A. (2019). The neuroendocrinological aspects of pregnancy and postpartum depression. *Acta Endocrinologica (Bucharest), 15*(3), 410–415. https://doi.org/10.4183/aeb.2019.410

United States Census Bureau. (2020, March). *Current population survey: PINC-05. Work experience-people 15 years old and over, by total money earnings, age, race, Hispanic origin, sex, and disability status*. Retrieved September, 2021, from www.census.gov/data/tables/time-series/demo/income-poverty/cps-pinc/pinc-05.html

United States Government Accountability Office. (2022). *Women in the workforce: The gender pay gap is greater for certain racial and ethnic groups and varies by education level*. www.gao.gov/products/gao-23-106041

Upadhyay, R. P., Chowdhury, R., Salehi, A., Sarkar, K., Singh, S. K., Sinha, B., . . . Kumar, A. (2017). Postpartum depression in India: A systematic review and meta-analysis. *Bulletin of the World Health Organization, 95*(10), 706–717C. https://doi.org/10.2471/BLT.17.192237

Vasquez, M. J. (2007). Cultural difference and the therapeutic alliance: An evidence-based analysis. *American Psychologist, 62*(8), 878. https://doi.org/10.1037/0003-066X.62.8.878

Veisani, Y., Delpisheh, A., Sayehmiri, K., & Rezaeian, S. (2013). Trends of postpartum depression in Iran: A systematic review and meta-analysis. *Depression Research and Treatment, 2013*, 291029. https://doi.org/10.1155/2013/291029

Veisani, Y., & Sayehmiri, K. (2012). Prevalence of postpartum depression in Iran: A systematic review and meta-analysis. *The Iranian Journal of Obstetrics, Gynecology and Infertility, 15*(14), 21–29. https://doi.org/10.22038/ijogi.2012.5689

Wallerstein, N., & Duran, B. (2010). Community-based participatory research contributions to intervention research: The intersection of science and practice to improve health equity. *American Journal of Public Health, 100*(Suppl), S40–S46. https://doi.org/10.2105/AJPH.2009.184036

Wang, Z., Liu, J., Shuai, H., Cai, Z., Fu, X., Liu, Y., Xiao, X., Yang, B. X. (2021). Mapping global prevalence of depression among postpartum women. *Translational Psychiatry, 11*(1), 543. https://doi.org/10.1038/s41398-021-01663-6

Wardrop, A. A., & Popadiuk, N. E. (2013). Women's experiences with postpartum anxiety: Expectations, relationships, and sociocultural influences. *The Qualitative Report, 18*(3), 1–24. https://doi.org/10.46743/2160-3715/2013.1564

Waters, A. (2022). Racism is "at the root" of inequities in UK maternity care, finds inquiry. *BMC.* https://doi.org/10.1136/bmj.o1300

Watson, H., Harrop, D., Walton, E., Young, A., & Soltani, H. (2019). A systematic review of ethnic minority women's experiences of perinatal mental health conditions and services in Europe. *PloS One, 14*(1), e0210587. https://doi.org/10.1371/journal.pone.0210587

Wells, S. J., Merritt, L. M., & Briggs, H. E. (2009). Bias, racism and evidence-based practice: The case for more focused development of the child welfare evidence base. *Children and Youth Services Review, 31*(11), 1160–1171. https://doi.org/10.1016/j.childyouth.2009.09.002

World Health Organization. (2015). *Thinking healthy: A manual for psychosocial management of perinatal depression*. https://apps.who.int/iris/handle/10665/152936

World Health Organization. (2022). *WHO guide for integration of perinatal mental health in maternal and child health services*. www.who.int/publications/i/item/9789240057142

Zayas, L. H., Cunningham, M., McKee, M. D., Jankowski, K. R. (2002). Depression and negative life events among pregnant African-American and Hispanic women. *Womens Health Issues, 12*, 16–21. https://doi.org/10.1016/s1049-3867(01)00138-4

Zegeye, A., Alebel, A., Gebrie, A., Tesfaye, B., Belay, Y. A., Adane, F., & Abie, W. (2018). Prevalence and determinants of antenatal depression among pregnant women in Ethiopia: A systematic review and meta-analysis. *BMC Pregnancy and Childbirth, 18*(1), 462. https://doi.org/10.1186/s12884-018-2101-x

Zlotnick, C., Tzilos, G., Miller, I., Seifer, R., & Stout, R. (2016). Randomized controlled trial to prevent postpartum depression in mothers on public assistance. *Journal of Affective Disorders, 189*, 263–268. https://doi.org/10.1016/j.jad.2015.09.059

32

PERINATAL MENTAL HEALTH DISORDERS IN MIGRANT WOMEN

Brieanne Kidd Kohrt, Gwen Vogel Mitchell,
and Gretchen Heinrichs

Globally, over 140 million women give birth annually, an experience shaped by medical systems, family traditions, and cultural norms. Women experience a host of conflicting beliefs and expectations throughout pregnancy and motherhood, which is heightened for immigrant and refugee women living in cultural contexts outside their own. In this chapter, we use the stories of two women, Iman and Xitlaly, to highlight the unique challenges immigrant and refugee women experience as they navigate the perinatal period and consider how this impacts psychosocial well-being.

Iman

Iman is an 18-year-old woman who grew up in Somaliland. She is a devout Muslim from a family that practices religious and traditional ceremonies for important milestones. She grew up in a large family surrounded by siblings, grandparents, aunties, and cousins. At 17, she was married to Filsan, a 28-year-old engineer who has a green card to work in the United States and lives in Minneapolis. Iman's cousins in Minneapolis helped arrange their marriage. The couple had a traditional ceremony where Iman was celebrated by her female relatives with the decoration of henna. Iman underwent a virginity inspection by Filsan's aunt, and the couple then consummated the marriage, which Iman found painful and distressing ("I froze and left my body"). Following the ceremony, her family displayed the bloodied sheets as proof of her worth as a bride. Iman became pregnant on her wedding night, and in anticipation of the birth, Iman and her family organized a ceremony where they engaged in dances and incense burning. Iman gave birth to a boy, Abel, with the assistance of a midwife at a health facility.

Iman and Abel joined Filsan in Minnesota when Abel was one-year-old. Iman struggled to adjust to the large city and felt isolated due to her lack of English. Iman's family began pressuring her to send money home, so she took a part-time job at a meat-packing plant. She was four months pregnant with her second child and was concerned about how the hard labor might impact her baby. At her first prenatal check-up in the United States, she received a pelvic

---

DOI: 10.4324/9781003206903-38

exam, something she had never experienced before. When the practitioner realized Iman had had female circumcision, she called in a psychologist to consult on the case, which caused Iman great embarrassment and confusion.

Xitlaly

Xitlaly is a 20-year-old Guatemalan woman who identifies as Tz'utujil Mayan. She immigrated to the United States three years ago with the help of a coyote, with the goal of sending remittances to her family for her younger sibling's education. She moved in with her maternal aunt and got a job cleaning office buildings at night. She is undocumented and often works long shifts with no breaks. When Xitlaly was 18 years old, she became pregnant. Her partner, Manuel, is also Guatemalan. His mother insisted that Xitlaly come to live with her (the "suegra," or mother-in-law). Xitlaly's suegra forbid her from eating or drinking cold beverages or foods to protect the baby and found her a comadrona (midwife), who provided prenatal massage and advice. When Xitlaly was five months pregnant, she began to have sharp abdominal pains and bleeding while at work. Xitlaly's suegra urged her not to go to the hospital, stating, "when preparing to bring life, stay away from death." Her aunt rushed her to the hospital anyway, where Xitlaly was told she had a miscarriage. Xitlaly's aunt told her that the loss was God's will and that God would bless her with another child.

One year later, Xitlaly became pregnant again. She felt fearful and anxious throughout the pregnancy and often found herself daydreaming about what her first child would have been like. Xitlaly's daughter, Rosario, was born at home, with the assistance of Xitlaly's aunt, suegra, and the comadrona. Xitlaly and her daughter began the 40-day quarantine period (i.e., la cuarentena), during which her suegra and cousins tended to her and took care of the household responsibilities so Xitlaly could adjust to being a new mother. However, she struggled to feel a deep connection to Rosario, who cried "constantly." Her suegra told her that since Xitlaly was sad and distressed during her pregnancy, these feelings were passing to her daughter through her breastmilk. At Rosario's two-month check-up, Xitlaly became very overwhelmed and started crying. The nurse validated her distress, comforted her, and referred her to a nearby community mental health center.

Grounding Concepts

Migrant, Immigrant, Asylum Seeker, and Refugee

The terms *migrant, immigrant, asylum seeker*, and *refugee* are used throughout this chapter. These terms are primarily differentiated based on the motivators for leaving one's country and the status granted upon arrival. A *migrant* moves from one place to another; this movement can be within one's borders or to another country. The term, migrant, can also be used to encapsulate the larger group of all individuals living outside their country of birth, including immigrants, refugees, and asylum seekers (Anderson et al., 2017). For simplicity, we utilize the term migrant in this way throughout this chapter.

Individuals who decide to leave their country for a "better life," such as educational opportunities, higher-paid jobs, or access to specialized healthcare, and who can, in theory, return to their home country safely, are called *immigrants*. Individuals who flee their home country for their own safety, whether due to war, ethnic or tribal conflicts, climate disasters, or persecution based on their identity, status, or beliefs, can apply for international protection in another country. While awaiting this protected status, they are known as *asylees* or *asylum seekers*. If the government to whom they are petitioning decides their fear is credible (i.e., that it is not safe for them to go back to their home country), they are granted *refugee* status (International Rescue Committee, 2018).

What all migrant persons have in common is that they are living away from their home country and, thus, are isolated from familiar people, places, and practices. In the process of displacement, they experience the loss of cultural anchors, like religion, language, weather, holidays, food, and shared value systems. During the perinatal period, and especially for first-time mothers, the lack of these cultural anchors as they enter a sacred but stressful time can be the catalyst for perinatal mental health disorders (PMHDs).

Western, Eastern, Global South, and Global North

In this chapter, we employ the phrase *Global South* to refer to the regions where most migrant persons are leaving and *Global North* to describe where they typically migrate (see Figure 32.1). Global North is used instead of western, high-income, developed, or First World, though there is decidedly no perfect term for these distinctions (Litonjua, 2012). Global North countries are more likely to be democratic, capitalist, and individualistic, and offer more economic and educational opportunities. The Global North places a high value on personal freedom, achievement, and innovation. Countries in the Global South (previously referred to as Third World, developing, or low and middle income) tend to have more robust informal support networks due to a more collectivist worldview and sense of interdependence and connectedness (Hofstede, 2011). Conformity, humility, and individual sacrifice for the needs of the group are valued. Many Global South countries carry the legacy of oppression and exploitation from previous colonization by countries in the Global North (Badru, 2010; Crook et al., 2018).

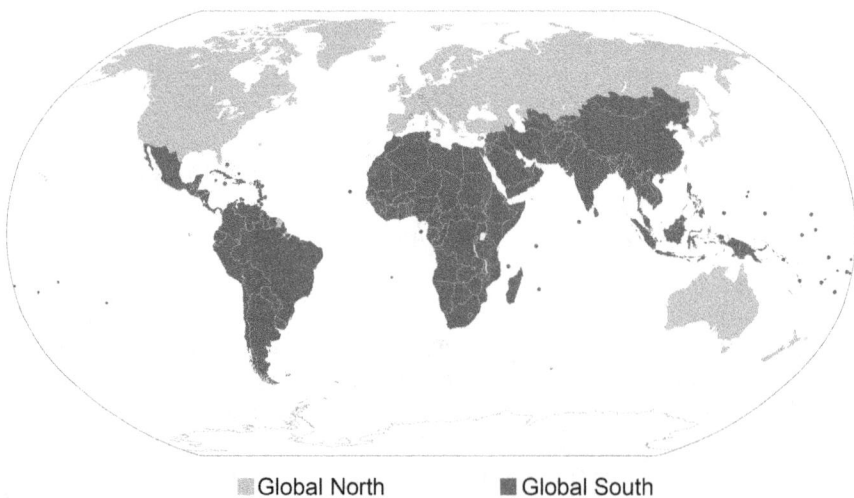

Global North   Global South

Figure 32.1 The Global North and South. Kingj123/Public Domain

Depression or Mala Leche? Considering Idioms of Distress and Explanatory Models of Illness

When describing perinatal psychological distress in women, clinicians in the Global North typically utilize diagnostic terms, such as depression, anxiety, or posttraumatic stress disorder (PTSD). However, these concepts often do not exist, are not culturally relevant, or carry significant stigma in the Global South. It is important that providers be aware of *idioms of distress*, or culturally resonant ways of experiencing, understanding, and communicating unpleasant emotions, troubling thoughts, or confusing behaviors (Nichter, 2010). Idioms of distress may be derived from salient metaphors or cultural explanatory models and allow members of sociocultural groups to convey suffering, pain, or imbalance to others in their community (Hinton & Lewis-Fernández, 2010). The *Diagnostic and Statistical Manual of Mental Disorders*, 5th edition (DSM-5; American Psychiatric Association, 2013) includes an appendix of cultural constructs and culture-bound syndromes that can be consulted when working with migrant patients. Here we will consider three that are significant for perinatal migrant women: *thinking too much, evil eye,* and *mala leche.*

"Thinking too much" has been documented across countries in Africa, Asia, Latin American and the Caribbean (Kaiser et al., 2015). Ethnographic studies of thinking too much in perinatal women in Indonesia (Widiana et al., 2018), Nigeria (Adeponle et al., 2017), Uganda (Sarkar et al., 2018), Nicaragua (Yarris, 2014), and Guatemala (Kohrt et al., 2022) find descriptions akin to rumination, with resulting symptoms of loss of appetite, trouble sleeping, sadness, low self-esteem, and social withdrawal. In South Africa, symptoms of thinking too much in perinatal women can also include headaches, stress, and muscle tension (Davies et al., 2016). Thinking too much may be reflective of unresolved trauma, as was found in a study of perinatal migrant Cambodian women (Hinton & Lewis-Fernández, 2010). In assessing for psychological distress in migrant women, it may be useful to start with a question such as "Have you noticed that recently you have been thinking too much?" and consider the impact of this experience on their well-being.

Another important idiom related to perinatal mental health is evil eye or *mal de ojo*, a widespread belief among Middle Eastern, Southeast Asian (especially Pakistan, India, and Bangladesh) and Latin American migrants. It is most common among people who identify as Muslim or practice Indigenous faiths (Khalifa et al., 2011). According to this belief, if someone gazes at someone else with envy, whether that be due to their health, beauty, or economic status, the envied person can become mentally or physically ill. Pregnant women, babies, and young children are especially vulnerable (Khalifa et al., 2011). Believers in evil eye may go to great lengths to ward off its powers with religious rituals or cultural practices. In Nepal, women might put their baby in a used or torn sari to make the baby seem less fortunate (Sharma et al., 2016). In Guatemala, babies deemed attractive and healthy often have garlic rubbed on their body or wear a garlic clove to ward off mal de ojo (Kohrt et al., 2022). Mothers may fear taking the baby out of the home because of evil eye, leading to a potential for increased anxiety and social isolation among postpartum migrant women. They may be labeled as noncompliant or neglectful by Global North providers if they miss required vaccinations or appointments due to this fear, leading to further disenfranchisement with the medical system. Those afflicted with evil eye will typically seek treatment from a religious or indigenous healer, thus integrating spiritual practice with medical care will be the most effective and relevant for perinatal women with this explanatory model of distress.

A final important idiom for consideration is *mala leche,* a term used in communities in Latin America, including Peru, Bolivia, Panama, Guatemala, and southern Mexico (Kohrt et al., 2022; Martínez et al., 2021), as well as in the Pacific Islands (Team et al., 2009). As seen in the case of Xitlaly, mala leche has various cultural interpretations and causes, with the central idea being that a mother's physical or psychological suffering can be transmitted to the baby during breastfeeding. Sadness during the perinatal period can cause the milk to go "bad" (mala), leading to such afflictions as colic, diarrhea, skin rashes, sadness, or anxiety in the baby. In the Philippines, there is a similar idea that a woman who is sad or angry should not breastfeed, as these moods are transmitted to the baby through breastmilk (*gatas*), and can cause diarrheal episodes (Team et al., 2009). This concept is important to understand in our discussion of perinatal depression in migrant women, as it can be another source of guilt for the mother, or may impact the desire to breastfeed, impacting attachment.

In some migrant women, it is less a specific idiom or cultural concept used to describe an experience akin to perinatal depression, but rather that sadness or distress might manifest somatically (Evagorou et al., 2016). This may be related to the shame and the stigma associated with mental illness, unfamiliarity with mental health diagnoses or psychosocial terminology, or a lack of differentiation between the experiences of the brain and body (Davies et al., 2016). Assessing for persistent pain or somatic complaints should be a routine part of psychosocial assessment with perinatal migrant women.

Providers can find it challenging to address the well-being of their migrant patients in a culturally grounded way due to a lack of a common language to describe distress. A thorough understanding of the key terms and concepts summarized earlier is a great starting point for all professionals seeking to be culturally affirming, and can help them connect with the lived experiences of their patients.

Prevalence of Perinatal Mental Health Disorders in Migrant Women

Rates of PMHDs in the Global South are double those of the Global South (Chowdhary et al., 2014; Clarke et al., 2013; Premji, 2014). A 2015 meta-analysis of 53 studies of perinatal migrant women living in the Global North found that approximately 20% of migrant women met criteria for a PMHD, suggesting that increased risk continues even after migration (Anderson et al., 2017). However, the range across studies was vast; prenatal depression prevalence ranged from 12% to 45%, and postpartum from 1% to 59%. This may be due to threats to cross-cultural validity, as migrant women may be unfamiliar with common diagnostic terms like depression and anxiety, and the symptoms found on behavioral health measures may not be culturally meaningful (Kohrt et al., 2011). Stigma may also contribute to underreporting, as expressing depression or anxiety symptoms can violate norms related to the sacred role of the mother (Tobin et al., 2018).

Across studies, higher depression scores were seen among migrants with low perceived levels of social support, marital strain, socioeconomic difficulty, precarious legal status, limited English proficiency, higher levels of acculturation, and higher stressful life events. Asylum-seeking women were 1.86 times more likely to meet criteria for PMHDs than immigrant or refugee women and also more likely to meet criteria for PTSD, with 48% meeting diagnostic criteria as compared to 34% among refugees and 15% among immigrants (Anderson et al., 2017).

In sum, migrant women appear to be at increased risk for PMHDs when compared to their nonmigrant counterparts, with rates higher for asylum-seeking women and for those facing additional stressors associated with acculturation, partner conflict, and socioeconomic strain. Further complicating migrant maternal well-being are the high rates of PTSD, especially given burgeoning research regarding how traumatic stress symptoms, especially those related to sexual trauma, can be activated during childbirth (Halvorsen et al., 2013).

Correlates and Risk Factors of PMHDs in Migrant Women

Although migrants are provided with opportunities not available in their home countries (e.g., job opportunities, family reunification, and upward mobility), they are also far from home, separated from social support systems, and may have endured traumatic experiences on their journey (e.g., Cook et al., 2015; Rettger et al., 2016). Loss of cultural traditions and community and confrontation with various forms of discrimination further complicate their ability to resettle. In this section, we explore how migration-related stressors impact perinatal mental health.

Pre-Migration Experiences

The factors that shape motives for relocation can influence the nature and complexities of migrant mental health. Reactive (push) migrants are forced to relocate and are pushed out of their home country due to political turmoil, conflict, war, natural disasters or religious persecution (Papademetriou & Fratzke, 2016). This may lead to a sense of powerlessness and helplessness, both risk factors for depression. Reactive migrants may be fleeing recruitment into gangs, and many have witnessed the death of close relatives. Migrant girls and women in particular may experience additional trauma, including forced sterilizations, female genital mutilation/cutting, sexual violence, forced marriage, forced prostitution and trafficking. Trauma experienced during the migration journey complicates their experience of escape. They may hide this trauma from their loved ones back home due to shame and guilt, and the expectation that if they survived the journey, they should be grateful.

Adjustment to the Host Country

After settling in the host country, most new-arrivals continue to experience migration-related stressors, such as documentation status, loss of power and primary identity, lack of language proficiency, and difficulty navigating day-to-day life in their new environment. People are most likely to migrate in their reproductive years (Desiderio, 2020), and pregnancy during this time serves as an additional obstacle to integration. For women who are newly arrived in the country, the loss of family and friends can result in the loss of connectedness and practical support, something we see in the case of Iman. Iman is deeply connected to and loves her country, culture, and community, but she also believes that raising her children in the United States is the best thing for their future. Her emotional state after arriving in the United States can be understood using the term *cultural bereavement*, which describes the "grief experience of the uprooted person resulting from loss of social structures, cultural values and self-identity" (Bhugra & Becker, 2005, p. 19). An examination of cultural bereavement using the *Cultural Formulation Interview* (CFI; Lewis-Fernández et al., 2015), described in more detail at the end of this chapter, can be useful when working with migrant women demonstrating psychosocial distress.

Pregnant migrant women, especially those who are undocumented, may also face unemployment, jeopardizing their ability to attain health insurance and appropriate prenatal care. If they can find work, it might be in positions that require a high degree of physical labor or have harsh working conditions such as excessive heat or exposure to toxic chemicals, long hours without breaks, and high production quotas (i.e., meat and poultry plants, as we saw in the case of Iman). They may experience gender-based discrimination in the workplace, such as policies limiting regular access to restroom facilities. The manner in which a person is able to manage bodily functions is at the core of human dignity (Stauffer, 2019). Furthermore, many cultures, including Japan, India, and Samoa, prohibit hard labor during pregnancy, especially in the third trimester. Pregnant migrants may find themselves forced to go against their cultural beliefs for economic survival, or, as in Iman's case, to be able to send remittances to their family back home. Women in the mosque have told Iman that working would be too stressful and cause harm to the baby, increasing her anxiety, and creating stress in her relationship with her husband.

Migrant women often keep the symptoms of depression private, which compounds their suffering (Tobin et al., 2018). Furthermore, stigma and structural barriers related to language, insurance, and navigating a foreign health system, make migrant women less likely to seek out or receive adequate mental health services. This increases the risk for severe illness, prolonged suffering, and functional impairment (Bohr et al., 2021).

Sexual and Reproductive Experiences

The mental health of women and girls cannot be separated from the cultural and societal expectations placed upon them. Gendered ideas and cultural practices surrounding virginity, female genital mutilation/cutting, early marriage, and unwanted or unplanned pregnancy may impact perinatal mental health in migrant women. Expectations for onset of intimate relationships vary greatly by culture. Certain ceremonies that celebrate the onset or transition to womanhood generally occur around ages 12 to 15, following the onset of menstruation. In some communities in the Global South, this milestone is marked by female genital mutilation/cutting (FGM/C), a practice involving alteration or partial removal of the external genitalia of the girl, usually the clitoral structures, labia minora or labia majora. Typically, the procedure is performed in childhood by traditional practitioners and without anesthesia. FGM/C can have a significant impact on the mental health of migrant women. One study estimates that a third of women with FGM/C meet criteria for depression, PTSD, or anxiety disorders (Knipscheer et al., 2015). Iman, for example, was circumcised as a child and has grown up hearing of "the three feminine sorrows," referring to the cultural expectation of pain due to FGM/C throughout life (the original cutting, the wedding night, and childbirth). Iman experienced pain and embarrassment as a child at her circumcision and on her wedding night, undergoing an exam by her husband's aunt and suffering through her first intercourse. She is also fearful of judgment by medical providers due to her FGM/C and concern they will not know how to manage it at delivery. This fear can present as somatization or generalized anxiety to a provider trained in the Global North. The discourse around women who have experienced FGM/C as "injured" or "mutilated" contributes to women feeling judged, ashamed, or embarrassed when interacting with providers. Medical visits requiring pelvic exams, discussions about sexual function, pregnancy care, labor and delivery, and pap smear or contraceptive visits may leave the woman feeling particularly anxious or traumatized and contribute to negative body image and poor sexual self-esteem (Johnsdotter, 2018; Palm et al., 2019).

Migrant girls who experience adolescence in a Global North country may encounter significant cultural dissonance regarding sexuality and dating in school, where they feel like outsiders. They fear repercussions from their traditional families, who venerate virginity and arranged marriages, if they engage in what their peers may consider normal adolescent sexual exploration. Moreover, migrant girls are particularly at risk for unintended pregnancy given that they are less likely to have access to or knowledge about reproductive healthcare, including contraception and abortion services (Deeb-Sossa & Billings, 2014; Ostrach, 2013). Unintended pregnancy increases the risk for perinatal depression, and threatens maternal psychological well-being and life satisfaction (Bahk et al., 2015).

Child marriage (marriage prior to age 18) is another important correlate of perinatal mental health. Each year, 14 million girls worldwide marry before age 18, a practice intimately linked to gender inequality and poverty. Societies that practice child or forced marriage may marry a girl to her future husband shortly after her first menstruation to ensure virginity (i.e., Afghanistan, India, parts of East and West Africa). Child marriage is associated with increased rates of physical and sexual intimate partner violence (Kidman, 2017), and concomitantly, depression, anxiety, and PTSD (Kennedy & Prock, 2018). Fleeing the violence may degrade the family's reputation and the girl may be disowned by her family or community. This shame and separation from support structures may contribute to depressive episodes, and has been linked to suicidal ideation (Forte et al., 2018). Behavioral health and medical providers should inquire about the mother's age at the time of marriage and first pregnancy using a neutral and nonjudgmental tone, and integrate screening for partner violence into routine prenatal care. Importantly, these practices do not just occur in the Global South. Since 2000, more than 200,000 children were married in the United States, most of whom were girls married to older men (Bohr et al., 2021; Tahirih Justice Center, 2017). While illegal in the United States, FGM/C is still practiced, usually in secret within religious sects, or girls are sent abroad in an illegal practice known as "vacation cutting" (Litonjua, 2012). Thus, when working with migrant women, even if they have been in the United States since childhood, it is still important to explore these issues.

Incongruence Between Traditional Beliefs and Host Country Beliefs

Childbirth is a socially marked and shaped experience, with each culture and subculture being ripe with "shoulds" and "should nots" for a woman during the perinatal period (Gottlieb & DeLoache, 201). In this section, we present questions about the key beliefs regarding the perinatal period across cultural groups, and consider how the discounting of these beliefs by providers in the Global North can lead to increased psychological distress for migrant women.

How Does the Community Conceptualize Pregnancy? In the Global North, pregnancy is often approached from a perspective of risk, which can be confusing and contradictory for pregnant migrant women. In the traditional medical model, prenatal care educates the woman and her family around pregnancy, birth, and the postpartum period, while screening for medical complications of pregnancy that put the fetus and woman at risk. In contrast, in many Global South communities, pregnancy is seen as a spiritual and natural event. The integration of medical care might be seen as unnecessary. In Mayan Guatemala, where Xitlaly and her suegra are from, pregnant women should avoid hospitals at all costs, as these are places of death and spiritual contamination, and may avoid traditional prenatal care for this reason. The reduced likelihood for accessing prenatal care is an important consideration when addressing PMHDs, as screening is typically conducted during prenatal check-ups. Clinics that are away from hospitals may be more approachable for migrant patients (Withers et al., 2018).

What Does the Community Believe Impacts the Baby's Well-being During the Perinatal Period? In many societies, the pregnant woman's body is highly valued and sacred, as the role of carrying a child is revered (Gottlieb & DeLoache, 2016). Religious beliefs may venerate the role of the mother as primordial, such as the idealization of the Virgin Mary in the value of *marianismo* among many Latin American Catholic migrants (Lara-Cinisomo et al., 2019). In countries where Buddhism is practiced, an unborn baby is seen as a sacred gift and as part of the cycle of birth, death, and rebirth. Significant responsibility is placed on the mother to protect the unborn baby from harm, including ghosts or demons, contamination (such as exposure to blood), or "malicious emotions" (Hopgood, 2012, p. 156). Across cultures, the pregnant woman's spiritual and psychological state is important, and maternal distress is perceived as causing negative outcomes for the unborn child. Team et al. (2009) described how, in Filipino tradition, birthmarks, physical defects, or genetic problems in newborns are typically attributed to unpleasant emotions experienced by mothers during pregnancy. In a study conducted among Tz'utujil Mayan women in Guatemala, "deep sadness" and "thinking too much" were said to result in colic or health concerns in babies (Kohrt et al., 2022). As we saw in the case of Xitlaly, the beliefs about the strong connection between a mother's emotional state and the baby's well-being can offer a sense of bonding for some, but may increase feelings of guilt, shame, or hopelessness for others. Inquiring about how the mother understands the relationship between her well-being and that of the baby's will be important when working with migrant women.

Migrant women and their families may process and understand adverse pregnancy outcomes or anomalies very differently than healthcare providers. For example, in Oaxaca, Mexico, pregnant women attach safety pins in the sign of a cross to their underwear during eclipses or full moons to prevent cleft palate (Marazita, 2012). Because unborn babies and infants are seen as especially vulnerable to evil spirits, developmental delays or genetic disorders may be attributed to supernatural causes, which in turn affects decisions about treatments and maintenance of pregnancy or termination. These traditional beliefs and practices might be dismissed by maternal health providers in the Global North. Receiving conflicting advice from family versus providers can be stressful and overwhelming for migrant women, which can increase conflict within the family. Xitlaly experienced this when she chose to go to the hospital after suffering a miscarriage, despite her mother-in-law's warnings.

Another important prenatal care belief seen across many communities outside the United States and Europe is related to what medical anthropologists refer to as the hot-cold theory of illness. While an oversimplification, this theory generally describes certain illnesses, foods, medications, and conditions as either "hot" or "cold." To restore balance in the body, hot foods, drinks, and medications are used to treat cold conditions, and vice versa. Traditionally, people in Latin America, The Philippines, China, Japan, and Taiwan view pregnancy as a cold condition, and, thus, cold drinks or foods, or foods with cold energy (such as dark foods in Taiwan), should be avoided. In many cultures, the immediate postpartum period is often seen as a cold state, wherein the concept of being vulnerable to either cold or wind is common. This can lead to prohibitions against showering to avoid exposure to cold and wind, a postpartum practice that can be confusing or contradictory for medical providers in the Global North (Small et al., 2014). In urging women to shower, or encouraging the consumption of foods or drinks discouraged culturally, perinatal women find themselves unanchored and forced to choose between respecting their cultural traditions or pleasing the medical authorities, causing anxiety and distress. A thorough assessment of perinatal beliefs (see the recommendations section of this chapter) will be a helpful starting point for providers working with migrant women.

Finally, for many migrant women from Asia, Latin America, and the Pacific Islands, the first 30 to 40 days postpartum are viewed as both a period of heightened spiritual and physical vulnerability for both mother and the baby and a crucial time for developing the maternal-infant bond. Female relatives may take over the housework, as we saw with Xitlaly's relatives, and provide the mother with a specific diet of foods believed to improve milk production, cleanse the womb, and "purge" impurities. Adherence to this time period of rest, referred to in Latin America as *cuarentena*, is thought to help prevent postpartum depression (Blackmore & Chaudron, 2014). A lack of universal paid maternity leave in the United States and strict infant vaccination timelines may jeopardize the ability of the mother and baby to respect this important cultural practice, which is tied to increased rates of perinatal depression for migrant women (Chen et al., 2012).

Who Supports the Woman During the Perinatal Period? The combination of the sacredness, spiritual vulnerability, and potential for humoral imbalance associated with pregnancy leads to the importance of community guidance and support during this period, a role almost exclusively taken on by other females in the community. In traditional patriarchal cultures that otherwise limit a woman's decision-making, pregnancy and birth are where women can assert their autonomy (Higginbottom et al., 2013). Women across the globe regularly consult with or are accompanied by different types of pregnancy guides. These can be spiritual guides, such as *shamans* in Hmong culture, or as we saw in the case of Xitlaly, the *comadronas* (midwives) in Central America and Mexico. Navaho tribes carry out blessing gatherings, where a pregnant woman receives massage and symbolic gifts from other women in the community, creating a sense of connectedness that prepares her emotionally, physically, and spiritually for childbirth (Pordié & Kloos, 2021). Within medical decision-making, if the voice and opinion of the expert support person(s) within the familial or community system is not elicited, migrant women may avoid or discount formal medical or mental healthcare. As seen in the case studies of Iman and Xitlaly, the presence of support women during birth is crucial to their well-being. When familial separation, restrictive hospital visitation, or family leave policies prevent her from receiving culturally necessary support, it can increase anxiety and depression.

What Are Their Beliefs About Medical Intervention During Birth? In the context of labor and delivery, the medical system in the Global North values minimizing maternal and fetal morbidity and mortality over optimizing patient experience. This leads to differing priorities for medical professionals compared to those of the expectant migrant mother and her family, increasing the likelihood for traumatic birth experiences (Watson et al., 2021). The most prominent risk factors for experiencing a traumatic birth include a lack of support in labor, negative subjective birth experience, operative delivery and dissociation (Ayers, 2017). Additionally, for those women who have experienced sexual trauma in their home country or during migration, birth can cause sensations of loss of bodily control that can be triggering (Muzik et al., 2016).

A collaborative patient/provider relationship may be undermined by a family's profound distrust of the medical system due to prior experience either in their home country or the Global North related to their migration status, inadequate insurance, lack of common language, or racism. Additionally, a belief that the pregnancy and its outcome are preordained or in the hands of a higher power may conflict with medical decision-making. Language barriers and health literacy gaps contribute to poor communication around medical recommendations, especially in the setting of obstetric emergencies. Many women worry about being subjected to unnecessary or unwanted interventions without consent, such as induction of labor, episiotomy, forceps or vacuum delivery, or cesarean delivery (Withers et al., 2018). These unfamiliar interventions may cause additional stress and anxiety.

Cesarean birth is another important consideration in the discussion of perinatal mental health of migrant women. Rates of postpartum depression increase when someone has a cesarean rather than a vaginal birth, with emergency cesarean associated with the highest postpartum depression scores on the *Edinburgh Postpartum Depression Scale* (EPDS; Meky et al., 2020). Furthermore, the migrant woman—and her community—may feel her identity as a woman is tied to her ability to deliver vaginally, increasing the risk for a sense of worthlessness and low self-esteem if a cesarean birth is required. Migrant patients may also fear forced or coerced sterilization at the time of surgery, a documented practice in much of the world. Given these perceived hidden risks of surgery, patients may be willing to accept fetal death or disability when a cesarean is offered or recommended, and the result may be a traumatic birth, perinatal loss, or other grief-inducing experience. Traumatic birth experiences such as these can profoundly impact maternal child bonding, and have been linked to anxiety, relationship and sexual dysfunction and fear of subsequent birth (Ayers, 2017).

Fertility, Infertility, and Perinatal Loss

Fertility is valued by most cultures as a means to promote and continue the lineage of ancestry, and is important in the preservation of cultural practices and traditions. *Infertility*, which is experienced by 10% to 14% of women worldwide, is defined as the inability to attain pregnancy after at least a year of regular sexual intercourse without contraception (Ombelet, 2020). For women all over the world, motherhood is essential to their identity and place in society; however for many women in the Global South, the inability to conceive is often seen as a "sin," or judgment on the couple (Cui, 2010; Inhorn & Van Balen, 2002). Women who do not have children may be ostracized, even if the underlying medical cause lies in their male partners. Infertility causes a loss of social status and can be grounds for divorce, returning of bride wealth, or to the man fathering a child with another woman. Infertility in migrant women has been tied to increased rates of anxiety and depression (Kazemi et al., 2021; Massarotti et al., 2019). Furthermore, concepts of fertility and "woman-ness" are strongly tied to organs such as the uterus, fallopian tubes, and ovaries. Many migrant women who require the removal of female organs for health reasons experience social stigmatization, and may also experience profound grief at the loss of their childbearing identity (Bakare & Gentz, 2020). This is an important area for clinical exploration when working with migrant women.

Pregnancy loss is another significant risk factor for psychological distress. Rates of pregnancy loss are higher among migrant women living in Europe and the United States as compared to their nonmigrant counterparts. The highest rates are seen in refugees and asylum seekers from North Africa, Asia, and the Middle East (Heslehurst et al., 2018). Whether the loss is due to a miscarriage, stillbirth, or abortion, the loss of a child in utero causes a significant grief reaction. How a migrant woman and her community define or understand what a baby *is* has an impact on what this reaction might look like. For example, in Uganda, a stillborn is referred to as *empuna* or *ekintu* (a thing, not fully human;

Kiguli et al., 2015), and because a stillborn has never cried, it cannot be buried in a cemetery because it cannot communicate with the spirit world. A mock grave might be created outside the mother's home, but the mother typically cannot attend the burial. One mother described this practice as a way to "taunt families rather than honor the baby's memory" (Kiguli et al., 2015, p. 19). The mother is to grieve silently to show that she is strong enough to be blessed with another baby; she is often urged to forget and avoid intense grief. The lack of social validation of this loss can lead to complicated grief, a powerful correlate of depression (Grauerholz et al., 2021).

This idea of "weeping in silence" has been echoed in studies from Africa and the Middle East (Haws et al., 2010; Sisay et al., 2014), where women are typically not allowed to see or hold their deceased baby (Kuti & Ilesanmi, 2011). Soon after the loss, the mother is not to talk about the deceased child anymore, as this is seen as jeopardizing her physical and spiritual recovery. This contrasts with many Global North countries where there has been a push to break the silence regarding pregnancy loss, and where the practice of holding, naming, and sharing photos of a stillborn child have been found to be fundamental to healthy grieving (Leon, 2017). According to contemporary grief theories, seeing the body of the deceased is crucial to accepting the reality of the loss, and that experiencing the pain of grief is necessary to adaptation and healing. The stifling of this reaction, as may be required by cultural norms for some migrant women, correlates with impaired psychosocial functioning long-term (Worden, 2015). Practitioners should ask the woman and her support system what is normative in their community or religious tradition after perinatal loss while also offering the same options for both migrant and nonmigrant mothers. Providing information about the cause of death to the mother and support system can help reduce the potential for blame being placed on the mother (Team, et al., 2009). This blame can lead to a loss of social support, a significant risk factor across cultures for perinatal depression (Fellmeth et al., 2021; Racine et al., 2020).

Finally, in considering pregnancy loss, grief, and perinatal mental health, we must consider how bereavement is a deeply cultural experience. Culture, religion, stage of pregnancy, and social scripts all impact how grief is expressed. Whereas crying is an "expected" reaction, some women may engage in behaviors that do not align with Anglican expectations for emotional control and restraint. Women may shout, scream, rock, pull at their hair, bite their hands, or be completely silent. Family members may chant or recite passages from the Quran or bible. All grief reactions are valid; however, in working with migrant women, there can be a tendency for providers from the Global North to be alarmed by "extreme" grief reactions, or "loud" bereavement practices. This can result in measures like calling security or reducing the number of family allowed in a patient's room. This experience of having your grief punished, rather than witnessed, has been termed "suffocated grief," and is rooted in systems of oppression and discrimination. The suffocated griever silences themselves to avoid penalty, at the expense of their own well-being (Bordere, 2019). This has been tied to depression in Black women in the United States and is a concept that practitioners should keep in mind when supporting migrant mothers who have experienced perinatal loss.

Impact of PMHDs in Migrant Women on Their Children and Families

The economic and human costs of PMHDs are particularly alarming because they extend to the next generation. In the Global South, infants of mothers with PMHDs are more likely to be born premature and of low birth weight, have more diarrheal episodes, have lower rates of vaccination, and have higher rates of stunting (Premji, 2014; Chowdhary et al., 2014). As they get older, these same children often show deficits in social, cognitive, and psychological domains, and they are at increased risk for both internalizing and externalizing disorders (Premji, 2014). Migrant women with PMHDs may have difficulty breastfeeding, are less likely to seek treatment for infant medical needs, and have more inconsistent and avoidant parenting styles, increasing the risk for insecure attachment. The presence of another healthy and reliable adult figure in the children's lives such as a father, grandmother, auntie, or older sibling can help buffer this risk; unfortunately, migrant women are less likely to have this extended family support. Father involvement in newborn care was found to have a positive impact on maternal mental health in studies conducted in Korea, Taiwan, Pakistan, Bangladesh, Peru, India, Ethiopia, Kenya, and Taiwan, and appears to buffer the relation between maternal depression and negative child developmental outcomes (Duan et al., 2020; Knopp, 2017; Laurenzi et al., 2021). Unfortunately, the reverse was also found to be true. In a study conducted in Pakistan; increased duration of poor maternal mental health predicted lower levels of father involvement (Maselko et al., 2019).

Increased marital discord and conflict can occur within families of depressed women, and can lead to paternal depression (Fillo et al., 2015). For example, a 2020 study from Wuhan, China found a correlation between maternal postpartum depression, mother-in-law and daughter-in-law relationship satisfaction, maternal and paternal marital satisfaction, and paternal depression (Duan et al., 2020). These findings suggest that it is important for future PMHD interventions to target both maternal and paternal mental health. Doing so through a parenting program that also teaches skills for play, interaction, and newborn care may reduce stigma and buffer the impact of PMHDs on child development.

Culturally Affirming Treatment Recommendations

Clinicians working with perinatal migrant women are not expected to be experts on all the cultural practices and traditions of the migrant woman's host culture that may be affecting her psychosocial well-being; in fact, assuming belief systems and potential concerns based on identity is antithetical to patient-centered culturally affirming practice. However, doing some background research on a specific cultural group demonstrates interest, respect, and a genuine desire to connect. This type of information can be found in the Refugee Health Profiles published by the Centers for Disease Control and Prevention (United States): www.cdc.gov/immigrantrefugeehealth/profiles/index.html the Cultural Profiles published by Queensland Health (Australia): www.health.qld.gov.au/multicultural/health_workers/cultdiver_guide, the Best Practices for Treating Diverse Populations from the American Psychiatric Association: www.psychiatry.org/psychiatrists/cultural-competency/education/best-practice-highlights, and the Refugee Background resources developed by the Cultural Orientation Resource Center: www.culturalorientation.net/learning/backgrounders. Another option for learning more about a specific cultural group is to speak with a cultural broker, defined as someone who is well immersed in both mainstream culture and in his or her own ethnic culture (Brar-Josan & Yohani, 2014). Many interpreter networks also provide cultural brokering services.

After learning more about the specific identity group and country the client is from, there are additional practices that a clinician can engage in to improve access, quality, and appropriateness of psychosocial services for migrant women. Figure 32.2 is a noncomprehensive list that can serve as a starting point to becoming a culturally affirming practitioner.

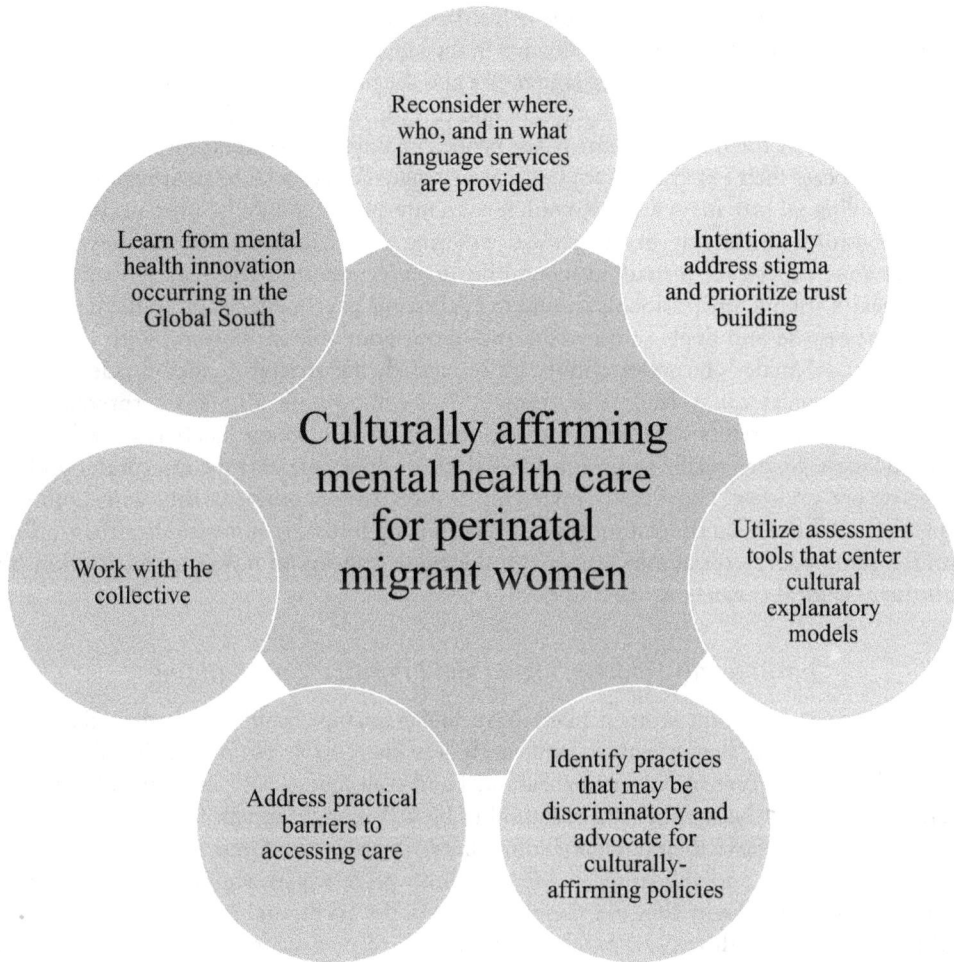

Figure 32.2   Culturally affirming mental healthcare for perinatal migrant women

Reconsider Where, Who, and in What Language Services Are Provided

Many migrant women may be hesitant to access prenatal health services that are hospital-based, in part due to potential superstitious beliefs about hospitals being associated with death. Providing options for in-home, telehealth, or integrated health services may be ideal in reaching migrant women. Connecting with immigrant and refugee-serving agencies and religious institutions in your community is a good first step, whether to provide referral information, or offer to host workshops or support groups at their locations. When individuals are in a trusted space, and are presented to the provider by someone they know and trust, they may be more likely to share, engage, and seek additional support.

After addressing the *where*, it is important to consider *who* is providing the service. Providers who are bilingual in the migrant woman's language and the language of the host country can provide the highest level of care. Second language competencies are lowest when one is stressed, sick, or emotionally distraught (Altarriba, 2002; Caldwell-Harris, 2015). Furthermore, memories for events are often encoded in the language in which they occurred, and the neural pathways connecting the language center and the limbic system is stronger when one is speaking in their native language (Ayçiçegi-Dinn & Caldwell-Harris, 2009; Caldwell-Harris, 2015). Thus, even for migrant women are proficient English speakers, the ability to code-switch or process their experiences in their native language is crucial to treatment success.

When bilingual providers are not available, an interpreter should be present. It is important to consult with the interpreter prior to entering the treatment space, as they may not have previous experience providing mental health interpretation and may have their own mental health stigma. Professionals should provide some psychoeducation to the interpreter about the purpose and goals of the visit, and about your role in working with the client. If available, a female interpreter should be requested; the stricter gender divide in many migrant communities may lead to discomfort in speaking with a male interpreter. When working with interpreters who speak a rare or uncommon language, such as an indigenous or tribal language, or specific geographical dialect, it is possible that the interpreter and client know one another. Thoroughly reviewing and revisiting confidentiality with both parties will be useful. Given the importance of relationship building in mental health, working with the same interpreter across sessions (if the client appears to have a good relationship with them) is ideal (Leanza et al., 2014).

Intentionally Address Stigma and Prioritize Trust Building

Whereas perinatal migrant women likely have higher mental health needs than their non-migrant counterparts, they are also significantly less likely to access mental health services, or only do so in the case of emergency. Schmied and colleagues (2017) described how many migrant women fear being labeled a bad mother by accessing treatment for perinatal depression or bringing shame to their family or community. One way to address this stigma is to start by explicitly naming and validating it. Mental health professionals should provide psychoeducation on their role, why they are there to speak to the client, and acknowledge that there might be some fear or distrust of psychologists and allied professionals. Utilizing the *Coping and Help-Seeking* and the *Patient-Clinician Relationship* sections of the *Cultural Formulation Interview* (Lewis-Fernández et al., 2015) can be a good way to open this conversation to determine if seeing a mental health provider might cause ostracization within the community. Furthermore, migrants from countries with internal conflict, ongoing war, or severe economic inequality may not trust health professionals, as they may be viewed as representatives of corrupt governments. The explanation of who ones work for and what one's work entails an important part of this psychoeducation when working with migrant women and families.

Other minor linguistic adaptations can help reduce stigma; for example, replacing the term "therapist" with "helper," "teacher," or "companion" increases buy-in in culturally adapted evidence-based treatments. Similarly, changing the word "therapy" to "training," "consults," or "visits" can also be helpful (Domenech Rodríguez et al., 2011; McCabe et al., 2005). Finally, trust building with migrant women, especially those from collectivist cultures in the Global South, may require a loosening of rigid "professional" ideas from the Global North prohibiting self-disclosure and prioritizing strict boundaries in therapeutic settings. Informal chatting, appropriate levels of self-disclosure, especially as it relates to one's family, and acceptance of small gestures or gifts can be fundamental to engagement in treatment (Duden & Martins-Borges, 2021; Phiri et al., 2019).

Utilize Assessment Tools That Center Cultural Explanatory Models

The authors of this chapter highly recommend two excellent tools for engaging in culturally affirming clinical interviewing with migrant women: The first is called the *Cultural Formulation Interview* (CFI; Lewis-Fernández et al., 2015), a semi-structured interview for systematically assessing cultural factors in the clinical encounter. Questions cluster around themes of identity (and how intersectional identities contribute to their current psychological state), cultural conceptualizations of distress, sociocultural risk and resilience factors, and cultural features of the relationship between the individual and the clinician. Clinicians are prompted to consider the client's experiences of racism and discrimination in the larger society and how this may impede trust building. The CFI section, *Cultural Definition of the Problem*, can be used to gather idioms of distress or assess for culture-bound syndromes. In the context of perinatal migrant women, clinicians may also ask specific questions about "thinking too much," evil eye, and mala leche. Such questions as, "Have you noticed that recently you have been thinking too much?" "how has your body been reacting to the problems you are experiencing right now?" and "How do you think these feelings might be impacting your unborn child/baby? Do you have any concerns about the impact on breastfeeding?" might be especially relevant. The CFI is available in 23 languages, https://nyculturalcompetence.org/resources/cfi-translations/. Supplementary modules have also been developed for specific populations, such as children and adolescents, elderly individuals, and immigrants and refugees, the latter of which is especially relevant for this chapter.

The second indispensable resource is called *Cultural Dimensions of Pregnancy, Birth and Postnatal Care*, developed by Queensland Health (Team et al., 2009). The guide addresses key factors influencing the health and illness experiences of patients from multicultural backgrounds, including language and communication styles, explanatory models of health and illness, knowledge and familiarity with health system and procedures within health services, complementary and alternative treatments, spirituality and religion, family and community, gender and modesty, diet and food preferences, pain and disability, and the impact of trauma on expression of illness and distress. This handbook has specific resources dedicated to working with Muslim, Hindu, or Sikh patients, provides a thorough list of languages spoken by country, and has a chapter dedicated to cultural dimensions of pregnancy, birth, and postpartum care.

Identify Practices That May Be Discriminatory Toward Migrant Families and Advocate for Culturally Affirming Policies

The culturally affirming clinician recognizes that their role goes beyond the therapeutic space and requires advocating for policy change. This can be at the organization level, such as advocating for more flexible visitation policies in labor and delivery spaces, or at the local or national government level. For example, providers in the United States can advocate for paid parental leave or for increased employment protections for undocumented workers. Becoming part of the policy task forces of one's jurisdiction's professional organization is a good starting place for this work. On a micro level, providers can re-examine their settings with a critical eye in terms of potential barriers to culturally affirming care. Something as simple as providing access to video technology in post-birth suites to assist new mothers in connecting with family back home can make a substantial difference in reducing a sense of isolation. In the case of perinatal loss and associated grief experiences, providers working in hospital settings can educate hospital staff about the concept of suffocated grief, and ensure that all families are supported, rather than punished, during their grief process. Small steps like these can make a huge difference.

Work with the Collective

As mentioned throughout this chapter, many migrant women come from collectivist societies where existence is interdependent. Even if a migrant woman is interested in services, her partner or extended family may discourage or prohibit this. It is important from the start to provide services to the collective, rather than the individual, with starts with identifying and consulting with the migrant woman's support network. The CFI supplementary module on *Social Network* can guide this process. Support persons can be integrated into psychoeducation regarding services and enlisted as collaborative treatment partners.

Group-based or peer support models may also be more appropriate for perinatal migrant women. One example of this is the ALMA peer support model from the University of Colorado, which trains mothers who have faced depression in their own lives to be "acompañantes" (companions) to perinatal Latinx women experiencing sadness, loneliness, anxiety, or depression. Acompañantes learn simple behavioral activation techniques and basic helping skills, which are delivered over the course of six to eight sessions done in the client's home. Presently this program is delivered in English and Spanish only, but a similar model could be replicated in other settings and communities. Because the facilitators are mothers who themselves faced depression, the participants see a story of recovery and relatability. Initial studies of the ALMA program have found high acceptability for the peer-delivered model from both mothers and healthcare providers (Vanderkruik & Dimidjian, 2019). More information about the ALMA program and the ongoing pilot studies of efficacy can be found here: https://valleysettlement.org/programs/alma/

Another evidence-based program for perinatal depression is called the *Thinking Healthy Program* (World Health Organization, 2015). Initially developed in Pakistan and now piloted in numerous countries in the Global South, this 16-session in-home program is delivered by local community health workers. The program builds buy-in by focusing on the well-being of the baby, emphasizing how maternal mental health is crucial to optimal physical and socioemotional development. It is based in cognitive behavioral therapy (CBT) and includes instruction in relaxation techniques, attachment-promoting behaviors, and skills for improving one's support system. Family members are invited to participate in sessions. The program has shown efficacy in reducing depressive symptoms, increasing maternal functioning, increasing birth spacing, and increasing paternal involvement in childcare (Turner et al., 2016). It is simple and visual and gives women the tools to heal themselves in a manner congruent with collectivist values.

Group-based programs, such as the *Mothers and Babies Course* (Muñoz et al., 20), may also be especially feasible and beneficial for migrant women. This program is described as a course, rather than group therapy to reduce stigma, and focuses on enhancing mood-management skills and maternal self-efficacy in mothers-to-be, while also creating a supportive community of other expecting mothers. A randomized control trial of the program found reduced depressive symptoms and increased social support (Le et al., 2011).

Workshops or programs specifically directed at the family members or kinship networks of migrant perinatal women is another important consideration. An ethnographic study of Middle Eastern migrant women revealed how participants desired educational programming for their close family about postpartum depression. One migrant woman in the study described "*I hope that they will include husbands and especially my mother and mother-in-law in this education program so that they will also know about this condition. They will be more understanding, and they will not call me crazy or bad mother*" (Schmied et al., 2017, p. 17).

Address Practical Barriers to Accessing Care

Once perinatal migrant women have accepted or sought out care, their ability to complete treatment can be jeopardized by a number of practical and economic barriers. Migrant women may be preoccupied with obtaining visas, securing employment and housing, learning English, and ensuring their children have access to education and healthcare services. Their own mental health is likely at the bottom of the to-do-list, if it is present at all. To increase motivation for and retention in psychosocial services, providers can consider changing the focus. Women and their families can rally around the well-being of the child, even when significant distrust of mental health or stigma is present. This is a good starting place for buy-in to mental health treatment. Providing psychoeducation about the impact on the child's well-being (in a nonshaming way) is important. Models for how to do this can be found in the *Thinking Healthy Program* or the *Mothers and Babies Course* mentioned previously.

In addition to building engagement and commitment from the family, reducing practical barriers is necessary. Providers should speak with their agencies about securing transportation and caregiving services for mothers when accessing mental health support. The simplest way to do this is through group interventions, where childcare providers can serve multiple families at once. Providing documentation showing that a person was receiving services so that they can be excused from work, and small incentives to help offset the cost of lost work when attaining services (like grocery store coupons or international calling cards) also improves treatment retention.

Learn From Mental Health Innovation Occurring in the Global South

Often, working with immigrants, refugees, and cultural or ethnic minorities in the Global North has focused too much on trying to adapt interventions developed in the WEIRD world (White, Educated, Industrial, Rich, Democratic; Li et al., 2021) to non-WEIRD people. However, this approach discounts all the incredible work being done in the Global South to promote mental health, including stigma reduction campaigns, play-based approaches, participatory models, and task-sharing paradigms. Clinicians working with migrant and refugee clients are encouraged to review existing perinatal mental health interventions with evidence in the migrant's host community or culture. This information can be accessed through the Mental Health Innovations website: www.mhinnovation.net/innovations.

Closing

We hope that this chapter has provided some insight into the challenges, strengths, and cultural considerations that can arise when working with migrant women during the perinatal period. The sustained presence of distress in perinatal migrant women and the expression of their symptoms should be understood, in part, as a function of the cultural, structural, and racial dynamics of the contexts of daily life and one's environment. Treatment should be informed by examining the intersections of personhood, culture, and context, as well as the congruence (or incongruence) between these and the host environment. When working with perinatal migrant women, it is crucial to examine both positive and negative aspects of one's homeland and host culture, while also exploring how cultural bereavement impacts mental health. We close this chapter by revisiting the case studies of Iman and Xitlaly to provide specific ideas for how clinicians could have provided culturally affirming care.

Iman

One of the best ways to promote the mental health and psychosocial well-being of Iman is by focusing on her healthcare team. One of Iman's first encounters with the U.S. health system is when she presented with is a pelvic exam. For someone from a traditional Muslim community, the discussion of sex is potentially taboo. Her care team needs to slow down the typical examination and care process and start by building trust and providing psychoeducation about the U.S.-based medical system, especially as it relates to perinatal care. Thoroughly explaining and assessing for understanding and consent for each procedure will help reduce anxiety. Providers may also engage in culturally affirming self-disclosure regarding their identity status and previous experience (or lack of) in working with someone from her community. They can help Iman to understand that they want to learn from her about common perinatal practices and beliefs, but also about her anxieties and fears regarding this process. The use of the Multicultural Clinical Support Resource chapter entitled "Cultural Dimensions of Pregnancy, Birth, and Postnatal Care" mentioned previously can help to guide this conversation.

It is important for mental health providers consulting with medical professionals to highlight the importance of addressing FGM/C directly. Above all, providers should aim to provide respectful, patient-centered care without perpetuating victimization. Due to the social and cultural stigma surrounding this practice, many women have difficulty bringing up the subject, fearing practitioners' ignorance, reactions, and judgment. Working with an interpreter can exacerbate this fear, as they may also be concerned about the interpreter telling others in their community. Conversations about limits of confidentiality should be ongoing with Iman and her interpreter.

In discussing her FGM/C, symptoms of trauma from the procedure itself, or from other aspects of her migration and acculturation process, might surface in Iman. Linkages to mental health providers should be done via "warm hand-offs" and should include significant normalization of the role of mental health in prenatal care in the United States to reduce stigma. Mental health providers should seek consultation around FGM/C and may start by reviewing the article, *Psychological and counseling interventions for female genital mutilation* (Smith & Stein, 2017).

Clinicians should explore Iman's explanatory models for mental distress and any cultural idioms of distress and resilience that capture her lived experience. The use of the CFI in the initial encounter with Iman can facilitate this conversation in a culturally affirming way. The social and cultural stigma surrounding depression, grief, and mental illness in her country suggests it may take time and the establishment of a therapeutic alliance to truly get to the root of her distress. It will be helpful to incorporate strategies discussed in the previous section to reduce stigma, such as by replacing mental health terms, taking time to build a relationship through chatting and appropriate self-disclosure, and providing psychoeducation that normalizes and validates her experience.

Furthermore, Iman is moving from a place where she was surrounded by support from other women, and where cultural traditions helped to mark life transitions. She may be feeling rootless and overwhelmed in the host country and may demonstrate symptoms consistent with cultural bereavement. She may benefit especially from treatments that help her to rebuild her support system, such as working with peer mentors who can connect her to others in her community, or group interventions for new mothers.

Xitlaly

Xitlaly may encounter the mental health system if she were to receive a nurse home visit at two weeks postpartum, as is common in many hospital systems in the Global North. This may include a screening for postpartum depression. It is unlikely that Xitlaly will be alone for this conversation, and she may not feel comfortable discussing her emotional state in front of her mother-in-law or other family members. Furthermore, given that Xitlaly identifies as Guatemalan, it is likely that clinicians working with her will request the services of a Spanish interpreter; however, Xitlaly may be most comfortable speaking in Tz'utujil, her Mayan language. The CFI supplementary module on cultural identity would be an excellent place to start, as it includes an in-depth discussion of language preferences and identity.

If a referral is made for mental health follow-up, the inclusion of Xitlaly's mother-in-law and aunt in this process is crucial. These women, more than Xitlaly, are the primary decision makers with regard to seeking care and will likely have the final say on whether Xitlaly should attain mental health services. The clinician should provide in-depth psychoeducation on the role of mental health and who benefits from services (addressing myths about these services being for "crazy" people) and center the discussion around a shared goal: the development and health of the newborn baby. Utilizing the Explanatory Model section of the CFI with Xitlaly and her mother-in-law and aunt could be a way to facilitate a discussion among the women, and build trust by showing respect for their worldview.

Xitlaly would likely benefit from a group treatment approach, perhaps focusing on stress relief, newborn care, and fundamentals of attachment. Individual therapy, where she could share openly her fears and feelings of disconnection without fear of being judged by others, and address the unresolved grief related to her pregnancy loss, would also be useful. She may benefit from grief-oriented exercises, like making a memory box for her lost pregnancy, or creating an oral or written letter to the child she lost. Spending time with Xitlaly to understand Mayan beliefs around perinatal loss and bereavement rituals will also be important, as well as encouraging dialectical feeling (e.g., she can both mourn for her lost baby and feel excitement about her life with Rosario). A gentle and supportive discussion regarding *mala leche* can be approached from a starting point of asking how she thinks her current emotional state might be impacting her daughter.

Conclusion

While the learning curve in providing support to perinatal migrant women may be steep, the growth potential as a clinician, and as a person, is immeasurable. Being invited into someone's story of migration, and helping them to heal as they embark on the journey of motherhood, is an honor.

Positionality Statements

We offer these positionality statements so that the reader can understand that the information summarized and interpreted in this chapter is not without bias. We welcome feedback on our paths to decolonizing mental health and improving psychosocial care for perinatal migrant women.

Brieanne Kidd Kohrt:	I am a White, Cisgender woman from a rural community. I was raised by parents who both work in health professions, who value biomedical sources of knowledge, and who are members of the L.G.B.T.Q. community. I am a child clinical psychologist who works primarily with Spanish-speaking families, and I engage in community-based research focused on improving mental health services for Latinx immigrants to the United States. I have been involved in mental health capacity building projects in Guatemala and Peru since 2010, with a focus on perinatal depression and interpersonal trauma. Given that I am not a member of the community that I serve, I strive to be culturally responsive, but am acutely aware of how the deep roots of White Privilege and the long legacy of Colonialism influence my ideas. In contributing to this chapter, I hope to highlight the experience of marginalized migrant voices, while recognizing the inherent flaw in this task being undertaken by a person of my identity.
Gwen Vogel Mitchell:	I am a Euro-American White cisgender woman who has worked in hospitals, private practice spaces and community-based organizations around the world in positions of authority as a clinical psychologist engaged in mental health and psychosocial support and capacity building. As an outsider to the communities I have aimed to serve, I want to acknowledge there have been times I have overlooked my personhood including my membership status in relation to clients our projects have aimed to serve. I am committed to making up for that, and I am working toward decolonizing my practice and centering the voices of historically marginalized individuals and healing practices. As a mother, I would like to center and celebrate all the ceremonies and traditions that honor women during pregnancy and childbirth. The Global North can learn much from these practices and traditions.

Gretchen Heinrichs:	I am a Euro-American White cisgender woman and first-generation physician. I have worked my whole professional career as an obstetrician/gynecologist in a safety net institution in Denver Colorado, while working in global health to learn from students, residents, colleagues, and patients in India, Mexico, Rwanda, Nigeria, Guatemala, and The Philippines. I have sought to correct disparities and inequality in education, knowledge transfer, access to quality healthcare, and the immigration systems through my clinical and global health work. My work conducting medical asylum evaluations with women who have experienced FGM/C has been humbling, and illuminated the value of rejecting stereotypes and expectations related to gender, culture, race, and ethnicity. I am committed to correcting my biases, learning from each patient, and addressing the cultural dominance that I have benefitted from. I offer this chapter as a tribute to the lessons learned from my teachers along this path.

References

Adeponle, A., Groleau, D., Kola, L., Kirmayer, L. J., & Gureje, O. (2017). Perinatal depression in Nigeria: Perspectives of women, family caregivers and health care providers. *International Journal of Mental Health Systems, 11*(1), 1–13.

Altarriba, J. (2002). Bilingualism: Language, memory, and applied issues. *Online Readings in Psychology and Culture, 4*(2), 1–10.

American Psychiatric Association. (2013). *Diagnostic and statistical manual of mental disorders* (5th ed.). American Psychiatric Association. https://doi.org/10.1176/appi.books.9780890425596

Anderson, F. M., Hatch, S. L., Comacchio, C., & Howard, L. M. (2017). Prevalence and risk of mental disorders in the perinatal period among migrant women: A systematic review and meta-analysis. *Archives of Women's Mental Health, 20*(3), 449–462.

Ayçiçegi-Dinn, A., & Caldwell-Harris, C. L. (2009). Emotion-memory effects in bilingual speakers: A levels-of-processing approach. *Bilingualism: Language and Cognition, 12*(3), 291–303.

Ayers, S. (2017). Birth trauma and post-traumatic stress disorder: The importance of risk and resilience. *Journal of Reproductive and Infant Psychology, 35*(5), 427–430.

Badru, P. (2010). Ethnic conflict and state formation in post-colonial Africa: A comparative study of ethnic genocide in the Congo, Liberia, Nigeria, and Rwanda-Burundi. *Journal of Third World Studies, 27*(2), 149–169.

Bahk, J., Yun, S.-C., Kim, Y., & Khang, Y.-H. (2015). Impact of unintended pregnancy on maternal mental health: A causal analysis using follow up data of the Panel Study on Korean Children (PSKC). *BMC Pregnancy and Childbirth, 15*(1), 85.

Bakare, K., & Gentz, S. (2020). Experiences of forced sterilisation and coercion to sterilise among women living with HIV (WLHIV) in Namibia: An analysis of the psychological and socio-cultural effects. *Sexual and Reproductive Health Matters, 28*(1), 335–348.

Bhugra, D., & Becker, M. A. (2005). Migration, cultural bereavement and cultural identity. *World Psychiatry, 4*(1), 18–24.

Blackmore, E. R., & Chaudron, L. (2014). Psychosocial and cultural considerations in detecting and treating depression in Latina perinatal women in the United States. In S. Lara-Cinisomo and K. L. Wisner (Eds.), *Perinatal depression among Spanish-speaking and Latin American women* (pp. 83–96). Springer.

Bohr, Y., Bimm, M., Bint Misbah, K., Perrier, R., Lee, Y., Armour, L., & Sockett-DiMarco, N. (2021). The crying clinic: Increasing accessibility to infant mental health services for immigrant parents at risk for peripartum depression. *Infant Mental Health Journal*, 42(1), 140–156.

Bordere, T. C. (2019). Suffocated grief, resilience and survival among African American families. In M. H. Jacobsen & A. Petersen (Eds.) *Exploring Grief* (pp. 188–204). Routledge.

Brar-Josan, N., & Yohani, S. C. (2014). A framework for counsellor-cultural broker collaboration. *Canadian Journal of Counselling and Psychotherapy*, 48(2), 81–99.

Caldwell-Harris, C. L. (2015). Emotionality differences between a native and foreign language: Implications for everyday life. *Current Directions in Psychological Science*, 24(3), 214–219.

Chen, T.-L., Tai, C.-J., Wu, T.-W., Chiang, C.-P., & Chien, L.-Y. (2012). Postpartum cultural practices are negatively associated with depressive symptoms among Chinese and Vietnamese immigrant mothers married to Taiwanese men. *Women & Health*, 52(6), 536–552.

Chowdhary, N., Sikander, S., Atif, N., Singh, N., Ahmad, I., Fuhr, D. C., . . . Patel, V. (2014). The content and delivery of psychological interventions for perinatal depression by non-specialist health workers in low and middle income countries: A systematic review. *Best Practice & Research Clinical Obstetrics & Gynaecology*, 28(1), 113–133.

Clarke, K., King, M., & Prost, A. (2013). Psychosocial interventions for perinatal common mental disorders delivered by providers who are not mental health specialists in low-and middle-income countries: A systematic review and meta-analysis. *PLoS Medicine*, 10(10), e1001541.

Cook, T. L., Shannon, P. J., Vinson, G. A., Letts, J. P., & Dwee, E. (2015). War trauma and torture experiences reported during public health screening of newly resettled Karen refugees: A qualitative study. *B.M.C. International Health and Human Rights*, 15(1), 1–13.

Crook, M., Short, D., & South, N. (2018). Ecocide, genocide, capitalism and colonialism: Consequences for indigenous peoples and glocal ecosystems environments. *Theoretical Criminology*, 22(3), 298–317.

Cui, W. (2010). Mother or nothing: The agony of infertility. *World Health Organization: Bulletin of the World Health Organization*, 88(12), 881.

Davies, T., Schneider, M., Nyatsanza, M., & Lund, C. (2016). "The sun has set even though it is morning": Experiences and explanations of perinatal depression in an urban township, Cape Town. *Transcultural Psychiatry*, 53(3), 286–312.

Deeb-Sossa, N., & Billings, D. L. (2014). Barriers to abortion facing Mexican immigrants in North Carolina: Choosing folk healers versus standard medical options. *Latino Studies*, 12(3), 399–423.

Desiderio, R. (2020). The impact of international migration on fertility: An empirical study. *Knomad Paper*, 36, World Bank.

Domenech Rodríguez, M. M., Baumann, A. A., & Schwartz, A. L. (2011). Cultural adaptation of an evidence based intervention: From theory to practice in a Latino/a community context. *American Journal of Community Psychology*, 47(1–2), 170–186.

Duan, Z., Wang, Y., Jiang, P., Wilson, A., Guo, Y., Lv, Y., . . . Wu, Z. (2020). Postpartum depression in mothers and fathers: A structural equation model. *B.M.C. Pregnancy and Childbirth*, 20(1), 1–6.

Duden, G. S., & Martins-Borges, L. (2021). Psychotherapy with refugees–supportive and hindering elements. *Psychotherapy Research*, 31(3), 402–417.

Evagorou, O., Arvaniti, A., & Samakouri, M. (2016). Cross-cultural approach of postpartum depression: Manifestation, practices applied, risk factors and therapeutic interventions. *Psychiatric Quarterly*, 87(1), 129–154.

Fellmeth, G., Plugge, E., Fazel, M., Nosten, S., Oo, M. M., Pimanpanarak, M., . . . McGready, R. (2021). Perinatal depression in migrant and refugee women on the Thai–Myanmar border: Does social support matter? *Philosophical Transactions of the Royal Society B*, 376(1827), 20200030.

Fillo, J., Simpson, J. A., Rholes, W. S., & Kohn, J. L. (2015). Dads doing diapers: Individual and relational outcomes associated with the division of childcare across the transition to parenthood. *Journal of Personality and Social Psychology*, 108(2), 298–316.

Forte, A., Trobia, F., Gualtieri, F., Lamis, D. A., Cardamone, G., Giallonardo, V., . . . Pompili, M. (2018). Suicide risk among immigrants and ethnic minorities: A literature overview. *International Journal of Environmental Research and Public Health*, 15(7), 1438.

Gottlieb, A., & DeLoache, J. S. (2016). *A world of babies: Imagined childcare guides for eight societies* (2nd ed). Cambridge University Press.

Grauerholz, K. R., Berry, S. N., Capuano, R. M., & Early, J. M. (2021). Uncovering prolonged grief reactions subsequent to a reproductive loss: Implications for the primary care provider. *Frontiers in Psychology, 12*(673050), 1–12.

Halvorsen, L., Nerum, H., Øian, P., & Sørlie, T. (2013). Giving birth with rape in one's past: A qualitative study. *Birth, 40*(3), 182–191.

Haws, R. A., Mashasi, I., Mrisho, M., Schellenberg, J. A., Darmstadt, G. L., & Winch, P. J. (2010). "These are not good things for other people to know": How rural Tanzanian women's experiences of pregnancy loss and early neonatal death may impact survey data quality. *Social Science & Medicine, 71*(10), 1764–1772.

Heslehurst, N., Brown, H., Pemu, A., Coleman, H., & Rankin, J. (2018). Perinatal health outcomes and care among asylum seekers and refugees: A systematic review of systematic reviews. *BMC Medicine, 16*(1), 1–25.

Higginbottom, G. M., Safipour, J., Mumtaz, Z., Chiu, Y., Paton, P., & Pillay, J. (2013). "I have to do what I believe": Sudanese women's beliefs and resistance to hegemonic practices at home and during experiences of maternity care in Canada. *BMC Pregnancy and Childbirth, 13*(1), 1–10.

Hinton, D. E., & Lewis-Fernández, R. (2010). Idioms of distress among trauma survivors: Subtypes and clinical utility. *Culture, Medicine, and Psychiatry, 34*(2), 209–218.

Hofstede, G. (2011). Dimensionalizing cultures: The Hofstede model in context. *Online Readings in Psychology and Culture, 2*(1), 2307–0919.

Hopgood, M.-L. (2012). *How Eskimos keep their babies warm: And other adventures in parenting (from Argentina to Tanzania and everywhere in between)*. Algonquin Books.

Inhorn, M., & Van Balen, F. (Eds.). (2002). *Infertility around the globe: New thinking on childlessness, gender, and reproductive technologies*. University of California Press.

International Rescue Committee. (2018, June 22). *Migrants, asylum seekers, refugees and immigrants: What's the difference?* www.rescue.org/article/migrants-asylum-seekers-and-immigrants-whats-difference.

Johnsdotter, S. (2018). The impact of migration on Attitudes to female genital cutting and experiences of sexual dysfunction among migrant women with FGC. *Current Sexual Health Reports, 10*(1), 18–24.

Kaiser, B. N., Haroz, E. E., Kohrt, B. A., Bolton, P. A., Bass, J. K., & Hinton, D. E. (2015). "Thinking too much": A systematic review of a common idiom of distress. *Social Science & Medicine, 147*, 170–183.

Kazemi, A., Torabi, M., & Abdishahshahani, M. (2021). Adjustment toward infertility mediates the relationship between coping, depression and anxiety in men: A confirmatory analysis. *European Journal of Obstetrics, Gynecology, and Reproductive Biology, 258*, 48–52.

Kennedy, A. C., & Prock, K. A. (2018). "I still feel like I am not normal": A review of the role of stigma and stigmatization among female survivors of child sexual abuse, sexual assault, and intimate partner violence. *Trauma, Violence & Abuse, 19*(5), 512–527.

Khalifa, N., Hardie, T., Latif, S., Jamil, I., & Walker, D. M. (2011). Beliefs about Jinn, black magic and the evil eye among Muslims: Age, gender and first language influences. *International Journal of Culture and Mental Health, 4*(1), 68–77.

Kidman, R. (2017). Child marriage and intimate partner violence: A comparative study of 34 countries. *International Journal of Epidemiology, 46*(2), 662–675.

Kiguli, J., Namusoko, S., Kerber, K., Peterson, S., & Waiswa, P. (2015). Weeping in silence: Community experiences of stillbirths in rural eastern Uganda. *Global Health Action, 8*(1), 24011.

Knipscheer, J., Vloeberghs, E., van der Kwaak, A., & van den Muijsenbergh, M. (2015). Mental health problems associated with female genital mutilation. *BJPsych Bulletin, 39*(6), 273–277.

Knopp, Y. M. (2017). *The relationship between level of social support and the development of postpartum depression among women in Pumwani Maternity Hospital in Nairobi County* [Unpublished doctoral dissertation/master's thesis]. United States International University-Africa.

Kohrt, B. A., Jordans, M. J., Tol, W. A., Luitel, N. P., Maharjan, S. M., & Upadhaya, N. (2011). Validation of cross-cultural child mental health and psychosocial research instruments: Adapting the Depression Self-Rating Scale and Child PTSD Symptom Scale in Nepal. *BMC Psychiatry, 11*(1), 1–17.

Kohrt, B. K., Saltiel, M. M., Rosen, E. L., & Cholotio, M. (2022). The use of formative research to culturally adapt a psychosocial support program for perinatal Mayan women in Guatemala. *SSM-Mental Health, 2*, 100078.

Kuti, O., & Ilesanmi, C. E. (2011). Experiences and needs of Nigerian women after stillbirth. *International Journal of Gynecology & Obstetrics, 113*(3), 205–207.

Lara-Cinisomo, S., Wood, J., & Fujimoto, E. M. (2019). A systematic review of cultural orientation and perinatal depression in Latina women: Are acculturation, Marianismo, and religiosity risks or protective factors? *Archives of Women's Mental Health, 22*(5), 557–567.

Laurenzi, C. A., Hunt, X., Skeen, S., Sundin, P., Weiss, R. E., Kosi, V., . . . Tomlinson, M. (2021). Associations between caregiver mental health and young children's behaviour in a rural Kenyan sample. *Global Health Action, 14*(1), 1861909.

Le, H. N., Perry, D. F., & Stuart, E. A. (2011). Randomized controlled trial of a preventive intervention for perinatal depression in high-risk Latinas. *Journal of Consulting and Clinical Psychology, 79*(2), 135.

Leanza, Y., Miklavcic, A., Boivin, I., & Rosenberg, E. (2014). Working with interpreters. In L. J. Kirmayer, J. Guzder, & C. Rousseau (Eds.) *Cultural consultation* (pp. 89–114). Springer.

Leon, I. G. (2017). Empathic psychotherapy for pregnancy termination for fetal anomaly. *Psychotherapy, 54*(4), 394–399.

Lewis-Fernández, R., Aggarwal, N. K., Hinton, L., Hinton, D. E., & Kirmayer, L. J. (Eds.). (2015). *DSM-5® handbook on the cultural formulation interview*. American Psychiatric Publishing.

Li, X., Hu, Y., Huang, C. S., & Chuang, S. S. (2021). Beyond W.E.I.R.D. (Western, educated, industrial, rich, democratic)-centric theories and perspectives: Masculinity and fathering in Chinese societies. *Journal of Family Theory & Review, 13*(3), 317–333.

Litonjua, M. D. (2012). Third world/Global South: From modernization, to dependency/liberation, to postdevelopment. *Journal of Third World Studies, 29*(1), 25–56.

Marazita, M. L. (2012). The evolution of human genetic studies of cleft lip and cleft palate. *Annual Review of Genomics and Human Genetics, 13*, 263–283.

Martínez, N. N., Wallenborn, J., Mäusezahl, D., Hartinger, S. M., & Ribera, J. M. (2021). Sociocultural factors for breastfeeding cessation and their relationship with child diarrhea the rural high-altitude Peruvian Andes–a qualitative study. *International Journal for Equity in Health, 20*(1), 1–12.

Maselko, J., Hagaman, A. K., Bates, L. M., Bhalotra, S., Biroli, P., Gallis, J. A., . . . Rahman, A. (2019). Father involvement in the first year of life: Associations with maternal mental health and child development outcomes in rural Pakistan. *Social Science & Medicine, 237*, 112421.

Massarotti, C., Gentile, G., Ferreccio, C., Scaruffi, P., Remorgida, V., & Anserini, P. (2019). Impact of infertility and infertility treatments on quality of life and levels of anxiety and depression in women undergoing in vitro fertilization. *Gynecological Endocrinology, 35*(6), 485–489.

McCabe, K. M., Yeh, M., Garland, A. F., Lau, A. S., & Chavez, G. (2005). The GANA program: A tailoring approach to adapting parent child interaction therapy for Mexican Americans. *Education and Treatment of Children, 26*(2), 111–129.

Meky, H. K., Shaaban, M. M., Ahmed, M. R., & Mohammed, T. Y. (2020). Prevalence of postpartum depression regarding mode of delivery: A cross-sectional study. *Journal of Maternal-Fetal & Neonatal Medicine, 33*(19), 3300–3307.

Muñoz, R. F., Le, H. N., Ippen, C. G., Diaz, M. A., Urizar Jr., G. G., Soto, J., . . . Lieberman, A. F. (2007). Prevention of postpartum depression in low-income women: Development of the Mamás y Bebés/Mothers and Babies Course. *Cognitive and Behavioral Practice, 14*(1), 70–83.

Muzik, M., McGinnis, E. W., Bocknek, E., Morelen, D., Rosenblum, K., Liberzon, I., . . . Abelson, J. L. (2016). PTSD symptoms across pregnancy and early postpartum among women with lifetime PTSD diagnosis. *Depression and Anxiety, 33*(7), 584–591.

Nichter, M. (2010). Idioms of distress revisited. *Culture, Medicine, and Psychiatry, 34*(2), 401–416.

Ombelet, W. (2020). WHO fact sheet on infertility gives hope to millions of infertile couples worldwide. *Facts, Views & Vision in ObGyn, 12*(4), 249–251.

Ostrach, B. (2013). "Yo No Sabía . . ."–immigrant women's ese of national health systems for reproductive and abortion care. *Journal of Immigrant and Minority Health, 15*(2), 262–272.

Palm, C., Essén, B., & Johnsdotter, S. (2019). Sexual health counselling targeting girls and young women with female genital cutting in Sweden: Mind-body dualism affecting social and health care professionals' perspectives. *Sexual and Reproductive Health Matters, 27*(1), 192–202.

Papademetriou, D. G., & Fratzke, S. (2016). *Beyond care and maintenance: Rebuilding hope and opportunity for refugees*. Migration Policy Institute. www.migrationpolicy.org/sites/default/files/publications/TCM_Dev-CouncilStatement-FINAL.pdf

Phiri, P., Rathod, S., Gobbi, M., Carr, H., & Kingdon, D. (2019). Culture and therapist self-disclosure. *The Cognitive Behaviour Therapist*, 12(25), 1–12.

Pordié, L., & Kloos, S. (Eds.). (2021). *Healing at the periphery: Ethnographies of Tibetan medicine in India*. Duke University Press.

Premji, S. (2014). Perinatal distress in women in low- and middle-income countries: Allostatic load as a framework to examine the effect of perinatal distress on preterm birth and infant health. *Maternal and Child Health Journal*, 18(10), 2393–2407.

Racine, N., Zumwalt, K., McDonald, S., Tough, S., & Madigan, S. (2020). Perinatal depression: The role of maternal adverse childhood experiences and social support. *Journal of Affective Disorders*, 263, 576–581.

Rettger, J. P., Kletter, H., & Carrion, V. (2016). Trauma and acculturative stress. In S. Patel & D. Reicherter (Eds.), *Psychotherapy for immigrant youth* (pp. 87–105). Springer.

Sarkar, N. D., Bardaji, A., Peeters Grietens, K., Bunders-Aelen, J., Baingana, F., & Criel, B. (2018). The social nature of perceived illness representations of perinatal depression in rural Uganda. *International Journal of Environmental Research and Public Health*, 15(6), 1197–1209.

Schmied, V., Black, E., Naidoo, N., Dahlen, H. G., & Liamputtong, P. (2017). Migrant women's experiences, meanings and ways of dealing with postnatal depression: A meta-ethnographic study. *PLoS One*, 12(3), e0172385.

Sharma, S., van Teijlingen, E., Hundley, V., Angell, C., & Simkhada, P. (2016). Dirty and 40 days in the wilderness: Eliciting childbirth and postnatal cultural practices and beliefs in Nepal. *BMC Pregnancy and Childbirth*, 16(147), 1–12.

Sisay, M. M., Yirgu, R., Gobezayehu, A. G., & Sibley, L. M. (2014). A qualitative study of attitudes and values surrounding stillbirth and neonatal mortality among grandmothers, mothers, and unmarried girls in rural Amhara and Oromiya regions, Ethiopia: Unheard souls in the backyard. *Journal of Midwifery & Women's Health*, 59(s1), S110–S117.

Small, R., Roth, C., Raval, M., Shafiei, T., Korfker, D., Heaman, M., . . . Gagnon, A. (2014). Immigrant and non-immigrant women's experiences of maternity care: A systematic and comparative review of studies in five countries. *BMC Pregnancy and Childbirth*, 14(1), 1–17.

Smith, H., & Stein, K. (2017). Psychological and counselling interventions for female genital mutilation. *International Journal of Gynecology & Obstetrics*, 136, 60–64.

Stauffer, B. (2019, September 4). *"When we're dead and buried, our bones will keep hurting": Workers' rights under threat in U.S. meat and poultry plants*. www.hrw.org/report/2019/09/04/when-were-dead-and-buried-our-bones-will-keep-hurting/workers-rights-under-threat

Tahirih Justice Center. (2017). *Falling through the cracks: How laws allow child marriage to happen in today's America*. www.tahirih.org/wp-content/uploads/2017/08/TahirihChildMarriageReport-1.pdf

Team, V., Vasey, K., & Lenor, M. (2009). *Cultural dimensions of pregnancy, birth, and post-natal care* (Multicultural Clinical Support Resource, p. 69). Queensland Health. www.health.qld.gov.au/__data/assets/pdf_file/0035/158669/14mcsr-pregnancy.pdf

Tobin, C. L., Di Napoli, P., & Beck, C. T. (2018). Refugee and immigrant women's experience of postpartum depression: A meta-synthesis. *Journal of Transcultural Nursing*, 29(1), 84–100.

Turner, E. L., Sikander, S., Bangash, O., Zaidi, A., Bates, L., Gallis, J., . . . Maselko, J. (2016). The effectiveness of the peer delivered Thinking Healthy Plus (THPP+) Programme for maternal depression and child socio-emotional development in Pakistan: Study protocol for a three-year cluster randomized controlled trial. *Trials*, 17, 1–11.

Vanderkruik, R., & Dimidjian, S. (2019). Perspectives on task-shifting depression care to peers for depressed Latina mothers. *Journal of Latinx Psychology*, 7(1), 22–38.

Watson, K., White, C., Hall, H., & Hewitt, A. (2021). Women's experiences of birth trauma: A scoping review. *Women and Birth*, 34(5), 417–424.

Widiana, H. S., Manderson, L., & Simpson, K. (2018). Experiences of depression in Yogyakarta, Indonesia. *Mental Health, Religion & Culture*, 21(5), 470–483.

Withers, M., Kharazmi, N., & Lim, E. (2018). Traditional beliefs and practices in pregnancy, childbirth and postpartum: A review of the evidence from Asian countries. *Midwifery*, 56, 158–170.

Worden, J. W. (2015). Theoretical perspectives on loss and grief. In J. M. Stillion & T. Attig (Eds.), *Death, dying, and bereavement: Contemporary perspectives, institutions, and practices* (91–103). Springer Publishing Company.

World Health Organization. (2015). *Thinking healthy: A manual for psychosocial management of perinatal depression, WHO generic field-trial version 1.0, 2015* (No. WHO/MSD/MER/15.1). World Health Organization.

Yarris, K. E. (2014). "Pensando mucho" ("thinking too much"): Embodied distress among grandmothers in Nicaraguan transnational families. *Culture, Medicine, and Psychiatry, 38*(3), 473–498.

CONCLUSION

Next Steps for the Field of Perinatal Mental Health Disorders

Amy Wenzel

The Routledge International Handbook of Perinatal Mental Health Disorders is truly a tour de force of current scholarship in the field of perinatal mental health—a tribute to the distinguished experts who contributed chapters to this volume. The material contained in these pages allows for a rich and sophisticated framework for researchers, clinicians, and trainees who encounter perinatal clients in their work to understand and help with the experiences these clients have and the issues that they face. What is clear from these chapters is the passion and commitment that these individuals bring to the highest quality research and to provide the highest quality care to this population. I believe that the field of perinatal mental health stands out among fields devoted to the understanding and treatment of mental health disorders in specific populations for these reasons and can serve as a model for burgeoning fields to emulate.

In this brief conclusion, I revisit the three themes that I highlighted in the Introduction to this volume, this time with an eye toward future directions that the field can take. First, as has been evidenced throughout this volume, much attention has been devoted over the past decade to the study of perinatal mental health disorders other than depression. The chapters in Parts II and III of this volume presented invaluable information on the nature, prevalence, and course of perinatal anxiety disorders, obsessive-compulsive disorder (OCD), posttraumatic stress disorder (PTSD), eating disorders, alcohol and drug use disorders, bipolar disorder, and psychosis. Knowledge in these areas will undoubtedly help perinatal women who might, otherwise, have been overlooked if depression was not a prominent part of their clinical presentation. In the next decade, I am eager to see screening, prevention, and intervention approaches designed and evaluated for these mental health disorders.

One curious omission in the literature is the study of perinatal social anxiety. In my own program on the nature and prevalence of postpartum anxiety disorders, my students and I found that although the absolute prevalence of social anxiety disorder was lower than would be expected in women representative of the general population, there was a striking group of new onset cases (Wenzel et al., 2005). Social anxiety disorder has the potential to be quite debilitating, as it is associated with lowered quality of life and functional impairment (Wittchen et al., 1999), particularly in the area of close relationships (Whisman et al., 2000). New onset cases in our study described ways in which their social anxiety

DOI: 10.4324/9781003206903-39

unexpectedly interfered with marital adjustment and the maintenance of friendships (particularly with friends who did not have children), which were experienced as extremely upsetting. It will be important for future research to incorporate assessments of social anxiety into their batteries and examine the degree to which they affect the quality of existing relationships, parents' ability to form new relationship with other parents as their children grow up, life choices such as whether to resume work at pre-pregnancy levels, their child's social and emotional development, and comorbidity with other mental health disorders such as depression.

I also hope to see more in the literature on a reformulated diagnostic category, illness anxiety disorder. A brief literature search on this topic (using the outdated diagnostic category, hypochondriasis) yielded two brief articles published over 30 years ago by the same research group (Fava et al., 1990; Savron et al., 1989). Although some aspects of illness anxiety disorder in pregnancy are captured in samples who score high on measures of pregnancy anxiety and who are diagnosed with a fear of childbirth (i.e., tokophobia), it would behoove researchers to examine this condition systematically, as pregnancy brings much health-related uncertainty and feelings of general unwell. Clinically, we see many women who have a foundation of high health anxiety who struggle mightily during pregnancy—physically, cognitively, and emotionally. Many of the interventions described in this volume would have much applicability to pregnant women with health anxiety and/or who are diagnosed with illness anxiety disorder, including cognitive behavioral therapy (CBT) to manage catastrophic thoughts of illness, interpersonal psychotherapy (IPT) to address the effects of such anxiety on close relationships (especially the partner relationship), and mindfulness-based interventions to develop tolerance and acceptance of whatever bodily sensations are being experienced in the moment.

Finally, I expect that there will be more attention given to the experience of pregnancy and postpartum adjustment in people with borderline personality disorder (BPD). Transitions, in general, are difficult for people with BPD due to emotion dysregulation, emotional volatility, and the idealization-devaluation cycle that many of these patients have toward people and situations. At times, people with BPD self-regulate and self-soothe through harmful activities, such as excessive alcohol and drug use or self-harm, which could obviously be detrimental to the unborn child or infant's health and well-being. Fortunately, dialectical behavioral therapy (DBT) was originally developed to meet this exact clinical presentation (Linehan, 1993), and, at present, we are beginning to see pilot exploration of the efficacy of CBT for emotion dysregulation, the hallmark feature of BPD (Agako et al., 2022).

Second, as mentioned in the Introduction, the number of intervention options for perinatal clients has proliferated greatly over the past decade (including the innovative pharmacological agent, brexanolone). A decade ago, it was primarily IPT, CBT, and psychotropic medications that received attention in the literature. Now, the field has expanded, as there is a developing evidence base for mindfulness-based interventions, and the field of Internet interventions has simply exploded. Moreover, other aspects of intervention were referenced in a number of chapters in this volume, even if those chapters were not the subject of full chapters in and of themselves, such as integrative services involving both the mother and infant and complementary and alternative approaches, such as yoga. It is not difficult to conclude that an expanded array of intervention options for perinatal women suffering from mental health disorders, as well as increased accessibility through the Internet, will allow for even more women to be reached and obtain relief from their suffering.

I call on researchers to begin to evaluate the "third-wave" evidence-based psychotherapies for perinatal mental health disorders. "Third-wave" psychotherapies have an emphasis on acceptance and tolerance, focusing less on cognitive and behavior change than does traditional cognitive behavioral therapy (CBT), and emphasize the function of various manifestations of symptoms rather than their form or content (Hayes & Hofmann, 2017). As mentioned in my chapter in this volume on CBT, not only do I believe that "third-wave" psychotherapies will be extraordinary beneficial for perinatal clients, I believe that CBT practiced in a "contemporary" manner, in which each course of treatment is informed by current literature and thinking in the field, as well as by the individual client's case formulation, needs, and preferences; Wenzel, 2017), incorporates strategies and principles from "third-wave" psychotherapies. The mindfulness-based interventions described in Chapter 25 of this volume constitute one example of a "third-wave" psychotherapy. In the next decade, I hope to see evaluations of DBT and acceptance and commitment therapy (ACT; Hayes et al., 1999, 2012), as well as their integration into a contemporary, case-formulation driven, CBT package.

I am also eager to see more research on the treatment of fathers who struggle with the transition to parenthood. As Holmberg and Pappa noted in Chapter 27, at present, there are only two studies that have evaluated treatment options for fathers. This issue is close to my heart, as I think about a father who was referred to me in my clinical practice approximately ten years ago. He came to me after he and his wife experienced a horrific pregnancy loss when his wife was very late into her third trimester. When he presented for treatment, I had recently published a book through the American Psychological Associations LifeTools division on pregnancy loss and infertility (Wenzel, 2014), and my initial reaction was that I was grateful for that came to me at that time, as I thought I had much I could offer him. How incredibly wrong I was. I certainly had a great deal to offer him about what his wife was experiencing and what she might need. In fact, I was passionate and invested in that which I thought I had to offer him, as someone who also experienced a late pregnancy loss. I distinctly remember him taking a pause and telling me that "No one takes the time to understand the fathers' experience" and that he was "suffering in silence" as he cared for his wife. I now understand, ten years later and upon much reflection, with this father never returning to treatment and not responding to my subsequent efforts of connection, that I did not understand it either, no matter what scholarly and personal experience I had that I thought I was offering. Systematic research and scholarship on fathers' experiences and interventions for fathers will help to prevent these unfortunate occurrences.

The third theme that I highlighted in the Introduction is the impressive and admirable drive within the field of perinatal mental health disorders to understand cultural experiences of perinatal mental health disorders, consider ways in which validated interventions can be adapted in a sensitive, respectful way, and disseminate the interventions in a way that they are sustainable. When I reference culture, not only am I referring to ethnic minorities and people who live in Global South countries, but also people who do not identify as heteronormative and who might be transitioning or have transitioned. Nearly every chapter in this volume speaks to these cultural considerations, and they are the focus of many chapters in the final part of this volume.

There were also many case studies throughout the volume that highlighted a case of someone who was of an ethnic or sexual minority. What stood out in some of these cases were the microaggressions made by members of the obstetric team, often in the form of misguided assumptions about their family composition. Perhaps the most salient message that I take away from these chapters, collectively, is the need to (a) conduct myself as an ally of perinatal people who experience these microaggressions and (b) speak out to my colleagues and fellow care providers when I see them occurring. Moreover, research into the prevalence of microaggressions and their association with perinatal mental health disorders would be welcomed so that we can use data to be the catalyst of change.

In all, I will say that it has been my distinct privilege to edit such a powerful volume. My scholarship and clinical practice have grown tremendously from it, and I hope that this is the case for the contributors and readers, alike. If my experience is similar to that of the contributors and readers, I know that I am continually called upon to treat perinatal clients, to train and supervise clinicians who hope to specialize in this area, and to provide commentary for the media on relevant issues that receive attention. It is my sincerest hope that this volume will help to guide us as we field these requests, as we continue to advocate for perinatal mental health and the people who are affected by them.

References

Agako, A., Burckell, L., McCabe, R. E., Frey, B. N., Barrett, E., Silang, K., & Green, S. M. (2022). A pilot study examining the effectiveness of a short-term DBT informed skills group for emotion dysregulation during the perinatal period. *Psychological Services, 20*, 697–707.

Fava, G. A., Grandi, S., Michelacci, L., Saviotti, F., Conti, S., Bovicelli, L., . . . Orlandi, C. (1990). Hypochondriacal beliefs and fears in pregnancy. *Acta Psychiatrica Scandinavica, 82*, 70–72.

Hayes, S. C., & Hofmann, S. G. (2017). The third wave of cognitive behavioral therapy and the rise of process-based care. *World Psychiatry, 16*, 245–246.

Hayes, S. C., Strosahl, K. D., & Wilson, K. G. (1999). *Acceptance and commitment therapy: An experiential approach to behavior change.* Guilford Press.

Hayes, S. C., Strosahl, K. D., & Wilson, K. G. (2012). *Acceptance and commitment therapy: The process and practice of mindful change* (2nd ed.). Guilford Press.

Linehan, M. M. (1993). *Cognitive behavioral treatment of borderline personality disorder.* Guilford Press.

Savron, G., Grandi, S., Michelacci, L., Saviotti, F. M., Bartolucci, G., Conti, S., . . . Fava, G. A. (1989). Hypochondriacal symptoms in pregnancy. *Psychotherapy and Psychosomatics, 52*, 106–109.

Wenzel, A. (2014). *Coping with infertility, miscarriage, and neonatal loss: Finding perspective and creating meaning.* American Psychological Association (LifeTools Division).

Wenzel, A. (2017). *Innovations in cognitive behavioral therapy: Strategic interventions for creative practice.* Routledge.

Wenzel, A., Haugen, E. N., Jackson, L. C., & Brendle, J. R. (2005). Anxiety disorders at eight weeks postpartum. *Journal of Anxiety Disorders, 19*, 295–311.

Whisman, M. A., Sheldon, C. T., & Goering, P. (2000). Psychiatric disorders and dissatisfaction with social relationships: Does type of relationship matter? *Journal of Abnormal Psychology, 109*, 803–808.

Wittchen, H. U., Fuetsch, M., Sonntag, H., Muller, N., & Liebowitz, M. (1999). Disability and quality of life in pure and comorbid social phobia: Findings from a controlled study. *European Psychiatry, 14*, 118–131.

INDEX

Note: Page numbers in *italics* indicate a figure and page numbers in **bold** indicate a table on the corresponding page.

For Product Safety Concerns and Information please contact our EU
representative GPSR@taylorandfrancis.com
Taylor & Francis Verlag GmbH, Kaufingerstraße 24, 80331 München, Germany

www.ingramcontent.com/pod-product-compliance
Lightning Source LLC
Chambersburg PA
CBHW081207220326
41598CB00037B/6704